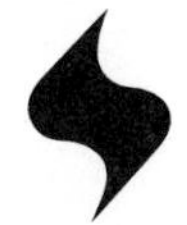

Stedman's

NEUROLOGY & NEUROSURGERY WORDS

THIRD EDITION

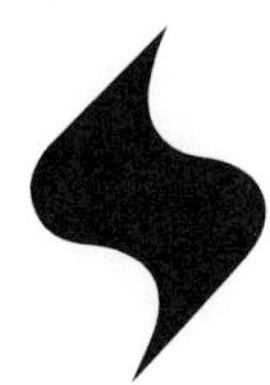

Stedman's

NEUROLOGY & NEUROSURGERY WORDS

THIRD EDITION

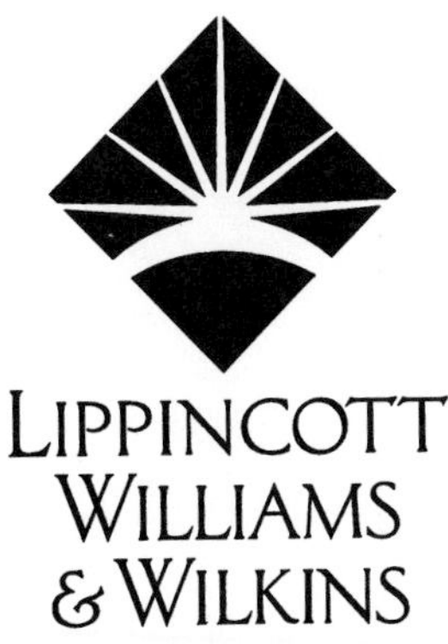

LIPPINCOTT
WILLIAMS
& WILKINS

Publisher: Julie K. Stegman
Series Managing Editor: Trista A. DiPaula
Art Program Project Manager: Jennifer Clements
Assistant Production Manager: Kevin Iarossi
Typesetter: Peirce Graphic Services, LLC.
Printer & Binder: Malloy Litho, Inc.

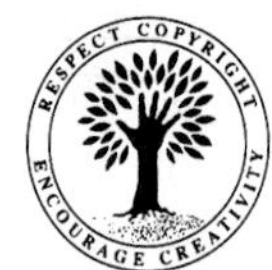

Printed in the United States of America

Third Edition, 2003

Library of Congress Cataloging-in-Publication Data

Stedman's neurology & neurosurgery words.-- 3rd ed.
p. ; cm.
Rev. ed. of: Stedman's psychiatry/neurology/neurosurgery words. c1999.
Includes bibliographical references.
ISBN 0-7817-4405-9 (alk. paper)
1. Neurology—Dictionaries. 2. Neurosurgery–Dictionaries.
[DNLM: 1. Neurology—Terminology—English. 2. Neurosurgery—Terminology—English. WL 15 S8115 2003] I. Title: Neurology & neurosurgery words. II. Title: Stedman's neurology and neurosurgery words. III. Stedman, Thomas Lathrop, 1853–1938. IV. Stedman's psychiatry/neurology/neurosurgery words.

RC334.S74 2003
616.8′003—dc21

2003004778
03
1 2 3 4 5 6 7 8 9 10

Contents

Acknowledgments

An important part of our editorial process is the involvement of medical transcriptionists—as advisors, reviewers, and/or editors.

We extend special thanks to Sandy Kovacs, CMT, and Sandy Enlow, for editing the manuscript, helping resolve many difficult questions, and contributing material for the appendix sections. We are grateful to our MT Editorial Advisory Board members, including Carol Aten, CMA Transcription; Jo-Ann Clarke; Penny Doyle, CMT; Katherine Duggins; Alisha Henri; Judy Lichtenberger, CMT; Lori Mae, MT, QA; Peg Nelson, CMT; Cheryl Rittschoff, MLS; and Anne Thorpe, who were instrumental in the development of this reference. They recommended sources and shared their valuable judgment, insight, and perspective.

We also extend thanks to Jeanne Bock, CSR, MT, for working on the appendix. Additional thanks to Helen Littrell for performing the final prepublication review. Other important contributors to this edition include Marty Cantu, CMT; Shemah Fletcher; Patricia Gibson; Jaimee A. Givens; Robin Koza; Diana L. Krug, CMT; Beverly S. Oberline, CMT; Donna Perez; Wendy Ryan, RHIT; Gail Schoolcraft, CMT; Harriet R. Stewart, CMT, FAAMT ; Diann Velovitch; Jenifer F. Walker, MA; and Sandra Wideburg, CMT.

And, as always, Barb Ferretti played an integral role in the process by reviewing the content files for format, updating the content, and providing a final quality check. Special thanks also goes to Lisa Fahnestock for her assistance as well.

As with all our *Stedman's* word references, this resource incorporates the suggestions and expertise of our many contacts in the medical transcriptionist community. Thanks to all of our advisory board participants, reviewers, and editors; AAMT meeting attendees; and others who have written us with requests and comments—keep talking, and we'll keep listening.

Editor's Preface

How do you define a challenge? To a newlywed bride, a challenge is preparing their first meal. To a toddler, a challenge is attempting to take those first steps. To a medical transcriptionist, a challenge is when a complicated dictation comes up next in the cue. How do you approach a complex report? One of the best tools is a comprehensive reference book, and I believe the *Stedman's Neurology & Neurosurgery Words, Third Edition* is just the reference you will reach for when transcribing an EEG or EMG interpretation, a ventriculoperitoneal shunt implantation, or a neurological consultation.

Stedman's Neurology & Neurosurgery Words, Third Edition contains comprehensive neurology and neurosurgery terminology, as well as new terminology relating to sleep studies, EMGs, EEGs, neurosurgical procedures, and equipment. The appendix has been expanded and includes new sample reports, common terms listed by procedure, a listing of types of brain cancers, drugs by indication, and sleep medicine terminology. Also featured are anatomical illustrations and a table of nerves. Make sure you avail yourself of the valuable information that can be found in the appendix. We have carefully selected material that we believe will benefit you the most. Understanding what you are transcribing can be another challenge, and the appendix will help answer your questions.

I would like to thank Sandy Enlow, who took on the task of the second editor and did a superb job. This book would not be as comprehensive without the assistance of those who submitted terminology, the editorial advisory board, the research editor, the format editor, and the online editor. It definitely takes a team to create a great reference book, and I thank each of you for sharing your expertise.

As with any new word book or new edition, our challenge was to compile the most useful and current information regarding neurology and neurosurgery. I believe we have accomplished this task.

Sandy Kovacs, CMT

Publisher's Preface

Stedman's Neurology & Neurosurgery Words, Third Edition, offers an authoritative assurance of quality and exactness to the wordsmiths of the healthcare professions—medical transcriptionists, medical editors and copyeditors, health information management personnel, court reporters, and the many other users and producers of medical documentation.

Previously combined with *Stedman's Psychiatry Words,* we determined due to the advancement and sheer volume of medical terminology related to these specialties, that the titles would be separated and be presented in two distinct titles. *Stedman's Neurology & Neurosurgery Words, Third Edition* is the presentation of such advancement and evolution of the terminology associated with the neurology and neurosurgery specialties, featuring related topics such as child neurology, neuroanatomy, and neurologic therapeutics. In this new edition, we have expanded all terminology, particularly in the areas of sleep medicine, Parkinson's and Alzheimer's disease, as well as radiosurgical and stereoactic techniques.

In *Stedman's Neurology & Neurosurgery Words, Third Edition,* users will find protocols, diagnoses, and therapeutic procedures, new techniques, lab tests, clinical research terms, as well as abbreviations with their expansions pertinent to neurology and neurosurgery. The appendix sections, substantially enhanced over the previous edition, provide anatomical illustrations with useful captions and labels; a table of nerves; types of brain cancers; sample reports; common terms by procedure; and drugs by indication.

This new edition, including more than 100,000 entries, includes the Stedman's Word Book Series trademarks: fully cross-indexed by first and last word, A-Z format with main entries and subentries, and appendix material for additional comprehension and application of the terminology.

We at Lippincott Williams & Wilkins strive to provide you with the most up-to-date and accurate word references available. Your use of this Word Book will prompt new editions, which we will publish as often as updates and revisions justify. We welcome your suggestions for improvements, changes, corrections, and additions—whatever will make this *Stedman's* product more useful to you. Please complete the postage-paid card in this book for future suggestions and recommendations, or visit us online at www.stedmans.com.

Explanatory Notes

Medical transcription is an art as well as a science. Both approaches are needed to correctly interpret the dictation of a physician, whose language is a product of education, training, and experience. This variety in medical language means that there are several acceptable ways to express certain terms, including jargon. *Stedman's Neurology & Neurosurgery Words, Third Edition,* provides variant spellings and phrasings for many terms. These elements, in addition to complete cross-indexing, make *Stedman's Neurology & Neurosurgery Words, Third Edition,* a valuable resource for determining the validity of terms as they are encountered.

Alphabetical Organization

Alphabetization of main entries is letter by letter as spelled, ignoring punctuation, spaces, prefixed numbers, or other characters. For example:

hydroxyl radical
4-hydroxynonenal
hydroxyproline

Terms beginning or ending with Greek letters show the Greek letters spelled out and listed alphabetically. For example:

beta, β
b. activity

In subentry alphabetization, the abbreviated singular form or the spelled-out plural form of the noun main entry word is ignored.

Format and Style

All main entries are in **boldface** to expedite locating a sought-after term, to enhance distinction between main entries and subentries, and to relieve the textual density of the pages.

Irregular plurals and variant spellings are shown on the same line as the singular or preferred form of the word. For example:

colliculus, pl. colliculi
facet, facette

Hyphenation

As a rule of style, multiple eponyms (e.g., Mears-Rubash approach) are hyphenated. Also, hyphens have been added between a manufacturer and one or more eponyms (e.g., Vital-Metzenbaum dissecting scissors). Please note that in many cases, hyphenation is a question of style, not of accuracy, and thus is a matter of choice.

Possessives

Possessive forms have been dropped in this reference for the sake of consistency and conformance with the guidelines of the American Association for Medical Transcription (AAMT) and other groups. Please note, however, that in many cases, retaining the possessive, like hyphenating, is a question of style, not of accuracy, and thus is a matter of choice. To form the possessive of a word, simply add the apostrophe or apostrophe "s" to the end of the word.

Cross-indexing

The word list is in an index-like main entry-subentry format that contains two combined alphabetical listings:

(1) A *noun* main entry-subentry organization, which is typical of the A-Z section of medical dictionaries like *Stedman's:*

gland
  basal g.
  eccrine g.
  estopic pituitary g.

hemorrhage
  brainstem h.
  central nervous system h.
  cerebellar h.

(2) An *adjective* main entry-subentry organization, which lists words and phrases as you hear them. The main entries are the adjectives or modi-

fiers in a multiword term. The subentries are the nouns around which the terms are constructed and to which the adjectives or modifiers pertain:

dynamic
d. bed
d. block
d. compression plate

intraspinal
i. adenoma
i. drug infusion system
i. epidural pressure

This format provides the user with more than one way to locate and identify a multiword term. For example:

corpuscle
Krause c.

Krause
K. corpuscle

outer
o. plexiform layer

layer
outer plexiform l.

It also allows the user to see together all terms that contain a particular descriptor, as well as all types, kinds, or variations of a noun entity. For example:

hypoglycemic
h. coma
h. encephalopathy
h. peripheral neuropathy

maleable
m. endoscope
m. microsurgical suction device
m. multipore suction tube

Wherever possible, abbreviations are separately defined and cross-referenced. For example:

ICP
intracranial pressure

intracranial
i. pressure (ICP)

pressure
intracranial p. (ICP)

References

In addition to the manufacturers' literature we gather at various medical meetings, scientific reports from hospitals, and the lists of our MT Editorial Advisory Board members (from their daily transcription work), we used the following sources for new terms in *Stedman's Neurology & Neurosurgery Words, Third Edition.*

Books

The AAMT Book of Style, 2nd Edition. Modesto, CA: AAMT, 2002.

Agur AM, Lee MJ. Grant's Atlas of Anatomy, 10th Edition. Baltimore: Lippincott Williams & Wilkins, 1999.

Arnoff G. Evaluation and Treatment of Chronic Pain. Philadelphia: Lippincott Williams & Wilkins, 1998.

Bear M, Connors B, Paradiso M. Neuroscience, Exploring the Brain, 2nd Edition. Baltimore: Lippincott Williams & Wilkins, 2000.

Biller J. Practical Neurology, 2nd Edition. Philadelphia: Lippincott Williams & Wilkins, 2002.

Brazis PW, Masdeu JC, Biller J. Localization in Clinical Neurology, 4th Edition. Baltimore: Lippincott Williams & Wilkins, 2001.

Browne TR, Holmes GL. The Handbook of Epilepsy, 2nd Edition. Baltimore: Lippincott Williams & Wilkins, 1999.

Campbell WW, Pridgeon RM. Practical Primer of Neurology. Philadelphia: Lippincott Williams & Wilkins, 2001.

Dorland's Neurology Word Book for Medical Transcriptionists. Philadelphia: Saunders, 2001.

Drake E. Sloane's Medical Word Book, 4th Edition. Philadelphia: Saunders, 2001.

Fairbanks DNF, Mickelson SA, Woodson BT. Snoring and Obstructive Sleep Apnea. Philadelphia: Lippincott Williams & Wilkins, 2002.

Howard MA, III. Clinical Neurosurgery: A Publication of the Congress of Neurological Surgeons. Philadelphia: Lippincott Williams & Wilkins, 2001.

Lance LL. Quick Look Drug Book. Baltimore: Lippincott Williams & Wilkins, 2002.

Levy RH, Mattson RH, Meldrum BS, Perucca E. Antiepileptic Drugs, 5th Edition. Baltimore: Lippincott Williams & Wilkins, 2002.

Mazzoni P, Rowland LP. Merritt's Neurology Handbook. Philadelphia: Lippincott Williams & Wilkins, 2001.

Menkes JH, Sarnat HB. Child Neurology. Philadelphia: Lippincott Williams & Wilkins, 2000.

Orthopedic/Neurology Words and Phrases, 2nd Edition. Modesto, CA: Health Professions Institute, 2000.

Pillitteri A. Maternal and Child Health Nursing, 3rd Edition. Philadelphia: Lippincott Williams & Wilkins, 1998.

Rosdahl DB. Textbook of Basic Nursing, 7th Edition. Philadelphia: Lippincott Williams & Wilkins, 1999.

Samuels MA. Manual of Neurologic Therapeutics, 6th Edition. Baltimore: Lippincott Williams & Wilkins, 1999.

Sirven JI, Malamut BL. Clinical Neurology of the Older Adult. Philadelphia: Lippincott Williams & Wilkins, 2002.

Stedman's Medical Dictionary, 27th Edition. Baltimore: Lippincott Williams & Wilkins, 2000.

Stedman's Psychiatry/Neurology/Neurosurgery Words, 2nd Edition. Baltimore: Lippincott Williams & Wilkins, 1999.

Vera Pyle's Current Medical Terminology, 8th Edition. Modesto, CA: Health Professions Institute, 2000.

Wyllie E. The Treatment of Epilepsy, 3rd Edition. Baltimore: Lippincott Williams & Wilkins, 2001.

Journals

Current Opinion in Neurology. Baltimore: Lippincott Williams & Wilkins, 2002.

Journal of Cerebral Blood Flow and Metabolism. Baltimore: Lippincott Williams & Wilkins, 2002.

Latest Word. Philadelphia: Saunders, 1999–2002.

The Neurologist. Baltimore: Lippincott Williams & Wilkins, 2002.

NeuroReport. Baltimore: Lippincott Williams & Wilkins, 2001.

Neurosurgery. Baltimore: Lippincott Williams & Wilkins, 1999–2002.

Neurosurgery Quarterly. Baltimore: Lippincott Williams & Wilkins, 2002.

Perspectives on the Medical Transcription Profession. Modesto, CA: Health Professions Institute, 2001.

Stroke. Baltimore: Lippincott Williams & Wilkins, 2002.

CDs

LifeART Emergency Collection 2, CD-ROM. Baltimore: Lippincott Williams & Wilkins.

LifeART Nursing Collection 1, CD-ROM. Baltimore: Lippincott Williams & Wilkins.

LifeART Nursing Collection 2, CD-ROM. Baltimore: Lippincott Williams & Wilkins.

LifeART Pediatrics Collection 1, CD-ROM. Baltimore: Lippincott Williams & Wilkins.

LifeART Super Anatomy Collection 3, CD-ROM. Baltimore: Lippincott Williams & Wilkins.

LifeART Super Anatomy Collection 7, CD-ROM. Baltimore: Lippincott Williams & Wilkins.

LifeART Super Anatomy Collection 8, CD-ROM. Baltimore: Lippincott Williams & Wilkins.

LifeART Super Anatomy Collection 9, CD-ROM. Baltimore: Lippincott Williams & Wilkins.

MediClip Human Anatomy Collection 1–3, CD-ROM. Baltimore: Lippincott Williams & Wilkins.

Websites

http://emedicine.com/neuro

http://www.americanspine.com

http://www.biomedcentral.com

http://www.centerwatch.com/patient/drugs/druglist.html

http://www.medtronicssofamordanek.com

http://www.mtdesk.com/lstpsych.shtml

http://www.mtdesk.com/psychdef.shtml

http://www.promedproducts.com

http://www.thejns-net.org

http://www.thesaundersgroup.com

A
A band
A fiber
A wave
a
a posteriori
a priori criterion
1a
interferon-beta 1a
10a
Cerebrograph 10a
A2 segment of anterior cerebral artery
AA
amino acid
anterograde amnesia
AAAS
Triple A syndrome gene
AADC
aromatic amino acid decarboxylase
A1 adenosine receptor
AADPRT
American Association of Directors of Psychiatric Residency Training
AAGP
American Association for Geriatric Psychiatry
aaNAT1gene
AANS/CNS
American Association of Neurological Surgeons/Congress of Neurological Surgeons
AANS/CNS Joint Committee of Military Neurosurgeons
AANS/CNS Joint Section Lumbar Disc Herniation Study
AANS/CNS Outcomes Committee
AAO
alert and oriented
Aarskog-Scott syndrome (AAS)
AAS
Aarskog-Scott syndrome
A1, A2 segment of anterior cerebral artery
AB
alertness behavior
Abadie
A. sign
A. sign of tabes dorsalis
ABaer
automated brainstem auditory evoked response
abaptiston
abarognosis
abase
abasement
abash
abasia
atactic a.
ataxic a.
choreic a.
frontal a.
spastic a.
abasia-astasia
abasic, abatic
abatardissement
abaxial, abaxile
abaxonal
Abbokinase
Abbott fluorescence polarization immunoassay technique
Abboxapam
abbreviated
A. Injury Score
A. Life Event Questionnaire
ABC
angry backfiring C
atomic, biologic, chemical
ABC anterior cervical plating system
ABC syndrome
ABC warfare
abciximab
abdomen
anterior cutaneous nerves of a.
carinate a.
navicular a.
abdominal
a. aortic plexus
a. aura
a. brain
a. epilepsy
a. migraine
a. neuralgia
a. reflex
a. trauma
abdominalis
plexus aorticus a.
abdominocardiac reflex
abdominopelvic splanchnic nerve
abducens
a. eminence
a. nerve
a. nerve palsy
a. nerve paralysis
a. nerve paresis
nervus a. [CN VI]
a. nucleus
a. pathway

abducentis
eminentia a.
nucleus nervi a.
abducent nerve [CN VI]
abduction
a. nystagmus
a. weakness
abductor pollicis brevis
Abercrombie neuronal cell count formula
aberrant
a. artery
a. autocrine control
a. bundle
a. carotid
a. gamma burst pattern
a. ganglion
a. laboratory parameter
a. motor behavior
a. regeneration
aberration
intersegmental a.
Abeta
amyloid beta
Abeta fibril
Abeta molecule
Abeta peptide
Abeta protein
AbetaB fibrillogenesis
Abeta-centered neuritic plaque
abetalipoproteinemia
ABG
arterial blood gas
ABI
acquired brain injury
auditory brainstem implant
Multichannel ABI
abidance
abient
Abilitator
Change A.
ability
abstracting a.
bathing and dressing a.
conceptual a.
construction a.
constructional a.
fluid a.
intellectual a.
nonverbal abstractive a.
nonverbal synthesizing a.
Porch Index of Communicative A.
positive a.
premorbid a.
response generalization general learning a.
a. test
verbal a.
visuoconstructional a.
abirritation
ablation
choroid plexus a.
stereotactic surgical a.
thermal a.
total pituitary a.
ablative central neurosurgical procedure
ablienation
ablution
abnegate
abnerval
abneural
abnormal
a. epileptic neuron
a. illness behavior
A. Involuntary Movement Scale
A. Involuntary Movement Score
a. metabolism
a. muscle response
a. nocturnal respiratory reflex
a. personality
a. reaction
a. respiratory drive
a. sleep-wake schedule disorder
a. tactile sensation
a. thinking
a. trait
a. ventilation
a. waveform
abnormality
behavioral a.
bony a.
branchial cleft a.
bulbar a.
central nervous system a.
C-nociceptor filter-evoked central a.
CNS a.
concordant interictal epileptiform a.
convergence a.
cranial nerve a.
cytoarchitectonic a.
cytoskeletal a.
endogenous a.
filter-evoked central a.
focal slow-wave a.
frontal plane growth a.
gain-of-function a.
gait a.
G protein a.
hallucal a.
ictal epileptiform a.
immunologic a.
interictal epileptiform a.
mesocorticolimbic dopaminergic a.
mesostriatal system a.

metabolic a.
migration a.
morphometric a.
motor a.
motoric a.
neuritic cytoskeletal a.
neuronal migration a.
oculomotor a.
personality a.
polysomnographic a.
posture reflex a.
psychomotor a.
pupillary a.
radiologic a.
saccadic a.
sleep hygiene a.
slow-wave a.
soft tissue a.
spinal cord injury without radiographic a. (SCIWORA)
striatal dopaminergic a.
structural a.
subcortical-frontal lobe a.
torsional a.
trait-level region a.'s
transient signal a.
white matter signal a.
X-linked a.

ABO antigen compatibility

aboiement

abolic syndrome

abolition
concentration-dependent a.

aboriginal

abortive
a. neurofibromatosis
a. poliomyelitis
a. therapy

abortus
Brucella a.

aboulia (*var. of* abulia)

ABPN
American Board of Psychiatry and Neurology

ABR
auditory brainstem-evoked response
auditory brainstem response

abract set

abradant

Abrams heart reflex

Abramson catheter

abreact

abrineurin

Abrodil

abrogate

abrupt loss of vision

abscess
actinomycotic brain a.
arthrifluent a.
Aspergillus brain a.
Aspergillus cerebral a.
bacterial brain a.
brain a.
cerebellar a.
cerebral a.
cranial epidural a.
daughter a.
encapsulated brain a.
epidural a.
extradural a.
frontal lobe a.
intracranial epidural a.
intradural a.
nocardial brain a.
otic a.
otitic a.
parasitic brain a.
periapical a.
pituitary a.
Pott a.
psoas a.
pyogenic brain a.
retropharyngeal a.
spinal cord a.
spinal epidural a.
sterile a.
subdural a.
subgaleal a.
temporal lobe a.
thecal a.
tuberculous a.

absence
atonic a.
a. attack
atypical a.
automatic a.
complex a.
a. of emotional responsiveness
enuretic a.
epilepsy with myoclonic a.
epileptic a.
hypertonic a.

NOTES

absence *(continued)*
muscle a.
myoclonic a.
protein induced by vitamin K a. (PIVKA)
pure a.
retrocursive a.
a. seizure
simple a.
a. status epilepticus
sternutatory a.
subclinical a.
tussive a.
vasomotor a.
absent
a. ataxia
a. pupil
a. speech
a. spinous process
a. state
absentia
epileptica a.
***Absidia* infection**
absolute
a. agraphia
a. band amplitude
a. construction of phase
a. EP amplitude
a. flow
a. metabolic activity
a. neutrophil count (ANC)
a. refractory period
a. scale
a. terminal innervation ratio
a. threshold
absorbable
a. gelatin film
a. gelatin sponge
absorbefacient
absorptiometry
dual-energy x-ray a. (DEXA, DXA)
absorption
cerebrospinal fluid a.
erratic a.
intramuscular a.
a. velocity
abstemious
abstract
a. behavior
a. versus representational
abstracting
a. ability
a. disability
abstraction
level of a.
a. skill
abstract-versus-representational dimension
abstruse
abterminal
abubble
abulia, aboulia
abulic mental change
abundancy motive
abuse
a. field
a. potential
abysm
AC
alternating current
AC133 antigen
ACA
acute cerebellar ataxia
academic
academician
acalculia
aphasic a.
visual-spatial a.
acamprosate
acanthamebiasis
Acanthamoeba
A. infection
A. meningitis
acanthesthesia
acanthocytosis with chorea
acapnia
acarbose
acarinatum syndrome
ACAT
acyl-CoA
acatamathesia
acataphasia (*var. of* akataphasia)
acathectic
acathexia
acathisia (*var. of* akathisia)
acaudal
acaudate
accelerans
accelerating center
acceleration-deceleration forces in craniocerebral trauma
acceleration extension injury
accelerator
Bevatron a.
a. fiber
isocentric linear a.
linear a. (LINAC)
a. nerve
Philips linear a.
racetrack Microtron MM50 a.
stereotactic linear a.
accentuation
acceptance strategy

access
arterial a.
lexical a.
accession
accessorii
nervi phrenici a.
nuclei oculomotorii a.
nucleus spinalis nervi a.
pars spinalis nervi a.
pars vagalis nervi a.
radix cranialis nervi a.
radix spinalis nervi a.
rami musculares rami externi nervi a.
ramus externus nervi a.
ramus internus nervi a.
truncus nervi a.
accessorius
nervus obturatorius a.
nervus peroneus profundus a.
nucleus cuneatus a.
a. willisii
accessory
a. basal amygdaloid nucleus
a. conduction pathway (ACP)
a. cramp
a. cuneate nucleus
a. flocculus
Isola spinal implant system a.
a. middle cerebral artery
a. nerve [CN XI]
a. nerve lymph node
a. nerve paresis
a. nerve trunk
a. nucleus of optic tract
a. oculomotor nucleus
a. olivary nucleus
a. olive
a. phrenic nerve
a. portion of spinal cord
accident
a. behavior
cerebrovascular a. (CVA)
a. neurosis
vascular a.
accidental
a. image
a. injury
accident-prone
acclimation
cold a.
acclimatize
accommodation
a. curve
a. disorder
a. of nerve
accompaniment
late-life migraine a.
psychopathologic a.
accompanying vein of hypoglossal nerve
accompli
accoucheur's hand
accretion
accrual
Accu-Flo
A.-F. CSF reservoir
A.-F. dura film
A.-F. polyethylene bur hole cover
A.-F. silicone rubber bur hole cover
A.-F. ventricular catheter
Acculink stent
acculturate
acculturation difficulty
accumbens
nucleus a.
accumbentis
pars lateralis nuclei a.
pars medialis nuclei a.
accumulation
cholesterol a.
galactose-1-phosphate a.
galactosylsphingosine a.
glucosylsphingosine a.
ketoacid a.
psychosine a.
sulfatide a.
accuracy of memory
Accura shunt
Accuray
A. CyberKnife
A. Neurotron 1000 machine
Accusway balance measurement system
Ace
A. halo-cast assembly
A. halo pelvic girdle
A. Hershey halo jig
A. low profile MR halo
A. Mark III halo
A. Trippi-Wells tong cervical traction
A. universal tong cervical traction

NOTES

acebutolol
acedia
0-2A cell
acellular human dermal graft
acenesthesia
acephalgic migraine
acephaly
ACER
  A. Advanced Test B40
acerbate
acerbic, acerb
acerbophobia
aceruloplasminemia
acervuline
acervulus
acetaldehyde
acetamidobenzoate
  deanol a.
acetaminobenzoate
  deanol a.
acetate
  butyl a.
  cortisone a.
  Cortone a.
  desmopressin a.
  desoxycorticosterone a.
  ethylene-vinyl a. (EVAc)
  glatiramer a.
  Hydrocortone A.
  leuprolide a.
  medroxyprogesterone a.
  methylprednisolone a.
  potassium a.
  sodium a.
  zinc a.
acetazolamide
acethycholinesterase
acetohexamide
acetonemia
acetonemic
acetonide
acetrizoate
acetrizoic acid
acetyl
  a. cholinesterase inhibitor
  a. coenzyme A
  a. coenzyme A carboxylase
***N*-acetylaspartate**
acetylcholine (ACH, ACh)
  a. esterase
  a. receptor (AChR)
acetylcholine-binding protein
acetylcholinesterase (AChE)
10% acetylcysteine 0.05% isoproterenol hydrochloride solution
***N*-acetylgalactosamine-4-sulfate sulfatase**
acetylmethadol
acetylphosphate
acetylsalicylic
  a. acid
  a. acid patch
acetyltransferase
  choline a.
ACF
  asymmetrical crying facies
ACH, ACh
  acetylcholine
  ACH receptor
AChA
  anterior choroidal artery
***achaete-scute* gene**
achalasia
  cricopharyngeal a.
  esophageal a.
AChE
  acetylcholinesterase
acheiria, achiria
Achilles
  A. reflex
  A. tendon reflex time
achlorhydria
achondroplasia
AChR
  acetylcholine receptor
achromasia
  neuronal a.
achromatic response
achromatopsia
achromia
  cortical a.
achromians
  incontinentia pigmenti a.
acid
  acetrizoic a.
  N-acetylaspartic a.
  N-acetylneuraminic a.
  acetylsalicylic a.
  adenosine monophosphate a. (AMPA)
  alpha-amino-3-hydroxy-5-methylisoxazole-4-proprionic a.
  amidotrizoic a.
  amino a. (AA)
  aminocaproic a.
  arachidonic a.
  atractylic a.
  benzoic a.
  carbonic a.
  cerebrospinal fluid lactic a.
  chenodeoxycholic a.
  cis-parinaric a.
  cis-retinoic a. (CRA)
  13-*cis*-retinoic a. (CRA, 13-CRA)
  clavulanic a.

complementary deoxyribonucleic a. (cDNA)
cyclic deoxyribonucleic a.
deoxyribonucleic a. (DNA)
diatrizoic a.
diethylenetriaminepentaacetic a. (DTPA)
diethylene triamine pentaacetic acid (DTPA)
differential display of messenger ribonucleic a.
dihomogammalinolenic a.
docosahexaenoic a. (DHA)
double-stranded deoxyribonucleic a. (dsDNA)
eicosapentaenoic a.
epsilon-aminocaproic a.
ethacrynic a.
ethylenediaminetetraacetic a.
excitatory amino a.
folic a.
folinic a.
gadolinium diethylenetriamine pentaacetic a. (Gd-DTPA)
gamma-aminobutyric a. (GABA)
gamma-aminobutyric a. type A (GABA-A)
gamma-aminolevulinic a.
gamma-linolenic a.
ganglioside monosialic a.
glucuronic a.
glutaric a.
a. hematoxylin
hepatoiminodiacetic a. (HIDA)
heteronuclear ribonucleic a. (hnRNA)
highly unsaturated fatty a. (HUFA)
homocysteine a.
homovanillic a. (HVA)
hyaluronic a.
5-hydroxyindoleacetic a.
hypochlorous a. (HOCl)
inhibitory amino a.
iobenzamic a.
iobutoic a.
iocarmic a.
iodamic a.
iodoalphionic a.
iodoxamic a.
ioglicic a.
ioglycamic a.
iopanoic a.
iophenoxic a.
ioprocemic a.
iopronic a.
iosefamic a.
ioseric a.
iosumetic a.
ioteric a.
iothalamic a.
iotroxic a.
ioxaglic a.
ioxithalamic a.
iozomic a.
ipodate a.
kainic a.
kynurenic a.
a. lipase
a. lipase deficiency
long-chain fatty a.
a. maltase deficiency
mefenamic a.
messenger ribonucleic a.
metrizoic a.
myristic a.
neuroactive amino a.
nitric a.
okadaic a.
Owsley a.
oxolinic a.
palmitic a.
paraisopropyliminodiacetic a. (PIPIDA)
plasma fatty a.
polyanhydride poly[bis(carboxyphenoxy-propane)-sebacic a.]
polyanhydroglucuronic a.
polylactic a.
potassium citrate and citric a.
quinolinic a.
quisqualic a.
retinoic a.
rho-aminosalicylic a.
ribonucleic a. (RNA)
serum folic a.
sialic a.
tolfenamic a.
tranexamic a.
tricarboxylic a. (TCA)
triiodobenzoic a.
tyropanoic a.

NOTES

acid *(continued)*
uric a.
valerianic a.
valproic a.
acid-base
a.-b. disturbance
a.-b. imbalance
acidemia
methylmalonic a.
organic a.
propionic a.
acid-fast
a.-f. bacilli smear
a.-f. stain
acidophil adenoma
acidophilic pituitary tumor
acidosis
extracellular a.
hypokalemic metabolic a.
lactic a.
metabolic a.
myoclonus epilepsy with ragged red fibers-lactic a. (MERRLA)
respiratory a.
acid-Schiff
periodic a.-S. (PAS)
aciduria
alpha-aminoadipic a.
alpha-ketoadipic a.
alpha-methylacetoacetic a.
argininosuccinic a.
ethylmalonic a.
glutaric a. type I, II
4-hydroxybutyric a.
2-hydroxyglutaric a.
3-hydroxyisobutyric a.
3-hydroxy-3-methyl-glutaric a.
isovaleric a.
3-methylglutaconic a.
methylmalonic a.
mevalonic a.
organic a.
pipoglutamic a.
propionic a.
acinesia
acinetic
Acinetobacter calcoaceticus
acinic cell carcinoma
Acland clip
ACM
acute cerebrospinal meningitis
acmesthesia
acnes
Propionibacterium a.
ACoA, AComA
anterior communicating artery
acolyte
aconative
aconite
aconitine
acoria, akoria
acorn
a. bit
a. drill
acoustic
a. agraphia
a. ambiguity
a. aphasia
a. area
a. bone window
a. crest
a. evoked potential
a. lemniscus
a. nerve
a. nerve complex
a. nerve disorder
a. nerve sheath tumor
a. neurilemoma
a. neurinoma
a. neuroma
A. Neuroma Association
A. Neuroma Registry
a. neuroma surgery
a. noise
a. nucleus
a. papilla
a. radiation
a. reflex
a. schwannoma
a. signature event (ASI)
a. spot
a. stria
a. tubercle
acoustica
acoustical shadowing
acousticofacial
a. crest
a. ganglion
acousticopalpebral reflex (APR)
ACP
accessory conduction pathway
AC-PC
anterior commissure-posterior commissure
AC-PC line
acquired
a. antibody
a. brain injury (ABI)
a. dementia
a. demyelinative neuropathy
a. drive
a. epileptic aphasia
a. epileptiform opercular syndrome
a. fluent aphasia

a. hepatocerebral degeneration
a. hepatocerebral syndrome
a. hydrocephalus
a. immunodeficiency syndrome (AIDS)
a. immunodeficiency syndrome dementia complex
a. nystagmus
a. reflex
a. spinal stenosis
a. toxoplasmosis
a. vertical diplopia

acquisita
myotonia a.

acquisition
EWACS system data a.
target a.
three-dimensional a.
a. time

Acraclip scalp clip system

Acra-Cut
A.-C. blade
A.-C. cranial perforator
A.-C. cranioblade
A.-C. wire pass drill

Acragun system

acral

Acremonium alabamensis

acrid

acrimicria

acrimonious

acrimony

acroagnosis

acroanesthesia

acroasphyxia

acroataxia

acrobrachycephaly

acrocallosal syndrome

acrocephalia

acrocephalic

acrocephalosyndactyly

acrocephalous

acrocephaly

acrocinesia

acrodermatis chronica atrophicans

acrodynia

acrodysesthesia

acroedema

acroesthesia

AcroFlex disk prosthesis

acrognosis

acrohypothermia

acrolect

acromegalia

acromegalic neuropathy

acromegaloid-hypertelorism-pectus
a.-h.-p. carinatum syndrome

acromegaly
hypothalamic a.

acromelalgia

acromial
a. dimple
a. reflex

acromicria

acronarcotic

acroneurosis

acroparalysis

acroparesthesia syndrome

acropathy
mutilating a.

acrophase

acrosclerosis

acrotrophodynia

acrotrophoneurosis

acrylaldehyde

acrylamide
a. monomer
a. peripheral neuropathy

acrylic
a. cranioplasty
a. glue
a. prosthesis

act
Individuals with Disabilities Education A. (IDEA)
instrumental a.
Terazoff A.

ACTH
adrenocorticotropic hormone

Acthar

ACTH-producing adenoma

ACTH-secreting
A.-s. pituitary tumor
A.-s. tumor

Actigraph

actigraphy

actin filament

Actinomadura madurae

Actinomyces

actinomycetoma

actinomycosis lymphocytic meningitis

actinomycotic brain abscess

NOTES

actinoneuritis
action
drug a.
dual mechanism of a.
a. dystonia
hypnotic a.
local vasoconstrictive a.
a. potential
pseudoirreversible mechanism of a.
reflex a.
scotomata of a.
a. tremor
vasoconstrictive a.
viscoelastic a.
Activa
A. Tremor Control System
A. Tremor Control System implant
A. Tremor Control Therapy
activated
a. epilepsy
a. estrogen receptor
a. macrophage
activating condition
activation
amygdala a.
anterior hippocampal a.
ascending reticular a.
brain a.
brainstem a.
cerebellar a.
complement a.
a. defect
EEG a.
electroencephalogram a.
emotion-related a.
enzyme a.
face-graded a.
face-preferential a.
functional a.
GFAP a.
glial fibrillary acidic protein activation a.
hippocampal a.
latency of tibialis anterior a.
limbic a.
metabolic a.
neural a.
neuronal a.
nociceptor a.
parahippocampal a.
peripheral nociceptor a.
posterior hippocampal a.
prefrontal cortex a.
a. procedure
right ventricular a. (RVA)
activator
plasminogen a. (PA)
recombinant tissue plasminogen a. (RTPA)
a. table
tissue plasminogen a. (TPA, t-PA)
urokinase-type plasminogen a. (u-PA)
active
a. integral range of motion (AIROM)
a. metabolite
a. pathophysiologic process
a. state
a. surface electrode
a. technique
a. zone
active-phase
activity
absolute metabolic a.
adrenal nerve a.
adrenomedullary a.
alpha frequency a.
antimuscarine cholinergic a.
anxiolytic a.
asymmetrical generalized epileptiform a.
background a.
barbiturate-induced spindle-like a.
beta a.
bilateral a.
bimanual neuronal a.
biochemical a.
blocking a.
burst of delta a.
calmodulin-independent neuronal nitric oxide synthase a.
cerebral antioxidant a.
C fiber a.
cholinergic a.
cortical a.
a.'s of daily living (ADL)
decreased interest in a.
delta a.
desynchronization a.
diffuse distribution of a.
disruption of normal a.
dopaminergic a.
efferent sympathetic a.
electrical a.
electrocerebral a.
electrographic seizure a.
endplate a.
epileptiform a.
excessive diffuse low and medium wave beta a.
extracellular calcium a.
extracerebral a.
fad a.

focal delta slow wave a.
focal epileptiform a.
frenzied psychomotor a.
frontal intermittent rhythmic delta a. (FIRDA)
gamma-aminolevulinic acid dehydratase a.
high-frequency a.
high voltage slow and sharp a.
hypersynchronous a.
hypnotic a.
ictal epileptiform a.
insertional a.
intensive motor a.
interictal EEG a.
interictal epileptiform a.
intermittent rhythmic delta a. (IRDA)
lambdoid a.
lateralized a.
level of a.
Lewis blood group a.
A. Loss Assessment
low-amplitude a.
low-frequency a.
low physical a.
low-voltage a.
lysosomal enzymatic a.
metabolic a.
MFD a.
monomorphic a.
monorhythmic frontal delta a.
monorhythmic sinusoidal delta a.
motor a.
muscle a.
myorelaxant a.
neuronal spike a.
noncerebral a.
nonepileptiform a.
occipital dominant intermittent rhythmic delta a.
occipital intermittent rhythmic delta a. (OIRDA)
orbitofrontal a.
oscillatory brain a.
paroxysmal alpha a.
pathologic spontaneous a.
peripheral cholinergic a.
peripheral electromyographic a.
photic-induced epileptiform a.
physical a.
polymorphic delta a. (PDA)
polyrhythmic a.
pontogeniculooccipital spike-inhibiting a.
posterior dominant a.
posttraumatic epileptiform a.
progestational a.
propagation of a.
pseudoepileptiform a.
reflex neurologic a.
rhythmic delta a.
rhythmic spindle-shaped a.
runs of a.
scalp-derived EEG a.
scattered dysrhythmic slow a.
sedative a.
seizure a.
seizurelike a.
semipurposeful a.
serotonergic a.
sigma a.
sleep a.
slow wave a. (SWA)
spectral peak frequency of a.
spiking a.
spontaneous a.
synaptic a.
synchronous epileptiform a.
thermoeffector a.
theta a.
tonic-clonic a.
triphasic slow wave a.
unilateral epileptiform a.
unilateral focus of a.
widespread beta a.
widespread distribution of a.

Actron

ACT system

actylate

ACU-dyne antiseptic

acuity
central vision a.
temporal processing a. (TPA)

acuology

acupuncture anesthesia

acustica
area a.
radiatio a.

acusticae
striae medullares a.

NOTES

acusticae *(continued)*
taeniae a.
teniae a.
acustici
trigonum nervi a.
acusticus
nervus a. [CN VIII]
nucleus a.
porus a.
acute
a. acquired hemiplegia
a. African sleeping sickness
a. angular kyphosis
a. anoxia
a. anterior poliomyelitis
a. aphonia
a. ascending paralysis
a. atrophic paralysis
a. axonal motor neuropathy
a. brachial radiculitis
a. brain syndrome
a. bulbar poliomyelitis
a. burst injury
a. central cervical spinal cord injury
a. cerebellar ataxia (ACA)
a. cerebellar hemispheric lesion
a. cerebrospinal meningitis (ACM)
a. change in mental status
a. chorea
a. confusional migraine
a. confusional state
a. decubitus ulcer
a. delirium
a. disconnection syndrome
a. disseminated encephalomyelitis (ADE)
a. disseminating encephalomyelitis
a. dystonic reaction (ADR)
a. epidemic leukoencephalitis
a. febrile polyneuritis
a. foot-shock stress
a. fulminating meningococcemia
a. genomic response
a. hemorrhagic encephalitis
a. hydrocephalus
a. idiopathic demyelinating polyradiculoneuritis (AIDP)
a. idiopathic polyneuritis
a. inclusion body encephalitis
a. infective polyneuritis
a. inflammatory demyelinating polyradiculoneuropathy
a. inflammatory demyelinating polyradiculopathy
a. inflammatory polyneuropathy
a. intermittent porphyria
a. ischemic brachial neuropathy
a. lateral poliomyelitis
a. lateral sclerosis (ALS)
a. Marchiafava-Bignami disease
a. motor-sensory axonal sensory neuropathy
a. mountain sickness (AMS)
a. necrotizing encephalitis
a. necrotizing hemorrhagic encephalomyelitis
a. necrotizing hemorrhagic leukoencephalitis
a. necrotizing myelitis
a. neuronal damage
a. neuronal toxicity
a. neuropsychologic disorder
a. nociceptive response
a. organic brain syndrome
a. organic reaction
a. pain disorder
a. painful polyneuropathy
a. pandysautonomia
a. paralytic poliomyelitis
a. partial myelopathy
a. perivascular myelinoclasis
a. physiologic assessment and chronic health evaluation (APACHE)
A. Physiology Score
a. posterior multifocal placoid pigment
a. postinfectious polyneuropathy
a. postinfective polyneuritis
a. posttraumatic neurosis
a. primary hemorrhagic meningoencephalitis
a. psychoorganic syndrome
a. purulent meningitis
a. reflex bone atrophy
a. sensory-motor axonal neuropathy
a. severe hypotension
a. steroid quadriplegic myopathy
a. stroke
a. subdural hematoma
a. thrombosis
a. transverse myelitis
a. transverse myelopathy
a. trypanosomiasis
a. tubular necrosis
a. whiplash
acutely acquired hemiplegia
acute-onset paraparesis
acyclovir
acyl-CoA (ACAT)
a.-C. dehydrogenase deficiency
a.-C. oxidase deficiency
palmitoyl a.-C.

AD
Alzheimer disease
autonomic dysreflexia
AD-related dementia
Ad7C cerebrospinal fluid test
adamantinoma
pituitary a.
Adamkiewicz artery
Adams-Stokes
A.-S. disease
A.-S. syncope
A.-S. syndrome
adaptation
a. dynamic
fascicular a.
adaptational approach
adapter
Brown-Roberts-Wells ring a.
halo-ring a.
MicroSeal a.
Telestill photo a.
adaptive
a. control of thought system
a. equipment
a. functioning
ADAS
Alzheimer Disease Assessment Scale
A. noncognitive subscale
ADC
AIDS dementia complex
Alzheimer Disease Center
apparent diffusion coefficient
axiodistocervical
Adcon-L
A.-L. adhesion control in a barrier gel
Adderall XR
Addison disease
addisonia
encephalopathia a.
additive
a. neurotoxicity
a. W
add-on drug
adduction weakness
adductor
a. dysphonia
a. foot reflex
a. thigh reflex
ADE
acute disseminated encephalomyelitis
A-delta fiber
adendric
adendritic
adenine arabinoside
adenocarcinoma
mucin-secreting a.
adenohypophyseal, adenohypophysial
a. cell
a. compromise
a. neoplasia
adenohypophysectomy
adenohypophyseos
intermedia a.
pars distalis a.
pars intermedia a.
adenohypophysial (*var. of* adenohypophyseal)
adenohypophysis
agranular chromophobe cell in a.
intermediate part of a.
adenohypophysitis
allergic a.
lymphocytic a.
adenoid cystic carcinoma
adenoid-type adenoma
adenoma
acidophil a.
ACTH-producing a.
adenoid-type a.
basophil a.
basophilic a.
choroid plexus a.
chromophil a.
chromophobe a.
chromophobic a.
cutaneous a.
ectopic pituitary a. (EPA)
endocrine-inactive pituitary a.
eosinophil a.
fetal a.
follicle-stimulating/luteinizing hormone a.
giant pituitary a.
glycoprotein-secreting a.
gonadotropin-producing a.
growth hormone-producing a.
growth hormone-secreting a.
hypersecretory a.
intraspinal a.
invasive pituitary a.
islet cell a.

NOTES

adenoma *(continued)*
mammosomatotroph cell a.
mixed growth hormone-prolactin cell a.
nonfunctioning a.
null-cell a.
pituitary a.
pleomorphic a.
prolactin-producing a.
prolactin-secreting pituitary a.
sebaceous a.
a. sebaceum
suprasellar a.
thyrotropin-producing a.
undifferentiated cell a.
adenomatoid odontogenic tumor
adenomectomy
transsphenoidal selective a.
adenoneural
adenopathy
hilar a.
adenopituicyte
adenosine
a. 3′,5′-cyclic monophosphate (cAMP)
a. diphosphate (ADP)
endogenous a.
a. monophosphate acid (AMPA)
nucleoside a.
a. 5′-phosphosulfate (APS)
a. receptor
a. triphosphatase (ATPase)
a. triphosphate
a. 5′-triphosphate (ATP)
a. triphosphate-dependent potassium channel
a. triphosphate synthesis
adenosylcobalamin
adenovirus
adenylate cyclase
adenyl cyclase
adenylosuccinase deficiency
adenylyl cyclase
adequate stimulus
ADH
antidiuretic hormone
Adhalin
adhesio, pl. **adhesiones**
a. interthalamica
a. interthalamica tumor
adhesion
arachnoid a.
interthalamic a.
matrix a.
a. molecule
motility a.
neuronal a.
VLA-4 a.
adhesive arachnoiditis
adiabatic fast passage
adiadochokinesis, adiadochocinesia, adiadochocinesis
adiaphoria
Adie
A. tonic pupil
A. tonic pupil syndrome
Adie-Holmes pupil
adipiodone
adipocellular
adipogenic
adipogenous
adiposalgia
adipose
a. graft
a. tissue
adiposis cerebralis
adiposity
cerebral a.
pituitary a.
adiposogenital
a. degeneration
a. dystrophia
a. dystrophy
a. syndrome
adiposogenitalis
dystrophia a.
aditus
a. ad aqueductum cerebri
a. ad infundibulum
adjacent level disease
adjunct
neuroleptic a.
adjunctive
a. amphetamine
a. medication
a. screw fixation
a. strategy
adjuration
adjustability
3D positional a.
adjustable pedicle connector
adjuvant
a. therapy
a. whole-brain radiation therapy
adjuvanticity
Adkins spinal fusion
ADL
activities of daily living
extended ADL
ADL index
instrumental ADL
ADL test
Adlone Injection

ADmark Assay
administration
chronic a.
compulsive drug a.
drug a.
intracisternal a.
intramuscular a.
leptomeningeal enhancement postcontrast a.
long-standing corticosteroid a.
methylphenidate a.
oral a.
standard dose a.
systematic drug a.
admonition
ADMSEP
Association of Directors of Medical Student Education in Psychiatry
adnerval
adneural
adolescence
myoclonic epilepsy of a.
adolescent-onset epilepsy
adonadism
ADP
adenosine diphosphate
ADPR
Alzheimer Disease Patient Registry
ADP-ribosylation
pertussis-toxin-catalyzed A.-r.
ADR
acute dystonic reaction
ADRC
Alzheimer Disease Research Center
adrenal
a. androgen
a. androgen production
a. androstenedione
a. axis
a. body transplant
a. chromaffin cell
a. cortex
a. cortical hyperfunction
a. crisis
a. gland
a. insufficiency
a. leukodystrophy
a. medulla graft
a. medulla transplantation
a. nerve activity
a. segment
adrenaline-Mecholyl test
adrenergic
a. blockade
a. fiber
a. hyperstimulation
a. innervation
a. neuronal blocking agent
a. neurotransmission
a. neurotransmitter
a. receptor
a. system
2-adrenergic
alpha 2-a.
adrenoceptive
adrenoceptor
adrenochrome
adrenocortical
a. coma
a. insufficiency
adrenocorticotrophic hormone-secreting pituitary tumor (ACTH-secreting pituitary tumor)
adrenocorticotropic
a. compromise
a. hormone (ACTH)
adrenocorticotropin
adrenoleukodystrophy (ALD)
neonatal a.
adrenoleukodystrophy/adrenomyeloneuropathy (ALD-AMN)
a.-a. complex
adrenoleukomyeloneuropathy
adrenolytic
adrenomedullary
a. activity
a. component
adrenomimetic
adrenomyelodystrophy (AMD)
adrenomyeloneuropathy
adrenoreceptor
adromania
adromia
ADRS
Alzheimer Disease Rating Scale
Adson
A. bipolar forceps
A. brain-exploring cannula
A. brain-extracting cannula
A. brain suction tip
A. brain suction tube
A. clip-introducing forceps

Adson *(continued)*
A. conductor
A. cranial rongeur
A. cup forceps
A. dissecting hook
A. dressing forceps
A. dural hook
A. dural knife
A. dural needle holder
A. dural protector
A. dural protector guide
A. elevator
A. enlarging bur
A. ganglion scissors
A. hemilaminectomy retractor
A. hemostatic forceps
A. hypophysial forceps
A. knot tier
A. laminectomy chisel
A. modified maneuver
A. needle
A. nerve hook
A. perforating bur
A. right-angle knife
A. scalp clip
A. test
A. tissue forceps
A. wire saw
Adson-Anderson cerebellar retractor
Adson-Brown forceps
Adson-Mixter neurosurgical forceps
Adson-Rogers cranial bur
AdTech
A. electrode guide
A. electrode strip
A. Spencer platinum depth electrode
adterminal
adult
a. acid maltase deficiency
General Ability Measure for A.'s (GAMA)
a. granulosa cell tumor (AGCT)
hemispheric asymmetry reduction in older a.'s (HAROLD)
a. lipofuscinosis
a. polyglucosan body disease
a. pseudohypertrophic muscular dystrophy
a. respiratory distress syndrome
a. Reye syndrome (ARS)
a. scoliosis
a. scoliosis patient
a. scoliosis surgery
subclinical rhythmic EEG discharge of a.'s (SREDA)
subclinical rhythmic epileptiform discharge of a.
a. unit
a. Wada testing
adultomorphic
a. behavior
a. behavior role
a. stance
adult-onset
a.-o. combined methylmalonic aciduria and homocystinuria
a.-o. dystonia
a.-o. epilepsy
a.-o. myasthenia gravis
a.-o. spinal muscular atrophy
advanced
a. cortical disease
a. design LINAC radiosurgery
a. glycation end-product (AGE)
a. sleep-phase syndrome (ASPS)
a. wakefulness theory
advancement
bimaxillary a.
frontoorbital a.
genioglossus a.
hyoid a.
monobloc a.
transcranial frontofacial a.
advantage
psychometric a.
right ear a.
therapeutic a.
adventitial neuritis
adverse
a. autonomic response
a. negative immunosuppressive effect
a. neurologic complication
a. side effect
adynamia episodica hereditaria
Aeby plane
AED
antiepileptic drug
Aedes aegypti
AEEG
ambulatory electroencephalogram
ambulatory electroencephalography
aegypti
Aedes a.
aerasthenia
aerocele
epidural a.
intracranial a.
aerophilus
Haemophilus a.
aerosolized droplet nucleus

aeruginosa
Pseudomonas a.
Aesculap
A. bipolar cautery
A. skull perforator
aestheticism
aesthetics
afebrile seizure
affability
surface a.
affect
cognitive generation of a.
a. elicitation
evoked a.
generation of a.
hyperactive a.
hypoactive a.
a. spasm
a. trauma model
affective
a. arousal theory
permissive hypothesis of a.
a. process
a. processing
a. prodrome of epilepsy
a. prodrome of migraine
a. property
a. reaction
a. schematic mental model
a. state
a. symptom
a. symptom of seizure
affectomotor
affect-related
a.-r. processing
a.-r. schematic mental model
affectualization
afferent
a. digital lesion
a. digital nerve
excitatory a.
general somatic a. (GSA)
general visceral a. (GVA)
a. input
a. limb
a. motor unit
a. nerve fiber
a. nerve lesion
a. neurofiber
a. neuron
a. pathway
a. pupillary defect
a. relation
special somatic a. (SSA)
a. thermosensory information
afferentes
neurofibrae a.
affiliation drive
affiliative drive
affinal
affinin
affinity
receptor a.
affinous
affixa
lamina a.
affix afflict
afflict
affix a.
A-fiber evoked response
afibrinogenemia
AFP
alpha-fetoprotein
A-frame electrode
African
A. sleeping sickness
A. trypanosomiasis
AFT
attractor field therapy
afterbrain
aftercontraction
aftercurrent
afterdischarge
amygdala-kindled a.
myotonic a.
photic a.
a. threshold
afterhyperpolarization
afterimage
afterimpression
afterloading catheter
aftermovement
afternystagmus
cycles of a.
optokinetic a. (OKAN)
afterperception
afterpotential
negative a.
positive a.
aftersensation
aftersound
aftertaste

NOTES

aftertouch
aftervision
afunction
agalactiae
Streptococcus a.
aganglionic
aganglionosis
agapism
agarose
a. gel electrophoresis
low-melt temperature a.
agastroneuria
AGCT
adult granulosa cell tumor
AGE
advanced glycation end-product
arterial gas embolism
age-appropriate strategy
age-associated
a.-a. memory failure
a.-a. memory impairment
a.-a. sensitivity
age-dependent
a.-d. epilepsy
a.-d. epilepsy syndrome
a.-d. length
a.-d. slowing
Agee technique
agenesia corticalis
agenesis
callosal a.
carotid artery a.
corpus callosum a.
a. of corpus callosum
nuclear a.
Pang type a.
partial a.
sacral a.
sacrococcygeal a.
total a.
agent
adrenergic neuronal blocking a.
alkylating a.
alpha-adrenergic blocking a.
anticholinergic a.
antidipsotropic a.
antidyskinetic a.
antifibrinolytic a.
antimicrobial a.
antiparkinsonism a.
beta-adrenergic receptor blocking a.
calcium channel blocking a.
cerebral blood flow a.
cerebral vasodilating a.
chemosensitivity enhancing a.
chimpanzee coryza a. (CCA)
conventional neuroleptic a.
dibenzoxozepine a.
disease-modifying a. (DMA)
endogenous neuroprotective a.
fast-acting a.
fibrinolytic a.
FloSeal hemostatic a.
ganglionic blocking a.
5-HT releasing a.
hyperosmotic a.
hypnotic a.
monoamine oxidase inhibitor-serotonergic a.
mood-stabilizing a.
natural chemotherapy a.
N-butyl 2-cyanoacrylate with lipiodol adhesive a.
neuromuscular blocking a.
neuronal stabilizing a.
nonionic contrast a.
noxious a.
Onyx liquid embolic a.
oral antiviral a.
pharmacologic a.
pharmacological a.
Proceed hemostatic a.
psychopharmacologic a.
psychotomimetic a.
psychotropic a.
reinforcing a.
second-line a.
serotonergic a.
short-acting hypnotic a.
susceptibility a.
sympathomimetic a.
tantalum powder contrast a.
therapeutic a.
traditional neuroleptic a.
tumor differentiating a.
in utero teratologic a.
age-related
a.-r. brain change
a.-r. comorbidity
a.-r. deterioration process
a.-r. developmental process
a.-r. epileptogenesis
a.-r. memory impairment
a.-r. pharmacodynamic change
a.-r. pharmacokinetic change
age-specific
a.-s. cumulative incidence
a.-s. risk factor
Ages and Stages Questionnaires
ageusia
ageusic aphasia
ageustia
agger nasi cell

agglutination
latex a.
agglutition
aggrandize
aggrecan proteoglycan
aggregate
epileptic neuronal a.
fibrillary a.
gaze coordinating a.
neuronal a.
aggregated
technetium 99m albumin a.
Aggrenox
aggressive papillary middle ear tumor
aggrieved
aging
amyloidosis of a.
brain a.
neuroanatomy of a.
agitans
Hunt juvenile paralysis a.
paralysis a.
spasmus a.
agitata
amentia a.
cephalea a.
melancholia a.
agitated
a. delirium syndrome
a. reaction
agitation
Caitlin a.
a. level
marked motor a.
nocturnal a.
overlapping a.
overt a.
a. response
agitator
agitolalia
agitophasia
aglomerular
agnate
agnea
agnesis
Kaplan a.
Toriello-Carey a.
Wilson a.
AgNOR
silver-staining nucleolar organizer region
agnosia
apperceptive visual a.
associative visual a.
auditory a.
autotopagnosia a.
color a.
corporal a.
facial a.
finger a.
generalized auditory a.
ideational a.
localization a.
object a.
optic a.
position a.
posture a.
selective auditory a.
somatagnosia a.
tactile a.
topographical a.
verbal auditory a.
visual a.
visual-spatial a.
agonism
GABA a.
gamma aminobutyric acid a.
agonist
dopamine a.
D_2-selective dopamine a.
ergot-derivative dopamine a.
high-dose dopaminergic a.
5-HT a.
low-dose dopaminergic a.
M1 a.
a. muscle
serotonin 5-HT receptor a.
vasopressin receptor a.
agrammatica
agrammatism agraphia
agrammatologia
agranular
a. chromophobe cell in adenohypophysis
a. cortex
agranulocytosis
agraphia
absolute a.
acoustic a.
agrammatism a.
a. alexia
alexia with a.

NOTES

agraphia *(continued)*
alexia without a.
amnemonic a.
aphasic a.
apraxic a.
atactic a.
atactica a.
cerebral a.
constructional a.
lexical a.
literal a.
mental a.
motor a.
musical a.
paretic a.
perseverative a.
phonological a.
pure a.
spatial a.
verbal a.
agraphic
agrypnodal coma
agyria
agyric
AH
autonomic hyperreflexia
AHI
apnea-hypopnea index
AHSCT
autologous hematopoietic stem cell transplantation
ahylognosia
ahypnia, ahypnosia
AI
apnea index
AI adenosine receptor (AIAR)
AI, AII area
AIAR
AI adenosine receptor
AICA
anterior inferior cerebellar artery
Aicardi-Goutieres
A.-G. disease
A.-G. syndrome
Aicardi syndrome
aid
ergogenic a.'s
external memory a.
walking a.
AIDP
acute idiopathic demyelinating polyradiculoneuritis
autoimmune demyelinating polyneuropathy
AIDS
acquired immunodeficiency syndrome
A. dementia
A. dementia complex (ADC)
A. encephalopathy
A. neuropathy
AIDS-associated vacuolar myelopathy
AIDS-related
A.-r. myelopathy
A.-r. toxoplasmosis
AIF
apoptosis-inducing factor
aigu
delire a.
AION
anterior ischemic optic neuropathy
air
a. blade
a. blast
a. cell
a. conduction test
a. contrast study
a. drill
a. embolism
a. embolus
intracranial a.
a. plasma spray
a. plethysmography
a. tube
a. ventriculography
air-bone gap
airborne arthroconidia
air-brain interface
airflow
air-fluid level
Airlife MediSpacer
AIROM
active integral range of motion
air-powered drill
air-stepping
airstream mechanism
airway
artificial a.
a. control
a. edema
esophageal a.
a. muscle tone
pharyngeal a.
a. protection
upper a.
akari
Rochalimaea a.
akataphasia, acataphasia
akathisia, acathisia
treatment-emergent a.
akinesia
a. algera
a. amnestica
early morning a.
akinesic

akinesis
akinesthesia
akinetic
a. apraxia
a. drop attack
a. drop spell
a. epilepsy
a. mutism
a. patient
akinetic-rigid syndrome
Akineton
akoria (*var. of* acoria)
Akros
A. extended care mattress
A. pressure mattress
AK-Taine
aktamathesia
Akureyri disease
ala, pl. **alae**
a. of central lobule
a. cerebelli
a. cinerea
alae lingulae cerebelli
a. lobuli centralis
a. lobulis centralis
alabamensis
Acremonium a.
Alagille syndrome
Alajouanine syndrome
alalia
alalic
alanine
a. transaminase
a. tRNA
alanyl
alanyl-tRNA synthetase
alar
a. lamina of neural tube
a. ligament
a. plate
a. plate of neural tube
a. screw
alaris
lamina a.
alarm
ventilator a.
alarm-clock headache
alba
commissura ventralis a.
substantia a.
Albee
A. lumbar spinal fusion
A. olive-shaped bur
A. shelf procedure
albendazole therapy
Albenza
Albert Grass Heritage PSG
albicans
Candida a.
Cryptococcus a.
albocinereous
Albright syndrome
albumin
low serum a.
a. metabolism
serum a.
technetium 99m macroaggregated a.
a. transfusion
albuminocytologic dissociation
albuterol
Alcadd Test, Revised Edition
Alcar
alchemy
Alcock test
alcohol
allyl a.
a. dehydrogenase
intermediate brain syndrome due to a.
a. metabolism
a. neurolysis
a. persisting dementia
polyvinyl a.
saliva screen for a.
a. toxicity
a. withdrawal seizure
alcoholic
a. amblyopia
a. amnesia
a. classification
a. coma
a. delirium tremens
a. encephalopathy
a. epilepsy
a. myopathy
a. peripheral neuropathy
a. poisoning
a. polyneuropathy
a. withdrawal tremor
alcoholica
amblyopia a.

NOTES

alcohol-induced
a.-i. depression
a.-i. peripheral neuropathy
alcoholism
Collaborative Study on the Genetics of A. (COGA)
alcohol-precipitated epilepsy
alcohol-related
a.-r. phenotype
a.-r. seizure
ALD
adrenoleukodystrophy
ALD-AMN
adrenoleukodystrophy/adrenomyeloneuropathy
ALD-AMN complex
aldehyde
a. dehydrogenase
aldose reductase
aldosterone deficiency
Aldrich syndrome
alemmal
alemtuzumab humanized monoclonal antibody
alendronate
alert
oriented and a.
a. and oriented (AAO)
Alertec
alerting
a. maneuver on electroencephalogram
a. stimulus on electroencephalogram
alertness
a. behavior (AB)
level of a.
mental a.
phasic a.
state of a.
Alexander disease
alexia
agraphia a.
a. allocheiria
anterior a.
central a.
incomplete a.
motor a.
musical a.
optical a.
posterior a.
pure a.
sensory a.
tactile a.
visual a.
a. with agraphia
a. without agraphia
alexic
alexithymic
alfentanil
algera
akinesia a.
dyskinesia a.
algesia
algesic
algesichronometer
algesimeter (*var. of* algesiometer)
algesimetry
algesiogenic
algesiometer, algesimeter
Aly a.
Björnström a.
Boas a.
algesthesia
algesthesis
algetic
algica
synesthesia a.
algiomotor
algiomuscular
algodystrophy
algogenesia
algogenesis
algogenic
algologist
algology
algometer
pressure a.
algometry
algoneurodystrophy
algophobia
algorithm
bone a.
Fourier transform a.
hydrophobicity a.
interpolation a.
algospasm
ALI
argon laser iridotomy
aliasing on electroencephalogram
Alice in Wonderland syndrome
aliele
alielism
alielomorph
alien
a. hand sign
a. hand syndrome
a. limb phenomenon
a. limb sign
alienation
body a.
sense of a.
alignment
ocular a.
sagittal anatomic a.

alimentary
a. edema
a. seizure
alimentation
parenteral a.
alinjection
aliphatic
aliquorrhea
aliquot
alkaline phosphatase
alkaloid
a. neuropathy
vinca a.
alkalosis
metabolic a.
respiratory a.
tetany of a.
alkaptonuria
Alksne iron suspension
alkylamine
alkylating
a. agent
a. chemotherapy
alkylguanine alkyltransferase
alkyltransferase
alkylguanine a.
allachesthesia
allantoic bladder
allantoidean
allantois
allele
ApoE e4 a.
a. A2 of TaqIA
e4 a.
wild-type a.
allelic
a. heterogeneity
a. loss
allelism
allemande
vice a.
Allen
A. maneuver
A. picture
A. rule
A. test
allergic
a. adenohypophysitis
a. angiitis
a. encephalomyelitis
a. reaction
allesthesia, alloesthesia
visual a.
Allevyn dressing
Allgrave syndrome
alliance
contractual a.
relational a.
allied reflex
alligator
a. cup forceps
a. MacCarty scissors
alliterate
alliteration
all-median nerve hand
allocheiria, allochiria
alexia a.
allochesthesia
allochiral
allochiria (*var. of* allocheiria)
allocinesia
allocortex
Alloderm
allodynia
brush-evoked a.
brush-induced a.
cold-induced a.
static a.
alloesthesia (*var. of* allesthesia)
allograft
a. bone grafting
fibular a.
a. iliac bone
Puros Accugraft a.
A. spacer
a. strut
Tutoplast processed a.
allokinesis
allokinetic
allolalia
Allomatrix bone substitute
allomeric function
allonomous
allopath
allopathist
allopatric species
allophasis
allophone tabulation
alloplastic
a. cranioplasty
a. material
allosteric manner

NOTES

allotriosmia
allotropic
Allport
all-ulnar nerve hand
allurement
allyl
a. alcohol
a. isothiocyanate
allylgycine
almond nucleus
almotriptan malate
Alnico
A. Magneprobe magnet
A. Magneprobe magnet alpha
alobar holoprosencephaly
alogia
alopecia
a. capitis totalis
a. disseminata
a. follicularis
Johnston a.
a. liminaris frontalis
lipedematous a.
moth-eaten a.
a. neurotica
patterned a.
a. prematura
a. triangularis congenitalis
alosetron
Alpers disease
alpha
a. 2-adrenergic
Alnico Magneprobe magnet a.
a. beta peptide
a. blocking
a. cell of anterior lobe of hypophysis
a. coefficient
Cronbach a.
a. ET
a. ethyltryptamine
a. fetoprotein
a. fiber
a. frequency activity
a. frequency band
a. frequency coma
a. frequency range
a. index
a. interferon
a. mannosidosis
a. motoneuron
a. motor neuron
obsessional compulsive inventory a.
occipital a.
a. pattern
a. response
a. rhythm
a. rhythm frequency
a. secretase
a. spindle
a. state
a. test
a. tocopherol
a. transient
a. wave
a. wave strain
alpha-1 adrenergic antagonist
alpha2 globulin
alpha-*N*-acetyl-galactosaminidase
alpha-*N*-acetyl-glucosaminidase
alpha-adrenergic
a.-a. blocking agent
a.-a. receptor
alpha-2 adrenergic receptor
alpha-adrenoceptor antagonist
alpha-aminoadipic aciduria
alpha-amino-3-hydroxy-5-methylisoxazole-4-proprionic acid
alpha-arc
alpha, beta, gamma hypothesis
***dl*-alpha-difluoromethylornithine**
alpha-fetoprotein (AFP)
alpha-galactoside A
alpha-galactoside B
alpha-glucosidase
alpha-*L*-iduronidase
alpha-ketoadipic aciduria
alpha-ketoglutarate oxidation
alpha-lactrotoxin
alpha-mannosidase
alpha-methylacetoacetic aciduria
alphamimetic
alphaprodine hydrochloride
alpha-synuclein
a.-s. protein
Alphavirus
Alport syndrome
alprazolam
ALS
acute lateral sclerosis
amyotrophic lateral sclerosis
ALS-like syndrome
ALS-PD
amyotrophic lateral sclerosis-Parkinson dementia
ALS-PD complex
Alstrom-Hallgren syndrome
alteplase
alteration
behavior a.
cyclic a.
genomic a.
language a.
a. of memory structure

neurocognitive a.
selective speech perception a.
speech processing a.
speech tracking a.
altered
a. cognition
a. consciousness
a. function
a. mental status
a. sleep schedule
a. spatial perception
a. tau processing
a. time perception
alternans
hemiplegia a.
alternate
a. binaural loudness balance
a. binaural loudness balance test
a. hemianesthesia
a. motion rate (AMR)
alternating
a. current (AC)
a. hemiplegia of childhood
a. hypoglossal hemiplegia
a. mydriasis
a. nystagmus
a. skew deviation
a. tremor
alternation
genetic a.
alternative
graft material a.
a. occipital artery middle cerebral artery
a. tremor
althesin
altitude insomnia
altitudinal
a. hemianopia
a. visual field defect
altophobia
altricial
altricious
Altropane
altruism
aluminum
brain a.
a. contouring template set
a. cranioplasty
a. glycinate
a. hydroxide with magnesium hydroxide and simethicone
a. intoxication
a. master rod
a. toxicity
alvear fasciculus
alvei (*pl. of* alveus)
alveolar
a. hypoventilation syndrome
a. nerve
alveolus, pl. **alveoli**
alveus, pl. **alvei**
a. of hippocampus
Aly algesiometer
Alzheimer
A. atrophic dementia
A. basket
A. cell
A. disease (AD)
A. Disease Assessment Scale (ADAS)
A. Disease Center (ADC)
A. disease neuropathology
A. disease noncognitive subscale
A. Disease Patient Registry (ADPR)
A. Disease Rating Scale (ADRS)
A. disease-related dementia
A. Disease and Related Disorders Association
A. Disease Research Center (ADRC)
A. neurofibrillary degeneration
A. precursor protein (APP)
A. sclerosis
A. senile dementia (ASD)
A. survivor
A. type I, II astrocyte
Alzheimer-type senile dementia
amacrine cell
Amanita
amanitin
amantadine hydrochloride
amarilla
barba a.
amativeness
amaurosis
cat's eye a.
central a.
a. centralis
cerebral a.

NOTES

amaurosis *(continued)*
a. fugax
gaze-evoked a.
Leber congenital a.
uremic a.
amaurotic idiocy
ambageusia
ambenonium
ambidexterity
ambidextrism
ambidextrous
Ambien
ambiens
cisterna a.
ambient cistern
ambiguity
acoustic a.
diagnostic a.
ambiguous
a. external stimulus
a. nucleus
ambiguus
a. nucleus
nucleus a.
ambilevosity
ambilevous
AmBisome
ambitieux
delire a.
amblyaphia
amblygeustia
amblyogenic period
amblyope
amblyopia
alcoholic a.
a. alcoholica
a. ex anopsia
tobacco-alcohol a.
toxic a.
ambon
ambulation
brace-free a.
a. skill
ambulatory
a. automatism
a. EEG recording
a. electroencephalogram (AEEG)
a. electroencephalography (AEEG)
AMD
adrenomyelodystrophy
AME
aseptic meningoencephalitis
AME microcurrent TENS unit
amebiasis
cerebral a.
Entamoeba histolytica cerebral a.
Iodamoeba buetschlii cerebral a.
amebic
a. aneurysm
a. infection
a. meningoencephalitis
ameboid
a. astrocyte
a. cell
ameboidism
ameloblastoma
pituitary a.
ameloblastomatous craniopharyngioma
amenorrhea
hypothalamic a.
primary a.
amentia
a. agitata
eclamptic a.
nevoid a.
amential
America
Huntington Disease Society of A. (HDSA)
American
A. Academy of Cerebral Palsy
A. Academy of Sleep Medicine
A. Association of Directors of Psychiatric Residency Training (AADPRT)
A. Association for Geriatric Psychiatry (AAGP)
A. Association of Neurological Surgeons/Congress of Neurological Surgeons (AANS/CNS)
A. Association for the Psychophysiological Study of Sleep
A. Board of Psychiatry and Neurology (ABPN)
A. Brain Tumor Association
A. College of Neuropsychiatrists
A. Council for Headache Education
A. Musculoskeletal Tumor Society rating scale
A. Optical Hardy-Rand-Rittler color plate
A. Pain Society
A. silk suture
A. Sleep Disorders Association
A. Spinal Cord Injury Association classification
A. Spinal Injury Association/International Medical Society of Paraplegia (ASIA/IMSOP)
A. Spinal Injury Association/International Medical

Society of Paraplegia Impairment Scale
A. Sterilizer operating table
A. Thoracic Society
Ames demonstration
A-methaPred Injection
Amicar
amiculum, pl. **amicula**
a. olivare
amidotrizoic acid
Amikin
amimia
amnesiac a.
amine
biogenic a.
a. precursor uptake decarboxylase (APUD)
amineptine
aminergic
amino
a. acid (AA)
a. acid metabolic disorder
a. acid neurotransmitter
a. acid transporter
aminoacidopathy
aminoaciduria
arginase deficiency a.
argininosuccinic a.
Baló a.
carnosinemia a.
cystathioninuria a.
a. deficiency
Devic a.
histidinemia a.
hydroxyisovaleric a.
hyperbetaalaninemia a.
hyperlysinemia a.
hyperprolinemia a.
isovaleric acidemia a.
Marchiafava-Bignami a.
methylmalonic a.
neonatal tyrosinemia a.
primary a.
Schilder a.
sulfite oxidase deficiency a.
tyrosinemia a.
aminobenzoate
butyl a.
sodium a.
aminocaproic acid
aminoglutethimide
aminoglycoside
aminopenicillin
4-aminopyridine
21-aminosteroid U74006F
aminotransferase
aspartate a. (AST)
kynurenine a.
ornithine-ketoacid a.
Amipaque
Amitone
amitriptyline
a. hydrochloride
a. hydrochloride and chlordiazepoxide
amixia
AML
amyotrophic lateral sclerosis
Ammon
A. horn
A. horn sclerosis
ammonia
a. blood level
a. intoxication
ammonis
cornu a.
subiculum cornu a.
ammonium
a. chloride
a. chloride delirium
a. tetrathiomolybdate
ammonotelic
amnemonic
a. agraphia
a. aphasia
amnesia
alcoholic a.
amnesic a.
antegrade a.
anterograde a. (AA)
auditory a.
basal forebrain a.
Broca a.
circumscribed a.
concussion a.
confabulatory a.
continuous a.
dissociative a.
emotional a.
episodic a.
executive (or frontal) deficit transient global a.

NOTES

amnesia *(continued)*
frontal dysexecutive a.
functional retrograde a.
generalized a.
global a.
hippocampal a.
hysterical a.
ictal a.
infantile a.
Korsakoff a.
korsakoffian a.
lacunar a.
localized a.
olfactory a.
organic a.
patchy retrograde a.
postconcussion a.
postconcussive a.
posthypnotic a.
posttraumatic a.
pretraumatic a.
psychogenic a.
retroactive a.
selective a.
shrinking retrograde a.
tactile a.
transient global a. (TGA)
a. for trauma
traumatic a.
verbal a.
visual a.
amnesiac amimia
amnesic
a. amnesia
a. memoration
a. patient
a. syndrome
amnestic
a. aphasia
a. apraxia
a. disorder
a. disorder due to a general medical condition
a. dysnomia
a. state
a. syndrome
amnestica
akinesia a.
amniocentesis
amniote
amobarbital-induced hemiparesis
amobarbital test
amodiaquine
amoral personality
amorphagnosia
amorphosynthesis
amorphous fraction of adrenal cortex
Amostat
amotivation
amount
maximum tolerable a.
amour-propre
amoxapine
AMPA
adenosine monophosphate acid
AMPA receptor
AMPA receptor-mediated response
ampakine CX-516
Ampalex
amperometric response
Amphedroxyn
amphetamine
adjunctive a.
a. and dextroamphetamine
gamma hydroxybutyrate and a.
a. sulfate
amphetamine/methamphetamine
analog of a.
phencyclidine and a.
amphicrania
amphicyte
amphotonia, amphotony
amp joint
Amplatz exchange length wire
amplification
a. reaction
symptom a.
amplifier
Botox injection a.
compression a.
DAM-80 a.
gradient a.
power a.
Ampligen
amplitude
absolute band a.
absolute EP a.
asymmetry a.
CMAP a.
compound muscle action potential a.
high a.
local reduction in a.
peak-to-peak a.
percentage of error in a. (PEA)
reduction of a.
relative band a.
sensory compound action potential a.
sensory nerve action potential a.
SNAP a.
very low a.
waveform a.

ampullaria
crura membranacea a.
a. ductuum
ampullaris
crista a.
cupula cristae a.
neuroepithelium cristae a.
ampullar nerve
ampullary
a. crest
a. cupula
a. limb of semicircular duct
amputation neuroma
AMR
alternate motion rate
AMS
acute mountain sickness
Amsler grid testing
AMTR
anterior mesial temporal resection
amurakh
amusia
instrumental a.
motor a.
sensory a.
vocal motor a.
AMY
amylase
AMY plaque
amyelencephalia
amyelia
amyelic
amyelinated
amyelination
amyelinic
amyeloic, amyelonic
amyelous
amygdala, pl. **amygdalae**
a. activation
a. atrophy
a. cerebelli
a. damage
a. kindling
nucleus amygdalae
a. nucleus group
a. response
a. seizure
a. subnucleus
a. volume
a. volumetric loss
amygdala-fear circuitry
amygdala-kindled afterdischarge
amygdala-prefrontal cortex-locus ceruleus interaction
amygdalar epilepsy
amygdaline
amygdaloclaustral area
amygdaloclaustralis
area a.
amygdalofugal
a. fiber
a. pathway
amygdalohippocampectomy
amygdaloid
a. body
a. complex
a. nucleus
a. tubercle
amygdaloidectomy
amygdaloidei
pars basolateralis corporis a.
pars corticomedialis corporis a.
pars olfactoria corporis a.
rami corporis a.
amygdaloideum
corpus a.
amygdalopiriformis
area transitionis a.
amygdalopiriform transition area
amygdalotomy
amyl
a. hydrate
a. nitrite
amylase (AMY)
amylene
a. chloral
a. hydrate
amyloid
a. angiopathy
a. angiopathy cerebral
a. beta (Abeta)
a. beta peptide
a. beta-protein
a. body
congophilic a.
a. deposition
a. neuropathy
a. polyneuropathy
a. precursor protein (APP)
a. precursor protein gene
amyloidoma

NOTES

amyloidosis
a. of aging
cerebrovascular a.
familial a.
hereditary neuropathic a.
heredofamilial a.
a. peripheral neuropathy
skeletal a.
transthyretin-associated neuropathic a.
amyloidosis-Dutch type
amyoesthesia, amyoesthesis
amyoplasia congenita
amyotonia congenita
amyotrophia
amyotrophic
a. lateral sclerosis (ALS, AML)
a. lateral sclerosis-Parkinson dementia (ALS-PD)
a. lateral sclerosis-Parkinson dementia complex
a. type of spongiform encephalopathy
amyotrophy
Aran-Duchenne a.
asthmatic a.
benign focal a.
brachial a.
diabetic a.
dystonic a.
hemiplegic a.
juvenile a.
monomelic a.
neuralgic a.
a. parkinsonism
primary progressive a.
progressive nuclear a.
progressive spinal a.
syphilitic a.
amyotrophy-parkinsonism
amytal
sodium a.
anacamptometer
anacatesthesia (*var. of* anakatesthesia)
anachronism
EEG a.
anacoluthon
anacusis
Anadenanthera
Anadrol
Anadrol-50
anaglyphoscope
anagoge
anagogic
anakatesthesia, anacatesthesia
anal
a. nerve
a. reflex
a. sphincter
a. verge
a. wink
analectrotonic zone
analeptic
analgesia
a. dolorosa
interpleural a. (IPA)
intrathecal morphine a.
paretic a.
patient-controlled a. (PCA)
reverse a.
analgesic
a. cuirass
migraine-neuralgia a.
a. rebound headache
analgesimeter
analgetic
analgosedation
analog, analogue
a. of amphetamine/methamphetamine
a. domain
a. filter
I-labeled cocaine a.
meperidine a.
a. of phencyclidine thiophene
prion a.
analogous brain mechanism
analog-to-digital converter
analogue (*var. of* analog)
analysis, pl. **analyses**
autoregressive model for signal a.
behavior a.
best-fit a.
bioelectrical impedance a.
biomechanical a.
cephalometric a.
cluster a.
complex segregation a.
compressed spectral a.
computer-aided image a.
computer-assisted EEG signal a.
computerized EEG signal a.
conventional factor a.
Courtship A.
Cox regression a.
deformity a.
densitometric a.
digital signal a.
DNA a.
3D relationship a.
electrooculographic a.
Fourier a.
functional a.
group a.
haplotype a.

high resolution chromosome a.
a. of homonomy
immunocytochemical a.
imprinting center mutation a.
intent-to-treat a.
interaction process a.
Kaplan-Meier survival a.
linear least-square regression a.
linear regression a.
linkage a.
mitochondrial deoxyribonucleic acid a.
morphometry a.
Northern blot a.
percept a.
perception a.
post hoc a.
power spectral a.
preliminary a.
principal-components a.
a. procedure
quantitative EEG a.
quantitative motor unit potential a.
Sassouni a.
shape a.
short EEG epoch FFT a.
signal a.
spatiotemporal source a.
SPECT a.
spectral a.
spinal fluid a.
state-of-the-art a.
taxometric a.
three-dimensional a.
total body neutron activation a.
a. of variance (ANOVA)
volumetric a.
voxel-by-voxel a.
voxel-wise a.
Western blot a.

analytic
a. therapy
thoroughness, reliability, efficiency, a.

analytical therapy

analyzer, analyzor
Axon sentinel-4 a.
fast Fourier transformation spectrum a.
immunoturbidimetry a.
IVEC-10 neurotransmitter a.
octopus visual field a.
wave a.

Anametrin

anamnestic

ananastasia

anapeiratic

anaphia, anhaphia

anaphylactic
a. shock
a. shock prophylaxis

anaphylactogenesis

anaphylactoid reaction

anaphylaxis

anaplasia

anaplastic
a. astrocytoma
a. ependymoma
a. focus
a. glioma
a. meningioma
a. oligodendroglioma

Anaprox

anaptic

anaptyxis

anarithmia

anarthria

anastomosing fiber

anastomosis, pl. **anastomoses**
carotid-basilar a.
carotid-vertebral a.
cross-facial nerve graft a.
end-to-end a.
excimer laser-assisted nonocclusive a. (ELANA)
extradural a.
faciofacial nerve a.
faciohypoglossal a.
Galen a.
grafting a.
hypoglossal-facial nerve a.
Hyrtl a.
intradural a.
intraterritorial a.
leptomeningeal a.
Martin-Gruber a.
microneurovascular a.
microvascular a.
persistent primitive carotid-basilar artery a.
persistent trigeminal artery a.
primary end-to-end a.

NOTES

anastomosis *(continued)*
Riche-Cannieu a.
spinal accessory nerve-facial nerve a.
STA-MCA a.
superior temporal artery-middle cerebral artery a.
temporal-cerebral arterial a.
traumatic a.
anastomotic
a. fiber
a. leak
anatomic
a. hook
a. pathology
anatomical
a. correlate
a. evidence
a. snuffbox
a. variant
anatomic-functional
anatomicoclinical syndrome
anatomy
cervicothoracic pedicle a.
MRI-based brain a.
pedicle a.
surgical a.
anaudia
anaxon
anaxone
ANC
absolute neutrophil count
ANCA
antineuronal cytoplasmic autoantibody
ANCA-positive granulomatous giant-cell arteritis
anchor
Isola spinal implant system a.
traction a.
anchorage-dependent signal
anchoring point
ancillary test
Ancylostoma ceylanicum
ancyroid
Andermann syndrome
Andersch
A. ganglion
A. nerve
Andersen syndrome
Anderson
A. disease
A. syndrome
Anderson-Adson scalp retractor
Andrade syndrome
André
A. anatomical hook
A. Thomas sign
Andrews frame
androgen
adrenal a.
circulating a.
a. receptor
a. secretion
androgenic property
androgenous
androgynous
androstenedione
adrenal a.
anecdotal
a. data
a. evidence
anecdote
clinical a.
anechoic chamber
anelectrotonic state
anelectrotonus
Anel method
anemic
a. anoxia
a. hypoxia
a. polyneuritis
a. polyneuropathy
anemometer
warm-wire a.
anencephalia
anencephalic
anencephalous
anencephaly screening
anepia
anergasia
anergastic
anergic
anergy
anesthekinesia, anesthecinesia
anesthesia
acupuncture a.
angiospastic a.
barbiturate burst-suppression a.
bulbar a.
compression a.
conduction a.
continuous intravenous regional a. (CIVRA)
contralateral a.
corneal a.
crash induction of a.
crossed a.
diagnostic a.
dissociated a.
dissociative a.
doll's head a.
a. dolorosa
facial a.
gauntlet a.

general endotracheal a.
general orotracheal a.
girdle a.
glove a.
gustatory a.
halothane a.
hysterical a.
intravenous regional a. (IVRA)
isoflurane a.
local a.
Mayo block a.
muscular a.
nausea a.
olfactory a.
painful a.
perineural a.
pharyngeal a.
pressure a.
ring block a.
SAB a.
saddle-shaped a.
segmental a.
sevoflurane a.
spinal a.
splanchnic a.
stocking a.
stocking-and-glove a.
tactile a.
thalamic hyperesthetic a.
thermal a.
thermic a.
unilateral a.
visceral a.

anesthesimeter

anesthetic

dissociative a.
a. leprosy
a. monitoring
short-acting local a.

anethopathy, anetopathy

anetic

aneuploidy

aneurogenic

aneuroid chest bellows

aneurolemmic

aneurysm

amebic a.
anterior circulation intracranial a.
anterior communicating artery a.
arterial a.
arteriosclerotic intracranial a.
arteriovenous a.
aspergillotic a.
atherosclerotic a.
bacterial a.
basilar apex a.
basilar artery trunk a.
basilar bifurcation a.
basilar tip a.
berry a.
bilobed a.
blister-like a.
blood blister-like a.
brain a.
carotid artery a.
carotid cave a.
carotid-ophthalmic artery a.
cavernous carotid a.
cavernous sinus a.
cerebral arterial a.
cerebral artery a.
cerebrovascular a.
Charcot-Bouchard intracerebral a.
circle of Willis a.
cirsoid a.
classic dissecting a.
clinoidal a.
a. clip
a. clip applicator
clip ligation of a.
a. clipping
coating of a.
congenital cerebral a.
cranial a.
de novo a.
dissecting a.
distal anterior cerebral artery a.
dolichoectatic a.
dome of a.
extracerebral a.
extracranial a.
familial intracranial a. (FIA)
feeding artery of a.
fundus of a.
fusiform a.
a. of Galen vein
giant cervical carotid artery a.
great cerebral vein of Galen a.
hunterian ligation of a.
Hunt-Kosnik classification of a.
hypophysial a.
incidental a.

NOTES

aneurysm *(continued)*
infectious a.
infraclinoid a.
internal carotid artery a.
International Study of Unruptured Intracranial A.'s (ISUIA)
intracavernous carotid a.
intracerebral a.
intracranial a.
intranidal a.
lower basilar a.
luetic a.
miliary a.
M1 segment a.
multiple intracranial a.
mycotic intracranial a.
neck of a.
a. neck dissector
a. needle
neoplastic a.
a. occlusion
ophthalmic artery a.
ophthalmic segment a.
paraclinoid internal carotid artery a.
a. of persistent trigeminal artery
PICA a.
posterior fossa a.
posterior inferior communicating artery a.
precursor sign to rupture of a.
prerupture of a.
rebleeding of a.
rerupture of a.
ruptured a.
saccular a.
sellar a.
serpentine a.
spirochetal a.
supraclinoid a.
suprasellar a.
a. surgery
thrombosed giant a.
a. trapping
trapping of a.
traumatic intracranial a. (TICA)
unruptured a.
unspecified a.
vein of Galen a.
venous a.
vertebrobasilar a.
wide-necked a.
Willis circle a.
wrapping of a.

aneurysmal
a. bleeding
a. bone cyst
a. bruit
a. bulging
a. clipping operation
a. dilation
a. dome
a. rebleed
a. rest
a. rupture
a. subarachnoid hemorrhage

aneurysmectomy

aneurysmoplasty

aneurysmorrhaphy

aneurysmotomy

aneusomy syndrome

Anexsia

Angeles
University of California Los A. (UCLA)

Angell James dissector

Angelman syndrome (AS)

Angelucci syndrome

angiitis
allergic a.
granulomatous a.
isolated a.
necrotizing a.
primary a.

angioblastic meningioma

angioblastoma

angiocentric immunoproliferative lesion

Angioconray

angiodysgenetic myelomalacia

angioedema

angioendothelioma
malignant endovascular papillary a.

angioendotheliomatosis
neoplastic a.

angiofibroma
juvenile a.
nasopharyngeal a.
Vogt triad of seizures, mental retardation, and facial a.

angiogenesis
glioma a.

angiogenic
a. inducer
a. inhibitor
a. response

angioglioma

angiogliomatosis

angiogliosis

angioglomoid tumor

Angiografin

angiogram
blush of dye on a.
carotid a.
cerebral digital a.
digital subtraction a.

four-vessel cerebral a.
innominate a.
intercostal artery a.
internal carotid a.
intraarterial digital subtraction a.
magnetic resonance a.
MR a.
postembolization a.
postoperative a.
preoperative a.
Seldinger a.
small angle double incidence a.
vertebral a.

angiogram-negative SAH

angiographic

a. catheter
a. finding
a. recanalization
a. reference system
a. road-mapping technique
a. targeting
a. targetry
a. vasospasm

angiographically

a. confirmed
a. occult intracranial vascular malformation (AOIVM)
a. visualized vascular malformation (AVVM)

angiography

baseline a.
cerebral a.
cerebrovascular a.
closed a.
contrast a.
contrast echocardiography magnetic resonance a. (CE MRA)
contrast-enhanced MR a. (CE MRA)
cut-film a.
2DFT time-of-flight MR a.
digital intravenous a.
digital subtraction a. (DSA)
digital subtraction venous a.
gadolinium-enhanced MR a. (Gd-MRA)
helical CT a.
intraarterial digital subtraction a. (IADSA)
intracranial MR a.
intraoperative a.
magnetic resonance a. (MRA)
nuclear cerebral a. (NCA)
open a.
orthogonal a.
phase contrast magnetic resonance a. (PCMRA)
preoperative a.
spinal a.
stereomagnification a.
stereotactic a.
superselective a.
three-dimensional computed tomographic a. (3D-CTA)
time-of-flight a.
transradial cerebral a.
vertebral a.

angioid streak

angio image

AngioJet rapid thrombectomy system

angiokeratoma corporis diffusum

angiokinetic

angiolipoma

epidural a.
spinal epidural a.

angiolithic sarcoma

angioma, pl. **angiomata**

arteriovenous interhemispheric a.
capillary a.
cavernous a.
cerebral cavernous a.
cerebral vein a.
cerebrovascular a.
cutaneous a.
encephalic a.
extracerebral cavernous a.
intracranial cavernous a.
intradermal a.
leptomeningeal venous a.
pontine a.
retinal a.
spinal cord a.
supratentorial cavernous a.
venous a.
vertebral a.

angiomatosis

cephalotrigeminal a.
cerebral a.
cerebroretinal a.
congenital dysplastic a.
corticomeningeal a.
cutaneomeningospinal a.

NOTES

angiomatosis *(continued)*
Divry-van Bogaert familial corticomeningeal a.
encephalofacial a.
encephalotrigeminal a.
leptomeningeal capillary-venous a.
meningeal a.
mesencephalooculofacial a.
neurocutaneous a.
neuroretinal a.
oculoencephalic a.
Rendu-Osler a.
retinocerebral a.
telangiectatic a.
angionecrosis
angioneurectomy
angioneuredema
angioneuropathic
angioneuropathy
angioneurosis
angioneurotic edema
angioneurotomy
angioparalysis
angioparalytic neurasthenia
angioparesis
angiopathic
a. neurasthenia
a. vertigo
angiopathy
amyloid a.
cerebral amyloid a. (CAA)
congenital dysplastic a.
congophilic amyloid a.
radiation a.
angiophacomatosis, angiophakomatosis
angioplastic meningioma
angioreticuloma
angiosarcoma
Angio-Seal closure device
angiospastic anesthesia
angiostatin
angiostrongyliasis
Angiostrongylus costaricensis
angiotensin III
angiotomomyelography
angiotropic lymphoma
angle
cephalic a.
cephalomedullary a.
cephalometric a.
cerebellopontine a. (CPA)
cervicothoracic pedicle a.
Citelli a.
craniofacial a.
flip a.
a. meningioma
pedicle axis a.
phase a.
pontine a.
a. position potentiometer
pulse flip a.
Rolando a.
sagittal pedicle a.
Schmidt-Fischer a.
sinodural a.
sylvian a.
Sylvius a.
tentorial a.
transverse pedicle a.
venous a.
angled
a. aneurysm clip
a. awl
a. needle
a. nerve root retractor
angled-lens endoscope
angled-shaft endoscope
anglophile
anglophilia
angophrasia
angry
a. backfiring C (ABC)
a. backfiring C nociceptor (ABC syndrome)
angular
a. bundle
a. convolution
a. frequency
a. gyrus
a. gyrus syndrome
a. knife
a. momentum
a. position
angularis
gyrus a.
angulation
radius of a.
screw a.
angulus pontocerebellaris
anhaphia (*var. of* anaphia)
anhidrosis
anhidrotic ectodermal dysplasia
anhydrase
carbonic a.
anhydration
anhydrous
anhypnia
ani (*pl. of* anus)
anion
peroxynitrite a.
superoxide a.
aniridia
anisocoria
anisodont

anisomastia
anisonucleosis
anisotrophy
chemical shift a.
anisotropic
a. band
a. 3DFT
a. diffusion
anisotropy
fractional a. (FA)
a. of white matter
ankle
a. clonus
a. jerk
a. reflex
ankle-brachial index
ankyloglossia
ankylosing spondylitis
ankylosis
cricoarytenoid a.
Ankylostoma
ankyroid
Annamese
annectent gyrus
annular
a. radial rupture
a. tear
annulospiral
a. ending
a. fiber
a. organ
annulus, pl. **annuli**
a. fibrosus
a. fibrous disci intervertebralis
fissure of a.
a. tendineus
a. of Vieussens
a. of Zinn
annuracetam
anochlesia
anociassociation
anococcygeal nerve
anococcygeus
nervus a.
anodal block
anodmia
anoesis
anoetic
anoexigenic
anoia
anomalous
a. branching
a. cerebral artery
a. innervation
a. nonrecurrent right inferior laryngeal nerve
a. origin
a. parental vocal pattern
a. result
anomaly
Aristotle a.
autosomal chromosomal a.
coloboma, heart disease, atresia choanae, retarded growth, genital anomalies, ear a.'s (CHARGE)
congenital a.
cranial a.
duplication a.
facial nerve congenital a.
megadolichobasilar a.
megadolichovertebrobasilar a.
multiple congenital a.
Willis circle developmental a.
anomia
color a.
finger a.
tactile a.
word-selection a.
anomic aphasia
anomie
anophthalmia
X-linked a.
anopsia
amblyopia ex a.
anorexia nervosa
anorthography
anosmia
essential a.
functional a.
a. gustatoria
hypogonadism with a.
ipsilateral a.
mechanical a.
preferential a.
reflex a.
respiratory a.
true a.
anosmic aphasia
anosodiaphoria
anosognosia

NOTES

anosognosic
a. epilepsy
a. seizure
anospinal center
anosteoplasia
anostosis
ANOVA
analysis of variance
global ANOVA
anovulation
anovulatory cycle
anoxemia
anoxia
acute a.
anemic a.
birth a.
cerebral a.
corneal a.
perinatal a.
perioperative a.
terminal a.
anoxic
a. damage
a. hypoxia
a. ischemia
anoxic-ischemic encephalopathy
ANP
atrial natriuretic peptide
ANS
autonomic nervous system
ansa, pl. **ansae**
a. cervicalis
Haller a.
a. hypoglossi
lenticular a.
a. lenticularis
ansae nervorum
ansae nervorum spinalium
peduncular a.
a. peduncularis
Reil a.
a. sacralis
a. subclavia
Vieussens a.
ansate
anserinus
pes a.
ansiformis
crus primum lobuli a.
ansiform lobule
ansoparamedian fissure
ansotomy
Anspach
A. craniotome
A. 65K drill
A. 65K instrument system
A. 65K neuro system
Anstie test
antagonism
central dopaminergic a.
pharmacological a.
physiological a.
antagonist
alpha-1 adrenergic a.
alpha-adrenoceptor a.
beta-adrenoreceptor a.
calcium channel a.
dopaminergic a.
a. drug
excitotoxic neurotransmitter a.
Glu-receptor a.
glutamate receptor a.
5HT1A a.
N-methyl-D-aspartate receptor a.
a. muscle
NMDA receptor a.
serotonin a.
serotonin/dopamine a.
antagonistes
gestes a.
antagonistic
a. effect
a. reflex
a. thermoeffector
antalgic limp
antapoplectic
antebrachial cutaneous nerve
antebrachium
antegrade amnesia
antephialtic
anterior
a. abdominal cutaneous branch of intercostal nerve
a. acoustic stria
a. alexia
a. ampullary nerve
a. amygdaloid area
a. antebrachial nerve
a. aphasia
a. apraxia
area amygdaloidea a.
arteria cerebelli inferior a.
arteria cerebri a.
arteria choroidea a.
arteria spinalis a.
a. auricular nerve
a. basal encephalocele
a. branch of axillary nerve
a. branch of thoracic nerve
a. bulb syndrome
a. callosotomy
a. canaliculus of chorda tympani
a. cavernous sinus space
a. C1-C2 screw approach

a. C1-C2 screw fixation
a. central convolution
a. central gyrus
a. cerebellar notch
a. cerebral artery
a. cerebral artery plexus
a. cerebral vein
a. cervical approach to cervicothoracic junction
a. cervical cord syndrome
a. cervical discectomy and fusion
a. cervical spine surgery
a. cervical surgery vocal cord damage
a. cervicothoracic junction surgery
a. cheek electrode
a. choroidal artery (AChA)
a. cingulate cortex
a. cingulate flow
a. cingulate gyrus
a. cingulate gyrus tumor
a. cingulate prefrontal syndrome
a. circulation intracranial aneurysm
a. circulation stroke
a. clinoid
a. clinoid process
a. colliculus
columna a.
a. column disruption
a. column of medulla oblongata
a. column osteosynthesis
a. column of spinal cord
commissura alba a.
commissura grisea a.
a. commissure-posterior commissure (AC-PC)
a. commissure-posterior commissure line
a. commissure-posterior commissure reference point
a. communicating artery (ACoA, AComA)
a. communicating artery aneurysm
a. communicating artery distribution infarction
a. construct
a. cord impingement
a. cord syndrome
a. cornual syndrome
a. corpectomy
a. correction
a. cortex penetration
a. corticospinal tract
a. cranial base
a. cranial fossa
a. cranial fossa surgery
a. craniofacial resection
a. cutaneous branch of femoral nerve
a. cutaneous branch of iliohypogastric nerve
a. cutaneous branch of intercostal nerve
a. cutaneous nerves of abdomen
a. decompression
decussatio tegmentalis a.
a. discectomy
a. distraction
a. distraction instrumentation
a. dorsal nucleus
ductus semicircularis a.
a. ethmoidal nerve
a. external arcuate fiber
a. extradural clinoidectomy
a. extremity of caudate nucleus
fasciculus corticospinalis a.
fasciculus proprius a.
a. fasciculus proprius
fasciculus pyramidalis a.
a. femoral cutaneous nerve
forceps a.
a. fossa skull base glabellar
a. fovea
a. frontal
a. funiculus
a. gray column
a. gray commissure
a. ground bundle
gyrus paracentralis a.
gyrus temporalis transversus a.
a. head region
a. hippocampal activation
a. horn
a. horn cell
a. horn cell disease
a. horn cell isolation
a. horn cell motor impairment
a. horn index
a. hypothalamic area
a. hypothalamic nucleus
a. hypothalamic region
a. hypothalamus

NOTES

anterior *(continued)*
incisura cerebelli a.
a. inferior cerebellar
a. inferior cerebellar artery (AICA)
a. inferior cerebral artery
a. inferior communicating artery
a. insula region
a. intercavernous sinus
a. interhemispheric approach
a. intermediate groove
a. intermediate sulcus
a. internal fixation device
a. internal stabilization
a. interosseous nerve
a. interosseus syndrome
a. interpositus nucleus
a. ischemic optic neuropathy (AION)
a. jugular vein
a. Kostuik-Harrington distraction system
a. limbic association area
a. limb of internal capsule
a. lobe of hypophysis
a. longitudinal ligament
a. lower cervical spine surgery
a. lumbar spine interbody fusion
a. lunate lobule
a. median fissure of medulla oblongata
a. median fissure of spinal cord
a. medullary velum
a. meningeal artery
a. mesial temporal resection (AMTR)
a. metallic fixation
nervus ampullaris a.
nervus ethmoidalis a.
nervus interosseus antebrachii a.
a. neuropore
a. neutralization
a. notch of cerebellum
a. nuclei of thalamus
a. nucleus
nucleus cochlearis a.
nucleus hypothalamicus a.
nucleus interpositus a.
nucleus olfactorius a.
a. nucleus of thalamus
a. nucleus of trapezoid body
nucleus ventralis a.
a. occipital artery-middle cerebral artery bypass
a. olfactory nucleus
a. paracentral gyrus
a. paracentral lobule
a. parietal lesion
a. parolfactory sulcus
pars a.
a. part of anterior commissure of brain
a. part of pons
a. pectoral cutaneous branch of intercostal nerve
a. peduncle of thalamus
a. perforated substance
a. periventricular nucleus
a. pillar of fornix
a. piriform gyrus
a. pituitary hormone
a. pituitary insufficiency
a. plate fixation
a. polar-amygdalar epilepsy
a. poliomyelitis
a. pontomesencephalic vein
a. primary division
a. pulmonary branch of vagus nerve
a. pyramid
a. pyramidal fasciculus
a. pyramidal tract
a. quadrigeminal body
radiatio thalami a.
radix a.
a. ramus of cervical nerve
a. ramus of lateral sulcus of cerebrum
a. ramus of lumbar nerve
a. ramus of sacral nerve
a. ramus of spinal nerve
a. ramus of thoracic nerve
a. raphespinal tract
a. recess
a. recess of interpeduncular fossa
recessus a.
regio hypothalamica a.
a. rhizotomy
a. root
a. root of spinal nerve
a. scalene muscle
a. screw fixation
a. serratus muscle
a. short-segment stabilization
sinus intercavernosus a.
a. skull base malignancy
spina bifida a.
a. spinal artery
a. spinal artery syndrome
a. spinal cord syndrome
a. spinal fixation
a. spinal plating
a. spinocerebellar tract
a. spinothalamic tract
a. stabilization procedure

stria cochlearis a.
substantia perforata a.
sulcus intermedius a.
sulcus lateralis a.
sulcus parolfactorius a.
a. superior alveolar branches of infraorbital nerve
a. surgical exposure
a. tegmental decussation
a. temporal artery
a. temporal atrophy
a. temporal branch
a. temporal focal spike
a. temporal lobectomy
a. temporobasal vein
a. thalamic radiation
a. thalamic tubercle
a. thalamotomy
a. tibialis sign
tractus corticospinalis a.
tractus pyramidalis a.
tractus raphespinalis a.
tractus reticulospinalis a.
tractus spinocerebellaris a.
tractus spinothalamicus a.
tractus trigeminothalamicus a.
a. transverse temporal gyrus
a. triangle approach
a. trigeminothalamic tract
truncus vagalis a.
a. tubercle of thalamus
a. vagal trunk
a. vein of septum pellucidum
vena cerebri a.
vena pontomesencephalica a.
vena septi pellucidi a.
ventralis oralis a. (Voa)
a. vermis
a. vermis syndrome
a. white commissure

anteriores
fibrae arcuatae externae a.
nervi auriculares a.
nervi labiales a.
nervi scrotales a.
nuclei tegmentales a.
rami temporales a.

anterioris
nuclei interstitiales hypothalami a.
pars anterior commissurae a.
pars anterior lobuli quadrangularis a.
pars dorsalis lobuli qudrangularis a.
pars posterior commissurae a.
pars posterior lobuli quadrangularis a.
pars precommunicalis arteriae cerebri a.
pars ventralis lobuli quadrangularis a.
rami gastrici anteriores trunci vagalis a.
rami hepatici trunci vagalis a.
rami nasales interni laterales nervi ethmoidalis a.
rami nasales interni mediales nervi ethmoidalis a.
rami nasales nervi ethmoidalis a.
ramus nasalis externus nervi ethmoidalis a.

anterior-posterior
a.-p. fusion with segmental spinal instrumentation
a.-p. fusion with SSI

anterius
cornu a.
corpus quadrigeminum a.
tuber a.

anterochiasmatic lesion

anterocollis dystonia

anterodorsal
a. nucleus of thalamus
a. thalamic nucleus

anterodorsalis
nucleus a.

anterograde
a. amnesia (AA)
a. axonal transport
a. fast component neuropathy
a. memory

anteroinferior cerebellar artery

anterolateral
a. central artery
a. column
a. column of spinal cord
a. cordotomy
a. groove
a. sulcus
a. system
a. tract
a. tractotomy

NOTES

anterolaterales
arteriae thalamostriatae a.
tractus a.
anterolateralis
nucleus a.
sulcus a.
anteromedial
a. central branch
a. nucleus of thalamus
a. retropharyngeal approach
a. temporal lobe resection
a. thalamic nucleus
anteromediales
arteriae thalamostriatae a.
rami centrales a.
anteromedialis
nucleus a.
ramus frontalis a.
anteromedian groove
anteromesial temporal lobectomy
anteroposterior (AP)
a. projection
a. talocalcaneal
anteroventralis
nucleus a.
anteroventral thalamic nucleus
anthophilous
anthrax
cerebral a.
meningeal a.
anthropomorphic face
anthroponomy
anthroposcopy
anthroposomatology
anthroposophy
anthypnotic
anti-33-kDa antibody
antiabsence antiepileptic drug
antiacetylcholine receptor antibody
anti-AChE
antiactin antibody
antiadrenergic
antiadrenogenic
antialias filtering
antianalytic
antianaphylaxis
antiapoptotic protein
antibiotic
intrathecal a.
a. neurotoxicity
a. penetration
a. powder
antibody
acquired a.
alemtuzumab humanized monoclonal a.
antiacetylcholine receptor a.
antiactin a.
anti-GFP polyclonal a.
anti-Hu a.
anti-human a.
anti-I-kBa a.
anti-33-kDa a.
anti-MAG a.
antineuronal a.
antinuclear a.
antiphospholipid a.
anti-Ri a.
anti-tau monoclonal a.
antitoxoplasmic a.
anti-Yo a.
disease-associated a.
human antimouse a. (HAMA)
IgM GM-1 antiganglioside a.
influenza A a.
monoclonal a.
OKT3 monoclonal a.
polyclonal a.
antibody-mediated disorder
anticatalyst
anticipatory a.
anticataplectic
anticephalalgic
Anticept
anticholinergic
a. agent
a. dose
a. drug
a. effect
a. medication
anticholinesterase
anticipatory
a. anticatalyst
a. vomiting (AV)
anticoagulant
lupus a.
anticoagulation therapy
anticonvulsant
a. effect
a. intoxication
a. medication-induced postural tremor
a. prophylaxis
a. therapy
anticonvulsant-induced dyskinesia
anticonvulsive
anticus
locus perforatus a.
a. reflex
scalenus a.
a. sign
tetanus a.
antidipsotropic agent
antidiuretic hormone (ADH)

antidopaminergic
a. effect
a. potency
antidote
BAL a.
a. drug
antidromic
a. conduction
a. response
a. stimulation
a. volley
antidyskinetic agent
antiepilepsirine
antiepileptic
a. drug (AED)
a. drug hypersensitivity syndrome
a. drug-induced bone disease
enzyme-inducing a.
antiepileptogenesis
antiferromagnetism
antifibrinolytic
a. agent
a. therapy
antiganglioside
antigen
AC133 a.
bacterial a.
carcinoembryonic a. (CEA)
CD44 a.
cryptococcal a.
DR15DR2 a.
histocompatibility a.
histoplasma polysaccharide a.
HLA-CW2 a.
HLA-DR2 a.
human lymphocyte a. (HLA)
33-kDa a.
prostate-specific a. (PSA)
tuberculous a.
varicella-zoster virus a.
antigen-antibody complex
anti-GFP polyclonal antibody
antiglial fibrillary acidic protein
anti-GM$_1$ antibody test
antigravity reflex
antihelix
double a.
antihemophilic
a. factor A, C
antihistamine
a. neurotoxicity
sedative a.
antihistaminergic effect
anti-Hu antibody
anti-human
a.-h. antibody
a.-h. transferrin
anti-I-kBa antibody
antikinesia
antilethargic
anti-Lewisite
British a.-L.
anti-MAG antibody
antimetabolite
antimicrobial
a. agent
a. prophylaxis
a. susceptibility test
a. therapy
antimigraine therapy
antimongoloid slant
antimuscarine cholinergic activity
antimuscarinic
a. drug
a. effect
antimyasthenic
antineuralgic
antineuritic
antineurofilament
antineuronal
a. antibody
a. cytoplasmic autoantibody (ANCA)
antinociceptive effect
antinodal behavior
antinomian
antinomianism
antinuclear
a. antibody
a. antibody test
antioncogene
antioxidant
a. effect
endogenous a.
a. system
a. therapy
antiparasympathomimetic
antiparkinsonian response
antiparkinsonism agent
antipersonnel

NOTES

antiphospholipid
a. antibodies in stroke study
a. antibody
a. syndrome
antiplatelet
a. drug
a. therapy
antipyrine
antiretroviral
a. medication
a. therapy
anti-Ri antibody
antiseizure
a. effect
a. medication
antisense
a. oligonucleotide
a. strategy
antiseptic
ACU-dyne a.
antiserum
nerve growth factor a.
antisiphon device
antispasmodic
antistrophe
antisympathetic
anti-tau monoclonal antibody
antitetanic
antithesis
antithetical
antithrombin
a. III (AT III)
a. III deficiency
antitonic
antitoxin
botulinum a.
tetanus a.
antitoxoplasmic antibody
antitrismus
Antivert
antiviral
chemotherapy a.
a. medication
a. therapy
antivivisection
anti-Yo antibody
Antley-Bixler syndrome
Anton
A. symptom
A. syndrome
Anton-Babinski syndrome
Antoni
A. A, B cell
A. A, B tissue
A. pattern (type A & B)
A. type A, B neurilemoma
Antoni-A neurinoma classification
Antopol disease
antra (*pl. of* antrum)
Antrizine
antrochoanal polyp
antrophose
antrostomy
antrum, pl. **antra**
mastoid a.
maxillary a.
Anturane
Antyllus method
anular plexus
anus, pl. **ani**
Bartholin a.
a. cerebri
anvil
Hurteau skull plate a.
anxietas tibiarum
anxiety control training
anxiogenic stimulus
anxiolytic
a. activity
a. drug
a. property
a. stimulus
anxiolytic-induced
anxiolytic/sedative
anxious
a. delirium
a. somatic depression
AO
AO dynamic compression plate
AO dynamic compression plate construct
AO fixateur interne
AO fixateur interne instrumentation
AO gouge
AO group
AO guide pin
AO internal fixator
AO notched instrumentation
AO reconstruction plate
AO scale
AO stopped-drill guide
AO/ASIF fixateur interne
AOIVM
angiographically occult intracranial vascular malformation
aorta, pl. **aortae**
pars thoracica aortae
thoracic part of a.
aortic
a. arch syndrome
a. body
a. body tumor
a. insufficiency
a. nerve

aorticorenal ganglion
aorticorenalia
ganglia a.
aorticum
corpus a.
glomus a.
aortobifemoral bypass graft
aortocranial disease
AP
anteroposterior
Apacet
APACHE
acute physiologic assessment and chronic health evaluation
APACHE II measure of disease severity
apallesthesia
apallic
a. state
a. syndrome
APAP
auto-PAP
APAP Plus
aparalytic
apastic
apathetic
a. akinetic mutism
a. hyperthyroidism
a. thyrotoxicosis
apathism
APB
wrist-to-abductor pollicis brevis
ape
a. fissure
a. hand
a. hand of syringomyelia
aperiodic
a. complex
a. wave
aperta
rhinolalia a.
spina bifida a.
Apert syndrome
apertura, pl. **aperturae**
a. aqueductus cerebri
a. aqueductus mesencephali
a. lateralis ventriculi quarti
a. mediana ventriculi quarti
aperture
lateral a.
median a.
apex, pl. **apices**
a. cornus dorsalis medullae spinalis
a. cornus posterioris
a. cornus posterioris medullae spinalis
a. of dorsal horn of spinal cord
petrous a.
a. of posterior horn
a. of posterior horn of spinal cord
Apfelbaum retractor
aphagia
aphagopraxia
aphanisis
aphasia
acoustic a.
acquired epileptic a.
acquired fluent a.
ageusic a.
amnemonic a.
amnestic a.
anomic a.
anosmic a.
anterior a.
associative a.
ataxic a.
auditory a.
Benson-Geschwind classification of a.
Broca a.
cerebrovascular a.
combined a.
commissural a.
conduction a.
contiguity disorder a.
cortical a.
crossed a.
A. Diagnostic Profiles
dynamic a.
dysnomic a.
Examining for A.
expressive a.
expressive-receptive a.
fluent a.
frontocortical a.
frontolenticular a.
functional a.
gibberish a.
global a.

NOTES

aphasia *(continued)*
graphic a.
graphomotor a.
Grashey a.
hypophonic a.
impressive a.
induced a.
intellectual a.
jargon a.
Kussmaul a.
A. Language Performance Scale
lenticular a.
a. lethica
Lichtheim a.
major motor a.
mixed a.
motor a.
nominal a.
nonfluent a.
optic a.
partial nominal a.
pathematic a.
pictorial a.
posterior a.
primary progressive a. (PPA)
progressive nonfluent a.
psychosensory a.
pure a.
receptive a.
semantic a.
sensory a.
subcortical motor a.
subcortical sensory a.
syntactical a.
tactile a.
temporoparietal a.
thalamic a.
total a.
transcortical a.
true a.
visual a.
Wernicke a.

aphasiac

aphasic
a. acalculia
a. agraphia

aphasiologist

aphasiology

aphemesthesia

aphemia

aphonia
acute a.
functional a.
hysterical a.
nonorganic a.
a. paralytica
spastic a.

aphonic

aphonogelia

aphonous

aphoria

aphorism
Hippocratic a.

aphorize

aphrasia

apical
a. dendrite
a. distraction
a. ectodermal ridge
a. process
a. turn of the cochlea

apices (*pl. of* apex)

apicis

apicoectomy

apiculate waveform

apiospermum
Scedosporium a.

apituitarism

aplasia
cerebellar a.
cerebral a.
cochlear a.
a. cutis congenita
labyrinthine a.
nuclear a.
vertebral a.

APLD
automated percutaneous lumbar discectomy

aplomb

Aplysia californica

apnea-hypopnea
a.-h. index (AHI)
obstructive sleep a.-h. (OSAH)

apnea index (AI)

apnea-like spell

apneic pause

apneusis

apneustic
a. breathing
a. center
a. period

apocalyptic

apocamnosis (*var. of* apokamnosis)

apocarteresis

apoceruloplasm deficiency

apocleisis

apocope

apocrine
a. cystadenoma
a. gland

apodemialgia

APOe4
apolipoprotein epsilon 4

ApoE
apolipoprotein E
ApoE e4 allele
ApoE genotype
apoenzyme
apoferritin
Apofix interlaminar clamp
apogeotropic nystagmus
apokamnosis, apocamnosis
apokemnophilia
apolar cell
apolegamic
apolipoprotein
a. E (ApoE)
a. E genotype
a. epsilon
a. epsilon 4 (APOe4)
a. gene cluster
apomorphine
aponeurectomy
aponeurorrhaphy
aponeurotica
galea a.
aponeurotic reflex
aponia
apophysary point
apophysial, apophyseal
a. joint
a. point
apophysis cerebri
apoplectic
a. coma
a. cyst
a. hemorrhage
a. vertigo
apoplecticus
habitus a.
apoplectiform
apoplectoid
apoplexia
apoplexy
bulbar a.
cerebellar a.
cerebral a.
chiasmal a.
delayed a.
embolic a.
functional a.
ingravescent a.
labyrinthine a.
neonatal a.
pituitary a.
pontile a.
pontine a.
posttraumatic a.
Raymond a.
serous a.
spasmodic a.
spinal a.
thrombotic a.
apopnixis
apoptosis
neuronal cell a.
a. suppression
thymocyte a.
apoptosis-inducing factor (AIF)
apoptosome
apoptotic
a. body
a. cell death
aporioneurosis
aposematic
apotentiality
cerebral a.
apothanasia
APP
Alzheimer precursor protein
amyloid precursor protein
apparatus
Brown-Roberts-Wells a.
C-arm fluoroscopic a.
halo a.
heat-loss a.
Horsley-Clarke stereotactic a.
Kandel stereotactic a.
Leksell a.
Mayfield-Kees skull fixation a.
mitotic spindle a.
Perroncito a.
Reichert-Mundinger a.
Spiegel-Wycis human a.
subneural a.
sucker a.
Todd-Wells a.
vestibular a.
Wells stereotactic a.
apparent
a. diffusion coefficient (ADC)
a. origin
appearance
axon torpedo a.
beaten-metal a.

NOTES

appearance *(continued)*
de novo a.
meningothelial a.
pearl-chain a.
ping-pong a.
posterior beaten copper a.
thumbprinting a.
tuberous sclerosis railroad track a.
Appedrine
appendicular
apperceptive
a. disorder
a. visual agnosia
appestat qualitative approach
appetitive
a. disturbance
a. state
appliance
Herbst a.
Klearway oral a.
monobloc-type a.
oral a.
application
clip a.
force a.
Harrington rod instrumentation force a.
Isola spinal implant system a.
paraspinal rod a.
transverse fixator a.
vertebral plate a.
applicator
aneurysm clip a.
NeuroAvitene a.
scalp clip a.
applied
A. Biosystems Perkin-Elmer
a. relaxation
applier
bayonet clip a.
clip a.
Crockard transoral clip a.
Ligaclip a.
Mayfield miniature clip a.
Mayfield temporary aneurysm clip a.
mini a.
Olivecrona clip a.
Raney scalp clip a.
Sano clip a.
Vari-Angle clip a.
approach
adaptational a.
anterior C1-C2 screw a.
anterior interhemispheric a.
anterior triangle a.
anteromedial retropharyngeal a.
appestat qualitative a.
Bailey-Badgley anterior cervical a.
basal interhemispheric a.
basal pterional a.
basal subfrontal a.
bottom-up a.
buccopharyngeal a.
cerebellopontine angle a.
cholinergic a.
Cloward cervical disk a.
combined anterior and posterior a.
combined low cervical and transthoracic a.
combined presigmoid-transtransversarium intradural a.
combined transsylvian and middle fossa a.
computer-assisted volumetric stereotactic a.
condylar a.
continuous a.
contralateral transcallosal a.
costotransversectomy a.
empirical a.
extended subfrontal a.
extreme lateral inferior transcondylar a.
extreme lateral transcondylar a.
far lateral inferior suboccipital a.
foraminal a.
frontotemporal a.
functional a.
glabellar a.
"go slow" a.
Hardy a.
Harmon cervical a.
holistic a.
inferior extradural a.
inferior-lateral endonasal transsphenoidal a.
inferior transvermian a.
infratemporal a.
infratentorial lateral supracellular a.
integrative a.
interfascial a.
interforniceal a.
interhemispheric transcallosal-subchoroidal transvelum interpositum a.
intradural a.
intraforaminal a.
intratentorial supracerebellar a.
ipsilateral a.
Kanavel a.
labioglossomandibular a.
labiomandibular a.
lateral extracavitary a.

lateral extracavity a.
lateral intradural a.
low cervical a.
medial extradural a.
middle cranial fossa a.
middle fossa craniotomy a.
middle fossa transtentorial translabyrinthine a.
midline spinal a.
mini-open a.
molecular a.
multimodal therapeutic a.
multiple-tracer a.
multisystemic therapy a.
neuroimaging a.
oblique transcorporeal a.
occipital interhemispheric a.
occipito-subtemporal a.
orbital venous a.
orbitofrontal a.
orbitozygomatic temporopolar a.
partial labyrinthectomy petrous apicectomy a.
patient-centered a.
petrosal a.
pharmacological a.
posterior fossa a.
posterior occipitocervical a.
posterolateral a.
presigmoid a.
primary pharmacological a.
psychotherapeutic a.
pterional a.
resection of pituitary tumor, transfacial a.
retrolabyrinthine-presigmoid a.
retrolabyrinthine-transsigmoid a.
retromastoid a.
retroperitoneal a.
retropharyngeal a.
retrosigmoid a.
rhinoseptal a.
sacral foraminal a.
screw plate a.
sensate focus a.
stabilization a.
standard retroperitoneal flank a.
stereotactic microsurgical a.
sternum-splitting a.
subchoroidal a.
subfrontal transbasal a.
subfrontal translamina terminalis a.
sublabial midline rhinoseptal a.
sublabial transseptal transsphenoidal a.
suboccipital posterior fossa a.
suboccipital transmeatal a.
subtemporal basal a.
subtemporal infratemporal a.
subtemporal keyhole a.
superior intradural a.
superior ophthalmic vein a.
suprabrow a.
supracerebellar a.
supraclavicular a.
supraorbital pterional a.
supratentorial a.
sylvian a.
targeted a.
therapeutic a.
thoracoabdominal a.
thoracolumbar retroperitoneal a.
transantral ethmoidal a.
transcallosal interforniceal-transforaminal microsurgical a.
transcallosal transforaminal a.
transcavernous transpetrous apex a.
transcerebellar hemispheric a.
transchoroidal a.
transcochlear a.
transcortical transventricular a.
transcranial frontotemporoorbital a.
transcubital a.
transfacial transclival a.
transfrontal a.
transfrontonasoorbital a.
translabyrinthine and suboccipital a.
translabyrinthine transotic a.
transmandibular glossopharyngeal a.
transmaxillosphenoidal a.
transnasal a.
transnasoorbital a.
transoral a.
transpalatal a.
transpedicular a.
transperitoneal a.
transpetrosal a.
transsinus a.
transsphenoidal a.
transsylvian a.
transtemporal a.
transtentorial a.

NOTES

approach *(continued)*
transthoracic a.
transtorcular a.
transuncodiscal a.
transvenous a.
transventricular a.
transzygomatic a.
ultrasound-guided transfrontal transventricular a.
Wiltberger anterior cervical a.
Wiltse paraspinal a.
zygomatic resection a.
approachable
approbation
approximating closure
approximation
method of successive a.
vocal fold a.
approximator
Neuromeet nerve a.
appurtenance
APR
acousticopalpebral reflex
apractagnosia
apractic
apraxia
akinetic a.
amnestic a.
anterior a.
a. battery
Bruns gait a.
buccofacial a.
callosal a.
cerebral mapping of a.
classic a.
Cogan oculomotor a.
congenital ocular motor a.
construction a.
constructional a.
cortical a.
developmental articulatory a.
diagnostic a.
disconnection a.
dressing a.
facial a.
gait a.
ideational a.
ideatory a.
ideokinetic a.
ideomotor a.
innervation a.
innervatory a.
left-sided a.
Liepmann a.
limb-kinetic a.
magnetic a.
motor a.
ocular motor a.
oral a.
A. Profile: A Descriptive Assessment Tool for Children
pure limb a.
sensory a.
speech a.
transcortical a.
verbal a.
visual spatial constructional a.
apraxia-ataxia
truncal a.-a.
apraxic
a. agraphia
a. disorder
a. dysarthria
apraxic-ataxic
apraxis
constructional a.
aprepitant
Apresazide
Apresoline
aprobarbital
aproctia
aprophoria
aprosencephaly
aprosexia
aprosodia
aprosody
speech a.
a. of speech
aprotinin
APS
adenosine 5′-phosphosulfate
APS hydroxyapatite
aptiganel hydrochloride
APUD
amine precursor uptake decarboxylase
APUD cell
apurinic
apyknomorphous
apyretic tetanus
apyrimidinic
AQP
aquaporin
AquaMEPHYTON Injection
aquaporin (AQP)
AquaSens
Aquatensen
aquatic rehabilitation
aqueduct
cerebral a.
a. cerebrum
cochlear a.
Cotunnius a.
forking of sylvian a.
gliosis of a.

mesencephalon a.
a. of midbrain
Monro a.
opening of cerebral a.
sylvian a.
a. of Sylvius
a. veil
ventricular a.
vestibular a.

aqueductal
a. gliosis
a. intubation
a. occlusion
a. plasty
a. stenosis

aqueductoplasty

aqueductus
a. cerebri
a. cochlea
a. cotunnii
a. mesencephali
a. sylvii
a. vestibuli

aqueous
a. humor deficiency
a. povidone-iodine

arabinoside
adenine a.
cytosine a. (ara-C)

ara-C
cytosine arabinoside

arachidonic
a. acid
a. acid cascade
a. acid metabolism

arachnitis

arachnodactyly
congenital a.
contracture a.

arachnoid
a. adhesion
a. of brain
a. canal
a. cell
cranial a.
a. cyst
a. fibrosis
a. foramen
a. granulation
a. granulation villi
a. knife
a. mater cranialis
a. mater encephali
a. membrane
a. nerve root sheath dilation
a. plane
a. sheath
a. sleeve
a. space
spinal a.
a. of spinal cord
a. trabecula
a. of uncus
a. villi

arachnoidal
a. gliomatosis
a. granulation
a. hyperplasia
a. root sleeve

arachnoidea, arachnoides
a. mater cranialis
a. mater encephali
a. mater spinalis

arachnoideae
granulationes a.

arachnoideales
granulationes a.

arachnoides (*var. of* arachnoidea)

arachnoiditis
adhesive a.
basilar a.
chiasmal a.
chronic adhesive a.
cysticerotic a.
fibrosing a.
neoplastic a.
obliterative a.
a. of opticochiasmatic cistern
ossifying a.
postoperative a.
spinal cord a.

arachnoid-shape Beaver blade

Aramine

Arana-Iniquez
A.-I. intracranial cyst removal
A.-I. intracranial cyst removal technique

Aran-Duchenne
A.-D. amyotrophy
A.-D. disease
A.-D. muscular atrophy
A.-D. muscular dystrophy

NOTES

Arantius ventricle
araphia
ARAS
ascending reticular activating system
arbor, pl. **arbores**
dendritic a.
a. vitae
a. vitae cerebelli
arborescent
a. white substance of cerebellum
arborization
dendrite a.
arbovirus, arborvirus
a. meningoencephalitis
arc
dynamic reference a.
a. guidance system
Leksell a.
monosynaptic reflex a.
neural a.
a. radius system
reflex a.
Sceratti a.
spinal reflex a.
stereotactic a.
Y-shaped reference a.
arcade of Frohse
arc-centered guidance system
arch
lamina of vertebral a.
archaeocerebellum, archeocerebellum, archicerebellum
archaeocortex
archaeopsychic
archaism
archeocerebellum (*var. of* archaeocerebellum)
archeokinetic
archicerebellum (*var. of* archaeocerebellum)
archicortex
Archimedes spiral
archipallial
archipallium
archistriatalis
nucleus robustus a.
robustus a. (RA)
architectonics
architecture
sleep a.
arciform wave
Arclite 20,000 light source
arc-quadrant stereotactic system
arcuate
a. eminence
a. fasciculus
a. fiber
a. fiber of cerebrum
a. nucleus
a. nucleus of thalamus
a. visual field defect
arcuati
nuclei a.
arcuatus
nucleus a.
arcus parietooccipitalis
ardanesthesia
arduous
area, pl. **areae**
acoustic a.
a. acustica
AI, AII a.
amygdaloclaustral a.
a. amygdaloclaustralis
a. amygdaloidea anterior
amygdalopiriform transition a.
anterior amygdaloid a.
anterior hypothalamic a.
anterior limbic association a.
Assessment of Adaptive Areas
association a.
auditory association a.
auditory cortical a.
Betz cell a.
bilateral contralateral primary sensorimotor a.
bilateral secondary sensorimotor a.
brain a.
Broca motor speech a.
Broca parolfactory a.
Brodmann a. 6,7,9,24,32,34,41,43,44,46
Brodmann cortical a.
a. CA4-1
callosal a.
a. centralis
a. cerebrovasculosa
cingulate motor a. (CMA)
cortical a.
cross-sectional a. (CSA)
dermatomic a.
diencephalic transition a.
dominant hemisphere parietal a.
dominant hemisphere temporal a.
dorsal hypothalamic a.
dorsolateral prefrontal cortical a.
eloquent versus noneloquent a.
entorhinal a.
excitable a.
a. of facial nerve
first somatosensory a.
first visual a.
Flechsig a.
a. of Forel

frontal cortical a.
frontoorbital a.
fusiform face a. (FFA)
gasserian ganglion a.
gray matter a.
gustatory receiving a.
Head a.
high density a.
hypothalamic a.
a. hypothalamica dorsalis
a. hypothalamica intermedia
a. hypothalamica lateralis
a. hypothalamica posterior
a. hypothalamica rostralis
inferior vestibular a.
insular a.
intermediate hypothalamic a.
Jarman Underprivileged A.
language a.
lateral hypothalamic a.
lateral rostral supplementary motor a.
low-density a. (LDA)
medial preoptic a.
medial rostral supplementary motor a.
a. medullovasculosa
mesencephalic transition a.
mesial prefrontal cortical a.
motor speech a.
neocortical association a.
a. nervi facialis
neuropsychologic a.
noneloquent a.
nucleus arcuatus of intermediate hypothalamic a.
occipital association cortical a.
olfactory a.
orbitofrontal a.
paraolfactory cortical a.
parastriate a.
parietal neocortical association a.
parietotemporal a.
a. parolfactoria
a. parolfactoria Brocae
parolfactory a.
periamygdaloid a.
perifornical a.
peristriate a.
periventricular gray matter a.
piriform a.
postcentral a.
posterior hypothalamic a.
a. postrema
postrolandic a.
precentral a.
precommissural septal a.
prefrontal cortical a.
premotor a.
preoptic a.
a. preoptica
prestriate a.
pretectal a.
a. pretectalis
primary motor a.
primary receiving a.
primary receptive a.
primary somatomotor a.
primary somatosensory a.
primary visual a.
processing a.
projection a.
pyriform a.
receptive a.
retrochiasmatic a.
a. retrochiasmatica
a. retroolivaris
retroolivary a.
rolandic a.
Rolando a.
rostral supplementary motor a.
sclerotic a.
sclerotome a.
secondary somatosensory a.
secondary visual a.
second somatosensory a.
second visual a.
sensorial a.
sensorimotor a.
sensory association a.
sensory processing a.
septal a.
silent a.
SI, SII a.
somatesthetic a.
somatosensory a.
somesthetic a.
striate a.
stripe a.
a. subcallosa
subcallosal a.
subcortical gray matter a.

NOTES

area *(continued)*
superior temporal auditory cortical a.
superior vestibular a.
supplementary motor a. (SMA)
suppressor a.
suprasellar a.
taste receiving a.
temporal neocortical association a.
temporoparietal association a.
third visual a.
a. transitionis amygdalopiriformis
trigger a.
a. under the curve
vagus a.
ventral regimental a.
ventral tegmental a. (VTA)
vestibular a.
a. vestibularis
a. vestibularis inferior
a. vestibularis superior
visual association a.
visual cortical a.
visual receiving a.
visuopsychic a.
visuosensory a.
watershed a.
Wernicke second motor speech a.
areal stimulation
arecholine
areflexia
detrusor a.
upper limb a.
arena
association a.
arenacea
corpora a.
arenavirus infection
Arenberg-Denver inner-ear valve implant
areolar tissue
Argentinian hemorrhage fever
arginase
a. deficiency
a. deficiency aminoaciduria
arginine
a. vasopressin
a. vasotocin
argininemia
arginine-vasopressin (AV, AVP)
argininosuccinic
a. acid synthase deficiency
a. aciduria
a. aminoaciduria
argininosuccinicaciduria
arginosuccinate lyase deficiency
argon
a. ion
a. laser
a. laser iridotomy (ALI)
argument
sylleptic a.
Argyll
A. Robertson pupil
A. trocar catheter
argyrophil
a. organizer region protein
a. plaque
arhinencephaly (*var. of* arrhinencephaly)
Aricept
Ariel computerized exercise system
aripiprazole
Aristotle anomaly
arithmetica
epilepsia a.
AR-JP
autosomal recessive juvenile parkinsonism
Arlin
arm
a. dystonia
fixed dosing a.
phantom a.
a. phenomenon
a. weakness
Yasargil Leyla retractor a.
armamentarium
clinical a.
pharmacological a.
Armstrong disease
Army-Navy retractor
Arnold
A. bundle
A. canal
A. ganglion
A. nerve
A. nerve reflex cough syndrome
A. tract
Arnold-Chiari
A.-C. deformity
A.-C. malformation
A.-C. syndrome
arobrea
Datura a.
aromatic
a. amino acid decarboxylase (AADC)
a. hydrocarbon
aromatization
peripheral a.
arousal
a. category
a. component of consciousness

cortical a.
a. defect
a. mechanism
mental a.
physiological a.
psychological/physiological a.
a. reaction
respiratory effort-related a.
respiratory event a.
respiratory-related a.
sleeplessness associated with conditional a.
a. symptom
a. threshold

array
compressed spectral a.
density-modulated spectral a. (DSA)
percutaneous electrode a.
rostrocaudal contact a.
rostrocaudal epidural a.
star a.
subdural electrode a.
surface coil a.
a. of symptom
transverse tripolar epidural a.

arrest
deep hypothermic circulatory a.
speech a.

arrested hydrocephalus
arrhaphia
arrhigosis
arrhinencephaly, arhinencephaly, arrhinencephalia
arrhythmia
cardiac a.
fatal a.
torsades de pointes a.

arrhythmogenic
arrhythmokinesis
arriere-pensee
ARS
adult Reye syndrome

arsenic
a. peripheral neuropathy
a. poisoning
a. polyneuropathy

arsenical
a. polyneuropathy
a. tremor

Artane
artefacta
self-induced dermatitis a.

artemether
artemisinin
arterenol
arteria, pl. **arteriae**
a. basilaris
a. calcarina
a. cerebelli inferior anterior
a. cerebelli inferior posterior
a. cerebelli superior
a. cerebri anterior
a. cerebri media
a. cerebri posterior
a. choroidea
a. choroidea anterior
a. choroidea posterior
arteriae encephali
a. inferior anterior cerebelli
a. inferior posterior cerebelli
a. occipitalis
a. occipitalis lateralis
a. occipitalis medialis
a. orbitofrontalis lateralis
a. orbitofrontalis medialis
arteriae parietooccipitalis
a. precunealis
a. radicularis magna
a. recurrens
a. spinalis anterior
a. spinalis posterior
a. superior cerebelli
a. temporalis posterior
arteriae thalamostriatae anterolaterales
arteriae thalamostriatae anteromediales

arterial
a. access
a. aneurysm
a. biopsy
a. blood gas (ABG)
a. border zone
a. bruit
a. circle of cerebrum
a. circle of Willis
a. dissection
a. gas embolism (AGE)
a. groove
a. hemorrhage
a. inflammation

NOTES

arterial *(continued)*
a. occlusive disease
a. oxygen saturation
a. photothrombosis
a. plasma input
a. thoracic outlet syndrome
a. thrombosis
a. vasospasm
arterialization
arterialized leptomeningeal vein
arterial-occlusive retinopathy
arteriograph bath
arteriography
carotid a.
cerebral a.
spinal a.
arteriolar infarction
arteriolopathy
retinocochleocerebral a.
arteriolosclerosis
arteriopalmus
arteriopathy
autosomal-dominant a.
arteriosclerosis
cerebral a.
eccentric a.
hyaline a.
arteriosclerotic
a. brain disease
a. encephalopathy
a. intracranial aneurysm
paranoid-type a.
subcortical a.
uncomplicated a.
a. vertigo
arteriosus
truncus a.
arteriovenous (AV)
a. aneurysm
a. fistula
a. interhemispheric angioma
a. malformation (AVM)
a. malformation nidus definition
a. malformation radiosurgery
arteritica
polymyalgia a.
arteritis, pl. **arteritides**
ANCA-positive granulomatous giant-cell a.
Aspergillus a.
a. cardiovascular disease (ASCVD)
cranial a.
extracranial a.
giant cell a. (GCA)
granulomatous a.
Heubner a.
Horton giant cell a.
intracranial granulomatous a.
necrotizing granulomatous systemic a.
neurocranial granulomatous a.
obliterative a.
rheumatoid a.
spinal a.
spinal cord a.
Takayasu a.
temporal a.
viral intracerebral a.
artery
A1, A2 segment of anterior cerebral a.
aberrant a.
accessory middle cerebral a.
Adamkiewicz a.
alternative occipital artery middle cerebral a.
aneurysm of persistent trigeminal a.
anomalous cerebral a.
anterior cerebral a.
anterior choroidal a. (AChA)
anterior communicating a. (ACoA, AComA)
anterior inferior cerebellar a. (AICA)
anterior inferior cerebral a.
anterior inferior communicating a.
anterior meningeal a.
anterior spinal a.
anterior temporal a.
anteroinferior cerebellar a.
anterolateral central a.
ascending cervical a.
ascending frontoparietal a.
A2 segment of anterior cerebral a.
auditory a.
axillary a.
basal cerebral a.
basilar a.
Bernasconi-Cassinari a.
a. of brain
calcarine a.
callosomarginal a.
caroticotympanic a.
carotid a.
a. of central sulcus
cerebellar a.
cerebral a.
a. of cerebral hemorrhage
Charcot a.
choroidal pericallosal a.
cingulothalamic a.
collicular a.
common carotid a. (CCA)
communicating branch of fibular a.

communicating branch of peroneal a.
contralateral temporary a.
costocervical a.
cranial a.
distal medial striate a.
dolichoectatic internal carotid a.
dynamic entrapment of vertebral a.
en passage feeder a.
external carotid a.
extracranial carotid a. (ECA)
extradural vertebral a.
facial a.
friable a.
frontal a.
frontopolar a. (FPA)
giant tortuous basilar a.
Global Utilization of Streptokinase and t-PA for Occluded Coronary A.'s (GUSTO-1)
great anterior medullary a.
a. of Heubner
inferior cerebellar a.
inferolateral pontine a.
innominate a.
intercostal a.
internal carotid a. (ICA)
intracranial a.
ipsilateral middle cerebral a.
lateral occipital a.
lateral posterior choroidal a.
left common carotid a.
lenticulostriate a. (LSA)
lumbar a.
maxillary a.
maxillomandibular a.
medial occipital a.
medial striate a.
medullary a.
meningeal a.
middle cerebral a. (MCA)
middle meningeal a. (MMA)
M2 segment of right middle cerebral a.
nodular induration of temporal a.
occipital a.
ophthalmic a.
paramedian thalamopeduncular a.
parent a.
periarterial plexus of choroid a.
pericallosal azygos a.
petrous carotid a.
pial a.
plexus of choroid a.
plexus of medial cerebral a.
polar a.
pontine a.
popliteal a.
a. of postcentral sulcus
posterior cerebellar a.
posterior cerebral a.
posterior choroidal a.
posterior communicating a. (PComA)
posterior inferior cerebellar a. (PICA)
posterior inferior communicating a. (PICA)
posterior spinal a.
posteroinferior cerebellar a.
posterolateral spinal a.
a. of precentral sulcus
primitive otic a.
primitive trigeminal a.
primordial inferior hypophysial a.
radial a.
radiculospinal a.
recurrent perforating a.
spinal cord a.
splenial a.
stapedial a.
subclavian a.
sulcocommissural a.
superficial temporal a. (STA)
superficial temporal artery-middle cerebral a. (STA-MCA)
superficial temporal artery to middle cerebral a. (STA-MCA)
superficial temporal artery-posterior cerebral a. (STA-PCA)
superficial temporal artery-superior cerebellar a. (STA-SCA)
superior cerebellar a.
superior hypophysial a.
superior laryngeal a.
superior temporal artery-middle cerebral a. (STA-MCA)
superior thyroid a.
supraclinoid internal carotid a.
supreme intercostal a.
telencephalic ventriculofugal a.
temporal a.

NOTES

artery *(continued)*
temporopolar a. (TPA)
thalamocaudate a.
thalamogeniculate a.
thalamoperforating a.
thyrocervical trunk of subclavian a.
trifurcation of middle cerebral a.
trigeminocerebellar a.
ventriculofugal a.
vermian a.
vertebral a. (VA)
vertebrobasilar a.
vidian a.
zygomaticoorbital a.
artery-to-artery embolism
artery-to-vein shunt
Artha-G
arthralgia
migratory a.
subtalar a.
temporomandibular joint a.
arthresthesia
arthrifluent abscess
arthritic general pseudoparalysis
arthritidis
Mycoplasma a.
arthritis, pl. **arthritides**
cervical spine a.
degenerative a.
enteropathic a.
gouty a.
hypertrophic a.
juvenile rheumatoid a.
neuropathic a.
psoriatic a.
rheumatoid a.
arthroconidia
airborne a.
arthrodesis
atlantoaxial a.
Brooks atlantoaxial a.
C1-C2 posterior a.
cervical a.
Cloward cervical a.
extension injury posterior atlantoaxial a.
flexion injury posterior atlantoaxial a.
occipitocervical a.
posterior atlantoaxial a.
arthrogryposis congenita multiplex
arthropathy
calcium pyrophosphate dihydrate a.
Charcot a.
diabetic a.
neurogenic a.
neuropathic a.
sensory neurogenic a.
tabetic a.
Arthus reaction
arthyreosis
articular
a. branch of deep fibular nerve
a. corpuscle
a. cortex
a. leprosy
a. mass separation
a. mass separation fracture
a. sensibility
articulare
corpusculum a.
articularia
corpuscula a.
articularis
nervus a.
ramus a.
articulating disk prosthesis
articulation
atlantoaxial a.
a. disorder
Vermont spinal fixator a.
articulatory
artifact
asymmetric a.
ballistocardiographic a.
beam hardening a.
blink a.
cardiac pacemaker a.
chemical shift a.
edge a.
electrode-popping a.
electromyographic a.
eye blink a.
eye movement a.
ferromagnetic a.
fried-egg a.
Gibbs a.
glossokinetic a.
impedance a.
lateralized a.
line a.
machine a.
magnetic susceptibility a.
motion a.
movement a.
nonbiological a.
nonphysiologic a.
oculographic a.
a. on x-ray
paper stop a.
perspiration a.
physiological a.
pulsation a.
pulse wave a.

rhythmic a.
spikelike a.
statistical a.
stimulus a.
susceptibility a.
tissue magnetic susceptibility a.
truncation a.
artificial
a. airway
a. blood substrate
a. spinal disk
a. vertebral body
artificialism
artiodactylous
artuum
tremor a.
aryepiglottic fold neurofibroma
arylsulfatase
a. A
a. A deficiency
AS
Angelman syndrome
ascending
a. cervical artery
a. current
a. degeneration
a. frontal convolution
a. frontal gyrus
a. frontoparietal (ASFP)
a. frontoparietal artery
a. myelitis
a. neuritis
a. neurotransmitter system
a. paralysis
a. parietal convolution
a. parietal gyrus
a. pharyngeal plexus
a. poliomyelitis
a. ramus of lateral sulcus of cerebrum
a. reticular activating system (ARAS)
a. reticular activation
a. reticular arousal system
a. tract
ascension phase
ascorbate
quinine a.
sodium a.
ASCVD
arteritis cardiovascular disease
atherosclerotic cardiovascular disease
ASD
Alzheimer senile dementia
asemasia, asemia
Asendin
asepsis
aseptic
a. meningeal reaction
a. meningoencephalitis (AME)
a. necrosis
a. uremic meningitis
ASFP
ascending frontoparietal
ashen
a. tuber
a. tubercle
a. wing
Asher physical build assessment technique
ash-leaf
a.-l. s. spot
a.-l. s. spot in tuberous sclerosis
Ashworth
A. scale
A. score of muscle spasticity
ASI
acoustic signature event
ASIA/IMSOP
American Spinal Injury Association/International Medical Society of Paraplegia
Asian alcohol flush reaction
ASIF
A. broad dynamic compression
A. broad dynamic compression bone plate
A. T plate
Aslan endoscopic scissors
asomatognosia
aspartate aminotransferase (AST)
aspartic proteinase
aspartoacylase deficiency
aspartylglycosaminidase
aspartylglycosaminuria
aspect
associative a.
diagnostic a.
immunologic a.
laminar cortex posterior a.

NOTES

aspect *(continued)*
marche a petits plantar a.
normative a.
perceptual a.
Aspen
A. electrocautery
A. laparoscopy electrode
A. ultrasound system
Asperger syndrome
aspergilloma
aspergillosis
aspergillotic aneurysm
Aspergillus
A. arteritis
A. brain abscess
A. cerebral abscess
A. flavipes
A. fumigatus
A. glaucus
A. nidulans
A. niger
A. terreus
A. ustus
asphyxia
lactic acid production in perinatal a.
Myers model of perinatal a.
neonatal a.
neonate a.
perinatal a.
aspiny neuron
aspiration
bone plate a.
Integra Selector ultrasonic a.
needle a.
negative a.
stereotactic needle a.
aspirator
Cavitron Ultrasonic Surgical A. (CUSA)
Selector ultrasonic a.
Sharplan Ultra ultrasonic a.
Sonocut ultrasonic a.
ultrasonic surgical a.
Aspir-code
ASPS
advanced sleep-phase syndrome
assault
brain a.
assaultive
assay
ADmark A.
B_2-TFn a.
a. buffer
CH50 a.
clonogenic cell a.
enzyme-linked immunosorbent a. (ELISA)
5-HT receptor a.
5-hydroxytryptamine receptor a.
immunocytochemical a.
immunofluorescence a.
involuntary repetitive movement disorder antineuronal antibody a.
Limulus amebocyte lysate a.
MAO spectrophotometric a.
nephelometric a.
plaque reduction a.
serotonin receptor a.
spectrophotometric a.
tissue-based monoamine oxidase a.
assembly
Ace halo-cast a.
Brown-Roberts-Wells arc-ring a.
cryocooler a.
multiple hook a.
tubulin a.
assessment
Activity Loss A.
A. of Adaptive Areas
A. of Aphasia and Related Disorders, Second Edition
Baycrest Neurocognitive A.
Behavioural Neurology A. (BNA)
closed-chain functional a.
cognitive function a.
competency a.
complement symptom-focused a.
comprehensive a.
cross-sectional a.
A. of Dementia
diagnostic a.
environmental a.
Fugl-Meyer a.
functional a.
longitudinal a.
a. method
Moire topographic scoliosis a.
multidimensional a.
neuroimaging a.
objective a.
outcome a.
Performance Oriented Balance and Mobility A.
A. for Persons Profoundly or Severely Impaired
presurgical a.
a. procedure
risk-benefit a.
Rivermead Motor A.
SQUID array for reproductive a. (SARA)
standardized a.

symptom a.
vision a.
in vivo stereological a.
ASSI coagulator
assiduity
assimilable
assimilating
assimilation
assimilative factor
assisted ventilation
assistive technology device
associated movement
association
Acoustic Neuroma A.
Alzheimer Disease and Related Disorders A.
American Brain Tumor A.
American Sleep Disorders A.
a. area
a. arena
clang a.
conditioned fear a.
contextual a.
a. cortex
A. of Directors of Medical Student Education in Psychiatry (ADMSEP)
fear a.
a. fiber
laws of a.
a. mechanism
multiple a.
National Aphasia A. (NAA)
National Mental Health A. (NMHA)
National Rehabilitation A.
a. neurofiber
occipital a.
A. of Sleep Disorder Center
Stroke and the Alzheimer Disease and Related Disorders A.
a. system
a. time
a. tract
associationis
neurofibra a.
associative
a. aphasia
a. aspect
a. visual agnosia
associativity
criterion of a.
assumption
Hodgkin-Huxley a.
AST
aspartate aminotransferase
astasia
astasia-abasia
astatic seizure
astereognosis
asterion
asterixis
asteroides
Nocardia a.
asthenia
myalgic a.
neurocirculatory a.
treatment-emergent a.
asthenic type
asthenopia
nervous a.
asthma
sleep-related a.
asthmatic amyotrophy
astigmatism
astragalectomy
astral body
astroblast
astroblastoma
astrocyte
Alzheimer type I, II a.
ameboid a.
fibrillary a.
fibrous a.
gemistocytic a.
peripapullar a.
plasmatofibrous a.
protoplasmic a.
reactive a.
stellate a.
suspended embryonic a.
wedge-shaped a.
astrocytic
a. change
a. end foot
a. gliosis
a. reaction
a. signal
a. tumor
astrocytoma
anaplastic a.

NOTES

astrocytoma *(continued)*
brainstem a.
cerebellar a.
cerebral anaplastic a.
chiasmatic-hypothalamic pilocytic a.
cystic a.
desmoplastic cerebral a.
diencephalic a.
diffuse cellular a.
fibrillary a.
gemistocytic a.
giant cell a.
grade I–IV a.
hypothalamic a.
intracranial a.
juvenile cerebellar a.
juvenile pilocytic a. (JPA)
low-degree a.
low-grade a.
malignant a.
optic nerve a.
pilocytic juvenile a.
piloid a.
pilomyxoid a.
a. protoplasmaticum
protoplasmic a.
pseudopalisading a.
subcortical protoplasmic a.
subependymal giant cell a.
subependymal glomerate a.
supratentorial a.
thalamic a.
astrocytosis cerebri
astroependymoma
astroglia cell
astrogliosis
astrotactin
asyllabia
asylum
asymbolia
pain a.
asymmetric
a. artifact
a. hyperreflexia
a. motor neuropathy
a. nystagmus
a. tonic neck reflex
asymmetrical
a. crying facies (ACF)
a. generalized epileptiform activity
asymmetry
a. amplitude
cytoarchitectural a.
encephalic a.
left-right a.
nasal-temporal a.
planum temporale a.
Wada memory a.
asymptomatic
a. carotid artery stenosis
a. carotid atherosclerosis study
a. carotid bruit
a. hydrocephalus
a. neck bruit
a. neurosyphilis
a. visual field defect
asynchronism
asynchrony
impulse a.
asynergia
asynergic
asynergy
AT
ataxia-telangiectasia
AT III deficiency
AT III
antithrombin III
atactic
a. abasia
a. agraphia
a. ataxia
atactica agraphia
atactiform
atactilia
ataractic
Atarax
ataraxic
Atavi atraumatic spine fusion system
atavistic
ataxia
absent a.
acute cerebellar a. (ACA)
atactic a.
autosomal dominant cerebellar a.
Biemond a.
Briquet a.
Bruns frontal a.
buccolingual a.
cerebellar a.
cerebral a.
chronic a.
crural a.
early-onset a.
echovirus infection a.
episodic a. type 2 (EA-2)
equilibratory a.
familial paroxysmal kinesigenic a.
familial spastic a.
Ferguson-Critchley a.
Friedreich hereditary a.
gluten a.
Greenfield classification of spinocerebellar a.

hand a.
hereditary cerebellar a.
hereditary posterior column a.
hereditary spinal a.
hysterical a.
infantile X-linked a.
inherited a.
ipsilateral cerebellar a.
kinesigenic a.
kinetic a.
late-onset a.
Leyden a.
locomotor a.
Marie a.
Menzel a.
motor a.
multiple sclerosis a.
ocular motor a.
optic a.
pancerebellar a.
periodic vestibular a. (PVA)
pes cavus in Friedreich a.
respiratory a.
Sanger Brown a.
sensory a.
spastic a.
spinal a.
spinocerebellar a.
spinocerebellar a. type 1
sporadic a.
static a.
a. telangiectasia
a. telangiectasia syndrome
truncal a.
trunk a.
vasomotor a.
vestibulocerebellar a.

ataxiadynamia
ataxiagram
ataxiagraph
ataxiameter
ataxiaphasia
ataxia-telangiectasia (AT)
ataxic
a. abasia
a. aphasia
a. breathing
a. cerebral palsy
a. dysarthria
a. gait
a. hemiparesis
a. lymphopathy
a. paramyotonia
a. paraplegia
a. respiration

ataxin 1, 2
ataxiophemia
ataxy
Ateles
cerebral cortex of A.

atheroembolism
diffuse disseminated a.

atheroma
atheromatosis
atheromatous disease
atherosclerosis
carotid a.
cerebral a.
coronary a.
vertebrobasilar a.

atherosclerotic
a. aneurysm
a. cardiovascular disease (ASCVD)
a. infarction
a. plaque

atherothromboembolism
athetoid
a. dysarthria
a. spasm

athetosic
a. dysarthria
a. dystonia
a. idiocy

athetosis, athetotic
double congenital a.
posthemiplegic a.

athymic
athyreosis
Ativan
atlantal fracture
Atlantis anterior cervical plate system
atlantoaxial
a. arthrodesis
a. articulation
a. dislocation
a. fixation
a. fusion
a. instability
a. interval
a. joint
a. separation

NOTES

atlantoaxial *(continued)*
a. stabilization
a. subluxation
atlantodental
atlantoepistrophic ligament
atlantomastoid
atlantooccipital
a. joint
a. separation
a. stabilization
atlas
a. burst fracture
A. of polysomnography
Schaltenbrand-Wahren stereotactic a.
stereotactic a.
a. of Talairach and Tournoux
atlas-axis combination fracture
ATL real-time Neurosector scanner
atomic, biologic, chemical (ABC)
atonia
choreatic a.
muscle a.
atonic
a. absence
a. bladder
a. cerebral palsy
a. drop attack
a. epilepsy
a. seizure
atonic-astatic diplegia
atopognosia, atopognosis
atopy
atorvastatin
ATP
adenosine 5′-triphosphate
ATPase
adenosine triphosphatase
sodium-potassium A.
atractylic acid
atracurium besylate
atraumatic Sprotte needle
atresia
aural a.
choanal a.
laryngeal a.
oral a.
atrial
a. myxoma
a. natriuretic peptide (ANP)
a. ring
atrobrunneum
Chaetomium a.
atrocity
atrophedema
atrophia
atrophic
a. lesion
a. neuroarthropathy
atrophica
myotonia a.
atrophicans
acrodermatis chronica a.
atrophoderma neuriticum
atrophy
acute reflex bone a.
adult-onset spinal muscular a.
amygdala a.
anterior temporal a.
Aran-Duchenne muscular a.
Behr complicated optic a.
cerebellar vermian a.
Charcot-Marie-Tooth a.
circumscribed cerebral a.
congenital cerebellar a.
cortical a.
corticospinal a.
Cruveilhier a.
Dejerine-Sottas a.
Dejerine-Thomas a.
denervated muscle a.
dentatorubral a.
dentatorubropallidoluysian a. (DRPLA)
diffuse brain a.
disuse a.
dorsum sellae a.
Duchenne-Aran spinal muscular a.
Eichhorst a.
entorhinal cortex a.
Erb a.
facial progressive a.
facioscapulohumeral a.
familial spinal muscular a.
Fazio-Londe a.
focal muscular a.
frontal temporal a.
Gudden a.
gyral a.
Gyralor superficial a.
hereditary cerebellar a.
hippocampal formation a.
Hoffmann muscular a.
Hunt a.
idiopathic muscular a.
infantile progressive spinal muscular a.
intermediate spinal muscular a.
intratentorial a.
ischemic muscular a.
juvenile spinal muscular a.
Kugelberg-Welander juvenile spinal muscle a.

Landouzy-Dejerine a.
Leber hereditary optic a.
lobar a.
Marie-Foix-Alajouanine cerebellar a.
Menzel olivopontocerebellar a.
monomelic muscular a.
multiple system a.
multisystem a. (MSA)
muscle a.
muscular a.
myelopathic muscular a.
myopathic a.
neuritic muscular a.
neurogenic a.
neuromuscular a.
neuropathic a.
neurotrophic a.
nutritional type cerebellar a.
olivopontocerebellar a.
optic nerve a.
pallidal a.
parenchymatous a.
perifascicular a.
peroneal muscular a.
Pick a.
postneuritic a.
primary optic a.
progressive circumscribed cerebral a.
progressive infantile spinal muscular a.
progressive neuromuscular a.
progressive neuropathic muscle a.
progressive postpolio muscle a. (PPPMA)
progressive spinal muscular a.
pseudohypertrophic muscular a.
scapulohumeral a.
scapuloperoneal muscular a.
segmental sensory disassociation with brachial muscular a.
spinal muscular a. type 1–4 (SMA)
subcortical a.
Sudeck a.
sulcal a.
temporal horn a.
temporal lobe a.
testicular a.
tooth a.
transneuronal a.
trophoneurotic a.
urogenital a.
vermian a.
Vulpian a.
Vulpian-Bernhardt spinal muscular a.
Welander distal muscular a.
Werdnig-Hoffmann spinal muscular a.
white a.
whole brain a.
X-linked recessive spinobulbar muscular a.
Zimmerlin a.

atropine

AT/RT
atypical teratoid/rhabdoid tumor

attached
a. cranial section
a. craniotomy

attachment
cerebellar a.
collodion a.
dural a.
a. dynamic
Hardy a.
Hudson cerebellar a.
Mayfield-Kees table a.
a. relationship
University Plate spinal a.
a. versatility

attack
absence a.
akinetic drop a.
atonic drop a.
brain a.
cataleptic a.
cephalgic a.
crescendo transient ischemic a.
cryptogenic drop a.
drop a.
epileptic drop a.
factitious a.
jackknife a.
kinesigenic a.
limited symptom a.
masticatory a.
motor jacksonian a.
oxygen radical a.
physical a.
position of a.

NOTES

attack *(continued)*
psychomotor a.
recurrent panic a.
salaam a.
sensory jacksonian a.
sleep a.
spontaneous panic a.
Stokes-Adams a.
tonic drop a.
transient hemisphere a.
transient ischemic a. (TIA)
uncinate a.
vagal a.
vasospastic a.
vasovagal a.
vertebrobasilar transient ischemic a.
Attenade
attenuation
a. of alpha rhythm on EEG
a. coefficient on MRI scan
intraaural a.
a. reflex
shame a.
a. value on MRI scan
attitudinal
a. reflex
a. risk factor
attitudinize
attonita
cephalea a.
attractor
a. field therapy (AFT)
A. retrieval device
atypical
a. absence
a. absence seizure
a. cleft
a. facial neuralgia
a. facial pain
a. giant cell tumor
a. lymphocytosis
a. meningioma
a. petit mal seizure
a. somatoform disorder
a. stereotyped movement disorder
a. teratoid/rhabdoid tumor (AT/RT)
a. teratoma
a. tic disorder
a. trigeminal neuralgia
au courant
audiofrequency eddy current
audiogenic
a. epilepsy
a. seizure
audiometry
average evoked response a.
brainstem electrical response a.
cortical a.
impedance a.
pure-tone a.
audiovisual
a. electroencephalogram
a. stimulation
audio-visual-tactile stimulation
audition
chromatic a.
gustatory a.
auditivae
ostium tympanicum tubae a.
auditooculogyric reflex
auditory
a. agnosia
a. amnesia
a. aphasia
a. arteriovenous malformation
a. artery
a. association area
a. association cortex
a. aura
a. brainstem-evoked response (ABR)
a. brainstem implant (ABI)
a. brainstem response (ABR)
a. canal
a. compound actional potential
a. continuous performance task
a. cortical area
a. cue
a. evoked potential
a. evoked response
a. fatigability
a. ganglion
a. hair
a. hallucination
a. hyperalgesia
a. hyperesthesia
a. illusion
a. koniocortex
a. lemniscus
a. nerve
a. neuropathy
a. nucleus
a. oculogyric reflex
a. organ
a. pathway
a. perception
a. perceptual disorder
a. prosthesis
a. radiation
a. receptor cell
a. region
a. seizure
a. span
a. spatial precueing

a. stria
a. synesthesia
a. system
a. three-stimuli oddball task
a. threshold
a. tract
a. transfer deficit
a. tubercle
a. visual-evoked response
a. vocabulary
a. word center

auditus
organum a.

Auerbach
A. ganglion
A. plexus

augmentor
a. fiber
a. nerve

aura, pl. **aurae**
abdominal a.
auditory a.
complex intellectual a.
consistent a.
déjà vu a.
epigastric a.
epileptic a.
experiential a.
gustatory a.
intellectual a.
jamais vu a.
kinesthetic a.
migraine with a.
migraine without a. (MwoA)
migrainous a.
motor a.
olfactory a.
painless a.
a. procursiva
psychical a.
reminiscent a.
residual a.
sensory a.
shimmering light with a.
simple primitive a.
somatosensory a.
status a.
tactile pricklings with a.
tingling with a.
uncinate a.
vertiginous a.
visceral a.
visual shimmering with a.
visual shining with a.
visual sparkling with a.
wavering light with a.

aural
a. atresia
a. vertigo

aureus
Staphylococcus a.

auricular
a. branch of vagus nerve
a. ganglion
a. lesion

auricularis
ramus anterior nervi a.

auriculopalpebral reflex

auriculotemporal
a. nerve
a. nerve syndrome

auriculotemporali
ramus communicans nervi glossopharyngei cum nervo a.

auriculotemporalis
nervus a.
rami parotidei nervi a.
rami temporales superficiales nervi a.
ramus membranae tympani nervi a.

auriculoventricular (AV)

aurique
grippe a.

auropalpebral reflex

Australian
A. Council for Education Research
A. X disease
A. X encephalitis

Autley-Bixler syndrome

autoantibody
antineuronal cytoplasmic a. (ANCA)
a. assay testing
striational a.

autoathography

autocerebral cooling

autochthonous graft

autocovariant

autoecholalia

autofluorescence focal fluorescence

autogenous
a. bone graft

NOTES

autogenous *(continued)*
a. cable graft interposition VII-VII neuroanastomosis
a. iliac bone
autograft
a. bone
a. bone grafting
autoimmune
a. demyelinating polyneuropathy (AIDP)
a. disease
a. illness
a. process
a. reaction
a. thyroiditis
autoimmunity
pituitary a.
autoinduction
enzyme a.
autokinesia, autokinesis
autokinetic
autologous
a. adrenal medullary tissue
a. blood transfusion
a. bone marrow rescue
a. fat graft
a. fibrin sealant glue
a. hematopoietic stem cell transplantation (AHSCT)
automate computed axial tomography
automated
a. brainstem auditory evoked response (ABaer)
a. percutaneous lumbar discectomy (APLD)
a. test target calibration
automatic
a. absence
a. auditory brainstem response
a. chorea
a. decompensation EMG
a. epilepsy
a. positioning system
automatism
ambulatory a.
chewing a.
epileptic a.
facial expression a.
gestural a.
ictal a.
immediate posttraumatic a.
lip smacking a.
mumbling a.
oral alimentary a.
patting a.
scratching a.
spinal a.
swallowing a.
automaton
automotor seizure
autonomic
a. affective law
a. arousal disorder
a. column of spinal cord
cranial a.
a. denervation
a. disruption
a. division of nervous system
a. dysfunction
a. dysreflexia (AD)
a. epilepsy
a. function
a. ganglion
a. hyperreflexia (AH)
a. hyperventilation
a. imbalance
a. impairment
a. instability
a. motor neuron
a. nerve
a. nerve fiber
a. nervous system (ANS)
a. neurofiber
a. neurogenic bladder
a. neuropathy
a. oculomotor nucleus
a. part
a. part of peripheral nervous system
a. plexus
a. seizure
a. varicosity
a. visceral motor nucleus
autonomica
pars abdominalis a.
pars pelvica a.
pars thoracica a.
autonomicae
neurofibrae a.
autonomici
nuclei oculomotorii a.
pars pelvica partis parasympatheticae systematis nervosi a.
pars pelvica systematis a.
pars thoracica systematis a.
plexus a.
autonomicorum
ganglia plexuum a.
autonomicum
systema nervosum a.
autonomicus
nervus a.

plexus a.
ramus a.
autonomotropic
autonomous
a. function
a. functional component
autonomy
bodily a.
patient a.
auto-PAP (APAP)
autophagy
autophony
autoplastic
autopsy-based neurochemical study
autopsychic
autoradiographic
a. image
a. localization
a. study
autoradiography
DAT a.
dopamine transporter a.
quantitative receptor a.
autoreceptor
autoregressive model for signal analysis
autoregulation
a. of cerebral blood flow
cerebral pressure a.
pressure a.
autoscope
autoscopy
Auto Segmentation software tool
autosomal
a. chromosomal anomaly
a. dominant cerebellar ataxia
a. dominant febrile convulsion
a. dominant inheritance
a. dominant migraine
a. dominant movement disorder
a. dominant nocturnal frontal lobe epilepsy
a. dominant temporal lobe epilepsy
a. dominant transmission
a. recessive inheritance
a. recessive juvenile parkinsonism (AR-JP)
a. recessive syndrome of encephalopathy
autosomal-dominant
a.-d. arteriopathy
a.-d. genetic defect
autosomatognosis
autosomatognostic
autosympathectomy secondary to neuropathy
Autotechnicon
autotopagnosia agnosia
AV
anticipatory vomiting
arginine-vasopressin
arteriovenous
auriculoventricular
AV shunt
avalanche
a. conduction
a. theory
Avanti sheath
avarice
avatar
AVE GFX stent
Avellis
palatopharyngeal paralysis of A.
A. paralysis
A. syndrome
Aventyl
average
a. evoked response
a. evoked response audiometry
pure-tone a.
a. velocity
Avicor
avidin-biotin
a.-b. peroxidase complex
a.-b. stain technique
avidin-biotin-complex-peroxidase method
avifauna
avis
calcar a.
nidus a.
unguis a.
avitaminosis B_{12} peripheral neuropathy
Avitene
A. microfibrillar collagen
A. microfibrillator collagen hemostat
A. packing
A. powder
AVM
arteriovenous malformation
AVM nidus definition
Avonex (IFN-B1a)

NOTES

AVP
arginine-vasopressin
avulsion
brachial plexus a.
bypass coaptation for cervical nerve root a.
cauda equina a.
conus medullaris root a.
a. injury
nerve root a.
peripheral a.
root a.
sacral plexus a.
third nerve a.
AVVM
angiographically visualized vascular malformation
awake, alert, and oriented
awakening
early a.
epilepsy with grand mal seizures on a.
nighttime a.
nocturnal a.
awl
angled a.
hemostat a.
pointed a.
reaming a.
rectangular a.
Swanson scaphoid a.
T-handle bone a.
axes (*pl. of* axis)
axial
a. compression
a. gradiometer
a. gripping strength
a. load
a. loading
a. loading fracture
a. magnetic resonance image
a. manual traction test
a. musculature
a. myopia
a. neuritis
a. pattern scalp flap
a. plane angular deformity biomechanics
a. posturing
a. projection
a. section
a. spinal system
a. spin-echo image
a. stiffness
a. traction
axial-occipital ligament
axifugal
axile corpuscle
axilemma
axilla, pl. **axillae**
axillaris
nervus a.
axillary
a. artery
a. nerve
a. sheath
AxioCam camera
axiodistocervical (ADC)
axiom
axiomatic
axion
axioplasm
axipetal
axiramificate
axis, pl. **axes**
adrenal a.
basicranial a.
cerebrospinal a.
a. corpuscle
corticotrophic a.
a. cylinder
encephalomyelonic a.
endocrine a.
a. function
hypothalamic hypophysial gonadal a.
hypothalamic-pituitary a.
hypothalamic-pituitary-adrenal a.
neural a.
thyrotrophic a.
time a.
visual a.
axis-atlas combination fracture
axoaxonic synapse
Axocet
axodendritic synapse
axodendrosomatic synapse
axofugal
axogenesis
axoid
Axokine
axolemma
axolemmal ion channel
axolysis
axon
bifurcating a.
cervix of the a.
corticospinal a.
a. degeneration
extending a.
a. flare
fusimotor a.
giant a.
granule cell a.

a. guidance
a. hillock
hypocretin a.
intracortical a.
a. loss polyneuropathy
motor unit a.
myelinated a.
myelination of a.
naked a.
a. reaction
a. reflex
a. reflex test
a. regeneration
a. regrowth
a. response
rostral spinal a.
sensory a.
A. sentinel-4 analyzer
swollen a.
a. terminal
thalamocortical a.
a. torpedo appearance
unmyelinated a.
a. wave

axonal
a. cytoskeleton
a. damage
a. degeneration
a. diameter
a. growth
a. lesion
a. loss
a. neuropathy
a. plasticity
a. polyneuropathy
a. process
a. reaction
a. regeneration
a. shearing injury
a. terminal bouton
a. transport

axone

axonography

axonopathic neurogenic thoracic outlet syndrome

axonopathy
distal a.
multifocal acquired motor a.
proximal a.

axonotmesis

axonotmetic injury

axopetal

axophage

axoplasm degeneration

axoplasmic
a. flow
a. flow and papilledema
a. transport

axosomatic synapse

Axostim nerve stimulator

axotomize

axotomy
delayed a.
instantaneous a.
peripheral nerve a.
primary a.
secondary a.

Axsain

ayahuasca

Ayala
A. disease
A. index
A. quotient

Ayers needle holder

Ayer test

Ayer-Tobey test

aypnia

azacyclonol hydrochloride

azamethonium bromide

azaperone

azaspirodecanedione

azidothymidine

aziridinylbenzoquinone

Azorean disease

Azorean-Joseph-Machado disease

aztreonam

azurophilic granule

azygous vein

NOTES

B
B amyloid protein
B cell
B fiber
B vitamin deficiency neuropathy
2B
limb girdle muscular dystrophy type 2B (LGMD2B)
B40
ACER Advanced Test B40
B_{12}
serum vitamin B_{12}
vitamin B_{12}
B_1
vitamin B_1
B_6
vitamin B_6
1b
interferon-beta 1b
36B10 glioma cell
Babcock forceps
Babès
B. node
B. nodule
B. tubercle
Babinski
B. percussion hammer
B. phenomenon
B. reflex
B. sign
B. syndrome
B. test
Babinski-Nageotte syndrome
bacampicillin
bacchanal
bacchant
bacillary layer
***Bacilles anthracis* meningitis**
bacilliformis
Bartonella b.
bacillus
gram-negative b.
tubercle b.
back
b. of foot reflex
b. pain
backache
backbone
background (BG)
b. activity
b. alpha frequency
b. disorganization
b. factor
b. rhythm
Backhaus towel clip
Backlund
B. biopsy needle
B. stereotactic instrument
backout
screw b.
backpack
b. palsy
b. paralysis
backward
digit span b. (DSB)
b. progression
spatial span b. (SSB)
baclofen
Bacon cranial rongeur
bacterial
b. aneurysm
b. antigen
b. brain abscess
b. cell wall component
b. encephalitis
b. infection
b. meningitis
b. meningitis treatment
b. meningoencephalitis
b. peripheral neuropathy
b. toxin
Bacteroides
B. fragilis
B. non-fragilis
Bactiseal antimicrobial impregnated catheter system
baculovirus infection
baculum
Baddeley model
Badgley
B. iliac wing resection
B. laminectomy retractor
badinage
BAEP
brainstem auditory evoked potential
BAER
brainstem auditory evoked response
bag
nuclear b.
Bahał
bahnung
Bailey
B. conductor
B. rib spreader
Bailey-Badgley
B.-B. anterior cervical approach
B.-B. cervical spine fusion

Baillarger
B. band
exterior band of B.
external band of B.
external line of B.
inner band of B.
inner line of B.
interior band of B.
internal band of B.
internal line of B.
B. line
outer band of B.
outer line of B.
B. sign
Bailliart ophthalmodynamometer
BAK cage
BAK/Cervical Interbody Fusion System
BAK/C Interbody Fusion System
baked brain phenomenon
Baker point
BAL
blood alcohol level
BAL antidote
balance
alternate binaural loudness b.
Clinical Test of Sensory Interaction and B. (CTSIB)
b. disorder
b. disturbance
dopaminergic-cholinergic b.
dynamic ambulatory b.
dynamic standing b.
fluid b.
genic b.
homeostatic b.
magnesium b.
B. Master-training and assessment system
measure of b.
sitting b.
standing b.
static and dynamic sitting b.
static and dynamic standing b.
static standing b.
B. subscale of the Fugl-Meyer test (FM-B)
balancer
MMS-900 microscope b.
balancing subdural hematoma
balbuties
Balint syndrome
ball
Marchi b.
B. operation
b. up
Ballantine hemilaminectomy retractor
Baller-Gerold syndrome
Ballet disease
ball-in-cone valve
ballism
ballismus
ballistic material
ballistocardiographic artifact
balloon
b. catheter
b. compression
detachable silicone b.
elastomeric b.
electrodetachable b.
Endeavor b.
Goldvalve detachable latex b.
latex b.
Magic B1 b.
metrizamide-filled b.
nondetachable endovascular b.
nondetachable occlusive b.
b. occlusion-aspiration emboli entrapment device
occlusion balloon catheter with silicone b.
b. occlusion test
silicone b.
Solstice b.
Spiegelberg epidural b.
Symmetry angioplasty b.
b. test occlusion
Worlpass Ninja b.
ballooned floor of ventricle
ballooning
b. of the sella
b. of vertebral interspace
ball-tip nerve hook
ball-type disk prosthesis
Baló
B. aminoaciduria
B. concentric sclerosis
B. disease
Baltic
B. myoclonus
B. myoclonus disease
B. myoclonus epilepsy
B. syndrome
Bamberger
B. disease
B. sign
Bamberger-Pins-Ewart sign
bamboo spine
Bancaud
B. phenomenon on EEG
B. phenomenon on electroencephalogram
band
A b.
alpha frequency b.

anisotropic b.
Baillarger b.
Bechterew b.
b. of Broca
Broca diagonal b.
Büngner b.
dentate b.
diagonal b.
Essick cell b.
furrowed b.
Gennari b.
b. of Giacomini
b. heterotopia
I b.
isofrequency b.
isotropic b.
b. of Kaes-Bechterew
b. keratopathy
normal-frequency b.
oligoclonal b.
Osborn b.
peritumoral b.
reelin immunoreactive b.
Reil b.
transcallosal b. (TCB)
Vicq d'Azyr b.

bandage
Comperm tubular elastic b.
Dressinet netting b.
fibrin b.
hammock b.

Band-Aid medicine
bandaletta diagonalis
banding
Giemsa b.
quinacrine fluorescent b.

bandwagon effect
bandwidth
data acquisition b.
receiver b.

banewort
bank
Traumatic Coma Data B.

Bankson Language Test 2
Bannayan syndrome
Bannister disease
Bannwarth syndrome
Banthine
bantiana
Cladophialophora b.

bar
distraction b.
Dynamic mesh pre-angled connecting b.
Greenberg-type b.
Leyla self-retaining tractor b.
longitudinal spinal b.
screw alignment b.

baragnosis, barognosis
Bárány
B. chair
B. maneuver
B. pointing test
positional vertigo of B.

Barb
Day B.

barba amarilla
barber chair syndrome
Barbidonna No. 2
Barbita
barbitalism
barbiturate
b. burst-suppression anesthesia
b. peripheral neuropathy
b. poisoning

barbiturate-induced
b.-i. spindle-like activity

Barbour technique
Bardeen disk
Bardet-Biedl syndrome
baresthesia
baresthesiometer
barium
b. ferrite
b. sulfate

Barker point
Barkman reflex
Barlow syndrome
Barnes
B. dystrophy
B. global score

baroceptor
barognosis (*var. of* baragnosis)
baroreceptor nerve
baroreflex
barostat
barotrauma
Barouk microstaple
barrage
Barratt scale
Barr body

NOTES

barrel
b. bur
b. field
b. staved graft
Barré-Lieou syndrome
Barré pyramidal sign
barrier
blood-brain b. (BBB)
blood-brain tumor b. (BBTB)
blood-cerebral b.
blood-cerebrospinal fluid b.
blood-CSF b.
blood-thymus b.
hematoencephalic b.
intrablood-brain b. (IBBB)
barrio
Bartel criteria
Bartelmez
club ending of B.
Barthel Activities of Daily Living Scale
Bartholin
B. anus
B. gland
Barth syndrome
Bartonella bacilliformis
bartonellosis
Bartter syndrome
bas
de haut en b.
basal
b. cell nevus syndrome
b. cerebral artery
b. cistern
b. encephalocele
b. endothelium-derived relaxing factor
b. forebrain amnesia
b. forebrain cholinergic pathway
b. forebrain region
b. ganglia classification
b. ganglia syndrome
b. ganglia-thalamocortical motor circuit
b. ganglion
b. ganglionic lesion
b. gland
b. interhemispheric approach
b. joint reflex
b. lamella
b. lamina
b. lamina of choroid
b. lamina of cochlear duct
b. lamina of neural tube
b. layer of choroid
b. line
b. meningoencephalocele
b. nucleus
b. nucleus of Ganser
b. nucleus of Meynert
b. plate
b. plate of neural tube
b. pterional approach
b. skull fracture
b. subfrontal approach
b. substantia
b. vein
b. vein of Rosenthal (BVR)
basales
nuclei b.
basalis
cisterna b.
lamina b.
substantia b.
vena b.
base
anterior cranial b.
b. of brain
data b.
b. of dorsal horn of spinal cord
lateral skull b.
phantom b.
b. of posterior horn of spinal cord
skull b.
baseborn
Basedow pseudoparaplegia
baseline
b. angiography
b. cognitive functioning
b. EEG
b. measure
b. rating
Reid b.
b. scan
b. severity
b. test
b. visit
baseline-to-endpoint change
basement
b. laboratory
b. membrane
b. membrane protein
bases (*pl. of* basis)
basiarachnitis
basiarachnoiditis
basic
b. brain mechanism
b. brain pathway
b. fibroblast growth factor
b. impairment
B. Living Skills Scale
b. skill
basicranial
b. axis
b. flexure

basilar
b. apex aneurysm
b. arachnoiditis
b. artery
b. artery migraine
b. artery migraine headache
b. artery thrombosis syndrome
b. artery trunk aneurysm
b. bifurcation
b. bifurcation aneurysm
b. crest of cochlear duct
b. ectasia
b. impression
b. invagination
b. lamina
b. leptomeningitis
b. membrane
b. membrane of cochlear duct
b. meninges
b. meningitis
b. part of pons
b. pontine sulcus
b. skull fracture
b. tip aneurysm
basilaris
arteria b.
glandula b.
membrana b.
sulcus b.
basilar-vertebral artery disease
basiocciput tumor
basis, pl. **bases**
compassionate use b.
b. cornus dorsalis medullae spinalis
b. cornus posterioris medullae spinalis
empirical b.
genetic b.
idiosyncratic b.
pathophysiological b.
b. pedunculi cerebri
b. pedunculus
b. pontis
presumptive b.
basket
Alzheimer b.
b. cell
fibrillar b.
Moss-Harms b.
basolateral amygdaloid nucleus
basomedial amygdaloid nucleus
basophil
b. adenoma
b. substance
basophilia
Cushing b.
pituitary b.
substantia b.
basophilic
b. adenoma
b. pituitary tumor
b. substance
basophilism
Cushing b.
Bassen-Kornzweig
B.-K. disease
B.-K. peripheral neuropathy
B.-K. syndrome
Basser syndrome
Bassett electrical stimulation device
Bastian-Bruns
B.-B. law
B.-B. sign
Bastian law
bastion
bath
arteriograph b.
bathesthesia, bathyesthesia
bathing and dressing ability
bathmotropic
negatively b.
positively b.
bathmotropism
bathyanesthesia
bathyesthesia (*var. of* bathesthesia)
bathyhyperesthesia
bathyhypesthesia
batimastat protease inhibitor
Batson plexus
Batten disease
Batten-Mayou disease
battery
apraxia b.
brief cognitive test b.
cognitive test b.
Dementia Assessment B.
Diagnostic Screening B.'s
Komet medical replacement b.'s
Rand Functional Limitations B.
Rand Physical Capacities B.
Rivermead Perceptual Assessment B.

NOTES

battledore incision
Battle sign
BAVM
brain arteriovenous malformation
Baxter disease
Baycrest Neurocognitive Assessment
Bayesian technique
Bayle disease
bayonet
b. aneurysm clip
b. clip applier
b. forceps
b. handle
BB5416
marimastat B.
BBB
blood-brain barrier
BBBD
blood-brain barrier disruption
BBS
Berg Balance Scale
BBTB
blood-brain tumor barrier
BCI X9digitX Cardial Imaging
***bcl-2* gene**
***Bcl-xL* gene**
BCNU
1,3-bis(2-chlorethyl)-1-nitrosourea
bischloroethylnitrosourea
bischloronitrosourea
BCNU-impregnated polymer wafer
BD
brain damage
brain dead
brain death
BDNF
brain-derived neurotrophic factor
BEAM
brain electrical activity method
brain electrical activity monitoring
beam
b. hardening artifact
high energy X-ray b.
laser b.
particle b.
proton b.
radiation b.
beaten
b. copper cranium
b. copper pattern
beaten-metal appearance
beating heart brain-dead donor
Beaver
B. discission blade
B. keratome blade
Bechterew
B. band
B. disease
layer of B.
line of B.
B. nucleus
B. sign
Bechterew-Mendel reflex
Becker
B. disease
B. myotonia
B. variant
B. variant of Duchenne dystrophy
Becker-Kiener dystrophy
Becker-type tardive muscular dystrophy
Beckman-Adson laminectomy blade
Beckman-Eaton
B.-E. laminectomy
B.-E. laminectomy blade
B.-E. laminectomy retractor
Beckman retractor
Beckman-Weitlaner
B.-W. laminectomy
B.-W. laminectomy retractor
bed
BioDyne b.
Burke Bariatric b.
Cardiopulmonary Paragon 8500 b.
CircOlectric b.
Clinitron air b.
dynamic b.
Flexicair b.
high-air-loss b.
high muscular resistance b.
Keane Mobility b.
KinAir b.
Lapidus b.
low-air-loss b.
Magnum 800 b.
Medicus b.
Mega-Air b.
Mega Tilt and Turn b.
b. nucleus of stria terminalis
Pulmonair 40 b.
Restcue b.
Skytron b.
SMI 5000 b.
Stryker b.
Thera Pulse b.
Tilt and Turn Paragon b.
tumor b.
bedside
B. Evaluation Screening Test, Second Edition
b. multimodality monitoring
Beery Developmental Test of Visuomotor
Beevor sign
Begbie disease

BEHAB
brain derived by hyaluronic acid binding
brain-enriched hyaluronan binding
behavior
aberrant motor b.
abnormal illness b.
abstract b.
accident b.
adultomorphic b.
alertness b. (AB)
b. alteration
b. analysis
antinodal b.
catatonic motor b.
Center for Ecology, Evolution and B. (CEEB)
chain b.
B. Change Inventory
chewing b.
chronic illness b.
b. deficit
b. disorder
drive b.
estrous b.
frontal lobe seizure with complex b.
hyperenergetic b.
interictal b.
b. mapping
b. modification therapy
molar b.
molecular b.
multidetermined b.
nonfunctional and repetitive motor b.
B. Pathology in Alzheimer's Disease Rating Scale
pattern of repetitive b.
perplexing b.
Positive Attention B.
rapid eye movement sleep b.
b. reflex
REM-sleep b.
semipurposeful b.
sensory-motor b.
Society for Quantitative Analyses of B.
sundowning b.
b. system
B. Therapy and Research Society
visuomotor b.
behavioral
b. abnormality
b. assessment measure
b. desensitization
b. difference
b. disorder
b. effect
b. function
b. inactivity
b. input
b. manifestation
b. neuroscience
b. perspective
b. symptom
b. trajectory
b. undercontrol
behavior-orientation
Behavioural Neurology Assessment (BNA)
Behçet
B. disease
B. syndrome
Behr
B. complicated optic atrophy
B. disease
beigelii
Trichosporon b.
Beimer-Clip aneurysm clip
Bekhterev
B. deep reflex
B. layer
B. reaction
B. test
B. tract
Bekhterev-Mendel reflex
Bell
B. law
B. nerve
B. Object Relations and Reality Testing Inventory
B. palsy
B. phenomenon
B. sign
B. spasm
Bellatal
Bell-Magendie law
bellows
aneuroid chest b.
bellwether
belly dancer dyskinesia
Belmont collar

NOTES

bemar
jinjinia b.
Ben-Allergin-50 Injection
benazepril and hydrochlorothiazide
Bence Jones protein
Bench Mark Measures
bender
French rod b.
B. Gestalt Visual Motor test
bending
rod b.
b. strength
bendroflumethiazide
beneceptor
Benedek reflex
benediction hand
Benedikt
B. ipsilateral oculomotor paralysis
B. syndrome
Benemid
benign
b. adult familial myoclonic epilepsy
b. capillary hemangioblastoma
b. childhood epilepsy with centrotemporal spike
b. childhood partial epilepsy
b. coital cephalalgia
b. congenital hypotonia
b. cranial nerve tumor
b. epileptiform transient of sleep
b. epileptiform variant
b. exertional headache
b. familial chorea
b. familial essential tremor
b. familial myoclonic epilepsy
b. familial neonatal convulsion
b. fasciculation with cramp
b. focal amyotrophy
b. focal of childhood epilepsy
b. functional vertigo
b. infantile familial convulsion
b. infantile familial convulsions plus paroxysmal choreoathetosis
b. infantile myoclonus
b. intracranial hypertension
b. lymphocytic choriomeningitis
b. lymphocytic meningitis
b. lymphoepithelial parotid tumor
b. maturation delay
b. meningioma
b. monoclonal gammopathy
b. myalgic encephalitis
b. myalgic encephalomyelitis
b. neonatal convulsion
b. neonatal sleep myoclonus
b. occipital epilepsy
b. paroxysmal positional vertigo
b. paroxysmal torticollis
b. paroxysmal vertigo of childhood
b. partial epilepsy of childhood
b. partial epilepsy with centrotemporal spike (BPECTS)
b. positional paroxysmal vertigo
b. postural vertigo
b. rolandic epilepsy
b. senescent forgetfulness
b. stupor
b. tetanus
b. X-linked recessive muscular dystrophy
benserazide
benserazide-L-dopa
Benson-Geschwind classification of aphasia
benthamism
Benton
B. Visual Form Discrimination Test
B. Visual Retention Test (BVRT)
Bentson exchange-length wire
Bentyl
benzamide
substituted b.
Benzedrine
benzenepropanamine
benzilate
quinuclidinyl b.
benznidazole
benzoate
rizatriptan b.
benzodiazepine
b. discontinuation syndrome
b. postsynaptic receptor
short-acting b.
benzoic acid
benzothiadiazide
benzothiazine
dibenzepin b.
benzoylecgonine
benztropine mesylate
Beradinelli syndrome
berdache
berdachism
bereitschaftspotential
Berenstein guiding catheter
Berg Balance Scale (BBS)
Berger
B. paresthesia
B. rhythm
B. sign
Bergeron chorea

Bergman
B. glia
B. rule
Bergmann
B. cord
B. fiber
B. glial cell
bergsonian
bergsonism
Bergstrom cannula
beriberi, beri beri
cerebral b.
dry b.
infantile b.
wet b.
Berliner percussion hammer
Bernard
B. puncture
B. syndrome
Bernard-Horner syndrome
Bernard-Soulier disease
Bernasconi-Cassinari artery
Bernhardt
B. disease
B. paresthesia
Bernhardt-Roth syndrome
Bernoulli law
Bero Test
berry aneurysm
Bertillon cephalometer
Bessman-Baldwin syndrome
best-fit
b.-f. analysis
b.-f. curve
best registration error
besylate
atracurium b.
beta
b. activity
amyloid b. (Abeta)
b. amyloid protein
b. B-sheet conformation
b. carboline
b. fiber
b. glucuronidase
b. hemolytic streptococcus meningitis
b. histine
b. hydroxybutyrate
b. mannosidosis
b. motoneuron
b. rhythm
b. secretase
transforming growth factor b.
b. wave
beta-1a
interferon b.
beta-adrenergic
b.-a. receptor blocking agent
beta-adrenoreceptor antagonist
beta-amyloid processing
beta-aspartyl(acetylglucosamine)
beta-1b
interferon b.
beta-blocker
beta-B-structure sheet
beta-B-TP
betaB-Trace protein
laser-nephelometric assay for beta-B-TP
betaB-Trace protein (beta-B-TP)
beta-emitting radiation
Betaferon (IFN-B1b)
beta-galactosidase
beta-HCG
beta-subunit of human chorionic gonadotropin
beta-human chorionic gonadotropin
beta-hydroxylase
plasma dopamine b.-h.
beta-lactam antibiotic neurotoxicity
beta-lactrotoxin
beta-mannosidase
betamethasone
beta-methylcrotonylglycinuria
beta$_2$ microglobulin
beta-pleated sheet
beta-protein
amyloid b.-p.
Betaseron needle-free delivery system
beta-subunit of human chorionic gonadotropin (beta-HCG)
bete noire
bethanechol
between-brain
Betz
B. cell
B. cell area
Beuren syndrome
Bevan-Lewis cell
Bevatron accelerator
Beyer laminectomy rongeur

NOTES

Bezold ganglion
Bezold-Jarisch reflex
BG
background
BHI
brain-heart infusion
breath-holding index
bias-free evidence
bibrachial paresis
BICAP
Bipolar Circumactive Probe
BICAP cautery
BICAP unit
bicarbonate
potassium b.
serum b.
sodium b.
bicaudate ratio
biceps
b. femoris reflex
b. jerk
bicerebral infarction
Bichat
B. canal
B. fissure
B. foramen
bicisate
technetium 99m b.
Bickerstaff
B. migraine
B. migraine headache
BiCNU
carmustine
bicoronal scalp flap
Bidder organ
bidentate
bidirectionally
Biedl-Moon-Laurence syndrome
Bielschowsky
B. disease
B. head tilt test
B. maneuver
Bielschowsky-Jansky disease
Biemond
B. ataxia
B. disease
B. syndrome
biennis
Oenothera b.
Bier
B. block
B. lumbar puncture needle
B. saw
Biernacki sign
bifid
b. cranium
b. hook
b. uvula
bifida
cranial b.
spina b.
bifidum
cranium b.
bifilar needle electrode
bifrontal
b. craniotomy
b. headache
b. incision
b. malignant meningioma
bifunctional
b. protein
b. protein deficiency
bifurcating axon
bifurcation
basilar b.
carotid b.
cervical carotid b.
b. cone
Bigelow calvarium clamp
bigemina
corpora b.
bigeminal body
bigeminum
biglycan proteoglycan
bihemispheral insult
bilateral
b. acoustic neuroma syndrome
b. activity
b. arachnoid cyst
b. centrocecal scotoma
b. choroid plexus cyst
b. contralateral primary sensorimotor area
b. craniectomy
b. eyelid blinking
b. gaze palsy
b. hemisphere dysfunction
b. homonymous hemianopia
b. hydrocephalus
b. hyperreflexia
b., independent, periodic, lateralized, epileptiform discharge (BIPLED)
b. ligamentectomy
b. medial orbital ecchymosis
b. mesial temporal lobe epilepsy
b. motor phenomenon
b. occipital infarction
b. periventricular nodular heterotopia
b. secondary sensorimotor area
b. spastic hemiplegia
b. synchrony

b. temporary tarsorrhaphy
b. temporoparietal emphasis
b. tonic stiffening
b. upper brain stem infarction
b. vagotomy
b. variable screw placement system
b. ventral rhizotomy
bilaterally synchronous epileptic discharges
bilayer
lipid b.
lipid-protein b.
bilevel
b. PAP (BiPAP)
b. positive airway pressure (BiPAP)
bilharziasis
biliary dyskinesia
Biligrafin
Biligram
Biliodyl
bilious headache
bilirachia
bilirubin
b. encephalopathy
b. serum level
Bilivistan
Billroth disease
bilobed aneurysm
Bilopaque
bilophodont
Biloptin
bimanual
b. coordination deficit
b. neuronal activity
bimastoid line
bimaxillary advancement
bimedial frontal leukotomy
binaural distorted speech test
binding
brain derived by hyaluronic acid b. (BEHAB)
brain-enriched hyaluronan b. (BEHAB)
H-imipramine b.
protein b.
serum protein b.
b. site
in vivo benzodiazepine receptor b.
Bing-Horton syndrome
Bing-Neel syndrome
Bing reflex
binocular
b. acuity change
b. flash stimulus
b. loupe
Binswanger
B. dementia
B. disease
B. encephalopathy
B. type
bioamine
bioaminergic
bioavailability
neuroleptic b.
Biobond
bioccipital headache
bioceramic
calcium phosphate b.
biochemical
b. activity
b. change
b. genetics
b. information
b. oxygen demand (BOD)
b. pathway
b. phenotypic marker
b. study
b. tumor marker
Biocoral graft material
biocycle
BioDyne bed
bioelectrical impedance analysis
bioelectricity
bioenergetic deficiency
bioethics bionics
biofeedback
EMG b.
Biogel Sensor surgical glove
biogenic amine
biohydraulic
Biojector 2000 needle-free injection management system
biolinguistic
biologic
b. correlate
b. determinant
b. dysregulation
b. evidence
b. intervention
b. marker
b. pathogenesis

NOTES

biologic *(continued)*
b. perspective
b. reductionism
b. research
b. response modifier
b. risk factor
b. substrate
b. time
b. training
b. windows on CNS function
biologically quiescent glioma
biomagnetometer
BTi b.
37-channel b.
biomechanical
b. analysis
b. factor
b. testing
biomechanics
axial plane angular deformity b.
distraction instrumentation b.
Dwyer instrumentation b.
posterior fixation system b.
Roy-Camille posterior screw plate fixation b.
biomedical model
biometal
biometric result
bionic
bionics
bioethics b.
bionomics
biopercular syndrome
Biopharmaceuticals
Keryx B.
biophysical study
biophysiology
bioplastic
biopotentiality
biopsy
arterial b.
brain b.
contralateral b.
CT-guided b.
endoscopic sphenoidal b.
image-guided stereotactic brain b.
leptomeningeal/wedge cortical b.
lumbar spine b.
meningeal b.
muscle b.
nerve b.
PET-guided stereotactic b.
quadriceps muscle b.
stereotactic b.
sural nerve b.
targeted brain b.
temporal artery b.
thoracic spine b.
transnasal b.
Tru-Cut needle b.
vastus lateralis muscle b.
biopterin deficiency
biosynthesis
heme b.
Biot
B. breathing
B. breathing sign
B. respiration
Bio-Thesiometer
biotin
b. holocarboxylase synthetase deficiency
b. metabolic disorder
biotinidase deficiency
BioTrainer exercise meter
BIOWARE software for Biodex isokinetic exercise system
BiPAP
bilevel PAP
bilevel positive airway pressure
biparietal
b. hypoperfusion
b. lesion
bipedal walking
biperiden
biphasic
b. action potential
b. locomotor response
Biphetamine
biplane roentgenogram
BIPLED
bilateral, independent, periodic, lateralized, epileptiform discharge
BIPLED on EEG
bipolar
b. bayonet forceps
b. cautery
b. cautery probe
b. cautery scissors
B. Circumactive Probe (BICAP)
b. coagulating forceps
b. coagulator
b. diathermy forceps tip
b. diathesis
b. electrocautery
b. electrocautery forceps
b. gradient
b. long-shaft forceps
b. montage
b. needle electrode
b. neuron
b. patient
b. retinal cell

b. stimulating electrode
b. vertebral traction
bipole
narrow b.
wide b.
biportal technique
Birbeck granule
birdcage resonator
birdlike facies
birefringence
crystalline b.
flow b.
form b.
intrinsic b.
strain b.
streaming b.
birefringent
birth
b. anoxia
b. palsy
1,3-bis(2-chlorethyl)-1-nitrosourea (BCNU)
bischloroethylnitrosourea (BCNU)
bischloronitrosourea (BCNU)
Bischof myelotomy
bisection
vertical line b.
bis(guanylhydrazone)
methylglyoxal b.
Bishop putty
bispectral EEG monitor
bisphosphonate
bisulfate
clopidogrel b.
bit
acorn b.
cannulated drill b.
diamond b.
drill guide with drill b.
Howmedica Microfixation System drill b.
Leibinger Micro System drill b.
Luhr Microfixation System drill b.
Storz Microsystems drill b.
Synthes Microsystem drill b.
bitartrate
metaraminol b.
bitemporal
b. headache
b. hemianopia
b. hypoperfusion
biundulant meningoencephalitis
bivalved speculum
biventer
b. lobule
lobulus b.
biventralis
lobulus b.
biventral lobule
bizarre
b. asynchronous movement
b. high-frequency discharge
b. high-frequency potential
b. posturing
b. repetitive discharge
b. variant
Björeson syndrome
Björnström algesiometer
black
b. box warning
b. eye
b. mass
B. Max high-speed drill
b. substance
Blacky picture
bladder
allantoic b.
atonic b.
autonomic neurogenic b.
cord b.
nervous b.
neurogenic b.
b. reflex
reflex neurogenic b.
stammering of the b.
uninhibited neurogenic b.
blade
Acra-Cut b.
air b.
arachnoid-shape Beaver b.
Beaver discission b.
Beaver keratome b.
Beckman-Adson laminectomy b.
Beckman-Eaton laminectomy b.
double-vector b.
Komet K-2000 surgical saw b.
K-2000 surgical saw b.
Meyerding laminectomy b.
Meyerding-Scoville b.
Micro-Aire b.
retractor b.
ribbon b.

NOTES

blade *(continued)*
Scoville b.
tapered b.
Blair-Ivy loop
Blake pouch
Blandin ganglion
bland myopathy
blank
Strong Vocational Interest B. (SVIB)
blast
air b.
b. effect
stoma b.
blastocyte
blastoderm
Blastomyces dermatitidis
blastomycosis
nasopharyngeal b.
spinal b.
blastomyocotic meningitis
Blastoplasma capsulatum
bleeding
aneurysmal b.
gastrointestinal b.
intraabdominal b.
intracranial b.
intrathoracic b.
b. time
blennorrhagic swelling
blennorrhagicum
keratoderma b.
Blenoxane
bleomycin sulfate
blepharocardiac reflex
blepharoconjunctivitis
blepharophimosis
blepharoplasts
blepharoptosis
blepharospasm, blepharospasmus
essential b.
blepsopathia
Blessed-Roth Dementia Scale
bleulerian type 2
blind
b. headache
b. spot
b. test
blindness
cerebral b.
cortical b.
gaze-evoked b.
hysterical b.
ipsilateral monocular b.
letter b.
mind b.
monocular b.
object b.
psychic b.
sight b.
sign b.
smell b.
syllabic b.
taste b.
text b.
total monocular b.
transient monocular b. (TMB)
word b.
blindsight
blink
b. artifact
eye b.
b. reflex
b. reflex latency
b. response
blinking
bilateral eyelid b.
eye b.
rapid eye movement onset b.
REM onset b.
blister-like aneurysm
bloater
blue b.
blob
b. cell
b. channel
bloc
en b.
Bloch equation
Bloch-Sulzberger syndrome
block
anodal b.
Bier b.
cervical steroid epidural nerve b.
clonic b.
conduction b.
depolarization b.
diagnostic b.
dynamic b.
epidural b.
exit b.
intracellular calcium b.
left bundle branch b.
local diagnostic b.
methylmethacrylate b.
monolithic adult b.
motor conduction b.
motor point b.
nerve root b.
neurolytic b.
phenol motor point b.
sham b.
short-acting b.
somatic b.

BUSINESS REPLY MAIL

FIRST CLASS PERMIT NO. 724 BALTIMORE, MD

POSTAGE WILL BE PAID BY ADDRESSEE

ATTN: JULIE STEGMAN
LIPPINCOTT WILLIAMS & WILKINS
351 WEST CAMDEN STREET
BALTIMORE MD 21201-2436

spinal subarachnoid b.
stellate ganglion b.
subarachnoid b. (SAB)
sugar b.
tonic b.
ventricular b.
b. vertebra
voltage-sensitive b.

blockade
adrenergic b.
D_2 b.
dopamine receptor b.
intravenous regional sympathetic b.
muscarinic cholinergic b.
neuromuscular b.
pharmacological b.
reuptake b.
sympathetic b.

blockage
shunt b.

blocker
calcium channel b.
dopamine receptor b.
voltage-gated sodium channel b.

blocking
b. activity
alpha b.
EEG alpha b.

Blocq disease

blood
b. alcohol level (BAL)
b. blister-like aneurysm
b. cell
b. culture
b. donor
b. feud
b. flow
b. flow change
b. flow measurement
b. flow velocity
b. flow volume
b. loss
b. oxygenation level dependent (BOLD)
b. oxygenation level-dependent contrast technique
b. oxygen level dependent (BOLD)
b. oxygen level-dependent functional magnetic resonance imaging (BOLD f-MRI)
b. pool imaging
b. and thunder retina
b. urea nitrogen (BUN)
b. velocity
b. vessel
b. viscosity

blood-brain
b.-b. barrier (BBB)
b.-b. barrier disruption (BBBD)
b.-b. barrier disruption chemotherapy
b.-b. transcytosis
b.-b. tumor barrier (BBTB)

blood-cerebral barrier

blood-cerebrospinal fluid barrier

blood-CSF barrier

blood-gas exchange

blood/injection phobia

bloodless decerebration

blood-thymus barrier

blood-tissue exchange

bloody tap

Bloom
B. disease
B. syndrome

Bloomer Learning Test

blot
Southern b.

Blount laminar spreader

blown pupil

blow-out fracture

blue
b. diaper syndrome
b. edema
Histacryl B.
methylene b.

blue bloater

blue-stained
toluidine b.-s.

Blumenau nucleus

Blumenbach clivus

blunt
b. nerve hook
b. spike-and-wave complex on EEG
b. suction tube

blunt-ring curette

blurring
visual b.

blush
choroidal b.
b. of dye on angiogram

NOTES

BMI
body mass index
B-mode
B.-m. image
B.-m. ultrasonography
BMP
bone morphogenetic protein
bone morphogenic protein
BNA
Behavioural Neurology Assessment
BNCT
boron neutron capture therapy
Boas algesiometer
Bobath response
bobbing
inverse ocular b.
ocular b.
reverse ocular b.
bobble-head doll syndrome
Bobechko
B. sliding barrel hook
B. spreader
Bochdalek
flower basket of B.
B. ganglion
B. pseudoganglion
Bock
B. ganglion
B. nerve
BOD
biochemical oxygen demand
Bodian silver impregnation
bodily
b. autonomy
b. symptom
body
b. alienation
amygdaloid b.
amyloid b.
anterior nucleus of trapezoid b.
anterior quadrigeminal b.
aortic b.
apoptotic b.
artificial vertebral b.
astral b.
Barr b.
bigeminal b.
carotid b.
b. of caudate nucleus
b. of cerebellum
b. coil
b. concept
b. of corpus callosum
cortical Lewy b.
Cowdry inclusion b. type A, B
Cowdry-type intranuclear inclusion b.
cytoid b.
dementia with Lewy b. (DLB)
dorsal nucleus of trapezoid b.
b. ego damage
foreign b.
b. of fornix
geniculate b.
glomus b.
Golgi b.
habenular b.
Harting b.
Herring b.
Hirano b.
hookean b.
b. image
inclusion b.
infundibular b.
juxtarestiform b.
Kelvin b.
Lafora b.
lateral geniculate b.
lateral nucleus of mammillary b.
lateral nucleus of trapezoid b.
b. of lateral ventricle
Lewy b.
Luys b.
b. of Luys syndrome
mamillary b.
mammary b.
b. mass index (BMI)
medial geniculate b.
medial nucleus of trapezoid b.
metallic foreign b.
b. modification
myelin b.
Negri b.
nerve cell b.
neuronal ceroid lipofuscinosis curvilinear b.
newtonian b.
Nissl b.
nucleus of lateral geniculate b.
nucleus of mamillary b.
nucleus of medial geniculate b.
nucleus of trapezoid b.
olivary b.
pacchionian b.
paraphysial b.
paraterminal b.
parietal b.
parolivary b.
PAS-positive circular b.
peduncle of mamillary b.
pedunculus of pineal b.
Pick b.
pineal b.
pontobulbar b.

posterior quadrigeminal b.
psammoma b.
pseudopsammoma b.
quadrigeminal b.
Reilly b.
Renaut b.
restiform b.
rhinencephalic mamillary b.
b. righting reflex
sand b.
b. schema
Schwann cell b.
b. sense
serotoninergic cell b.
b. spatial orientation
striate b.
tigroid b.
Todd b.
trapezoid b.
Vater-Pacini b.
ventral nucleus of trapezoid b.
Verocay b.
Weibel-Palade b.
b. weight-supported treadmill training
b. weight unloading
Wolf-Orton b.
zebra b.

body-image distortion

body-related obsessive-like symptom

Boehme disease

Bogaert-Bertrand spongy dystrophy

Bohlman

B. anterior cervical vertebrectomy
B. cervical fusion technique

Bohr effect

Bohr-Haldane effect

Bolam Principle

BOLD

blood oxygenation level dependent
blood oxygen level dependent
BOLD f-MRI

Bolivian hemorrhagic fever

Bollinger

posttraumatic apoplexy of B.

bolt

Camino microventricular b.
Camino ventricular b.
ICP Camino b.
Philly b.
Richmond b.
subarachnoid b.

Boltzmann

B. distribution
B. distribution law

bolus dosing

bombesin

Bondek suture

bone

b. algorithm
allograft iliac b.
autogenous iliac b.
autograft b.
bone in b.
calvarial b.
cancellous b.
b. conduction
b. curette
b. cyst
b. density scan
b. density screening
b. dissection
b. flap
b. graft
b. graft collapse
b. graft decompression
b. graft extrusion
b. grafting
b. graft placement
b. health
hyoid b.
increased Wormian b.
b. loss
magic b.
b. marrow
b. marrow rescue
b. marrow stromal cell
b. marrow suppression
b. marrow transplantation
b. marrow transplantation graft-versus-host disease
b. matrix formation
b. mineral density
b. morphogenetic protein (BMP)
b. morphogenic protein (BMP)
occipital b.
b. occipital malformation
b. pain
petrous b.
b. plate
b. plate aspiration

NOTES

bone *(continued)*
b. plate selection
b. punch
b. reflex
b. remodeling
b. screw
b. sensibility
spongy b.
b. stock
temporal b.
trabecular b.
trigeminal impression of temporal b.
b. tumor
Tutoplast b.
b. wax
wormian b.
bone-biting rongeur
bone/ligament dissection
bone-screw interface strength
BoneSource hydroxyapatite cement
bone-window CT scan
Bonferroni-Dunn procedure
Bonhoeffer
B. sign
B. symptom
B. syndrome
Bonnet-Dechaume-Blanc syndrome
Bonnet sign
Bonnevie-Ullrich syndrome
Bonnier syndrome
Bontril PDM
bony
b. abnormality
b. canal
b. dissection
b. dysplasia
b. element destruction
b. endplate
b. exposure
b. facet
b. overhang
b. purchase
Bookwalter retractor
booster clip
boost irradiation technique
boot
thigh-high alternating compression air b.
Borchardt olive-shaped bur
border
b. cell
vermilion b.
borderline
b. pathology
b. patient
borderzone infarction
Bordier-Frequentänkel sign
boric acid neurotoxicity
Börjeson-Forssman-Lehmann syndrome
Bornholm disease
boron neutron capture therapy (BNCT)
boronophenylalanine
Borrelia
B. burgdorferi
B. hermsii
borreliosis
Lyme b.
Bosin disease
bossing
occipital b.
Boston
B. Classification System
B. Diagnostic Aphasia Exam
B. Diagnostic Aphasia Exam-Cookie Theft Card
B. LINAC
B. neurosurgical couch
Bosworth spinal fusion
Botox
B. injection amplifier
B. injection amplifier brace
Böttcher
B. cell
B. ganglion
bottom-up approach
botulinum
b. antitoxin
b. A toxin
Clostridium b.
b. toxin injection
b. toxin type A, B
botulism
human b.
infantile b.
b. peripheral neuropathy
b. toxin
bouche de tapir
Bouchet-Gsell sign
Bouin-Hollande fixative
boulimia
boundary
diagnostic b.
whole brain b.
Bourneville
B. disease
B. tuberous sclerosis
Bourneville-Pringle disease
bouton
axonal terminal b.
b. en passage
synaptic b.
terminal b.
b. terminaux

bovine
b. chromaffin cell
b. percardium dural graft
b. spongiform encephalopathy
Bowditch law
Bower model of mood-congruent memory
bowing reflex
bow-tie nystagmus
box
Box and Block timed manipulation test
BTE Bolt B.
cyclin b.
boxcar effect
boydii
Pseudallescheria b.
BP
Imagent BP
BPECTS
benign partial epilepsy with centrotemporal spike
BPI
brain perfusion index
BPS spinal angiographic catheter
Braak stage
brace
Botox injection amplifier b.
halo b.
Hudson b.
kyphosis b.
Milwaukee b.
SOMI Jr. b.
Yale b.
brace-free ambulation
bracelet
Nageotte b.
brachial
b. amyotrophy
b. birth palsy
b. cutaneous nerve
b. diplegia
b. locomotion
b. plexitis
b. plexopathy
b. plexus
b. plexus avulsion
b. plexus avulsion injury
b. plexus exploration
b. plexus lesion
b. plexus neuritis
b. plexus neuropathy
brachial-basilar insufficiency syndrome
brachialgia
b. and cord syndrome
b. statica paresthetica
brachialis
divisiones anteriores plexus b.
divisiones posteriores plexus b.
fasciculus lateralis plexus b.
pars infraclavicularis plexus b.
pars supraclavicularis plexus b.
plexus b.
radices plexus b.
trunci plexus b.
truncus inferior plexus b.
truncus medius plexus b.
truncus superior plexus b.
brachiocephalic vein
brachiocephaly
brachiofacial cortical hypesthesia
brachioradialis
b. reflex
b. transfer for wrist extension
brachioradial reflex
brachium
b. of caudal colliculus
b. colliculi caudalis
b. colliculi inferioris
b. colliculi rostralis
b. colliculi superioris
b. conjunctivum cerebelli
b. of inferior colliculus
b. of the inferior colliculus
inferior quadrigeminal b.
b. opticum
b. pontis
b. quadrigeminum inferius
b. quadrigeminum superius
b. of rostral colliculus
b. of superior colliculus
superior quadrigeminal b.
Brachmann-de Lange syndrome
brachybasia
brachycephalia
brachycephalic
brachycephalism
brachycephalous
brachycephaly
brachycranic

NOTES

brachytherapy
high-energy b.
interstitial b.
remote afterloading b. (RAB)
b. seed implantation
stereotactic b.
volumetric interstitial b.
bracing
external b.
postoperative b.
Bracken Basic Concept Scale, Revised
Brackmann suction-irrigator
Bradbury-Eggleston syndrome
Braden flushing reservoir
bradyarthria
bradycinesia (*var. of* bradykinesia)
bradyesthesia
bradyglossia
bradykinesia, bradycinesia
end-of-dose b.
bradykinesia/akinesia
bradykinesis
bradykinetic
bradykinin
bradylalia
bradylexia
bradylogia
bradyphagia
bradyphasia
bradyphemia
bradyphrenia
bradypnea
bradypragia
bradypsychia
bradyteleokinesis, bradyteleocinesia
Bragard
B. sign
B. sign test
Bragg
B. ionization peak
B. peak proton beam therapy
B. peak radiation
B. peak radiosurgery
Brahmanism
braided
b. occlusion device
b. Spectra UHMWPE surgical cable
b. titanium cable
brain
abdominal b.
b. abscess
b. activation
b. aging
b. aluminum
b. aneurysm
anterior part of anterior commissure of b.
arachnoid of b.
b. area
b. arteriovenous malformation (BAVM)
artery of b.
b. assault
b. attack
base of b.
b. biopsy
b. biopsy needle
b. blood flow
b. central pain
b. cicatrix
b. circuitry
b. clip forceps
compression of b.
b. concussion
b. congestion
contrecoup injury of b.
b. contusion
b. cooling
b. cooling system
coup injury of b.
b. cryolesion
b. cyst
b. damage (BD)
b. dead (BD)
b. death (BD)
b. derived by hyaluronic acid binding (BEHAB)
b. development
b. differentiation
b. disease
b. disorder
b. dopamine
b. dopaminergic pathway
b. dopaminergic system
dura mater of b.
b. dysfunction
b. dysplasia
b. edema
b. electrical activity map
b. electrical activity mapping
b. electrical activity method (BEAM)
b. electrical activity monitoring (BEAM)
b. engorgement
enlarged b.
fetal b.
b. functional failure
b. function disruption
b. functioning
b. gene therapy
glucose metabolism in the b.

b. glucose metabolism
hemangioma of the b.
hemosiderin-stained b.
b. herniation
hypoxic-ischemic b.
b. illness
b. imaging
b. imaging method
b. infarction
b. infusion
injured b.
b. injury
b. involvement
b. ischemia
b. isoform
b. laceration
b. lactate
lateral fossa of b.
b. lesion
b. location
b. mantle
B. Matters Stroke Initiative Edinburgh Artery Study
medullary artery of b.
b. metabolic effect
b. metabolic mechanism
b. metabolic response
b. metastasis
b. morphometry
b. MRI
b. murmur
b. natriuretic peptide
b. neurochemical system
olfactory b.
b. oxygen consumption
b. parenchyma
b. perfusion index (BPI)
b. perfusion study
Planar Stereotaxic Atlas of the Human B.
b. potential
b. potential study
prefrontal cortex of the b.
b. process
b. prolyl oligopeptidase
b. puncture
b. purpura
b. reflex
respirator b.
b. retention
b. retraction
b. retractor
b. revascularization
b. sand
b. shift
smell b.
softening of b.
somatosensory cortices of the right hemisphere of the b.
b. space
b. spatula
b. spatula forceps
b. SPECT scan
split b.
b. spoon
b. stem
b. stimulation
b. structure
b. structure study
b. substrate
supratentorial b.
b. swelling
b. synaptic membrane
b. synaptosome
b. target
tight b.
b. tissue
b. transplantation
b. trocar
b. tumor
b. tumor forceps
B. Tumor Registry
B. Tumor Study Group (BTSG)
ventricle of b.
ventromedial prefrontal cortex of the b.
Virchow-Robin space of the b.
visceral b.
b. volume
b. voyager 4.0
b. wart
b. wave
b. wave complex
b. wave cycle
wet b.

Brain-Age Quotient

brain-behavior relationship

brain-blood partition

braincase

brain-derived

b.-d. HVA concentration

B

NOTES

brain-derived *(continued)*
b.-d. neurotrophic factor (BDNF)
b.-d. neurotropic factor
brain-enriched
b.-e. hyaluronan binding (BEHAB)
b.-e. hyaluronan binding protein
brain-heart infusion (BHI)
BrainLAB VectorVision neuronavigational system
BrainMap
Couples B.
BrainSCAN
B. II
B. computer planning system
B. Linac radiosurgery system
brainstem
b. activation
b. astrocytoma
b. auditory evoked potential (BAEP)
b. auditory evoked response (BAER)
b. cavernous malformation
b. compression
b. diencephalic mapping
b. edema
b. electrical response audiometry
b. encephalitis
b. evoked potential
b. evoked response
b. glioma
b. hemorrhage
b. infarction
b. injury (BSI)
b. ischemia
b. lesion
b. neuron
b. reticular formation
reticular nuclei of the b.
rostral b.
b. syndrome
b. tumor
BrainVoyager software
branch
anterior temporal b.
anteromedial central b.
b. artery occlusion
b. of auriculotemporal nerve to tympanic membrane
callosal marginal b.
carotid sinus b.
choroid b.
circumferential b.
communicating b.
b. to coracobrachialis
descending b.
frontal polar b.
b. of glossopharyngeal nerve to stylopharyngeus muscle
b. to internal capsule, genu
b. to internal capsule, posterior limb
b. to internal capsule, retrolentiform limb
b. of internal carotid artery to trigeminal ganglion
b. of lingual nerve to isthmus of fauces
M2 b.
meningohypophyseal b.
b. of ocular motor nerve to ciliary ganglion
peripheral trigeminal nerve b.
b. to sternocleidomastoid
superior laryngeal nerve external b.
trigeminal b.
branched-chain ketoaciduria
brancher enzyme deficiency disease
branchial
b. cleft
b. cleft abnormality
b. efferent column
branching
anomalous b.
branchiomotor nucleus
Brasdor method
brasiliensis
Paracoccidioides b.
Brauch-Romberg
B.-R. symptom
B.-R. syndrome
Braun-Yasargil right-angle clip
Bravais-jacksonian epilepsy
Brawner decision
BrDu, BrdU
bromodeoxyuridine
B. immunoactive cell
B. immunohistochemistry
B. immunolabeling cell
BrDu-positive cell
breach rhythm
break
major b.
b. shock
breakage
pedicle screw b.
screw b.
breakdown
myelin b.
breakpoint
sequencing deletion b.
breakthrough
depressive b.

normal perfusion pressure b. (NPPB)
b. phenomenon

breath-holding
b.-h. index (BHI)
b.-h. spell

breathing
apneustic b.
ataxic b.
Biot b.
Cheyne-Stokes b.
cluster b.
b. retraining
underlying sleep-disordered b.

breathy dystonia

bredouillement

bregma

bregmocardiac reflex

Bremer
B. AirFlo halo vest
B. halo
B. halo crown
B. halo crown system
B. halo crown traction
B. halo crown traction set
B. torque-limiting cap

Breschet sinus

Brescia-Cimino fistula

breves
fibrae associationes b.
nervi ciliares b.

Brevibloc

brevican proteoglycan

breviradiate

brevis
abductor pollicis b.
fibrae associationis b.
wrist-to-abductor pollicis b. (APB)

Brevital

Bricklin Perceptual Scale

bridegroom's palsy

bridge
caudolenticular gray b.
b. region
transcapsular gray b.

bridging vein

brief
B. Cognitive Rating Scale
b. cognitive test battery
B. Neuropsychological Mental Status Examination
B. Pain Inventory
B. Symptom Inventory
B. Test of Head Injury

Brigance
B. Diagnostic Comprehensive Inventory of Basic Skills
B. Diagnostic Comprehensive Inventory of Basic Skills, Revised
B. Diagnostic Inventory of Basic Skills
B. Diagnostic Inventory of Essential Skills
B. Diagnostic Life Skills Inventory

bright
b. light therapy
b. thalamus syndrome

Brill-Zinsser disease

brim sign

Briquet
B. ataxia
B. disease
B. syndrome

Brissaud
B. disease
B. reflex
B. syndrome

Brissaud-Marie syndrome

Brissaud-Sicard syndrome

Bristol
B. disk prosthesis
B. disk replacement

British
B. Ability Scale
B. anti-Lewisite

broad
b. AO dynamic compression plate
b. phonemic transcription

Broadbent law

Brobdingnagian disorder of visual perception in migraine

Broca
B. amnesia
B. aphasia
band of B.
B. center
B. convolution
B. diagonal band
B. dysphasia
B. field
B. fissure
B. gyrus

NOTES

Broca *(continued)*
B. motor speech area
B. parolfactory area
B. region
B. syndrome
Brocae
area parolfactoria B.
Brodie disease
Brodmann
B. area 6,7,9,24,32,34,41,43,44,46
B. classification
B. cortical area
B. cytoarchitectonic field
broken existing implant
bromfenac sodium capsule
bromide
azamethonium b.
calcium b.
ethidium b. (EB)
b. intoxication
ipratropium b.
pancuronium b.
perfluorooctyl b.
potassium b.
pyridostigmine b.
serum b.
sodium b.
vecuronium b.
brominized oil
bromisoval
bromocriptine
b. mesylate
b. test
bromodeoxyuridine (BrDu, BrdU)
bromzepan
Bronx Aging Study
brooding personality
Brooks
B. atlantoaxial arthrodesis
B. cervical fusion
B. technique
Brooks-Gallie cervical operation
Brooks-Jenkins
B.-J. atlantoaxial fusion
B.-J. cervical operation
brow-down position
Brown-Adson forceps
Brown-Goodwin scale
brownian motion
Browning vein
Brown-Roberts-Wells
B.-R.-W. apparatus
B.-R.-W. arc-ring assembly
B.-R.-W. arc system
B.-R.-W. base ring
B.-R.-W. computer
B.-R.-W. computerized tomography stereotactic guidance
B.-R.-W. floor stand
B.-R.-W. head frame
B.-R.-W. headrest
B.-R.-W. head ring halo
B.-R.-W. ring adapter
B.-R.-W. stereotactic system
B.-R.-W. technique
Brown-Séquard
B.-S. paralysis
B.-S. sign
B.-S. syndrome
Brown syndrome
Brown-Vialetto-van Laere syndrome
brow pang
brucei
Trypanosoma b.
Brucella
B. abortus
B. melitensis
brucellosis
cerebral b.
b. peripheral neuropathy
Bruce tract
Bruch membrane discontinuity
Brudzinski
B. reflex
B. sign
Brueghel syndrome
bruit
aneurysmal b.
arterial b.
asymptomatic carotid b.
asymptomatic neck b.
carotid b.
intracranial b.
Bruker
B. Biospec system
B. S 200 MR system
Brunner modified incision
Bruns
B. frontal ataxia
B. gait apraxia
B. nystagmus
B. sign
B. syndrome
brush
Cragg thrombolytic b.
brush-evoked allodynia
Brushfield spot
Brushfield-Wyatt
B.-W. disease
B.-W. syndrome
brush-induced allodynia

bruxism
sleep b.
SSRI-induced b.
Bryan
B. Cervical Disc System
B. cervical disk prosthesis
BSI
brainstem injury
BTE
BTE Bolt Box
BTE Work Simulator
B_2-TFn
B.-T. assay
BTi biomagnetometer
B_2-transferrin
BTSG
Brain Tumor Study Group
bubbly bone lesion
buccal
b. frenulum
b. nerve
buccalis
nervus b.
buccal-lingual dyskinesia
buccinator nerve
buccofacial apraxia
buccolingual
b. ataxia
b. dyskinesia
buccopharyngeal approach
Bucholz bipolar cauterizer
Buck
B. neurological hammer
B. percussion hammer
buckling sign
buckthorn polyneuropathy
bucrylate
Bucy
B. cordotomy knife
B. laminectomy rongeur
Bucy-Frazier
B.-F. coagulation cannula
B.-F. suction cannula
bud
gustatory b.
taste b.
Budde
B. halo retractor system
B. halo ring
B. halo ring retractor
B. surgical system
Budde-Greenberg-Sugita stereotactic head frame
Budge center
buffer
assay b.
Buffex
bulb
b. dynamometer
end b.
glomerular layer of olfactory b.
Held end b.
jugular b. (JB)
Krause end b.
Krause terminal b.
molecular layer of olfactory b.
b. of occipital horn
b. of occipital horn of lateral ventricle
olfactory b.
b. of posterior horn of lateral ventricle
bulbar
b. abnormality
b. anesthesia
b. apoplexy
b. cephalic pain tractotomy
b. corticonuclear fiber
b. dysfunction
b. hereditary motor neuropathy
b. involvement
b. muscle weakness
b. musculature
b. myelitis
b. nucleus
b. palsy
b. paralysis
b. poliomyelitis
b. syndrome
b. tract
bulbi (*pl. of* bulbus)
bulbocavernosus
b. reflex
b. reflex evaluation
bulboid corpuscle
bulboidea
corpuscula b.
bulboidum
corpusculum b.
bulbomimic reflex
bulbonuclear
bulbopontine sulcus

NOTES

bulbopontis
sulcus b.
bulboreticulospinalis
tractus b.
bulboreticulospinal tract
bulborum
pars intermedia commissura b.
bulbosacral system
bulbospinal
bulbospongiosus reflex
bulbothalamic tract
bulbus, pl. **bulbi**
b. cornus occipitalis ventriculi lateralis
b. cornus posterioris
b. cornus posterioris ventriculi lateralis
b. encephali
fibrae corticonucleares b.
b. olfactorius
phthisis b.
pyramis b.
stratum pigmenti b.
bulging
aneurysmal b.
bulk
b. flow transcytosis
tumor b.
bulldog response
bull's
b. eye deformity
b. eye rash
bullying
b. culture
b. target
Bumke pupil
BUN
blood urea nitrogen
bunamiodyl
bundle
aberrant b.
angular b.
anterior ground b.
Arnold b.
cingulum b.
comb b.
b. of fibril
Flechsig ground b.
Gierke respiratory b.
Gowers b.
ground b.
Held b.
Helweg b.
Hoche b.
Krause respiratory b.
lateral ground b.
lateral proprius b.
Lissauer b.
Loewenthal b.
longitudinal medial b.
longitudinal pontine b.
maculoneural b.
medial forebrain b.
medial longitudinal b.
Meynert retroflex b.
Monakow b.
olfactory b.
olivocochlear b.
b. of Oort
Pick b.
posterior longitudinal b.
precommissural b.
predorsal b.
Probst b.
b. of Rasmussen
Rasmussen olivocochlear b.
Schultze b.
Schütz b.
solitary b.
thalamomamillary b.
tumor-nerve b.
Türck b.
Vicq d'Azyr b.
bundle-nailing method
Büngner band
Bunnell
B. dissecting probe
B. forwarding probe
bunyavirus encephalitis
buphthalmia
buphthalmos, buphthalmus
bupivacaine
buprenorphine HCl
bupropion
b. hydrochlorothiazide
b. metabolite
bur, burr
Adson enlarging b.
Adson perforating b.
Adson-Rogers cranial b.
Albee olive-shaped b.
barrel b.
Borchardt olive-shaped b.
Cushing cranial b.
dermabrasion b.
D'Errico enlarging drill b.
D'Errico perforating drill b.
diamond b.
Doyen cylindrical b.
Doyen spherical b.
enlarging b.
finish b.
flame tip b.
high-torque b.

b. hole
b. hole cover
b. hole drainage
b. hole neuroendoscopic fenestration
b. hole transducer
Hudson brace b.
Lindermann b.
McKenzie enlarging b.
pear b.
perforating b.
right-ankle b.
Rosen b.
Rotablator rotating b.
round b.
Shannon b.
spherical b.
Stille b.

Burdach
B. column
B. cuneate fasciculus
B. fiber
B. fissure
B. nucleus
B. tract

Burdick Eclipse ECG machine
Burford-Finochietto rib spreader
Burford retractor
burgdorferi
Borrelia b.
burgeoning
Burke Bariatric bed
burner
b. injury
b. syndrome
burning
b. feet syndrome
b. hands syndrome
Burn and Rand theory
Burns Brief Inventory of Communication and Cognition
burr (*var. of* bur)
burst
b. of delta activity
epileptiform b.
epileptogenic b.
b. fracture
b. injury
b. suppression
b. temporal lobe
bursting
b. cell
epileptiform b.
paroxysmal b.
burst-suppression
electroencephalographic b.-s.
Burundanga intoxication
Buschke
B. disease
B. Free and Cued Selective Reminding Procedure
B. Free and Cued Selective Reminding Test
Buschke-Fuld Selective Memory Test
Buss-Durkee scale
Busse-Buschke disease
butaclamol hydrochloride
Butalan
butalbital
Butcher Treatment Planning Inventory
butethal
Butisol
butorphanol
b. tartrate
b. tartrate nasal spray
butterfly
b. coil
b. distribution
b. needle
b. rash
b. vertebra
butterfly-shaped
b.-s. monoblock
b.-s. monobloc vertebral plate
butterfly-type glioma
button
mescal b.
rubber b.
subdural b.
buttress response
butyl
b. acetate
b. aminobenzoate
b. chloride
b. formate
b. hydride
b. nitrate
butylcholinesterase
butyrophenone
Buzzard maneuver
buzz group
BVR
basal vein of Rosenthal

NOTES

BVRT
Benton Visual Retention Test

bypass
anterior occipital artery-middle cerebral artery b.
b. coaptation for cervical nerve root avulsion
ECIC arterial b.
extracranial-intracranial b.
Fukushima cavernous b.
b. graft
IC-IC b.
intracranial-intracranial b.
STA-MCA b.
STA-PCA b.
STA-SCA b.
superficial temporal artery to middle cerebral artery b.
superficial temporal artery to posterior cerebral artery b.
superficial temporal artery to superior cerebral artery b.
vertebral plate b.

bystander effect

C
angry backfiring C (ABC)
C fiber
C fiber activity
C2
medial branch C2
C2 syndrome
C4
fourth cervical nerve
c
cytochrome *c*
C2-C3 cervical disk excision
C5b-9 complex
C6-C7 dislocation
CA4-1
area C.
CA3 pyramidal cell
CAA
cerebral amyloid angiopathy
cabal
cabergoline
c. monotherapy
c. study
cabin
magnetic shielded c.
cable
braided Spectra UHMWPE surgical c.
braided titanium c.
coaxial c.
c. graft
SecureStrand c.
Songer c.
titanium c.
UHMWPE c.
ultra-high molecular weight polyethylene fiber c.
cabling
percutaneous c.
cachectic
cachexia
diabetic neuropathic c.
hypophysial c.
c. hypophysiopriva
pituitary c.
c. pituitary
cacosmia
CADASIL
cerebral autosomal dominant arteriopathy with subcortical infarcts and leukoencephalopathy
Ca^{2+}-dependent
cadherin
calcium-dependent c.
Cadwell
C. 5200A somatosensory evoked potential unit
C. 5200A somatosensory evoked potential unit device
CAE
childhood absence epilepsy
caecum
Vicq d'Azyr foramen c.
caeruleospinalis
tractus c.
caeruleun nucleus
caeruleus
locus c.
caerulospinal tract
café au lait spot
Cafergot
caffeine
ergotamine tartrate and c.
c. holiday
c. metabolism
c. response
c. sequela
c. toxicity
c. use disorder
c. withdrawal
caffeine-induced
c.-i. anxiety disorder
c.-i. contracture
c.-i. sleep disorder
c.-i. vasoconstriction
caffeine-related sequela
Caffey hyperostosis
CagA
cytotoxin-associated gene A
CAGE
Lumbar I/F CAGE
cage
BAK c.
Ray threaded fusion c.
threaded fusion c. (TFC)
CAI
carboxyaminoimidazole
Caitlin agitation
Cajal
horizontal cell of C.
C. horizontal cell
interstitial nucleus of C.
nucleus of C.
Cajal-Retzius cell
calamus scriptorius
Calan
calbindin
calcaneal gait

calcar avis
Cal Carb-HD
calcareous granule
calcarina
- arteria c.
- fissura c.

calcarine
- c. artery
- c. complex
- c. cortex
- c. cortex infarction
- c. fasciculus
- c. fissure
- c. spur
- c. sulcus

calcarinus
- sulcus c.

calcaroid
Calcibind
calcifediol
Calciferol
- C. Injection
- C. Oral

calcification
- c. of the basal ganglion
- dystrophic c.
- gyriform intracranial c.
- idiopathic c.
- intracranial c.

calcifying vasopathy
Calcijex
Calcimar Injection
Calci-Mix
calcinosis
- cerebral c.
- c. intervertebralis
- c., Raynaud phenomenon, esophageal motility disorders, sclerodactyly, and telangiectasia (CREST)
- tumoral c.

calcitonin
- c. gene-related peptide (CGRP)
- c. gene-related polypeptide
- c. receptor-like receptor (CRLR)

calcitriol
calcium
- c. bromide
- c. carbonate
- cerebrospinal fluid c.
- c. channel antagonist
- c. channel blocker
- c. channel blocking agent
- c. chloride
- c. citrate
- c. disodium edetate
- c. disodium versenate
- c. embolus
- c. glubionate
- c. gluceptate
- c. gluconate
- intracellular c.
- c. ion
- c. ionophore
- c. lactate
- low c.
- c. metabolism imbalance
- c. paradox
- c. phosphate bioceramic
- c. pyrophosphate dihydrate (CPPD)
- c. pyrophosphate dihydrate arthropathy
- c. pyrophosphate dihydrate decomposition disease
- serum c.

calcium-ATPase
calcium-calmodulin kinase II
calcium-dependent cadherin
calcoaceticus
- *Acinetobacter c.*

calculus, pl. **calculi**
- cerebral c.

Caldwell
- C. High Speed Magnetic stimulator
- C. projection

Caldwell-Luc
- C.-L. incision
- C.-L. procedure

calibration
- automated test target c.
- low-voltage c.

caliciform ending
caliculus, pl. **calicali**
- c. ophthalmicus

California encephalitis
californica
- *Aplysia c.*

caligo
calisthenics
Calleja
- island of C.
- C. islet

Call-Fleming syndrome
callosal
- c. agenesis
- c. apraxia
- c. area
- c. commissure
- c. commissurotomy
- c. convolution
- c. gyrus
- c. lesion
- c. marginal branch
- c. section

c. splenium
c. sulcus

callosi
genu corporis c.
pars frontalis corporis c.
pars occipitalis corporis c.
pedunculus corporis c.
radiatio corporis c.
raphe corporis c.
rostrum corporis c.
splenium corporis c.
stria longitudinalis lateralis corporis c.
stria longitudinalis medialis corporis c.
sulcus corporis c.
taeniola corporis c.
tapetum corporis c.
teniola corporis c.
truncus corporis c.
tuber corporis c.
vena dorsalis corporis c.
vena posterior corporis c.

callosomarginal
c. artery
c. fissure
c. sulcus

callosomarginalis
sulcus c.

callosotomy
anterior c.
corpus c.
posterior c.

callosum
agenesis of corpus c.
body of corpus c.
corpus c.
dorsal vein of corpus c.
frontal part of corpus c.
genu of corpus c.
hypogenetic corpus c.
occipital part of corpus c.
peduncle of corpus c.
posterior vein of corpus c.
radiation of corpus c.
rostrum of corpus c.
splenium of corpus c.
sulcus of corpus c.
transverse striae of corpus c.
trunk of corpus c.

calm
c. hypotonic coma
c. wakefulness state

Calman carotid clamp

calming effect

calmodulin dysfunction

calmodulin-independent neuronal nitric oxide synthase activity

calmodulin-regulated event

caloric
c. nystagmus
c. test
c. testing

calorifacient

calorimetry

calpain inhibitor

calvaria, pl. **calvariae**

calvarial
c. bone
c. hemangioma
c. hook
c. metastasis
c. tuberculosis

calyciform

CAM
cell adhesion molecule
computer-assisted myelography

camera
AxioCam c.
CTI-Siemens 933/08-12 PET c.
GE Maxicamera gamma c.
Multispect 3 c.
scintillation c.
time-of-flight positron emission tomographic c.

Camino
C. fiberoptic ICP monitor
C. intracranial catheter
C. intracranial pressure monitoring system
C. intraparenchymal fiberoptic device
C. microventricular bolt
C. OLM ICP monitor
C. subdural screw
C. transducer catheter
C. ventricular bolt

cAMP
adenosine 3′,5′-cyclic monophosphate
cAMP receptor protein (CRP)
cAMP response element

NOTES

cAMP *(continued)*
cAMP response element binding protein
Campath
C. IV
C. subcu injection
Campbell nerve root retractor
campi foreli
campotomy
camptocormia
camptospasm
Camptothecin
Campylobacter
C. jejuni
C. jejuni infection
Camurati-Engelmann
C.-E. disease
C.-E. syndrome
Canadian
C. Cognitive Abilities Test, Form 7
C. Test of Basic Skills, Forms 7 and 8
C. Test of Cognitive Skills
canal
arachnoid c.
Arnold c.
auditory c.
Bichat c.
bony c.
caudal c.
central c.
Cotunnius c.
craniopharyngeal c.
Dorello c.
Guyon c.
haversian c.
Hensen c.
Hunter c.
internal auditory c.
c. knife
lateral semicircular c. (LSC)
limbs of bony semicircular c.
Löwenberg c.
neural c.
optic c.
c. paresis
posterior semicircular c. (PSC)
semicircular c.
spinal c.
c. stenosis
superior semicircular c. (SSC)
uniting c.
c. of Vesalius
vidian c.
canaliculus, pl. **canaliculi**
c. reuniens
canalis, pl. **canales**
c. centralis medullae spinae
c. centralis medullae spinalis
c. reuniens
canalium semicircularium
canalolithiasis
canarc 1 gene
Canavan
C. disease
C. leukodystrophy
C. sclerosis
Canavan-van Bogaert-Bertrand disease
cancellation
fat/water signal c.
phase c.
cancellous
c. bone
c. screw
cancer-associated myositis
Candida
C. albicans
C. infection
candidal
c. meningitis
c. microabscess
candidate gene
candidate-gene strategy
Candidate Profile Record
candidiasis
Cane
Thera C.
canine spasm
caninus
risus c.
spasmus c.
canis
Toxocara c.
Cannon-Bard theory
Cannon theory
cannula
Adson brain-exploring c.
Adson brain-extracting c.
Bergstrom c.
Bucy-Frazier coagulation c.
Bucy-Frazier suction c.
Dorsey ventricular c.
Dyonics c.
Elsberg brain c.
Elsberg ventricular c.
Frazier brain-exploring c.
Frazier ventricular c.
Fujita suction c.
Haynes brain c.

large-egress c.
McCain TMJ c.
Portnoy ventricular c.
Scott c.
Sedan c.
side-cutting c.
Sluijter-Mehta SMK-C10 c.
SMK C5 with a 2-mm exposed tip c.
straightening c.
c. with locking dilator
cannulated drill bit
cannulation
unilateral pedicle c.
canonical neuron
canopy ventilation monitor
Cantelli sign
Canto-Rapin syndrome
CANVAS
Computer-Aided Neurovascular Analysis and Simulation protocol
canyon
Jamestown C. (JC)
CAO
carotid artery occlusion
cap
c. of the ampullary crest
Bremer torque-limiting c.
Navigus cranial base and c.
Quickcap electrode c.
Remind C.
c. sign
capability
cognitive c.
metabolic c.
capacitance
membrane c.
capacity
cognitive c.
cranial c.
empathic c.
forced vital c. (FVC)
functional c.
intrinsic c.
metacognitive c.
neural c.
paranormal c.
vital c.
volitional c.
capillariomotor
capillary
c. angioma
c. fracture
c. hemangioma
c. telangiectasia
capistratus
trismus c.
CAPIT
core assessment program for intracerebral transplantation
capita (*pl. of* caput)
capitis
dolor c.
semispinalis c.
capitium
capitus
splenius c.
caplet
Keep GOing c.
Mytelase C.
Symax-SR c.
TripTone C.'s
capnography
capnometer
MicroSpan C. 8800
Capozide
capreomycin
capsaicin
Capsin
capsula, pl. **capsulae**
crus anterius capsulae
crus posterius capsulae
c. externa
c. extrema
c. ganglii
c. interna
c. nuclei dentati
capsulae nuclei lentiformis
capsular infarction
capsulatum
Blastoplasma c.
Histoplasma c.
capsule
anterior limb of internal c.
bromfenac sodium c.
c. cell
Depakote Sprinkle C.
Duradrin c.
Exelon c.
external c.
extreme c.

NOTES

capsule *(continued)*
Fastlene c.
gabapentin c.
ganglion c.
genu of internal c.
Indochron E-R c.
internal c.
Kadian sustained-release morphine c.
Keep Alert c.
Metadate CD extended-release c.
methylphenidate HCl extended-release c.
Molie c.
Nimotop c.
otic c.
posterior limb of internal c.
Pro-Fast HS c.
Pro-Fast SR c.
retrolenticular limb of internal c.
retrolenticular part of internal c.
retrolentiform limb of internal c.
Ritalin LA extended-release c.
sublenticular limb of internal c.
sublenticular part of internal c.
sublentiform limb of internal c.
suprasellar c.
Zonegran c.
zonisamide c.
capsulocaudate infarction
capsulolabral complex
capsuloputaminal infarction
capsuloputaminocaudate infarction
capsulotomy
gamma c.
captation
captious
captopril
capture
IgM antibody c.
caput, pl. **capita**
c. cornus
c. nuclei caudati
c. succedaneum
CARASIL
cerebral autosomal recessive arteriopathy with subcortical infarcts and leukoencephalopathy
carbachol
carbamazepine
carbamylation
carbamylcholine chloride
carbamyl phosphate synthetase deficiency
carbapenem
Carbatrol
carbenicillin disodium
Carbex
Carb-HD
Cal C.-H.
carbidopa
levodopa and c.
carbidopa-levodopa
Carbocaine with Neo-Cobefrin
carbocyanine dye
carbohydrate
c. metabolism
c. metabolism disorder
carbohydrate-deficient
c.-d. glycoprotein
c.-d. transferrin
carboline
beta c.
carbon
c. dioxide (CO_2)
c. dioxide arterial pressure
c. dioxide chemoreceptor
c. dioxide laser
c. monoxide poisoning
c. tetrachloride poisoning
carbonate
calcium c.
lithium c.
magnesium c.
carbonic
c. acid
c. anhydrase
c. anhydrase inhibitor
carboxyaminoimidazole (CAI)
carboxylase
acetyl coenzyme A c.
3-methylcrontyonyl-CoA c.
propionyl-CoA c.
pyruvate c.
sylaminoimidazole c.
carboxyl-terminal region
carboxypenicillin
carbromal
carcinoembryonic antigen (CEA)
carcinoma, pl. **carcinomata**
acinic cell c.
adenoid cystic c.
choroid plexus c.
embryonal cell c.
leptomeningeal c.
meningeal c.
neuroendocrine c. (NEC)
pancreatic c.
c. peripheral neuropathy
c. in situ
small cell c.
squamous cell c.

carcinomatosis
leptomeningeal c.
meningeal c.
carcinomatosum
coma c.
carcinomatous
c. encephalomyelopathy
c. meningitis
c. myelopathy
c. neuromyopathy
c. neuropathy
c. polyneuropathy
card
Boston Diagnostic Aphasia Exam-Cookie Theft C.
diary c.
Personnel Identification C. (PIC)
cardiac
c. arrhythmia
c. catheterization
c. embolism
c. function test
c. ganglion
c. gating
c. glycoside
c. monitoring
c. nerve
c. pacemaker artifact
c. plexus
c. rhythm
c. risk index
c. syncope
cardiaca
ganglia c.
cardiacus
plexus c.
cardinal direction of gaze
cardioaccelerating center
Cardiocap II pressure monitor
Cardio-Conray
cardioembolic stroke
cardiofacial syndrome
cardiogenic
c. embolism
c. shock
Cardiografin
cardioinhibitory center
Cardiolite
technetium-gagged C.
cardioneural
Cardiopulmonary Paragon 8500 bed
CardioSearch sensor
cardiospasm
CardioTec
cardiovascular control center
carditis
rheumatic c.
care
end-of-life c.
K+ C.
pattern of c.
postoperative c.
respite c.
standard c.
standard of c.
caregiver depression
CARE-MEDICO
carezza
carina, pl. **carinae**
c. fornicis
carinate abdomen
carinii
Litmosoides c.
Pneumocystis c.
C-arm
C-a. fluoroscopic apparatus
C-a. fluoroscopy
reversible C-a.
carmabis
carmine
indigo c.
carmustine (BiCNU)
carnitine
c. muscle metabolism
c. palmitoyltransferase
c. palmitoyltransferase deficiency
c. serum level
L-carnitine
Carnitor Injection
carnosinemia aminoaciduria
carotic
carotici
ramus sinus c.
caroticocavernous fistula
caroticojugular spine
caroticooculomotor membrane
caroticotympanic
c. artery
c. nerve
caroticotympanici
nervi c.

NOTES

caroticum
rete mirabile c.
carotid
aberrant c.
c. ablative procedure
c. Amytal procedure
c. angiogram
c. arteriography
c. artery
c. artery agenesis
c. artery aneurysm
c. artery angioplasty and stent placement
c. artery disease
c. artery dissection
c. artery occlusion (CAO)
c. artery sacrifice
c. artery stenosis
c. atherosclerosis
c. baroceptor stimulation
c. bifurcation
c. body
c. body transplant
c. body tumor
c. branch of glossopharyngeal nerve [CN IX]
c. bruit
Carotid Artery Stenosis with Asymptomatic Narrowing: Operation Versus Aspirin Study (CASANOVA)
c. cave aneurysm
c. circulation
c. content
distal c.
c. endarterectomy
c. ganglion
c. plaque hematoma
c. plexus
c. preservation
c. preservation technique
c. pulsation
c. rete
c. ring
c. sheath
c. sinus branch
c. sinus hypersensitivity
c. sinus massage
c. sinus nerve
c. sinus reflex
c. sinus syncope
c. sinus syndrome
c. vein
carotid-basilar anastomosis
carotid-cavernous sinus fistula
carotid-dural fistula
carotid-ophthalmic artery aneurysm
carotid-sinus hypersensitivity-induced syncope
carotid-vertebral
c.-v. anastomosis
c.-v. vein bypass graft
carotodynia, carotidynia
carpal tunnel syndrome (CTS)
Carpenter-Philappart syndrome
Carpenter syndrome
carpopedal
c. contraction
c. spasm
carpoptosia
carpoptosis
carposcope
carrageenan, carragheenin
carrier
Yasargil ligature c.
Carrow Auditory-Visual Abilities Test
Carr-Purcell-Meiboom-Gill sequence
Carr-Purcell sequence
Carter immobilization cushion
Cartesian coordinate representation
cartilage
c. cranioplasty
c. inflammation
c. plate
thyroid c.
Tutoplast costal c.
cartilaginis thyroideae
cartilaginous
c. end plate
c. tumor
caryochrome
caryothecae
cisterna c.
Casal necklace appearance in pellagra
CASANOVA
Carotid Artery Stenosis with Asymptomatic Narrowing: Operation Versus Aspirin Study
cascabel
cascade
arachidonic acid c.
central injury c.
coagulation c.
immediate early gene c.
ischemic c.
pathophysiological c.
case
c. control experimental study design
c. formulation
c. study
caseating granuloma
casein kinase Ie gene
caseness definition

caseous necrosis
Caspar
C. anterior cervical plate
C. anterior plate fixation
C. cervical retractor
C. cervical screw
C. craniotome
C. disk space spreader
C. drill
C. headholder
C. plating
C. retraction post
C. trapezoidal plate
caspase-activated DNAse
caspase-independent mechanism
caspase inhibitor
CASS
computer-assisted stereotactic surgery
CASS digital read-out floorstand
CASS TrueTaper collimator
CASS whole-brain mapping system
cassava plant tropical myeloneuropathy
cast
endocranial c.
hinged c.
Risser-Cotrel body c.
Castellani-Low sign
Castleman disease
Castroviejo eye suture forceps
CAT
chloramphenicol acetyl transferase
computed axial tomography
CAT scan
CAT scanning
catabolic pathway
cataclysm
cataclysmic headache
catalepsy
cataleptic attack
cataleptoid, cataleptiform
catamenial
c. epilepsy
c. migraine
c. migraine headache
c. seizure
c. seizure pattern
cataphasia
cataphora
cataplectic
cataplecticus
status c.
cataplexy, cataplexis
Catapres
cataract-oligophrenia syndrome
catastrophic
c. effect
c. event
c. migraine
catathymic
catatonia protracta
catatonic
c. motor behavior
c. patient
c. rigidity
c. stupor
catchment
CAT/CLAMS
Clinical Adaptive Test/Clinical Linguistic and Auditory Milestone Scale
catecholamine
peripheral c.
c. receptor
catecholamine-induced
c.-i. change
c.-i. thermogenesis
catecholaminergic
c. nucleus
c. pathway
catechol-*O*-methyltransferase (COMT)
catechol-*O*-methyltransferase inhibitor
catechol-methyl-transferase inhibitor
categorization
symptom c.
category
arousal c.
diagnostic c.
disorder c.
dysphoric c.
early-onset c.
c. fluency test
Functional Ambulation C. (FAC)
late-onset c.
somatic c.
c. specific semantic impairment
category-specific naming
catelectrotonic state
catelectrotonus
cathepsin B, G
catheter
Abramson c.
Accu-Flo ventricular c.
afterloading c.

C

NOTES

catheter *(continued)*
angiographic c.
Argyll trocar c.
balloon c.
Berenstein guiding c.
BPS spinal angiographic c.
Camino intracranial c.
Camino transducer c.
cisterna magna c.
Codman ventricular silicone c.
c. coil
Cook mini-compression balloon c.
Cordis Brite Tip guiding c.
cup c.
delivery c.
distal c.
double-lumen Swan-Ganz c.
dummy seed c.
Ekos ultrasound c.
Endeavor nondetachable silicone balloon c.
Envoy guide c.
ePTFE ventricular shunt c.
Fasguide c.
FasTracker-18 infusion c.
Fogarty embolectomy c.
Heplock c.
Hickman c.
Hinck c.
ICP c.
ICP-T fiberoptic ICP intracranial temperature c.
ICP-T fiberoptic ICP monitoring c.
intracranial pressure c.
intraventricular c.
ITC radiopaque balloon c.
Lapras c.
lumbar c.
micro-Soft Stream sidehole infusion c.
Micro-Vac suction c.
Mikaelsson c.
monorail aspiration c.
MTC Ventcontrol ventricular c.
1505 NDSB occlusion balloon c.
nondetachable silicone balloon c.
peripherally inserted central c. (PICC)
peritoneal c.
Phoenix Anti-Blok ventricular c.
polyethylene intravenous c.
Portnoy ventricular c.
Prowler Plus c.
Pudenz ventricular c.
Racz Tun-L-Kath c.
Raimondi peritoneal c.
Raimondi spring c.
Raimondi ventricular c.
Rapid Transit c.
rheolytic c.
Scott silicone ventricular c.
Shaw c.
Shiley c.
Silastic c.
Simmons c.
Simpson c.
Soaker c.
spinal c.
Swan-Ganz c.
thin-wall introducer c.
toposcopic c.
Tracker-10 c.
Tracker-18 c.
Tracker infusion c.
transducer-tipped c.
transfemoral c.
Tun-L-Kath epidural c.
tunnelable ventricular ICP c.
Turbo Tracker c.
USCF II diagnostic c.
ventriculostomy c.
Ventrix SD fiberoptic subdural ICP c.

catheter-induced subclavian vein thrombosis

catheterization
cardiac c.
superselective c.

catheter/pump
DuPen c.

catochus

catscratch
c. disease (CSD)
c. fever

cat's eye amaurosis

cauda, pl. **caudae**
c. equina
c. equina avulsion
c. equina compression
c. equina incarceration
c. equina syndrome
c. fasciae dentatae
c. nuclei caudati
c. striati

caudal
c. canal
c. cerebellar peduncle (CCP)
c. colliculus
c. colliculus commissure
c. hook
c. lamina resection
c. neuropore
c. olivary nucleus
c. peduncle of thalamus

c. pontine reticular nucleus
c. regression syndrome
c. to rostral
c. stroke
c. transtentorial herniation
caudales
nuclei olivares c.
caudalis
brachium colliculi c.
colliculus c.
hilum nuclei olivaris c.
lobulus semilunaris c.
nuclei colliculi c.
nucleus reticularis pontis c.
nucleus tegmenti pontis c.
nucleus vestibularis c.
pars c.
pedunculus cerebellaris c.
subnucleus c.
caudate
c. cell
dorsolateral c.
c. nucleus
postinduction c.
c. tissue
c. volume
caudati
caput nuclei c.
cauda nuclei c.
corpus nuclei c.
rami caudae nuclei c.
venae nuclei c.
caudatolenticular
caudatum
caudatus
colliculus c.
nucleus c.
caudolenticulares
pontes grisei c.
caudolenticular gray bridge
caumesthesia
causal-attributional theory
causalgia
causalgic pain
causality
phenomenalistic c.
reverse c.
causal mechanism
causative
c. mechanism
c. organism
cause
contextual c.
neurobiological c.
cauterizer
Bucholz bipolar c.
cautery
Aesculap bipolar c.
BICAP c.
bipolar c.
Concept hand-held c.
c. hook
Mira c.
monopolar c.
right-angle bipolar c.
suction c.
cava
inferior vena c.
Cavalieri direct estimator method
cave
Meckel c.
septum pellucidum c.
trigeminal c.
cavernoma
cavernoma-related epilepsy
cavernosa
corpora c.
cavernosal nerve
cavernosus
sinus c.
cavernous
c. angioma
c. carotid aneurysm
c. hemangioma
c. malformation (CM)
c. nerve
c. plexus
c. sinus
c. sinus aneurysm
c. sinus fistula
c. sinus lesion
c. sinus meningioma
c. sinus syndrome
c. sinus thrombophlebitis
c. sinus thrombosis
c. sinus tumor
cavitas
c. epiduralis
c. septi pellucidi
c. subarachnoidea
c. subarachoidealis
c. trigeminalis

NOTES

Cavitron
C. dissector
C. laser
C. Ultrasonic Surgical Aspirator (CUSA)
cavity
epidural c.
head c.
nasal c.
oral c.
c. of septum pellucidum
sinonasal c.
subarachnoid c.
subdural c.
syringomyelic c.
syrinx c.
trigeminal c.
tympanic c.
cavum
c. epidurale
c. meckelii
c. psalterii
c. septi pellucidi
c. septum pellucidum
c. subarachnoideum
c. subdurale
c. trigeminale
c. veli interpositi
c. vergae
Cawthorne-Cooksey vestibular exercise
Cayler syndrome
CBC
complete blood count
CBF
cerebral blood flow
C. reduction
C. study
CBI
closed brain injury
C. stereotactic head holder
CBV
cerebral blood volume
C1-C2
C.-C. cable fixation
C.-C. posterior arthrodesis
CCA
chimpanzee coryza agent
common carotid artery
CCA clamp
C_2-ceramide
CCI
chronic constrictive injury
CCK
cholecystokinin
CCK-4
cholecystokinin tetrapeptide
CCK-8
cholecystokinin octapeptide
CCNU
lomustine
CCP
caudal cerebellar peduncle
CCSEQ
Community College Student Experiences Questionnaire
CCTV-EEG
continuous video-EEG monitoring
CD
CD Horizon Sextant percutaneous screw-rod system
Metadate CD
CD track
C-D
Cotrel-Dubousset
C-D instrumentation
C-D instrumentation device
C-D instrumentation fixation strength
C-D instrumentation rigidity
C-D rod insertion
C-D screw modification
CD4
CD4 cell
CD4 lymphocyte
CD95
cluster of differentiation 95
CD29+ memory cell
CD34 staining
CD44 antigen
CD4+CD45RA+ cell
CD4/CD8 ratio
CDK2NA gene
cDNA
complementary deoxyribonucleic acid
CDR
Clinical Dementia Rating
C. Scale
CEA
carcinoembryonic antigen
CEA-Tc 99m
cebocephaly
cecocentral scotoma
CED
chondroectodermal dysplasia
CEEB
Center for Ecology, Evolution and Behavior
cefalothin sodium
cefepime
cefuroxime
CEI
continuous extravascular infusion
converting enzyme inhibitor

Celexa
celiac
c. ganglion
c. nerve
c. plexus
celiaca
ganglia c.
celiacus
plexus nervosus c.
cell
0-2A c.
adenohypophyseal c.
c. adhesion molecule (CAM)
adrenal chromaffin c.
agger nasi c.
air c.
Alzheimer c.
amacrine c.
ameboid c.
anterior horn c.
Antoni A, B c.
apolar c.
APUD c.
arachnoid c.
astroglia c.
auditory receptor c.
B c.
basket c.
Bergmann glial c.
Betz c.
Bevan-Lewis c.
36B10 glioma c.
bipolar retinal c.
blob c.
blood c.
bone marrow stromal c.
border c.
Böttcher c.
bovine chromaffin c.
BrDu immunoactive c.
BrDu immunolabeling c.
BrDu-positive c.
bursting c.
Cajal horizontal c.
Cajal-Retzius c.
capsule c.
CA3 pyramidal c.
caudate c.
CD4 c.
CD4+CD45RA+ c.
CD29+ memory c.
cerebellar granular c.
cerebellar granule c.
chandelier c.
chief c.
chromaffin c.
Clarke c.
cochlear hair c.
color-opponent c.
column c.
commissural c.
compound granule c.
Corti c.
corticotroph c.
cuboidal c.
c. cycle
dark c.
c. death
Deiters c.
c. division
Dogiel c.
dorsal horn c.
dorsal root ganglion c.
down-gaze paralysis, ataxia/athetosis and foam c. (DAF syndrome)
effector c.
ependymal c.
epithelioid c.
erisynaptic glial c.
ethmoid air c.
excitable c.
external pillar c.
Fañanás c.
fatty granule c.
foam c.
forebrain c.
ganglion c.
gemästete c.
gemistocytic c.
giant Dopamine-containing c. (GDC)
giant pyramidal Betz c.
Gierke c.
gitter c.
glial c.
glitter c.
globoid c.
globose c.
Golgi epithelial c.
gonadotroph c.
grandmother c.
granule c.

NOTES

cell *(continued)*
gustatory c.
gyrochrome c.
hair c.
hamster c.
hecatomeral c.
hemosiderin-laden c.
Hensen c.
heteromeric c.
hilar c.
HNK c.
horn c.
Hortega c.
human adult bone marrow mesenchymal stem c. (hMSCs)
human brain microvascular endothelial c. (HBMEC)
human neonatal kidney c.
human Purkinje c.
hypothalamic pacemaker c.
internal pillar c.
interstitial c.
intracarotid marrow c.
karyochrome c.
lactotroph c.
Langerhans c.
large polymorphic ganglion c.
Leydig tumor c.
c. line
lipid-laden stromal c.
c. loss
lupus erythematosus c.
lymphokine-activated killer c.
macroglia c.
macrophage-derived c.
mammalian c.
Martinotti c.
mastoid air c.
Mauthner c.
MBP-reactive T c.
c. membrane lipid
meningothelial arachnoid c.
Merkel tactile c.
mesoglial c.
Meynert solitary c.
microglia c.
midget bipolar c.
migratory c.
mitral c.
mononuclear c. (MNC)
mossy c.
motor c.
Müller radial c.
multipolar c.
multipotential c.
myelin-producing c.
myxomatous c.
Nageotte c.
natural killer c.
c. necrosis
nerve c.
neural crest c.
neural hamster c.
neural progenitor c.
neural stem c.
neural tube floor plate c.
neurilemma c.
neuroendocrine transducer c.
neuroepithelial c.
neuroglia c.
neurolemmal sheath c.
neuroprogenitor c.
neurosecretory c.
nigral TH-positve c.
non-neural c.
NT2 c.
olfactory receptor c.
olfactory sheathing c.
oligodendrocyte-like c. (OLC)
oligodendrocyte lineage c.
oligodendroglia c.
Opalski c.
parafollicular c.
PC12 c.
periglomerular c.
peripheral blood mononuclear c. (PBMC)
perivascular mononuclear c.
phalangeal c.
physaliphorous c.
pia-arachnoid c.
Pick c.
pillar c.
pineal c.
porcine dopaminergic c.
primary neuronal c.
c. processing
progenitor c.
c. proliferation
proliferative malignant glial c.
pseudounipolar ganglion c.
Purkinje c.
PV positive c.
pyramidal c.
radial glial c.
reactive c.
Renshaw c.
resting T c.
retinal ganglion c. (RGC)
Rolando c.
Sala c.
satellite c.
C. Saver
Schaffer collateral c.

Schultze c.
Schwann c.
sensory c.
Sertoli c.
SK-N-SH c.
small intensely fluorescent c.
somatotroph c.
S phase c.
spider c.
spindle c.
stem serotonergic c.
c. survival
SV40 tumor antigen immortalized c.
syncytiotrophoblastic giant c. (STGC)
T c.
tactile c.
taste c.
tau-negative nerve c.
tautomeral c.
thymic myoid c.
thyrotroph c.
touch c.
transducer c.
tuberous sclerosis monster c.
tufted c.
TUNEL-positive c.
tunnel c.
unipolar c.
vector-producing c. (VPC)
ventral mesencephalic dopaminergic c.
vestibular hair c.
visual receptor c.
VZV-specific T c.
wandering c.
white blood c. (WBC)
xenogeneic chromaffin c.

cella, pl. **cellae**
c. media
Rohon-Beard c.

cell-mediated immunity

cell-permeable

cellular
c. brain edema
c. immune function
c. ion homeostasis
c. kinetics
c. layers of cortex
c. macromolecule
c. organelle
c. prion protein (PrP^c)
c. respiratory function
c. store
c. system
c. therapy

cellulosa
vagina c.

cellulose
c. acetate polymer
oxidized regenerated c.

Celontin

CEM
C. handswitching nosecone

cement
BoneSource hydroxyapatite c.

CE MRA
contrast echocardiography magnetic resonance angiography

cenesthesia, coenesthesia

cenesthesic, cenesthetic

Cenestin

Cenolate

center
accelerating c.
Alzheimer Disease C. (ADC)
Alzheimer Disease Research C. (ADRC)
anospinal c.
apneustic c.
Association of Sleep Disorder C.
auditory word c.
Broca c.
Budge c.
cardioaccelerating c.
cardioinhibitory c.
cardiovascular control c.
ciliospinal c.
communal residential c.
coughing c.
defecation c.
deglutition c.
C. for Ecology, Evolution and Behavior (CEEB)
ejaculatory c.
eupraxic c.
expiratory c.
feeding c.
gaze pontine c.
genital c.
genitospinal c.

center *(continued)*
glossokinesthetic c.
heat-regulating c.
higher c.
imprinting c. (IC)
inspiratory c.
Kronecker c.
Lumsden c.
medullary c.
micturition c.
Minnesota Regional Sleep Disorders C.
motor speech c.
nerve c.
panting c.
pneumotaxic c.
polypneic c.
pontine lateral gaze c.
regulatory c.
respiratory c.
retrovesical c.
satiety c.
semioval c.
sensory speech c.
sex-behavior c.
sleep-generating c.
speech c.
sudorific c.
swallowing c.
sweat c.
thermoregulatory c.
thirst c.
UCLA Brain Mapping C.
vasoconstrictor c.
vasodilator c.
vasomotor c.
vesical c.
vesicospinal c.
vital c.
vomiting c.
Wernicke c.

centra (*pl. of* centrum)

central
c. alexia
c. alveolar hypoventilation syndrome
c. amaurosis
c. amygdaloid nucleus
c. anticholinergic syndrome
c. anticholinergic toxicity
c. auditory pathway
c. benzodiazepine receptor
c. canal
c. caudate nucleus
c. cerebral sulcus
c. chemosensitivity
c. cholinergic system
c. chromatolysis
c. cord injury syndrome
c. core disease
c. dazzle
c. deafness
c. direct current bright spot
c. dopamine content
c. dopaminergic antagonism
C. European encephalitis
C. European tick-borne encephalitis virus
C. European tick-borne fever
c. excitatory state
c. facial paresis
c. ganglioneuroma
c. gelatinous substance of spinal cord
c. gray
c. gray matter region
c. gray substance
c. gyrus
c. hypoventilation syndrome
c. inflammatory demyelination
c. injury cascade
c. and lateral intermediate substance
c. lateral nucleus of thalamus
c. lesion
c. lobule
c. lobule of cerebellum
c. lobule wing
c. nervous system (CNS)
c. nervous system abnormality
c. nervous system hemorrhage
c. nervous system hypersomnolence
c. nervous system influenza virus infection
c. nervous system leukemia
c. nervous system lymphoma
c. nervous system malformation
c. nervous system myelination
c. nervous system nocardiosis (CNS nocardiosis)
c. nervous system stimulant, nonamphetamine
c. nervous system tumor
c. neuritis
c. neurocytoma
c. nystagmus
c. paralysis
c. paraphasia
c. part of lateral ventricle
c. peduncle of thalamus
c. pontine myelinolysis
c. post-stroke pain
c. respiratory chemoreception
c. respiratory neuron

c. retinal fovea
c. role
c. sacral line
c. sensitization
c. sensory loss
c. sleep apnea syndrome
c. somatosensory conduction time
c. sulcus of insula
c. tegmental fasciculus
c. tegmental tract
c. thalamic radiation
c. timing process
c. transactional core
c. transtentorial herniation
c. type neurofibromatosis
c. venous channel
c. venous pressure
c. vertigo
c. vestibular system
c. vision acuity

centrale
systema nervosum c.

centralis
ala lobuli c.
ala lobulis c.
amaurosis c.
area c.
nucleus amygdalae c.
nucleus caudalis c.
nucleus cuneatus pars c.
pars inferior alae lobuli c.
pars superior ali lobuli c.
radiatio thalami c.
substantia gelatinosa c.
substantia grisea c.
substantia intermedia c.
sulcus c.
tractus tegmentalis c.

centralization phenomenon
Centrax
centre médian de Luys
centrencephalic
c. epilepsy
c. integrating system

centrencephalon
centrifugal
c. current
c. nerve

centripetal
c. current
c. nerve
c. spread

centroblastic B-cell lymphoma
centrocecal visual field
centrofacial lentiginosis
centrokinesia
centrokinetic
centromedian thalamic nucleus
centromedianus
nucleus c.

centronuclear myopathy
centrophose
centrotemporal
c. paroxysmal focus
c. sharp wave

centrotemporoparietal lesion
centrum, pl. **centra**
c. medianum
c. medullare
c. ovale
c. semiovale
Vieussens c.

cephalad
cephalalgia, cephalgia
benign coital c.
histamine c.
histaminic c.
Horton histamine c.
pharyngotympanic c.

cephalea
c. agitata
c. attonita
epileptic c.

cephaledema
cephalemia
cephalexin
cephalgia (*var. of* cephalalgia)
cephalgic attack
cephalhematocele
Stromeyer c.

cephalhematoma (*var. of* cephalohematoma)
cephalhydrocele traumatica
cephalic
c. angle
c. flexure
c. tetanus

cephalitis
cephalocele
orbital c.

cephalocentesis

NOTES

cephalochordate
cephalocranial disproportion
cephalodynia
cephalogyric
cephalohematocele
cephalohematoma, cephalhematoma
c. deformans
cephalohemometer
cephalomedullary angle
cephalomeningitis
cephalometer
Bertillon c.
cephalometric
c. analysis
c. angle
c. measurement
cephalometrography
cephalomotor
cephalooculocutaneous telangiectasia
cephalopalpebral reflex
cephalopathy
cephaloplegia
cephalopolysyndactyly
Greig c.
cephaloridine
cephalorrhachidian index
cephalosporin
fourth-generation c.
third-generation c.
cephalosporin-resistant *Staphylococcus pneumoniae*
cephalostat
cephalothin
cephalotrigeminal angiomatosis
cephapirin
cephradine
ceptor
chemical c.
contact c.
distance c.
ceramic vertebral spacer
ceramidase
ceramide
c. dihexoside
c. trihexoside
trihexosyl c.
ceramidosis
Ceratite ceramic implant
Ceraxon
c-erbB-2-encoded oncoprotein
cercopithecoid
cerea flexibilitas
cerebella (*pl. of* cerebellum)
cerebellae
ramus tonsillae c.
cerebellar
c. abscess
c. activation
c. aggregation culture
c. aggregation culture for teratogenicity testing
anterior inferior c.
c. aplasia
c. apoplexy
c. arachnoid cyst
c. artery
c. artery infarction
c. astrocytoma
c. ataxia
c. attachment
c. cerebral palsy
c. cognitive affective syndrome
c. cortex
c. cortical degeneration
c. degeneration paraneoplastic
c. dysmetria
c. ectopia
c. encephalitis
c. ependymoma
c. fit
c. fit seizure
c. folium
c. fossa
c. frenulum
c. gait
c. gliosarcoma
c. granular cell
c. granule cell
c. granule neuron
c. hematoma
c. hemisphere
c. hemisphere syndrome
c. hemorrhage
c. hemorrhage syndrome
c. hypoperfusion
c. hypoplasia
c. malaria
c. mass
c. metabolism
c. mutism
c. nucleus
c. nystagmus
c. pathway
c. peduncle
c. pressure cone
c. pyramid
c. region
c. retraction
c. retractor
c. rigidity
c. speech
c. sulcus
c. tentorium
c. tonsil

c. decortication
c. degenerative disorder
c. diataxia
c. digital angiogram
c. disease
c. dominance
c. dyschromatopsia
c. dysfunction
c. dysgenesis
c. dysplasia
c. dysrhythmia
c. edema
c. embolus
c. fissure
c. flexure
c. fluid marker
c. foreign body embolization
c. formed-element embolism
c. gaze paresis
c. gigantism
c. glioblastoma
c. glioma
c. gumma
c. gyrus
c. hemianesthesia
c. hemicorticectomy
c. hemidecortication
c. hemisphere
c. hemodynamic
c. hemodynamics and oxygenation
c. hemorrhage
c. hemosiderosis
c. hernia
c. herniation
c. hydatid
c. hyperesthesia
c. hypertension
c. hypoperfusion
c. hypoxia
c. impairment
c. infection
c. intermittent claudication
c. ischemia
c. ischemia steal
c. laceration
c. lacuna
c. layer of retina
c. lesion
c. lipidosis
c. lobe
c. localization
c. lymphoma
c. malaria
c. mantle
c. mapping of apraxia
c. metabolic rate
c. metabolic rate of glucose (CMRglc)
c. metabolic rate of oxygen ($CMRO_2$)
c. metastasis
c. microembolism
c. nerve
c. neuroblastoma
c. nocardiosis
c. palsy
c. palsy infant stimulation program
c. peduncle
c. perfusion
c. perfusion pressure
c. poliodystrophy
c. poliomyelitis
c. porosis
c. potential
c. pressure autoregulation
progressive c.
c. protection
c. protective therapy
c. ptosis
c. radiation necrosis
c. region
c. revascularization
c. salt wasting
c. salt wasting syndrome
c. sclerosis
c. sensory input
c. sinus
c. sphingolipidosis
c. stalk
c. steal syndrome
c. sulcus
c. tetanus
c. toxoplasmosis
c. tremor
c. trigone
c. tuberculosis
c. vasodilating agent
c. vasoreactivity
c. vasospasm
c. vein
c. vein angioma
c. vein thrombosis

NOTES

cerebral *(continued)*
c. venous malformation (CVM)
c. venous thrombosis
c. ventricle
c. ventriculography
c. vertigo
c. vesicle
c. vomiting

cerebrale
tache c.
trigonum c.

cerebrales
sulci c.
sulci c.

cerebralgia

cerebralia
juga c.

cerebralis
adiposis c.
cortex c.
mycetism c.
pedunculus c.

cerebration

cerebri
aditus ad aqueductum c.
anus c.
apertura aqueductus c.
apophysis c.
aqueductus c.
astrocytosis c.
basis pedunculi c.
circulus arteriosus c.
cisterna fossae lateralis c.
cisterna venae magnae c.
commissura magna c.
commissura posterior c.
commotio c.
contusio c.
cortex c.
crus c.
epiphysis c.
facies inferior hemispherii c.
facies medialis et inferior hemispherii c.
facies medialis hemispherii c.
facies superolateralis hemispherii c.
falx c.
familial gliomatosis c.
fibrae arcuatae c.
fissura longitudinalis c.
fissura transversa c.
formatio reticularis pedunculi c.
fossa lateralis c.
fungus c.
glioblastosis c.
gliomatosis c.
gyri c.
gyrus transitivi c.
hemiseptum c.
hemispherium c.
hypophysis c.
labium c.
lacuna c.
lamina molecularis corticis c.
lamina plexiformis corticis c.
lamina terminalis c.
lobi c.
lobus frontalis c.
lobus occipitalis c.
lobus parietalis c.
margo inferior c.
margo inferolateralis hemispherii c.
margo inferomedialis hemispherii c.
margo medialis c.
margo superomedialis c.
medial sulcus of crus c.
membrana c.
pars anterior pedunculi c.
pars dorsalis pedunculi c.
pars ventralis pedunculi c.
pedunculus c.
poliodystrophia c.
polus frontalis hemispherii c.
polus occipitalis hemispherii c.
polus temporalis c.
pseudomotor c.
pseudotumor c.
ramus anterior sulci lateralis c.
ramus ascendens sulci lateralis c.
ramus posterior sulci lateralis c.
sulci interlobares c.
sulcus centralis c.
sulcus lateralis pedunculi c.
sulcus lunatus c.
sulcus medialis cruris c.
tutamina c.
unguis ventriculi lateralis c.
venae anteriores c.
venae inferiores c.
venae internae c.
venae profundae c.
venae superficiales c.
venae superiores c.
vena magna c.
vena media profunda c.
vena media superficialis c.
ventriculus dexter c.
ventriculus lateralis c.
ventriculus quartus c.
ventriculus sinister c.
ventriculus tertius c.
zero cerebral pseudotumor c.

cerebrifugal

cerebripetal

cerebritis
lupus c.
suppurative c.
cerebroatrophic hyperammonemia
cerebrocerebellar projection
cerebrocortical nerve terminal
cerebrofaciothoracic dysplasia syndrome
Cerebrograph 10a
cerebrohepatorenal syndrome
cerebrology
cerebroma
cerebromacular
c. degeneration
c. dystrophy
cerebromalacia
cerebromedullary cistern
cerebromeningeal
cerebromeningitis
cerebropathia psychica toxemia
cerebropathy
cerebrophysiology
cerebropontile
cerebroretinal
c. angiomatosis
c. degeneration
cerebrosclerosis
cerebroside
c. lipidosis
c. lipoidosis
c. reticulocytosis
c. sulfatase
cerebrosidosis
cerebrosis
cerebrospinal
c. axis
c. fever
c. fluid (CSF)
c. fluid absorption
c. fluid calcium
c. fluid ferritin level
c. fluid fistula
c. fluid formation
c. fluid glucose
c. fluid lactic acid
c. fluid leak
c. fluid leakage
c. fluid leukocyte
c. fluid otorrhea
c. fluid pathway
c. fluid pleocytosis
c. fluid pressure
c. fluid protein
c. fluid rhinorrhea
c. fluid shunt
c. fluid volume
c. index
c. meningitis
c. syphilis
c. system
cerebrospinalis
liquor c.
cerebrospinant
cerebrostomy
cerebrotendinous
c. cholesterolosis
c. xanthomatosis
cerebrotomy
CEREBROTRAC 2500
cerebrovascular
c. accident (CVA)
c. accident dementia
c. amyloidosis
c. aneurysm
c. angiography
c. angioma
c. aphasia
c. arterial dissection
c. arterial thrombosis
c. computed tomography
c. disease
c. embolism
c. embryonic development
c. hemorrhage
c. infarction
c. ischemia
c. lesion
c. magnetic resonance imaging
c. malformation
c. morphology
c. neurosyphilis
c. pathology
c. regulation
c. syndrome
c. ulceration
c. venous thrombosis
cerebrovasculosa
area c.
cerebrovasospasm
cerebrum, pl. **cerebra**
anterior ramus of lateral sulcus of c.
aqueduct c.

NOTES

cerebrum *(continued)*
arcuate fiber of c.
arterial circle of c.
ascending ramus of lateral sulcus of c.
cistern of great vein of c.
cistern of lateral fossa of c.
frontal lobe of c.
great transverse fissure of c.
gyri of c.
lamina terminalis of c.
lobe of c.
longitudinal fissure of c.
occipital lobe of c.
occipital pole of c.
parietal lobe of c.
superolateral surface of c.
temporal pole of c.
transverse fissure of c.
Cerebyx
Cereport
Ceresine
CERESPECT brain imager
Cerestat
Ceretec imaging kit
cerium
cerivastatin
ceroid lipofuscinosis
cerulean
locus c.
ceruleus
nucleus c.
perilocus c.
ceruloplasmin
c. deficiency
serum c.
c. serum level
ceruminoma
cerveau isolé
cervical
c. aortic knuckle
c. arthrodesis
c. carotid bifurcation
Cloward double-hinge c.
c. collar
c. compression syndrome
c. cord lesion
c. corpectomy
c. decompression surgery
c. discectomy
c. disk excision
c. disk herniation
c. disk syndrome
c. dystonia
c. enlargement
c. enlargement of spinal cord
c. fibrositis
c. flexure
c. fusion syndrome
hypertrophic c.
c. immobilization device (CID)
c. intersegmental vein
c. interspace
c. intramedullary tumor
c. muscle spasm
c. myelography
c. myospasm
c. nerve
c. nerve root injury
c. neural foramen
c. nucleus
c. part of spinal cord
c. perivascular sympathectomy
c. plate
c. plexus
c. radiculopathy
c. rib and band syndrome
c. root distribution
c. screw insertion technique
c. segments of spinal cord [C1–C8]
c. spinal stenosis
c. spine
c. spine arthritis
c. spine atlantoaxial instability
c. spine basilar impression
c. spine decompression
c. spine injury
c. spine internal fixation
c. spine kyphotic deformity
c. spine laminectomy
c. spine posterior fusion
c. spine posterior ligament disruption
c. spine rheumatoid disease
c. spine screw-plate fixation
c. spine stabilization
c. spine stabilization procedure
c. spine trauma
c. spondylosis
c. spondylosis without myelopathy
c. spondylotic myelopathy
c. spondylotic myelopathy fusion technique
c. spondylotic myelopathy vertebrectomy
c. steroid epidural nerve block
c. subluxation
c. sympathetic chain location
c. syringomyelia
c. tension myositis
c. tension syndrome
c. vertebra

c. vertigo
c. vessel compression
cervicales
nervi c.
cervicalia
segmenta c. 1–8
segmentum medullae spinalis c.
cervicalis
ansa c.
descendens c.
inferior root of ansa c.
intumescentia c.
nervus transversus c.
plexus c.
posterior root of ansa c.
radix anterior ansae c.
radix inferior ansae c.
radix posterior ansae c.
radix superior ansae c.
ramus lateralis rami posterioris nervi c.
ramus medialis rami posterioris nervi c.
ramus thyrohyoideus ansae c.
root of ansa c.
superior limb of ansa c.
superior root of ansa c.
cervicalium
rami anteriores nervorum c.
rami dorsales nervorum c.
rami posteriores nervorum c.
rami ventrales nervorum c.
cervices (*pl. of* cervix)
cervicis
descendens c.
c. muscle
splenius c.
cervicobrachialgia
cervicobrachial syndrome
cervicocephalic arterial dissection
cervicocollic reflex
cervicodynia
cervicogenic headache
cervicolumbar phenomenon
cervicomedullary
c. deformity
c. junction
c. junction compression
c. kink
c. tumor
cervicooccipital fusion
cervicothoracic
c. ganglion
c. junction
c. junction stabilization
c. junction surgery
c. orthosis
c. pedicle anatomy
c. pedicle angle
cervicothoracicum
ganglion c.
cervix, pl. **cervices**
c. of the axon
c. columnae posterioris
c. cornus dorsalis medullae spinalis
c. cornus posterioris medullae spinalis
cesium fluoride scintillation detector
Cestan-Chenais syndrome
Cestan-Raymond syndrome
Cestan syndrome
cesticidal
cestode infection
ceylanicum
Ancylostoma c.
CF
climbing fiber
C-factor
CFE
chronic focal encephalitis
CFI
"cut-flow" index
C-fiber
C.-f. nociceptor
C.-f. reflex
C-fiber evoked response
c-fos gene
7C Gold test
CGRP
calcitonin gene-related peptide
CH
cluster headache
crown-heel length
CH50 assay
Chaddock
C. reflex
C. sign
Chaetomium atrobrunneum
Chagas disease
chain
c. behavior
electron transport c.

C

NOTES

chain *(continued)*
human neurofilament light c.
immunoglobulin kappa light c.
kappa light c.
lambda light c.
nuclear c.
oligosaccharide c.
c. reflex
respiratory c.
Sno-Traks wheelchair c.
sympathetic c.
variable heavy c. (VH)

chair
Bárány c.
Combisit surgeon's c.

chamber
anechoic c.
drip c.
flush c.
Monoplace hyperbaric c.
Multiplace c.
Sechrist monoplace hyperbaric c.

Chamberlain palatooccipital line

chameleon tongue

chamomile
German c.

champagne-bottle leg

Champion Trauma Score

Chance fracture

chancre
hard c.

chandelier cell

change
C. Abilitator
abulic mental c.
age-related brain c.
age-related pharmacodynamic c.
age-related pharmacokinetic c.
astrocytic c.
baseline-to-endpoint c.
binocular acuity c.
biochemical c.
blood flow c.
catecholamine-induced c.
chronic c.
circadian rhythm c.
circumscribed c.
Clinical Global Impression of C.
Clinician's Interview-Based Impression of C.
cognitive c.
Crooke hyaline c.
deep white matter hyperintensity c.
degenerative discogenic vertebral c.
degenerative spine c.
electrical c.
electrolyte c.
electrophysiologic c.
c. in energy
Fairbanks c.
Frisén-grade c.
global c.
hormonal c.
hyperintensity c.
interictal behavior c.
Interview Based Impression of C.
intrapsychic c.
maturational c.
mental status c.
metabolic c.
methylphenidate-induced c.
morphologic c.
negative c.
neurochemical c.
neuropeptide c.
newly emergent categorical c.
nutritional c.
onion bulb c.
pathological c.
perivascular c.
personality c.
polyneuropathy, organomegaly, endocrinopathy, monoclonal gammopathy, skin c.'s (POEMS)
polyneuropathy, organomegaly, endocrinopathy, myeloma, and skin c.
pressure-gradient c.
reflex c.
c. in sleep pattern
stoichiometric c.
structural c.
subjective mood c.
telangiectatic c.
trophic c.
vascular c.
vasomotor c.
visual c.
white matter c.

channel
adenosine triphosphate-dependent potassium c.
axolemmal ion c.
blob c.
central venous c.
chloride c.
glutamate-gated NMDA receptor c.
grasp c.
ion c.
ligand-gated ion c.
L-type calcium c.
membrane ion c.
potassium c.
PQ calcium c.

transmitter-gated ion c.
T-type calcium c.
voltage-gated calcium c. (VGCC)
voltage-gated potassium c.
voltage-gated sodium c.
voltage-regulated calcium c.
20-channel Beckman EEG instrument
37-channel biomagnetometer
channelopathy
epileptogenic c.
4-channel Transcranial Doppler monitor
8-channel whole-head magnetometer
Chapman Scale
characteristic
clinical c.
comorbid c.
core c.
demographic c.
electrical c.
environment c.
c. manifestation
neuropsychologic c.
objective trauma c.
c. pattern of motivation
phenomenological c.
predictive c.
receiver operating c. (ROC)
signal-noise c.
temporal c.
trait c.
trauma c.
CharcoAid
Charcocaps
Charcot
C. artery
C. arthropathy
C. disease
C. gait
C. joint
C. sign
C. triad
C. vertigo
Charcot-Bouchard intracerebral aneurysm
Charcot-Marie syndrome
Charcot-Marie-Tooth
C.-M.-T. atrophy
C.-M.-T. disease
C.-M.-T. disease type 1, 2
Charcot-Weiss-Baker syndrome
CHARGE
coloboma, heart disease, atresia choanae, retarded growth, genital anomalies, ear anomalies
CHARGE syndrome
charged particle radiosurgery
charger
KM universal battery c.
Charité disk prosthesis
Charles Bonnet syndrome
Charlevoix-Saguenay syndrome
charley horse
Charlin syndrome
Charnley suction drain
chasing spike
Chaslin gliosis
Chassaignac tubercle
Chatillon dolorimeter
Chaussier line
Chealamide
checkerboard field
Checklist-90
Symptom C.
Chediak-Higashi syndrome
cheek phenomenon
cheese reaction headache
cheilophagia
cheiloschisis
cheiralgia paresthetica
cheirobrachialgia, chirobrachialgia
cheirognostic
cheirokinesthesia, chirokinesthesia
cheirokinesthetic
cheirospasm, chirospasm
chelation therapy
chemical
c. aseptic meningitis
atomic, biologic, c. (ABC)
c. ceptor
c. denervation
c. hemostasis
c. injury
c. neurolysis
psychoactive c.
c. rhizotomy
c. shift
c. shift anisotrophy
c. shift artifact
c. signaling
c. sympathectomy
chemically-induced seizure

C

NOTES

chemical-mechanical transduction
chemical-shift imaging
chemiluminescence
chemoattractant
  c. axonal outgrowth
  T-cell alpha c. (ITAC)
chemoceptor
chemoconvulsant
chemodectoma
  petrous ridge c.
chemodenervation
chemoneurolysis
  glycerol c.
  percutaneous retrogasserian glycerol c.
chemonucleolysis
chemopallidectomy
chemopallidothalamectomy
chemopallidotomy
chemoperception
chemoreception
  central respiratory c.
chemoreceptor
  carbon dioxide c.
  medullary c.
  peripheral c.
  c. tumor
chemoreflex
chemosensitive zone
chemosensitivity
  central c.
  c. enhancing agent
chemosensory
  c. receptor
  c. stimulus
chemosignal
chemosis
  orbital c.
chemothalamectomy
chemothalamotomy
chemotherapy
  alkylating c.
  c. antiviral
  blood-brain barrier disruption c.
  combination c.
  cyclohexylchloroethylnitrosurea c.
  glioma c.
  intratumoral c.
  PCV c.
chemotransmitter
chenodeoxycholic acid
Cherry
  C. brain retractor
  C. laminectomy retractor
  C. osteotome
  C. traction tongs
Cherry-Kerrison
  C.-K. laminectomy forceps
  C.-K. laminectomy rongeur
cherry-red
  c.-r. spot
  c.-r. spot myoclonus syndrome
chevaux de frise
chewing
  c. automatism
  c. behavior
Cheyne disease
Cheyne-Stokes
  C.-S. breathing
  C.-S. respiration
Chiari
  C. II syndrome
  C. deformity
  C. formation
  C. malformation (I–IV)
chiaroscuro
chiasm
  cistern of c.
  glioma of optic c.
  optic c.
  prefixed c.
chiasma, pl. **chiasmata**
  c. opticum
  c. syndrome
chiasmal
  c. apoplexy
  c. arachnoiditis
  c. compression
  c. epidermoid
  c. lesion
  C. syndrome
chiasmapexy
  transsphenoidal c.
chiasmata (*pl. of* chiasma)
chiasmatic
  c. cistern
  c. defect
  c. glioma
  c. lesion
  c. recess
  c. sulcus
  c. syndrome
  c. tumor
chiasmatic-hypothalamic pilocytic astrocytoma
chiasmaticus
  ramus c.
chiasmatis
  cisterna c.
  sulcus c.
chicken-wire vascular pattern

chief
c. cell
c. cell of corpus pineale
childhood
c. absence epilepsy (CAE)
c. absence epilepsy evolving to juvenile myoclonic epilepsy
c. absence epilepsy with generalized tonic-clonic seizure
alternating hemiplegia of c.
c. ataxia with cerebral hypomyelination
c. benign focal epilepsy
benign paroxysmal vertigo of c.
benign partial epilepsy of c.
C. Brain Tumor Consortium
C. Brain Tumor Consortium database
c. epilepsy with occipital paroxysm
c. moyamoya disease
c. muscular dystrophy
c. myositis
c. optic glioma
polymorphic epilepsy of c.
c. primitive neuroectodermal tumor
progressive bulbar palsy of c.
progressive bulbar paralysis of c.
c. stressor
torsion disease of c.
transient tic disorder of c.
childhood-onset
c.-o. dystonia
c.-o. epilepsy
c.-o. Tourette syndrome
children
Apraxia Profile: A Descriptive Assessment Tool for C.
subclinical status epilepticus induced by sleep in c.
Children's
C. Coma Score
C. Hospital brain spatula
C. Hospital clip
C. Silapap
chill
nervous c.
chimeric stimulant
chimpanzee coryza agent (CCA)
chin
c. jerk
c. reflex
Chinese paralytic syndrome
Chippaux-Smirak arch index
chirobrachialgia (*var. of* cheirobrachialgia)
chirognostic
chirokinesthesia (*var. of* cheirokinesthesia)
chirospasm (*var. of* cheirospasm)
chisel
Adson laminectomy c.
D'Errico lamina c.
Freer c.
Hajek c.
chi-square test
chloral
amylene c.
chloralose
chlorambucil
chloramphenicol
c. acetyl transferase (CAT)
c. sodium succinate
chlordiazepoxide
amitriptyline hydrochloride and c.
c. hydrochloride
chlorhexidine shampoo
chloride
ammonium c.
butyl c.
calcium c.
carbamylcholine c.
c. channel
c. conductance
edrophonium c.
magnesium c.
manganese c.
Mytelase c.
oxybutynin c.
potassium c.
serum c.
sodium c.
^{201}Tl c.
2,3,5-triphenyltetrazolium c. (TTC)
chlorimipramine
chlormethiazole
chloroethylnitrosourea
lipophilic c.
chloroform
chloroma
Chloromycetin
chloroquine
chlorothiazide

NOTES

Chlorpazine
chlorpheniramine maleate
chlorphenoxamine
chlorproethazine
chlorpromazine
c. HCl
c. hydrochloride
chlorprothixene
chlorthalidone
chlorthiazide
Chlor-Trimeton
choanal atresia
Chodzko reflex
Choice
C. PT exchange wire
C. PT guidewire
choked disk
Cholebrine
cholecystokinin (CCK)
c. octapeptide (CCK-8)
c. tetrapeptide (CCK-4)
choleotopic
cholera
cholera-toxin-catalyzed densitometry
choleric constitutional type
choleromania
cholestanol
cholesteatoma
congenital c.
intracranial c.
cholesteatomatous
cholesterol
c. accumulation
c. crystal
c. cyst
c. embolism
c. ester storage disease
c. granuloma
c. metabolism
c. serum level
cholesterolosis, cholesterinosis
cerebrotendinous c.
cholestyramine
choline acetyltransferase
choline:*N*-acetyl-aspartate (Cho:NAA)
choline:*N*-acetyl-aspartate ratio
cholinergic
c. activity
c. approach
c. crisis
c. dysfunction
c. effect
c. fiber
c. input
c. neuron
c. neurotransmission
c. system
c. therapy
c. transmission
cholinesterase
c. inhibitor
c. inhibitory poisoning
cholinoceptive
cholinoceptor
cholinomimetic therapy
Chlolografin
Cholovue
Cho:NAA
choline:*N*-acetyl-aspartate
Cho:NAA ratio
chondritis
nasal c.
chondroblastoma
chondrocalcinosis
chondrodystrophic
myotonia c.
c. myotonia
chondrodystrophy
chondroectodermal dysplasia (CED)
chondrohypoplasia
chondroitin-4-sulfate
chondroitin-6-sulfate
chondroitin sulfate proteoglycan
chondroma
juxtacortical c.
chondromatous tumor
chondromyxoid fibroma
chondroosteodystrophy
chondrosarcoma
chondroskeleton
CHOP frame
Chopper-Dixon hybrid imaging
chorda
c. magna
c. spinalis
c. tympani
c. tympani nerve
chordae willisii
chord length
chordoblastoma
chordocarcinoma
chordoma
clival c.
chordosarcoma
chordotomy
chorea
acanthocytosis with c.
acute c.
automatic c.
benign familial c.
Bergeron c.
chronic progressive hereditary c.
chronic progressive nonhereditary c.

c. cordis
c. corpuscle
dancing c.
degenerative c.
c. dimidiata
Dubini c.
electric c.
c. festinans
fibrillary c.
c. gravidarum
habit c.
hemilateral c.
Henoch c.
hereditary nonprogressive c.
Huntington c. (HD)
hysterical c.
c. immune
c. insaniens
juvenile c.
kinesigenic c.
laryngeal c.
c. magna
c. major
malleatory c.
methodical c.
mimetic c.
c. minor
c. mollis
Morvan c.
c. nocturna
c. nutans
one-sided c.
oral contraceptive-induced c.
paralytic c.
phenytoin-induced c.
posthemiplegic c.
prehemiplegic c.
procursive c.
rheumatic c.
rhythmic c.
c. rotatoria
c. sailatoria
c. saltatory
Schrötter c.
senile c.
simple c.
Sydenham c.
tetanoid c.
thyrotoxicosis-induced c.
unilateral c.

chorea-acanthocytosis

choreal

choreathetosis

choreatic atonia

choreic
c. abasia
c. dyskinesia
c. movement
c. syndrome

choreicus
status c.

choreiform
c. disorder
c. movement

choreoacanthocytosis

choreoathetoid cerebral palsy

choreoathetosis
benign infantile familial convulsions plus paroxysmal c.
congenital c.
dystonic c.
familial benign c.
familial paroxysmal c.
kinesigenic c.
paroxysmal kinesigenic c.
phenytoin-induced c.
psychotic c.
thyrotoxicosis-induced c.

choreoid

choreophrasia

choriocarcinoma
pineal regional c.

choriomeningitis
benign lymphocytic c.
lymphocytic c.

chorionic
c. gonadotropin
c. villus sampling (CVS)

chorioretinitis

choristoma
intrasellar neuroadenohyphophyseal c.
c. nest

choroid
basal lamina of c.
basal layer of c.
c. branch
c. detachment
c. enlargement
c. fissure
c. glomus
c. line

NOTES

C

choroid *(continued)*
c. membrane
c. plexus
c. plexus ablation
c. plexus adenoma
c. plexus carcinoma
c. plexus extirpation
c. plexus of fourth ventricle
c. plexus hemangioma
c. plexus hemorrhage
c. plexus of lateral ventricle
c. plexus papilloma
c. plexus of third ventricle
c. plexus villi
c. plexus water hammer effect
c. skein
c. tela of fourth ventricle
c. tela of third ventricle
c. vein
choroidal
c. blush
c. detachment
c. fissure
c. fold
lateral posterior c.
medial posterior c.
c. metastasis
c. osteoma
c. pericallosal artery
c. xanthoma
choroidal-hippocampal
c.-h. fissure
c.-h. fissure complex
choroidea
arteria c.
fissura c.
lamina c.
plica c.
taenia c.
tela c.
tenia c.
choroideae
lamina basalis c.
choroidectomy
choroidei
rami c.
choroideum
glomus c.
choroideus
plexus c.
choroidopathy
CHP
chronic paroxysmal hemicrania
Christensen-Krabbe disease
Christmas disease
Christoferson disk bony implant
CHRNA4 gene
CHRNA7 gene
chromaffin
c. cell
c. cell transplant
c. tumor
chromaffinoma
chromaffinopathy
chromatic
c. audition
c. granule
chromatin-negative
chromatinolysis
chromatin-positive
chromatolysis
central c.
retrograde c.
transsynaptic c.
chromatolytic
chromesthesia
chromium
chromogranin A
chromolysis
chromophil
c. adenoma
c. corpuscle
c. granule
c. substance
chromophobe
c. adenoma
c. cells of anterior lobe of hypophysis
chromophobic adenoma
chromophose
chromosomal banding technique
chromosome
c. 13, 14, 15, 17, 18, 21
human c. 20
linear c.
loss of heterozygosity c. 10 (LOH10)
marker c.
c. (9_p) monosomy
c. 1p
c. 6p
c. 8pter-23
c. 2q
c. 2q21-33
c. 2q24
c. 6q24
c. 8q
c. 8q13-21
c. 8q24
c. 10q22-24
c. 15q14
c. 15q24
c. 16q
c. 19q11-13

c. 19q13.3
c. 20q
c. 20q13.2
c. 20q13.3
c. 21q22.1
c. 21q22.3
ring c.
c. study
c. walking
X c.

chronic
c. adhesive arachnoiditis
c. administration
c. African sleeping sickness
c. angle-closure glaucoma
c. anterior poliomyelitis
c. ataxia
c. basal meningitis with cranial nerve paralysis
c. change
c. cluster headache
c. communicating hydrocephalus
c. constrictive injury (CCI)
c. corticosteroid therapy
c. course
c. delirium
c. dysthymia
c. effect
c. familial polyneuritis
c. fatigability
c. fatigue
c. fatigue and immune dysfunction syndrome
c. focal encephalitis (CFE)
c. hepatic failure peripheral neuropathy
c. hyperventilation syndrome
c. illness behavior
c. inflammatory demyelinating polyneuropathy (CIDP)
c. inflammatory demyelinating polyradiculoneuropathy (CIDP)
c. inflammatory demyelinating polyradiculopathy
c. inflammatory demyelinating sensorimotor neuropathy
c. insomnia
c. intractable pain
c. migrainous neuralgia
c. motor tic disorder
c. neuropsychologic disorder
c. occlusion
c. ocular ischemia
c. paranoid reaction
c. paraparesis
c. paroxysmal hemicrania (CHP, CPH)
c. paroxysmal hemicrania-tic syndrome (CPH-tic syndrome)
c. partial epilepsy
c. pattern
c. progressive external ophthalmoplegia (CPEO)
c. progressive hereditary chorea
c. progressive myelopathy
c. progressive nonhereditary chorea
c. progressive syphilitic meningoencephalitis
c. relapsing polyneuropathy
c. relapsing polyradiculoneuropathy
c. response
c. sleep disorder
c. spinal epidural infection
c. spinal intradural infection
c. subdural hematoma
c. thrombus
c. tic
c. traumatic encephalopathy
c. trypanosomiasis
c. vertigo

chronica
encephalitis subcorticalis c.

chronometric and force generation task

chuck
T-handle Jacob c.

Churg-Strauss
C.-S. syndrome
C.-S. vasculitis

Chvostek sign

Chvostek-Weiss sign

chylous leakage

Chymodiactin

chymopapain

Cibacalcin Injection

Cibalith

Cibalith-S

cicaprost

cicatrix, pl. **cicatrices**
brain c.
meningocerebral c.

C

NOTES

CID
cervical immobilization device
CID Picture SPINE
CIDP
chronic inflammatory demyelinating polyneuropathy
chronic inflammatory demyelinating polyradiculoneuropathy
cigar-shaped diffusion ellipsoid
ciguatera
cilia (*pl. of* cilium)
ciliare
ganglion c.
ramus nervi oculomotorii ganglii ad c.
ciliari
ramus communicans nervi nasociliaris cum ganglio c.
ciliaris
radix brevis ganglii c.
radix longa ganglii c.
radix nasociliaris ganglii c.
radix oculomotoria ganglii c.
radix parasympathica ganglii c.
radix sympathica ganglii c.
ramus sympathicus ganglii c.
ciliary
c. ganglion
c. ganglionic plexus
c. migraine
c. migraine headache
c. nerve
c. neuralgia
c. neurotrophic factor (CNF)
ciliochoroid detachment
ciliospinal
c. center
c. reflex
ciliotomy
cilium, pl. **cilia**
cilostazol
cimbia
cimetidine
cinanesthesia
cinclisis
cincture sensation
cine phase contrast magnetic resonance imaging
cinerea
ala c.
commissura c.
fascia c.
fasciola c.
lamina c.
substantia c.
cinereae
nucleus alae c.
cinereal
cinerei
rami tuberis c.
cinereum
hamartoma of the tuber c.
tuber c.
tuberculum c.
cinereus
locus c.
cineritious
cinesalgia
cineseismography
cingula (*pl. of* cingulum)
cingularis
ramus c.
cingulate
c. convolution
c. epilepsy
c. gyrus
c. gyrus dysgenesis
c. gyrus eversion
c. herniation
c. motor area (CMA)
c. operation
posterior c.
c. response
c. sulcus
c. tissue
cingulectomy
cinguli
fasciola cinerea c.
gyrus c.
isthmus gyri c.
isthmus of gyrus c.
sulcus c.
cingulothalamic artery
cingulotomy
rostral c.
stereotactic c.
cingulum, pl. **cingula**
c. bundle
sulcus of c.
cingulumotomy
cinnarizine
cinoxacin
cinq
folie á c.
circadian
c. clock
c. modulator
c. pacemaker
c. rhythm
c. rhythm change
c. rhythmicity
c. timing

circannual
c. cycle
c. rhythm
circle
cerebral arterial c.
Haller c.
Papez c.
Ridley c.
c. of Willis
c. of Willis aneurysm
Zinn vascular c.
CircOlectric bed
circuit
basal ganglia-thalamocortical motor c.
cortex c.
cortical-striatal-pallidal-thalamic neural c.
dysfunctional neural c.
error detection c.
frontal subcortical brain c.
frontostriatal-pallidalothalamic c.
frontothalamic c.
lateral orbitofrontal c.
neuroanatomic c.
Papez c.
reflex c.
reverberating c.
traditional limbic c.
circuitry
amygdala-fear c.
brain c.
cortical language c.
dysfunctional c.
frontal-cerebellar-thalamic c.
limbic c.
normal c.
reciprocal c.
reward c.
striatofrontal c.
circulaire
folie c.
circular
c. fiber
c. laminar hook with offset top
c. nystagmus
c. sinus
c. sulcus of insula
c. sulcus of Reil
circulares
fibrae c.
circularis
sinus c.
circulating
c. androgen
c. leptin level
circulation
carotid c.
cerebral c.
collateral c.
intracranial c.
macro-eCVR-FV c.
micro-eCVR-FV c.
thalamic c.
vertebrobasilar c.
circulus, pl. **circuli**
c. arteriosus cerebri
c. arteriosus halleri
c. vasculosus nervi optici
c. venosus halleri
c. venosus ridleyi
circumcallosal
circumduction gait
circumferential branch
circumferentially aortofemoral graft
circumflex
c. nerve
c. nerve trauma
circumgemmal
circuminsular
circumlocution
circumplex
multifacet c.
circumscribed
c. amnesia
c. cerebral atrophy
c. change
c. craniomalacia
c. edema
c. lesion
c. pyocephalus
c. region
circumscribing incision
circumscripta
meningitis serosa c.
osteoporosis c.
circumstantiality
circumventricular organ
cirsoid aneurysm
cisapride

NOTES

***cis*-parinaric acid**
13-*cis*-retinoic acid (CRA, 13-CRA)
***cis*-retinoic acid (CRA)**
cissa
cistern
ambient c.
arachnoiditis of opticochiasmatic c.
basal c.
cerebellomedullary c.
cerebellopontine angle c.
cerebromedullary c.
c. of chiasm
chiasmatic c.
crural c.
fossa of Sylvius c.
great c.
c. of great cerebral vein
c. of great vein of cerebrum
insular c.
interpeduncular c.
c. of lamina terminalis
lateral cerebellomedullary c.
c. of lateral cerebral fossa
c. of lateral fossa of cerebrum
lumbar c.
mesencephalic c.
c. of nuclear envelope
obliterated basal c.
opticochiasmatic c.
parasellar c.
pericallosal c.
perimesencephalic c.
pontine c.
posterior cerebellomedullary c.
premedullary c.
prepontine c.
quadrigeminal c.
subarachnoid c.
subarachnoidal c.
superior c.
suprasellar c.
sylvian c.
c. sylvii
c. of Sylvius fossa
trigeminal c.
cisterna, pl. **cisternae**
c. ambiens
c. basalis
c. caryothecae
c. cerebellomedullaris
c. cerebellomedullaris lateralis
c. cerebellomedullaris posterior
c. chiasmatis
c. cruralis
c. fossae lateralis
c. fossae lateralis cerebri
c. fossae sylvii
c. intercruralis profunda
c. interpeduncularis
c. laminae terminalis
c. lumbalis
c. lumbar
c. magna
c. magna catheter
c. magna enlargement
c. pericallosa
c. pontis
c. pontocerebellaris
c. quadrigeminalis
c. retrothalamica
cisternae subarachnoideae
cisternae subarachnoideales
c. sulci lateralis
c. superioris
c. venae magnae
c. venae magnae cerebri
cisterna-atrial shunt
cisternal
c. clot
c. puncture
cisternal-peritoneal shunt
cisternal-pleural shunt
cisternogram
indium c.
isotope c.
radioisotope c.
cisternography
cerebellopontine c.
computed tomographic c.
isotope c.
isotopic c.
perioperative c.
radioisotope c.
radionuclide c.
citalopram HBr
Citanest Plain
Citelli angle
citolopram
Citracal
citrate
calcium c.
potassium acetate, potassium bicarbonate, and potassium c.
potassium bicarbonate, potassium chloride, and potassium c.
sufentanil c.
citric acid cycle
***Citrobacter* meningitis**
citrullinemia
citrullinuria
citta, cittosis
CIVRA
continuous intravenous regional anesthesia

CJD
Creutzfeldt-Jakob disease
c-jun
c.-j. gene
c.-j. N-Terminal kinase
CK
creatine kinase
CK-MB
creatine kinase MB fraction
cladiosic
Cladophialophora bantiana
cladosporiosis
cerebral c.
cladribine
clamp
Apofix interlaminar c.
Bigelow calvarium c.
Calman carotid c.
CCA c.
Crile c.
Crutchfield carotid artery c.
Dandy c.
Diethrich bulldog c.
Duvol lung c.
Gardner neurosurgical skull c.
Halifax interlaminar c.
head c.
interlaminar c.
Jacobson-Potts vascular c.
Javid carotid c.
Kindt carotid c.
Kocher c.
Kocher-Lovelace c.
Mayfield head c.
Mayfield neurosurgical skill c.
mosquito c.
Olivecrona aneurysm c.
Péan c.
Poppen-Blalock carotid c.
Roosen c.
Salibi carotid artery c.
Schnidt c.
Schwartz temporary intracranial artery c.
Selverstone c.
Sugita head c.
suture c.
Thompson carotid c.
three-point skull c.
Thumb-Saver introducer c.
Yasargil carotid c.
clamping mechanism
clang association
Clarke
C. cell
C. column
C. nucleus
nucleus dorsalis of C.
C. stereotactic instrument
Clark electrode
Clarus spinescope
clasp-knife
c.-k. effect
c.-k. phenomenon
c.-k. reflex
c.-k. response
c.-k. rigidity
c.-k. spasticity
clasp knife
class
Gardner-Robertson c.
c. I–III evidence
pyranocarboxylic acid c.
classic
c. apraxia
c. brain tumor headache
c. cervical rib syndrome
c. dissecting aneurysm
c. migraine
classification
alcoholic c.
American Spinal Cord Injury Association c.
Antoni-A neurinoma c.
basal ganglia c.
Brodmann c.
Daumas-Duport c.
empirical c.
Engel postoperative seizure c.
Fränkel c.
Functional Ambulation C.
Hannover c.
Hunt-Hess aneurysm c.
Hunt-Hess neurological c.
Hunt and Kosnik c.
International Working Formulation c.
Kernohan system of glioma c.
Kiel c.
Kistler subarachnoid hemorrhage c.
LeFort c.
Melmon and Rosen c.

C

NOTES

classification *(continued)*
modified Fischer c.
Newcastle c.
Nordstadt c.
Paykel c.
Ratliff avascular necrosis c.
Russell-Rubinstein cerebrovascular malformation c.
Spetzler-Martin c.
Sunderland c.
Sundt carotid ulceration c.
Suzuki c.
c. system
Universal Spine C.
WHO astrocytoma c.
Claude-Bernard syndrome
Claude syndrome
claudication
cerebral intermittent c.
intermittent neurogenic c.
jaw c.
mental c.
neurogenic c. (NC)
visual c.
claustral layer
claustrum, pl. **claustra**
clava
claval
clavate
clavi (*pl. of* clavus)
Claviceps purpurea
clavulanic acid
clavus, pl. **clavi**
c. clinical grouping
c. hystericus
clawed pedicle hook
clawhand deformity
clay shoveler's fracture
clearance
creatinine c.
dopamine c.
c. rate
clear cell ependymoma
clearheaded
clearheadedness
clear-sighted
clear-sightedness
cleft
atypical c.
branchial c.
Lanterman c.
pharyngeal c.
primary synaptic c.
Schmidt-Lanterman c.
secondary synaptic c.
c. spine
subneural c.
synaptic c.
cleidocranial dysostosis
Cleocin
Clerambault syndrome
clericorum
dysphonia c.
Clevenger fissure
click stimulation
Click'X
climbing fiber (CF)
clinical
C. Adaptive Test/Clinical Linguistic and Auditory Milestone Scale (CAT/CLAMS)
c. anecdote
c. armamentarium
c. characteristic
c. comparison study
c. conceptualization
c. condition
c. correlate
c. criterion
c. data
c. dementia
C. Dementia Rating (CDR)
C. Dementia Rating Scale
c. difference
c. effect
c. efficacy
c. electromagnetic flowmeter
c. electromagnetic flowmeter clip
c. formulation
C. Global Impression of Change
C. Global Improvement Scale
c. heterogeneity
c. ictal event
c. improvement
c. intervention
c. intervention program
C. Linguistic Auditory Milestone Scale
c. manifestation
c. method
c. monitoring
c. monitoring technique
c. neurology
c. neuropsychology
c. neuroscientist
C. Observations of Motor and Postural Skills
c. phenomenology
c. phenomenon
c. phenotype
c. procedure
c. progression
c. relevance

c. response
c. seizure
c. sequela
c. sign
c. stability
c. subtype
c. symptom
c. syndrome
C. Test of Sensory Interaction and Balance (CTSIB)
c. theory
c. thinking
c. trial
c. understanding
c. validity
c. variable
c. visit

clinically
c. adverse sequela
c. isolated syndrome

clinician
C. Global Rating Scale
C. Rated Overall Life Impairment
c. rating
c. rating scale

clinician-rated
c.-r. cognitive symptom
c.-r. scale

Clinician's Interview-Based Impression of Change

clinicopathological

clinicopathologic study

Clinitron air bed

clinodactyly

clinoid
anterior c.
c. process

clinoidal
c. aneurysm
c. meningioma
c. segment

clinoidectomy
anterior extradural c.
extradural c.

Clinoril

ClinSeg

clioquinol

clip
Acland c.
Adson scalp c.
aneurysm c.
angled aneurysm c.
c. application
c. applier
Backhaus towel c.
bayonet aneurysm c.
Beimer-Clip aneurysm c.
booster c.
Braun-Yasargil right-angle c.
Children's Hospital c.
clinical electromagnetic flowmeter c.
Codman aneurysm c.
Cologne pattern scalp c.
crankshaft c.
cross-legged c.
Delrin plastic scalp c.
distal basilar temporary c.
Drake fenestrated c.
Drake-Kees c.
Elgiloy c.
fenestrated aneurysm c.
ferromagnetic intracerebral aneurysm c.
c. force meter
c. graft
heavy-duty straight c.
Heifetz c.
Heifetz-Weck c.
Housepian aneurysm c.
Ingraham-Fowler tantalum c.
Iwabuchi c.
Kerr c.
LeRoy-Raney scalp c.
Ligaclip c.
c. ligation of aneurysm
L-shaped aneurysm c.
Mayfield aneurysm c.
McFadden cross-legged c.
McFadden-Kees c.
McKenzie hemostasis c.
McKenzie silver c.
Michel scalp c.
microvascular c.
mini-Sugita c.
nonferromagnetic c.
Olivecrona c.
c. placement
plastic scalp c.
primary c.
Raney scalp c.
right-angle booster c.

NOTES

clip *(continued)*
scalp c.
Schwartz aneurysm c.
Scoville c.
Slimline c.
Spetzler titanium aneurysm c.
straight aneurysm c.
Sugita aneurysm c.
Sugita cross-legged c.
Sugita-Ikakogyo c.
Sugita side-curved bayonet c.
Sugita temporary straight c.
Sundt booster c.
Sundt cross-legged c.
Sundt-Kees encircling patch c.
Sundt-Kees graft c.
Sundt-Kees Slimline c.
Sundt straddling c.
temporary c.
titanium aneurysm c.
Vari-Angle aneurysm c.
Weck c.
Yasargil-Aesculap spring c.
Yasargil cross-legged c.
Yasargil titanium aneurysm c.
Yasargil vessel c.
Zimmer c.
clip-induced stricture
clipping
aneurysm c.
microsurgical neck c.
proximal c.
shank c.
clip-reinforced cotton sling
clip-type electrode
clitoral
clitoridis
nervi cavernosi c.
nervus dorsalis c.
clival
c. chordoma
c. meningioma
c. mucocele
clivales
rami c.
clivus, pl. **clivi**
Blumenbach c.
c. canal line
lobulus clivi
lobus clivi
lower c.
c. meningioma
c. monticulus
mucopyocele of the c.
***CLN1* gene**
***CLN2* gene**
***CLN3* gene**
***CLN5* gene**
***CLN8* gene**
cloaca therapy
clock
circadian c.
internal circadian c.
clodanolene
clofazimine
Clofen
clomethiazole
clomipramine
clonal
c. evolution hypothesis
c. expansion
clonazepam
clonic
c. block
c. contraction
c. convulsion
c. seizure
c. spasm
clonicity
clonicotonic seizure
clonidine
c. hydrochloride
topical c.
clonogenic cell assay
clonospasm
clonus
ankle c.
foot c.
patellar c.
persistent c.
subsultus c.
sustained ankle c.
toe c.
wrist c.
clopenthixol
clopidogrel bisulfate
Clopixol
Cloquet
C. ganglion
C. pseudoganglion
clorazepam
clorazepate dipotassium
clorazepic
clordiazepoxide
clorgyline
clorhexidine gluconate
closed
c. angiography
c. brain injury (CBI)
c. circuit television monitoring
c. Cotrel-Dubousset hook
c. disk space infection
c. galea
c. head injury

C. Head Injury Screener
c. head syndrome
c. loop reflex
c. skull fracture
c. transverse process TSRH hook
closed-chain functional assessment
closed-circuit-television electroencephalographic telemetry
close-sightedness
clostridial infection
Clostridium
C. botulinum
C. difficile
C. tetani
closure
approximating c.
neural tube c.
premature c.
c. pressure
scalp c.
watertight c.
clot
cisternal c.
cobweb-like c.
clotrimazole
clotting
c. disorder
c. factor deficiency
clouded-state epilepsy
cloudy cornea
cloverleaf
c. skull
c. skull syndrome
Cloward
C. back fusion
C. blade retractor
C. bone graft impactor
C. brain retractor
C. cautery hook
C. cervical arthrodesis
C. cervical disk approach
C. cervical dislocation reducer
C. cervical retractor
C. cervical vertebra spreader
C. disk rongeur
C. double-hinge cervical
C. double-hinge cervical retractor handle
C. dural hook
C. dural retractor
C. elevator
C. instrument
C. lamina spreader
C. lumbar lamina retractor
C. nerve root retractor
C. operation
C. procedure
C. skin retractor
C. small cervical retractor
C. spinal fusion osteotome
C. surgical saddle
C. technique
C. tissue retractor
Cloward-Cone ring curette
Cloward-Cushing vein retractor
Cloward-English laminectomy rongeur
Cloward-Hoen laminectomy retractor
clozapine therapy
Clozaril
cloze procedure
CLS
Coffin-Lowry syndrome
club ending of Bartelmez
clumsy
c. child syndrome
c. hand syndrome
cluneal nerve
cluster
c. A, B, C disorder
c. analysis
apolipoprotein gene c.
c. breathing
c. B trait
c. C, D symptom
diagnostic c.
c. of differentiation 95 (CD95)
dissociative symptom c.
DSM c.
eccentric A c.
emotional B c.
fearful C c.
c. headache (CH)
microglial c.
c. period
c. of symptom
cluster-tic syndrome
cluttering
c. in speech
speech and language c.
Clymer-Barrett Readiness Test, Revised
Clysodrast

C

NOTES

CM
cavernous malformation
CMA
cingulate motor area
CMAP
compound motor action potential
compound muscle action potential
C. amplitude
C. on electromyogram
CMC-III
Malis irrigating bipolar C.-I.
CMRglc
cerebral metabolic rate of glucose
$CMRO_2$
cerebral metabolic rate of oxygen
CMS
congenital myasthenic syndrome
CMS AccuProbe 450 system
CMV
controlled mechanical ventilation
cytomegalovirus
C. encephalitis
C. meningitis
C. polyradiculomyelitis
CMV-PRAM
cytomegalovirus polyradiculomyelitis
CNAP
compound nerve action potential
CNAP on electromyogram
CNCD
Consortium of Neurology Clerkship Director
CNF
ciliary neurotrophic factor
C-nociceptor filter-evoked central abnormality
***cnot* gene**
CNR
contrast-to-noise ratio
CNS
central nervous system
C. abnormality
granulomatous angiitis of the C.
C. insult
C. lymphoma
C. nocardiosis
primary angiitis of the C.
C. vasculature
CO_2
carbon dioxide
end-tidal CO_2
CO_2 inhalation
CO_2 narcosis
co-activation
coactive strategy
Coag
Rapidpoint Access/Rapidpoint C.
coagulase-negative staphylococci
coagulation
c. cascade
c. disorder
disseminated intravascular c. (DIC)
coagulative necrosis
coagulator
ASSI c.
bipolar c.
Concept bipolar c.
Fukushima monopolar malleable c.
Malis CMC-II bipolar c.
Malis solid state c.
Polar-Mate c.
solid-state c.
coagulopathy
consumptive c.
coagulum
cryoprecipitate c.
coaptation
direct end-to-end c.
coarse
c. nystagmus
c. tremor
coating of aneurysm
Coats disease
coaxial
c. cable
c. needle electrode
cobalamin
c. metabolism disorder
c. reductase deficiency
cobalt
c. Gray equivalent
c. samarium magnet
cobalt-60
collimated c.
Cobb
C. method of measuring kyphosis
C. periosteal elevator
C. syndrome
C. technique
cobblestone degeneration
Coblation-based spinal surgery system
cobweb-like clot
cocaine-induced choreoathetoid movement
coccidioidal
c. complement fixation of cerebrospinal fluid
c. meningitis
Coccidioides
C. immitis
C. infection
coccidioidomycosis

coccygea
segmentum c. 1–3
segmentum medullae spinalis c.
coccygeal
c. ganglion
c. ligament
c. nerve
c. part of spinal cord
c. plexus
c. segment of spinal cord
coccygei
ramus anterior nervi c.
ramus dorsalis nervi c.
ramus posterior nervi c.
ramus ventralis nervi c.
coccyges (*pl. of* coccyx)
coccygeus
nervi sacrales et nervus c.
nervus c.
plexus c.
coccygodynia
coccyx, pl. **coccyges**
posterior surgical exposure of sacrum and c.
cochlea, pl. **cochleae**
apical turn of the c.
aqueductus c.
cupula c.
ganglion spirale c.
lamina basilaris c.
membranous c.
spiral ganglion of c.
vestibular fissure of c.
cochlear
c. aplasia
c. aqueduct
c. duct
c. ganglion
c. hair cell
c. implant
c. microphonic potential
c. nerve examination
c. nucleus
c. part of vestibulocochlear nerve
c. recess
c. response time
c. root of eighth nerve
c. root of vestibulocochlear nerve
c. vascular supply
cochleare
ganglion c.
cochleares
nuclei c.
cochlearis
crista basilaris ductus c.
ductus c.
nervus c.
nuclei nervi c.
paries vestibularis ductus c.
pars c.
radix c.
recessus c.
cochleogram
cochleoorbicular reflex
cochleopalpebral reflex
cochleopupillary reflex
cochleosacculotomy
cochleostapedial reflex
cochleovestibular compression syndrome
cochornis
Cochrane Collaboration
Cockayne syndrome
Cockgraft-Gault equation
cocktail
c. chatter in hydrocephalus
Viñuela c.
coconut sound
code
multimodal c.
c. substitution-immediate recall-accuracy
codeine
Empracet with c.
c. neurotoxicity
Codman
C. aneurysm clip
C. anterior cervical plate system
C. Bactiseal antimicrobial impregnated catheter system
C. cranioblade
C. drill
C. Hakim programmable valve
C. IC
C. neurological headrest system
C. scissors
C. slit valve
C. ventricular silicone
C. ventricular silicone catheter
Codman-Harper laminectomy rongeur
Codman-Kerrison laminectomy rongeur
Codman-Leksell laminectomy rongeur
Codman-Medos programmable valve

NOTES

Codman-Schlesinger
C.-S. cervical laminectomy rongeur
C.-S. laminectomy rongeur
coefficient
alpha c.
apparent diffusion c. (ADC)
contingency c.
familiar correlation c.
high alpha c.
low alpha c.
olfactory c.
scoring c.
Spearman correlation c.
c. of variation (COV)
coeliaca
ganglia c.
coeliaci
rami renales plexus c.
coeliacus
plexus c.
coenesthesia (*var. of* cenesthesia)
coenzyme
acetyl c. A
coercion program
coeruleus
locus c. (LC)
nucleus c.
Coffin-Lowry syndrome (CLS)
Coffin-Siris syndrome
COGA
Collaborative Study on the Genetics of Alcoholism
Cogan
C. lid twitch
C. oculomotor apraxia
C. syndrome
Cogentin
COGENTLIGHT
Cogent microillumination technology
Cognex
Cognistat (The Neurobehavioral Cognitive Status Examination)
cognition
altered c.
Burns Brief Inventory of Communication and C.
constriction of c.
c. disorder
frontally based c.
impaired c.
premorbid c.
social c.
visuospatial constructive c.
cognitive
C. Abilities Scale
C. Abilities Test, Form 5
C. Adaptive Computer Help
c. analytic therapy
c. behavioral group therapy
c. capability
c. capacity
c. change
c. decline
c. deficit
c. deterioration
c. difficulty
c. disorder
c. disturbance
c. domain
c. dysfunction
c. dysmetria
c. enhancement therapy
C. Failures Questionnaire
c. fatigue
c. function
c. function assessment
c. function deficiency
c. function development
c. function immaturity
c. functioning
c. generation of affect
c. impairment
c. impairment of depression
c. impairment, no dementia
c. improvement
c. intervention
c. maturity
c. measure
c. mechanism
c. method
c. neuropsychology
c. neuroscience
c. pathology
c. performance
c. restricting
c. score
C. Skills Assessment Battery, Second Edition
c. slowing
c. state
c. status
c. subsystem
c. symptom
c. task
c. technique
c. tendency
c. test battery
c. testing
c. therapy
c. trajectory
cognitively intact
cognizance
CogScreen Aeromedical Edition

cogwheel
c. phenomenon
c. rigidity
c. sign
Cohen syndrome
coherence
phase c.
coherent
c. motion
c. negative picture-caption pair
c. positive picture-caption pair
coil
body c.
butterfly c.
catheter c.
crossed c.
Dacron fibered platinum c.
detachable c.
Dixon radiofrequency c.
electrodetachable platinum c.
c. embolization
endovascular c.
Golay gradient c.
gradient c.
Guglielmi detachable c. (GDC)
head c.
Helmholtz c.
Hilal c.
Ivalon wire c.
occlusion c.
orthogonal square Helmholtz c.
phased-array c.
platinum c.
quadrature head c.
radiofrequency head c.
receiver c.
RF c.
saddle c.
shim c.
solenoid c.
surface c.
three axis gradient c.
thrombogenic c.
transverse gradient c.
Yasargil-Leyla brain retractor z-gradient c.
z-gradient c.
coiled spring
coiling procedure
coital headache
Col-3
Colace
colchicine
cold
c. acclimation
c. effector
c. receptor
c. sensitivity
c. stimulus headache
cold-induced allodynia
cold-sensitive neuron
Coleman method
coli
Escherichia c.
colic lead
colla (*pl. of* collum)
Collaboration
Cochrane C.
Collaborative Study on the Genetics of Alcoholism (COGA)
collagen
Avitene microfibrillar c.
intercellular c.
microfibrillar c.
c. vascular disease
Vitrogen 100 c.
collagenase
c. activating factor
c. inhibition
collagen-impregnated Dacron
collapse
bone graft c.
c. delirium
hemispheric c.
interspace c.
upper airway c.
vertebral c.
collapsible tissue retractor
collar
Belmont c.
cervical c.
Exo-Static c.
Miami Acute Care cervical c.
Miami J c.
Newport c.
Philadelphia c.
plastic c.
Plastizote cervical c.
collateral
c. blood flow
c. blood supply
c. circulation

NOTES

collateral *(continued)*
c. eminence
c. fissure
c. nerve sprouting
Schaffer c.
c. sprouting neuron
c. sulcus
c. trigone
c. vessel
collaterale
trigonum c.
collateralis
eminentia c.
fissura c.
sulcus c.
collector
common venous c.
Collet-Sicard syndrome
Collet syndrome
colli
nervus transversus c.
rami inferiores nervi transversi c.
rami superiores nervi transversi c.
collicular artery
colliculorum
commissura c.
colliculus, pl. **colliculi**
anterior c.
brachium of caudal c.
brachium of inferior c.
brachium of the inferior c.
brachium of rostral c.
brachium of superior c.
caudal c.
c. caudalis
c. caudatus
commissure of inferior c.
commissure of superior c.
deep gray layer of superior c.
deep white layer of superior c.
facial c.
c. facialis
gray layer of superior c.
c. inferior
inferior nasal c.
intermediate white layer of superior c.
middle gray layer of superior c.
nuclei of caudal c.
nuclei of inferior c.
rostral c.
c. rostralis
superficial gray layer of superior c.
superior c.
zonal layer of superior c.
Collier
C. sign
C. tract
collimated cobalt-60
collimation
collimator
CASS TrueTaper c.
external c.
c. helmet
multileaf c.
stereoguide c.
Collins law of survival after brain tumor
collision
electron c.
c. tumor
collodion attachment
colloid
c. cyst
c. cyst of third ventricle
c. oncotic pressure
technetium albumin c.
technetium 99m sulfur c.
collum, pl. **colla**
c. distortum
coloboma, heart disease, atresia choanae, retarded growth, genital anomalies, ear anomalies (CHARGE)
colocalization
Cologne pattern scalp clip
Colonna shelf procedure
colony-forming efficiency
color
c. agnosia
c. anomia
c. taste
c. velocity imaging quantification
c. vision
c. vision loss
Colorado
C. MicroDissection needle
C. MicroNeedle
C. tick fever viral encephalitis
color-flow
c.-f. Doppler
c.-f. Doppler sonography
c.-f. imaging
color-opponent cell
colpocephaly
column
anterior gray c.
anterolateral c.
branchial efferent c.
Burdach c.
c. cell
Clarke c.
dorsal gray c.

forniceal c.
c. of fornix
fundamental c.
general somatic afferent c.
general somatic efferent c.
general visceral afferent c.
general visceral efferent c.
Goll c.
Gowers c.
gray c.
intermediate c.
intermediolateral cell c.
lateral c.
Lissauer c.
Rolando c.
special somatic afferent c.
special visceral efferent c.
spinal c.
Spitzka-Lissauer c.
c. of Spitzka and Lissauer
Stilling c.
striomotor c.
thoracic c.
Türck c.
ventral white c.
vertebral c.

columna, pl. **columnae**
c. anterior
c. anterior medullae spinalis
c. dorsalis medullae spinalis
c. fornicis
columnae griseae
columnae griseae medullae spinalis
c. intermedia
c. intermedia medullae spinalis
c. intermediolateralis medullae spinalis
c. lateralis
c. posterior
c. posterior medullae spinalis
c. thoracica
c. ventralis medullae spinalis
c. vertebralis

coma
adrenocortical c.
agrypnodal c.
alcoholic c.
alpha frequency c.
apoplectic c.
calm hypotonic c.
c. carcinomatosum
diabetic c.
hepatic c.
c. hepaticum
hyperosmolar (hyperglycemic) nonketotic c.
hypoglycemic c.
hypopituitary c.
hypoventilation c.
Kussmaul c.
metabolic c.
myxedema c.
nonketotic hyperglycemic hyperosmolar c.
pentobarbital c.
postanoxic c.
c. scale
spindle c.
thyrotoxic c.
uremic c.
c. vigil

comatose

comb bundle

combination
c. chemotherapy
fabulized c.
c. headache
Isola spinal implant system plate-rod c.
muscle-fascia-Gelfoam c.
c. needle electrode
orthogonal c.
paradoxical c.
c. strategy

combined
c. anterior and posterior approach
c. aphasia
c. flexion-distraction injury and burst fracture
c. low cervical and transthoracic approach
c. predictive power
c. presigmoid-transtransversarium intradural approach
c. sclerosis
c. system disease
c. transsylvian and middle fossa approach

Combisit surgeon's chair

Combitrans transducer

Combivir

comedication

NOTES

comma
c. bundle of Schultze
c. tract of Schultze
comme il faut
commensalism
comminuted skull fracture
commissura, pl. **commissurae**
c. alba anterior
c. alba anterior medullae spinalis
c. alba posterior
c. alba posterior medullae spinalis
c. anterior grisea
c. cinerea
c. colliculi inferioris
c. colliculi rostralis
c. colliculi superioris
c. colliculorum
c. epithalamica
c. fornicis
c. grisea anterior
c. grisea anterior medullae spinalis
c. grisea anterior/posterior medullae spinalis
c. grisea posterior
c. grisea posterior medullae spinalis
c. habenularum
c. hippocampus
c. magna cerebri
c. olivarum
c. posterior cerebri
c. posterior grisea
c. supraoptica dorsalis
commissurae supraopticae
c. supraoptica ventralis
c. ventralis alba
commissural
c. aphasia
c. cell
c. fiber
c. myelotomy
c. neurofiber
c. plate
commissuralis
fibra c.
neurofibra c.
commissure
anterior commissure-posterior c. (AC-PC)
anterior gray c.
anterior white c.
callosal c.
caudal colliculus c.
cerebral c.
c. of cerebral hemisphere
dorsal supraoptic c.
epithalamus c.
c. of fornix
Ganser c.
gray c.
Gudden c.
habenular c.
hippocampal c.
c. of inferior colliculus
Meynert c.
nucleus of posterior c.
posterior cerebral c.
posterior gray c.
rostral colliculus c.
c. of superior colliculus
supraoptic c.
ventral white c.
Wernekinck c.
white c.
commissurotomy
callosal c.
percutaneous balloon c.
committee
AANS/CNS Outcomes C.
common
c. basal vein
c. carotid artery (CCA)
c. carotid nervous plexus
c. central process
c. crus
c. fibular nerve
c. iliac artery injury
c. limb of membranous semicircular duct
c. membranous limb of membranous semicircular duct
c. migraine
c. peroneal nerve
c. sensibility
c. venous collector
c. venous confluence
commotio
c. cerebri
c. spinalis
communal residential center
commune
crus membranaceum c.
Schizophyllum c.
sensorium c.
communicans
macula c.
ramus c.
communicantes
rami c.
white rami c.
communicating
c. branch
c. branch of anterior interosseous nerve with ulnar nerve

c. branch of auriculotemporal nerve with facial nerve
c. branch of chorda tympani with lingual nerve
c. branch of facial nerve with glossopharyngeal nerve
c. branch of facial nerve with tympanic plexus
c. branch of fibular artery
c. branch of intermediate nerve with tympanic plexus
c. branch of lacrimal nerve with zygomatic nerve
c. branch of lingual nerve with hypoglossal nerve
c. branch of median nerve with ulnar nerve
c. branch of nasociliary nerve with ciliary ganglion
c. branch of otic ganglion to auriculotemporal nerve
c. branch of otic ganglion to chorda tympani
c. branch of otic ganglion with chorda tympani
c. branch of otic ganglion with medial pterygoid nerve
c. branch of peroneal artery
c. branch of radial nerve with ulnar nerve
c. branch of spinal nerve
c. branch of superficial radial nerve with ulnar nerve
c. branch of sympathetic trunk
c. branch of tympanic plexus with auricular branch of vagus nerve
c. branch with nasociliary nerve
c. hydrocephalus

communication
C. Activities of Daily Living
c. disorder
emotional c.
facilitation of c.
c. function
functional c. (FC)
c. impairment
pathological c.
C.'s Profile Questionnaire
c. skill
C. Skills Profile
c. tool

Communicative Abilities in Daily Living

communis
nervus fibularis c.
plexus caroticus c.
ramus communicans fibularis nervi fibularis c.
ramus communicans peroneus nervi peronei c.
sacculus c.

community-acquired bacterial meningitis

Community College Student Experiences Questionnaire (CCSEQ)

Community-Oriented Programs Environment Scale

comorbid
c. characteristic
c. condition
c. dementia
c. disease
c. illness

comorbidity
age-related c.
medical c.

compacta
pars c.
substantia nigra pars c. (SNc)

company
neurologic c.

compartment
extradural c.
infratentorial c.
lateral sellar c.
c. syndrome

Compass
C. arc-quadrant stereotactic system
C. frame-based stereotactic system
C. stereotactic phantom

compassionate use basis

compatibility
ABO antigen c.
MRI c.

compensated hydrocephalus

compensation
gradient c.

compensatory
c. innervation
c. scoliosis

Comperm tubular elastic bandage

competency
c. assessment
high degree of c.

NOTES

C

competency *(continued)*
low threshold of c.
maternal c.
competent
mentally c.
competition
hemisphere c.
intermodal c.
complainant-listener relationship
complement
c. activation
c. fixation antibody test
c. fixation antibody titer
c. fixation inhibition
c. symptom-focused assessment
complementary
c. deoxyribonucleic acid (cDNA)
c. medicine
complete
c. blood count (CBC)
c. iridoplegia
c. lateral hemilaminectomy
c. tetanus
c. transverse myelitis
c. visual loss
completed stroke
completus
tetanus c.
complex
c. absence
acoustic nerve c.
acquired immunodeficiency syndrome dementia c.
adrenoleukodystrophy/adrenomyeloneuropathy c.
AIDS dementia c. (ADC)
ALD-AMN c.
ALS-PD c.
amygdaloid c.
amyotrophic lateral sclerosis-Parkinson dementia c.
antigen-antibody c.
aperiodic c.
avidin-biotin peroxidase c.
brain wave c.
calcarine c.
capsulolabral c.
C5b-9 c.
choroidal-hippocampal fissure c.
Dandy-Walker c.
discoligamentous c.
c. disease
disorganized symptom c.
c. febrile convulsion
c. febrile seizure
c. finger routine
c. fracture
Guam parkinsonism-dementia c.
c. hand routine
heteromultimeric c.
hippocampal c.
hippocampal-amygdala c.
histocompatibility c.
homomultimeric c.
immune c.
inferior olivary c.
inferior orbitofrontal c.
c. intellectual aura
interictal c.
K c.
major histocompatibility c. (MHC)
mastoid c.
membrane attack c.
c. meningioma
c. motor seizure
occipitoatlantoaxial c.
oculomotor nuclear c.
omphalocele-exstrophy-imperforate anus-spinal defects c.
c. paradigm
Parkinson disease and lateral sclerosis-dementia c.
c. partial nocturnal seizure
c. partial status
c. partial status epilepticus
PDH c.
perihypoglossal nuclear c.
periodic sharp wave c.
plasmin-antiplasmin c.
polyspike-wave c.
c. precipitated epilepsy
pyruvate dehydrogenase c.
c. regional pain syndrome
c. relationship
c. repetitive discharge (CRD)
Rey-Osterrieth c.
Sakoda c.
c. segregation analysis
sharp-wave c.
slow wave c.
Sokoda c.
spike-and-wave c.
spike-wave c.
superior olivary c.
syringomyelia-Chiari c.
Tag c.
c. task
troponin-tropomyosin c.
urethral c.
ventrobasal nuclei c.
ventrolateral nuclear c.
vertebrogenic symptom c.
c. visual perception
complexus olivaris inferior

compliance
intracranial c.
c. rate
sustained c.
treatment c.
complicated
c. fracture
c. migraine
complication
adverse neurologic c.
drug-induced medical c.
iatrogenic c.
Isola spinal implant system c.
mumps vaccination c.
neurologic c.
perioperative c.
rubella vaccination c.
smallpox vaccination c.
transsphenoidal c.
ventilatory support neurologic c.
component
adrenomedullary c.
autonomous functional c.
bacterial cell wall c.
cross-sectional c.
endogenous electrophysiological c.
functional c.
genetic c.
hypermetabolic tumor c.
inotropic c.
Isola spinal implant system c.
physiological c.
prominent phobic anxiety c.
signal transducing receptor c.
somatic motor c.
somatic sensory c.
splanchnic motor c.
splanchnic sensory c.
sudomotor c.
thermogenic c.
true c.
vasomotor c.
visceral motor c.
visceral sensory c.
composite
c. addition technique
c. disk prosthesis
c. index
compound
disease-modifying c.
c. granular corpuscle
c. granule cell
lipophilic c.
c. motor action potential (CMAP)
c. muscle action potential (CMAP)
c. muscle action potential amplitude
c. nerve action potential (CNAP)
ovabain-like c.
porphyrin c.
primary active c.
c. skull fracture
comprehensive
c. assessment
c. evaluation
C. Identification Process, Revised
C. Level of Consciousness Scale
C. Qualifying Examination
c. treatment planning
compressed
c. spectral analysis
c. spectral array
compression
c. amplifier
c. anesthesia
ASIF broad dynamic c.
axial c.
balloon c.
c. of brain
brainstem c.
cauda equina c.
cerebral aqueduct c.
cervical vessel c.
cervicomedullary junction c.
chiasmal c.
epidural cord c.
c. fracture
Harrington rod instrumentation c.
c. instrumentation posterior construct
intervertebral disk c.
nerve c.
c. neuropathy
c. ophthalmodynamometer
optic chiasm c.
optic tract c.
c. paralysis
percutaneous trigeminal nerve c.
c. rod
c. rod treatment
spinal cord c.
c. spring

compression *(continued)*
c. syndrome
thecal sac c.
c. U-rod
c. U-rod instrumentation
ventral medullary c.
compression-rarefaction strain in craniocerebral trauma
compressive
c. mass lesion
c. myelopathy
c. neuropathy
c. rod
c. trigeminal nerve lesion
compromise
adenohypophyseal c.
adrenocorticotropic c.
endocrinological c.
Compton scattering
compulsive
c. drug administration
c. quality
c. reaction
c. spasms and tics
compurgation
computed
c. axial tomography (CAT)
subtraction ictal ethyl cysteinate dimer single photon emission c.
c. tomographic cisternography
c. tomographic metrizamide myelography
c. tomography (CT)
computer
Brown-Roberts-Wells c.
Licox partial pressure of oxygen measuring c.
computer-aided
c.-a. image analysis
c.-a. therapy
Computer-Aided Neurovascular Analysis and Simulation protocol (CANVAS)
computer-assisted
c.-a. EEG signal analysis
c.-a. image-guided system
c.-a. myelography (CAM)
c.-a. neuroendoscopy
c.-a. stereotactic surgery (CASS)
c.-a. volumetric stereotactic approach
c.-a. volumetric stereotactic lesionectomy
computer-controlled
c.-c. neurological stimulation system
c.-c. neurological stimulation system cone
computer-guided therapy
computerized
c. axial tomography
c. axial tomography scanning
c. EEG signal analysis
c. infrared telethermographic imaging
c. tomography scan
COMT
catechol-*O*-methyltransferase
COMT inhibitor
conarium
concealed reflex
concentrate
factor IX complex c.
GABA c.
gamma-aminobutyric acid c.
concentration
brain-derived HVA c.
elevated protein c.
glucose c.
hippocampal monoamine c.
homovanillic acid c.
HVA c.
hydrogen ion c.
impaired c.
interstitial serotonin c.
ligand c.
maximal plasma c.
minimal alveolar c. (MAC)
minimum effective c.
motion c.
plasma glutamate c.
protein c.
serum lipid c.
supratherapeutic c.
concentration-dependent abolition
concentric
c. herniation
c. needle electrode
c. sclerosis
c. visual field defect
concentrica
encephalitis periaxialis c.
leukoencephalitis periaxialis c.
concept
C. bipolar coagulator
body c.
C. hand-held cautery
Heidelberg c.
c. of spiritual coping
three-column c.
von Monakow diaschisis c.
c. of will
Winslow c.
Zanarini c.
conceptual
c. ability

c. limitation
c. planning
c. problem
c. system
conceptualization
clinical c.
Lindamood Auditory C.
spatial c.
conceptualizing
concernment
Concerta
concordant
c. interictal epileptiform abnormality
c. result
concrete
c. operation
c. operational development
c. operational stage
concupiscence
concurrent video-EEG recording
concussion
c. amnesia
brain c.
c. myelitis
spinal cord c.
Standardized Assessment of C.
condensation
mitochondrial c.
c. stimulation
condition
activating c.
amnestic disorder due to a general medical c.
clinical c.
comorbid c.
craniofacial c.
degenerative spine c.
dementia due to hepatic c.
experimental c.
haloperidol c.
heterogeneous c.
hypomyelinating c.
neuromuscular c.
neuropsychiatric c.
noise c.
nonprogressive myoclonus c.
proband c.
respondent c.
REST c.
stimulation c.
c. stimulus (CS)
subcortical c.
treatment c.
underlying c.
conditioned
c. drug response
c. fear association
c. insomnia
c. reflex (CR)
c. stimulation
c. stimulus
conductance
chloride c.
voltage-activated c.
conduction
c. anesthesia
antidromic c.
c. aphasia
avalanche c.
c. block
bone c.
c. delay
ephaptic c.
motor c.
saltatory c.
speed of c.
synaptic c.
c. testing
c. time
c. velocity
conductor
Adson c.
Bailey c.
Davis c.
conduit
peripheral nerve regeneration c.
condylar
c. approach
c. hypoplasia
condyle
c. dissection
c. resection
condylectomy
mandibular c.
cone
bifurcation c.
c. cell of retina
cerebellar pressure c.
computer-controlled neurological stimulation system c.
c. fiber
growth c.

NOTES

cone *(continued)*
implantation c.
C. laminectomy retractor
layer of rods and c.'s
medullary c.
pressure c.
retinal c.
C. ring curette
C. scalp retractor
C. skull punch
C. skull punch forceps
C. skull traction tongs
spinal cord terminal c.
C. suction biopsy curette
C. suction tube
C. ventricular needle
C. wire-twisting forceps
Cone-Grant technique
confabulatory
c. amnesia
c. amnestic state
configuration
Cotrel-Dubousset hook claw c.
triangular base transverse bar c.
venous lake c.
confirmed
angiographically c.
conflict
escalating c.
horizontal c.
intermanual c.
vertical c.
visual-vestibular c.
confluence
common venous c.
c. of sinus
confluens sinuum
confocal laser scanning
conformation
beta B-sheet c.
confrontation
premature c.
c. stage
c. testing
confusion
nocturnal c.
postoperative c.
right-left c.
confusional
c. migraine
c. state
congenita
amyoplasia c.
amyotonia c.
aplasia cutis c.
myotonia c.
paramyotonia c.
congenital
c. anomaly
c. arachnodactyly
c. atonic pseudoparalysis
c. bilateral perisylvian syndrome
c. central hypoventilation syndrome
c. cerebellar atrophy
c. cerebral aneurysm
c. cholesteatoma
c. choreoathetosis
c. cytomegalovirus infection
c. dilation
c. dysplastic angiomatosis
c. dysplastic angiopathy
c. facial diplegia
c. hamartomatosis
c. herpes simplex virus infection
c. hippocampal sclerosis
c. Horner syndrome
c. hydrocephalus
c. hypomyelination neuropathy
c. hypothesis
c. hypothyroidism
c. infratentorial disorder
c. kyphosis
c. malformation
c. muscular dystrophy
c. myasthenia gravis
c. myasthenic syndrome (CMS)
c. myopathy
c. neurosyphilis
c. nystagmus
c. ocular motor apraxia
c. pain c.
c. paramyotonia
c. porencephaly
c. rubella
c. scoliosis
c. sensory neuropathy
c. spastic paraplegia
c. suprabulbar paresis
c. toxoplasmosis
c. tumor
c. varicella
c. virilizing adrenal hyperplasia
congenitalis
alopecia triangularis c.
congestion
brain c.
neurotonic c.
congophilic
c. amyloid
c. amyloid angiopathy
congruence
congruous hemianopia
coni (*pl. of* conus)

conjoined
c. nerve root
c. twins
conjugal
c. tension
c. visitation
conjugate
c. contraversive eye movement
c. fixed gaze
c. horizontal gaze
c. nystagmus
c. paralysis
conjugated eye movement
conjunctiva, pl. **conjunctivae**
decussation of brachia c.
fornix c.
conjunctival
c. cul-de-sac
c. injection
conjunctivi
decussatio brachii c.
conjunctivitis
connection
intracortical c.
monosynaptic c.
neuroanatomic c.
patterning synaptic c.
reciprocal c.
synaptic c.
thalamocortical c.
therapeutic c.
connective
c. tissue
c. tissue disease
connector
adjustable pedicle c.
dual bypass c.
intrinsic transverse c.
longitudinal member to anchor c.
stepdown c.
straight c.
tandem c.
transverse c.
connexin
c. gene
c. 32 protein
connexus interthalamicus
Conradi-Hünermann syndrome
Conradi syndrome
consciously
consciousness
altered c.
arousal component of c.
c. impaired
level of c.
loss of c.
c. stress reaction
threshold of c.
conscious simulation
consensual
c. gaze
c. response pupil
c. understanding
consequence
neurobehavioral c.
psychological c.
conservation
energy c.
conservative cutoff score
consistent
c. aura
c. delivery
c. response
console
Dissectron ultrasonic neurosurgical aspirator c.
Marconi Medical Systems c.
consolidation
memory c.
Consortium
Childhood Brain Tumor C.
C. to Establish a Registry for Alzheimer's Disease
European Brain Injury C.
C. of Neurology Clerkship Director (CNCD)
North American Brain Tumor C. (NABTC)
Consta
Risperdal C.
constant
c. current stimulator
relaxation c.
T_1 relaxation c.
T_2 relaxation c.
time c.
Constantinidis-Wisniewski syndrome
constitutional medicine
constrained induced therapy
constraint-induced therapy
constrastimulus

NOTES

constriction of cognition
construct
anterior c.
AO dynamic compression plate c.
c. AO fixateur interne
compression instrumentation posterior c.
double-rod c.
Edwards modular system bridging sleeve c.
Edwards modular system compression c.
Edwards modular system distraction-lordosis c.
Edwards modular system kyphoreduction c.
Edwards modular system neutralization c.
Edwards modular system rod-sleeve c.
Edwards modular system scoliosis c.
Edwards modular system spondylo c.
Edwards modular system standard sleeve c.
Guiot-Talairach c.
hook-to-screw L4-S1 compression c.
iliosacral and iliac fixation c.
pedicle screw c.
posterior c.
psychological c.
c. research
rod-hook c.
screw-to-screw compression c.
segmental compression c.
single-rod c.
spondylo c.
Texas Scottish Rite Hospital double-rod c.
titanium c.
TSRH double-rod c.
TSRH pedicle screw-laminar claw c.
upper cervical spine anterior c.
upper cervical spine posterior c.
Wiltse system double-rod c.
Wiltse system H c.
Wiltse system single-rod c.
construction
c. ability
c. apraxia
endocentric c.
visuospatial c.
constructional
c. ability
c. agraphia
c. apraxia
c. apraxis
c. impairment
Constulose
consumption
brain oxygen c.
nervous c.
consumptive coagulopathy
contact
c. ceptor
c. compressive forceps
c. receptor
c. sense
contained disk
container exercise
containing
dopa-decarboxylase c.
content
carotid c.
central dopamine c.
context
space c.
spatial-temporal c.
time c.
contextual
c. association
c. cause
C. Memory Test
contiguity disorder aphasia
contiguous
c. nonoverlapping axial CT
c. supramarginal gyrus
c. voxel
continence
fecal c.
urine c.
contingency coefficient
contingent negative variation
continua
epilepsia partialis c.
hemicrania c.
continuous
c. amnesia
c. anatomical passive exerciser
c. approach
c. cognitive testing
c. daytime drowsiness
c. electromyographic recording
c. extravascular infusion (CEI)
c. inflammatory process
c. intrathecal baclofen infusion
c. intravenous infusion
c. intravenous regional anesthesia (CIVRA)
c. maintenance medication
c. muscle activity syndrome
c. muscle fiber activity syndrome

c. on-line recording
c. performance task-accuracy
c. performance task-efficiency
c. positive airway pressure (CPAP)
c. tremor
c. variable
c. venous oximetry
c. video-EEG monitoring (CCTV-EEG)
C. Visual Memory Test, Revised
c. wave (CW)

continuous-wave
c.-w. Doppler
c.-w. Doppler imaging
c.-w. technique

contour
Cupid's bow c.
C. Emboli artificial embolization device
field c.
illusionary c. (IC)
pitch c.
real c. (RC)

contoured
c. anterior spinal plate
c. anterior spinal plate drill guide
c. anterior spinal plate technique

contouring
Isola spinal implant system longitudinal member c.

contraception

contraction
carpopedal c.
clonic c.
c. fasciculation
fibrillary c.
maximal voluntary c.
maximum voluntary c. (MVC)
myotatic c.
nonepileptic myoclonic c.
paradoxical c.
Rossolimo c.
tetanic c.
tonic c.
twitch c.

contractual alliance

contracture
c. arachnodactyly
caffeine-induced c.
Dupuytren c.
fixed c.
functional c.
myotatic c.
organic c.
Skoog release of Dupuytren c.
Volkmann c.

contrafissura

contralateral
c. anesthesia
c. biopsy
c. eye
c. facial paralysis
c. hemiparesis
c. hemiplegia
c. homonymous hemianopia
c. loss
c. monocular nystagmus
c. reflex
c. routing of signal
c. routing of sound
c. sign
c. somatosensory cortex
c. straight leg raising test
c. tactical hypesthesia
c. temporary artery
c. transcallosal approach

contralesional
c. hand
c. hemifield

contrapulsion of saccade

contrast
c. angiography
c. density
c. dye reaction
c. enhancement
c. enhancement imaging
gadolinium c.
inherent c.
iodinated radiographic c.
c. media
paramagnetic c.
c. sensitivity reduction
soft-tissue c.
spontaneous echo c.

contrast echocardiography magnetic resonance angiography (CE MRA)

contrast-enhanced
c.-e. CT
c.-e. CT scan
c.-e. MR angiography (CE MRA)
c.-e. MRI

NOTES

contrast-enhanced · convexobasia

contrast-enhanced *(continued)*
c.-e. MR image
c.-e. MR imaging
contrast-to-noise ratio (CNR)
Contraves
C. stand
C. type floorstand
contrecoup
c. contusion
fracture by c.
c. injury
c. injury of brain
contretemps
contribution
extracellular c.
intracellular c.
therapeutic c.
control
aberrant autocrine c.
airway c.
c. cell proliferation
diffuse noxious inhibitory c. (DNIC)
double visual c.
3D positional c.
Engel classification system for postoperative seizure c. class I–IV
feeling of c.
FlexDial stimulus c.
graphomotor c.
idiodynamic c.
immediate c.
impaired c.
inadequate impulse c.
motor c.
c. picture-caption pair
reflex c.
sense of c.
synergic c.
televised radiofluoroscopic c.
tonic c.
tonic inhibitor c.
vestibuloequilibratory c.
controlled
c. hypothermia
c. mechanical ventilation (CMV)
c. medication trial
C. Oral Word Association (COWA)
C. Oral Word Association test
Contugno disease
contumacious
contumacy
contumelious
contusio cerebri
contusion
brain c.
cerebral c.
contrecoup c.
facial c.
gliding c.
hemorrhagic c.
scalp c.
spinal cord c.
wind c.
conus, pl. **coni**
c. medullaris
c. medullaris lesion
c. medullaris root avulsion
c. medullaris syndrome
c. perimedullary arteriovenous fistula
c. terminalis
convection-enhanced drug delivery
conventional
c. factor analysis
c. fractionated irradiation
c. neuroleptic
c. neuroleptic agent
c. neuroleptic drug
c. neuroleptic treatment
c. pharmacotherapy
convergence
c. abnormality
c. insufficiency
c. nucleus of Perlia
c. spasm
convergence-divergence pattern
convergence-evoked nystagmus
convergence-projection theory
convergence-retraction nystagmus
convergent
c. beam irradiation
c. strabismus
Conversational Skills Rating Scale
converse ocular dipping
conversion
metabolic c.
c. reaction
c. V profile
converter
analog-to-digital c.
digital-to-analog c.
converting enzyme inhibitor (CEI)
Convery polyarticular disability index
convexity
cerebral c.
cortical c.
c. meningioma
c. metastatic tumor
convexobasia

convolution
angular c.
anterior central c.
ascending frontal c.
ascending parietal c.
Broca c.
callosal c.
cingulate c.
first temporal c.
Heschl c.
hippocampal c.
inferior frontal c.
inferior temporal c.
middle frontal c.
middle temporal c.
occipitotemporal c.
posterior central c.
second temporal c.
superior frontal c.
superior temporal c.
supramarginal c.
third temporal c.
transitional c.
transverse temporal c.
Zuckerkandl c.
convulsant threshold
convulsion
autosomal dominant febrile c.
benign familial neonatal c.
benign infantile familial c.
benign neonatal c.
clonic c.
complex febrile c.
coordinate c.
eclamptic c.
epileptiform c.
ether c.
febrile c.
generalized tonic-clonic c.
GTC c.
hysterical c.
hysteroid c.
immediate posttraumatic c.
infantile c.
mimetic c.
mimic c.
paroxysmal c.
salaam c.
static c.
tetanic c.
tonic c.
uremic c.
convulsive
c. reflex
c. seizure
c. state
c. status epilepticus
c. syncope
c. therapy
c. tic
convulsivus
status c.
Cook
C. mini-compression balloon catheter
C. stereotactic guide
cooling
autocerebral c.
brain c.
c. helmet
nasopharyngeal c.
whole-body c.
CoolLine intravascular device
Coombs test
cooperativity
criterion of c.
Cooper method
coordinate
c. convulsion
MEG sensorimotor mapping c.
Z c.
coordinated reflex
coordination
fluid c.
interlimb c.
c. testing
coordinatus
spasmus c.
Copaxone
coping
concept of spiritual c.
maladaptive c.
c. response
copodyskinesia
copolymer-1
glatirama c.
glatiramer c.
copper
c. deposition
serum c.

C

NOTES

copper *(continued)*
c. sulfate hydrogel
c. wire effect
copper-constantan thermocouple
coprodaeum, coprodeum
coprolalia
tic convulsive with c.
coprophemia
coproporphyria
hereditary c.
urine c.
copropraxia
copula
coracobrachialis
branch to c.
coral
madreporic c.
scleractinian c.
cord
accessory portion of spinal c.
anterior column of spinal c.
anterior median fissure of spinal c.
anterolateral column of spinal c.
apex of dorsal horn of spinal c.
apex of posterior horn of spinal c.
arachnoid of spinal c.
autonomic column of spinal c.
base of dorsal horn of spinal c.
base of posterior horn of spinal c.
Bergmann c.
c. bladder
central gelatinous substance of spinal c.
cervical enlargement of spinal c.
cervical part of spinal c.
cervical segments of spinal c. [C1–C8]
coccygeal part of spinal c.
coccygeal segment of spinal c.
cornu of spinal c.
dentate ligament of spinal c.
dorsal column of spinal c.
dorsal funicular column of spinal c.
dorsal median fissure of spinal c.
dura mater of spinal c.
c. embarrassment
fiber tract of spinal c.
gelatinous substance of posterior horn of spinal c.
glioma of the spinal c.
gracile fasciculus of spinal c.
intermediate column of spinal c.
intermediate zone of spinal c.
intermediolateral cell column of spinal c.
lateral column of spinal c.
lateral funiculus of spinal c.
Lissauer tract of spinal c.
lumbar enlargement of spinal c.
lumbar part of spinal c.
lumbosacral enlargement of spinal c.
phrenic nucleus of anterior column of spinal c.
posterior column of spinal c.
posterior median fissure of spinal c.
posterior median sulcus of spinal c.
posteromedian column of spinal c.
postmortem spinal c.
segment of spinal c.
spinal c.
subacute combined degeneration of the spinal c.
c. syndrome
tethered spinal c.
thoracic part of spinal c.
ventral column of spinal c.
ventral fasciculus proprius of spinal c.
ventral median fissure of spinal c.
vocal c.
Weitbrecht c.
white column of spinal c.
white commissure of spinal c.
white substance of spinal c.
Wilde c.
Willis c.
cordectomy
cordis
C. Brite Tip guiding catheter
chorea c.
C. implantable drug reservoir device
C. Secor implantable pump
Cordis-Hakim
C.-H. shunt system
C.-H. valve
cordopexy
cordotomy
anterolateral c.
c. hook holder
open c.
percutaneous c.
posterior column c.
spinothalamic c.
stereotactic c.
core
c. assessment program for intracerebral transplantation (CAPIT)
central transactional c.

c. characteristic
c. cognitive disturbance
c. consensual understanding
c. pain
c. problem
c. temperature
c. temperature fluctuation
corectopia
coregistered image
coregistration
multimodality image c.
coreoathetoid movement
Corgard
corkscrew dural hook
cornea
cloudy c.
corneal
c. anesthesia
c. anoxia
c. reflex
c. reflex testing
c. respiration
Cornell Scale for Depression in Dementia
corneomandibular reflex
corneomental reflex
corneopterygoid reflex
corn-picker's pupil
cornu, pl. **cornua**
c. ammonis
c. anterius
c. anterius medullae spinalis
c. anterius ventriculi lateralis
c. dorsalis medullae spinalis
c. frontale ventriculi lateralis
c. inferius
c. inferius cartilaginis thyroideae
c. inferius hiatus saphenus
c. inferius marginis
c. inferius ventriculi
c. inferius ventriculi lateralis
c. laterale
c. laterale medullae spinalis
cornua of lateral ventricle
c. occipitale ventriculi lateralis
c. posterius
c. posterius medullae spinalis
c. posterius ventriculi
c. posterius ventriculi lateralis
c. of spinal cord
c. temporale ventriculi lateralis
c. ventrale medullae spinalis
cornucommissural
cornuradicular zone
cornus
caput c.
corona, pl. **coronae**
c. radiata
Zinn c.
coronal
c. cleft vertebra
c. craniectomy
c. insonation plane
c. orientation
c. plane deformity
c. plane deformity sagittal translation
c. scalp incision
c. section
c. suture
c. synostosis
coronary
c. artery bypass grafting
c. atherosclerosis
coronata
Cryptococcus c.
coronavirus
corpectomy
anterior c.
cervical c.
median c.
c. model
Stackable Cage c.
vertebral body c.
corpora (*pl. of* corpus)
corporal agnosia
corporeal
corporis
corpses
corpulence
corpus, pl. **corpora**
c. amygdaloideum
c. aorticum
corpora arenacea
corpora bigemina
c. callosal impingement
c. callosotomy
c. callosum
c. callosum agenesis
c. callosum dysgenesis
corpora cavernosa

NOTES

corpus *(continued)*
c. dentatum
c. fimbriatum
c. fimbriatum hippocampus
c. fornicis
c. geniculatum externum
c. geniculatum internum
c. geniculatum laterale
c. geniculatum mediale
c. juxtarestiforme
c. luteum
c. luysii
c. mamillare
c. medullare cerebelli
c. nuclei caudati
c. olivare
c. paraterminale
c. pineale
c. pontobulbare
corpora quadrigemina
c. quadrigeminum anterius
c. quadrigeminum posterius
c. restiforme
c. striatum
c. striatum syndrome
c. subthalamicum
c. trapezoideum
corpuscallostomy
corpuscle
articular c.
axile c.
axis c.
bulboid c.
chorea c.
chromophil c.
compound granular c.
Dogiel c.
genital c.
Gluge c.
Golgi c.
Golgi-Mazzoni c.
Herbst c.
Krause c.
lamellated c.
lingual c.
Mazzoni c.
Meissner c.
Merkel c.
oval c.
pacchionian c.
Pacini c.
pacinian c.
Purkinje c.
Ruffini c.
Schwalbe c.
tactile c.
taste c.
terminal nerve c.
Timofeew c.
touch c.
Valentin c.
Vater c.
Vater-Pacini c.
corpusculum, pl. **corpuscula**
c. articulare
corpuscula articularia
corpuscula bulboidea
c. bulboidum
c. genitale
corpuscula lamellosa
c. lamellosum
corpuscula nervosa terminalia
c. nervosum terminale
corpuscula tactus
c. tactus
correction
anterior c.
King type IV curve posterior c.
kyphosis c.
mechanism of c.
rotational c.
small volume c. (SVC)
surgical c.
correctitude
correlate
anatomical c.
biologic c.
clinical c.
differential c.
correlation
image c.
intraclass c.
item-total c.
c. method
potential c.
c. time
corridor
transcallosal interforniceal c.
corset, corsette
lumbosacral c.
Warm 'n Form lumbosacral c.
CORT
corticosteroid
Cor-Tech guidance to stereotatic head frame
Cortef
cortex, pl. **cortices**
adrenal c.
agranular c.
amorphous fraction of adrenal c.
anterior cingulate c.
articular c.
association c.
auditory association c.

calcarine c.
cellular layers of c.
cerebellar c.
c. cerebellaris
c. cerebelli
cerebral c.
c. cerebralis
c. cerebri
c. circuit
contralateral somatosensory c.
dorsal premotor c.
dorsolateral prefrontal c.
dysgranular c.
eloquent c.
entorhinal c.
epileptogenic c.
excitomotor c.
extrastriate visual c.
extrastriate V5/MT c.
frontotemporal c.
fusiform cell of cerebral c.
ganglionic layer of cerebellar c.
ganglionic layer of cerebral c.
granular layer of cerebellar c.
granular layer of cerebral c.
gustatory c.
hemispheric hippocampal c.
heteromodal association c.
heterotypic c.
homotypic c.
inferior anterocaudal cingulate c.
inferior prefrontal c.
inferior temporal c.
insular c.
ipsilateral somatosensory c.
ipsilateral temporal c.
lamina of the cerebral c.
laminated c.
language associated c.
lateral orbitofrontal c.
layer of cerebellar c.
layer of cerebral c.
limbic c.
medial frontal c.
medial orbitofrontal c.
medial prefrontal c. (mPFC)
medial temporal c.
mesial epileptogenic c.
mesial-frontal c.
molecular layer of cerebellar c.
molecular layer of cerebral c.
motor c.
multiform layer of cerebral c.
multimodal association c.
nonolfactory c.
occipital c.
occipitotemporal c.
olfactory c.
opercular c.
orbital prefrontal c.
orbitofrontal c.
paralimbic c.
parastriate c.
parietal c.
periamygdaloid c.
perilesional inhibitory c.
perirolandic parietal c.
peristriate c.
perisylvian c.
piriform c.
plexiform layer of cerebral c.
posterior language c.
posterior parietal c. (PPC)
postinduction occipital c.
prefrontal c.
preinduction occipital c.
premotor c.
prepiriform c.
primary auditory c.
primary sensorimotor c.
primary sensory c.
primary somatosensory c.
primary visual c.
primates motor c.
pyriform c.
right basilar mesial
 temporoparietal c.
rolandic c.
rostral medial prefrontal c.
secondary sensory c.
secondary somatosensory c.
secondary visual c.
sensory c.
somatic sensory c.
somatosensory c.
somesthetic c.
stellate cell of cerebral c.
striate c.
subcortical band
 heterotopia/double c.
subcortical ectopic c.
sulcal prefrontal c.

C

NOTES

cortex *(continued)*
supplementary motor c.
temporal c.
unimodal association c.
ventromedial prefrontal c.
vertebral body anterior c.
visual association c.
zonal layer of cerebral c.
Cortexplorer cerebral blood flow monitor
Corti
C. cell
C. ganglion
C. organ
C. pillar
pillar cell of C.
C. rod
cortical
c. achromia
c. activity
c. amygdaloid nucleus
c. aphasia
c. apraxia
c. area
c. arousal
c. atrophy
c. audiometry
c. blindness
c. convexity
c. deafness
c. dementia
c. disconnection syndrome
c. dysgenesis
c. dysplasia
c. epilepsy
c. epileptogenic focus
c. functioning
c. gray matter
c. gray matter deficit
c. gray region
c. hamartoma
c. incision coronary dilator
c. infarction
c. input
c. language circuitry
c. lesion
c. Lewy body
c. malformation
c. mapping
c. mapping of memory function
c. metabolism
c. microcirulatory flow
c. microdysgenesia
c. motor output
c. myoclonus
c. neuritic plaque
c. obliteration
c. organization
c. pathology
c. plasticity
c. plate
c. pyramidal neuron
c. reorganization
c. resection
c. screw
c. seizure focus
c. sensibility
c. sensory loss
c. somatosensory evoked potential
c. spreading depression (CSD)
c. structure
c. substance of cerebellum
c. sulcus
c. syndrome
c. tissue
c. transient ischemia
c. tuber
c. undercutting
c. vein
c. venous thrombosis
c. volume
cortical-basal ganglionic degeneration
corticalis
agenesia c.
nucleus amygdalae c.
pars c.
corticalization
cortical-striatal-pallidal-thalamic neural circuit
corticectomy
frontal c.
occipital c.
parietal c.
cortices (*pl. of* cortex)
corticifugal
corticipetal
corticis
corticoafferent
corticoautonomic
corticobasal
c. ganglia-cortical parallel loop
c. ganglion degeneration
c. ganglionic degeneration
c. ganglionic-thalamocortical loop
corticobasilar ganglionic degeneration
corticobasoganglionic degeneration
corticobulbar
c. deficit
c. fiber
c. motor neuron
c. pathway
c. tract
corticobulbaris
tractus c.

corticocancellous strut
corticocerebellum
corticodiencephalic
corticoefferent
corticofugal pathway
corticography
corticohypothalamic tract
corticomedial
corticomeningeal angiomatosis
corticomesencephalic
c. fiber
c. tract
corticomesencephalicae
fibrae c.
corticonucleares
fibrae c.
corticopeduncular
corticopetal
corticopontinae
fibrae c.
corticopontine
c. fiber
c. tract
corticopontini
tractus c.
corticopontocerebellar
corticoreticulares
fibrae c.
corticorubral
c. fiber
c. tract
corticorubrales
fibrae c.
corticospinal
c. atrophy
c. axon
c. disease
c. fiber
c. motor neuron
c. motor pathway
c. motor system dysfunction
c. pathway lesion
c. tract
corticospinales
fibrae c.
corticospinalis
tractus c.
corticosteroid (CORT)
oral c.
postoperative c.
c. therapy
corticostriatal slice
corticostriatopallidothalamocortical (CSPTC)
corticothalamicae
fibrae c.
corticothalamic fiber
corticotomy
Ilizarov c.
subperiosteal c.
corticotroph cell
corticotrophic axis
corticotropin
corticotropin-releasing
c.-r. factor
c.-r. hormone (CRH)
cortisol
c. level
c. and sodium succinate
cortisone acetate
cortistatin
Cortone acetate
Corynebacterium diphtheriae
cosegregate
Cosman-Roberts-Wells
C.-R.-W. stereotactic frame
C.-R.-W. stereotactic ring
C.-R.-W. stereotactic system
cosmology
costal arch reflex
costaricensis
Angiostrongylus c.
Costen syndrome
costimulatory
c. signal
c. stimulus
costocervical artery
costoclavicular syndrome
costopectoral reflex
costotransversectomy
c. approach
posterolateral c.
costotransverse ligament
costovertebral ligament
cosyntropin
cotinine
serum c.
cotransmitter
peptide c.
Cotrel
C. pedicle screw

NOTES

Cotrel *(continued)*
C. pedicle screw fixation strength
C. pedicle screw rigidity
Cotrel-Dubousset (C-D)
C.-D. distraction system
C.-D. dynamic transverse traction device
C.-D. fixation
C.-D. hook claw configuration
C.-D. pedicle screw instrumentation
C.-D. pedicular instrumentation
C.-D. rod
C.-D. rod flexibility
C.-D. screw-rod system
C.-D. spinal instrumentation
co-trimoxazole
Cotte
C. operation
C. presacral neurectomy
Cottle
C. elevator
C. knife
Cottle-Neivert retractor
cotton
oxidized c.
c. pad
c. paddies
c. pledget
c. wool sign
c. wrap
cottonoid
c. covering
c. pledget
cotton-wool spot
cotunnii
aqueductus c.
Cotunnius
C. aqueduct
C. canal
C. disease
C. nerve
couch
Boston neurosurgical c.
Siemens c.
couch-mounted head frame
cough
habit c.
c. headache
c. reflex
c. syncope
trigeminal c.
coughing
c. center
c. sign
council
Medical Research C. (MRC)
count
absolute neutrophil c. (ANC)
complete blood c. (CBC)
platelet c.
radioactive c.
white blood cell c.
counteracting impulsivity
countercurrent immunoelectrophoresis test
counterintuitive relationship
Counterpoint electromyograph
countertransference
counting disruption
coup injury of brain
Couples BrainMap
coupling
excitation-contraction c.
G-protein c.
spin-spin c.
courage
Dutch C.
courant
au c.
courbe
Cournand arteriogram needle
Cournand-Grino arteriogram needle
course
chronic c.
developmental c.
Functional Obstacle C.
c. of illness measure
long-term c.
rapid fluctuating c.
recurrent c.
temporal c.
Courtship Analysis
couvade crapulent
COV
coefficient of variation
covariation
intersegmental c.
cover
Accu-Flo polyethylene bur hole c.
Accu-Flo silicone rubber bur hole c.
bur hole c.
c. test
titanium mini bur hole c.
coverage
neocortical c.
covering
cottonoid c.
titanium mini bur hole c.
COWA
Controlled Oral Word Association
Cowden disease
Cowdry inclusion body type A, B

Cowdry-type intranuclear inclusion body
CO_2-withdrawal seizure test
COX
cyclooxygenase
COX-1
cyclooxygenase-1
COX-2
cyclooxygenase-2
COX-2 inhibitor
***Coxiella burnetii* infection**
Cox regression analysis
coxsackie encephalitis
coxsackievirus
c. A, B
c. infection paralytic syndrome
c. meningitis
CP
cerebellopontine
CPA
cerebellopontine angle
CPAP
continuous positive airway pressure
nasal C.
CPEO
chronic progressive external ophthalmoplegia
CPH
chronic paroxysmal hemicrania
CPH-tic syndrome
CPPD
calcium pyrophosphate dihydrate
CPT
current perception threshold
CR
conditioned reflex
Sinemet CR
CRA
cis-retinoic acid
13-*cis*-retinoic acid
13-CRA
13-*cis*-retinoic acid
cracked pot sign
crack-like vessel
crackling
parchment c.
craft palsy
Cragg thrombolytic brush
Craig vertebral body biopsy instrument
cramp
accessory c.
c. benign fasciculation
benign fasciculation with c.
intermittent c.
miner's c.
muscle c.
musician's c.
nocturnal leg c.
pianist's c.
seamstress's c.
shaving c.
stoker's c.
tailor's c.
violinist's c.
waiter's c.
watchmaker's c.
writer's c.
crania (*pl. of* cranium)
cranial
c. aneurysm
c. anomaly
c. arachnoid
c. arachnoid mater
c. arteritis
c. artery
c. autonomic
c. autonomic symptom
c. bifida
c. bone fixation plate
c. bone graft
c. capacity
c. cerebellar peduncle
c. computed tomography
c. cracked pot sign
c. cuff
c. dermal sinus
c. dysmorphia
c. epidural abscess
c. extension
c. flexure
c. fracture
c. ganglion
c. insufflation
c. Jacobs hook
c. motor nucleus
c. muscle
c. nerve
c. nerve abnormality
c. nerve congenital disorder
c. nerve damage
c. nerve deficit
c. nerve dissection
c. nerve examination

NOTES

cranial *(continued)*
c. nerve heredodegenerative disease
c. nerve manipulation
c. nerve monitoring
c. nerve neoplasm
c. nerve palsy
c. nerve postinfectious disorder
c. nerve regeneration
c. nerve repair
c. nerve trauma
c. neuralgia
c. neuropathy
c. olivary nucleus
c. osteomyelitis
c. osteopetrosis
c. osteosynthesis
c. osteosynthesis system
c. perforator
c. perfusion pressure
c. pia mater
c. plating system
c. polyneuritis
c. puncture
c. radiosurgery
c. reflex
c. rongeur
c. rongeur forceps
c. root
c. settling
c. suture
c. synostosis
c. ultrasonography
c. ultrasound
c. vault
c. vault trephination
c. venous obstruction
craniales
nervi c.
radices c.
cranialis
arachnoidea mater c.
arachnoid mater c.
frenulum veli medullaris c.
ganglion sensorium nervi c.
nucleus nervi c.
nucleus olivaris c.
pia mater c.
cranialium
nuclei nervorum c.
cranialization
craniamphitomy
craniectomy
bilateral c.
coronal c.
decompressive c.
linear c.
metopic c.
partial-thickness c.
retromastoid suboccipital c.
retrosigmoid c.
suboccipital c.
cranii
osteoporosis circumscripta c.
periostitis interna c.
pneumatocele c.
cranioblade
Acra-Cut c.
Codman c.
Spiral Flute c.
craniobuccal cyst
CranioCap custom-made cranial orthosis
craniocardiac reflex
craniocele
craniocerebellocardiac syndrome
craniocerebral
c. drug trauma
trauma c.
craniocervical
c. junction
c. plate
c. region
craniofacial
c. angle
c. condition
c. dysjunction
c. dysostosis
c. dysraphism
c. malformation
c. osteotomy
c. reconstruction
c. remodeling
c. resection
c. surgery
craniofrontonasal dysplasia
craniognomy
craniolacunia
craniology
Gall c.
craniomalacia
circumscribed c.
craniomaxillofacial plating system
craniomeningocele
craniometaphyseal dysplasia
craniometry
cranioorbital
c. deformity
c. zygomatic craniotomy
craniopathy
craniopharyngeal
c. canal
c. duct tumor
craniopharyngioma
ameloblastomatous c.
cystic papillomatous c.

intrasellar c.
monocystic c.
cranioplasty
acrylic c.
alloplastic c.
aluminum c.
cartilage c.
metallic c.
methylmethacrylate c.
c. plate
rib c.
tantalum c.
vascularized split calvarial c.
craniopuncture
craniorachischisis
craniosacral
c. nervous system
c. vault (CV)
c. vault four (CV4)
cranioschisis
craniosclerosis
cranioscopy
craniosinus fistula
craniospinal
c. meningioma
c. sensory ganglion
c. space
craniostenosis
craniosynostosis
lambdoid c.
sagittal c.
craniotabes
craniotome
Anspach c.
Caspar c.
Freiberg c.
Hall neurosurgical c.
Midas Rex c.
Mira Mark V c.
Smith air c.
craniotomy
attached c.
bifrontal c.
cranioorbital zygomatic c.
CT-assisted stereotactic c.
c. cut
detached c.
endoscope-assisted c.
c. flap
frontal c.
frontoorbitozygomatic c.
frontotemporal c.
frontotemporoparietal c.
keyhole c.
open stereotactic c.
orbital zygomatic c.
osteoplastic c.
parietal c.
parietooccipital c.
posterior fossa c.
pterional c.
radical decompressive c.
retromastoid c.
right parietal occipital vertex c.
right temporoparietal c.
stereotactic-guided c.
stereotactic microsurgical c.
subfrontal c.
suboccipital c.
suprabrow transorbital roof c.
supratentorial c.
temporooccipital c.
trephine c.
Yasargil c.
craniotonoscopy
craniotopography
craniotrypesis
craniovertebral junction
cranium, pl. **crania**
beaten copper c.
bifid c.
c. bifidum
c. bifidum cysticum
c. bifidum occultum
cranium-affixed fiducial
crankshaft clip
crapulent
couvade c.
crapulous
crash induction of anesthesia
Crawford dural elevator
CRD
complex repetitive discharge
CRD on electromyogram
C-reactive
C.-r. protein
C.-r. protein test
crease
hand palmar c.
palmar c.
simian c.

NOTES

creatine
c. kinase (CK)
c. kinase equilibrium
c. kinase MB fraction (CK-MB)
c. phosphokinase
creatinine
c. clearance
c. deficiency syndrome
c. kinase serum level
urinary c.
creation
kyphosis c.
lordosis c.
creative
C. Behavior Inventory
C. Reasoning Test
C. Styles Inventory
CREB binding protein
Cre + Cho ratio
Creed dissector
creeping palsy
Cree Questionnaire
cremasteric reflex
crepitance
crepuscular state
crescendo
c. sleep
c. transient ischemic attack
crescentic lobule of cerebellum
CREST
calcinosis, Raynaud phenomenon, esophageal motility disorders, sclerodactyly, and telangiectasia
CREST syndrome
crest
acoustic c.
acousticofacial c.
ampullary c.
cap of the ampullary c.
falciform c.
ganglionic c.
neural c.
neuroepithelium of ampullary c.
supramastoid c.
transverse c.
triangular c.
trigeminal c.
vestibular c.
c. of vestibule
Creutzfeldt-Jakob disease (CJD)
CRF knockout mice
CRH
corticotropin-releasing hormone
cribalis
status c.
criblé
état c.
cribriform plate
cribrosa
lamina c.
macula c.
cribrosae
maculae c.
cribrosus
status c.
Crichton-Browne sign
cricoarytenoid ankylosis
cricoid ring
cricopharyngeal achalasia
cricothyrotomy
cri du chat syndrome
Crigler-Najjar
C.-N. disease
C.-N. syndrome
Crile
C. artery forceps
C. clamp
C. gasserian ganglion knife
C. gasserian ganglion knife and dissector
C. head traction
C. hemostat
C. needle holder
C. nerve hook
C. nerve hook and dissector
C. retractor
crisis, pl. **crises**
adrenal c.
cholinergic c.
gastric c.
laryngeal c.
myasthenic c.
nephralgic c.
oculocephalogyric c.
oculogyric c.
parkinsonian c.
spondylolisthetic c.
tabetic c.
tumarcin c.
tyramine-induced hypertensive c.
visceral c.
crisnatol
crispation
crista, pl. **cristae**
c. ampullaris
c. basilaris ductus
c. basilaris ductus cochlearis
c. galli
c. quarta
c. transversa
c. transversalis
c. transversa meatus acustici interni

c. triangularis
c. vestibuli
criterion, pl. **criteria**
c. of associativity
Bartel criteria
clinical c.
c. of cooperativity
dependence c.
diagnostic c.
c. F
field-tested c.
Hunt and Hess criteria
c. level
level-of-care c.
Marsden and Harrison criteria
Mulholland and Gunn criteria
Nyquist sampling criteria
patient placement c.
a priori c.
criteria of Rechtschaffen
criteria of Rechtschaffen and Kales
restrictive c.
criteria of Rowland
c. of specificity
traditional circulatory criteria (TCC)
c. validity
Volpe criteria
White and Panjabi criteria
***Crithidia* IFA test**
critical
c. illness myopathy
c. illness polyneuropathy
c. perfusion
Criticare
criticus
status c.
Crixivan
CRLR
calcitonin receptor-like receptor
crocidismus
Crockard
C. retractor
C. transoral clip applier
crocodile tears syndrome
Crohn disease
Cronbach alpha
Crooke
C. granule
C. hyaline change
C. hyalinization
cross
Ranvier c.
cross-aggregation
cross-bracing
spinal rod c.-b.
Wiltse system c.-b.
crossed
c. adductor jerk
c. adductor reflex
c. adductor sign
c. anesthesia
c. aphasia
c. coil
c. extension reflex
c. eye
c. hemianesthesia
c. hemiplegia
c. knee jerk
c. knee reflex
c. laterality
c. lens
c. paralysis
c. phrenic phenomenon
c. pyramidal tract
c. reflex of pelvis
c. spinoadductor reflex
crossed immunoelectrophoresis
crossed-screw fixation
cross-facial nerve graft anastomosis
cross-flow reserve
crossing
Mistichelli c.
cross-legged
c.-l. clip
c.-l. progression
crosslink
Edwards modular system rod c.
Galveston fixation with TSRH c.
c. gamma
Texas Scottish Rite Hospital c.
cross-modal fluency
cross-over study
cross-sectional
c.-s. area (CSA)
c.-s. assessment
c.-s. component
c.-s. evaluation
c.-s. experimental study design
c.-s. image
c.-s. research

C

NOTES

cross-sectional *(continued)*
c.-s. snapshot
c.-s. study
crossway
sensory c.
Crouzon
C. disease
C. syndrome
CR/OV
OncoScint C.
Crowe sign
Crow-Fukase syndrome
crown
Bremer halo c.
radiate c.
crown-heel length (CH)
crown-rump length
CRP
cAMP receptor protein
CRS-39
cruciata
hemianesthesia c.
hemiplegia c.
cruciate
c. eminence
c. ligament
cruciform
c. eminence
c. slit valve
cruciformis
eminentia c.
crura (*pl. of* crus)
crural
c. ataxia
c. cistern
c. interosseus nerve
c. monoplegia
c. paresis
c. plexus
cruralis
cisterna c.
cruris
nervus interosseus c.
tegmen c.
crus, pl. **crura**
c. anterius capsulae
c. anterius capsulae internae
cerebellum superior c.
c. cerebri
common c.
c. fornicis
c. of fornix
c. II
internal capsule anterior c.
internal capsule posterior c.
crura membranacea
crura membranacea ampullaria
c. membranaceum commune
c. membranaceum commune ductus semicircularis
c. membranaceum simplex
c. membranaceum simplex ductus semicircularis
crura ossea
crura ossea canales semicirculares
c. posterius capsulae
c. posterius capsulae internae
c. primum lobuli ansiformis
crush injury
crusotomy
crutch
c. palsy
c. paralysis
Crutchfield
C. carotid artery clamp
C. drill point
C. hand drill
C. skeletal traction tongs
C. skull traction tongs
Crutchfield-Raney skull traction tongs
Cruveilhier
C. atrophy
C. disease
C. paralysis
C. plexus
cruzi
Trypanosoma c.
Cruz trypanosomiasis
CRW
CRW arc system
CRW base frame
CRW head frame
CRW stereotactic system
CRx Diamond valve
cry
epileptic c.
c. reflex
cryalgesia
cryanesthesia
cryesthesia
crying-cat syndrome
crymodynia
cryoanalgesia
cryocooler assembly
Cryocup ice massager
cryoglobulinemia
cryoglobulinemic vasculitis
cryohypophysectomy
transphenoidal c.
cryolesion
brain c.
cryomagnet
cryomicrotome sectioning
cryopallidectomy

cryoprecipitate coagulum
cryopreserved tissue
cryoprobe
cryopulvinectomy
cryospasm
cryostat
cryosurgery
cryothalamectomy
cryothalamotomy
cryptic
c. arteriovenous malformation
c. cerebrovascular malformation
c. vascular malformation
cryptococcal
c. antigen
granuloma c.
c. infection
c. meningitis
c. organism
c. polysaccharide antigen test
c. spondylitis
cryptococcoma
cryptococcosis
intracranial c.
Cryptococcus
C. albicans
C. coronata
C. infection
C. neoformans
cryptogenic
c. drop attack
c. hemifacial spasm
c. infarction
c. infection
c. late-onset epilepsy
c. myoclonic epilepsy
c. partial epilepsy
cryptomerorachischisis
cryptotia
crystal
cholesterol c.
crystallin
crystalline birefringence
crystallization
symptom c.
crytotetany
CS
condition stimulus
CSA
cross-sectional area
CSD
catscratch disease
cortical spreading depression
CSF
cerebrospinal fluid
CSF bacterial culture
CSF Gram stain
CSF outflow pathway
CSF shunt
CSF-pressure syndrome
CSF-to serum glucose ratio
C-shaped
C-s. incision
C-s. microplate
C-s. resistive magnet
C-s. scalp flap
CSPTC
corticostriatopallidothalamocortical
CSTB
cystatin B
CSTB gene
CT
computed tomography
CT bone window
contiguous nonoverlapping axial CT
contrast-enhanced CT
dynamic CT
metrizamide-enhanced CT
PemADD CT
CT scan
serial CT
stable xenon CT
xenon CT
xenon-enhanced CT
CT-assisted stereotactic craniotomy
C-Tek anterior cervical plate system
C-terminal fragment
C-terminus
CT-guided
CT-g. biopsy
CT-g. stereotactic evacuation
CTI-Siemens
CTI-S. 933/08-12 PET camera
CTI-S. 933 tomograph
CTS
carpal tunnel syndrome
CTSIB
Clinical Test of Sensory Interaction and Balance
C-type natriuretic peptide
Cuban epidemic neuropathy

NOTES

cubital
c. nerve
c. tunnel
c. tunnel syndrome
cuboidal cell
cuboidodigital reflex
cue
auditory c.
c. effect
environmental c.
external c.
interoceptive c.
nonverbal c.
response-produced c.
semantic c.
specific sensory c.
trauma c.
verbal c.
cued
cue-induced subjective effect
cueing
semantic c.
Cueva cranial nerve electrode
cuff
cranial c.
Finapres finger c.
perivascular c.
cuffing
perivascular c.
cuirass
analgesic c.
tabetic c.
cul-de-sac
conjunctival c.-d.-s.
Culler hook
culmen, pl. **culmina**
c. cerebelli
culminis
lobulus c.
culture
blood c.
bullying c.
cerebellar aggregation c.
CSF bacterial c.
forebrain cell c.
fungal c.
immortalized primary cell c.
c. medium
tissue c.
culture-specific intervention
Cummins disk prosthesis
cumulative
c. action
c. dose
c. effect
c. medication reduction
c. stressor
c. trauma disorder
cuneate
c. fasciculus
c. funiculus
c. nucleus
c. tubercle
cuneati
nucleus funiculi c.
tuberculum nuclei c.
cuneatum
tuberculum c.
cuneatus
fasciculus c.
nucleus c.
cunei (*pl. of* cuneus)
cuneiform
c. lobe
c. nucleus
cuneiformis
lobulus c.
nucleus c.
cuneocerebellar
c. fiber
c. tract
cuneocerebellares
fibrae c.
cuneospinales
fibrae c.
cuneospinal fiber
cuneus, pl. **cunei**
cup
c. catheter
c. ear
c. forceps
ocular c.
optic c.
Cupid's
C. bow contour
C. bow sign
Cuprimine
cupula, pl. **cupulae**
ampullary c.
c. cochlea
c. cristae ampullaris
cupular
c. part
c. part of epitympanic recess
cupularis
pars c.
cupulate part
cupulolithiasis
cura
curanderismo
curare poisoning
curarization-induced flaccidity

curette, curet
- blunt-ring c.
- bone c.
- Cloward-Cone ring c.
- Cone ring c.
- Cone suction biopsy c.
- disk c.
- downbiting Epstein c.
- Epstein c.
- flat back c.
- Halle bone c.
- Hardy c.
- Hibbs spinal c.
- Hibbs-Spratt spinal fusion c.
- Howard spinal c.
- Jansen bone c.
- Malis c.
- Marino transsphenoidal c.
- Mayfield spinal c.
- pituitary c.
- Raney stirrup-loop c.
- Ray pituitary c.
- reverse-angled c.
- Rhoton blunt-ring c.
- Rhoton loop c.
- Rhoton spoon c.
- Richards c.
- ring c.
- Scoville ruptured disk c.
- secret c.
- Semmes c.
- straight ring c.
- transsphenoidal c.
- vertical ring c.
- Yasargil micro c.

current
- alternating c. (AC)
- ascending c.
- audiofrequency eddy c.
- centrifugal c.
- centripetal c.
- demarcation c.
- c. depression
- descending c.
- direct c. (DC)
- eddy c.
- electrotonic c.
- hyperpolarization-activated cationic c.
- hyperpolarization-activated chloride c.
- hyperpolarizing c.
- inhibitory postsynaptic c.
- c. of injury
- nerve-action c.
- c. perception threshold (CPT)
- radiofrequency eddy c.
- receptor-mediated c.

Curschmann-Steinert
- C.-S. disease
- C.-S. syndrome

curse
- Ondine c.

cursiva
- epilepsia c.

curtailed sleep

curve
- accommodation c.
- area under the c.
- best-fit c.
- developmental c.
- double thoracic c.
- frequency dispersion c.
- isodose c.
- Kaplan-Meier survival c.
- King type I–V c.
- low single thoracic c.
- lumbar c.
- nonlinear developmental c.
- right thoracic c.
- rigid c.
- severe rigid right thoracic c.
- signal intensity c.
- specific c.
- strength-duration c.
- thoracolumbar c.
- time-density c.

curved
- c. cannula with locking dilator
- c. conventional microscissors
- c. electrode
- c. incision
- c. knot-tying forceps
- c. microneedle holder

curved-tipped spatula

CUSA

Cavitron Ultrasonic Surgical Aspirator
- CUSA CEM system
- CUSA electrosurgical module
- CUSA system 200 straight autoclavable handpiece
- CUSA tip

C

NOTES

Cushing
C. basophilia
C. basophilism
C. bayonet forceps
C. bipolar forceps
C. bivalve retractor
C. brain forceps
C. brain spatula
C. brain spatula spoon
C. cranial bur
C. cranial perforator
C. cranial rongeur
C. decompressive retractor
C. disease
C. dressing forceps
C. dural hook
C. dural hook knife
C. effect
C. gasserian ganglion hook
C. intervertebral disk rongeur
C. Little Joker elevator
C. monopolar forceps
C. nerve hook
C. nerve retractor
C. periosteal elevator
C. phenomenon
C. pituitary elevator
C. pituitary scoop
C. pituitary spoon
C. reflex
C. response
C. saw
C. saw guide
C. staphylorrhaphy elevator
C. subtemporal retractor
C. syndrome
C. technique
C. tissue forceps
C. triad in brain tumor
C. ulcer
C. vein retractor
C. ventricular needle
Cushing-Landolt speculum
cushingoid
cushion
Carter immobilization c.
custom implant
cut
craniotomy c.
Panama c.
visual field c.
cutaneomeningospinal angiomatosis
cutaneon histamine-sensitive fiber
cutaneous
c. adenoma
c. angioma
c. electrical stimulation
external auditory canal c.
c. horn
c. mechanoreceptor
c. meningioma
c. nerve
c. neurofibromatosis
c. nociceptor
c. pupil reflex
c. receptor
c. sensation
cutaneus
nervus c.
ramus c.
cut-film angiography
"cut-flow" index (CFI)
cutis
neuroma c.
cutoff score
cutter
dowel c.
Howmedica Microfixation System plate c.
Leibinger Micro System plate c.
CV
craniosacral vault
CV4
craniosacral vault four
CVA
cerebrovascular accident
CVM
cerebral venous malformation
CVS
chorionic villus sampling
CW
continuous wave
CX-516
ampakine C.
cyanide poisoning
cyanoacrylate
c. glue
N-butyl c.
cyanophilous
cyanopia
CyberKnife
Accuray C.
C. robotic radiosurgery system
C. stereotactic radiosurgery/radiotherapy system
cybermedicine
cybernetics
Cyberonics vagus nerve stimulator electrode
CyberPager
Cyberware 3030RGB digitizer
CyberWatch
Cybon surgical navigation

cyclase
adenyl c.
adenylate c.
adenylyl c.
guanylate c.
guanylyl c.
cycle
c.'s of afternystagmus
anovulatory c.
brain wave c.
cell c.
circannual c.
citric acid c.
disturbed sleep-wake c.
fusion-defusion c.
Hodgkin c.
introjective-projective c.
late luteal phase of menstrual c.
menstrual c.
sleep c.
sleep-awake c.
sleep-wake c.
urea c.
cyclic
c. adenosine monophosphate
c. alteration
c. deoxyribonucleic acid
c. depression
c. endoperoxide
c. guanosine monophosphate
c. vomiting
cyclicity
sleep-wake c.
cyclin box
cyclin-dependent kinase inhibitory protein
cycling
futile c.
phase c.
cyclizine
cyclobarbital
cyclobenzaprine hydrochloride
cyclohexylchloroethylnitrosurea chemotherapy
cyclooxygenase (COX)
c. enzyme
c. inhibitor
cyclooxygenase-1 (COX-1)
cyclooxygenase-2 (COX-2)
Cyclopan
cyclopentolate
cyclophosphamide
cyclopia
cycloplegia
cyclops lesion
cycloserine
cyclosporin A
cyclosporine
cyclothyme
cyclothymic PD
cyclotorsion
eye c.
Cygnus PFS Image-Guided system
cylinder
axis c.
Ruffini c.
terminal c.
cylindraxis
cylindroma
Cymbalta
cynic spasm
Cyon nerve
cyproheptadine hydrochloride
cyst
aneurysmal bone c.
apoplectic c.
arachnoid c.
bilateral arachnoid c.
bilateral choroid plexus c.
bone c.
brain c.
cerebellar arachnoid c.
cerebellopontine angle arachnoid c.
cholesterol c.
colloid c.
craniobuccal c.
Dandy-Walker c.
daughter c.
dentigerous c.
dermoid c.
endodermal c.
enteric c.
enterogenous c.
ependymal c.
epidermoid c.
extradural c.
extraforaminal synovial c.
c. fenestration
foramen magnum c.
foregut c.
frontoparietal convexity c.
giant sacral perineural c.

C

NOTES

cyst *(continued)*
glial parenchymal c.
hydatid c.
interhemispheric c.
intracerebral hydatid c.
intracranial arachnoid c.
intradiploic epidermoid c.
intramedullary epidermoid c.
intraneural ganglion c.
intraparenchymal c.
intrapituitary c.
intrasellar Rathke cleft c.
juxtaarticular c.
leptomeningeal c.
lumbar synovial c.
middle cranial fossa c.
mucous retention c.
nasopharyngeal mucus retention c.
neural c.
neuroenteric c.
neuroepithelial c.
nonenteric c.
paraphysial c.
paraventricular c.
perineurial c.
pineal c.
pontine hydatid c.
pontomedullary epidermoid c.
porencephalic c.
posttraumatic leptomeningeal c.
primary epidural c.
quadrigeminal arachnoid c.
radicular c.
Rathke cleft c.
Rathke pouch c.
recurrent enteric c.
retinal c.
sacral nerve root c.
sellar c.
soapsuds c.
solitary hydatid c.
spinal canal hydatid c.
spinal cord arachnoid c.
spinal endodermal c.
spinal neurenteric c.
spinal synovial c.
spindle-shaped c.
subarachnoid-ependymal c.
subperiosteal c.
suprasellar c.
synovial c.
Tarlov c.
temporal arachnoid c.
thyroglossal duct c.
Tornwaldt c.
xanthogranulomatous c.
xanthomatous Rathke cleft c.

cystadenoma
apocrine c.
cystine c.
eccrine c.
c. lymphomatosum

cystathionine synthetase deficiency

cystathioninuria aminoaciduria

cystatin B (CSTB)

cysteine
c. protease
c. protease inhibitor
c. proteinase
secreted protein acidic and rich in c.

cystic
c. astrocytoma
c. degenerative disorder
c. encephalomalacia
c. fibrosis
c. hydroma
c. intraparenchymal meningioma
c. lacunar infarction
c. medial necrosis
c. microadenoma
c. myelomalacia
c. papillomatous
c. papillomatous craniopharyngioma
c. periventricular leukomalacia

cystica
hydronephrosis in spinal bifida c.
spina bifida c.
urinary infection in spina bifida c.

cysticercal infection

cysticerci
subarachnoid c.

cysticercosis

cysticerotic arachnoiditis

cysticum
cranium bifidum c.

cystine cystadenoma

cystoatrial shunt

Cystografin

Cystokon

cystoma
papilliferous c.

cystoscope

cytarabine liposome

cytoarchitectonic abnormality

cytoarchitectonics

cytoarchitectural asymmetry

cytoarchitecture
neural c.

cytochrome
c. *c*
c. c oxidase
c. c oxidase deficiency
c. oxidase defect

c. P
c. P450 metabolism
cytodendrite
cytodistal
cytodomain
cytoid body
cytokeratin
c. c.
low molecular weight c.
cytokine
inflammatory c.
c. inhibitor
interacting c.
cytology
cytolysis
cytomegalic
c. inclusion disease
c. inclusion virus
cytomegalovirus (CMV)
c. meningitis
c. polyradiculomyelitis (CMV-PRAM)
c. ventriculoencephalitis
Cytomel
cytometry
flow c.
cyton
cytopathy
mitochondrial c.
cytophotometry
Feulgen c.
cytoplasm
neuronal c.
cytoplasmic
c. dynein
c. inclusion
c. microtubule
c. organelle
cytoprotective
cytoproximal
cytoreduction
cytoreductive surgery
cytosine
c. arabinoside (ara-C)
c. arabinoside therapy
cytoskeletal
c. abnormality
c. degradation
c. protein
cytoskeletal-membrane event
cytoskeleton
axonal c.
cytosol fluid
cytotoxic
c. drug
c. edema
c. lymphocyte
cytotoxin-associated gene A (CagA)
Cytoxan
C. Injection
C. Oral
Czarnecki sign
Czerny suture

C

NOTES

2D
two-dimensional
2D graphic localization
3D
three-dimensional
3D positional adjustability
3D positional control
3D relationship analysis
3D titanium mini bone plate
D_2
D_2 blockade
D_2 occupancy
D2 receptor
D3 receptor
DA
dopamine
***dab1* gene**
daboia
dacarbazine
d'accoucheur
main d.
DaCosta syndrome
Dacron
collagen-impregnated D.
D. fibered platinum coil
dacryoadenitis
dacryocystic epilepsy
dacryocystis
dacryocystitis
dacryocystocele
dactinomycin
d'action
folie d.
dactylospasm
DAF
D. syndrome
Dahlgren cranial rongeur
DAI
diffuse axonal injury
daily
D. Rating Scale
D. Record of Severity of Problems
D. Stress Inventory
Dalalone
daledalin tosylate
DAM-80 amplifier
damage
acute neuronal d.
amygdala d.
anoxic d.
anterior cervical surgery vocal cord d.
axonal d.
body ego d.
brain d. (BD)
cranial nerve d.
diencephalic d.
excitotoxic cell d.
frontal cortex d.
HI-induced brain d.
hypoxic brain d.
hypoxic-ischemic brain d.
insult-induced neuronal d.
intrinsic d.
ischemic brain d.
left hemisphere d. (LHD)
liver d.
neuronal d.
occipital cortex d.
parietal cortex d.
retraction-induced cerebral d.
temporal cortex d.
Damasio and Damasio template
dampened waveform
Dana
D. operation
D. posterior rhizotomy
Dana-Farber Cancer Institute protocol
danaparoid sodium
danazol
dance
Saint Anthony d.
Saint Guy d.
Saint Vitus d.
dancing
d. chorea
d. disease
d. eye
d. spasm
Dandy
D. clamp
D. maneuver
D. myocutaneous scalp flap
D. nerve hook
D. neurological scissors
D. neurosurgical scissors
D. operation
D. probe
D. scalp hemostatic forceps
D. suction tube
D. trigeminal nerve scissors
D. ventricular needle
Dandy-Walker
D.-W. complex
D.-W. cyst
D.-W. deformity
D.-W. malformation

Dandy-Walker *(continued)*
D.-W. phenomenon
D.-W. syndrome
Danek
Medtronic Sofamor D.
danger
physical d.
danger-laden schema vulnerability
dangerous image
Danielssen-Boeck disease
Danielssen disease
Danocrine
Dantrium
dantrolene sodium
dapsone neuropathy
DAP Test
Daraprim
dark
d. cell
D. Warrior epilepsy
Darkschewitsch
nucleus of D.
dartos reflex
darwinian reflex
darwinism
neural d.
Das-Naglieri Cognitive Assessment System
DAT
dementia Alzheimer type
dopamine transporter
DAT autoradiography
DAT gene
DAT for PCA
data, sing. **datum**
d. acquisition bandwidth
d. acquisition system
anecdotal d.
d. base
clinical d.
followup d.
functional imaging d.
longitudinal expert evaluation using all available d.
mental d.
narrative d.
nutraceutical d.
postmortem d.
quantitative d.
in vivo d.
databank
trauma coma d. (TCDB)
database
Childhood Brain Tumor Consortium d.
Odense Pharmacoepidemiological D. (OPED)
whole-brain mapping d.
DATATOP
deprenyl and tocopherol antioxidative therapy of parkinsonism
Datex infrared CO_2 monitor
Datril
datum (*sing. of* data)
Datura arobrea
daughter
d. abscess
d. cyst
Daumas-Duport
D.-D. classification
D.-D. system
DAVF
dural arteriovenous fistula
Davidenkow syndrome
davidis
lyra d.
Davidoff age stratification
Davidoff-Dyke-Masson syndrome
Davis
D. brain retractor
D. brain spatula
D. coagulating forceps
D. conductor
D. dura dissector
D. dural separator
D. monopolar forceps
D. nerve separator
D. nerve separator-spatula
D. nerve spatula
D. percussion hammer
D. rib spreader
D. saw guide
D. scalp retractor
Dawson encephalitis
Daxolin
Day Barb
Daypro
daytime
d. drowsiness
d. fatigability
d. fatigue
d. hallucination
d. napping
d. sleep hangover
d. sleepiness
d. somnolence
d. stupor
dazzle
central d.
DBD
dementia behavior disturbance
DBD Scale

DBF
distant brain failure
DBS
deep brain stimulation
DBS electrode
DBS electrode implantation
DC
direct current
DC SQUID sensor
DC SQUID sensor decompressive
3D-CTA
three-dimensional computed tomographic angiography
D-dimer
de
de haut en bas
De Mayo two-point discrimination device
De Monte grading
de Morsier syndrome
de novo
de novo aneurysm
de novo appearance
de novo development
de novo metachronous neoplasm
de novo nonconvulsive status epilepticus
de novo synthesis
de pensós echo
de Quervain disease
De Sanctis-Cacchione syndrome
De Toni-Fanconi syndrome
dead
brain d. (BD)
d. hand
d. space
deafferentation
hemispherical d.
d. pain
d. pain syndrome
deafness
central d.
cortical d.
high frequency d.
infantile X-linked d.
midbrain d.
nerve d.
neural d.
pure word d.
retrocochlear d.
sensorineural d.
word d.
dealkylation
deaminase
myoadenylate d.
porphobilinogen d.
3′-deamino-3′-morpholino-13-deoxo-10-hydroxycarminomycin
Deanar
deanol
d. acetamidobenzoate
d. acetaminobenzoate
deaquation
death
apoptotic cell d.
brain d. (BD)
cell d.
cerebral d.
ischemic neuronal cell d.
living d.
neuronal d.
programmed cell d. (PCD)
Deaver
D. method
D. retractor
DeBakey
D. endarterectomy scissors
D. forceps
D. rib spreader
DeBastiani
D. distractor
D. external fixator
D. frame
debilitating
d. dysphoric symptom
d. illness
Debrancher enzyme deficiency
Debré-Sémélaigne pseudomyotonia
Debre-Sémélaigne syndrome
debulking procedure
Decadron
decanoate
nandrolone d.
decarbamylation
decarboxylase
amine precursor uptake d. (APUD)
aromatic amino acid d. (AADC)
glutamate d.
glutamic acid d.
glutamine d. (GAD)
ornithine d.

D

NOTES

decarceration
decathexis
decay
free induction d. (FID)
decentration
decerebellation
decerebrate
decorticate and d.
d. posturing
d. rigidity
d. state
decerebration
bloodless d.
decerebrize
decision
Brawner d.
Decker
D. alligator forceps
D. alligator scissors
D. microsurgical forceps
D. microsurgical scissors
declarative
d. emotional memory processing
d. memory
d. memory process
decline
cognitive d.
functional d.
hormonal d.
inexorable d.
d. rate
declive
declivis
decomposition of movement
decompression
anterior d.
bone graft d.
cerebral d.
cervical spine d.
d. equipment
extensive posterior d.
foramen magnum d.
foraminal d.
hindbrain d.
interlaminar d.
internal d.
laser disk d. (LDD)
lumbar spine d.
microvascular d. (MVD)
nerve d.
d. operation
optic nerve sheath d. (ONSD)
orbital d.
posterior d.
sacral spine d.
d. sickness
simple d.
spinal d.
suboccipital d.
subtemporal d.
surgical d.
thoracic spine d.
thoracolumbar spine d.
timing of d.
transantral ethmoidal orbital d.
trigeminal d.
vascular d.
ventricular d.
vertebral body d.
decompressive
d. craniectomy
DC SQUID sensor d.
d. laminectomy
d. sickness
d. surgery
decorticate
d. and decerebrate
d. posturing
d. rigidity
d. state
decortication
cerebral d.
reversible d.
d. technique
decortization
decreased
d. interest in activity
d. need for sleep
d. respiratory drive
d. sleep efficiency
decremental response
decrementing response
decrescendo discharge
decubitus
d. paralysis
d. position
d. ulcer
decussate
decussatio, pl. **decussationes**
d. brachii conjunctivi
d. fibrarum nervorum trochlearium
d. fontinalis
d. lemnisci mediales
d. lemniscorum
d. motoria
d. nervorum trochlearis
d. pedunculorum cerebellarium superiorum
d. pyramidum
d. sensoria
decussationes tegmentales
d. tegmentalis anterior
d. tegmentalis posterior
decussationes tegmenti

decussationes tegmentorum
d. trochlearis
decussation
anterior tegmental d.
d. of brachia conjunctiva
dorsal tegmental d.
d. of the fillet
Forel d.
fountain d.
Held d.
d. of medial lemniscus
Meynert fountain d.
motor d.
optic d.
posterior tegmental d.
d. of pyramid
pyramidal d.
rubrospinal d.
d. of superior cerebellar peduncle
tectospinal d.
tegmental d.
d. of trochlear nerve
d. of trochlear nerve fiber
ventral tegmental d.
Wernekinck d.
dedifferentiation hypothesis
Deductive Reasoning Test
deefferentation
deefferented state
deep
d. abdominal reflex
d. brain extension
d. brain lead
d. brain microelectrode recording
d. brain stimulation (DBS)
d. brain stimulation for mood disorder
d. cerebellar nucleus
d. cerebral vein
d. gray layer of superior colliculus
d. hypothermic circulatory arrest
d. middle cerebral vein
d. origin
d. retractor
d. sensibility
d. tendon reflex (DTR)
d. transitional gyrus
d. vein thrombosis
d. venous thrombosis
d. white layer of superior colliculus
d. white matter
d. white matter hyperintensity
d. white matter hyperintensity change
d. white matter lesion (DWML)
d. white matter pathology
d. white matter region
defatigation
defecation center
defect
activation d.
afferent pupillary d.
altitudinal visual field d.
arcuate visual field d.
arousal d.
asymptomatic visual field d.
autosomal-dominant genetic d.
chiasmatic d.
concentric visual field d.
cytochrome oxidase d.
developmental d.
extradural d.
field d.
focal plaquelike d.
galactosidase d.
glycosphingolipid metabolic d.
hematopoietic stem cell d.
imprinting d.
methylene tetrahydrofolate reductase d.
midline fusion d.
mitochondrial d.
neural tube d. (NTD)
nonhomonymous field d.
partial homonymous field d.
postoperative skull d.
protrusio d.
pursuit d.
relative afferent pupillary d. (RAPD)
residual dense nasal d.
reversible ischemic neurologic d.
smooth pursuit d.
temporoparietal d.
visual field d.
defected eye
defective glucose transport
defense
egomechanism of d.
endogenous antioxidative d.
heat d.

NOTES

defense *(continued)*
normal heat d.
d. reflex
deferens
plexus of ductus d.
deferentialis
plexus d.
deferoxamine
deferred shock
deficiency
N-acetylglutamate d.
acid lipase d.
acid maltase d.
acyl-CoA dehydrogenase d.
acyl-CoA oxidase d.
adenylosuccinase d.
adult acid maltase d.
aldosterone d.
aminoaciduria d.
antithrombin III d.
apoceruloplasm d.
aqueous humor d.
arginase d.
argininosuccinic acid synthase d.
arginosuccinate lyase d.
arylsulfatase A d.
aspartoacylase d.
AT III d.
bifunctional protein d.
bioenergetic d.
biopterin d.
biotin holocarboxylase synthetase d.
biotinidase d.
carbamyl phosphate synthetase d.
carnitine palmitoyltransferase d.
ceruloplasmin d.
clotting factor d.
cobalamin reductase d.
cognitive function d.
cystathionine synthetase d.
cytochrome c oxidase d.
Debrancher enzyme d.
dementia due to vitamin d.
factor VII d.
factor VIII d.
factor IX d.
factor XII d.
folate d.
folic acid d.
fructose-1,6-diphosphatase d.
galactokinase d.
galactose-1-phosphate uridyltransferase d.
galactosylceramidase d.
glucuronidase d.
glutamyl cysteine synthetase d.
glutathione synthetase d.
glycerol kinase d.
glycogen debrancher d.
growth hormone d.
hereditary high-density lipoprotein d.
hexosaminidase d.
holocarboxylase synthetase d.
hypoxanthine guanine phosphoribosyltransferase d.
idiopathic growth hormone d.
infantile acid maltase d.
intellectual d.
intrinsic factor d.
iodine d.
iron d.
isoniazid-induced pyridoxine d.
lignoceroyl coenzyme A synthase d.
literacy d.
merosin d.
mevalonate kinase d.
molybdenum cofactor d.
multiple carboxylase d.
myelin basic protein d.
myoadenylate deaminase d.
myopathic carnitine d.
myophosphorylase d.
neuraminidase d.
ornithine-ketoacid aminotransferase d.
ornithine transcarbamylase d. (OTCD)
phenylalanine hydroxylase d.
phosphofructokinase transferase d.
phosphoglycerate kinase d.
phosphoglycerate mutase d.
phosphorylase d.
platelet glycoprotein Ia/IIa d.
protein C, S d.
protein S d.
purine nucleotide phosphorylase d.
pyridoxine d.
pyruvate carboxylase d.
pyruvate kinase d.
quantal release d.
respiratory chain complex I d.
riboflavin d.
sarcoglycan d.
sulfatase A d.
thiamine d.
thyroid d.
triosephosphate isomerase d.
vitamin B1 d.
vitamin B6 d.
vitamin B12 d.
vitamin D d.
vitamin E d.

deficient spinous process
deficit
auditory transfer d.
behavior d.
bimanual coordination d.
cognitive d.
cortical gray matter d.
corticobulbar d.
cranial nerve d.
delayed ischemia d.
delayed ischemic neurological d. (DIND)
emotional memory d.
executive function d.
expressive language d.
focal neurologic d.
frontal lobe-related d.
functional d.
gaze d.
general temporal processing d.
intellectual function d.
lexical-syntactic d.
magnocellular d.
memory function d.
motor d.
neurological d.
neuropsychologic d.
olfactory d.
Orgogozo score for neurological d.
osteoporosis with vertebral collapse and neurologic d.
perfusion d.
permanent cranial nerve d.
proprioception d.
proprioceptive sensory d.
radicular motor d.
resolving ischemic neurologic d. (RIND)
d. reversal
reversible ischemic neurologic d. (RIND)
reversible ischemic neurological d.
sensory d.
sleep d.
social relations d.
subcortical d.
d. syndrome
tactile transfer d.
transfer d.
unilateral d.
verbal d.
vestibular d.
visual field d.
volitional d.
definition
arteriovenous malformation nidus d.
AVM nidus d.
caseness d.
diagnostic d.
nidus d.
three-dimensional target d.
deflazacort
deflection
d. force
high-voltage d.
initial upward d.
deformans
cephalohematoma d.
dystonia musculorum d. (DMD)
musculorum d.
osteitis d.
recessive dystonia musculorum d.
spondylitis d.
spondylosis d.
deformation
morphological d.
shear-strain d.
trefoil tendon d.
deformity
d. analysis
Arnold-Chiari d.
bull's eye d.
cervical spine kyphotic d.
cervicomedullary d.
Chiari d.
clawhand d.
coronal plane d.
cranioorbital d.
Dandy-Walker d.
drop-finger d.
drop-thumb d.
flat back d.
hand d.
hindbrain d.
J-sella d.
Klippel-Feil d.
kyphotic d.
lumbar spine kyphotic d.
main en griffe d.
musculoskeletal d.
pes cavus d.
posttraumatic spinal d.

NOTES

D

deformity *(continued)*
saddle nose d.
sagittal d.
skeletal d.
spinal coronal plane d.
swan-neck d.
thoracic spine scoliotic d.
thoracolumbar gibbus d.
deformity/instability
spinal d.
deganglionate
degeneratio micans
degeneration
acquired hepatocerebral d.
adiposogenital d.
Alzheimer neurofibrillary d.
ascending d.
axon d.
axonal d.
axoplasm d.
cerebellar cortical d.
cerebelloolivary d.
cerebromacular d.
cerebroretinal d.
cobblestone d.
cortical-basal ganglionic d.
corticobasal ganglion d.
corticobasal ganglionic d.
corticobasilar ganglionic d.
corticobasoganglionic d.
dentatorubral d.
descending d.
disk d.
end-organ d.
fascicular d.
fibrinoid d.
frontal lobe d.
frontotemporal lobar d.
glistening d.
Gombault d.
granular d.
granulovacuolar d.
gray d.
hepatocerebral d.
hepatolenticular d.
Holmes cortical cerebellar d.
hyaline d.
hypertrophic olivary d.
infantile neuronal d.
lattice d.
lenticular progressive d.
Marchi d.
Menzel olivopontocerebellar d.
neurofibrillary d.
neuronal d.
Nissl d.
olivary d.
olivopontocerebellar d.
orthograde d.
oxidative d.
pallidal d.
paraneoplastic cerebellar d.
paraneoplastic cerebral d.
parenchymatous cerebellar d.
paving stone d.
pontosubicular d.
premature infant pontosubicular d.
primary neuronal d.
primary progressive cerebellar d.
Purkinje cell d.
Ramsay Hunt type of inherited dentatorubral d.
reaction of d.
retinal d.
retrograde d.
rim d.
Rosenthal d.
secondary d.
spinal disk d.
spinocerebellar d. (SCD)
spinopontine d.
spongy d.
striatonigral d.
subacute cerebellar d.
subacute combined d.
synaptic d.
transneuronal d.
transsynaptic d.
traumatic d.
Türck d.
uratic d.
vacuolar d.
wallerian d.
white matter d.
Wilson hepatolenticular d.
degenerative
d. arthritis
d. brain disease
d. cervical disk disease
d. cervical spine disease
d. cervical spine disorder
d. chorea
d. dementia
d. discogenic end-plate disease
d. discogenic vertebral change
d. hypothesis
d. lumbar scoliosis
d. lumbar spine fusion
d. narrowing
d. neuronal disorder
d. spine change
d. spine condition
d. spondylolisthesis
d. spondylosis

d. spondylosis decompression and fusion
d. subluxation
degloving
midface d.
deglutition
d. center
d. paralysis
d. reflex
deglycyrrhizinated licorice
Degos disease
degradable starch microspheres (DSM)
degradation
cytoskeletal d.
dopamine d.
elastin d.
leucine d.
myelin d.
NO-induced DNA d.
degustation
7-dehydrocholesterol
dehydroepiandrosterone (DHEA)
d. sulfate (DHEA-S, DHGA)
dehydrogenase
alcohol d.
aldehyde d.
flavoprotein d.
glutaryl-CoA d.
isovaleyl-CoA d.
lactate d.
phosphogluconate d. (PGD)
pyruvate d. (PDH)
deiterospinal tract
Deiters
D. cell
D. nucleus
D. process
déjà
d. vecu
d. voulu
d. vu
d. vu aura
Dejerine
D. anterior bulb syndrome
D. disease
D. hand phenomenon
D. onion peel sensory loss
D. percussion hammer
D. peripheral neurotabes
D. reflex
D. sign
Dejerine-Davis percussion hammer
Dejerine-Klumpke
D.-K. palsy
D.-K. paralysis
D.-K. syndrome
Dejerine-Landouzy dystrophy
Dejerine-Lichtheim phenomenon
Dejerine-Roussy syndrome
Dejerine-Sottas
D.-S. atrophy
D.-S. disease
D.-S. peripheral neuropathy
D.-S. syndrome
Dejerine-Thomas
D.-T. atrophy
D.-T. syndrome
DEL
delay
Delatestryl
delavirdine
delay (DEL)
benign maturation d.
conduction d.
developmental d.
interpeak d.
d. of kindling
macrocephaly with somatic and genital growth d.
psychomotor d.
readout d.
transcallosal conduction d.
delayed
d. after depolarization
d. apoplexy
d. axotomy
d. cerebral vasospasm
d. coma after hypoxia
d. computed tomographic myelography
d. hydrocephalus
d. hypersensitivity reaction
d. ischemia deficit
d. ischemic deterioration
d. ischemic neurological deficit (DIND)
D. List Recall Test
d. postischemic hypoperfusion
d. recall index
d. reflex
d. sensation
d. shock

D

NOTES

delayed *(continued)*
d. sleep phase
d. sleep-phase syndrome
d. traumatic intracerebral hematoma (DTICH)
d. traumatic intracerebral hemorrhage
delayed-onset postherpetic neuralgia
deleterious effect
deletion
d. mutation
15q11-q13 d.
deliberate infliction of pain
delire
d. aigu
d. ambitieux
d. chronique a evolution systematique
d. d'emblee
d. denormite
d. de toucher
d. ecmnesique
d. en partie double
d. oneirique
d. terminal
d. tremblant
d. vesanique
deliria (*pl. of* delirium)
deliriant
delirifacient
delirious
d. patient
d. shock
delirium, pl. **deliria**
acute d.
ammonium chloride d.
anxious d.
chronic d.
collapse d.
D., Dementia, and Amnestic and Other Cognitive Disorders
d. ebriosorum
eclamptic d.
low d.
d. mussitans
muttering d.
d. palingnosticum
pathophysiology of d.
phencyclidine d.
d. phenomenology
posttraumatic d.
D. Rating Scale (DRS)
secondary d.
senile d.
sine d.
substance induced d.
toxic d.
d. tremens (DT)
d. unit
d. verborum
delivery
d. catheter
consistent d.
convection-enhanced drug d.
gene therapy d.
d. guidewire
intraarterial drug d.
intraparenchymal drug d.
intraventricular drug d.
polymer drug d.
viral d.
DeLong Interest Inventory
Delrin
D. plastic scalp clip
D. plastic scalp clip Delta
D. rod
delta
d. activity
d. activity of stage
Delrin plastic scalp clip D.
d. fornicis
monorhythmic frontal d. (MFD)
d. rhythm
d. sleep
D. valve
D. valve in ventriculoperitoneal shunt
d. wave
delta-aminolevulinate dehydratase porphyria
delta-function arterial plasma
***delta* gene**
Deltasone
delta-9-tetrahydrocannabinol
deltoid-splitting incision
delusional
d. and hallucinatory syndrome
d. misidentification syndrome
Demadex
demand
biochemical oxygen d. (BOD)
functional d.
demarcation
d. current
d. potential
DeMartel
D. scalp flap forceps
D. wire saw
d'emblee
delire d.
demeclocycline
demented patient
dementia
acquired d.

AD-related d.
AIDS d.
alcohol persisting d.
Alzheimer atrophic d.
Alzheimer disease-related d.
Alzheimer senile d. (ASD)
D. of the Alzheimer's Type
d. Alzheimer type (DAT)
Alzheimer-type senile d.
amyotrophic lateral sclerosis-Parkinson d. (ALS-PD)
Assessment of D.
D. Assessment Battery
d. behavior disturbance (DBD)
Binswanger d.
cerebrovascular accident d.
clinical d.
cognitive impairment, no d.
comorbid d.
Cornell Scale for Depression in D.
cortical d.
degenerative d.
depressed-type presenile d.
depression in d.
depressive d.
dialysis d.
dialytica d.
diffuse Lewy body d. (DLBD)
d. due to hepatic condition
d. due to multiple etiologies
d. due to vitamin deficiency
epileptic d.
ethical aspects of d.
evolving d.
frontal lobe d.
d. frontal type
frontotemporal d. (FTD)
global d.
Gottfries-Brane-Steen Rating Scale for D.
hereditary dysphasic d.
HIV-associated d.
d. homozygous
hydrocephalic d.
hysterical d.
infarction d.
ischemic vascular d.
late-life d.
Lewy body d.
Manchester and Oxford Universities Scale for the Psychopathological Assessment of D. (MOUSEPAD)
mild d.
D. Mood Assessment Scale
multiinfarct d. (MID)
multiple sclerosis d.
non-Alzheimer frontal lobe type d.
paralytic d.
d. paralytica
d. paralytica juvenilis
paranoid-type arteriosclerotic d.
paranoid-type presenile d.
paranoid-type senile d.
d. paratonia progressiva
paretic d.
d. patient
pellagra d.
posttraumatic d.
d. praecox
preexisting d.
premorbid d.
presenile d.
primary senile d.
d. prodrome
d. progression
d. pugilistica
d. reversible
semantic d. (SD)
senile d.
d. severity
subcortical ischemic vascular d.
d. syndrome
d. syndrome of depression
toxic d.
uncomplicated arteriosclerotic d.
uncomplicated presenile d.
uncomplicated senile d.
vascular d.
vitamin B12 deficiency d.
Wernicke d.
d. with Lewy body (DLB)

dementia-aphonia
dementing illness
Demianoff sign
demimonde
demodulator
demographic
d. characteristic
d. feature

NOTES

demographic *(continued)*
d. risk factor
d. variable
demonstration
Ames d.
demyelinate
demyelinated myelitis
demyelinating
d. encephalopathy
d. neuropathy
d. polyneuropathy
d. polyradiculoneuropathy
d. procedure
d. trigeminal nerve lesion
d. white matter disease
demyelination
central inflammatory d.
multifocal subcortical d.
osmotic d.
segmental d.
demyelinative
d. disorder
d. spinal fluid profile
demyelinization
dendraxon
dendriform
dendrite
apical d.
d. arborization
d. proliferation
d. synaptogenesis
dendritic
d. arbor
d. plasticity
d. process
d. shaft
d. shape
d. spine
d. spine density
d. thorn
d. tree
d. tuft
dendrodendritic synapse
dendroid
dendron
dendrophagocytosis
dendrophilia, dendrophily
dendrotomy
denervate
denervated
d. fiber
d. muscle atrophy
denervation
autonomic d.
chemical d.
Krause d.
law of d.
muscle d.
d. neuronal hypersensitivity
d. pain syndrome
dengue
d. fever
d. viral encephalitis
d. virus
Denis
D. Browne neuropathy
D. Browne syndrome
D. forceps
Denny-Brown
D.-B. sensory radicular neuropathy
D.-B. syndrome
denormite
delire d.
de-novo Parkinson
dens, pl. **dentes**
d. anterior screw fixation
densa
macula d.
dense
d. hemianopia
d. hemiparesis
d. hemiplegia
d. sensory loss
densitometric analysis
densitometry
cholera-toxin-catalyzed d.
optical d.
density
bone mineral d.
contrast d.
dendritic spine d.
fiber d.
GFAP fiber d.
intraepidermal nerve fiber d.
lumbosacral junction bone d.
proton d.
receptor d.
relative optical d. (ROD)
spectral d.
spin d.
striatal dopamine transporter d.
synaptic d.
density-modulated spectral array (DSA)
dental
d. nerve
d. pathology
dentata
fissura d.
hilus of fascia d.
dentatae
cauda fasciae d.
dentate
d. band

d. fascia
d. fissure
d. gyrus
d. ligament
d. ligament of spinal cord
d. nucleus
d. nucleus of cerebellum
dentatectomy
dentated serration
dentati
capsula nuclei d.
hilum nuclei d.
strata gyri d.
dentatoolivary pathway
dentatorubral
d. atrophy
d. cerebellar atrophy with polymyoclonus
d. degeneration
d. fiber
dentatorubrales
fibrae d.
dentatorubropallidoluysian atrophy (DRPLA)
dentatorubrothalamic
dentatothalamic
d. fiber
d. tract
dentatum
corpus d.
dentatus
gyrus d.
nucleus d.
dentes (*pl. of* dens)
denticola
Treponema d.
denticulate ligament
denticulatum
ligamentum d.
dentiform
dentigerous cyst
dentinogenesis imperfecta
dentoliva
Denver
D. hydrocephalus shunt
D. valve
Denver-II Developmental screening test
deontologic theory
deoxygenation
deoxyhemoglobin
intracellular d.
deoxynucleside triphosphate
deoxyribonucleic acid (DNA)
Depacon
Depakene
Depakote
D. D.
D. ER
D. Sprinkle Capsule
depalatalization
dependence
d. criterion
d. trait
dependent
blood oxygenation level d. (BOLD)
blood oxygen level d. (BOLD)
dose d.
depigmentation of noradrenergic brainstem nucleus
depMedalone Injection
DepoCyt
Depoject Injection
depolarization
d. block
delayed after d.
early after d.
late after d.
primary afferent d. (PAD)
depolarization-dependent synaptic transmission
depolarize
depolarizer
Depo-Medrol Injection
Depopred Injection
deposit
intracellular insoluble protein d.
lipofuscinosis granular osmiophilic d.
deposition
amyloid d.
copper d.
hemosiderin d.
depot
Fluanxol D.
d. form
Depo-Testosterone
deprenyl and tocopherol antioxidative therapy of parkinsonism (DATATOP)
depressed
d. migraineur
d. skull fracture

NOTES

depressed *(continued)*
d. ventilatory response to hypercapnia
depressed-type presenile dementia
depression
alcohol-induced d.
anxious somatic d.
caregiver d.
cognitive impairment of d.
cortical spreading d. (CSD)
current d.
cyclic d.
d. in dementia
dementia syndrome of d.
drug-induced d.
drug-resistant d.
exaggerated d.
geriatric d.
headache, insomnia, and d. (HID)
hypersomnic d.
hysterical d.
later-life d.
Leão spreading d.
level of d.
manifestation of d.
myxedema d.
nuclear d.
paradoxical d.
paralyzing d.
postactivation d.
post stroke d.
post TIA d.
pseudodementia of d.
pure d.
reversible cognitive impairment of d.
ruminative d.
d. severity
somatic d.
d. spectrum disease
sporadic d.
spreading d.
subjective d.
subsyndromal d.
symptomatic d.
syndromal d.
syndromic d.
unspecified d.
visual field d.
depressive
d. auditory hallucination
d. breakthrough
d. dementia
d. disease
d. mixed state
d. olfactory hallucination
d. pseudodementia
d. psychoneurotic reaction
d. psychotic reaction
d. situational reaction
d. stupor
d. syndrome
d. visual hallucination
depressive-executive dysfunction
depressive-type
depressomotor
depressor
d. anguli oris muscle
d. fiber
d. nerve of Ludwig
d. reflex
deprivation
rapid eye movement d.
REM d.
sensory d.
sleep d. (SD)
volitional sleep d.
Deprol
depth
d. electrode
d. guard
d. recording
skin d.
wire penetration d.
depth-recorded electroencephalogram
DePuy
D. AcroMed DOC ventral cervical stabilization system
D. nerve hook
deramciclane
deranged neural development
derangement
metabolic d.
derby hat fracture
derivative
ergotamine d.
hematoporphyrin d.
tricyclic dibenzodiazepine d.
valproic acid and d.
derived
endothelium d.
dermabrasion bur
Dermaflex Gel
dermal
d. meningioma
d. sinus
dermatan sulfate
DermaTemp infrared thermographic sensor
dermatica
zona d.
dermatitidis
Blastomyces d.
dermatofibrosarcoma protuberans

dermatogenic torticollis
dermatoglyphic pattern
dermatome
d. pain
thoracic d.
trigeminal d.
dermatomic area
dermatomyositis
juvenile d.
dermatomyotome
dermatoneurology
dermatoneurosis
dermatosensory evoked potential
dermohygrometer
dermoid
d. cyst
d. tumor
dermometer
dermometry
dermoneurosis
dermoneurotropic
Derogatis
D. Affects Balance Scale
D. Affects Balance Scale, Revised
D. Stress Profile
D'Errico
D. bayonet pituitary forceps
D. brain spatula
D. enlarging drill bur
D. hypophysial forceps
D. lamina chisel
D. nerve root retractor
D. perforating drill
D. perforating drill bur
D. periosteal elevator
D. pituitary forceps
D. skull trephine
D. tissue forceps
D. ventricular needle
D'Errico-Adson retractor
desacralize
desamino-D-arginine vasopressin
desaturation index (DI)
descendens
d. cervicalis
d. cervicis
d. hypoglossi
descending
d. branch
d. current
d. degeneration
d. dyscontrol durable
d. motor pathway
d. neuritis
d. nucleus of the trigeminus
d. tract of trigeminal nerve
desensitization
behavioral d.
eye movement d.
deserpidine
desferrioxamine
desflurane
design
case control experimental study d.
cross-sectional experimental study d.
hook hollow-ground connection d.
hook V-groove connection d.
Isola spinal implant system d.
longitudinal experimental study d.
mechanical plate d.
naturalistic d.
pedicle screw linkage d.
prospective experimental study d.
retrospective experimental study d.
spinal implant d.
transpedicular fixation system d.
V-groove hollow-ground connection d.
d.'s for vision frame
d.'s for vision side shield
desipramine
desmethylclomipramine
desmin
d. storage myopathy
d. tumor marker
desmocytoma
desmodynia
desmoplastic
d. cerebral astrocytoma
d. infantile ganglioglioma
d. medulloblastoma
desmopressin
d. acetate
Desormaux endoscope
desoxycorticosterone acetate
desoxymorphine
desoxyphenobarbital
des penses echo
destruction
bony element d.

NOTES

destructive
d. interference technique
d. stereotactic lesion
desynchronization
d. activity
event-related d.
post-movement beta d.
desynchronized
d. discharge pattern
d. sleep
desynchronous
Desyrel
DET
diethyltryptamine
detachable
d. coil
d. silicone balloon
detached
d. cranial section
d. craniotomy
detachment
choroid d.
choroidal d.
ciliochoroid d.
dural d.
retinal d.
detail response to small white space
detection
signal d.
spike d.
detector
cesium fluoride scintillation d.
phase-sensitive d.
quadrature d.
deterioration
cognitive d.
delayed ischemic d.
end-of-dose d.
functional d.
memory d.
d. process
determinant
biologic d.
determination
fusion limit d.
serum enzyme d.
detoxicate
detrusor
d. areflexia
d. hyperreflexia
d. reflex
detrusor-external sphincter dyssynergia
detrusor-sphincter dyssynergia
detrusor-striated sphincter dyssynergia
deutencephalon
devascularized
developing
D. Cognitive Abilities Test, Second Edition
d. stroke
development
brain d.
cerebrovascular embryonic d.
cognitive function d.
concrete operational d.
de novo d.
deranged neural d.
dissociated motor d.
disturbance of intellectual d.
egocentric stage of d.
focal malformations of cortical d.
neonatal language d.
neurobiology of early childhood d.
perinatal d.
piagetian theory of moral reasoning d.
rhythms of lags and spurts in d.
spinal cord segmentation in embryonic d.
developmental
d. articulatory apraxia
D. Assessment of the Severely Handicapped
d. course
d. curve
d. defect
d. delay
d. disorder screening
d. effect
d. malformation
D. Observation Checklist System
d. perspective
d. process
d. quotient in Down syndrome
d. root
d. task
developmental-vulnerability model
deviation
alternating skew d.
disconjugate eye d.
eye-gaze d.
ipsilateral tonic d.
ocular d.
vertical ocular d.
wrong-way d.
Devic
D. aminoaciduria
D. disease
device
Angio-Seal closure d.
anterior internal fixation d.
antisiphon d.
assistive technology d.

Attractor retrieval d.
balloon occlusion-aspiration emboli entrapment d.
Bassett electrical stimulation d.
braided occlusion d.
Cadwell 5200A somatosensory evoked potential unit d.
Camino intraparenchymal fiberoptic d.
C-D instrumentation d.
cervical immobilization d. (CID)
Contour Emboli artificial embolization d.
CoolLine intravascular d.
Cordis implantable drug reservoir d.
Cotrel-Dubousset dynamic transverse traction d.
De Mayo two-point discrimination d.
DeWald spinal d.
Dunn d.
Dwyer d.
dynamic transverse traction d.
Edwards modular system sacral fixation d.
Egemen keyhole suction-control d.
endoscope lens cleansing d.
ferromagnetic monitoring d.
Fischer-Leibinger bur hole-mounted fixation d.
fixation d.
flow-controlled d.
fracture fixation d.
frameless stereotactic d.
Galtac d.
GDC SynerG detachment d.
gravitational d.
Harrington rod instrumentation distraction outrigger d.
head fixation d.
Heyer-Schulte antisiphon d.
inanimate learning d.
In-Exsufflator respiratory d.
InterFix RP threaded spinal fusion cage d.
intravascular d.
JACE-STIM electrotherapy stimulation d.
Kaneda anterior spine stabilizing d.
Kostuik-Harrington d.
Leksell adapter to Mayfield d.
malleable microsurgical suction d.
mandibular advancing d.
Mayfield/ACCISS stereotactic d.
Medelec five-channel neurophysiological d.
Microvena retrieval d.
MurphyScope neurologic d.
Neuromed Octrode implantable d.
newer-generation d.
Nicolet Pathfinder I recording d.
noise reduction d.
Novo-10a CBF measuring d.
optical d.
OssaTron d.
PDN d.
Perclose closure d.
Portnoy DPV d.
prosthetic disc nucleus d.
Quartzo d.
Roeder manipulative aptitude test d.
roentgen knife stereotactic radiosurgical d.
sequential compression d.
Silastic d.
SmartStent delivery d.
Snore Guard mandibular repositioning d.
Sofamor spinal instrument d.
Somanetics INVOS cerebral oximeter d.
SomaSensor d.
Sono-Stat Plus sound d.
superconducting quantum interference d. (SQUID)
SynchroMed drug administration d.
TACTICON peripheral neuropathy screening d.
Taylor halter d.
Texas Scottish Rite Hospital corkscrew d.
Texas Scottish Rite Hospital mini-corkscrew d.
tongue-locking d.
tongue-retaining d.
d. for transverse traction (DTT)
ultrasonic aspirating d.
VasoSeal closure d.
Viking II nerve monitoring d.
z-touch laser d.

Device/M2
Microcomputer Imaging D.
DeVilbiss
D. cranial rongeur
D. rongeur forceps
D. skull trephine
DeWald spinal device
Dewar posterior cervical fixation procedure
DEXA, DXA
dual-energy x-ray absorptiometry
dexamethasone suppression test
dexanabinol
dexclamol hydrochloride
dexmedetomidine
dexmethylphenidate HCl
Dexoval
dextran
dextroamphetamine
amphetamine and d.
d. neurotoxicity
dextrocerebral
dextromanual
dextropedal
dextrorotoscoliosis
dextroscoliosis
dextrosinistral
Dextrostix Uristix
Deyerle sciatic tension test
DFF
DNA fragmentation factor
2DFT
two-dimensional Fourier transform
2DFT gradient-echo imaging
2DFT GRASS
2DFT time-of-flight MR angiography
3DFT
three-dimensional Fourier transform
anisotropic 3DFT
3DFT gradient-echo MR imaging
3DFT GRASS
isotropic 3DFT
DGx
Thymatron DGx
DHA
docosahexaenoic acid
DHEA
dehydroepiandrosterone
DHEA-S
dehydroepiandrosterone sulfate
D.H.E. 45 Injection
DHGA
dehydroepiandrosterone sulfate
DI
desaturation index
diabetic
d. amyotrophy
d. arthropathy
d. coma
d. mononeuritis multiplex
d. myelopathy
d. neuropathic cachexia
d. neuropathy
d. neuropathy neuralgia pain
d. oculomotor palsy
d. polyradiculopathy
d. pseudotabes
d. sensorimotor polyneuropathy
d. third nerve palsy
d. thoracic radiculopathy
diabetica
tabes d.
Diabinese
diacele
Diaginol
diagnosis, pl. **diagnoses**
dimensional d.
headache differential d.
neurologic d.
pendulum of d.
diagnostic
d. ambiguity
d. anesthesia
d. apraxia
d. aspect
d. assessment
d. block
d. boundary
d. category
d. cluster
d. criteria
d. criterion
d. definition
d. impression
d. measure
d. method
d. monitoring
d. noise
d. process
d. profile
D. Screening Batteries
d. template
diagonal
d. band
d. nystagmus
diagonalis
bandaletta d.
d. stria
stria d.
diagram
pulse timing d.
vector d.

Dial Away Pain 400 electrotherapy unit
dialing
random digital d.
dialysis
d. dementia
d. dysequilibrium
d. dysequilibrium syndrome
d. encephalopathy syndrome
dialytica dementia
diamagnetism
diambista
diameter
axonal d.
effective pedicle d.
effective thread d.
fiber d.
horizontal pedicle d.
lumbar spine pedicle d.
midsagittal d.
pedicle d.
sagittal pedicle d.
thoracic spine pedicle d.
transcerebellar d.
transpedicular fixation effective pedicle d.
transverse pedicle d.
vertical pedicle d.
diamond
d. bit
d. bur
d. high-speed air drill
d. knife
D. valve flow-regulating shunt
Diamox challenge testing
diaphragm
lumbar part of d.
d. of sella
d. of sella turcica
sella turcica d.
diaphragma, pl. **diaphragmata**
d. sellae
diaphragmatic
d. nerve
d. plexus
d. tic
d. weakness
diaphragmatis
pars anterior facies d.
pars lumbalis d.
Diapid
diaplexus
diary
d. card
sleep d.
diaschisis
Diasonics magnetic resonance imaging
Diaspan
D. instrumentation system
D. screw-rod system
diastasis
suture d.
Diastat
diastatic skull fracture
diastematocrania
diastematomyelia
diastole-phased pulsatile infusion
diastolic blood pressure
diataxia
cerebral d.
d. cerebralis infantilis
diatela
diathesis
bipolar d.
epileptic d.
spasmodic d.
spasmophilic d.
diathesis-stress
diatrizoate meglumine
diatrizoic acid
diaxon
Diazemuls Injection
diazepam (DZ)
D. Intensol
d. rectal gel
diazoxide
dibasic
d. calcium phosphate
dibenzepin benzothiazine
dibenzodiazepine
dibenzoxozepine agent
Dibenzyline
dibromodulcitol
DIC
disseminated intravascular coagulation
dichloralphenazone
dichloroacetate
dichlorodifluoromethane and trichloromonofluoromethane
dichlorotetrafluoroethane
ethyl chloride and d.
dichlorphenamide
Dick AO fixateur interne

Dickman
method of D.
Dickson method
dicoumarol
dicyclomine
didanosine
diencephala (*pl. of* diencephalon)
diencephali
pars dorsalis d.
pars ventralis d.
diencephalic
d. astrocytoma
d. damage
d. epilepsy
d. glioma
d. lesion
d. membrane
d. syndrome of infancy
d. transition area
d. vein
diencephalohypophysial
diencephalon, pl. **diencephala**
ventricle of d.
Dieters tract
Diethrich bulldog clamp
diethylenetriaminepentaacetic acid (DTPA)
diethylene triamine pentaacetic acid (DTPA)
diethylstilbestrol
diethyltryptamine (DET)
DIF
diffuse interstitial fibrosis
Diferrante disease
difference
behavioral d.
cerebral arteriovenous oxygen content d.
clinical d.
dose-related d.
functional d.
genetic d.
gray/white matter d.
hormonal d.
interear d.
mean consecutive d.
mean sorted d.
metabolic d.
morphological d.
pharmacological d.
religious d.
true d.
differential
D. Ability Scale
d. beneficial effect
d. correlate
d. display of messenger ribonucleic acid
d. increase
d. interaction
d. pressure valve
d. threshold
differentiation
brain d.
cluster of d. 95 (CD95)
neuronal d.
retrogressive d.
Schwann cell d.
sexual d.
difficile
Clostridium d.
difficulty
acculturation d.
cognitive d.
index of d. (ID)
diffusa
encephalitis periaxialis d.
diffuse
d. axonal injury (DAI)
d. bilateral slowing
d. brain atrophy
d. brain injury
d. cellular astrocytoma
d. cerebral histiocytosis
d. cerebral sclerosis
d. disseminated atheroembolism
d. distribution of activity
d. electrodecrement
d. fibrillary astrocytic tumor
d. heteropsia
d. idiopathic skeletal hyperostosis (DISH)
d. infantile familial sclerosis
d. interstitial fibrosis (DIF)
d. intrinsic brainstem tumor
d. Lewy body dementia (DLBD)
d. Lewy body disease
d. necrotizing leukoencephalopathy
d. noxious inhibitory control (DNIC)
d. pontine glioma
d. pontine lesion
d. tension imaging (DTI)
d. white matter disease
d. white matter shearing injury
diffused reflex
diffusion
anisotropic d.
identity d.
normoxic d.
d. respiration
d. tension imaging
d. tensor imaging (DTI)

d. tensor magnetic resonance imaging (diffusion tensor MRI)
d. tensor MRI
d. transmission
diffusion-perfusion magnetic resonance imaging
diffusion-weighted
d.-w. echo plantar image (DW-EPI)
d.-w. imaging (DWI)
d.-w. magnetic resonance imaging
d.-w. scanning
diffusivity
transverse d.
diffusum
angiokeratoma corporis d.
diflavin free radical
diflunisal
difluoromethylornithin
digastric
d. line
d. muscle
d. nerve
DiGeorge syndrome
digit
d. span backward (DSB)
d. span forward (DSF)
digital
d. holography
d. intravenous angiography
d. nerve
d. pinch
d. radiography (DR)
d. reflex
d. signal analysis
d. subtraction angiogram
d. subtraction angiography (DSA)
d. subtraction venography
d. subtraction venous angiography
d. subtraction venous angiography slice
d. syncope
d. temple massage
d. vascular imaging (DVI)
d. vernier scale
digital-to-analog converter
digitationes hippocampus
digitized
d. instrument
d. spinography
digitizer
Cyberware 3030RGB d.
infrared d.
optical d.
three-dimensional sonic d.
digressed speech
dihexoside
ceramide d.
dihomogammalinolenic acid
dihydrate
calcium pyrophosphate d. (CPPD)
dihydrochloride
pramipexole d.
triethylene tetramine d.
dihydroergotamine
d. mesylate
d. mesylate nasal spray
dihydroindolone
dihydrolipoyldehydrogenase
dihydrolipoyltransacetylase
dihydromorphinone hydrochloride
dihydropteridine reductase
dihydrotachysterol
dihydroxyphenylalanine
3,4-dihydroxyphenylalanine
5,7-dihydroxytryptamine
dilantinization
Dilantin Kapseals
dilatans
pneumosinus d.
dilatation
infundibular d.
ventricular d.
dilated
d. intercavernous sinus
d. poorly reactive pupil
dilation
aneurysmal d.
arachnoid nerve root sheath d.
congenital d.
episcleral vascular d.
hypertensive d.
junctional d.
progressive ventricular d.
dilator
cannula with locking d.
cortical incision coronary d.
curved cannula with locking d.
Eder-Puestow metal olive d.
straight cannula with locking d.
dileptic seizure
dilute Russell Viper Venom time (DRVVT)

NOTES

DiMauro syndrome
dimeglumine
gadopentetate d.
dimenhydrinate
dimension
abstract-versus-representational d.
disorganization d.
Isola spinal implant system d.
micropsychotic d.
pedicle d.
personality d.
positive symptom d.
sensory d.
symptom d.
dimensional
d. diagnosis
d. rating
3-dimensional reconstruction wand
dimercaprol
dimerization
receptor d.
2,5-dimethoxy-4-methylamphetamine
4-dimethoxyphenylethylamine
dimethoxyquinazoline
dimethylamine sulfate (DMAS)
dimethylaminoethyl methacrylate
dimethyl sulfoxide (DMSO)
dimethyltryptamine
dimidiata
chorea d.
dimple
acromial d.
sacral d.
DIND
delayed ischemic neurological deficit
Dingman
D. mouth gag
D. oral retraction system
dinitrate
isosorbide d.
dinitrophenol peripheral neuropathy
dinucleotide
flavin adenine d. (FAD)
dioctyl sodium sulfosuccinate
diode
light-emitting d. (LED)
diodine
diodone
Diodrast
Dionosil
dioxide
carbon d. (CO_2)
partial arterial gas tension of carbon d.
thorium d.
diphasic
d. dyskinesia
d. milk fever
diphenhydramine hydrochloride
diphenoxylate neurotoxicity
diphenylbutyl
diphenylbutylpiperidine
diphenylhydantoin
diphenylhydramine
diphosphate
adenosine d. (ADP)
guanosine d.
diphtheria
d. peripheral neuropathy
d., tetanus toxoids, and pertussis vaccine
diphtheriae
Corynebacterium d.
diphtheric polyneuropathy
diphtheritic
d. neuropathy
d. paralysis
diplegia
atonic-astatic d.
brachial d.
congenital facial d.
facial d.
Förster d.
infantile d.
masticatory d.
spastic d.
diploë
diploic vein
diplomyelia
diplophonia
diplopia
acquired vertical d.
diploscope
dipole
equivalent current d.
d. field
d. localization
magnetic d.
d. tracing
dipole-dipole
d.-d. interaction
d.-d. relaxation
dipotassium
clorazepate d.
dipping
converse ocular d.
ocular d.
Diprivan
Diprotrizoate
direct
d. auditory compound actional potential

d. brain stimulation
d. cortical stimulation and somatosensory evoked potential (SSEP)
d. current (DC)
d. embolectomy
d. end-to-end coaptation
d. fracture
d. lateral vein
d. multiplanar imaging
d. pyramidal tract
d. screw fixation technique
d. thermogenic effect
d. vision surgery

direction
flow d.
phase-encoding d.

directive

Director
Consortium of Neurology Clerkship D. (CNCD)

dirigation

disability
abstracting d.
D. Adjusted Life Years
overall d.
partial d.
reversible ischemic neurologic d. (RIND)

disabling
d. headache
d. positional vertigo (DPV)

disarray
myofibrillary d.

disaster
d. stressor
d. trauma
d. work
d. worker

disaster-related
d.-r. avoidant symptom
d.-r. intrusive symptom

disc (*var. of* disk)

Discase

discectomy, diskectomy
anterior d.
automated percutaneous lumbar d. (APLD)
cervical d.
lumbar d.
microlumbar d.
microsurgery d.
microsurgical d. (MSD)
Robinson anterior cervical d.
thoracic d.
transthoracic d.

discharge
bilateral, independent, periodic, lateralized, epileptiform d. (BIPLED)
bilaterally synchronous epileptic d.'s
bizarre high-frequency d.
bizarre repetitive d.
complex repetitive d. (CRD)
decrescendo d.
double d.
EEG anteromesial temporal d.
epileptic d.
epileptiform burst d.
exercise-induced sympathetic d.
focal epileptiform d.
grouped d.
hippocampal seizure d.
hypersynchronous d.
ictal focal epileptiform d.
interictal bisynchronous d.
interictal focal epileptiform d.
interictal generalized spike-and-wave d.
interictal spike d.
iterative d.
monosynaptic reflex d.
motor unit d.
multiple d.
myokymic d.
myotonic d.
nervous d.
neural d.
neuromyotonic d.
notched appearance of spike-wave d.
paroxysmal epileptiform d.
d. pattern
periodic lateralizing epileptiform d. (PLED)
period lateralized epileptiform d.
polyspike-and-wave d.
polysynaptic d.
premature d.
psuedoperiodic d.
rate of recovery at d.
repetitive d.

NOTES

discharge *(continued)*
rhythmic d.
rhythmical midtemporal d.
rolandic epileptiform d.
spike d.
spike-and-wave electroencephalographic d.
spike-wave d.
subclinical rhythmic EEG d.
sympathetic d.
synchronized neuronal d.
synchronous corticofugal epileptic d.
synchronous spike-and-wave d.
triple d.
unilateral interictal focal epileptic d.
waning d.
discharging lesion
disci (*pl. of* discus)
discission knife
discitis, diskitis
iatrogenic d.
intervertebral d.
pyogenic d.
discogenic sclerosis
discogram
discography
discoid
d. marker
d. skin lesion
discoidectomy
discoligamentous
d. complex
d. injury
discomfiture
disconjugate eye deviation
disconnection
d. apraxia
d. syndrome
discontinuity
Bruch membrane d.
facial nerve d.
nerve d.
discopathy
traumatic cervical d.
discordance
d. of movement
d. of voice
discordant
discoscope
percutaneous d.
discotomy
discountenance
Discourse Comprehension Test
discrete
d. emotional response
d. symptom
discriminant stimulus
discrimination
pure tone d.
Sweet two-point d.
discus, pl. **disci**
d. lentiformis
disdiadochokinesia
disease
acute Marchiafava-Bignami d.
Adams-Stokes d.
Addison d.
adjacent level d.
adult polyglucosan body d.
advanced cortical d.
Aicardi-Goutieres d.
Akureyri d.
Alexander d.
Alpers d.
Alzheimer d. (AD)
Anderson d.
anterior horn cell d.
antiepileptic drug-induced bone d.
Antopol d.
aortocranial d.
Aran-Duchenne d.
Armstrong d.
arterial occlusive d.
arteriosclerotic brain d.
arteritis cardiovascular d. (ASCVD)
atheromatous d.
atherosclerotic cardiovascular d. (ASCVD)
Australian X d.
autoimmune d.
Ayala d.
Azorean d.
Azorean-Joseph-Machado d.
Ballet d.
Baló d.
Baltic myoclonus d.
Bamberger d.
Bannister d.
basilar-vertebral artery d.
Bassen-Kornzweig d.
Batten d.
Batten-Mayou d.
Baxter d.
Bayle d.
Bechterew d.
Becker d.
Begbie d.
Behçet d.
Behr d.
Bernard-Soulier d.

Bernhardt d.
Bielschowsky d.
Bielschowsky-Jansky d.
Biemond d.
Billroth d.
Binswanger d.
Blocq d.
Bloom d.
Boehme d.
bone marrow transplantation graft-versus-host d.
Bornholm d.
Bosin d.
Bourneville d.
Bourneville-Pringle d.
brain d.
brancher enzyme deficiency d.
Brill-Zinsser d.
Briquet d.
Brissaud d.
Brodie d.
Brushfield-Wyatt d.
Buschke d.
Busse-Buschke d.
calcium pyrophosphate dihydrate decomposition d.
Camurati-Engelmann d.
Canavan d.
Canavan-van Bogaert-Bertrand d.
carotid artery d.
Castleman d.
catscratch d. (CSD)
central core d.
cerebral d.
cerebrovascular d.
cervical spine rheumatoid d.
Chagas d.
Charcot d.
Charcot-Marie-Tooth d.
Charcot-Marie-Tooth d. type 1, 2
Cheyne d.
childhood moyamoya d.
cholesterol ester storage d.
Christensen-Krabbe d.
Christmas d.
Coats d.
collagen vascular d.
combined system d.
comorbid d.
complex d.
connective tissue d.
Consortium to Establish a Registry for Alzheimer's D.
Contugno d.
corticospinal d.
Cotunnius d.
Cowden d.
cranial nerve heredodegenerative d.
Creutzfeldt-Jakob d. (CJD)
Crigler-Najjar d.
Crohn d.
Crouzon d.
Cruveilhier d.
Curschmann-Steinert d.
Cushing d.
cytomegalic inclusion d.
dancing d.
Danielssen d.
Danielssen-Boeck d.
degenerative brain d.
degenerative cervical disk d.
degenerative cervical spine d.
degenerative discogenic end-plate d.
Degos d.
Dejerine d.
Dejerine-Sottas d.
demyelinating white matter d.
depression spectrum d.
depressive d.
de Quervain d.
Devic d.
Diferrante d.
diffuse Lewy body d.
diffuse white matter d.
Dorfman-Chanarin d.
drug-induced white matter d.
Dubini d.
Duchenne d.
Duchenne-Aran d.
Duchenne-Griesinger d.
Eales d.
early-onset familial Alzheimer d.
early-onset Parkinson d.
Ehlers-Danlos d.
Ehlers-Danlos d. type IV
Emery-Dreifuss d.
Engelmann d.
enterococcal d.
epidural hemorrhage epidural metastatic d.
Erb d.
Erb-Charcot d.

D

NOTES

disease *(continued)*
Erb-Goldflam d.
Erdheim-Chester d.
Escobar d.
d. etiology
Eulenburg d.
d. exacerbation
exophytic joint d.
extracranial carotid occlusive d.
extracranial occlusive vascular d.
extrapyramidal motor system d.
Fabry d.
Fahr d.
Falret d.
familial Alzheimer d.
familial Parkinson d.
familial paroxysmal choreoathetosis d.
familial startle d.
Farber d.
Fazio-Londe d.
Feer d.
Flatau-Schilder d.
Foix-Alajouanine d.
Folling d.
foot-and-mouth d. (FMD)
Forbes d.
Forbes-Cori d.
Forestier d.
Fothergill d.
Freiberg-Kohler d.
Friedmann d.
Friedreich d.
Fuerstner d.
Fukuyama d.
Gaucher d.
Gerhardt d.
Gerlier d.
Gerstmann-Sträussler-Scheinker d.
Gilles de la Tourette d.
Glanzmann d.
glial d.
glutamyl ribose-5-phosphate storage d.
glycogen storage d.
Goldflam d.
Goldflam-Erb d.
Gowers d.
Graefe d.
graft-versus-host d. (GVHD)
Graves d.
Greenfield d.
Guinon d.
Haglund d.
Hallervorden-Spatz d.
Hammond d.
Hand-Schüller-Christian d.
Hansen d.
Hartnup d.
Heidenhain d.
Heine-Medin d.
hemoglobin H d.
hemoglobin SC d.
hepatocerebral d.
hepatolenticular d.
hereditary striatopallidal d.
heredodegenerative d.
Hers d.
heterogeneous system d.
Heubner d.
Hippel d.
Hippel-Lindau d.
Hirschsprung d.
Hodgkin d.
Hoehn and Yahr staging of Parkinson d.
Holmes cerebellar degeneration d.
Hoppe-Goldflam d.
Horton d.
Hunt d.
Hunter d.
Huntington d.
Hurler d.
Hurler-Scheie d.
Hurst d.
hyalin inclusion d.
hydatid d.
iatrogenic d.
Iceland d.
I-cell d.
idiopathic Parkinson d.
inclusion cell d.
infantile Gaucher d.
infantile inflammatory multisystem d.
infantile multisystem inflammatory d.
infantile Refsum d.
inflammatory demyelinating d.
intracranial d.
intradural inflammatory d.
intraneuronal inclusion d.
intrinsic d.
ischemic cerebrovascular d.
Jakob-Creutzfeldt d.
Jansky-Bielschowsky d.
Jeep driver's d.
Joseph d.
jumper d.
jumping Frenchmen of Maine d.
juvenile nonneuropathic Niemann-Pick d.
Kawasaki d.
Kearns-Sayre d.

Kennedy d.
Kennedy-Fischbeck d.
kinky-hair d.
Kinnier-Wilson d.
Klippel d.
kok d.
konzo d.
Krabbe d.
Krabbe-Weber-Dimitri d.
Kraepelin-Morel d.
K's d.
Kufs d.
Kugelberg-Welander d.
labyrinthine d.
Lafora body d.
Lake-Cavanaugh d.
Landouzy-Dejerine d.
Lasègue d.
late-onset Werdnig-Hoffmann d.
L4-5 disk d.
Leber d.
Legg d.
Leigh d.
leptomeningeal neoplastic d.
Lesch-Nyhan d.
Letterer-Siwe d.
Lewy body d.
Lhermitte-Duclos d.
Lichtheim d.
Lindau d.
Lindau-von Hippel d.
Little d.
Lou Gehrig d.
lower motor neuron d.
L5-S1 disk d.
Luft d.
lumbar disk d.
lumbar facet d.
Lyme d.
Lyodura-associated Creutzfeldt-Jakob d.
lysosomal storage d.
Lytico-Bodig d.
Machado-Joseph d.
Machiafava-Bignami d.
Marchiafava-Bignami d.
Marie-Foix-Alajouanine d.
Marie-Strümpell d.
Marie-Tooth d.
Maroteaux-Lamy d.
McArdle d.
Medin d.
medullary cystic d. (MCD)
Meige d.
Ménière d.
Menkes d.
Merzbacher-Pelizaeus d.
metastatic d.
Milton d.
Minamata d.
Minor d.
Mitchell d.
mitochondrial d. (MD)
mixed connective tissue d. (MCTD)
Möbius d.
Morel-Kraepelin d.
Morgagni d.
Morquio d.
Morton d.
Morvan d.
motor neuron d. (MND)
motor pathways d.
motor system d.
moyamoya d.
multicore d.
Murray Valley d.
muscle-eye-brain d.
myelinoclastic d.
Nasu-Hakola d.
Neftel d.
neonatal hemorrhagic d.
neuro-Behçet d.
neurodegenerative d.
neurologic d.
neuromuscular d.
neurooncologic d.
new variant Creutzfeldt-Jakob d.
Niemann d.
Niemann-Pick d. (NPD)
Niemann-Pick d., type A, B, C
nonneoplastic d.
nonviral infectious d.
Norrie d.
occlusive cerebrovascular d.
oculocraniosomatic d.
Ollier d.
Oppenheim d.
orbital d.
organic brain d. (OBD)
Paget d.
paraneoplastic neurologic d.

NOTES

disease *(continued)*
paraneoplastic neurological d.
Parkinson d.
Parrot d.
Parry-Romberg d.
Parsonage-Turner d.
pediatric moyamoya d.
Pelizaeus-Merzbacher d.
peripheral nerve d.
peripheral vascular d.
periventricular d.
peroxisomal d.
Pette-Döring d.
Peyronie d.
Pick d.
polyglucosan storage d.
polyglutamine d.
Pompe d.
Pompe d., type 2
Portuguese-Azorean d.
Pott d.
Pringle d.
prion d.
pseudo-Hurler d.
pseudomyotonia d.
pulseless d.
pyramidal tract d.
Quincke d.
Rabot d.
Ragin' Cajun d.
Raynaud d.
Recklinghausen d.
Refsum d.
Rendu-Osler-Weber d.
reversible motor neuron d.
rigid spine d.
rippling muscle d.
Romberg d.
Rosai-Dorfman d. (RDD)
Roth d.
Roussy-Lévy d.
Rust d.
Salla d.
sanatorium d.
Sandhoff d.
Sanfilippo d.
Santavuori d.
Santavuori-Haltia d.
Santavuori-Haltia-Hagberg d.
Schaumberg d.
Scheie d.
Scheuermann d.
Schilder d.
Schindler d.
Schmitt d.
Scholz d.
Seitelberger d.
self-induced artefactual skin d.
self-perpetuated d.
Selter d.
severe degenerative disk d.
Shy-Drager d.
Siemerling-Creutzfeldt d.
Sly d.
small-vessel d.
Spielmeyer-Sjögren d.
Spielmeyer-Vogt d.
Spielmeyer-Vogt-Sjögren d.
spinal cord d.
spinal metastatic d.
startle d.
Steele-Richardson-Olszewski d.
Steinert d.
St. Martin d.
Stokes-Adams d.
storage d.
structural intracranial d.
Strümpell d.
Strümpell-Leichtenstern d.
Strümpell-Lorrain d.
Strümpell-Marie d.
Strümpell-Westphal d.
Sturge d.
Sturge-Weber d.
subcortical cerebrovascular d.
subcortical small vessel d.
Swash-Schwartz d.
Sweet d.
swineherd d.
Sydenham d.
symptomatic extrapulmonary d.
systemic inflammatory d.
Takayasu d.
Talma d.
Tangier d.
Tay-Sachs d.
Thomsen d.
thoracolumbar degenerative d.
Thornton-Griggs-Moxley d.
Tooth d.
Tourette d.
transmissible neurodegenerative d.
Trevor d.
Ulrich d.
Unverricht d.
Unverricht-Lafora d.
Unverricht-Lundborg d.
upper motor neuron d.
van Bogaert d.
van Bogaert-Canavan d.
vascular Parkinson d.
venous occlusive d.
venous thromboembolic d. (VTED)
vertebrobasilar d.

Virchow d.
Vogt d.
Vogt-Spielmeyer d.
von Economo d.
von Eulenberg d.
von Gierke d.
von Hippel d.
von Hippel-Lindau d.
von Recklinghausen d.
von Willebrand d.
Wartenberg d.
Weber-Christian d.
Welander d.
Werdnig-Hoffmann d.
Wernicke d.
Weston Hurst d.
Westphal d.
Whipple d.
white matter degenerative d.
Whytt d.
Wilson d.
Winkelman d.
Wohlfart-Kugelberg-Welander d.
Wolman d.
X-linked Charcot-Marie-Tooth d.
Ziehen-Oppenheim d.

disease-associated antibody

disease-modifying
d.-m. agent (DMA)
d.-m. agent therapy (DMA therapy)
d.-m. compound
d.-m. drug (DMD)
d.-m. therapy

disengagement mechanism

disequilibrium
neurochemical d.

DISH
diffuse idiopathic skeletal hyperostosis

dishpan fracture

disialyl ganglioside

disk, disc
artificial spinal d.
Bardeen d.
choked d.
contained d.
d. curette
d. degeneration
d. edema
embryonic d.
extruded d.
frayed d.
free fragment d.
herniated cervical d.
herniated intervertebral d.
d. herniation
injury of intervertebral d.
intervertebral d.
intraspinal herniated d.
Link SB Charité d.
magnetic d.
d. matrix proteoglycan
Merkel tactile d.
noncontained d.
optic d.
PDN prosthetic d.
plastic-covered hydrogel d.
d. prolapse
protruded d.
d. protrusion
d. punch
Ranvier tactile d.
d. replacement
d. rongeur
d. rupture
ruptured d.
Schiefferdecker d.
sequestrated d.
slipped d.
d. space
d. space infection
d. syndrome
tactile d.
vacuum d.
Z d.

diskectomy (*var. of* discectomy)

diskiform

diskitis (*var. of* discitis)

diskogenic

diskogram

diskography

disk-shaped diffusion ellipsoid

dislocation
atlantoaxial d.
C6-C7 d.
fracture d.
temporomandibular joint d.

dislodgement
hook d.

dismutase
superoxide d. (SOD)

Dismutec

NOTES

disodium
carbenicillin d.
d. etidronate
disofenin
technetium 99m d.
disomy
uniparental d.
disopyramide phosphate
disorder
abnormal sleep-wake schedule d.
accommodation d.
acoustic nerve d.
acute neuropsychologic d.
acute pain d.
amino acid metabolic d.
amnestic d.
antibody-mediated d.
apperceptive d.
apraxic d.
articulation d.
atypical somatoform d.
atypical stereotyped movement d.
atypical tic d.
auditory perceptual d.
autonomic arousal d.
autosomal dominant movement d.
balance d.
behavior d.
behavioral d.
biotin metabolic d.
brain d.
caffeine-induced anxiety d.
caffeine-induced sleep d.
caffeine use d.
carbohydrate metabolism d.
d. category
cerebral degenerative d.
choreiform d.
chronic motor tic d.
chronic neuropsychologic d.
chronic sleep d.
clotting d.
cluster A, B, C d.
coagulation d.
cobalamin metabolism d.
cognition d.
cognitive d.
communication d.
congenital infratentorial d.
cranial nerve congenital d.
cranial nerve postinfectious d.
cumulative trauma d.
cystic degenerative d.
deep brain stimulation for mood d.
degenerative cervical spine d.
degenerative neuronal d.
Delirium, Dementia, and Amnestic and Other Cognitive D.'s
demyelinative d.
drug-induced movement d.
drug-induced neuromuscular d.
dysmyelinating/hypomyelinating d.
electrolyte metabolism d.
environmental sleep d.
d. of excessive sleepiness
d. of excessive somnolence
extrapyramidal d.
extrinsic sleep d.
eye movement d.
frontal gait d.
functional voice d.
gait d.
genetic d.
global amnestic d.
global anterograde memory d.
glycoprotein degradation d.
glycoprotein storage d.
hereditary brachial plexus d.
hereditary sensory and autonomic d.
heterogenous d.
histidine metabolism d.
Hunting d. (HD)
hyperkinetic conduct d.
hyperkinetic impulse d.
hyperkinetic motor d.
hypnotic-dependent sleep d.
hysterical gait d.
hysterical movement d.
inherited global neurodegenerative d.
d. of initiation and maintenance of sleep
ion channel d.
jet lag sleep d.
labyrinthine d.
limb movement d.
limb psychogenic d.
limit-setting sleep d.
lipid metabolic d.
lipid metabolism d.
lipid storage d.
lipoprotein metabolic d.
low back pain psychogenic d.
lymphoproliferative d.
lysine metabolism d.
lysosomal storage d.
mastication d.
medical/neurological d.
medication-induced movement d.
metabolic d.
metal metabolic d.
mitochondrial metabolic d.

mixed receptive/expressive language d.
monogenetic d.
mood spectrum d.
motor neuron d.
motor psychogenic d.
motor retardation developmental delay d.
movement d.
multiple tic d. (MTD)
multisomatoform d.
muscle inflammatory d.
muscle myotonic d.
muscle psychogenic d.
musculoskeletal psychogenic d.
myeloproliferative d.
neural migration d.
neural tube development d.
neurocirculatory d.
neurodegenerative d.
neurogenic d.
neurologic d.
neurometabolic d.
neuromuscular junction d.
neuronal lysosomal storage d.
neuronal migraine d.
neuronal migration d.
neuroophthalmic d.
neuropsychiatric d.
neuropsychologic d.
occupational neurotic d.
ophthalmic d.
optokinetic d.
organic anxiety d.
organic brain d.
organic delusional d.
organic mental d.
organic mood d.
organic personality d.
organic psychiatric d.
overfocusing d.
pain d.
paralytic psychosomatic d.
paraneoplastic neurologic d.
paroxysmal sleep d.
periodic limb movement d. (PLMD)
peripheral nervous system d.
peroxisomal metabolic d.
peroxisome biogenesis d. (PBD)
pervasive developmental d.
physical comorbid d.
potential cumulative trauma d.
primary thought d.
psychoactive substance-induced organic mental d.
psychogenic learning d.
psychogenic limb d.
psychogenic motor d.
psychogenic muscle d.
psychogenic musculoskeletal d.
psychogenic neurocirculatory d.
psychogenic obsessional d.
psychogenic pain d.
psychogenic respiratory d.
psychogenic rheumatic d.
psychogenic sexual d.
psychogenic skin d.
psychogenic sleep d.
psychogenic stomach d.
purine metabolic d.
pyrimidine metabolic d.
recurrent mood d.
reflex d.
REM sleep behavior d. (RBD)
REM sleep-related d.
rhythmic movement d.
secondary d.
self-perceived cognitive d.
senile gait d.
serotonin excess d.
shift work-related sleep d.
shift work sleep d.
sleep-onset association d.
sleep psychogenic d.
sleep-related breathing d. (SRBD)
sleep-starts d.
sleeptalking d.
sleep terror d.
sleep-wake transition d.
smell d.
sodium channel d.
solitary aggressive type conduct d.
somatization d.
somatoform d.
spectrum d.
speech developmental d.
sphingolipid metabolism d.
spinal cord d.
spoken language d.
stereotyped movement d.
stimulant-dependent sleep d.

NOTES

disorder *(continued)*
substance-induced organic mental d.
substantia nigra d.
swallowing d.
systemic giant cell d.
taste d.
taxonomy of anger d.
temporary personality d.
tic-related obsessive-compulsive d.
toxin-induced sleep d.
transient d.
trauma spectrum d.
traumatic brachial plexus d.
triple repeat d.
tyrosine metabolism d.
urea cycle d.
vestibular d.
violent conduct d.
visceral d.
visual field d.
visual image movement d.
vocal tic d.
wakefulness d.
X-linked cortical migration d.
disordered personality function
disorganization
background d.
d. dimension
EEG background d.
segmental arterial d.
d. symptom
disorganized
d. speech
d. symptom complex
d. thinking
disorientation
visuospatial d.
Disotate
disparity
pupil size d.
dispersion
intravoxel phase d.
nuclear magnetic relaxation d.
temporal d.
displacement
d. of interhemispheric fissure
significant d.
spondylolisthesis with significant d.
traumatic d.
display
Virtual Vision heads-up d.
disposable Doppler-constant thermocouple sensor
dispositional
disproportion
cephalocranial d.
muscle fiber type d.
disputed neurogenic thoracic outlet syndrome
disruption
anterior column d.
autonomic d.
blood-brain barrier d. (BBBD)
brain function d.
cervical spine posterior ligament d.
counting d.
incudostapedial d.
level of d.
d. of normal activity
pedicle cortex d.
sleep d.
disruptive
d. impact
d. psychotic patient
dissecting
d. aneurysm
d. forceps
d. hook
dissection
arterial d.
bone d.
bone/ligament d.
bony d.
carotid artery d.
cerebral artery d.
cerebrovascular arterial d.
cervicocephalic arterial d.
condyle d.
cranial nerve d.
extracranial vascular d.
familial cervicocephalic arterial d.
hard palate d.
incisural d.
intracranial vascular d.
intradural d.
jugular vein d.
middle fossa floor/petrous d.
muscle d.
parotid d.
soft tissue d.
subperiosteal d.
subtemporal d.
suction d.
sylvian d.
vascular d.
vertebral d.
waterjet d.
dissector
aneurysm neck d.
Angell James d.
Cavitron d.
Creed d.
Crile gasserian ganglion knife and d.

Crile nerve hook and d.
Davis dura d.
Effler-Groves d.
endarterectomy d.
Field suction d.
Freer d.
golf-stick d.
Hajek-Ballenger d.
Hardy d.
hockey-stick d.
Jannetta aneurysm neck d.
joker d.
Kennerdell-Maroon d.
Kocher d.
MacDonald d.
Malis d.
Marino transsphenoidal d.
Maroon-Jannetta d.
Milligan d.
needle d.
neural d.
Oldberg d.
Olivecrona dura d.
Penfield d.
Rayport dural and knife d.
Rhoton ball d.
Rochester lamina d.
Schmieden-Taylor d.
Scoville d.
Smithwick d.
spatula d.
teardrop d.
tissue plane d.
Toennis-Adson d.
Toennis dura d.
ultrasonic d.
Yasargil micro d.

Dissectron ultrasonic neurosurgical aspirator console

disseminata

alopecia d.

disseminated

d. central nervous system histoplasmosis
d. CNS histoplasmosis
d. encephalomyelitis
d. intravascular coagulation (DIC)
d. leiomyosarcoma
d. sclerosis

dissimulation

dissociable mechanism

dissociated

d. anesthesia
d. motor development
d. nystagmus
d. sensory loss

dissociate-dysmnesic

dissociation

albuminocytologic d.
d. level
d. measure
nonpathological d.
pathological d.
pupil light-near d.
d. sensibility
sleep d.
d. symptom
syringomyelic d.
tabetic d.
visual-kinetic d.

dissociative

d. amnesia
d. anesthesia
d. anesthetic
d. patient
d. psychoneurotic reaction
d. response
d. symptom cluster
d. tendency

distal

d. anterior cerebral artery aneurysm
d. axonopathy
d. basilar temporary clip
d. carotid
d. catheter
d. catheter lengthening
d. medial striate artery
d. motor latency
d. motor paresis
d. muscle
d. muscular dystrophy
d. myopathy
d. occlusion
d. part of anterior lobe of hypophysis
d. sensory polyneuropathy (DSP)
d. stimulation generator
d. symmetric axonal sensorimotor neuropathy
d. symmetric polyneuropathy
d. sympathetic stump
d. tingling on percussion (DTP)

NOTES

D

distalis
pars d.
distance
d. ceptor
internodal d.
interpedicular d.
interuncal d.
d. sense
distant
d. brain failure (DBF)
d. metastasis
distensae
striae d.
distensible tissue
distinction
primary/secondary d.
distortion
body-image d.
eddy current d.
local field d.
reality d.
significant subjective d.
subjective d.
distortum
collum d.
distraction
anterior d.
apical d.
d. bar
d. force
Harrington d.
d. instrumentation
d. instrumentation biomechanics
d. laminoplasty
d. rod
distraction/compression scoliosis treatment
distractor
DeBastiani d.
distribution
Boltzmann d.
butterfly d.
cervical root d.
fixed d.
nervous d.
onion-skin d.
regional d.
sensory d.
stocking-and-glove d.
d. volume ratio (DVR)
disturbance
acid-base d.
appetitive d.
balance d.
cognitive d.
core cognitive d.
dementia behavior d. (DBD)
electrolyte d.
endocrine d.
focal neurologic d.
gait d.
global assessment of sensory d.
hemisensory d.
d. of intellectual development
language d.
memory d.
mood d.
ocular motor d.
perceptual d.
peripheral vasomotor d.
physical d.
psychomotor behavioral d.
sleep d.
sleep-related respiratory d.
sleep-wake schedule d.
speech d.
temporospatial orientation d.
transient emotional d.
visual d.
disturbed
emotionally d.
d. sleep
d. sleep-wake cycle
disulfiram
disuse
d. atrophy
d. osteoporosis
d. supersensitivity
Diurigen
Diuril
diurnal
d. epilepsy
d. mood variation
d. nap
d. sleepiness
divalproex sodium
divergence
d. insufficiency
synergistic d.
diverticula
meningeal d.
diverticularization
diving
d. reflex
d. spinal cord injury
divisio, pl. **divisiones**
divisiones anteriores plexus brachialis
d. autonomica systematis nervosi peripherici
divisiones posteriores plexus brachialis
division
anterior primary d.

cell d.
lobar d.
Divry-van
D.-v. Bogaert familial corticomeningeal angiomatosis
D.-v. Bogaert syndrome
Dix-Hallpike
D.-H. maneuver
D.-H. test
Dixon
D. method opposed imaging
D. radiofrequency coil
dizziness (DZ)
DKA
olanzapine-associated DKA
dl-alpha-difluoromethylornithine
DLB
dementia with Lewy body
DLBD
diffuse Lewy body dementia
DMA
disease-modifying agent
DMA therapy
DMAS
dimethylamine sulfate
DMD
disease-modifying drug
Duchenne muscular dystrophy
dystonia musculorum deformans
DMD gene
DMD phenotype
D-Med Injection
d-methylphenidate
DMSO
dimethyl sulfoxide
DNA
deoxyribonucleic acid
DNA analysis
double-stranded DNA
DNA fragmentation factor (DFF)
DNA marker
mitochondrial DNA
DNA protein kinase
DNA repair enzyme
DNA repletion syndrome
viral DNA
DNA virus
DNAse
caspase-activated D.
DNIC
diffuse noxious inhibitory control
dobutamine
docetaxel
docking
neurotransmitter vessel d.
docosahexaenoic acid (DHA)
documented pseudarthrosis
DOC ventral cervical stabilization system
Dogbone anterior cervical plate fixation system
Dogiel
D. cell
D. corpuscle
dolce
d. far niente
d. vita
Dolenc technique
Dolgic
dolichocephaly
dolichoectasia
intracranial arterial d.
dolichoectatic
d. aneurysm
d. internal carotid artery
doll's
d. eye maneuver
d. eye reaction
d. eye reflex
d. eye sign
d. eyes phenomenon
d. head anesthesia
d. head phenomenon
Dolophine
dolor capitis
dolore
dolorific
dolorificus
trismus d.
dolorimeter
Chatillon d.
dolorimetry
dolorogenic zone
dolorology
dolorosa
analgesia d.
anesthesia d.
hypalgesia d.
paraplegia d.
dolorosum
punctum d.

NOTES

domain
analog d.
cognitive d.
Fas-associated death d.
d. of functioning
microtubule-binding d.
neuropsychologic d.
particle d.
dome
d. of aneurysm
aneurysmal d.
double d.
dominance
cerebral d.
feeling of d.
lack of clear-cut cerebral d.
left hemisphere d.
left/right hemisphere d.
mixed cerebral d.
right hemisphere d.
dominant
d. frequency
d. hemisphere
d. hemisphere infarction
d. hemisphere lesion
d. hemisphere parietal area
d. hemisphere temporal area
domperidone
Donaghy angled suture needle holder
Donaldson line
donepezil hydrochloride
donor
beating heart brain-dead d.
blood d.
Doose syndrome
dopa
d. decarboxylase inhibitor
methyl d.
dopa-decarboxylase containing
dopamine (DA)
d. agonist
d. beta hydrolase (DPH)
brain d.
d. clearance
d. degradation
d. D_2 receptor
d. enhancement
d. hydrochloride
d. metabolism
d. neurotoxicity
d. neurotransmission
d. pathway
d. projection
d. receptor blockade
d. receptor blocker
d. release
d. stimulation
striatal d.
d. synthesis
d. system
d. transporter (DAT)
d. transporter autoradiography
d. uptake site
dopamine-acetylcholine imbalance
dopamine-innervated limbic region
dopamine-modulating transmitter system
dopaminergic
d. activity
d. antagonist
d. antagonists-related exacerbation
d. blocking drug
d. effect
d. inhibition
d. medication
d. modulation
d. neuron
d. projection
d. stimulant
d. system
d. therapy
d. tone
d. treatment
d. tuberoinfundibular pathway
dopaminergic-cholinergic balance
dopa-responsive dystonia
Dopascan injection
dopium
Doppelganger phenomenon
Doppler
color-flow D.
continuous-wave D.
D. effect
D. flowmetry
D. frequency spectrum
D. imaging
Mizuho surgical D.
multifrequency transcranial D.
Neuroguard transcranial D.
D. precordial end-tidal carbon dioxide monitoring
D. probe
D. pulsatility index
pulsed D.
pulse wave D.
D. sonography
transcranial D. (TCD)
D. ultrasonography
D. ultrasound
D. ultrasound monitor
Doral
Dorello canal
Dorfman-Chanarin disease
d'orient
mal d.

Dormarex Oral
dorsal
d. accessory olivary nucleus
d. anterior cingulate region
d. aponeurotic expansion hood
d. callosal vein
d. central gray
d. cochlear nucleus
d. column sensory pathway
d. column sensory tract
d. column of spinal cord
d. column stimulation
d. column stimulator
d. column syndrome
d. cord stimulation
d. enteric fistula
d. funicular column of spinal cord
d. funiculus
d. gray column
d. horn
d. horn cell
d. horn neuron
d. horn neuronal response
d. hypothalamic area
d. hypothalamic region
d. intermediate sulcus
d. lateral geniculate nucleus
d. limbic region
d. longitudinal fasciculus
d. median fissure of medulla oblongata
d. median fissure of spinal cord
d. median sulcus
d. mesencephalic syndrome
d. midbrain glioma
d. midbrain syndrome
d. motor nucleus of vagus
d. neocortical region
d. nucleus of thalamus
d. nucleus of trapezoid body
d. nucleus of vagus
d. pallidum
d. part of pons
d. plate of neural tube
d. premammillary nucleus
d. premotor cortex
d. ramus
d. raphe
d. raphe nucleus
d. reflex
d. rhizotomy
d. root entry zone (DREZ)
d. root entry zone lesion
d. root entry zone lesioning
d. root ganglion (DRG)
d. root ganglion cell
d. root of spinal nerve
d. scapular nerve
d. septal nucleus
d. spinal root
d. spine
d. spinocerebellar tract
d. spinocerebellar tract neuron
d. stream
d. stream dysfunction
d. stream structure
d. striatum
d. subcutaneous space
d. supraoptic commissure
d. tegmental decussation
d. thalamus
d. thoracic nucleus
d. trigeminothalamic tract
d. vagal nucleus
d. vein of corpus callosum
dorsale
pallidum d.
striatum d.
tuber d.
dorsalis
Abadie sign of tabes d.
area hypothalamica d.
commissura supraoptica d.
fasciculus longitudinalis d.
funiculus d.
hypertrophic pachymeningitis d.
lamina d.
nucleus campi d.
nucleus hypothalamicus d.
nucleus olivaris accessorius d.
nucleus paramedianus d.
nucleus premammillaris d.
nucleus thoracicus d.
nucleus vagalis d.
radix d.
ramus corporis callosi d.
regio hypothalamica d.
spina d.
tabes d.
tetanus d.
thalamus d.
tractus spinocerebellaris d.

NOTES

D

Dorsey
D. dural separator
D. ventricular cannula
dorsiflex
dorsolateral
d. caudate
d. fasciculus
d. nucleus
d. prefrontal cortex
d. prefrontal cortical area
d. prefrontal syndrome
d. region
d. resection
d. sulcus
d. tract
dorsolateralis
fasciculus d.
tractus d.
dorsomedial
d. hypothalamic nucleus
d. mesencephalic syndrome
d. nucleus of hypothalamus
d. thalamotomy
dorsomedialis
nucleus hypothalamicus d.
dorsopontomesencephalic lacunar infarction
dorsum
d. pedis reflex
d. sellae atrophy
d. sella erosion
dosage
medication d.
neuroleptic d.
steroid d.
total neuroleptic d.
dose
anticholinergic d.
cumulative d.
d. dependent
effective d. (ED)
equivalent d.
d. escalation
full d.
improper d.
lithium d.
marginally therapeutic d.
maximum tolerated d.
minimal lethal d. (MLD)
modal d.
neuroleptic d.
nominal standard d.
oral d.
periphery d.
priming d.
d. range
d. reduction
d. reduction method
d. reduction strategy
sequential d.
standard d.
steady-state d.
subtherapeutic d.
dose-dependent neurotoxicity
dose-limiting toxicity
Dosepak
Medrol D.
dose-related difference
dose-response
d.-r. relation
d.-r. relationship
dosimeter
thermoluminescent d.
dosimetry
dosing
bolus d.
energy d.
fixed d.
flexible neuroleptic d.
neuroleptic d.
Dospan
Tenuate D.
dot
line frequency noise d.
dothiepin hydrochloride
dot-probe task
double
d. antihelix
d. compartment hydrocephalus
d. congenital athetosis
delire en partie d.
d. discharge
d. dome
d. elevator palsy
d. fishhook retractor
d. fragment sign
d. hemiplegia
d. major curve pattern
d. major curve scoliosis
d. spring ball valve
d. step paradigm
d. taper
d. thoracic curve
d. thoracic curve scoliosis
d. vision
d. visual control
d. yoke
d. Zielke instrumentation
double-action rongeur
double-blind
d.-b. drug study
d.-b. placebo trial
***doublecortin* gene**
"double donut" system

double-L spinal rod
double-lumen Swan-Ganz catheter
double-point threshold
double-pore vent system
double-rod
d.-r. construct
d.-r. technique
double-stranded
d.-s. deoxyribonucleic acid (dsDNA)
d.-s. DNA
d.-s. DNA virus
double-vector
d.-v. blade
d.-v. brain spatula
douce
mort d.
douloureux
tic d.
doute
folie du d.
maladie du d.
dowel cutter
Dowling
D. intracranial cyst removal
D. intracranial cyst removal technique
down
d. gaze
D. syndrome
D. syndrome clinical feature
D. syndrome dermatoglyphic pattern
D. syndrome pathology
D. syndrome screening
downbeat nystagmus
downbiting Epstein curette
down-gaze paralysis, ataxia/athetosis and foam cell (DAF syndrome)
Downing retractor
down-moving optokinetic nystagmus
downsized circular laminar hook
downstream signaling
downturned corners of the mouth
downward gaze paresis
Dox
doxazosin mesylate
doxepin hydrochloride
Doxised
doxogenic
doxorubicin hydrochloride
Doyen
D. cylindrical bur
D. rib spreader
D. spherical bur
Doyère eminence
Doz
d-penicillamine
D-penicillamine treatment
DPH
dopamine beta hydrolase
DPV
disabling positional vertigo
DR
digital radiography
DR1
Somatom D.
DR15DR2 antigen
dracunculiasis
Drager MTC transducer
drain
Charnley suction d.
external ventricular d.
Hemovac Hydrocoat d.
Heyer-Schulte wound d.
Jackson-Pratt d.
lumbar d.
Red-O-Pack d.
Shirley d.
subgaleal d.
Surgivac d.
Wound-Evac d.
drainage
bur hole d.
epidural venous d.
external ventricular d.
infratentorial venous d.
lumbar d.
serial percutaneous needle d.
Spetzler-Martin grade III medium-size lesion with deep venous d.
Spetzler-Martin grade II small lesion with deep venous d.
spinal d.
stereotactic catheter d.
syrinx d.
ventricular d.
draining vein
Drake
D. fenestrated clip
D. tandem clipping technique
D. tourniquet

D

NOTES

Drake-Kees clip
Dramamine Less Drowsy Formula
dramatogenic
drape
NeuroDrape surgical d.
OPMI microscopic d.
Dravet syndrome
***DRD2* gene**
dreaming sleep
dreamlike state
dreamy state
Dressinet netting bandage
dressing
Allevyn d.
d. apraxia
dry sterile d.
DuoDerm d.
Fabco gauze d.
Flexinet d.
d. forceps
hour-glass d.
Inerpan flexible burn d.
Kaltostat d.
Kerlix d.
Mills d.
modified Robert Jones d.
Mother Jones d.
NeoDerm d.
OpSite d.
Owen gauze d.
Reston d.
Sof-Rol d.
Sof-Wick d.
Stimson d.
surgical d.
Surgicel Nu-Knit d.
Tubex gauze d.
DREZ
dorsal root entry zone
DREZ electrode
DREZ lesioning
DREZ procedure
DREZ surgery
DREZotomy
microsurgical DREZotomy
DRG
dorsal root ganglion
drift
EEG amplifier d.
genic d.
mesenchymal d.
drill
acorn d.
Acra-Cut wire pass d.
air d.
air-powered d.
Anspach 65K d.
Black Max high-speed d.
Caspar d.
Codman d.
Crutchfield hand d.
D'Errico perforating d.
diamond high-speed air d.
electric d.
Fisch d.
d. guide
d. guide with drill bit
Hall Surgairtome II d.
Hall UltraPower d.
Hall Versipower d.
high-speed air d.
Hudson d.
McKenzie perforating twist d.
MedNext high-speed d.
Midas Rex d.
Mira Mark III cranial d.
Phoenix cranial d.
power d.
powered automatic stopping d.
Quick Connect twist d.
right-angle d.
Stryker d.
Xpress 100 disposable perforator burr hole d.
drilling technique
drink
malternative d.
Drinker tank respirator
drinking
thymogenic d.
drip
d. chamber
perfusate d.
Drisdol Oral
drive
abnormal respiratory d.
acquired d.
affiliation d.
affiliative d.
d. behavior
decreased respiratory d.
kinetic d.
physiological d.
primary d.
secondary d.
sleep d.
stimulus d. (SD)
thermal d.
vestibulospinal d.
drivel
drivenness
organic d.
driver's thigh

driving
phōtic d.
dromedary gait
dromica
epilepsia d.
dromotropic
dromotropism
negative d.
positive d.
dronabinol
droopy shoulder syndrome
drop
d. attack
d. foot
d. hand
d. metastasis
d. seizure
toe d.
wrist d.
drop-entry (closed body) hook
droperidol
drop-finger deformity
dropfoot
dropped foot
drop-thumb deformity
drowsiness
continuous daytime d.
daytime d.
incapacitating d.
pathological d.
rhythmic midtemporal theta of d. (RMTD)
drowsy
DRPLA
dentatorubropallidoluysian atrophy
DRS
Delirium Rating Scale
DRSP
drug-resistant Streptococcus pneumoniae
drug
d. action
add-on d.
d. administration
antagonist d.
antiabsence antiepileptic d.
anticholinergic d.
antidote d.
antiepileptic d. (AED)
antimuscarinic d.
antiplatelet d.
anxiolytic d.
conventional neuroleptic d.
cytotoxic d.
disease-modifying d. (DMD)
dopaminergic blocking d.
d. efficacy
enzyme-inducing antiepileptic d.
d. fever
FK-506 d.
d. half-life
hypnotic d.
immunosuppressive d.
d. infusion pump
d. intervention
intramuscular administered d.
d. metabolism
neuroleptic d.
neuropsychiatric d.
oral administered d.
phenytoin interaction with other d.
platinum-based d.
psychostimulant d.
d. reaction
d. regimen
d. reinforcement
d. risk analysis message system
sympathomimetic d.
d. tapering
d. tetanus
d. toxicity
d. transporter
tricyclic d.
d. war
d. washout
drug-induced
d.-i. depression
d.-i. dystonia
d.-i. encephalopathy
d.-i. hallucination
d.-i. hallucinatory state
d.-i. medical complication
d.-i. movement disorder
d.-i. myoglobinuria
d.-i. negative symptom
d.-i. neuromuscular disorder
d.-i. nystagmus
d.-i. organic personality syndrome
d.-i. paranoid state
d.-i. semihypnotic state
d.-i. status epilepticus
d.-i. tremor
d.-i. white matter disease

D

NOTES

drug-like desire state
drug-resistant
d.-r. depression
d.-r. localization-related seizure
d.-r. Streptococcus pneumoniae (DRSP)
drug/toxin-induced tremor
Drummond
D. spinous wiring technique
D. wire
DRVVT
dilute Russell Viper Venom time
dry
d. beriberi
d. eye syndrome
d. leprosy
d. sterile dressing
d. up
DSA
density-modulated spectral array
digital subtraction angiography
DSB
digit span backward
dsDNA
double-stranded deoxyribonucleic acid
D_2-selective dopamine agonist
DSF
digit span forward
DSM
degradable starch microspheres
DSM cluster
DSP
distal sensory polyneuropathy
DT
delirium tremens
DTI
diffuse tension imaging
diffusion tensor imaging
DTI-015
stereotactic injection D.
DTICH
delayed traumatic intracerebral hematoma
DTP
distal tingling on percussion
DTPA
diethylenetriaminepentaacetic acid
diethylene triamine pentaacetic acid
gadolinium D.
DTR
deep tendon reflex
DTT
device for transverse traction
DTT implant
***DTY1* gene**
dual
d. bypass connector
d. compression scoliosis treatment
d. mechanism of action
d. octapolar lead
d. pathology
d. quadrapolar lead
D. Quattrode spinal cord stimulation system
dual-energy x-ray absorptiometry (DEXA, DXA)
dualism
mind/body d.
molecular d.
dual-isotope SPECT
dual-switch valve
Duane retraction syndrome
Dubini
D. chorea
D. disease
Duchenne
D. disease
D. paralysis
D. sign
D. syndrome
Duchenne-Aran
D.-A. disease
D.-A. spinal muscular atrophy
Duchenne-Davidoff-Masson syndrome
Duchenne-Erb
D.-E. paralysis
D.-E. syndrome
Duchenne-Griesinger disease
Duchenne-Landouzy dystrophy
Duchenne muscular dystrophy (DMD)
duck-billed anodized spatula
Duckworth
D. phenomenon
D. sign
duct
ampullary limb of semicircular d.
basal lamina of cochlear d.
basilar crest of cochlear d.
basilar membrane of cochlear d.
cochlear d.
common limb of membranous semicircular d.
common membranous limb of membranous semicircular d.
endolymphatic d.
Hensen d.
lacrimal d.
medullary collecting d. (MCD)
parotid d.
perilymphatic d.
semicircular d.
simple membranous limb of semicircular d.
Stensen d.
thoracic part of thoracic d.

uniting d.
utriculosaccular d.

ductus
d. cochlearis
crista basilaris d.
d. endolymphaticus
d. perilymphaticus
d. reuniens
d. semicirculares
d. semicircularis
d. semicircularis anterior
d. semicircularis lateralis
d. semicircularis posterior
d. utriculosaccularis

ductuum
ampullaria d.
d. semicircularium

Dulbecco modified Eagle medium
dull unremitting headache
duloxetine hydrochloride
Dumbach cranial titanium mesh
dumbbell
d. ganglioneuroma
d. lesion
d. neuroblastoma
d. neurofibroma
d. tumor

dumbbell-shaped
d.-s. neurinoma
d.-s. spinal cavernous hemangioma

dumbbell-type neuroblastoma
dummy seed catheter
Duncan
D. syndrome
D. ventricle

Dunn device
Dunnett test
DuoCet
Duo-Cline bed wedge
DuoDerm dressing
Duografin
DuPen catheter/pump
duplex
d. scanning
d. transmission

duplication anomaly
Dupuytren contracture
dura
endosteal d.
freeze-dried cadaveric d.
d. hook
lyophilized cadaveric d.
d. mater
d. mater of brain
d. mater encephali
d. mater of spinal cord
d. mater spinalis
d. propria
d. protecting forceps
supratentorial d.
Tisseel artificial d.
Tutoplast D.

durable
descending dyscontrol d.

durabolin
Duract
Duradrin capsule
duraencephalosynangiosis
DuraGen dural graft matrix
Duragesic Transdermal
Dura-Guard dural repair patch
Dura-Kold ice wrap
dural
d. arteriovenous fistula (DAVF)
d. arteriovenous malformation
d. attachment
d. detachment
d. ectasia
d. endothelioma
d. fibrosis
d. graft
d. hematoma
d. incision
d. margin
d. metastasis
d. part of filum terminale
d. punch
d. retractor
d. ring
d. sac
d. sac effacement
d. scissors
d. separator
d. sheath
d. sinus occlusion
d. tack-up suture
d. tail
d. terminal filament
d. venous fistula
d. venous sinus
d. venous sinus thrombosis

NOTES

durale
filum terminale d.
duralis
sinus venosi d.
duramatral
duraplasty
duration
minimum d.
movement d. (MD)
stimulus d.
d. tetany
Duret
D. hemorrhage
D. lesion
Durkan CTS gauge
duroarachnitis
durocutaneous fistula
Duroliopaque
Duros
durotomy
paramedian d.
Dutch Courage
duteplase
Duvol lung clamp
DVI
digital vascular imaging
DVR
distribution volume ratio
dwarf
dwarfism
hypothyroid d.
pituitary d.
DW-EPI
diffusion-weighted echo plantar image
DWI
diffusion-weighted imaging
DWML
deep white matter lesion
Dwyer
D. device
D. instrument
D. instrumentation biomechanics
DXA (*var. of* DEXA)
Dyazide
dye
carbocyanine d.
dying-back
d.-b. neuropathy
d.-b. polyneuropathy
Dyke-Davidoff-Mason syndrome
Dyke-Davidoff syndrome
Dyken-Edathodu syndrome
Dyken syndrome
Dyken-Wisniewski syndrome
Dymelor
dymethzine
DYNA-LOC anterior fixation system
dynamic
adaptation d.
d. ambulatory balance
d. aphasia
attachment d.
d. bed
d. block
d. compression plate instrumentation
d. CT
d. entrapment of vertebral artery
flow d.
d. formulation
d. gait index
hemispheric d.
intermediate hemispheric d.
lateral hemispheric d.
medial hemispheric d.
D. mesh pre-angled connecting bar
d. polarity
power d.
d. reference arc
d. referencing
religious d.
d. single photon emission computed tomography
d. standing balance
temporal d.
d. transverse traction device
d. variable
dynamogenesis
dynamogenic
dynamogeny
dynamometer
bulb d.
dynamopathic
dynamopsychism
Dynapen
dyne
dynein
cytoplasmic d.
d. protein
dynorphin
Dyonics
D. cannula
D. rod-lens endoscope
Dyrenium
dysacusis
dysangiogenesis
hemorrhagic d.
dysantigraphia
dysaphia
dysaphic
dysarthria
apraxic d.
ataxic d.
athetoid d.
athetosic d.

flaccid d.
hyperkinetic d.
hypokinetic d.
labial d.
laryngeal d.
d. literalis
lower motor neuron d.
parkinsonian d.
peripheral d.
progressive d.
rigid d.
sensual d.
somesthetic d.
spastic d.
d. syllabaris spasmodica
dysarthric
dysarthrosis
dysautonomia
familial d.
fungiform papillae in familial d.
histamine test in familial d.
dysautonomic feature
dysbasia lordotica progressiva
dyscalculia
dyscheiral, dyschiral
dyscheiria, dyschiria
dyschromatopsia
cerebral d.
dyscinesia (*var. of* dyskinesia)
dyscoimesis
dysconjugate
d. gaze
d. movement
dyscontrol
dysdiadochokinesia, dysdiadochocinesia
dysdiadochokinesis
dysdiadochokinetic
dysembryoplastic neuroepithelial tumor
dysequilibrium
dialysis d.
frontal d.
subcortical d.
dyserethism
dysergia
dysesthesia
facial d.
dysesthesic sensation
dysexecutive syndrome
dysferlinopathy
dysfibrous layer
dysfunction
autonomic d.
bilateral hemisphere d.
brain d.
bulbar d.
calmodulin d.
cerebellovestibular d.
cerebral d.
cholinergic d.
cognitive d.
corticospinal motor system d.
depressive-executive d.
dorsal stream d.
emptying d.
focal cortical d.
focal temporal lobe d.
frontal cortical d.
frontal lobe d.
global cognitive d.
higher cerebral d.
hypothalamic d.
hypothalamic-pituitary d.
immunologic d.
interictal physiologic d.
intraictal physiologic d.
lacrimal gland d.
lingual airway d.
lobar d.
lower motor neuron d.
magnocellular d.
maternal d.
memory d.
minimal brain d.
oculosympathetic d.
optokinetic reflex d.
organic d.
pituitary d.
postictal cognitive d.
refractory erectile d.
renal d.
salivary gland d.
sensory integration d.
small-fiber d.
somatosensory d.
striatofrontal d.
temporal lobe d.
trigeminal motor d.
dysfunctional
d. circuitry
d. dopamine system

NOTES

dysfunctional *(continued)*
d. neural circuit
socially d.
dysgenesis
cerebellar vermis d.
cerebral d.
cingulate gyrus d.
corpus callosum d.
cortical d.
hemispheric cerebral d.
macroscopic d.
dysgenetic syndrome
dysgerminoma
parasellar d.
dysgeusia
dysgnosia
dysgranular cortex
dysgraphia
dysimmune polyneuropathy
dysjunction
craniofacial d.
dysjunctive
d. gaze
d. nystagmus
dyskinesia, dyscinesia
d. algera
anticonvulsant-induced d.
belly dancer d.
biliary d.
buccal-lingual d.
buccolingual d.
choreic d.
diphasic d.
dystonic paroxysmal nonkinesigenic d.
extrapyramidal d.
faciobuccolingual d.
levodopa-induced d.
lingual-facial-buccal d.
ocular d.
oral d.
oral-buccal-lingual d.
orolingual-buccal d.
d. paroxysmal
paroxysmal exertional d.
paroxysmal kinesigenic d.
paroxysmal nonkinesigenic d. (PNKD)
peak-dose d.
tardive oral d.
tardive orobuccal d.
withdrawal-emergent d.
dyskinesis
dyskinetic
dyslogia
dysmegalopsia
dysmetria
cerebellar d.
cognitive d.
lower limb d.
ocular d.
truncal d.
dysmnesic syndrome
dysmorphia
cranial d.
dysmorphic
dysmyelinating/hypomyelinating disorder
dysmyelination
dysmyelinatus
status d.
dysmyelinisatus
status d.
dysmyotonia
dysnomia
amnestic d.
dysnomic aphasia
dysnystaxis
dysorthographia
dysostosis
cleidocranial d.
craniofacial d.
mandibulofacial d.
dyspallia
dysphagia
D. Evaluation Protocol
neurogenic d.
receptive d.
dysphasia
Broca d.
Wernicke d.
dysphasic
hereditary d.
dysphonia
adductor d.
d. clericorum
d. spastica
dysphoria
omnipresent d.
premenstrual d.
dysphoric
d. category
d. character structure
d. manic state
d. patient
dysphrasia
dysplasia
anhidrotic ectodermal d.
bony d.
brain d.
cerebral d.
chondroectodermal d. (CED)
cortical d.
craniofrontonasal d.

craniometaphyseal d.
fibromuscular d. (FMD)
fibrous d.
focal cortical d.
mullerian duct aplasia, renal aplasia, cervicothoracic somite d. (MURCS)
odontoid d.
septooptic d.
septooptic-pituitary d.
sphenoid wing d.

dysplastic
d. gangliocytoma
d. spondylolisthesis

dyspnea
functional d.
nocturnal d.
sighing d.

dyspraxia
ideomotor d.
innervatory d.
limb-kinetic d.
oromotor d.
speech d.

dysprosium-DTPA

dysprosody
expressive d.
receptive d.
sensory d.

dysraphia

dysraphicus
status d.

dysraphism
craniofacial d.
occult spinal d.
spinal d.
tectocerebellar d.

dysreflexia
autonomic d. (AD)

dysregulated
d. neurotransmission
d. stress response
d. T-cell function

dysregulation
biologic d.
hypothalamic d.
immune d.
neurologic d.
sleep-related respiratory d.

dysrhythmia
cerebral d.
electroencephalographic d.
paroxysmal cerebral d.

dysrhythmic

dyssomnia

dysspondylism

dysstatic

dyssynergia
d. cerebellaris myoclonica
d. cerebellaris progressiva
detrusor-external sphincter d.
detrusor-sphincter d.
detrusor-striated sphincter d.
vesico-sphincter d.

dystasia
hereditary areflexic d.
Monro-Kel Roussy-Lévy hereditary areflexic d.
Roussy-Lévy hereditary areflexic d.

dystaxia
sensory d.

dysthymia
chronic d.

dystonia
action d.
adult-onset d.
anterocollis d.
arm d.
athetosic d.
breathy d.
cervical d.
childhood-onset d.
d. deformans progressiva
dopa-responsive d.
drug-induced d.
end of dose d.
d. examination
facial d.
focal hand d.
generalized d.
d. lenticularis
d. musculorum
d. musculorum deformans (DMD)
myoclonic d.
nocturnal paroxysmal d.
nuchal d.
off-period d.
on-period d.
oromandibular d.
oropharyngeal d.
paradoxical phenomenon of d.
paroxysmal nocturnal d.

D

NOTES

dystonia *(continued)*
pathogenic d.
postanoxic d.
primary d.
psychogenic d.
retrocollis d.
secondary d.
segmental d.
spastic d.
symptomatic d.
tardive d.
torsion d.
transient d.
d. treatment
whispering d.
dystonic
d. amyotrophy
d. cerebral palsy
d. choreoathetosis
d. movement
d. paroxysmal nonkinesigenic dyskinesia
d. reaction
d. spasm
d. torticollis
d. tremor
dystopia
orbital d.
pituitary d.
dystrophia
adiposogenital d.
d. adiposogenitalis
d. musculorum progressiva
d. myotonica
dystrophic
d. calcification
d. neurite
d. neuron
dystrophica
myotonia d.
dystrophin
dystrophinopathy
dystrophoneurosis
dystrophy
adiposogenital d.
adult pseudohypertrophic muscular d.
Aran-Duchenne muscular d.
Barnes d.
Becker-Kiener d.
Becker-type tardive muscular d.
Becker variant of Duchenne d.
benign X-linked recessive muscular d.
Bogaert-Bertrand spongy d.
cerebromacular d.
childhood muscular d.
congenital muscular d.
Dejerine-Landouzy d.
distal muscular d.
Duchenne-Landouzy d.
Duchenne muscular d. (DMD)
Emery-Dreifuss muscular d.
Erb muscular d.
facioscapulohumeral muscular d.
FSH d.
Fukuyama congenital muscular d.
Fukuyama-type congential muscular d.
Gowers muscular d.
humeroperoneal muscular d.
infantile neuroaxonal d.
Kiloh-Nevin ocular form or progressive muscular d.
Landouzy d.
Landouzy-Dejerine muscular d.
Leyden-Möbius muscular d.
limb-girdle muscular d.
merosin-positive congenital muscular d.
muscular d.
myotonic muscular d.
neuroaxonal d.
oculogastrointestinal muscular d.
oculopharyngeal muscular d. (OPMD)
pelvofemoral muscular d.
progressive muscular d.
pseudohypertrophic muscular d.
reflex sympathetic d. (RSD)
scapulohumeral muscular d.
scapuloperoneal muscular d.
severe childhood autosomal recessive muscular d.
Simmerlin d.
Steinert myotonic d.
sympathetic reflex d.
Thomsen d.
Welander muscular d.
X-linked recessive muscular d.
dystropy
DZ
diazepam
dizziness

E1
ubiquitin-activating enzyme E1
E2
ubiquitin-conjugating enzyme E2
E3
ubiquitin-ligating enzyme E3
e4 allele
e4/e4 genotype
E9000 Power System
EA-2
episodic ataxia type 2
EAE
experimental allergic encephalitis
Eagle
E. minimum essential medium
E. syndrome
Eales disease
ear
e. cartilage inflammation
cup e.
e. forceps
Earle salts
early
e. after depolarization
e. awakening
e. morning akinesia
e. pharmacological intervention
e. posttraumatic epilepsy
e. right-anterior negativity
e. seizure
e. speech impairment
e. treatment diabetic retinopathy study
e. warning sign
early-onset
e.-o. ataxia
e.-o. category
e.-o. familial Alzheimer disease
e.-o. Parkinson disease
East
E. African sleeping sickness
E. African trypanosomiasis
eastern equine encephalomyelitis (EEE)
easy
e. fatigability
e. fatigue
EasyGuide Neuro image-guided surgery system
eating epilepsy
Eaton-Lambert syndrome
EB
ethidium bromide
Ebbinghaus test
ebriety
ebriose
ebriosorum
delirium e.
ebrious
EBRT
external beam radiotherapy
ebullience
ebullient
ebullition
EBV
Epstein-Barr virus
EBV encephalitis
ECA
extracranial carotid artery
ECA study
ECA-PCA bypass surgery
ecaudate
eccentric
e. A cluster
e. arteriosclerosis
ecchondrosis
ecchordosis physaliphora
ecchymosis, pl. **ecchymoses**
bilateral medial orbital e.
periorbital e.
posterior e.
eccrine
e. angiomatous hamartoma
e. cystadenoma
e. gland
ECF
epidermal growth factor
echeosis
echinacea
echinococcosis
Echlin laminectomy rongeur
Echlin-Luer rongeur
ECHO
enteric cytopathic human orphan
ECHO virus
echo
de pensós e.
des penses e.
gradient recalled e.
Hahn e.
e. planar diffusion- and perfusion-weighted imaging scan
e. planar image
e. planar imaging
radiofrequency-induced e.
rapid spin e. (RSE)
e. reaction
e. speech
spin e.

echo *(continued)*
spoiled gradient e.
e. time (TE)
T1-weighted spin e.
T2-weighted spin e.
echodensity
intraparenchymal periventricular e.
echoencephalography
echographia
echokinesis, echokinesia
echolalia
echomimia
echomotism
echopathy
echophrasia
echopraxia
echovirus
e. infection ataxia
e. meningitis
Echovist
ECI
electrocerebral inactivity
ECIC
extracranial-intracranial
ECIC arterial bypass
Ecker fissure
eclampsia
puerperal e.
eclamptic
e. amentia
e. convulsion
e. delirium
e. idiocy
e. seizure
e. symptom
eclamptogenic
eclamptogenous
ECL chemiluminescence system
Eclipse TENS unit
ECM
extracellular matrix
ecmnesique
delire e.
ECoG
electrocorticography
E. monitoring
ecologic framework
ecology
human e.
economic viewpoint
ECOScales
ECS
electrocerebral silence
ECST
European Carotid Surgery Trial
ectal origin
ectasia
basilar e.
dural e.
segmental e.
ectoderm
embryonic neural e.
neural e.
ectomorphic
ectopia
cerebellar e.
e. lentis
posterior pituitary gland e.
ectopic
e. ACTH syndrome
e. hormone
e. intracranial retinoblastoma
e. pinealoma
e. pituitary adenoma (EPA)
e. pituitary gland
ectoretina
ectropion
ED
effective dose
EDAS
encephaloduroarteriosynangiosis
EDAS procedure
eddy
e. current
e. current distortion
e. current heating
EDE
effective dose equivalent
edema
airway e.
alimentary e.
angioneurotic e.
blue e.
brain e.
brainstem e.
cellular brain e.
cerebral e.
circumscribed e.
cytotoxic e.
disk e.
focal e.
granulocytic brain e.
hereditary angioneurotic e. (HANE)
holohemispheric vasogenic e.
interstitial hydrocephalic e.
intraneural e.
ipsilateral vasogenic e.
ischemic brain e.
meningioma-associated cerebral e.
nerve root e.
neurogenic pulmonary e. (NPE)
orthostatic e.
perifocal e.

periodic e.
peritumoral brain e.
perocephalic e.
pulmonary e.
Quincke e.
reflect e.
retroauricular e.
vasogenic e.
Eder-Puestow metal olive dilator
edetate
calcium disodium e.
edge
e. artifact
e. enhancement
Edinburgh
E. 2 Coma Scale
E. Questionnaire
Edinger
E. fiber
E. nucleus
Edinger-Westphal nucleus
edipism
Edition
Alcadd Test, Revised E.
Assessment of Aphasia and Related Disorders, Second E.
Bedside Evaluation Screening Test, Second E.
Cognitive Skills Assessment Battery, Second E.
CogScreen Aeromedical E.
Developing Cognitive Abilities Test, Second E.
Edmonton extension tongs
EDRF
endothelial-derived relaxing factor
endothelium-derived relaxing factor
Edronax
edrophonium
e. chloride
e. chloride test
EDS
Ehlers-Danlos syndrome
excessive daytime sleepiness
EDSS
Expanded Disability Status Scale
education
American Council for Headache E.
educational
e. intervention
e. stressor
Edwards
E. instrumentation
E. modular system
E. modular system bridging sleeve construct
E. modular system compression construct
E. modular system construct selection
E. modular system distraction-lordosis construct
E. modular system dynamic loading
E. modular system kyphoreduction construct
E. modular system load sharing
E. modular system neutralization construct
E. modular system rod crosslink
E. modular system rod-sleeve construct
E. modular system sacral fixation device
E. modular system scoliosis construct
E. modular system spinal rod-sleeve
E. modular system spondylo construct
E. modular system standard sleeve construct
E. modular system universal rod
E. sacral screw
Edwards/Barbaro syringo-peritoneal shunt
Edwards-Levine rod
EEE
eastern equine encephalomyelitis
EEG
electroencephalogram
electroencephalography
EEG activating procedure
EEG activation
EEG alpha blocking
EEG alpha pattern
EEG alpha rhythm
EEG alpha spindle
EEG alpha wave
EEG amplifier drift
EEG anachronism

NOTES

EEG *(continued)*
EEG anteromesial temporal discharge
attenuation of alpha rhythm on EEG
EEG background disorganization
Bancaud phenomenon on EEG
baseline EEG
BIPLED on EEG
blunt spike-and-wave complex on EEG
frontal intermittent rhythmic delta activity on EEG
ictal pattern on EEG
low voltage EEG
mixed frequency EEG
scattered dysrhythmic slow activity on EEG
sleep-deprived EEG
waking background EEG
EEG with NP lead

EEG-electrogenesis

efavirenz

effacement
dural sac e.
nerve root sheath e.
sulcus e.
ventricle e.

effect
adverse negative immunosuppressive e.
adverse side e.
antagonistic e.
anticholinergic e.
anticonvulsant e.
antidopaminergic e.
antihistaminergic e.
antimuscarinic e.
antinociceptive e.
antioxidant e.
antiseizure e.
bandwagon e.
behavioral e.
blast e.
Bohr e.
Bohr-Haldane e.
boxcar e.
brain metabolic e.
bystander e.
calming e.
catastrophic e.
cholinergic e.
choroid plexus water hammer e.
chronic e.
clasp-knife e.
clinical e.
copper wire e.
cue e.
cue-induced subjective e.
cumulative e.
Cushing e.
deleterious e.
developmental e.
differential beneficial e.
direct thermogenic e.
dopaminergic e.
Doppler e.
empathogenic e.
enhanced e.
euphoric e.
extrapyramidal motor side e.
Féré e.
first night e.
flow-induced influx e.
frontal cortex damage e.
gastrointestinal side e.
genetic e.
genomic e.
Hawthorn e.
head trauma e.
heat e.
hypermetabolic e.
iatrogenic e.
IC e.
immunosuppressive e.
inflow e.
inhibitory e.
insulin e.
interactive e.
Lazarus e.
limbic e.
limited e.
long-lasting drug e.
magnetohydrodynamic e.
main e.
mass e.
maximal e.
measurement e.
medical e.
medication-related side e.
medication side e.
metabolic e.
Mierzejewski e.
missile e.
modified Stroop e.
Mozart e.
muscarinic side e.
muscle-relaxing e.
negative immunosuppressive e.
negative priming e.
neurochemical e.
neuroprotective e.
neurotropic e.
nonsignificant protective e.

noradrenergic e.
Orbeli e.
panicogenic e.
paradoxical e.
peak behavioral e.
peripheral antimuscarinic side e.
phase-shift e.
phenothiazine toxic e.
positive e.
primary e.
proconvulsant e.
progesterone e.
protective e.
psychiatric e.
psychodynamic e.
psychological e.
psychostimulant e.
putative e.
radiation e.
rebound e.
recency e.
reinforcing e.
salicylate toxic e.
secondary e.
serial position e.
serotonergic side e.
sexual side e.
e. size
specific e.
steal e.
stimulation-related adverse e.
stimulatory e.
subjective e.
sundowner e.
susceptibility e.
sympathectomy e.
thermogenic e.
time-of-flight e.
time-on-task e.
toxic side e.
treatment-emergent extrapyramidal side e.
tricyclic e.
undifferentiated e.
Vulpian e.
washboard e.
Wedensky e.
withdrawal e.

effectance motive

effected pain

effective
e. dose (ED)
e. dose equivalent (EDE)
e. half time (Te)
e. level
e. pedicle diameter
e. technique
e. thread diameter
vasoactive e.

effectiveness
long-term e.
relative biologic e. (RBE)
relative biological e.
treatment e.

effector
e. cell
cold e.
heat e.
e. organ
warm e.

efferent
e. fiber
gamma e.
e. limb
e. motor unit
e. nerve
e. neurofiber
e. pathway
postganglionic e.
preganglionic e.
e. relation
e. sympathetic activity

efferentes
neurofibrae e.

Effer-K

effervescent
K+ Care E.
K-Electrolyte E.
K-Gen E.
Klorvess E.
K-Lyte E.
potassium bicarbonate and potassium chloride, e.
potassium bicarbonate and potassium citrate, e.

efficacy
clinical e.
drug e.
lack of e.
relational e.
e. scale

NOTES

efficacy *(continued)*
e. study
therapeutic e.
efficiency
colony-forming e.
decreased sleep e.
index of forecasting e.
sleep e.
Effler-Groves dissector
effort syndrome
effusion
subdural e.
effusive
Egemen keyhole suction-control device
egersis
EGFR
epidermal growth factor receptor
eggcrate mattress
egg-shelling procedure
egocentric stage of development
egomechanism of defense
egosyntonic trait
EGPR-TKI
epidermal growth factor-tyrosine kinase inhibitor
***EGR2* gene**
Ehlers-Danlos
E.-D. disease
E.-D. disease type IV
E.-D. syndrome (EDS)
Ehrenritter ganglion
EIA
electroimmunoassay
MAC EIA
Eichhorst
E. atrophy
E. neuritis
eicosanoid production
eicosapentaenoic acid
eight-and-a-half syndrome
eight-ball hemorrhage
eight-channel muscle stimulator
eighth
e. cranial nerve [CN VIII]
e. nerve herpetic neuritis
e. nerve tumor
Eisenlohr syndrome
eisoptrophia
ejaculatio retardata
ejaculatory center
ejection fraction
Ekbom syndrome
Ekos ultrasound catheter
ELANA
excimer laser-assisted nonocclusive anastomosis
Elan-E electronic motor system
elantrine
elan vital
elastase
myeloid e.
plasma e.
Elastica-Masson stain
Elastica van Gieson stain
elastic-type
e.-t. disk prosthesis
e.-t. disk replacement
elasticum
pseudoxanthoma e.
elastin
e. degradation
e. gene
elastomeric balloon
Elavil
elbow
e. jerk
e. reflex
Eldepryl
electicism
elective mutism
electric
e. chorea
e. differential therapy
e. drill
General E. (GE)
e. knife
e. wine
electrical
e. activity
e. change
e. characteristic
e. cortical stimulation
e. evoked potential
e. injury
e. silence
e. status epilepticus
e. status epilepticus during slow sleep
e. status epilepticus of sleep
e. stimulation of centromedian thalamic nucleus
e. stimulation mapping
Electri-Cool cold therapy system
electroanalgesia
electroaxonography
electroblotting
electrocautery
Aspen e.
bipolar e.
Fox bipolar e.
monopolar e.
electrocerebral
e. activity
e. inactivator

e. inactivity (ECI)
e. silence (ECS)
electrocoagulation
RF e.
electrocochleogram
electrocontractility
electroconvulsive
e. seizure
e. therapy
electrocorticogram
electrocorticography (ECoG)
intraoperative e.
electrode
active surface e.
AdTech Spencer platinum depth e.
A-frame e.
anterior cheek e.
Aspen laparoscopy e.
bifilar needle e.
bipolar needle e.
bipolar stimulating e.
Clark e.
clip-type e.
coaxial needle e.
combination needle e.
concentric needle e.
Cueva cranial nerve e.
curved e.
Cyberonics vagus nerve stimulator e.
DBS e.
depth e.
DREZ e.
El-Naggar-Nashold right-angled nucleus caudalis DREZ e.
epidural peg e.
exploring e.
external auditory meatus e.
external canthus e.
flexible wire e.
foramen ovale e.
Goldmann-Offner reference of e.
ground e.
helical e.
e. impedance
indifferent e.
intracerebral depth e.
Levin thermocouple cordotomy e.
mandibular notch e.
metal e.
e. migration
monopolar needle e.
monopolar stimulating e.
multilead e.
Nashold TC e.
nasopharyngeal e.
needle e.
Nichrome cylindrical e.
noncephalic e.
percutaneous epidural e.
Pisces e.
Pisces-Quad e.
Quad e.
Ray RRE-TM thermistor e.
record e.
recording e.
reference e.
Resume e.
scalp e.
self-adhering e.
self-attaching e.
semiinvasive e.
Silverman placement of e.
silver-silver chloride e.
Sluyter-Mehta thermocouple e.
SMK e.
Somatics monitoring e.
Spencer probe depth e.
sphenoidal e.
spring-loaded e.
Stephenson-Gibbs reference e.
stimulating e.
straight needle e.
subdural grid e.
subdural strip e.
surface e.
temporary percutaneous SCS e.
thermistor e.
Thymapad stimulus e.
trigeminal e.
tripolar nerve cuff e.
Wolfram needle e.
Wyler cylindrical subdural e.
electrodecrement
diffuse e.
electrodecremental seizure
electrode-popping artifact
electrodermal
electrodetachable
e. balloon
e. platinum coil
electrodiagnosis

NOTES

electrodiagnostic
e. medicine
e. study
e. testing
electroencephalogram (EEG)
e. activation
alerting maneuver on e.
alerting stimulus on e.
aliasing on e.
ambulatory e. (AEEG)
audiovisual e.
Bancaud phenomenon on e.
e. BEAM technique
e. brain electrical activity method technique
e. burst suppression pattern
depth-recorded e.
flat e.
HFF on e.
hippocampal e.
hypersynchronous e.
interictal e.
intracranial e. (ICEEG)
IRDA on e.
isoelectric e.
Janz response on e.
Laplacian montage on e.
LFF on e.
MFD waves on e.
MSLT with e.
normal e. (NEEG)
OIRDA on e.
PDA on e.
POSTS on e.
quantitative e. (QEEG)
e. rhythm
RMTD on e.
SREDA on e.
SSS on e.
stereotactic depth e. (SDEEG)
e. study
surface scalp e.
electroencephalogram/ electroencephalography
electroencephalograph
electroencephalographer
electroencephalographic
e. burst-suppression
e. dysrhythmia
e. pattern
e. wave
electroencephalography (EEG)
ambulatory e. (AEEG)
electroencephalogram/ e.
intracranial e.
scalp ictal e.
scalp-sphenoidal e.
single fiber e. (SFEMG)
stereotactic depth e. (SDEEG)
subdural e.
electroencephalography-guided cortical resection
electroencephaloscope
electrogram
electrograph
electrographic
e. seizure
e. seizure activity
electrography
electrogustometry
electroimmunoassay (EIA)
electrolyte
e. change
e. disturbance
e. imbalance
e. metabolism disorder
electromagnetic
e. flowmeter
e. flow probe
e. focusing field
e. focusing field probe
e. interference (EMI)
e. radiation
electromicturation
electromuscular sensibility
electromyelogram
electromyelography
electromyogram (EMG)
CMAP on e.
CNAP on e.
CRD on e.
Erb point stimulation on e.
MUAP on e.
SNAP on e.
SSR on e.
electromyogram-triggered neuromuscular stimulation (EMG-triggered neuromuscular stimulation)
electromyograph
Counterpoint e.
electromyographic (EMG)
e. artifact
e. feedback
e. incomplete interference pattern
needle e.
e. potential
e. response
electromyography (EMG)
facial e.
needle e.
single-fiber e.
electron
e. collision
e. micrograph

e. microscopy
e. transport chain
e. transport particle (ETP)
electron-coupled nuclear spin-spin interaction
electroneurogram (ENoG)
electroneurography (ENoG)
facial e.
electroneurolysis
electroneuromyography
electronic
e. monitor
e. monitoring
e. stimulator
electronystagmography (ENG)
electrooculogram
electrooculographic analysis
electrooculography (EOG)
electropathology
electrophoresis
agarose gel e.
protein e.
pulsed-field gel e.
sodium dodecyl sulfate-polyacrylamide gel e.
thin-layer agarose gel e.
two-dimensional e.
electrophrenic respiration
electrophysiologic
e. change
e. integrity
e. study
e. test
electrophysiological
e. guidance
e. mapping
e. procedure
e. stimulation
electrophysiology test
electroplaque
Torpedo e.
electroretinogram
electroretinography (ERG)
electroshock seizure threshold
electrosleep
electrospectrogram
electrospectrography
electrospinogram
electrospinography
electrostimulation
electrotherapeutic
e. sleep
e. sleep therapy
electrothermal
intradiscal e.
electrothrombosis
electrotonic
e. current
e. junction
e. synapse
electrotonus
Elekta
E. Leksell rongeur
E. Robotic Surgical Microscope
E. stereotactic head frame
E. viewing wand
element
cAMP response e.
glioneuronal e.
identical e.'s
elephantiasis neuromatosa
eletriptan
Eleutherococcus senticosus
elevated
e. protein concentration
e. score
elevation
flap e.
ischemia-induced e.
mood e.
nonfocal e.
e. paresis
prolactin e.
T score e.
elevator
Adson e.
Cloward e.
Cobb periosteal e.
Cottle e.
Crawford dural e.
Cushing Little Joker e.
Cushing periosteal e.
Cushing pituitary e.
Cushing staphylorrhaphy e.
D'Errico periosteal e.
Frazier dural e.
Freer septal e.
Hajek-Ballenger septal e.
Jannetta duckbill e.
Jarit periosteal e.
Kennerdell-Maroon e.

NOTES

elevator *(continued)*
Key e.
Langenbeck periosteal e.
Malis e.
periosteal e.
round-tipped periosteal e.
Yasargil e.
elevatus
iatrogenic e.
eleventh cranial nerve [CN XI]
elfin
e. facies
e. facies syndrome
Elgiloy
E. clip
E. clip material
elicitation
affect e.
emotion e.
Elihorn Maze Test
ELISA
enzyme-linked immunosorbent assay
ELISA Quantikine kit
ELISA test
ellipsis
ellipsoid
cigar-shaped diffusion e.
disk-shaped diffusion e.
elliptical
e. incision
e. nystagmus
El-Naggar-Nashold right-angled nucleus caudalis DREZ electrode
eloquent
e. cortex
e. versus noneloquent area
Elsberg
E. brain cannula
E. test
E. ventricular cannula
elusive illness state
EM
extraordinary meridian
emarginate
emargination
embarrassment
cord e.
nerve root e.
respiratory e.
embedding
paraffin e.
embolalia, embololalia
embolden
embolectomy
direct e.
emboli (*pl. of* embolus)
embolic
e. apoplexy
e. infarction
e. source
e. stroke
emboliformis
nucleus e.
emboliform nucleus
emboligenic
embolism
air e.
arterial gas e. (AGE)
artery-to-artery e.
cardiac e.
cardiogenic e.
cerebral formed-element e.
cerebrovascular e.
cholesterol e.
fat e.
paradoxical air e.
paradoxical cerebral e.
pulmonary e.
retinal e.
rheumatic fever cerebral e.
spinal e.
therapeutic e.
venous e.
embolization
cerebral foreign body e.
coil e.
flow-directed e.
Histoacryl e.
particulate e.
percutaneous intraarterial e.
percutaneous transvenous coil e.
selective e.
staged e.
stent-supported coil e.
superselective e.
therapeutic e.
transarterial platinum coil e.
transtorcular e.
venous-side e.
embololalia (*var. of* embolalia)
embolophasia
embolophrasia
embolotherapy
embolus, pl. **emboli**
air e.
calcium e.
cerebral e.
fat e.
fibrin-platelet-fibrin e.
Gelfoam powder e.
organism e.
platelet-fibrin e.
septic e.

embolus-to-blood ratio
Embolyx liquid embolic system
embouchment
embryonal cell carcinoma
embryonic
e. cervical somite
e. disk
e. implant
e. isoform
e. neural ectoderm
e. tail
EMC
encephalomyocarditis
EMC encephalitis
EMD121974
EMDR
eye movement desensitization and reprocessing
Emery-Dreifuss
E.-D. disease
E.-D. muscular dystrophy
emetine peripheral neuropathy
EMG
electromyogram
electromyographic
electromyography
automatic decompensation EMG
EMG biofeedback
EMG examination
needle EMG
Nomad-LE EMG
Single-fiber EMG
single fiber EMG (SFEMG)
EMG stimulator
triggered EMG
EMG-triggered neuromuscular stimulation
EMI
electromagnetic interference
eminence
abducens e.
arcuate e.
collateral e.
cruciate e.
cruciform e.
Doyère e.
eminentia teres facial e.
facial e.
hypoglossal e.
malar e.
medial e.
median e.
olivary e.
postchiasmic e.
postfundibular e.
pyramidal e.
restiform e.
round e.
terete e.
thenar e.
trigeminal e.
eminentia, pl. **eminentiae**
e. abducentis
e. collateralis
e. cruciformis
e. facialis
e. hypoglossi
e. medialis
e. medialis fossae rhomboideae
e. mediana
e. pyramidalis
e. restiformis
e. teres
e. teres facial eminence
vagi e.
emissary
e. foramen
e. vein
emission computed tomography
Emitrip
Emory Functional Ambulation Profile
emotion
e. elicitation
e. production
emotional
e. amnesia
e. B cluster
e. communication
e. control therapy
e. excitability
e. functioning
e. information processing
e. input
e. instability
e. leukocytosis
e. mechanism
e. memory deficit
e. memory process
e. memory processing
e. memory score
e. neglect
e. numbness

NOTES

emotional *(continued)*
e. reactivity
e. regulation
e. release therapy
e. salience
e. stimulation
e. trajectory
e. undercontrol
e. upheaval
e. withdrawal
emotionally
e. disturbed
e. unavailable
e. ungiving
emotion-related activation
emotive
e. stimulus
e. theory
empacho
empathic
e. capacity
e. failure
empathogenic effect
emphasis
bilateral temporoparietal e.
emphrensy
emphysema
subgaleal e.
empirical
e. approach
e. basis
e. classification
e. finding
e. limitation
e. research
e. study
e. therapy
empiricism
scientific e.
Empracet with codeine
emprosthotonos position
empty
e. delta sign
e. sella
e. sella sign
e. sella syndrome
e. set
e. triangle sign
emptying dysfunction
empyema
subdural e.
E-M syndrome
emulsion
polyvinyl acetate e.
EMV
eye-motor-verbal
en
e. bloc
e. bloc laminoplasty
e. bloc resection
e. Neuroscience
e. passage feeder artery
e. plaque meningioma
enanthate
testosterone e.
enantiomer
encapsulated
e. brain abscess
e. end organ
encapsulation
polymer e.
encephala (*pl. of* encephalon)
encephalalgia
encephalatrophic
encephalatrophy
encephalauxe
encéphale isolé
encephalemia
encephali
arachnoidea mater e.
arachnoid mater e.
arteriae e.
bulbus e.
dura mater e.
pia mater e.
truncus e.
encephalic
e. angioma
e. asymmetry
e. nerve
e. trunk
e. vertigo
e. vesicle
encephalici
nervi e.
encephalicus
truncus e.
encephalitic
encephalitis, pl. **encephalitides**
acute hemorrhagic e.
acute inclusion body e.
acute necrotizing e.
Australian X e.
bacterial e.
benign myalgic e.
brainstem e.
bunyavirus e.
California e.
Central European e.
cerebellar e.
chronic focal e. (CFE)
CMV e.
Colorado tick fever viral e.

coxsackie e.
Dawson e.
dengue viral e.
EBV e.
EMC e.
enteroviral e.
epidemic e.
equine e.
experimental allergic e. (EAE)
Far East Russian e.
forest-spring e.
fulminant necrotizing e.
granulomatous e.
Hayem e.
e. hemorrhagica
herpes/herpetic e.
herpes simplex virus e. (HSVE)
herpesvirus e.
herpes zoster e.
HSV e.
hyperergic e.
Ilhéus e.
inclusion body e.
influenzal e.
Japanese B e.
e. japonica
Kozhevnikov spring-summer e.
La Crosse e.
lead e.
Leichtenstern e.
e. lethargica
limbic e.
lymphocytic choriomeningitis virus e.
lymphogranuloma venereum e.
Marie-Strümpell e.
measles e.
Mengo e.
metabolic e.
microglial nodular e.
mumps e.
Murray Valley e.
Mycoplasma pneumoniae e.
necrotizing e.
e. neonatorum
Nipah virus e.
e. periaxialis
e. periaxialis concentrica
e. periaxialis diffusa
postinfective e.
postvaccinal e.
Powassan e.
psittacosis e.
purulent e.
e. pyogenica
Rasmussen chronic focal e.
rotavirus e.
Russian autumn e.
Russian autumnal e.
Russian endemic e.
Russian forest-spring e.
Russian spring-summer e.
Russian spring-summer e. (Eastern subtype)
Russian spring-summer e. (Western subtype)
Russian tick-borne e.
Russian vernal e.
Saint Louis e.
Schilder e.
secondary e.
Semliki Forest e.
septic e.
St. Louis e.
Strümpell-Leichtenstern e.
subacute inclusion body e.
subacute measles e.
e. subcorticalis chronica
subcorticalis chronica e.
summer e.
suppurative e.
tick-borne e. (Central European subtype)
tick-borne e. (Eastern subtype)
toxoplasmic e. (TE)
van Bogaert e.
varicella e.
Venezuelan equine e.
vernal e.
vernoestival e.
Vienna e.
viral e.
von Economo e.
Western equine e.
West Nile e.
woodcutter's e.
yellow fever e.

encephalitogen

encephalitogenic protein

encephalization

encephalocele

anterior basal e.

NOTES

E

encephalocele *(continued)*
basal e.
frontal e.
frontoethmoidal e.
frontosphenoidal e.
nasoethmoidal e.
nasofrontal e.
nasoorbital e.
occipital e.
orbital e.
parietal e.
sphenoethmoidal e.
sphenoid e.
sphenoidal e.
sphenomaxillary e.
sphenoorbital e.
suboccipital e.
transethmoidal e.
transsphenoidal e.
encephaloclastic
e. microcephaly
e. porencephaly
encephalocystocele
encephalodialysis
encephaloduroarteriomyosynangiosis
encephaloduroarteriosynangiosis (EDAS)
encephaloduromyosynangiosis
ribbon e.
encephalodynia
encephalodysplasia
encephalofacial angiomatosis
encephalogaleosynangiosis
encephalogram
isoelectric e.
encephalography
encephaloid
encephalolith
encephalology
encephaloma
encephalomalacia
cystic e.
end-stage ischemic e.
multicystic e.
subcortical e.
encephalomeningitis
encephalomeningocele
encephalomeningopathy
encephalometer
encephalomyelitis
acute disseminated e. (ADE)
acute disseminating e.
acute necrotizing hemorrhagic e.
allergic e.
benign myalgic e.
disseminated e.
eastern equine e. (EEE)
epidemic myalgic e.
experimental allergic e.
experimental autoimmune e.
granulomatous e.
Leigh subacute necrotizing e.
necrotizing e.
paraneoplastic e.
postinfectious disseminated e.
postparainfectious e.
postvaccinal e.
subacute necrotizing e.
toxoplasmic e.
vaccination e.
varicella zoster e.
Venezuelan equine e. (VEE)
viral e.
virus e.
western equine e. (WEE)
zoster e.
encephalomyelocele
encephalomyeloneuropathy
nonspecific e.
encephalomyelonic axis
encephalomyelopathy
carcinomatous e.
epidemic myalgic e.
necrotizing e.
paracarcinomatous e.
paraneoplastic e.
postinfection e.
postvaccinal e.
subacute necrotizing e. (SNE)
encephalomyeloradiculitis
encephalomyeloradiculopathy
encephalomyocarditis (EMC)
encephalomyopathy
mitochondrial neurogastrointestinal e.
encephalomyosynangiosis
encephalon, pl. **encephala**
encephalonarcosis
encephalopathia addisonia
encephalopathic
encephalopathy
AIDS e.
alcoholic e.
amyotrophic type of spongiform e.
anoxic-ischemic e.
arteriosclerotic e.
autosomal recessive syndrome of e.
bilirubin e.
Binswanger e.
bovine spongiform e.
chronic traumatic e.
demyelinating e.
drug-induced e.
epileptic e.
familial e.

fulminant hepatic e.
Heidenhain type of spongiform e.
hemorrhagic e.
hepatic e.
HIV e.
hyperkinetic e.
hypernatremic e.
hypertensive e.
hypoglycemic e.
hyponatremic e.
hypoparathyroid e.
hypoxic-hypercarbic e.
hypoxic ischemic e. (HIE)
infantile subacute necrotizing e.
ischemic-hypoxic e.
lead e.
Leigh necrotizing e.
liver e.
Lyme e.
metabolic e.
mitochondrial e.
mitochondrial neurogastrointestinal e. (MNGIE)
multicystic e.
myoclonic e.
myoneurogastrointestinal e.
necrotizing e.
Nevin-Jones subacute spongiform e.
palindromic e.
pancreatic e.
pertussis vaccination e.
portal systemic e.
postanoxic e.
postcontusion syndrome e.
postvaccinal e.
progressive degenerative subcortical e.
progressive dialysis e.
progressive multifocal leuko-J e.
progressive spongiform e.
progressive subcortical e.
progressive traumatic e.
pulmonary e.
recurrent e.
saturnine e.
severe postanoxic e.
spongiform virus e.
subacute necrotizing e.
subacute spongiform e.
subcortical arteriosclerotic e.
subcortical vascular e.
thiamine deficiency e.
thyrotoxic e.
transmissible spongiform viral e.
traumatic progressive e.
uremic e.
vaccination e.
Wernicke e.
Wernicke-Korsakoff e.

encephalopsy
encephalopuncture
encephalopyosis
encephaloradiculitis
encephalorrhachidian
encephalorrhagia
pericapillary e.
encephaloschisis
encephalosclerosis
encephaloscope
encephaloscopy
encephalosepsis
encephalosis
encephalospinal
encephalothlipsis
encephalotome
encephalotomy
encephalotrigeminal
e. angiomatosis
e. angiomatosis seizure
e. vascular syndrome
enclosed
e. macroadenoma
e. space
encoding
frequency e.
phase e.
velocity e.
encotretic
encroachment
foraminal e.
encyprate
end
e. bulb
e. of dose dystonia
e. organ
e. plate
endarterectomy
carotid e.
e. dissector
endarteritis
Heubner e.
endbrain

NOTES

E

end-brush
end-bulb
Endeavor
E. balloon
E. Instructional Rating System
E. nondetachable silicone balloon catheter
endemic
e. hiccup
e. neuritis
e. paralytic vertigo
e. poliomyelitis
endemica
panneuritis e.
Endep
end-gaze physiologic nystagmus
ending
annulospiral e.
caliciform e.
epilemmal e.
flower-spray e.
free nerve e.
grape e.
hederiform e.
nerve e.
nonencapsulated nerve e.
presynaptic nerve e.
primary e.
Ruffini e.
secondary e.
sole-plate e.
sympathetic nerve e.
synaptic e.
end-ischemic
end-labeling
terminal deoxynucleotidyl transferase-mediated dUTP nick e.-l. (TUNEL)
transferase-mediated dUTP-digoxigenin nick e.-l. (TUNEL)
Endler
endoaneurysmoplasty
endoaneurysmorrhaphy
Endobile
endocathection
endoceliac
endocentric construction
endocept
endocranial cast
endocraniosis
endocranitis
endocranium
endocratic power
endocrine
e. axis
e. disturbance
e. function
e. gland
e. system
endocrine-inactive pituitary adenoma
endocrinologic
endocrinological compromise
endocrinopathy
endodermal
e. cyst
e. sinus
e. sinus tumor
endoesophageal pressure measurement
end-of-dose
e.-o.-d. bradykinesia
e.-o.-d. deterioration
end-of-life care
endogenesis
endogenous
e. abnormality
e. adenosine
e. antioxidant
e. antioxidative defense
e. benzodiazepine-like toxin
e. brain mechanism
e. chromosomal promoter
e. circadian rhythm
e. electrophysiological component
e. fiber
e. force
e. neuroprotective agent
e. oxidant
e. pyrogen (EP)
e. steroid hormone
e. thyrotoxicosis
e. transmitter
endoglycosidase
Endografin
endolemniscalis
nucleus e.
endolemniscal nucleus
endolymphatic
e. duct
e. hydrops
e. sac
endolymphaticus
ductus e.
endolymph production
endomeninx
endomysial
endomysium
endonasal skull-base endoscopy
endoneural tube
endoneurial fluid
endoneuritis
endoneurium
endoneurolysis
endonuclease
restriction e.

endopeduncularis
nucleus e.
endopeduncular nucleus
endoperineuritis
endoperoxide
cyclic e.
endoplasmic reticulum
endoprosthesis
Wallgraft e.
endopsychic perception
end-organ degeneration
endorphin
endorphinergic
endorrhachis
endosaccular
e. coil placement
e. packing
endoscope
angled-lens e.
angled-shaft e.
Desormaux e.
Dyonics rod-lens e.
flexible e.
Gaab e.
e. holder
Hopkins II e.
e. lens cleansing device
malleable e.
percutaneous spinal e.
Perneczky-designed microscope-assisting e.
rigid rod-lens e.
Tamaki e.
Wolf e.
endoscope-assisted craniotomy
endoscope-controlled microsurgery
endoscopic
e. sinus surgery
e. skull-base
e. skull-base surgery
e. sphenoidal biopsy
e. third ventriculostomy (ETV)
e. visualization
endoscopic-assisted
microscopic neurosurgery e.-a.
endoscopy
endonasal skull-base e.
heads-up adjunctive e.
intraventricular e.
laser-assisted spinal e.
transcranial skull-base e.
virtual e.
endostatin
endosteal dura
endothelial
e. adhesion molecule
e. cell-derived procoagulant
e. cell inhibitor
e. cell-stimulating angiogenesis factor
e. cell-stimulating glioma
e. injury
e. monolayer
e. nitric oxide synthase
endothelial-derived relaxing factor (EDRF)
endothelin (ET)
endothelin-1 (ET-1)
e. platinum-Dacron microcoil
e. platinum-Dacron microcoil endotracheal tube
endothelioma
dural e.
endotheliomatous meningioma
endothelium
e. derived
tight junctioned e.
vascular e.
endothelium-derived relaxing factor (EDRF)
endotherm
endothermic
endothermy
endotoxin
gram-negative e.
meningococcal e.
endotracheal tube
endovascular
e. balloon occlusion
e. carotid sacrifice
e. coil
e. technique
e. therapy
endovasculoscopy
endozepine
endplate, end-plate
e. activity
bony e.
e. instability
motor e.

NOTES

endplate *(continued)*
muscle e.
e. potential (EPP)
end-point
e.-p. CGI score
e.-p. nystagmus
end-product
advanced glycation e.-p. (AGE)
Endrate
endrin
end-stage ischemic encephalomalacia
end-state functioning
end-tidal
e.-t. carbon dioxide monitoring
e.-t. CO_2
e.-t. nitrogen monitoring
end-to-end anastomosis
Enduron
endyma
end-zone pain
enelicomorphism
energy
change in e.
e. conservation
e. dosing
intense e.
e. lack
Law of Specific Nerve E.
e. metabolism
e. requirement
enervation
enflurane
ENG
electronystagmography
Engel
E. classification system for postoperative seizure control class I–IV
E. postoperative seizure classification
E. Seizure Outcome Scale
Engelmann disease
***En* gene**
engorgement
brain e.
engrailed gene
engram
engraphia
enhanced
e. effect
e. physiologic tremor
e. sensitivity
enhancement
contrast e.
dopamine e.
edge e.
flow-related e.
gadolinium e.
MR imaging with gadolinium e.
nodular e.
paramagnetic contrast e.
postsynaptic e.
relaxation rate e.
selective relaxation e.
vertebral end-plate e.
enhancing
e. exophytic tumor
e. ring
enkephalinergic
enkephalins
Enker brain retractor
enlarged
e. brain
e. pupil
enlargement
cervical e.
choroid e.
cisterna magna e.
lumbosacral e.
moyamoya collateral e.
sulcal e.
tympanic e.
ventricular e.
enlarging bur
Enlon Injection
Ennis-Weir Critical Thinking Essay Test
ENoG
electroneurogram
electroneurography
enolase
neuron-specific e. (NSE)
serum neuron-specific e.
enophthalmos
Enovil
entacapone
ental origin
Entamoeba
E. histolytica
E. histolytica cerebral amebiasis
entasia, entasis
entatic
entendu
enteric
e. cyst
e. cytopathic human orphan (ECHO)
e. cytopathic human orphan virus
e. virus infection
entericus
plexus e.
entering root
Enterobacter
Enterobacteriaceae

enterococcal disease
enterocolitica
Yersinia e.
enterogastric reflex
enterogenous cyst
enteropathic arthritis
enteroviral encephalitis
enterovirus
e. infection
e. meningitis
enthesitis
enthesopathy
enthlasis
entity locative
entoptic pulse
entorbital fissure
entorhinal
e. area
e. cortex
e. cortex atrophy
entorhinal-hippocampal system
entrance
sellar e.
entrapment
median nerve e.
e. mononeuropathy
nerve e.
e. neuropathy
PIN e.
suprascapular nerve e.
ulnar nerve e.
entrapy
entropy
wavelet e.
entry
e. point
e. zone
e. zone lesion
entubulation technique
enucleation
tumor e.
enucleator
Hardy microsurgical e.
Marino transsphenoidal e.
enuresis
functional e.
nocturnal e.
primary e.
enuretic absence
envelope
cistern of nuclear e.
nuclear e.
environmental
e. assessment
e. cue
e. factor
e. impediment
e. neurology
e. press
e. process
e. sleep disorder
e. susceptibility
environment characteristic
Envision anterior cervical plate system
Envoy guide catheter
enzymatic binding site
enzyme
e. activation
e. autoinduction
cyclooxygenase e.
DNA repair e.
ET-converting e.
Fas-associated death domain-like interleukin-converting e.
hepatic e.
Hind III e.
interleukin-1 B-converting e.
lipolytic e.
neurotransmitter metabolic e.
porphyria synthesizing e.
rate-limiting e.
enzyme-inducing
e.-i. antiepileptic
e.-i. antiepileptic drug
enzyme-linked immunosorbent assay (ELISA)
EOF
oxygen extraction fraction
EOG
electrooculography
EOM
extraocular movement
eosinophil adenoma
eosinophilia-myalgia syndrome
eosinophilic
e. granuloma
e. granulomatosis
e. leukocyte
e. meningitis
e. meningoencephalitis

NOTES

eosinophilic *(continued)*
e. myeloencephalitis
e. myositis
eosin stain
EP
endogenous pyrogen
evoked potential
EPA
ectopic pituitary adenoma
epena
ependopathy
ependyma
ventricular e.
ependymal
e. cell
e. cyst
e. layer
e. tumor
e. zone
ependymitis
granular e.
e. granularis
ependymoblastoma
ependymocyte
ependymocytoma
ependymoma
anaplastic e.
cerebellar e.
clear cell e.
exophytic e.
intramedullary e.
myxopapillary e.
sacrococcygeal myxopapillary e.
spinal e.
subcutaneous sacrococcygeal myxopapillary e.
supratentorial lobar e.
ependymopathy
ephapse
ephaptic
e. conduction
e. transmission
ephebophilia
Ephedra sinica
ephedrine
e. sulfate
e., theophylline, phenobarbital
ephemera
ephemeral
epicerebral space
epicondylectomy
medial e.
epiconus syndrome
epicortical lesion
epicranium
epicritic
e. sensation
e. sensibility
epidemic
e. cerebrospinal meningitis
e. encephalitis
e. multiple sclerosis
e. myalgic encephalomyelitis
e. myalgic encephalomyelopathy
e. neuromyasthenia
e. poliomyelitis
e. tetany
e. typhus
e. vertigo
epidemica
myalgia cruris e.
tetania e.
epidemiological
E. Catchment Area Study
e. research
e. study
epidemiology
Multi-Institutional Research in Alzheimer Genetic E.
pandemic e.
epidermal
e. growth factor (ECF)
e. growth factor receptor (EGFR)
e. growth factor receptor gene
e. growth factor-tyrosine kinase inhibitor (EGPR-TKI)
e. necrolysis
e. nevus syndrome
epidermidis
Staphylococcus e.
epidermoid
chiasmal e.
e. cyst
e. lipoma
torcular e.
e. tumor
epidermoidoma
epidural
e. abscess
e. abscess evacuation
e. aerocele
e. angiolipoma
e. block
e. cavernous hemangioma
e. cavity
e. cord compression
e. fat
e. hematoma
e. hemorrhage
e. hemorrhage epidural metastatic disease
e. implant

e. infection
e. lipomatosis
e. meningioma
e. meningitis
e. needle
e. neuroplasty
e. peg electrode
e. pneumatosis
e. pneumocephalus
e. space
e. steroid injection
e. tumor
e. tumor evacuation
e. venography
e. venous drainage
e. venous plexus

epidurale
cavum e.
spatium e.

epiduralis
cavitas e.

epidurography

epiendoneurium

epifascicular epineurium

epigastric
e. aura
e. plexus
e. reflex

epilemma

epilemmal ending

epilepsia
e. arithmetica
e. cursiva
e. dromica
e. gravior
e. major
e. minor
e. mitior
e. nutans
e. partialis continua
e. tarda

epilepsy
abdominal e.
activated e.
adolescent-onset e.
adult-onset e.
affective prodrome of e.
age-dependent e.
akinetic e.
alcoholic e.
alcohol-precipitated e.
amygdalar e.
anosognosic e.
anterior polar-amygdalar e.
atonic e.
audiogenic e.
automatic e.
autonomic e.
autosomal dominant nocturnal frontal lobe e.
autosomal dominant temporal lobe e.
Baltic myoclonus e.
benign adult familial myoclonic e.
benign childhood partial e.
benign familial myoclonic e.
benign focal of childhood e.
benign occipital e.
benign rolandic e.
bilateral mesial temporal lobe e.
Bravais-jacksonian e.
catamenial e.
cavernoma-related e.
centrencephalic e.
childhood absence e. (CAE)
childhood absence epilepsy evolving to juvenile myoclonic e.
childhood benign focal e.
childhood-onset e.
chronic partial e.
cingulate e.
clouded-state e.
complex precipitated e.
cortical e.
cryptogenic late-onset e.
cryptogenic myoclonic e.
cryptogenic partial e.
dacryocystic e.
Dark Warrior e.
diencephalic e.
diurnal e.
early posttraumatic e.
eating e.
extratemporal lobe e.
familial adult myoclonic e.
familial mesial temporal lobe e.
familial progressive myoclonic e.
febrile e.
focal frontal lobe e.
frontal lobe e.
gelastic e.
e. gene

NOTES

E

epilepsy *(continued)*
generalized tonic-clonic e.
grand mal e.
haut mal e.
hemiconvulsion, hemiplegia, and e. (HHE)
hippocampal e.
hot water e.
idiopathic generalized e.
idiopathic partial e.
e. implant
impulsive petit mal e.
insular e.
intermittent myoclonus e.
International League Against E.
intractable grand mal e.
intractable psychomotor e.
Jackson e.
jacksonian e.
juvenile absence e.
juvenile myoclonic e.
Kojewnikoff e.
Kozhevnikov e.
Lafora familial myoclonic e.
laryngeal e.
late e.
latent e.
lateral-onset temporal lobe e.
local e.
localization-related e.
Lundborg myoclonic e.
major e.
malignant familial myoclonic e.
masked e.
matutinal e.
medial temporal lobe e.
medically intractable partial e.
menstrual e.
mesiobasal limbic e.
mixed-type e.
musicogenic e.
myoclonic astatic e.
myoclonus e.
National Society for E. (NSE)
neocortical e.
Nintendo e.
nocturnal e.
occipital lobe e.
opercular e.
orbitofrontal e.
parietal lobe e.
partial complex e.
partial temporal lobe e.
pattern-induced e.
pattern-sensitive e.
pediatric and adolescent e. (PAE)
petit mal e.
pharmacoresistent e.
photogenic e.
physiologic e.
postapoplectic e.
posttraumatic e.
prandic e.
primary generalized e.
primary rhinencephalic psychomotor e.
procursive e.
progressive familial myoclonic e.
progressive myoclonic e.
progressive myoclonus e. (PME)
psychogenic e.
psychomotor e.
quiritarian e.
reflex e.
refractory partial e.
resistant e.
rolandic e.
rotatory e.
secondary generalized e.
self-induced e.
sensory precipitated e.
sleep e.
sleep-related e.
somnambulic e.
startle e.
sudden unexplained death in e. (SUDEP)
supplementary motor area e.
e. surgery
E. Surgery Inventory-55
surgical e.
symptomatic partial e.
e. syndrome
tardy e.
television-induced e.
temporal lobe e.
temporolimbic e.
tonic e.
tornado e.
uncinate e.
Unverricht-Lundborg myoclonus e.
Unverricht myoclonus e.
vasomotor e.
vasovagal e.
vestibulogenic e.
video game e.
visceral e.
visual reflex e.
e. with continuous spikes and waves during sleep
e. with grand mal seizures on awakening

e. with multiple independent spike focus
e. with myoclonic absence

epileptic
e. absence
e. aura
e. automatism
e. cephalea
e. clouded state
e. cry
e. dementia
e. diathesis
e. discharge
e. drop attack
e. encephalopathy
e. event
e. focus
e. migraineur
e. negative myoclonus
e. neuron
e. neuronal aggregate
e. prodrome
e. seizure
e. spasm
e. twilight state

epileptica absentia
epilepticus
absence status e.
complex partial status e.
convulsive status e.
de novo nonconvulsive status e.
drug-induced status e.
electrical status e.
focal status e.
furor e.
generalized convulsive status e.
globus e.
ictus e.
nonconvulsive status e.
pentobarbital in status e.
refractory status e.
status e.
tonic-clonic status e.
tonic status e.

epileptiform
e. activity
e. burst
e. burst discharge
e. bursting
e. convulsion
e. neuralgia

epileptogenesis
age-related e.
progressive e.
secondary e.

epileptogenic
e. brain injury
e. burst
e. channelopathy
e. cortex
e. focus
e. stimulation
e. structural lesion
e. temporal lesion
e. zone

epileptogenicity
epileptogenous
epileptoid
orthostatic e.

epileptologist
epileptology
epileptosis
epiloia
epimysium
epinephrine-anesthetic mixture
epinephrine toxicity
epineural
epineurectomy
epineurial neurorrhaphy
epineurium
epifascicular e.

epineurolysis
epinosic
epinosis
epiphenomenon
epiphora
epiphysis cerebri
epipial
episcleral vascular dilation
episcleritis
episode
mitochondrial encephalomyopathy with lactic acidosis and strokelike e.'s (MELAS)
mitochondrial myopathy, encephalopathy, lactic acidosis, strokelike e.'s (MELAS)
nocturnal confusional e.
nocturnal hypotensive e.
psychoepileptic e.
strokelike e.

NOTES

E

episodic
e. amnesia
e. ataxia type 2 (EA-2)
e. cluster headache
e. dyscontrol syndrome
e. memory
e. memory function
e. nocturnal wandering
e. paroxysmal hemicrania
e. tension-type headache (ETTH)
e. vertigo
epispinal space
epistemic
epistemology
genetic e.
episthotonos
epistolary
epithalamic
epithalamica
commissura e.
epithalamus commissure
epithelial
e. choroid layer
e. hemangioendothelioma
e. lamina
e. membrane antigen tumor marker
epithelialis
lamina choroidea e.
epithelioid
e. cell
e. hemangioendothelioma
e. histiocyte
epithelioma
epitheliopathy
multifocal placoid pigment e.
placoid pigment e.
retinal pigment e.
epithelioserosa
zona e.
epithelium
olfactory e.
retinal pigment e.
sense e.
sensory e.
subcapsular e.
epitope
surface e.
epitympanici
pars cupularis recessus e.
epivaginal connective tissue
Epival
***EPM2A* gene**
EPO
evening primrose oil
epoch
Frequency Analysis of Consecutive E. (FACE)
epoxide hydrolase
epoxy-mounted preamplifier
EPP
endplate potential
EPS
exophthalmos-producing substance
extrapyramidal sign
extrapyramidal symptom
epsilon
apolipoprotein e.
apolipoprotein e. 4 (APOe4)
e. opiate receptor
epsilon-aminocaproic acid
EPSP
excitatory postsynaptic potential
Epstein
E. curette
E. neurological hammer
E. staging system
E. symptom
Epstein-Barr virus (EBV)
ePTFE
expanded polytetrafluoroethylene
ePTFE ventricular shunt catheter
Epworth Sleepiness Scale (ESS)
equal potential
Equanil
equation
Bloch e.
Cockgraft-Gault e.
Goldman constant field e.
Larmor e.
logistic regression e.
Nernst e.
Poiseuille e.
Solomon-Bloembergen e.
Equilet
equilibration
hanging-drop e.
equilibratory ataxia
equilibrium
creatine kinase e.
sense of e.
equina
cauda e.
equine
e. encephalitis
e. gait
Equinox EEG neuromonitoring system
equipment
adaptive e.
decompression e.
insertion e.
stainless steel e.
Vitallium e.
equipotential

equivalent
cobalt Gray e.
e. current dipole
e. dose
effective dose e. (EDE)
migraine e.
equivocal finding
ER
Depakote ER
Erb
E. atrophy
E. disease
E. injury
E. muscular dystrophy
E. palsy
E. point
E. point stimulation on electromyogram
E. sclerosis
E. sign
E. spinal paralysis
E. syphilitic spastic paraplegia
Erb-Charcot disease
Erb-Duchenne
E.-D. palsy
E.-D. paralysis
E.-D. syndrome
Erb-Duchenne-Klumpke
E.-D.-K. injury
E.-D.-K. injury to brachial plexus
Erben
E. phenomenon
E. reflex
E. sign
Erb-Goldflam disease
Erb-Westphal sign
Erdheim-Chester disease
Erdheim tumor
erector spinae reflex
erector-spinal reflex
erethism mercuralis
ERG
electroretinography
ERG theory
***ERG2* gene**
ergic trait
ergocalciferol
ergoesthesiograph
ergogenic aids
Ergomar
ergonovine
Ergostat
ergot
ergotamine
e. derivative
Medihaler e.
e. tartrate
e. tartrate and caffeine
ergot-derivative dopamine agonist
ergot-derived medication
ergotica
tabes e.
ergotropic
erigentes
nervi e.
Eriksen task
erisynaptic glial cell
erosion
dorsum sella e.
vascular e.
erosive sphenoid mucocele
erotique
monomanie e.
erratic
e. absorption
e. sleep
error
best registration e.
e. detection circuit
frequency e.
gross medical e.
line bisection e. (LBE)
measurement e.
perceptual e.
registration e.
root mean square e.
target localization e.
target registration e. (TRE)
volume-averaging e.
ERS
extended, rotated, sidebent
ERSL
extended, rotated, sidebent left
ERSR
extended, rotated, sidebent right
ERT
estrogen replacement therapy
ertotropid system
erudite
erudition

NOTES

eruption
palatal mucosal e.
vesicular e.
erythema
e. chronicum migrans
e. multiforme
e. multiforme-like
erythematosus
lupus e.
neuropsychiatric systemic lupus e.
systemic lupus e. (SLE)
erythredema polyneuritis
erythroblastosis fetalis
erythrocyte
e. protoporphyria
e. sedimentation rate (ESR)
erythromelalgia
head e.
erythroprosopalgia
escalating conflict
escalation
dose e.
escalative process
escape phenomenon
Escherich
E. reflex
E. sign
Escherichia coli
escitalopram oxalate
Escobar
E. disease
E. syndrome
E-selectin level
ESEP
excitatory postsynaptic potential
esmolol
esodeviation
esodic nerve
esoethmoiditis
esophageal
e. achalasia
e. airway
e. perforation
e. pH monitoring
e. plexus
e. pressure monitoring
esophagealis
plexus e.
esophageus
plexus e.
esophagi
pars cervicalis e.
pars thoracica e.
esophagosalivary reflex
esophagus
thoracic part of e.
esotropia
espiritismo
Espocan combined spinal/epidural needle
esprit
ESR
erythrocyte sedimentation rate
ESRRL
extension, sidebent right, rotated left
ESS
Epworth Sleepiness Scale
essential
e. anosmia
e. blepharospasm
e. headache
e. hypotonia
e. myoclonus
e. palatal tremor
e. thrombocytosis
Essex-Lopresti axial fixation
ESSF
external spinal skeletal fixation
Essick cell band
estazolam
esterase
acetylcholine e.
Esterom
esthematology
esthesia
esthesic
esthesiodic system
esthesiogenesis
esthesiogenic
esthesiography
esthesiology
esthesiometer
Semmes-Weinstein e.
Weber e.
esthesiometry
esthesioneure
esthesioneuroblastoma
olfactory e.
esthesioneurocytoma
esthesioneurosis
esthesionosus
esthesiophysiology
esthesioscopy
esthesodic
estimated cerebrovascular resistance
estradiol
ethinyl e.
estradiol-17 B
estrogen
e. level
e. receptor
e. replacement therapy (ERT)
e. withdrawal
estrogen-related protein
estrogen-to-progesterone ratio

estrous behavior
ET
endothelin
alpha ET
ET-1
endothelin-1
état
état criblé
état lacunaire
ET-converting enzyme
eternus
puer e.
eterobarb
ethacrynic acid
ethambutol
ethanol
e. treatment
e. withdrawal
ethaverine hydrochloride
ether convulsion
ethical aspects of dementia
Ethicon Ligaclip
ethidium bromide (EB)
ethinyl estradiol
Ethiodane
ethiodized oil
ethmoid
e. air cell
e. sinus
ethmoidal
e. meningoencephalocele
e. nerve
e. osteotomy
ethopropazine
ethosuximide
ethotoin
ethyl
e. alcohol peripheral neuropathy
e. chloride and dichlorotetrafluoroethane
e. loflazepate
ethylene
e. glycol poisoning
e. vinyl alcohol copolymer liquid
ethylenediaminetetraacetic acid
ethylene-vinyl acetate (EVAc)
ethylester
levodopa e.
ethylmalonic aciduria
ethyltryptamine
alpha e.
etidocaine
etidronate
disodium e.
technetium e.
etifoxine
etiological heterogeneity
etiologic role
etiology
dementia due to multiple e.'s
disease e.
multifactorial e.
organic e.
e. theory
etiopathogenesis
MS e.
etizolam
etodolac
etodroxizine
etomidate injection
Etomidate-Lipuro
etomidate-propylene glycol infusion
etoposide
ETP
electron transport particle
etretinate
etryptamine
ETTH
episodic tension-type headache
ETV
endoscopic third ventriculostomy
euhemerism
eukaryotic messenger
eulaminate
Eulenburg disease
eumetria
euphoric effect
eupractic
eupraxia
eupraxic center
European
E. Brain Injury Consortium
E. Carotid Surgery Trial (ECST)
E. Sleep Research Society
E. Society for Sleep Research
EuroQol visual analog scale
eurycephalic, eurycephalous
eurythmic
eurythmy
euthymic memory
eutychian

NOTES

EVAc
ethylene-vinyl acetate
evacuation
CT-guided stereotactic e.
epidural abscess e.
epidural tumor e.
hematoma e.
transsphenoidal e.
Evalose
evaluation
acute physiologic assessment and chronic health e. (APACHE)
bulbocavernosus reflex e.
comprehensive e.
cross-sectional e.
myasthenia gravis e.
neurologic e.
Neurometer CPT/C for nerve e.
pedicle e.
preoperative e.
seizure e.
Evaluation/Examination
Reitan-Klove Sensory Perceptual E.
evaluator
Recovery Attitude and Treatment E. (RAATE)
Evans
E. index
E. ratio
even-echo rephasing
evening
e. headache
e. primrose oil (EPO)
event
acoustic signature e. (ASI)
calmodulin-regulated e.
catastrophic e.
clinical ictal e.
cytoskeletal-membrane e.
epileptic e.
genomic e.
ischemic e.
e. memory
multifactorial e.
neurologic e.
nonepileptic e.
e. recall
e. recall score
transient focal neurologic e. (TFNE)
unilateral electrodecremental e.
event-related
e.-r. brain potential study
e.-r. desynchronization
e.-r. innocuous somatosensory stimulation paradigm
e.-r. potential
Evers diet for multiple sclerosis
Evershears surgical instrument
eversion
cingulate gyrus e.
evidence
anatomical e.
anecdotal e.
bias-free e.
biologic e.
class I–III e.
evidence-based medicine
evisceroneurotomy
evoked
e. affect
e. cortical response
e. potential (EP)
e. potential trending
e. seizure
Evolution 1 precision robot
evolving
e. dementia
e. hematoma
EWACS system data acquisition
Ewald-Hudson forceps
E wave
Ewing sarcoma
Ex
extra point
exacerbation
disease e.
dopaminergic antagonists-related e.
headache e.
e. rate
seizure e.
spontaneous e.
symptom e.
exaggerated
e. depression
e. response
exam
Boston Diagnostic Aphasia E.
PRO-ton Brain e. (PROBE)
examination
Brief Neuropsychological Mental Status E.
cochlear nerve e.
Cognistat (The Neurobehavioral Cognitive Status E.)
Comprehensive Qualifying E.
cranial nerve e.
dystonia e.
EMG e.
glossopharyngeal nerve e.
Hertel exophthalmometry e.
Lateral Dominance E.
motor development e.
muscle e.

Navy neurologic screening e.
needle electrode e. (NEE)
neurologic e. (NE)
neuropathologic e.
nystagmus e.
ocular motility e.
oculomotor nerve e.
olfactory nerve e.
ophthalmologic e.
optic nerve e.
posture e.
Sensory Perceptual E.
slit-lamp e.
soft sign in neurologic e.
sternocleidomastoid muscle testing in spinal accessory nerve e.
Stroke Data Bank Neurologic Rush Alzheimer Registry E.
tangent screen e.
vagus nerve e.
vestibular nerve e.

Examining for Aphasia

exanthem subitum

Ex-B
extra point on the back of the trunk

Excel double-tipped microcatheter

excessive
e. daytime sleepiness (EDS)
e. daytime somnolence
e. diffuse low and medium wave beta activity
e. exercise
e. fatigability
e. fatigue
e. speech

exchange
blood-gas e.
blood-tissue e.
e. force
plasma e. (PE)

excimer laser-assisted nonocclusive anastomosis (ELANA)

excision
C2-C3 cervical disk e.
cervical disk e.
extratemporal e.
retropulsed bone e.

excitability
emotional e.
membrane e.
neuronal e.
somatodendritic e.
e. test
thalamocortical e.

excitable
e. area
e. cell

excitation
glutamate e.
number of e.
postsynaptic e.
selective e.

excitation-contraction coupling

excitatory
e. afferent
e. amino acid
e. amino acid receptor
e. amino acid receptor inhibitor
e. irradiation
e. lesion
e. neurotransmitter
e. postsynaptic potential (EPSP, ESEP)
e. pyramidal neuron
e. stimulus

excitomotor cortex

excitoreflex nerve

excitor nerve

excitotoxic
e. cell damage
e. neuronal cell injury
e. neurotransmitter antagonist

excitotoxicity
glutamate e.
glutamatergic e.

excitotoxin inhibitor

excitoxic insult

excyclotorsion

executive
e. function
e. function deficit
e. (or frontal) deficit transient global amnesia
e. process

Exelon capsule

exencephalic

exencephalocele

exencephalous

exencephaly

exercise
Cawthorne-Cooksey vestibular e.
container e.

NOTES

exercise *(continued)*
excessive e.
intellectual e.
physical e.
PNF e.
verbal memory e.
exercise-induced
e.-i. myoglobinuria
e.-i. sympathetic discharge
exerciser
continuous anatomical passive e.
exertional headache
exhaustion
heat e.
postactivation e.
posttetanic e.
existential-humanistic theory
exit block
exiting segment
Exner
E. Comprehensive System
E. plexus
exodic nerve
exogenous
e. fiber
e. force
e. nitric oxide (GSNO)
e. reaction
exon splicing
exophthalmometer
Hertel e.
exophthalmos
exophthalmos-producing substance (EPS)
exophytic
e. brainstem glioma
e. ependymoma
e. joint disease
exorbitance
Exo-Static collar
exotoxin
Pseudomonas e.
exotropia
paralytic pontine e.
expanded
E. Disability Status Scale (EDSS)
e. polytetrafluoroethylene (ePTFE)
expansion
clonal e.
field e.
trinucleotide repeat e.
volume e.
expectancy
quality-adjusted life e. (QALE)
e. wave
experience-induced cortical plasticity
experiential
e. aura
e. factor
experimental
e. allergic encephalitis (EAE)
e. allergic encephalomyelitis
e. autoimmune encephalomyelitis
e. condition
e. intervention
e. study
expiratory center
exploding head syndrome
exploration
brachial plexus e.
stereotactic biopsy e.
therapeutic e.
transcranial orbital e.
exploratory incision
exploring electrode
explosive
e. psychotic state
e. speech
exposure
anterior surgical e.
bony e.
extradural e.
fetal mercury e.
fetal phenytoin e.
half-and-half e.
e. keratopathy
light e.
membrane phosphatidylserine e.
middle fossa e.
midline e.
neuroleptic e.
prolonged e.
radiation e.
surgical e.
thoracolumbar junction surgical e.
thoracolumbar spine anterior e.
toxic e.
e. to trauma
upper cervical spine anterior e.
vertebral e.
in vivo situational e.
x-ray e.
exposure-based intervention
expressed skull fracture
expression
e. level
neurofilament e.
neuronal NAHPH-diaphorase/NOS e.
neurotrophic factor e.
nontoxic gene e.
pattern of e.
phenotypic e.
RNA e.

expressive
e. aphasia
e. dysprosody
e. language deficit
expressive-receptive aphasia
Extencaps
Micro-K 10 E.
extended
e. ADL
e. phenytoin sodium
e., rotated, sidebent (ERS)
e., rotated, sidebent left (ERSL)
e., rotated, sidebent right (ERSR)
e. sector ultrasonic probe
e. subfrontal approach
extending axon
extension
brachioradialis transfer for wrist e.
cranial e.
deep brain e.
extrameatal tumor e.
e. injury
e. injury posterior atlantoaxial arthrodesis
intrasellar e.
neurite e.
Orascoptic loupe e.
paraplegia in e.
passive e.
radiolucent operating room table e.
e., sidebent right, rotated left (ESRRL)
subependymal e.
suprasellar e.
tumor e.
extension-type cervical spine injury
extensive
e. neoplasm
e. posterior decompression
e. seizure focus
extensor
e. plantar response
e. tetanus
e. toe response
exterior band of Baillarger
externa
capsula e.
glia limitans e.
globus pallidus e.
hematorrhachis e.
lamina medullaris thalami e.
lamina pyramidalis e.
ophthalmoplegia e.
pachymeningitis e.
externae
fibrae arcuatae e.
stria laminae granularis e.
external
e. acoustic meatus
e. arcuate fiber
e. auditory canal cutaneous
e. auditory canal mass
e. auditory meatus electrode
e. auditory meatus reflex
e. band of Baillarger
e. beam radiotherapy (EBRT)
e. bracing
e. canthus electrode
e. capsule
e. carotid artery
e. collimator
e. corticotectal tract
e. cue
e. cuneate nucleus
e. granular layer
e. hydrocephalus
e. intercostal muscle
e. line of Baillarger
e. malleolar sign
e. maxillary plexus
e. medullary lamina
e. memory aid
e. meningitis
e. nuclear layer of retina
e. oblique reflex
e. pillar cell
e. popliteal nerve
e. pyocephalus
e. rhinoplasty
e. sheath of optic nerve
e. source
e. speech
e. speech stimulus
e. spinal skeletal fixation (ESSF)
e. spinal skeletal fixator
e. support system
e. terminal filament
e. ventricular drain
e. ventricular drainage
e. vertebral venous plexus

NOTES

externi
nervi carotici e.
nervus meatus acustici e.
externum
corpus geniculatum e.
filum terminale e.
stratum limitans e.
stratum nucleare e.
stratum plexiforme e.
externus
nervus spermaticus e.
plexus caroticus e.
exteroceptive nervous system
exteroceptor
exterofective system
extirpate
extirpation
choroid plexus e.
tumor e.
extorsion
extra
e. point (Ex)
e. point on the back of the trunk (Ex-B)
extraaxial
e. cavernous hemangioma
e. lesion
extracanicular acoustic neuroma
extracellular
e. acidosis
e. action potential
e. calcium activity
e. contribution
e. matrix (ECM)
e. matrix protein
e. matrix proteoglycan
e. proteosome
e. signal-regulated protein
e. space
extracerebral
e. activity
e. aneurysm
e. cavernous angioma
e. hematoma
extraconal lesion
extracorporeal
e. membrane oxygenation
e. membrane oxygenation affecting cognitive function
extracorticospinal
e. system
e. tract
extracranial
e. aneurysm
e. arteritis
e. carotid artery (ECA)
e. carotid occlusive disease
e. ganglion
e. mass lesion
e. meningioma
e. occlusive vascular disease
e. pneumatocele
e. pneumocele
e. radiosurgery
e. vascular dissection
extracraniale
ganglion e.
extracranial-intracranial (ECIC)
e.-i. bypass
e.-i. bypass surgery
extracranial-to-intracranial bypass procedure
extract
kava e.
perchlorate e.
extradural
e. abscess
e. anastomosis
e. clinoidectomy
e. compartment
e. cyst
e. defect
e. exposure
e. hemangioma
e. hematoma
e. hematorrhachis
e. hemorrhage
e. infection
e. injection
e. meningioma
e. phase
e. space
e. spinal metastasis
e. tumor
e. vertebral artery
extradurale
spatium e.
extraforaminal
foraminal e.
e. lumbar disk herniation
e. synovial cyst
extrafusal fiber
extrageniculate
extrajunctional nucleus
extralemniscal
e. myelotomy
e. system
extralesional hippocampal resection
extraluminal
extrameatal
e. intracapsular tumor
e. tumor extension

extramedullary
e. hemangioma
e. spinal cord tumor
extrameningeal
e. tuberculous infection
extramesial temporal lesion
extraocular
e. motility
e. movement (EOM)
e. muscle involvement
e. muscle palsy
e. muscle paresis
e. paralysis
extraordinary meridian (EM)
extrapineal
e. pinealoma
e. pinealoma false neuroma
extrapolar region
extrapyramidal
e. cerebral palsy
e. disorder
e. dyskinesia
e. motor feature
e. motor side effect
e. motor system
e. motor system disease
e. nucleus
e. pathway
e. rigidity
e. sign (EPS)
e. symptom (EPS)
e. symptom potential
e. syndrome
e. syndrome symptom
extraspinal
e. leiomyoma
e. nerve stimulation
extrastriatal dopamine transmission
extrastriate
e. visual cortex
e. V5/MT cortex
extrasynaptic receptor
extratemporal
e. excision
e. lobe epilepsy
e. resection
e. seizure
extraterritorial spontaneous pain
extrathalamic pathway
extrema
capsula e.
extreme
e. capsule
e. lateral inferior transcondylar approach
e. lateral transcondylar approach
e. narrowing limit
e. range
e. somatosensory evoked potential
extremely low frequency magnetic field
extrinsic sleep disorder
extruded disk
extrusion
bone graft e.
wire e.
extubation
postoperative e.
ex vivo
eye
black e.
e. blink
e. blink artifact
e. blink conditioning test
e. blinking
contralateral e.
crossed e.
e. cyclotorsion
dancing e.
defected e.
glassy e.
e. lead
lusterless e.
e. movement artifact
e. movement desensitization
e. movement desensitization and reprocessing (EMDR)
e. movement disorder
e. muscle weakness
e. pain
paretic e.
raccoon e.
red e.
e. tracking
eye-blink response
eyebrow incision
eye-closure reflex
eye-gaze deviation
eyelash sign
eyelid
e. myoclonia

NOTES

eyelid *(continued)*
e. myokymia
e. ptosis
eye-motor-verbal (EMV)
e.-m.-v. profile
eyes, motor, voice/verbal
E-Z
E-Z Flap cranial bone plate
E-Z flap cranial flap fixation system
Ezide

F
F response
F wave
FA
fractional anisotropy
FaAct
Fabco gauze dressing
fabric
polyethylene terephthalate f.
Fabry disease
fabulized
f. combination
f. response
FAC
Functional Ambulation Category
FACE
Frequency Analysis of Consecutive Epochs
face
anthropomorphic f.
immobile f.
masklike f.
Mooney f.
upside-down Mooney f.
face-dominant hemisphere
face-evoked magnetic field
face-graded activation
face-nondominant hemisphere
face-preferential activation
facet, facette
bony f.
f. excision technique
f. fracture stabilization wiring
f. hypertrophy
f. joint
f. joint preparation
f. joint syndrome
locked f.
f. replacement
f. rhizotomy
f. subluxation stabilization wiring
f. syndrome
facetectomy
partial f.
facial
f. agnosia
f. anesthesia
f. apraxia
f. artery
f. colliculus
f. contusion
f. diplegia
f. dysesthesia
f. dystonia
f. electromyography
f. electroneurography
f. eminence
f. expression automatism
f. flushing
f. fracture
f. genu
f. habit spasm
f. hematoma
f. hemiatrophy of Romberg
f. hemiplegia
f. hemispasm
f. hillock
f. migraine
f. motor nucleus
f. myokymia
f. nerve [CN VII]
f. nerve congenital anomaly
f. nerve discontinuity
f. nerve function
f. nerve paralysis
f. nerve perinatal trauma
f. neuralgia
f. neuroma
f. neuropathy
f. numbness
f. osteosynthesis
f. pain
f. palsy
f. plexus
f. profiling
f. progressive atrophy
f. progressive hemiatrophy
f. reanimation
f. reflex
f. root
f. sign
f. tic
f. trophoneurosis
f. vision
f. weakness
faciali
rami communicantes nervi auriculotemporalis cum nervi f.
facialis
area nervi f.
colliculus f.
eminentia f.
ganglion geniculatum nervi f.
ganglion geniculi nervi f.
geniculum nervi f.
geniculum nervus f.
genu nervi f.
nervus f. [CN VII]

facialis *(continued)*
nucleus f.
nucleus nervi f.
f. phenomenon
radix nervi f.
rami buccales nervi f.
rami zygomatici nervi f.
ramus cervicalis nervi f.
ramus colli nervi f.
ramus digastricus nervi f.
ramus lingualis nervi f.
ramus marginalis mandibularis nervi f.
ramus stylohyoideus nervi f.

facies
asymmetrical crying f. (ACF)
birdlike f.
elfin f.
hatchet f.
Hutchinson f.
f. inferior hemispherii cerebelli
f. inferior hemispherii cerebri
mask f.
masked f.
masklike f.
f. medialis et inferior hemispherii cerebri
f. medialis hemispherii cerebri
moon f.
myasthenic f.
myopathic f.
myotonic f.
Parkinson f.
f. superior hemispherii cerebelli
f. superolateralis hemispherii cerebri

facilitation
f. of communication
intracortical inhibition and f.
postactivation f.
postspike f.
posttetanic f.
proprioceptive neuromuscular f. (PNF)
Wedensky f.

facioauriculovertebral

faciobuccolingual dyskinesia

faciocephalalgia

faciocephalic pain

faciofacial nerve anastomosis

faciohypoglossal anastomosis

faciolingual

facioplegia

facioplegic
f. migraine
f. migraine headache

facioscapulohumeral
f. atrophy
f. muscular
f. muscular dystrophy

faciostenosis

faciotelencephalopathy

FACScan-analysis
three-color F.-a.

factitious attack

factor
age-specific risk f.
antihemophilic f. A, C
apoptosis-inducing f. (AIF)
assimilative f.
attitudinal risk f.
background f.
basal endothelium-derived relaxing f.
basic fibroblast growth f.
biologic risk f.
biomechanical f.
brain-derived neurotrophic f. (BDNF)
brain-derived neurotropic f.
ciliary neurotrophic f. (CNF)
collagenase activating f.
corticotropin-releasing f.
demographic risk f.
DNA fragmentation f. (DFF)
endothelial cell-stimulating angiogenesis f.
endothelial-derived relaxing f. (EDRF)
endothelium-derived relaxing f. (EDRF)
environmental f.
epidermal growth f. (ECF)
experiential f.
Fiblast trafermin growth f.
fibroblastic growth f. (FGF)
fiddle f.
filling f.
fork head response f.
genetic risk f.
glial cell line-derived neurotrophic f.
glial-derived neurotrophic f. (GDNF)
glial line-derived neurotrophic f.
granulocyte-macrophage colony-stimulating f.
growth hormone-release inhibiting f. (GHRIF)
Hageman f.
helix-loop-helix response f.
hepatocyte growth f.
hepatocyte growth factor/scatter f. (HGF/SF)
HLH f.

homeodomain f.
human f.
hyperpolarize f.
hypothalamic-releasing f.
insulin growth f.
insulinlike growth f. (IGF)
ischemia-modifying f.
f. IX complex concentrate
f. IX deficiency
Leiden f. V
leukemia inhibitory f. (LIF)
melanocyte-inhibiting f.
melanotropin-releasing f. (MRF)
middle glial cell line-derived neurotrophic f.
midlife cardiovascular risk f.
motivation f.
motivational/behavioral f.
nerve growth f. (NGF)
neural growth f.
neurobiological f.
neurophysiological phenotypic f.
neurotic f.
neurotrophic f.
nonspecific neurotic f.
obsessional Q f.
orthogonal depression f.
pathogenic f.
pathophysiologic f.
pharmacologic f.
phenotypic f.
phenylketonuria genetic f.
plasma f.
platelet-activating f. (PAF)
platelet-derived growth f. (PDGF)
potential predisposing f.
predictive f.
pretraumatic risk f.
primary risk f.
prolactin-inhibiting f. (PIF)
prolactin-releasing f. (PRF)
Q f.
quality f.
radiolabeled neurotrophic f.
rheumatoid f.
f. score
serum von Willebrand f.
state f.
Stuart-Power f.
susceptibility f.
synthetic corticotropin-releasing f.
transcription f.
transforming growth f. (TGF)
tumor necrosis f. (TNF)
vascular endothelial growth f. (VEGF)
vascular growth f.
f. VII deficiency
f. VIII
f. VIII antigen tumor marker
f. VIII deficiency
vitamin K-dependent clotting f. II
vitamin K-dependent clotting f. VII
vitamin K-dependent clotting f. IX
vitamin K-dependent clotting f. X
von Willebrand f. (vWF)
f. XII deficiency

factor-1
redox f.

factor-alpha
recombinant human tumor necrosis f.-a.
tumor necrosis f.-a. (TNF-alpha)

factual memory

FAD
flavin adenine dinucleotide

fad activity

Fahn-Tolosa-Marin Tremor Rating Scale

Fahr
F. disease
F. syndrome

failed
f. back surgery syndrome
f. back syndrome (FBS)
f. back syndrome with documented pseudarthrosis

failure
age-associated memory f.
brain functional f.
distant brain f. (DBF)
empathic f.
fatigue f.
functional f.
Harrington rod instrumentation f.
instrumentation f.
isolated gait ignition f.
metal f.
poliomyelitis-induced respiratory f.
pure autonomic f.
recall f.
spinal implant load to f.

NOTES

Fairbanks
F. change
F. method
Fajersztajn crossed sciatic sign
FAK
focal adhesion kinase
FAK protein
falcate
falces (*pl. of* falx)
falcial
falciform
f. crest
f. lobe
falciformis
f. hiatus sapheni
lobus f.
falcine
falciparum
Plasmodium f.
Falconer lobectomy
falcotentorial meningioma
falcula
falcular
fallopian neuritis
Fallopio foramen
Falret disease
FALS
familial amyotrophic lateral sclerosis
false
f. localizing sign
f. neuroma
f. neurotransmitter
false-negative PCR
false-positive rate
falx, pl. **falces**
f. cerebelli
f. cerebri
f. hypoplasia
f. meningioma
parasagittal f.
F. sign
famciclovir
familial
f. adult myoclonic epilepsy
f. Alzheimer disease
f. amyloid neuropathy
f. amyloidosis
f. amyloidotic polyneuropathy
f. amyotrophic lateral sclerosis (FALS)
f. arteriovenous malformation
f. autosomal recessive idiopathic myoclonic epilepsy of infancy
f. benign choreoathetosis
f. centrolobar sclerosis
f. cervicocephalic arterial dissection
f. cortical tremor
f. dysautonomia
f. dysautonomia syndrome
f. encephalopathy
f. fatal insomnia
f. form of amyotrophic lateral sclerosis
f. glioma
f. gliomatosis cerebri
f. glycosuria
f. hemiplegic migraine (FHM)
f. hypercholesterolemia
f. hypokalemic periodic paralysis
f. intracranial aneurysm (FIA)
f. Mediterranean fever (FMF)
f. medulloblastoma
f. mesial temporal lobe epilepsy
f. neurovisceral lipidosis
f. neuroviscerolipidosis
f. Parkinson disease
f. paroxysmal choreoathetosis
f. paroxysmal choreoathetosis disease
f. paroxysmal kinesigenic ataxia
f. partial epilepsy with variable focus
f. progressive myoclonic epilepsy
f. restless leg syndrome
f. spastic ataxia
f. spastic paraplegia
f. spinal muscular atrophy
f. startle disease
f. transmission
familiar correlation coefficient
famille névropathique
family
leucine zipper f.
zinc-finger f.
fan
f. retractor
f. sign
Fañanás cell
Fanconi syndrome
far
F. East Russian encephalitis
f. lateral inferior suboccipital approach
Faraday shield
Farber
F. disease
F. lipogranulomatosis
farcinica
Nocardia f.
Farley retractor
farnesyl transferase inhibitor
FAS
fetal alcohol syndrome

Fas-associated
F.-a. death domain
F.-a. death domain-like interleukin-converting enzyme
fascia, pl. **fasciae**
f. cinerea
f. dentata hippocampus
dentate f.
infraspinous f.
f. lata sling
lumbodorsal f. (LDF)
Tarin f.
vertebral f.
fascia-muscle-fascia sandwich
fascicle
muscle f.
nerve f.
peripheral nerve f.
fascicular
f. adaptation
f. degeneration
f. graft
f. ophthalmoplegia
fasciculation
contraction f.
cramp benign f.
f. potential
fasciculitis
thalamic f.
fasciculus, pl. **fasciculi**
f. aberrans of Monakow
alvear f.
f. anterior proprius
anterior pyramidal f.
arcuate f.
Burdach cuneate f.
calcarine f.
central tegmental f.
f. circumolivaris pyramidis
f. corticospinalis anterior
f. corticospinalis lateralis
cuneate f.
f. cuneatus
dorsal longitudinal f.
dorsolateral f.
f. dorsolateralis
fasciculus subcallosus for superior occipitofrontal f.
Flechsig f.
Foville f.
frontooccipital f.
Gowers f.
gracile f.
f. gracilis
f. gracilis medullae oblongatae
f. gracilis medullae spinalis
hooked f.
inferior longitudinal f.
inferior occipitofrontal f.
interfascicular f.
f. interfascicularis (FI)
intersegmental f.
interstitial nucleus of medial longitudinal f.
f. lateralis plexus brachialis
f. lateralis proprius
lateral pyramidal f.
lenticular f.
f. lenticularis
Lissauer f.
fasciculi longitudinales pontis
f. longitudinalis dorsalis
f. longitudinalis inferior
f. longitudinalis medialis
f. longitudinalis posterior
f. longitudinalis superior
longitudinal pontine f.
macular f.
f. macularis
mamillotegmental f.
f. mamillotegmentalis
mamillothalamic f.
f. mamillothalamicus
mammillotegmental f.
mammillothalamic f.
marginal f.
f. marginalis
f. medialis telencephali
medial longitudinal f. (MLF)
median longitudinal f.
Meynert f.
f. of Meynert
nucleus of cuneate f.
oblique pontine f.
f. obliquus pontis
occipitofrontal f.
f. occipitofrontalis
f. occipitofrontalis inferior
f. occipitofrontalis superior
oval f.
f. pedunculomamillaris
pedunculomammillary f.

NOTES

fasciculus *(continued)*
perpendicular f.
proper f.
fasciculi proprii
f. proprius anterior
f. proprius anterior medullae spinalis
f. proprius dorsalis medullae spinalis
f. proprius lateralis
f. proprius lateralis medullae spinalis
f. proprius posterior medullae spinalis
f. pyramidalis anterior
f. pyramidalis lateralis
retroflex f.
f. retroflexus
f. rotundus
round f.
rubroreticular f.
fasciculi rubroreticulares
Schütz f.
semilunar f.
f. semilunaris
septomarginal f.
f. septomarginalis
slender f.
f. solitarius
solitary f.
subcallosal f.
f. subcallosus
subthalamic f.
f. subthalamicus
f. sulcomarginalis
superior longitudinal f.
superior occipitofrontal f.
thalamic f.
f. thalamicus
f. thalamomamillaris
f. thalamomammillaris
transverse f.
fasciculi transversi
Türck f.
unciform f.
f. uncinatus
f. uncinatus cerebelli
Vicq d'Azyr f.
wedge-shaped f.

fasciola, pl. **fasciolae**
f. cinerea
f. cinerea cinguli

fasciolar gyrus

fasciolaris
gyrus f.

FasDasher-14 microguidewire

Fasguide catheter

fast
f. axonal transport
F. Dasher 14 wire
f. field-potential rhythm
f. Fourier transformation spectrum analyzer
f. Fournier transform (FFT)
f. gradient recalled spectroscopic imaging technique
F. Health Knowledge Test, 1986 Revision
f. imaging
f. imaging with steady precession (FISP)
f. low-angle shot (FLASH)
f. low-angle shot sequence
f. motor unit
f. saccadic eye movement
f. spin-echo inversion recovery sequence
f. spin echo scan

fast-acting agent

fast-frequency repetitive transcranial magnetic stimulation

fastigatum

fastigial
f. nucleus
f. pressor response

fastigiatus
nucleus f.

fastigii
nucleus f.

fastigiobulbar
f. fiber
f. tract

fastigiobulbaris
tractus f.

fastigiospinal
f. fiber
f. tract

fastigiospinalis
tractus f.

fastigium

Fastlene capsule

FasTracker-18 infusion catheter

fast-scan magnetic resonance

fat
f. embolism
f. embolus
epidural f.
f. malabsorption

fatal
f. arrhythmia
f. familial insomnia
f. hypothermia

fat-free mass

fatigability
auditory f.
chronic f.
daytime f.
easy f.
excessive f.
nervous f.
psychogenic f.
stimulation f.
sustained f.
fatigue
chronic f.
cognitive f.
daytime f.
easy f.
excessive f.
f. failure
implant f.
metal f.
sense of f.
stapedius muscle f.
f. of systemic illness
fat-patch graft
fat-suppression
f.-s. MR imaging
f.-s. technique
fatty
f. acid oxidation
f. acid transport into mitochondria
f. degeneration in Reye syndrome
f. granule cell
f. streak
fat/water
f. chemical shift
f. signal cancellation
fauces
branch of lingual nerve to isthmus of f.
faucial
f. paralysis
f. reflex
fausse reconnaissance
faut
comme il f.
faute de mieux
Favaloro-Morse sternal spreader
FAV syndrome
Fazio-Londe
F.-L. atrophy
F.-L. disease
F.-L. syndrome
FBS
failed back syndrome
feedback signal
FC
functional communication
Fc
Fc fragment
FCR
flexor carpi radialis
FDG
fluorodeoxyglucose
FDG method
fear
f. association
ictal f.
lingering f.
FearFighter computer program tailored for specific fear therapy
fearful C cluster
FEAR program
feature
demographic f.
Down syndrome clinical f.
dysautonomic f.
extrapyramidal motor f.
gross pathological f.
junctural f.
leonine facial f.
narcissistic f.
neurobehavioral f.
neurologic f.
neuropsychiatric f.
paralinguistic f.
passive-aggressive f.
pathological f.
sleep f.
featureless headache
febarbamate
febrile
f. convulsion
f. epilepsy
f. seizure
fecal continence
feedback
electromyographic f.
negative f.
positive f.
f. projection
f. sensitivity
f. signal (FBS)
f. system

F

NOTES

feedforward projection
feeding
f. artery of aneurysm
f. center
f. difficulties in cerebral palsy
f. mean arterial pressure (FMAP)
feel-good molecule
feeling
f. of control
f. of dominance
f. of unworthiness
Feer disease
FEF
forced expiratory flow
Fehling TOP ejector punch
felbamate
Felbatol
feltwork
Kaes f.
Felty syndrome
FemBack
Femcet
femoral
f. cutaneous nerve
f. introducer sheath
f. nerve stretch test
f. neuropathy
f. reflex
femoralis
nervus f.
plexus f.
rami cutanei anteriores nervi f.
rami musculares nervi f.
femoris
nervus musculi quadrati f.
nervus quadratus f.
femoroabdominal reflex
fenestra
fenestrated
f. aneurysm clip
f. oculomotor nerve
fenestration
bur hole neuroendoscopic f.
cyst f.
fenisorex
fenobam
Fenton reaction
Féré effect
Féréol-Graux palsy
Fere phenomenon
Ferguson
F. brain suction tip
F. brain suction tube
F. suction
Ferguson-Critchley ataxia
ferpentetate
technetium 99m f.
Ferrein foramen
Ferris
F. Smith-Kerrison laminectomy rongeur
F. Smith-Kerrison punch
ferrite
barium f.
ferritin
serum f.
f. test
ferromagnetic
f. artifact
f. implant
f. intracerebral aneurysm clip
f. monitoring device
ferrous sulfate neurotoxicity
ferruginea
substantia f.
ferrugineus
locus f.
ferumoxide injectable solution
FESS shaver
festinans
chorea f.
festinating gait
fetal
f. adenoma
f. AIDS transmission
f. alcohol syndrome (FAS)
f. brain
f. brain transitory neuron
f. cell transplantation
f. cerebrovascular system
f. dopaminergic tissue implant
f. growth retardation
f. heart rate monitoring
f. hydrocephalus
f. mercury exposure
f. mesencephalic grafting
f. mesencephalic tissue
f. neural implant
f. neural transplant
f. phenytoin exposure
f. planum
f. planum temporal lateralization
f. position
f. response
f. shunt procedure
f. substantia nigra
f. tau
f. tissue transplant
f. transfusion
f. valproic acid syndrome
fetalis
erythroblastosis f.
fetoprotein
alpha f.

feud
blood f.
Feulgen cytophotometry
fever
Argentinian hemorrhage f.
Bolivian hemorrhagic f.
catscratch f.
f. caused by infection (FI)
Central European tick-borne f.
cerebrospinal f.
dengue f.
diphasic milk f.
drug f.
familial Mediterranean f. (FMF)
hemorrhagic f.
Jarisch-Herxheimer f.
Katayama f.
meningotyphoid f.
Q f.
relapsing f.
Rift Valley f.
Rocky Mountain spotted f.
saddleback f.
South African tick-bite f.
spotted f.
trypanosome f.
typhus f.
undulant f.
West Nile f.
yellow f.
Zika f.
Feverall
Infant's F.
FFA
fusiform face area
[^{18}F] fluoride solution
[^{18}F]fluoro-2-deoxy-D-glucose
[^{13}F]fluorodeoxyglucose
FFM
free-fat mass
FFT
fast Fournier transform
FGF
fibroblastic growth factor
FGFR2
fibroblast growth factor receptor 2
***FGFR3* gene**
FG syndrome
FHM
familial hemiplegic migraine
FI
fasciculus interfascicularis
fever caused by infection
FIA
familial intracranial aneurysm
fiber, fibre
A f.
accelerator f.
A-delta f.
adrenergic f.
afferent nerve f.
alpha f.
amygdalofugal f.
anastomosing f.
anastomotic f.
annulospiral f.
anterior external arcuate f.
arcuate f.
association f.
augmentor f.
autonomic nerve f.
B f.
Bergmann f.
beta f.
bulbar corticonuclear f.
Burdach f.
C f.
cerebellohypothalamic f.
cerebelloolivary f.
cerebellospinal f.
cholinergic f.
circular f.
climbing f. (CF)
commissural f.
cone f.
corticobulbar f.
corticomesencephalic f.
corticopontine f.
corticorubral f.
corticospinal f.
corticothalamic f.
cuneocerebellar f.
cuneospinal f.
cutaneon histamine-sensitive f.
decussation of trochlear nerve f.
denervated f.
f. density
dentatorubral f.
dentatothalamic f.
depressor f.
f. diameter

F

NOTES

fiber *(continued)*
f. dissection technique
Edinger f.
efferent f.
endogenous f.
exogenous f.
external arcuate f.
extrafusal f.
fastigiobulbar f.
fastigiospinal f.
frontopontine f.
gamma f.
geniculostriate f.
Goll f.
gracile spinal f.
Gratiolet radiating f.
gray f.
heterodesmotic f.
homodesmotic f.
hypothalamocerebellar f.
hypothalamospinal f.
inhibitory f.
inner cone f.
internal arcuate f.
internuncial f.
intersegmental f.
intraaxial f.
intracortical transverse f.
intraepidermal nerve f. (IENF)
intrafusal f.
intrasegmental f.
intrathalamic f.
intrinsic f.
layer of nerve f.
lemniscal f.
long association f.
longitudinal pontine f.
Mauthner f.
mechanoreceptor f.
medullated nerve f.
mesencephalic corticonuclear f.
Micro link f.
micro-thin plastic f.
Monakow f.
monoaminergic f.
mossy f.
motor f.
Müller f.
muscle f.
myelinated nerve f.
Myer f.
myoclonic epilepsy with ragged red f.
myoclonus epilepsy with ragged red f. (MERRF)
nerve f.
neuroglial f.
nigrostriate f.
nonmedullated f.
nuclear bag f.
nuclear chain f.
nucleocortical f.
oblique gastric f.
occipitopontine f.
occipitotectal f.
olivocerebellar f.
olivospinal f.
outer cone f.
parallel f.
paraventricular f.
parietopontine f.
parietotemporopontine f.
peptidergic f.
periventricular f.
pilomotor f.
pontine corticonuclear f.
pontocerebellar f.
postcommissural f.
posterior external arcuate f.
postganglionic nerve f.
preganglionic autonomic f.
preganglionic nerve f.
pressor f.
pretectoolivary f.
projection f.
pyramidal f.
radicular f.
ragged red f. (RRF)
raphespinal f.
Rasmussen nerve f.
reinnervated f.
Reissner f.
Remak f.
retinothalamic projection f.
Retzius f.
rod f.
Rosenthal f.
rubroolivary f.
sensory myelinated f.
f. sensory tract
short association f.
f. size
somatic afferent f.
somatic efferent f.
somatic nerve f.
spinocuneate f.
spinogracile f.
spinohypothalamic f.
spinomesencephalic f.
spinoolivary f.
spinoperiaqueductal f.
spinoreticular f.
spinotectal f.
spinothalamic f.

Stilling f.
stria terminalis f.
striatonigral f.
sudomotor f.
supraoptic f.
T f.
tangential nerve f.
tautomeric f.
tectoolivary f.
tectopontine f.
tectoreticular f.
temporopontine f.
tendril f.
thalamocortical f.
f. tract of spinal cord
f. tract transection
transverse pontine f.
trigeminothalamic f.
ultra high molecular weight polyethylene f.
ultraterminal f.
unmyelinated f.
varicose f.
vasomotor f.
visceral afferent f.
visceral efferent f.
visceral nerve f.
von Monakow f.

fiberoptics

fiberscope

superfine f.

Fiblast trafermin growth factor

fibra, pl. **fibrae**

fibrae arcuatae cerebri
fibrae arcuatae externae
fibrae arcuatae externae anteriores
fibrae arcuatae externae posteriores
fibrae arcuatae internae
fibrae associationes breves
fibrae associationes longae
fibrae associationis brevis
fibrae associationis telencephali
fibrae cerebelloolivares
fibrae circulares
fibrae commissurales telencephali
f. commissuralis
fibrae corticomesencephalicae
fibrae corticonucleares
fibrae corticonucleares bulbus
fibrae corticonucleares mesencephali
fibrae corticonucleares pontis
fibrae corticopontinae
fibrae corticoreticulares
fibrae corticorubrales
fibrae corticospinales
fibrae corticothalamicae
fibrae cuneocerebellares
fibrae cuneospinales
fibrae dentatorubrales
fibrae frontopontinae
fibrae gracilispinales
fibrae hypothalamospinales
fibrae intrathalamicae
fibrae occipitopontinae
fibrae occipitotectales
fibrae olivospinales
fibrae paraventriculares
fibrae paraventriculohypophysiales
fibrae parietopontinae
fibrae parietotemporopontinae
fibrae periventriculares
fibrae pontis longitudinales
fibrae pontis profundae
fibrae pontis superficialis
fibrae pontis transversae
fibrae pontocerebellares
fibrae postcommissurales
fibrae precommissurales
fibrae pretectoolivares
fibrae pyramidales
fibrae rubroolivares
fibrae spinocuneatae
fibrae spinograciles
fibrae spinohypothalamicae
fibrae spinomesencephalicae
fibrae spinoolivares
fibrae spinoperiaqueductales
fibrae spinoreticulares
fibrae spinotectales
fibrae striae terminalis
fibrae supraopticae
fibrae supraopticohypophysiales
fibrae tectoolivares
fibrae tectopontinae
fibrae tectoreticulares
fibrae temporopontinae
fibrae thalamoparietales

fibre (*var. of* fiber)

fibril

Abeta f.
bundle of f.
Golgi side f.

NOTES

fibril *(continued)*
nerve f.
thioflavin-positive f.
fibrillar basket
fibrillary
f. aggregate
f. astrocyte
f. astrocytoma
f. chorea
f. contraction
f. glia
f. myoclonia
f. neuroma
f. tremor
fibrillation
nonrheumatic atrial f.
paroxysmal atrial f.
f. potential
ventricular f.
fibrillinopathy
fibrillogenesis
AbetaB f.
fibrin
f. bandage
f. film
f. glue
f. glue-soaked Gelfoam
fibrinogen
fibrinoid degeneration
fibrinolysin
fibrinolysis
intracisternal f.
fibrinolytic agent
fibrin-platelet-fibrin embolus
fibroblast
f. growth factor receptor 2 (FGFR2)
senescent f.
transfected f.
fibroblastic
f. growth factor (FGF)
f. meningioma
f. proliferation
fibroblastoma
perineural f.
fibrodysplasia ossificans
fibrogliosis
fibrohistiocytoma
malignant f.
fibrolipoma
fibroma
chondromyxoid f.
ossifying f.
periungual f.
psammomatoid ossifying f.
sinonasal psammomatoid ossifying f.
subungual f.
fibromatosis
juvenile f.
fibromuscular
f. dysplasia (FMD)
f. hyperplasia
fibromyalgia
fibromyelinic plaque
fibronectin synthesis
fibroneuroma
fibroplasia
retrolental f.
fibropsammoma
fibrosa
meninx f.
fibrosarcoma
fibrosclerosis
multifocal f.
systemic multifocal f.
fibrosing arachnoiditis
fibrosis
arachnoid f.
cystic f.
diffuse interstitial f. (DIF)
dural f.
leptomeningeal f.
meningeal f.
muscle f.
postradiation f.
progressive leptomeningeal f.
f. radiation
retroperitoneal f.
root sleeve f.
fibrositic headache
fibrositis
cervical f.
fibrosum
molluscum f.
fibrosus
annulus f.
fibrous
f. astrocyte
f. dysplasia
f. mesothelioma
f. plaque
f. sarcoma
f. sheath of optic nerve
fibroxanthoma
fibroxanthosarcoma
fibular
f. allograft
f. grafting
f. nerve
f. peg
fictitious seizure

FID
free induction decay
repeated FID
fiddle factor
fiducial
cranium-affixed f.
inexact f.
f. marker
MKM f.
radiopaque f.
field
abuse f.
barrel f.
Broca f.
Brodmann cytoarchitectonic f.
centrocecal visual f.
checkerboard f.
f. contour
f. defect
dipole f.
electromagnetic focusing f.
f. expansion
extremely low frequency magnetic f.
face-evoked magnetic f.
f. of Forel
fringing f.
frontal eye f.
f. of gaze
Goldmann visual f.
f. gradient
gradient magnetic f.
H f.
harmonic error f.
f. homogeneity
Humphrey visual f.
f. independence-dependence
f. inhomogeneity
lateral central tegmental f.
lattice f.
f. magnet
magnetic f.
main f.
medial central tegmental f.
nerve f.
nucleus of dorsal f.
nucleus of medial f.
nucleus of perizonal f.
nucleus of prerubral f.
nucleus of ventral f.
occipital eye f.
f. pattern
prerubral f.
pulsating electromagnetic f.
pulsed electromagnetic f. (PEMF)
radiofrequency electromagnetic f.
f. shift
static magnetic f.
f. strength
F. suction dissector
supplementary eye f. (SEF)
vector f.
f. of view
Wernicke f.
z-gradient f.
Fielding membrane
field-tested criterion
FIENS
Foundation for International Education in Neurological Surgery
fifth
f. cranial nerve [CN V]
f. ventricle
Figueira syndrome
figure
fortification f.
myelin f.
figure-ground perception
fila (*pl. of* filum)
filament
actin f.
dural terminal f.
external terminal f.
filum terminale pial f.
glial f.
helical-like f.
internal terminal f.
meningeal f.
myosin f.
paired helical f.
pial terminal f.
root f.
sinal dura mater f.
spinal nerve root f.
straight f.
terminal f.
***filamin* 1 gene**
filial piety
filiformis
nucleus f.
filiform nucleus

NOTES

fillet
decussation of the f.
lateral f.
f. layer
medial f.
triangle of f.
trigone of f.
filling factor
film
absorbable gelatin f.
Accu-Flo dura f.
fibrin f.
Instat fibrin f.
orthogonal f.
filovaricosis
filter
analog f.
high-frequency f. (HFF)
high linear f.
low-frequency f. (LFF)
low-pass f.
Millipore f.
muscle f.
notch f.
Nucleopore f.
roll-off f.
shunt f.
filtered-back projection
filter-evoked central abnormality
filtering
antialias f.
perceptual f.
signal f.
filum, pl. **fila**
f. durae matris spinalis
fila olfactoria
olfactory f.
radicular f.
fila radicularia
fila radicularia nervi spinalis
f. spinale
terminal f.
f. terminale
f. terminale durale
f. terminale externum
f. terminale internum
f. terminale piale
f. terminale pial filament
f. terminale syndrome
fimbria, pl. **fimbriae**
f. of hippocampus
tenia f.
fimbria-fornix lesion
fimbriatum
corpus f.
fimbriodentate sulcus
fimbriodentatus
sulcus f.
final common pathway
Finapres finger cuff
finding
angiographic f.
empirical f.
equivocal f.
motor f.
obtained f.
pathological f.
postmortem f.
spurious f.
fine
f. motor function
f. rapid nystagmus
f. tremor
fine-cup forceps
fine-tipped up-and-down-angled bipolar forceps
finger
f. agnosia
f. anomia
f. fracture technique
f. indicator
jerk f.
lock f.
f. phenomenon
snap f.
spring f.
F. Tapping Test
trigger f.
finger-nose test
finger-thumb reflex
finger-to-finger test
finger-to-nose test
finish bur
Finnish
F. type familial amyloid polyneuropathy
F. variant of neuronal ceroid lipofuscinosis
Finochietto
F. retractor
F. rib spreader
Fiorgen PF
FIRDA
frontal intermittent rhythmic delta activity
firing
neuronal element f.
sustained high-frequency repetitive f. (SRF)
firma
terra f.
FIRO Awareness Scale

FIR.S.T.
first seizure study
first
f. cranial nerve [CN I]
f. night effect
f. seizure study (FIR.S.T.)
f. somatosensory area
f. temporal convolution
f. temporal gyrus
f. visual area
first-degree nystagmus
first-episode patient
first-line therapy
first-order
f.-o. elimination kinetics
f.-o. neuron
first-rank symptom
first-trimester maternal seizure
Fisch
F. drill
F. dural hook
F. micro hook
Fischer
F. grade
F. stereotaxy system
F. syndrome
Fischer-Leibinger bur hole-mounted fixation device
FISH
fluorescence in situ hybridization
Fisher
F. exact test
F. grading
F. syndrome
Fishgold line
fish vertebra
FISP
fast imaging with steady precession
fissura, pl. **fissurae**
f. calcarina
f. cerebri lateralis
f. choroidea
f. collateralis
f. dentata
f. hippocampus
f. horizontalis
f. horizontalis cerebelli
f. intercruralis cerebelli
f. intersemilunaris
f. intraculminalis
f. longitudinalis cerebri
f. mediana anterior medullae oblongatae
f. mediana anterior medullae spinalis
f. mediana ventralis medullae oblongatae
f. mediana ventralis medullae spinalis
f. parietooccipitalis
f. petrooccipitalis
f. posterior superior
f. posterolateralis
f. posterolateralis cerebelli
f. postpyramidalis
f. precentralis
f. preculminalis
f. prepyramidalis
f. prima cerebelli
f. secunda cerebelli
f. sphenooccipitalis
f. transversa cerebelli
f. transversa cerebri
fissure
f. of annulus
ansoparamedian f.
ape f.
Bichat f.
Broca f.
Burdach f.
calcarine f.
callosomarginal f.
cerebellomedullary f.
cerebral f.
choroid f.
choroidal f.
choroidal-hippocampal f.
Clevenger f.
collateral f.
dentate f.
displacement of interhemispheric f.
Ecker f.
entorbital f.
great horizontal f.
great longitudinal f.
hippocampal f.
inferior orbital f.
inferofrontal f.
intercrural f.
interhemispheric f.
intersemilunar f.
intraculminate f.

NOTES

F

fissure *(continued)*
lateral cerebral f.
longitudinal cerebral f.
lunate f.
Monro f.
optic f.
Pansch f.
paracentral f.
parietooccipital f.
postcentral f.
postclival f.
posterior median f.
posterior superior f.
posterolateral f.
posthippocampal f.
postlingual f.
postlunate f.
postpyramidal f.
postrhinal f.
precentral f.
preclival f.
preculminate f.
precuneal f.
prenodular f.
prepyramidal f.
presylvian f.
retrotonsillar f.
rhinal f.
f. of Rolando
Schwalbe f.
simian f.
subfrontal f.
subtemporal f.
superfrontal f.
superior orbital f. (SOF)
superior temporal f.
sylvian f.
f. of Sylvius
transtemporal f.
transverse cerebral f.
zygal f.

fistula, pl. **fistulae**
arteriovenous f.
Brescia-Cimino f.
caroticocavernous f.
carotid-cavernous sinus f.
carotid-dural f.
cavernous sinus f.
cerebrospinal fluid f.
conus perimedullary arteriovenous f.
craniosinus f.
dorsal enteric f.
dural arteriovenous f. (DAVF)
dural venous f.
durocutaneous f.
iatrogenic carotid-cavernous f.
intradural arteriovenous f.
intradural retromedullary arteriovenous f.
perilymph f. (PLF)
perilymphatic f.
posterior fossa dural arteriovenous f.
radiculomedullary f.
spinal dural arteriovenous f. (SDAVF)
trauma-induced f.
vertebrovenous f.
wall f.

fistula-induced sinus thrombosis

fistular
premedullary arteriovenous f.

fit
cerebellar f.
uncinate f.

Fite stain

fixateur interne

fixation
adjunctive screw f.
anterior C1-C2 screw f.
anterior metallic f.
anterior plate f.
anterior screw f.
anterior spinal f.
atlantoaxial f.
Caspar anterior plate f.
C1-C2 cable f.
cervical spine internal f.
cervical spine screw-plate f.
Cotrel-Dubousset f.
crossed-screw f.
dens anterior screw f.
f. device
Essex-Lopresti axial f.
external spinal skeletal f. (ESSF)
Galveston f.
Halifax clamp posterior cervical f.
Harrington rod f.
hook-plate f.
iliac f.
f. instability
intermaxillary f.
internal spinal f.
lumbar pedicle f.
lumbar spine segmental f.
lumbar spine transpedicular f.
Luque-Galveston f.
Luque loop f.
Magerl posterior C1-C2 screw f.
mandibular f.
Manual of Internal F.
Modulock posterior spinal f.
multiple-point sacral f.
f. nystagmus

occipitocervical f.
odontoid fracture internal f.
pedicle screw-rod f.
pedicular f.
pelvic f.
plate f.
plate-screw f.
posterior cervical f.
posterior segmental f.
reduction f.
ReFix noninvasive f.
rigid internal f.
Roy-Camille posterior screw plate f.
sacral pedicle screw f.
sacral spine f.
sacrum fusion screw f.
scoliotic curve f.
screw f.
segmental f.
Sofwire spinal f.
spinal f.
spinopelvic transiliac f. (STIF)
spondylolisthesis reduction f.
sublaminar f.
f. technique
Texas Scottish Rite Hospital rod f.
transarticular screw f.
transpedicular screw-rod f.
transverse f.
TSRH rod f.
visual f.

fixative
Bouin-Hollande f.

fixator
AO internal f.
DeBastiani external f.
external spinal skeletal f.
intermediate head f.
ReFix stereotactic head f.
Vermont spinal f.

fixed
f. contracture
f. distribution
f. dose stimulation
f. dosing
f. dosing arm
f. gaze
f. pupil
f. spasm
f. torticollis

fixed-action pattern

fixedness
functional f.

FK-506
F. drug
F. neurotoxicity

[^{18}F]-labeled
[^{18}F]-l. fluorodeoxyglucose
positron emission tomography with [^{18}F]-l.

flaccid
f. dysarthria
f. paralysis
f. paresis

flaccida
pars f.

flaccidity
curarization-induced f.

FLAIR
fluid-attenuated inversion recovery
FLAIR sequence magnetic resonance imaging

flame-shaped hemorrhage

flame tip bur

Flamm technique

Flanagan spinal fusion gouge

flap
axial pattern scalp f.
bicoronal scalp f.
bone f.
craniotomy f.
C-shaped scalp f.
Dandy myocutaneous scalp f.
f. elevation
free bone f.
horseshoe-shaped f.
I-shaped scalp f.
island pedicle scalp f.
liver f.
lumbar periosteal turnover f.
myocutaneous f.
neurovascular f.
osteoplastic bone f.
palatopharyngeal f.
pedicled pericranial f.
pericranial temporalis f.
scalp f.
sickle f.
skin f.
supraorbital pericranial f.

F

NOTES

flap *(continued)*
trap-door type f.
U-shaped scalp f.
flapping tremor
flare
axon f.
FLASH
fast low-angle shot
flash-frozen tumor specimen
flashing pain syndrome
Flashpoint 5000 3-D localizer
flat
f. back curette
f. back deformity
f. back syndrome
f. electroencephalogram
f. occiput
f. tire sign
f. top wave
Flatau law
Flatau-Schilder disease
flattening of gyrus
flavin
f. adenine dinucleotide (FAD)
f. mononucleotide (FMN)
flavin-containing mono-oxygenase metabolic system
flavipes
Aspergillus f.
Flavivirus
flavoprotein dehydrogenase
flavum
ligamentum f.
flecainide
Flechsig
F. area
F. bundle in cerebellum
F. fasciculus
F. ground bundle
oval area of F.
F. primordial zone
semilunar nucleus of F.
F. tract
fleece
Stilling f.
fleeting
f. auditory hallucination
f. visual hallucination
Flesh-Kincaid method
FlexDial stimulus control
Flexeril
Flex Foam orthosis
flexibilitas
cerea f.
flexibility
Cotrel-Dubousset rod f.
mental f.
flexible
f. arm microretractor
f. arm retractor
f. endoscope
f. neuroleptic dosing
f. wire electrode
Flexicair bed
Flexinet dressing
flexion
flicker thumb f.
forelimb f.
f. injury posterior atlantoaxial arthrodesis
paraplegia in f.
passive f.
f. reflex testing
spontaneous f.
flexion-compression spine injury stabilization
flexion-distraction injury
flexion-extension injury
flexion-extension-mediated injury
flexor
f. carpi radialis (FCR)
f. carpi radialis muscle
f. reflex
f. tetanus
flexura, pl. **flexurae**
flexure
basicranial f.
cephalic f.
cerebral f.
cervical f.
cranial f.
mesencephalic f.
pontine f.
telencephalic f.
transverse rhombencephalic f.
F.L. Fischer modular stereotaxy system
flicker
f. frequency grating
f. thumb flexion
Flickinger
formula of F.
flip angle
flittering scotoma
floating-forehead operation
floccule
flocculi (*pl. of* flocculus)
flocculonodular
f. arteriovenous malformation
f. lobe
f. lobule
f. node
flocculonodularis
lobus f.
flocculus, pl. **flocculi**

accessory f.
peduncle of f.
pedunculus f.
flomoxef
floor
fourth ventricle f.
lateral ventricle f.
f. plate
temporal fossa f.
third ventricle f.
floorstand
CASS digital read-out f.
Contraves type f.
floppy
f. head syndrome
f. infant syndrome
FloSeal
F. hemostatic agent
F. Matrix hemostatic sealant
flounder
Flouren law
flow
absolute f.
anterior cingulate f.
autoregulation of cerebral blood f.
axoplasmic f.
f. birefringence
blood f.
brain blood f.
cerebral blood f. (CBF)
collateral blood f.
cortical microcirulatory f.
f. cytometry
f. detection technique
f. direction
f. dynamic
forced expiratory f. (FEF)
global vertebral blood f. (gCBF)
hemispheric blood f.
hemispheric cross f.
hypothalamic blood f.
intraarterial f.
local cerebral blood f. (LCBF)
f. misregistration
orbital blood f.
prefrontal f.
regional cerebral blood f. (rCBF)
f. regulated suction tube
resting anterior cingulate f.
retrograde blood f.
spinal cord white matter blood f.
f. theory
f. tracer
f. velocity
whole brain blood f.
xenon CT cerebral blood f.
flow-controlled device
flow-directed embolization
flower basket of Bochdalek
flower-spray
f.-s. ending
f.-s. organ of Ruffini
flow-induced influx effect
flowmeter
clinical electromagnetic f.
electromagnetic f.
laser Doppler f. (LDF)
flowmetry
Doppler f.
laser Doppler f.
flow-related enhancement
flow-sensitive
f.-s. magnetic resonance imaging (FS MRI)
f.-s. MR imaging
FLP
Functional Limitation Profile
Fluanxol Depot
fluconazole
fluctuation
core temperature f.
motor f.
on-off motor f.
orthostatic f.
temperature f.
flucytosine
f. blood level
5-flucytosine
fludorex
fludrocortisone
flue-like
interferon f.-l.
fluency
cross-modal f.
fluent
f. aphasia
f. speech
FLUFTEX gauze roll
fluid
f. ability
f. balance
cerebrospinal f. (CSF)

NOTES

fluid *(continued)*
coccidioidal complement fixation of cerebrospinal f.
f. coordination
cytosol f.
endoneurial f.
hypoglycorrhachia of cerebrospinal f.
limulus lysate assay of cerebrospinal f.
lymphocyte:PMN ratio in cerebrospinal f.
lymphocytic pleocytosis-depressed glucose in cerebrospinal f.
mononuclear pleocytosis of cerebrospinal f.
f. percussion head injury
pleocytosis of cerebrospinal f.
f. retention
Sayk preparation of cerebrospinal f.
spinal f.
subglial cerebrospinal f.
Traube-Hering-Mayer waves in cerebrospinal f.
Tyndall effect seen in cerebrospinal f.
ventricular f.
xanthochromia of cerebrospinal f.
fluid-attenuated
f.-a. inversion recovery (FLAIR)
f.-a. inversion recovery sequence magnetic resonance imaging
fluidity
increased platelet membrane f.
f. of movement
flu-like syndrome
flumazenil
flumezapine
flummox
fluorescein
intrathecal f.
fluorescence
autofluorescence focal f.
f. in situ hybridization (FISH)
fluorescent treponemal antibody absorption test
fluorocytosine
fluorodeoxyglucose (FDG)
[^{18}F]-labeled f.
f. PET study
positron emission tomography-f. (PET-FDG)
fluorodopa
f. positron emission tomographic scan
f. positron emission tomography
fluorography
pulsed f.
fluorometer
FluoroNav
F. virtual fluoroscopic system
F. virtual fluoroscopy system
fluorophores
fluoroptic
f. thermometry probe
f. thermometry system
fluoroscopic
f. image guidance
f. imaging
fluoroscopy
C-arm f.
intraoperative lateral f.
fluorosis
5-fluorouracil
fluorouracil therapy
fluoxetine
f. intoxication
f. treatment
fluoxymesterone
fluphenazine hydrochloride
flurazepam
flurry of myoclonic jerk
flush chamber
flushing
facial f.
hemifacial f.
Flushmesh
F. panel
F. strap
flutamide
fluticasone
flutoprazepam
flutter
microsaccadic f.
ocular f.
fluvoxamine maleate
flux
ion f.
microcirculatory red cell f.
Flynn-Aird syndrome
FMAP
feeding mean arterial pressure
FM-B
Balance subscale of the Fugl-Meyer test
FMD
fibromuscular dysplasia
foot-and-mouth disease
FMF
familial Mediterranean fever
FMN
flavin mononucleotide
f-MRI
functional magnetic resonance imaging

BOLD f.-M.
blood oxygen level-dependent functional magnetic resonance imaging

foam
f. cell
gelatin f.
Ivalon f.
polyvinyl alcohol f.
PV f.

focal
f. adhesion kinase (FAK)
f. artery ischemia
f. brain syndrome
f. cerebral head injury
f. cerebral ischemia
f. cortical dysfunction
f. cortical dysplasia
f. delta slow wave activity
f. edema
f. epileptiform activity
f. epileptiform discharge
f. frontal lobe epilepsy
f. hand dystonia
f. infection
f. lesion
f. malformations of cortical development
f. motor seizure
f. muscular atrophy
f. neonatal hypotonia
f. neurologic deficit
f. neurologic disturbance
f. neuropathy
f. nodular heterotopia
f. plaquelike defect
f. pontine leukoencephaly
f. radiation
f. sclerosis
f. slowing
f. slowing of background rhythm
f. slow-wave abnormality
f. status epilepticus
f. stereotactic injection
f. temporal lobe dysfunction

focality

FocalSeal-S-surgical sealant

focus, pl. **foci**
anaplastic f.
centrotemporal paroxysmal f.
cortical epileptogenic f.
cortical seizure f.
epilepsy with multiple independent spike f.
epileptic f.
epileptogenic f.
extensive seizure f.
familial partial epilepsy with variable f.
f. of hemorrhage
inward f.
occult frontal f.
outward f.
restricted f.
rolandic paroxysmal f.
secondary epileptogenic f.
tuberculous f.

focused radiation therapy

fodrin

Fogarty embolectomy catheter

Foix-Alajouanine
F.-A. disease
F.-A. myelitis
F.-A. syndrome

Foix-Cavany-Marie syndrome

Foix syndrome

folate
f. deficiency
serum f.

fold
choroidal f.
interclinoid f.
medullary f.
neural f.
petroclinoid f.
postsynaptic f.
retrotarsal f.
f. of Veraguth

foldover
image f.

folia (*pl. of* folium)
f. cerebelli
f. of cerebellum

folic
f. acid
f. acid deficiency

folie
f. á cinq
f. circulaire
f. d'action
f. du doute
f. hypocondriaque

NOTES

folie *(continued)*
f. musculaire
f. paralytique
f. penitentiare
f. à pleusirs
f. raisonnante
f. simulee
f. simultanee
f. vaniteuse
folii
lobulus f.
folinic acid
folium, pl. **folia**
cerebellar f.
f. of vermis
f. vermis
follicle
hair f.
follicle-stimulating hormone (FSH)
follicle-stimulating/luteinizing hormone adenoma
follicularis
alopecia f.
Folling disease
following gaze
followup, follow-up
f. data
systematic f.
f. visit
fontanelle, fontanel
fonticulus nasofrontalis
fontinalis
decussatio f.
food allergy insomnia
foot
astrocytic end f.
f. clonus
drop f.
dropped f.
Friedreich f.
f. of hippocampus
Morton f.
perineuronal end f.
perivascular f.
perivascular end f.
precapillary end f.
f. reflex
f. slap
spastic equinus f.
sucker f.
foot-and-mouth disease (FMD)
footdrop
footplate of the stapes
foramen, pl. **foramina**
arachnoid f.
Bichat f.
f. caecum medullae oblongatae
f. caecum posterius
f. cecum medullae oblongatae
cervical neural f.
emissary f.
Fallopio f.
Ferrein f.
f. of Froesch
great f.
greater sciatic f.
Hyrtl f.
infrapiriform f.
interventricular f.
f. interventriculare
intervertebral f.
jugular f.
f. jugulare
f. of Key-Retzius
f. of Key and Retzius
f. lacerum
f. lateralis ventriculi quarti
f. of Luschka
f. of Magendie
f. magnum
f. magnum cyst
f. magnum decompression
f. magnum herniation
f. magnum line
f. of Monro
foramina of Monro
foramina nervosa
neural f.
open exit f.
f. ovale
f. ovale electrode
Pacchioni f.
pacchionian f.
parietal f.
posterior lacerate f.
Retzius f.
f. rotundum
Schwalbe f.
f. spinosum (FS)
stylomastoid f.
f. of Vesalius
Vicq d'Azyr f.
foraminal
f. approach
f. decompression
f. encroachment
f. extraforaminal
f. herniation
f. stenosis
foraminosus
tractus spiralis f.
foraminotomy
microendoscopic f.
microscopic f.

foraminulosus
tractus spiralis f.
foraminulum, pl. **foraminula**
Forbes-Cori disease
Forbes disease
force
f. application
F. 2 CEM generator
deflection f.
distraction f.
endogenous f.
exchange f.
exogenous f.
fraction maximal voluntary contraction f.
f. nucleus
shearing f.
societal f.
f. transducer
forced
f. choice of recognition test
f. expiratory flow (FEF)
f. grasping reflex
f. impulse
f. medication
f. relationship
f. vital capacity (FVC)
forceps
Adson bipolar f.
Adson-Brown f.
Adson clip-introducing f.
Adson cup f.
Adson dressing f.
Adson hemostatic f.
Adson hypophysial f.
Adson-Mixter neurosurgical f.
Adson tissue f.
alligator cup f.
f. anterior
Babcock f.
bayonet f.
bipolar bayonet f.
bipolar coagulating f.
bipolar electrocautery f.
bipolar long-shaft f.
brain clip f.
brain spatula f.
brain tumor f.
Brown-Adson f.
Castroviejo eye suture f.
Cherry-Kerrison laminectomy f.
Cone skull punch f.
Cone wire-twisting f.
contact compressive f.
cranial rongeur f.
Crile artery f.
cup f.
curved knot-tying f.
Cushing bayonet f.
Cushing bipolar f.
Cushing brain f.
Cushing dressing f.
Cushing monopolar f.
Cushing tissue f.
Dandy scalp hemostatic f.
Davis coagulating f.
Davis monopolar f.
DeBakey f.
Decker alligator f.
Decker microsurgical f.
DeMartel scalp flap f.
Denis f.
D'Errico bayonet pituitary f.
D'Errico hypophysial f.
D'Errico pituitary f.
D'Errico tissue f.
DeVilbiss rongeur f.
dissecting f.
dressing f.
dura protecting f.
ear f.
Ewald-Hudson f.
fine-cup f.
fine-tipped up-and-down-angled bipolar f.
Fox bipolar electrocautery f.
f. fracture
frontal f.
f. frontalis
Gerald f.
Gildenberg f.
Greenwood bipolar and suction f.
Gruenwald ear f.
Hajek-Koffler bone punch f.
Halsted artery f.
Halsted mosquito f.
Hardy bayonet dressing f.
Hardy microsurgical bayonet bipolar f.
Hardy sella punch f.
Heifetz cup serrated ring f.
hemostatic f.

F

NOTES

forceps *(continued)*
Hirsch hypophysis punch f.
Housepian f.
Howmedica Microfixation System plate-holding f.
Hudson f.
Hunt angled serrated ring f.
Hunt angled-tip f.
Hunt grasping f.
Hunt-Yasargil pituitary f.
Hurd bone-cutting f.
hypophysectomy f.
hypophysial f.
hypophysis punch f.
Ingraham skull punch f.
Jacobson mosquito f.
Jannetta alligator f.
Jannetta bayonet f.
Jansen-Middleton f.
Jansen monopolar f.
Jarell f.
Jarit brain f.
Jarit tendon-pulling f.
Jerald f.
jeweler's bipolar f.
Johnson brain tumor f.
Knight f.
laminectomy punch f.
Leibinger Micro System plate-holding f.
LeRoy scalp clip-applying f.
Love-Gruenwald intervertebral disk f.
Love-Gruenwald pituitary f.
Love-Kerrison rongeur f.
Luc ethmoid f.
MacCarty f.
major f.
Malis angled bayonet f.
Malis irrigation f.
Malis-Jensen microbipolar f.
Malis jeweler's bipolar f.
Maryland tissue grasping f.
McGill f.
McKenzie brain clip f.
McKenzie clip-applying f.
McKenzie clip-bending f.
McKenzie clip-introducing f.
microartery f.
microbipolar f.
microcup f.
microsurgery f.
Micro-Two f.
microvascular f.
Miles punch biopsy f.
minor f.
monopolar tissue f.
mosquito f.
Moynihan f.
Nicola f.
occipital f.
f. occipitalis
Oldberg pituitary f.
Olivecrona-Toennis clip-applying f.
Péan f.
peapod intervertebral disk f.
pituitary f.
plain f.
f. posterior
Preston ligamentum flavum f.
Raimondi infant scalp hemostatic f.
Raney coagulating f.
Raney rongeur f.
Raney scalp clip-applying f.
Rhoton-Cushing f.
Rhoton dissecting f.
Rhoton-Tew bipolar f.
Richter laminectomy punch f.
ringed formed f.
round-handled f.
scalp clip f.
scalp flap f.
Scharff microbipolar and suction f.
Scoville brain clip-applying f.
Scoville brain spatula f.
Scoville clip-applying f.
sella punch f.
Spencer biopsy f.
spinal perforating f.
sponge-holding f.
straight knot-tying f.
straight line bayonet f.
f. tip
tissue f.
Toennis tumor f.
transsphenoidal bipolar f.
tying f.
Yasargil artery f.
Yasargil bayonet f.
Yasargil clip-applying f.
Yasargil flat serrated ring f.
Yasargil hypophysial f.
Yasargil knotting f.
Yasargil micro f.
Yasargil tumor f.

forearm
f. jerk
f. sign

forebrain
f. cell
f. cell culture
magnocellular basal f.
f. vesicle

foregut cyst

forehead
remodeled f.
foreign
f. body
f. body granuloma
Forel
area of F.
F. decussation
field of F.
tegmental field of F.
foreli
campi f.
forelimb
f. flexion
f. kinematic
f. motor
Forestier disease
forest-spring encephalitis
forgetfulness
benign senescent f.
senescent f.
fork
Hardy 3-prong f.
f. head gene
f. head response factor
Jannetta f.
Sugita f.
forking of sylvian aqueduct
form
f. birefringence
depot f.
ICP wave f.
major f.
minor f.
PrP-C (normal f.)
PrP-Sc (abnormal f.)
scrapie f.
trimeric f.
wave f.
formate
butyl f.
formatio, pl. **formationes**
f. hippocampalis
f. reticularis
f. reticularis medullae oblongatae
f. reticularis medullae spinalis
f. reticularis pedunculi cerebri
f. reticularis tegmenti mesencephali
f. reticularis tegmenti pontis
formation
bone matrix f.
brainstem reticular f.
cerebrospinal fluid f.
Chiari f.
hemostatic plug f.
hippocampal f.
leukodystrophy with diffuse Rosenthal fiber f.
medulla oblongata reticular f.
meningioma f.
mesencephalic reticular f.
mesencephalon reticular f.
midbrain reticular f.
mucocele f.
neural plate f.
onion bulb f.
osteophyte f.
paramedian pontine reticular f. (PPRF)
pons reticular f.
pontine paramedian reticular f.
pontine parareticular f.
posttraumatic symptom f.
reticular f.
Rosenthal fiber f.
rouleaux f.
spinal cord reticular f.
spinal reticular f.
syrinx f.
formed visual hallucination
forme fruste, pl. **formes frustes**
formication sign
formula, pl. **formulae**
Abercrombie neuronal cell count f.
Dramamine Less Drowsy F.
F. EM oral solution
f. of Flickinger
parenteral f.
Penn cube function f.
formulation
case f.
clinical f.
dynamic f.
fornicate gyrus
fornicati
uncus gyri f.
fornicatus
gyrus f.
isthmus of gyrus f.
forniceal column
fornicis
carina f.

NOTES

fornicis *(continued)*
columna f.
commissura f.
corpus f.
crus f.
delta f.
stria f.
taenia f.
fornix, pl. **fornices**
anterior pillar of f.
body of f.
column of f.
commissure of f.
f. conjunctiva
crus of f.
pillar of f.
posterior pillar of f.
taenia of f.
transverse f.
Förster
F. diplegia
F. syndrome
fortification
f. figure
f. spectrum
forward
digit span f. (DSF)
f. modeling
spatial span f. (SSF)
fosazepam
fosphenytoin
FOS protein
fossa, pl. **fossae**
anterior cranial f.
anterior recess of interpeduncular f.
cerebellar f.
f. cerebellaris
cistern of lateral cerebral f.
cistern of Sylvius f.
hypophysial f.
f. incudis
inferior aperture of axillary f.
infratemporal f. (ITF)
interpeduncular f.
f. interpeduncularis
lateral cerebral f.
f. lateralis cerebri
limiting sulcus of rhomboid f.
middle cranial f.
f. ovalis
posterior cranial f.
posterior pituitary f.
posterior recess of interpeduncular f.
pterygoid f.
pterygopalatine f.
rhomboid f.
f. rhomboidea
f. of Rosenmüller
rostral posterior f.
sphenoidal f.
superior aperture of axillary f.
sylvian f.
f. of Sylvius
f. of Sylvius cistern
temporal f.
fossula, pl. **fossulae**
Foster
F. frame
F. Kennedy syndrome
FOT
functional occupational therapy
Fothergill
F. disease
F. neuralgia
Foundation for International Education in Neurological Surgery (FIENS)
fountain decussation
four
craniosacral vault f. (CV4)
four-channel Aesculap ventriculoscope
Fourier
F. analysis
F. pulsatility index
F. spectroscopy
F. synthesis
F. transform
F. transform algorithm
F. transformation zeugmatography
F. transform technique
four-poster frame
four-repeat isoform
fourth
f. cervical nerve (C4)
f. cranial nerve [CN IV]
f. nerve palsy
f. ventricle
f. ventricle floor
f. ventricle fovea
fourth-generation cephalosporin
four-vessel cerebral angiogram
fovea, pl. **foveae**
anterior f.
f. centralis maculae luteae
f. centralis retinae
central retinal f.
fourth ventricle f.
inferior f.
superior f.
foveal vision
foveola, pl. **foveolae**
Foville
F. fasciculus
F. syndrome

fowleri
Naegleria f.
Fox
F. bipolar electrocautery
F. bipolar electrocautery forceps
FPA
frontopolar artery
fractalkine
fraction
creatine kinase MB f. (CK-MB)
ejection f.
growth f.
f. maximal voluntary contraction force
oxygen extraction f. (EOF)
regional oxygen extraction f.
S-phase f.
fractional anisotropy (FA)
fractionated radiotherapy
fractionation protocol
fracture
articular mass separation f.
atlantal f.
atlas-axis combination f.
atlas burst f.
axial loading f.
axis-atlas combination f.
basal skull f.
basilar skull f.
blow-out f.
burst f.
capillary f.
Chance f.
clay shoveler's f.
closed skull f.
combined flexion-distraction injury and burst f.
comminuted skull f.
complex f.
complicated f.
compound skull f.
compression f.
f. by contrecoup
cranial f.
depressed skull f.
derby hat f.
diastatic skull f.
direct f.
dishpan f.
f. dislocation
expressed skull f.
facial f.
f. fixation device
forceps f.
growing skull f.
gutter f.
hairline f.
hangman's f.
indirect f.
Jefferson f.
LeFort f.
linear skull f.
low lumbar spine f.
lumbar spine burst f.
lumbosacral junction f.
maxillofacial f.
neurogenic f.
nondepressed skull f.
odontoid f.
open skull f.
orbital floor f.
perinatal clavicle f.
perinatal humerus f.
ping-pong f.
pond f.
f. reduction
rib f.
sagittal slice f.
seatbelt f.
sentinel spinous process f.
simple skull f.
skull f.
slice f.
slot f.
spinous process f.
f. stabilization
stellate skull f.
teardrop f.
thoracic spine f.
thoracolumbar burst f.
translational f.
vertebral f.
wedge-compression f.
f. with scoliosis
zygomatic f.
fracture-dislocation
f.-d. reduction
thoracolumbar spine f.-d.
f.-d. with anterior ligament
fragilis
Bacteroides f.

NOTES

F

fragility
vascular f.
fragment
C-terminal f.
Fc f.
free f.
proteolytic f.
tangle f.
fragmentary myoclonus
fragmentation
internucleosomal DNA f.
f. of nocturnal sleep
sleep f.
fragmented syndrome
frame
Andrews f.
Brown-Roberts-Wells head f.
Budde-Greenberg-Sugita stereotactic head f.
CHOP f.
Cor-Tech guidance to stereotatic head f.
Cosman-Roberts-Wells stereotactic f.
couch-mounted head f.
CRW base f.
CRW head f.
DeBastiani f.
designs for vision f.
Elekta stereotactic head f.
f. fixation-scanner assisted target localization
Foster f.
four-poster f.
gNomos head f.
Greenberg retractor f.
head f.
Horsley-Clarke stereotactic f.
Komai stereotactic head f.
Laitinen stereoguide 2000 arc-centered stereotactic f.
Laitinen stereotactic head f.
Leksell-Elekta stereotactic f.
Leksell Model G stereotactic f.
Lex-Ton spinal f.
Mayfield fixation f.
Mussen f.
OBT stereotactic f.
Olivier-Bertrand-Talairach stereotactic head f.
Olivier-Bertrand-Tipal f.
operative wedge f.
Patil stereotactic head f.
Pelorus stereotactic f.
Radionics CRW stereotactic head f.
Reichert-Mundinger-Fischer stereotactic head f.
Reichert-Mundinger stereotactic head f.
Relton-Hall f.
stereotactic f.
f. stereotaxy
Stryker f.
Sugita multipurpose head f.
Talairach stereotactic f.
Todd-Wells stereotactic f.
Wilson f.
ZD f.
frameless
f. and armless stereotactic neuronavigation
f. stereotactic device
f. stereotactic microsurgery
f. stereotactic technique
f. stereotaxy
f. stereotaxy system
framework
ecologic f.
multidimensional f.
Framingham
F. Eye Study
F. Heart Study
franca
lingua f.
frank
f. catatonic stupor
f. disk herniation
f. lesion
Fränkel
F. classification
F. classification of spinal cord injury
F. sign
Frankel scale
Frankenhäuser ganglion
Frankfurt Complaint Questionnaire
franklinic taste
frataxin gene PCR
frayed disk
Frazier
F. brain-exploring cannula
F. brain trocar
F. cordotomy knife
F. dural elevator
F. dural guide
F. dural hook
F. dural scissors
F. dural separator
F. laminectomy retractor
F. lighted brain retractor
F. nerve hook
F. pituitary knife
F. stylet
F. suction

F. suction tip
F. suction tube
F. ventricular cannula
F. ventricular needle
Frazier-Spiller
F.-S. operation
F.-S. rhizotomy
freckling
inguinal f.
free
f. bone flap
f. fragment
f. fragment disk
f. induction decay (FID)
f. induction signal
f. nerve ending
f. radical
f. radical homeostasis
f. radical hypothesis
f. radical scavenger
f. radical scavenging mechanism
free-fat mass (FFM)
free-hand
f.-h. injection
f.-h. ultrasound-guided intervention
Freehand neuroprosthetic system
Freer
F. chisel
F. dissector
F. septal elevator
Freer-Swanson ganglion knife
freeze-dried cadaveric dura
freezing phenomenon
Fregoli phenomenon/syndrome
Freiberg
F. craniotome
F. so-called infarction
Freiberg-Kohler disease
French
F. brain retractor
F. polio
F. rod bender
F. rod bender frontal
F. tip
Frenchay Aphasia Screening Test
Frenkel symptom
frenulum, pl. **frenula**
buccal f.
cerebellar f.
f. cerebelli
f. of Giacomini
multiple buccal f.
rostral medullary vellum f.
f. of superior medullary velum
f. veli medullaris cranialis
f. veli medullaris rostralis
f. veli medullaris superioris
f. veli medullaris superius
frenzied psychomotor activity
frequency
alpha rhythm f.
F. Analysis of Consecutive Epochs (FACE)
angular f.
background alpha f.
f. dispersion curve
dominant f.
f. encoding
f. error
high-filter f.
Larmor f.
low-filter f.
low linear f.
mean alpha f.
Nyquist f.
offset f.
precessional f.
f. range
resonant f.
f. shift
spatial f.
spectral edge f. (SEF)
spike f.
theta peak f.
frequency-encoding gradient
Fresnel paste-on prism
Frey
F. irritation hair
F. syndrome
friable artery
Friderichsen-Waterhouse syndrome
fried-egg artifact
Friedmann
F. disease
F. vasomotor syndrome
Friedreich
F. disease
F. foot
F. hereditary ataxia
F. tabes
fringe
radical f.

NOTES

fringing field
frise
chevaux de f.
Frisén
Lars F.
Frisén-grade change
Froesch
foramen of F.
Frohlich syndrome
Frohse
arcade of F.
Froin syndrome
Froment
F. paper sign
F. prehensile thumb sign
frontal
f. abasia
anterior f.
f. artery
f. brain region
f. convexity meningioma
f. cortex damage
f. cortex damage effect
f. cortical area
f. cortical dysfunction
f. cortical function
f. corticectomy
f. craniotomy
f. dysequilibrium
f. dysexecutive amnesia
f. encephalocele
f. eye field
f. forceps
French rod bender f.
f. gait disorder
f. groove
f. gyrectomy
f. gyrus
f. headache
f. horn
f. interhemispheric space
f. intermittent rhythmic delta activity (FIRDA)
f. intermittent rhythmic delta activity on EEG
f. lobe
f. lobe abscess
f. lobe of cerebrum
f. lobe degeneration
f. lobe dementia
f. lobe dysfunction
f. lobe epilepsy
f. lobe function
f. lobe impairment
f. lobe infarction
f. lobe lesion
f. lobe-related deficit
f. lobe seizure
f. lobe seizure with complex behavior
f. lobe syndrome
f. lobe tumor
f. lobe volume
f. lobotomy
f. metabolism
f. neoplasm
f. nerve
f. operculum
f. part of corpus callosum
f. phosphocreatinine
f. plane
f. plane growth abnormality
f. polar branch
f. pole
f. subcortical brain circuit
f. temporal atrophy
f. tuber
f. white matter lesion
frontal-cerebellar-thalamic circuitry
frontale
operculum f.
frontalis
alopecia liminaris f.
forceps f.
lobus f.
nervus f.
pars orbitalis ossis f.
polus f.
sulci orbitales lobi f.
sulcus olfactorius lobi f.
frontal-lobe abstraction/problem solving
frontally based cognition
frontocortical aphasia
frontoethmoidal
f. encephalocele
f. recess
frontolenticular aphasia
frontomarginalis
sulcus f.
frontonasomaxillary osteotomy
frontooccipital fasciculus
frontoorbital
f. advancement
f. area
f. osteotomy
frontoorbitozygomatic craniotomy
frontoparallel plane
frontoparietal
ascending f. (ASFP)
f. convexity cyst
f. operculum
frontoparietale
operculum f.

frontopolar
f. artery (FPA)
f. lead
frontopontinae
fibrae f.
frontopontine
f. fiber
f. tract
frontopontinus
tractus f.
frontopontocerebellar pathway
frontosphenoidal encephalocele
frontostriatal-pallidalothalamic circuit
frontostriatal pathway
frontotemporal
f. approach
f. cortex
f. craniotomy
f. dementia (FTD)
f. lobar degeneration
f. slowing
f. tract
frontotemporoparietal craniotomy
frontothalamic circuit
front tap
front-tap reflex
Froriep ganglion
frost
uremic f.
Frova
frovatriptan succinate
fructose-1,6-diphosphatase deficiency
fructose-1-phosphate
fruste, pl. **frustes**
forme f.
Fryns syndrome
FS
foramen spinosum
FS MRI
FSH
follicle-stimulating hormone
FSH dystrophy
FTD
frontotemporal dementia
ftorafur
Fuerstner disease
fugax
amaurosis f.
proctalgia f.
Fugl-Meyer assessment
Fujita
F. method
F. suction cannula
Fukase
Fukuhara syndrome
Fukushima
F. cavernous bypass
F. monopolar malleable coagulator
Fukuyama
F. congenital muscular dystrophy
F. disease
F. syndrome
Fukuyama-type congential muscular dystrophy
Fulci spherule
fulgurating migraine
full
f. dose
f. interepisode recovery
f. remission
f. syndrome
f. width at half maximum (FWHM)
full-blown syndrome
full-dose-treated patient
full-night polysomnography
full-width half maximum
fulminant
f. hepatic encephalopathy
f. hydrocephalus
f. necrotizing encephalitis
f. neuroleptic malignant syndrome
Fulton laminectomy rongeur
fulvius
fumarate
quetiapine f.
fumigatus
Aspergillus f.
function
allomeric f.
altered f.
autonomic f.
autonomous f.
axis f.
behavioral f.
biologic windows on CNS f.
cellular immune f.
cellular respiratory f.
cognitive f.
communication f.
cortical mapping of memory f.

F

NOTES

function *(continued)*
disordered personality f.
dysregulated T-cell f.
endocrine f.
episodic memory f.
executive f.
extracorporeal membrane oxygenation affecting cognitive f.
facial nerve f.
fine motor f.
frontal cortical f.
frontal lobe f.
GABA inhibitory f.
global f.
harmonic f.
higher cognitive f.
higher neural f.
impaired cerebral f.
impaired limbic-diencephalic f.
indolamine f.
intellectual f.
isomeric f.
left ventricular f.
Legendre f.
leukemia therapy affecting cognitive f.
level of cognitive f.
linear rate-response f.
LSUMC classification of motor and sensory f.
memory f.
motor f.
myelinated nerve fiber f.
neural f.
neuronal f.
nonlinear rate-response f.
noradrenergic system f.
ovarian f.
psychosocial f.
renal f.
reverse learning f.
secretory f.
semantic memory f.
sensory f.
f. of sleep
spectral density f.
T-cell f.
thermoeffector f.
thermoregulatory f.
f. type
urinary tract f.
vestibular f.
visuospatial f.
working memory f.

functional
f. activation
f. activation PET scanning
F. Ambulation Category (FAC)
F. Ambulation Classification
f. analysis
f. anosmia
f. aphasia
f. aphonia
f. apoplexy
f. approach
f. assessment
f. brain imaging
f. brain imaging study
f. capacity
f. communication (FC)
f. component
f. contracture
f. decline
f. deficit
f. demand
f. deterioration
f. difference
f. dyspnea
f. electrical stimulation
f. enuresis
F. Ergonomic Prolo Scale
f. failure
F. Fitness Assessment for Adults over 60 Years
f. fixedness
f. funnel
f. hearing impairment
f. hippocampal inactivation
f. imaging data
f. imaging technique
F. Independence Measure
F. Limitation Profile (FLP)
f. loss
f. magnetic resonance imaging (f-MRI)
f. MRI study
f. neuroimaging
f. neuromuscular stimulation
f. neuropharmacology
f. neurosurgery
f. object
F. Obstacle Course
f. occupational therapy (FOT)
f. pain
f. psychiatric syndrome
f. retrograde amnesia
f. spasm
f. status
F. Status Index
f. stereotaxy
f. terminal innervation ratio
f. vaginismus
f. voice disorder

functional/cognitive impairment

functionalism
functioning
adaptive f.
baseline cognitive f.
brain f.
cognitive f.
cortical f.
domain of f.
emotional f.
end-state f.
general verbal intellectual f.
global f.
impaired attentional f.
intellectual f.
level of f.
f. measure
measure of general cognitive f.
neuropsychologic f.
overall cognitive f.
physical f.
premorbid f.
verbal intellectual f.
visuospatial f.
in vivo brain f.
fundamental
f. cognitive process
f. column
f. conceptual problem
f. neural mechanism
f. predisposition
fundus of aneurysm
fungal
f. culture
f. infection
f. meningitis
f. smear
fungiform papillae in familial dysautonomia
fungus, pl. **fungi**
f. cerebri
f. isolation
funicular
f. graft
f. myelitis
f. myelosis
funiculitis
funiculus, pl. **funiculi**
anterior f.
cuneate f.
dorsal f.
f. dorsalis
f. gracilis
lateral f.
f. lateralis
f. lateralis medullae oblongatae
funiculi medullae spinalis
medulla oblongata lateral f.
posterior f.
f. posterior medullae oblongatae
f. separans
f. solitarius
spinal cord ventricular f.
f. teres
ventral f.
f. ventralis medullae spinalis
funnel
functional f.
pial f.
f. plot
f. vision
furcal nerve
furegrelate
furifosmin
technetium 99m f.
furor epilepticus
furosemide
furrowed band
fusiform
f. aneurysm
f. cell of cerebral cortex
f. face area (FFA)
f. gyrus
f. layer
fusiformis
gyrus f.
lobulus f.
fusimotor
f. axon
f. nerve
fusion
Adkins spinal f.
Albee lumbar spinal f.
anterior cervical discectomy and f.
anterior lumbar spine interbody f.
atlantoaxial f.
Bailey-Badgley cervical spine f.
Bosworth spinal f.
Brooks cervical f.
Brooks-Jenkins atlantoaxial f.
cervical spine posterior f.
cervicooccipital f.
Cloward back f.

NOTES

fusion *(continued)*
degenerative lumbar spine f.
degenerative spondylosis decompression and f.
Gallie cervical f.
Gallie spinal f.
Goldstein spinal f.
Harris-Smith cervical f.
Henry-Geist spinal f.
Hibbs-Jones spinal f.
interbody f.
interfacet wiring and f.
intertransverse process f.
f. limit determination
long segment spinal f.
lower cervical spine f.
lumbar interbody f.
lumbosacral f.
f. nonunion rate
occipitoatlantoaxial f.
occipitocervical f.
posterior interbody lumbar spinal f.
posterior-lateral lumbar spinal f.
posterior lumbar interbody f. (PLIF)
posterior spinal f.
posterolateral lumbosacral f.
Robinson anterior cervical f.
sacral spine f.
selective thoracic spine f.
short segment spinal f.
Simmons cervical spine f.
single-level spinal f.
in situ spinal f.
spinal f.
f. stiffness
f. technique
thoracic spinal f.
upper cervical spine f.
variable stereotactic image f.
vertebral f.
Wiltberger f.

fusion-defusion cycle

Fusobacterium

futile cycling

FVC
forced vital capacity

F-wave
F-w. monitoring
F-w. test

FWHM
full width at half maximum

G
G protein
G protein abnormality
G5
G5 Fleximatic massage/percussion unit
G5 Vibramatic massage/percussion unit
Gaab endoscope
GABA
gamma-aminobutyric acid
GABA agonism
GABA concentrate
GABA inhibitory function
GABA receptor
GABA transaminase
GABA-A
gamma-aminobutyric acid type A
GABAergic
GABAergic cortical interneuron
GABAergic inhibition
GABAergic neuron
GABA-mediated inhibitory synaptic transmission
gabapentin capsule
GABAR
$GABA_A$ receptor
$GABA_A$ receptor (GABAR)
$GABA_B$ receptor
$GABA_B$ receptor-mediated inhibition
GABAR-mediated inhibition
GABA-T
gamma aminobutyric acid transaminase
Gabitril
GAD
glutamine decarboxylase
gadodiamide
gadolinium
g. contrast
g. diethylenetriamine pentaacetate
g. diethylenetriamine pentaacetic acid (Gd-DTPA)
g. diethylenetriamine pentaacetic acid-enhanced MR
g. DTPA
g. enhancement
gadolinium-enhanced
g.-e. MR angiography (Gd-MRA)
g.-e. MRI
g.-e. MR imaging
gadopentetate dimeglumine
gadoteridol
GAD-specific intervention
Gaenslen test
GAG
glycosaminoglycan
gag
Dingman mouth g.
g. reflex
g. reflex loss
Gagel granuloma
gain-of-function abnormality
gait
g. abnormality
G. Abnormality Rating Scale
g. apraxia
ataxic g.
calcaneal g.
cerebellar g.
Charcot g.
circumduction g.
g. disorder
g. disorder, autoantibody, late-age onset, polyneuropathy
g. disturbance
dromedary g.
equine g.
festinating g.
gluteal g.
gluteus medius g.
helicopod g.
hemiplegic g.
high steppage g.
hip extensor g.
hysterical g.
intermittent double-step g.
maximus g.
myopathic g.
paraplegic spastic g.
parkinsonian g.
propulsive g.
quadriceps g.
scissors g.
small-step g.
spastic g.
steppage g.
tabetic g.
teddy bear g.
toppling g.
Trendelenburg g.
waddling g.
galactokinase deficiency
galactose-6-sulfate sulfatase
galactose-1-phosphate
g.-p. accumulation
g.-p. uridyltransferase deficiency
galactosialidosis
galactosidase defect

galactosylceramidase deficiency
galactosylceramide lipidosis
galactosylsphingosine accumulation
galanin
galantamine
g. HBr
g. hydrobromide
Galant reflex
Galassi
G. classification system
G. pupillary phenomenon
galea
g. aponeurotica
closed g.
galeatomy
Galen
G. anastomosis
great cerebral vein of G.
G. nerve
vein of G.
G. vein malformation
galenic draining group
gallamine triethiodide
Gall craniology
galli
crista g.
wing of crista g.
Gallie
G. cervical fusion
G. spinal fusion
G. wiring technique
Gallie-Rodgers technique
gallium
g. nitrate
g. scan
gallium-67
galloping tongue
Galtac device
Galt skull trephine
galvanic
g. skin reaction
g. skin reflex (GSR)
g. skin resistance (GSR)
g. skin response (GSR)
g. vertigo
g. vestibular stimulation
galvanogustometer
galvanometer
galvanopalpation
Galveston
G. fixation
G. fixation with TSRH
G. fixation with TSRH crosslink
G. Orientation and Awareness Test
GAMA
General Ability Measure for Adults
Gambian trypanosomiasis
Gambierdiscus toxicus
gamete
gamma
g. aminobutyric acid agonism
g. aminobutyric acid transaminase (GABA-T)
g. capsulotomy
g. carboxylated protein
crosslink g.
g. efferent
g. efferent system
g. fiber
g. globulin
g. glutamyl transpeptidase
g. hydroxybutyrate and amphetamine
g. irradiation
g. knife
G. knife instrument
g. knife radiosurgery (GKRS)
g. loop
G. Maxicamera
g. motoneuron
g. motor neuron
g. motor system
g. ray
g. rhythm
g. rigidity
g. secretase
g. thalamotomy
g. wave
gamma-acetylenic-GABA
gamma-aminobutyric
g.-a. acid (GABA)
g.-a. acid concentrate
g.-a. acid type A (GABA-A)
gamma-aminolevulinic
g.-a. acid
g.-a. acid dehydratase activity
gamma-glutamyltransferase
gamma-hydroxybutyrate
gamma-interferon treatment
gamma-linolenic acid
gamma-vinyl-GABA
gammopathy
benign monoclonal g.
monoclonal g.
ganaxolone
ganciclovir
ganglia (*pl. of* ganglion)
ganglial
gangliated nerve
gangliectomy
gangliform
ganglii
capsula g.
stroma g.

gangliitis
gangliocyte
gangliocytoma
dysplastic g.
sellar g.
ganglioformis
intumescentia g.
ganglioglioma
desmoplastic infantile g.
infantile g.
ganglioglioneurocytoma
ganglioglioneuroma
gangliolysis
percutaneous radiofrequency g.
ganglioma
intracerebral g.
ganglion, pl. **ganglia**
aberrant g.
acousticofacial g.
Andersch g.
aorticorenal g.
ganglia aorticorenalia
Arnold g.
auditory g.
Auerbach g.
auricular g.
autonomic g.
ganglia of autonomic plexus
basal g.
Bezold g.
Blandin g.
Bochdalek g.
Bock g.
Böttcher g.
branch of internal carotid artery to trigeminal g.
branch of ocular motor nerve to ciliary g.
calcification of the basal g.
g. capsule
cardiac g.
ganglia cardiaca
carotid g.
celiac g.
ganglia celiaca
g. cell
g. cell of dorsal spinal root
g. cell of retina
g. cervicale inferius
g. cervicale medium
g. cervicale superius
cervicothoracic g.
g. cervicothoracicum
g. ciliare
ciliary g.
Cloquet g.
coccygeal g.
cochlear g.
g. cochleare
ganglia coeliaca
communicating branch of nasociliary nerve with ciliary g.
Corti g.
cranial g.
ganglia craniospinalia sensoria
craniospinal sensory g.
dorsal root g. (DRG)
Ehrenritter g.
extracranial g.
g. extracraniale
g. of facial nerve
Frankenhäuser g.
Froriep g.
gasserian g.
geniculate g. (GG)
g. geniculatum nervi facialis
g. geniculi
g. geniculi nervi facialis
glossopharyngeal nerve jugular g.
glossopharyngeal nerve lower g.
glossopharyngeal nerve rostral g.
Gudden g.
g. habenula
g. hook
hypogastric g.
g. impar
inferior cervical g.
inferior mesenteric g.
inferior petrosal g.
g. inferius nervi glossopharyngei
g. inferius nervi vagi
inhibitory g.
intercrural g.
ganglia intermedia
intermediate g.
g. of intermediate nerve
interpeduncular g.
intervertebral g.
intracranial g.
g. isthmus
jugular g.
Laumonier g.

NOTES

ganglion *(continued)*
Lee g.
lenticular g.
Lobstein g.
long root of ciliary g.
Ludwig g.
ganglia lumbalia
lumbar g.
marbled appearance of basal g.
Meckel g.
Meckel lesser g.
Meissner g.
g. mesentericum inferius
g. mesentericum superius
middle cervical g.
motor root of ciliary g.
Müller g.
nasal g.
nerve g.
neural g.
g. nevi splanchnici
nodose g.
oculomotor root of ciliary g.
otic g.
g. oticum
parasympathetic root of ciliary g.
parasympathetic root of otic g.
parasympathetic root of pterygopalatine g.
parasympathetic root of sublingual g.
parasympathetic root of submandibular g.
paravertebral g.
pelvic g.
ganglia pelvica
ganglia pelvina
petrosal g.
petrous g.
phrenic g.
ganglia phrenica
ganglia plexuum autonomicorum
ganglia plexuum visceralium
posterior root g.
prevertebral g.
pterygopalatine g.
g. pterygopalatinum
radiocapitellar joint g.
Remak g.
renal g.
ganglia renalia
Ribes g.
root of otic g.
g. rostralis nervi glossopharyngei
g. rostralis nervi vagi
sacral g.
ganglia sacralia
Scarpa g.
Schacher g.
Schmiedel g.
semilunar g.
g. sensoriale
g. sensorium nervi cranialis
g. sensorium nervi spinalis
sensory root of ciliary g.
sensory root of otic g.
sensory root of submandibular g.
short root of ciliary g.
Soemmerring g.
solar g.
sphenomaxillary g.
sphenopalatine g.
spiral cochlear g.
g. spirale cochlea
splanchnic g.
stellate g.
g. stellatum
sublingual g.
g. sublinguale
submandibular g.
g. submandibulare
submaxillary g.
superior cervical g. (SCG)
superior mesenteric g.
g. superius nervi glossopharyngei
g. superius nervi vagi
suprarenal g.
sympathetic g.
ganglia of sympathetic trunk
g. of sympathetic trunk
g. sympatheticum
g. sympathicum
terminal g.
g. terminale
ganglia thoracica
thoracic splanchnic g.
g. thoracicum splanchnicum
trigeminal g.
g. trigeminale
ganglia trunci sympathici
g. of trunk of vagus
tympanic g.
g. tympanicum
vagus nerve jugular g.
vagus nerve rostral g.
Valentin tympanic g.
ventricular g.
vertebral g.
g. vertebrale
vestibular g.
g. vestibulare
Vieussens g.
g. viscerale
visceral plexuses g.

Walther g.
Wrisberg g.
ganglionare
ganglionaris
lamina pyramidalis g.
ganglionated
ganglionectomy
Meckel sphenopalatine g.
sphenopalatine g.
superior cervical g.
ganglioneuritis
ganglioneuroblastoma
ganglioneurocytoma
ganglioneurofibroma
ganglioneuroma
central g.
dumbbell g.
ganglioneuromatosis
ganglionic
g. blocking agent
g. cell layer of retina
g. crest
g. cyst in synovial tendon sheath
g. glioma
g. layer
g. layer of cerebellar cortex
g. layer of cerebral cortex
g. layer of optic nerve
g. layer of retina
g. motor neuron
g. stratum of optic nerve
ganglionicum
stratum g.
stroma g.
ganglionitis
gasserian g.
ganglionostomy
ganglioplegic
ganglioradiculitis
gangliosialidosis
ganglioside
disialyl g.
G_{M1} g.
g. lipidosis
g. monosialic acid
gangliosidosis
G_{M2} g.
generalized g.
infantile G_{M2} g.
type 1 G_{M1} g.
gangliosympathectomy
gangrene
trophic g.
Ganser
basal nucleus of G.
G. commissure
nucleus basalis of G.
gantry rotation
Gantzer muscle
Ganymede
gap
air-bone g.
g. junction
g. paradigm
treatment g.
Garcin syndrome
Gardner
G. headholder
G. meningocele repair
G. neurosurgical skull clamp
G. operation
G. and Robertson classification system
G. syndrome
Gardner-Robertson
G.-R. class
G.-R. hearing grade
Gardner-Wells
G.-W. headrest
G.-W. tongs
Garrett orientation line
gas
arterial blood g. (ABG)
g. chromatography mass spectrometry
Ga scintigraphy
Gaskell nerve
gasping
inspiratory g.
gasserian
g. ganglion
g. ganglion area
g. ganglionitis
g. ganglion neuroma
Gass syndrome
gastric
g. bypass surgery
g. coronary plexus
g. crisis
g. nerve
g. neurasthenia

NOTES

gastric *(continued)*
g. tetany
g. vertigo
gastrica
tetania g.
gastrici
plexus g.
gastrocolic reflex
gastrocytoma
gastroenteritis
gastroepiploic plexus
Gastrografin
gastroileac reflex
gastrointestinal
g. bleeding
g. secretion
g. side effect
g. symptom grouping
Gastrozepine
gate
g. control theory of pain
g. theory
gate-control
g.-c. hypothesis
g.-c. theory
gating
cardiac g.
g. mechanism
sensory g.
Gaucher disease
gauge
Durkan CTS g.
Padgett baseline pinch g.
pressure g.
strain g.
gauntlet anesthesia
gaussian noise
gaze
cardinal direction of g.
conjugate fixed g.
conjugate horizontal g.
consensual g.
g. coordinating aggregate
g. deficit
down g.
dysconjugate g.
dysjunctive g.
field of g.
fixed g.
following g.
horizontal g.
g. impairment
ipsilateral tonic conjugate g.
lateral g.
g. mechanism in brain stem
g. palsy
g. paralysis
g. paresis
periodic alternating g.
ping-pong g.
g. pontine center
g. preference
g. refixational shift
restriction of inward g.
vertical g.
gaze-evoked
g.-e. amaurosis
g.-e. blindness
g.-e. nystagmus
g.-e. visual loss
gaze-paretic nystagmus
gB
glycoprotein B
GBM
glioblastoma multiforme
GCA
giant cell arteritis
gCBF
global vertebral blood flow
GCS
Glasgow Coma Score
GDC
giant Dopamine-containing cell
Guglielmi detachable coil
G. SynerG detachment device
Gd-DTPA
gadolinium diethylenetriamine pentaacetic acid
Gd-DTPA-enhanced cranial MR imaging
Gd-MRA
gadolinium-enhanced MR angiography
GDNF
glial-derived neurotrophic factor
GDS
Global Deterioration Scale
GE
General Electric
GE 9800 CT system
GE Maxicamera gamma camera
GE Signa scanning
GE Vector scanning
gearshift probe
GEFS+
generalized epilepsy with febrile seizures plus
gegenhalten
Geigel reflex
gel
Adcon-L adhesion control in a barrier g.
Dermaflex G.
diazepam rectal g.
H.P. Acthar G.

gelastic
g. epilepsy
g. seizure
gelatin
g. foam
g. phantom
g. sponge
gelatinosa
substantia g.
gelatinosus
nucleus g.
gelatinous
g. hematoma
g. nucleus
g. substance
g. substance of posterior horn of spinal cord
Gelfoam
fibrin glue-soaked G.
G. pad
papaverine-soaked G.
G. pledget
G. powder embolus
thrombin-soaked G.
Gélineau syndrome
Gellman instrumentation
gelotripsy
Gelpi retractor
Gelusil
gemästete cell
gemistocyte
gemistocytic
g. astrocyte
g. astrocytoma
g. cell
g. reaction
gemistocytoma
gemma gustatoria
Gemnisyn
Gemonil
gene
achaete-scute g.
amyloid precursor protein g.
bcl-2 g.
Bcl-xL g.
canarc 1 g.
candidate g.
casein kinase Ie g.
CDK2NA g.
c-fos g.
CHRNA4 g.
CHRNA7 g.
c-jun g.
CLN1 g.
CLN2 g.
CLN3 g.
CLN5 g.
CLN8 g.
cnot g.
connexin g.
CSTB g.
cytotoxin-associated g. A (CagA)
dab1 g.
DAT g.
delta g.
DMD g.
doublecortin g.
DRD2 g.
DTY1 g.
EGR2 g.
elastin g.
En g.
engrailed g.
epidermal growth factor receptor g.
epilepsy g.
EPM2A g.
ERG2 g.
FGFR3 g.
filamin 1 g.
fork head g.
gooseberry g.
goosecoid g.
gox g.
GRIK1 g.
growth arrest-specific g.
gsc g.
hedgehog g.
hepatic apoprotein g.
homeodomain g.
homologous g.
housekeeping g.
Hox g.
immediate early g.
inverse polymerase chain reaction-based detection of frataxin g.
islet g.
kallikrein g.
KCNQ2 g.
KCNQ3 g.
krox g.
lamin a/c g. (LMNA)
leucine zipper g.

G

NOTES

gene *(continued)*
LIM g.
LIM-kinase g.
LIS1 g.
low penetrance-high frequency g.
math g.
MDM2 g.
MeCP2 g.
myotonic dystrophy g.
neuropeptide g.
nkx g.
noggin g.
notch g.
null g.
numb g.
organizer g.
otx g.
p53 g.
paired g.
patched g.
pax g.
persenilin g.
pigment g.
pitx g.
PMP-22 g.
polypeptide hormone g.
potassium channel g.
presenilin g.
g. product
PrP g.
ptc g.
reelin g.
reln g.
retinoblastoma g.
SCA g. (SCA 1-7)
SCN1B g.
seipin g.
shh g.
sialidase g.
slug g.
SMN g.
sonic hedgehog g.
sporadic fatal insomnia prion protein g.
structural g.
survival motor neuron g.
g. synergy
tau g.
TCOF1 g.
g. therapy
g. therapy delivery
g. therapy vector
TOAD-64 g.
Triple A syndrome g. (AAAS)
TSC1 g.
TSC2 g.
tumor suppressor g.
UBE3A g.
ubiquitin-ligase g.
unc-33 g.
wingless g.
wnt g.
zic g.
zinc-finger g.

GenePD study

genera (*pl. of* genus)

general
G. Ability Measure for Adults (GAMA)
g. cognitive status
G. Electric (GE)
G. Electric CT 9800 scanner
G. Electric Hi-Speed Advantage helical scanner
G. Electric Hi-Speed Spiral CT Scanner
G. Electric Signa 1.5-Tesla magnetic resonance scanner
g. endotracheal anesthesia
g. knowledge score
g. medical impairment
g. memory index
g. mood state
g. orotracheal anesthesia
g. paresis
g. paresis of the insane
g. sensation
g. somatic afferent (GSA)
g. somatic afferent column
g. somatic efferent column
g. temporal processing deficit
g. verbal intellectual functioning
g. visceral afferent (GVA)
g. visceral afferent column
g. visceral efferent column

generalized
g. amnesia
g. atypical absence seizure
g. auditory agnosia
g. convulsive status epilepticus
g. dystonia
g. epilepsy plus febrile seizure
g. epilepsy with febrile seizures plus (GEFS+)
g. gangliosidosis
g. headache
g. myokymia
g. paralysis
g. periodic sharp wave
g. polyneuropathy
g. slowing
g. social phobia
g. tetanus
g. tonic-clonic (GTC)

g. tonic-clonic convulsion
g. tonic-clonic epilepsy
g. tonic-clonic seizure (GTCS)

generandi
impotentia g.

generation
g. of affect
lesion g.
mitochondrial free radical g.
pericyte edema g.
slow-wave g.

generator
distal stimulation g.
Force 2 CEM g.
high-frequency g.
Itrel pulse g.
Medtronic 3470 pulse g.
model 100 pulse g.
model 101 pulse g.
Neuro N-50 lesion g.
pattern g.
g. potential
programmable pulse g.
pulse g.
radiofrequency g.
Radionics RF lesion g.

generic negative symptom

genetic
g. alternation
g. basis
g. component
g. difference
g. disorder
g. effect
g. epistemology
g. heterogeneity
g. mapping
g. relationship
g. risk factor
g. screening
g. strategy
g. susceptibility
g. tool
g. transmission
g. typing
g. viewpoint

genetics
biochemical g.
molecular g.

genic
g. balance
g. drift

genicula (*pl. of* geniculum)

geniculate
g. body
g. ganglion (GG)
g. herpes
g. neuralgia
g. nucleus
g. otalgia

geniculati
nucleus medialis magnocellularis corporis g.

geniculatus lateralis nucleus

geniculi
ganglion g.
gyrus g.

geniculocalcarine
g. radiation
g. tract

geniculocalvarium

geniculocortical pathway

geniculostriate
g. fiber
g. tract

geniculum, pl. **genicula**
g. of facial nerve
g. nervi facialis
g. nervus facialis

genioglossus
g. advancement
g. advancement-hyoid myotomy
g. advancement procedure

geniohyoid

genioplasty

genital
g. center
g. corpuscle
g. response
g. ulceration

genitale
corpusculum g.

genitofemoralis
ramus femoralis nervi g.
ramus genitalis nervi g.

genitofemoral nerve

genitospinal center

Gen-K

Gennari
G. band

NOTES

Gennari *(continued)*
G. line
line of G.
G. stria
stripe of G.
genome
herpes simplex virus g.
genomic
g. alteration
g. effect
g. event
g. imprinting
g. mechanism
genotype
ApoE g.
apolipoprotein E g.
e4/e4 g.
tryptophan hydroxylase allelic g.
genotypic
gentamicin
genu, pl. **genua**
branch to internal capsule, g.
g. capsulae internae
g. corporis callosi
g. of corpus callosum
facial g.
g. of the facial nerve
g. of internal capsule
g. nervi facialis
genus, pl. **genera**
Geodon
GeoMedica
Geopen
Gerald forceps
Gerbode-Burford rib spreader
Gerhardt disease
Gerhardt-Semon law
geriatric
g. depression
G. Depression Scale
g. neurology
Gerlier disease
germ
g. cell tumor
g. cell tumor with synchronous lesions in pineal and suprasellar region
German chamomile
germ-cell
germinal
g. matrix
g. matrix hemorrhage
germinoma
pineal g.
geromorphism
Gerson therapy
Gerstmann-Sträussler-Scheinker
G.-S.-S. disease
G.-S.-S. syndrome
Gerstmann-Sträussler syndrome
Gerstmann syndrome
Gesell Developmental Scale
GE-Signa
gestational polyneuropathy
gestes antagonistes
gestural automatism
GFAP
glial fibrillary acidic protein
GFAP activation
GFAP fiber density
GFAP-stained process
GFP
global field power
GFX II balloon and stent system
GG
geniculate ganglion
G_{M1} ganglioside
G_{M2} gangliosidosis
Ghajar guide
ghost
g. image
I/Q imbalance g.
GHRH
growth hormone-releasing hormone
GHRIF
growth hormone-release inhibiting factor
GI
Imagent GI
Giacomini
band of G.
frenulum of G.
uncus band of G.
giant
g. axon
g. axonal neuropathy
g. cell arteritis (GCA)
g. cell astrocytoma
g. cell glioblastoma
g. cell glioblastoma multiforme
g. cell granuloma
g. cell granulomatous hypophysitis
g. cell monstrocellular sarcoma of Zülch
g. cell tumor
g. cervical carotid artery aneurysm
g. Dopamine-containing cell (GDC)
g. glomus tumor
g. motor unit action potential
g. neuron
g. petroclival hemangiopericytoma
g. pituitary adenoma
g. pituitary tumor
g. pyramidal Betz cell

g. sacral perineural cyst
g. tortuous basilar artery
g. urticaria
giant-cell
Gianturco-Roubin II stent
gibberish aphasia
Gibbs
G. artifact
G. phenomenon
G. ring
GID
giddy headache
Giemsa banding
Gierke
G. cell
G. respiratory bundle
Giessing syndrome
Gifford reflex
gigans
urticaria g.
gigantea
urticaria g.
gigantism
cerebral g.
gigantocellular
g. glioma
g. nucleus of medulla oblongata
gigantocellularis
nucleus reticularis intermedius g.
Gigli
G. guide
G. saw
Gildenberg forceps
gill
G. laminectomy
G. procedure
G. Thomas locator
g. withdrawal reflex
Gilles
G. de la Tourette
G. de la Tourette disease
G. de la Tourette syndrome
Gilliat-Summer nerve-damaged hand
ginger paralysis
gingival hyperplasia
girdle
Ace halo pelvic g.
g. anesthesia
Hitzig g.
g. pain
g. sensation
Girdlestone laminectomy
githagism
gitter cell
gitterzelle
GKRS
gamma knife radiosurgery
glabella
glabella-inion
g.-i. line
g.-i. line landmark
glabellar
anterior fossa skull base g.
g. approach
g. exposure osteotomy
g. reflex
g. tap
glabrous skin
gland
adrenal g.
apocrine g.
Bartholin g.
basal g.
eccrine g.
ectopic pituitary g.
endocrine g.
hemal g.
lacrimal g.
master g.
neural lobe of pituitary g.
pacchionian g.
parathyroid g.
pineal g.
pituitary g.
posterior lobe of pituitary g.
salivary g.
thyroid g.
von Ebner g.
glandula, pl. **glandulae**
g. basilaris
g. pinealis
g. pituitaria
glandular lobe of hypophysis
Glanzmann disease
glare of light
Glaser automatic laminectomy retractor
Glasflex material
Glasgow
G. Assessment Schedule
G. Coma Score (GCS)
G. Outcome Scale
G. Outcome Score (GOS)

NOTES

Glasscock triangle
glassy eye
glatirama copolymer-1
glatiramer
g. acetate
g. copolymer-1
glaucoma
chronic angle-closure g.
low tension g.
low-tension g.
subacute angle closure g.
glaucus
Aspergillus g.
Glees
method of G.
glia
Bergman g.
fibrillary g.
g. limitans
g. limitans externa
radial g.
g. scar
gliacyte
Gliadel
G. implant
G. wafer
G. wafer treatment protocol
gliae
membrana limitans g.
glial
g. cell
g. cell line-derived
g. cell line-derived neurotrophic factor
g. cell maturation
g. disease
g. fibrillary acidic protein (GFAP)
g. fibrillary acidic protein activation activation
g. filament
g. limiting membrane
g. line-derived neurotrophic factor
g. metabolism
Müller g.
g. neuronal interaction
g. nodule
g. parenchymal cyst
g. reaction
g. scarring
g. tumor
g. tumorigenesis
glial-derived neurotrophic factor (GDNF)
glial-specific marker
GliaSite radiation therapy system
gliding contusion
glioblast
glioblastoma
cerebral g.
giant cell g.
g. multiforme (GBM)
occipital g.
g. xenograft
glioblastosis cerebri
gliocyte
gliocytoma
gliofibrillary
glioma
anaplastic g.
g. angiogenesis
biologically quiescent g.
brainstem g.
butterfly-type g.
cerebral g.
g. chemotherapy
chiasmatic g.
childhood optic g.
diencephalic g.
diffuse pontine g.
dorsal midbrain g.
endothelial cell-stimulating g.
exophytic brainstem g.
familial g.
ganglionic g.
gigantocellular g.
high-grade g.
hypothalamic g.
hypothalamic/chiasmatic g.
intracranial g.
low-grade g. (LGG)
malignant g.
medullary g.
mixed g.
multifocal g.
nasal g.
non-aplastic g.
g. of optic chiasm
optic nerve g.
optic pathway g.
pediatric brain stem g.
periaqueductal g.
peripheral g.
pontine g.
radiation-induced g.
rolandoparietal g.
g. of the spinal cord
subependymal mixed g.
supratentorial g.
tectal g.
tegmental g.
telangiectatic g.
g. telangiectodes
thalamic g.
glioma-polyposis syndrome

gliomatosis
arachnoidal g.
g. cerebri
leptomeningeal g.
meningeal g.
gliomatous
gliomyxoma
glioneuroma
glioneuronal element
gliophagia
gliopil
gliosarcoma
cerebellar g.
gliosis
g. of aqueduct
aqueductal g.
astrocytic g.
Chaslin g.
hemispheric g.
hemosiderin reactional g.
hypertrophic nodular g.
isomorphous g.
perivascular g.
piloid g.
progressive subcortical g.
reactive g.
unilateral g.
gliosome
glissando
glistening degeneration
glitter cell
global
g. AIMS score
g. amnesia
g. amnestic disorder
g. ANOVA
g. anterograde memory disorder
g. aphasia
g. assessment of sensory disturbance
g. brain lactate
G. Burden of Disease Study
g. cerebral ischemia
g. change
g. clinical impression score
g. clinician-rated scale
g. cognitive dysfunction
g. cognitive impairment
g. dementia
g. dementia rating scale
G. Deterioration Scale (GDS)
g. distress index
g. field power (GFP)
g. function
g. functioning
g. gene replacement therapy
g. ischemic neuronal injury
g. measure
g. measure of impairment
g. metabolism
g. outcome
g. paralysis
G. Tic Rating score
G. Utilization of Streptokinase and t-PA for Occluded Coronary Arteries (GUSTO-1)
g. vertebral blood flow (gCBF)
g. well-being
globi (*pl. of* globus)
globoid
g. cell
g. cell leukodystrophy
globose
g. cell
g. nucleus
globosus
nucleus g.
globule
Marchi g.
globulin
alpha2 g.
gamma g.
homologous tetanus immune g. (HTIG)
human tetanus immune g.
intravenous gamma g.
intravenous immune g.
sex hormone-binding g. (SHBG)
testosterone-estradiol-binding g.
zoster immune g.
globus, pl. **globi**
g. epilepticus
g. hystericus
g. pallidus
g. pallidus externa
g. pallidus external segment
g. pallidus interna
g. pallidus internalis (GPi)
g. pallidus internal segment
g. pallidus internus (GPi)
g. pallidus lateralis
g. pallidus medialis

NOTES

glome
glomectomy
glomera (*pl. of* glomus)
glomerular layer of olfactory bulb
glomerule
glomerulus, pl. **glomeruli**
nonencapsulated nerve g.
olfactory g.
stereoselective g.
synaptic g.
glomus, pl. **glomera**
g. aorticum
g. arteriovenous malformation
g. body
choroid g.
g. choroideum
intravagal g.
g. intravagale
jugular g.
g. jugulare
g. jugulare tumor
g. jugulotympanicum
g. pulmonale
pulmonary g.
g. tympanicum
g. vagale
g. vagale tumor
glossectomy
reduction g.
glossocinesthetic (*var. of* glossokinesthetic)
glossodontotropism
glossodyniotropism
glossokinesthetic, glossocinesthetic
g. center
glossokinetic
g. artifact
g. potential
glossolabiolaryngeal paralysis
glossolabiopharyngeal paralysis
glossolysis
glossopalatolabial paralysis
glossopharyngeal
g. cranial nerve [CN IX]
g. nerve examination
g. nerve jugular ganglion
g. nerve lower ganglion
g. nerve paralysis
g. nerve rostral ganglion
g. neuralgia (GPN)
g. neuropathy
g. tic
glossopharyngei
ganglion inferius nervi g.
ganglion rostralis nervi g.
ganglion superius nervi g.
nucleus nervi g.
rami linguales nervi g.
rami pharyngeal nervi g.
rami tonsillares nervi g.
ramus musculi stylopharyngei nervi g.
ramus sinus carotici nervi g.
glossopharyngeo
ramus communicans cum nervo g.
ramus communicans nervi facialis cum nervo g.
ramus communicans nervi vagi cum nervo g.
glossopharyngeolabial paralysis
glossopharyngeus
nervus g. [CN IX]
glossoplegia
glossoproptosis
glossospasm
glossotomy
labiomandibular g.
glossy skin
glottidospasm
glottis
glove
g. anesthesia
Biogel Sensor surgical g.
glubionate
calcium g.
glucagon
glucepate
technetium 99m g.
gluceptate
calcium g.
gluciphore
glucocerebrosidase
glucocorticoid
hypothalamic g.
glucocorticoid-induced
g.-i. bone loss
g.-i. osteoporosis
glucogenesis
glucomineralocorticoid
gluconate
calcium g.
clorhexidine g.
magnesium g.
potassium chloride and potassium g.
potassium citrate and potassium g.
glucophore
glucose
g. blood level
cerebral metabolic rate of g. (CMRglc)
cerebrospinal fluid g.
g. concentration
g. metabolism

g. metabolism in the brain
preischemic blood g.
g. transport
g. transporter molecule
glucose-6-phosphate transport system
glucose-6-phosphatase
glucosephosphate isomerase
glucosylsphingosine accumulation
glucuroconjugation
glucuronic acid
glucuronidase
beta g.
g. deficiency
glucuronidation
glucuronide
glue
acrylic g.
autologous fibrin sealant g.
cyanoacrylate g.
fibrin g.
Histoacryl g.
Gluge corpuscle
GluR1
glutamate receptor 1
Glu-receptor antagonist
glutamate
g. decarboxylase
g. excitation
g. excitotoxicity
g. metabolism
metabotropic g.
monosodium g.
g. neurotoxicity
g. plus glutamine
g. receptor
g. receptor 1 (GluR1)
g. receptor antagonist
g. receptor-mediated neurodegeneration
g. receptor subtype
g. toxicity
g. transporter
g. transport velocity
glutamate-containing neuron
glutamate-gated NMDA receptor channel
glutamate-mediated excitatory synaptic transmission
glutamatergic
g. excitotoxicity
g. hypoactivity
g. neuron
g. neurotransmission
g. pathway
g. response
g. synaptic transmission
glutamergic mechanism
glutamic acid decarboxylase
glutamide receptor subunit
glutamine
g. decarboxylase (GAD)
glutamate plus g.
glutamyl
g. cysteine synthetase deficiency
g. ribose-5-phosphate storage disease
g. transaminase
glutaraldehyde
glutaric
g. acid
g. aciduria type I, II
glutaryl-CoA dehydrogenase
glutathione (GSH)
g. peroxidase
g. persuades (GSHPx)
g. synthetase
g. synthetase deficiency
gluteal
g. gait
g. nerve
g. reflex
gluten ataxia
glutethimide group
gluteus medius gait
glycerol
g. chemoneurolysis
g. kinase deficiency
g. rhizotomy
g. test
glyceryl trinitrate
glycinate
aluminum g.
glycine
ketotic g.
nonketotic g.
g. supplementation
glycogen
g. debrancher deficiency
g. storage disease
glycogenosis (type I–VII)
glycogeusia
glycolipid

NOTES

G

glycolysis
glycoprotein
g. B (gB)
carbohydrate-deficient g.
g. degradation disorder
integral membrane g.
membrane-bound g.
myelin-associated g. (MAG)
myelin oligodendrocyte g. (MOG)
myelin/oligodendrocyte g.
p170 g.
platelet g. IIb/IIIa
g. storage disorder
variant surface g. (VSG)
glycoproteinosis
glycoprotein-secreting adenoma
glycopyrrolate
glycorrhachia
glycosaminoglycan (GAG)
glycoside
cardiac g.
glycosphingolipid metabolic defect
glycosuria
familial g.
glycosylase
glycosylation pattern
glycyl
GM
gray matter
Occip GM
occipital gray matter
GM-CSF
granulocyte-macrophage colony-stimulating factor immunogene therapy
GMFM
Gross Motor Function Measure
gnash
gnashing
gnathic
Gnathostoma
gnathostomiasis
gNomos
g. head frame
g. stereotactic system
gnosia
GnRH
gonadotropin-releasing hormone
Godtfredsen syndrome
Goebel syndrome
Golay gradient coil
Golda reflex
Goldberg-Shprintzen syndrome
Goldenhar-Gorlin syndrome
Goldenhar syndrome
Goldflam disease
Goldflam-Erb disease
Goldman
G. constant field equation
G. perimetry
Goldmann-Offner reference of electrode
Goldmann visual field
gold-myokymia syndrome
gold peripheral neuropathy
Goldscheider test
Goldstein
G. spinal fusion
G. toe sign
Goldthwait sign
Goldvalve detachable latex balloon
golf-stick dissector
Golgi
G. body
G. corpuscle
G. epithelial cell
G. reflex
G. side fibril
G. staining
G. system
G. tendon organ (GTO)
G. theory
G. type I, II neuron
vesiculation of the G.
Golgi-Mazzoni corpuscle
Goliath syndrome
Goll
G. column
G. column nucleus
G. fiber
nucleus of G.
tract of G.
Gombault
G. degeneration
G. neuritis
G. triangle
Gombault-Philippe triangle
gomitoli
Gomori
G. trichome stain
G. trichrome
gonadotroph cell
gonadotropin
beta-human chorionic g.
beta-subunit of human chorionic g. (beta-HCG)
chorionic g.
human chorionic g. (hCG)
gonadotropin-producing adenoma
gonadotropin-releasing hormone (GnRH, GRH)
gondii
Toxoplasma g.
gonioscopy
gonyalgia paresthetica

Goody's Body Pain
gooseberry gene
goosecoid gene
gooseneck rongeur
Gordon
G. Diagnostic System
G. reflex
G. sign
G. and Sweet silver reticulin stain
G. symptom
Gorlin
G. sign
G. syndrome
GOS
Glasgow Outcome Score
Gosling
G. pulsatility
G. pulsatility index
"go slow" approach
Gottfries-Brane-Steen Rating Scale for Dementia
Gottron sign
gotu kola
gouge
AO g.
Flanagan spinal fusion g.
Hibbs spinal fusion g.
Hoen lamina g.
Killian g.
spinal fusion g.
Goulet retractor
gout
tophaceous g.
gouty arthritis
Gowers
G. bundle
G. bundle in cerebellum
G. column
G. disease
G. fasciculus
G. maneuver
G. muscular dystrophy
G. phenomenon
G. sign
G. syndrome
G. tract
gown restriction
***gox* gene**
GPCR
G-protein-coupled receptor
GPi
globus pallidus internalis
globus pallidus internus
GPN
glossopharyngeal neuralgia
G-protein-coupled receptor (GPCR)
G-protein coupling
Gracely Pain Scale
gracile
g. fasciculus
g. fasciculus of medulla oblongata
g. fasciculus of spinal cord
g. lobule
g. nucleus
g. spinal fiber
g. tubercle
tuberculum g.
gracilis
fasciculus g.
funiculus g.
lobulus g.
nucleus fasciculi g.
nucleus funiculi g.
tubercle of nucleus g.
tuberculum nuclei g.
gracilispinales
fibrae g.
grade
Fischer g.
Gardner-Robertson hearing g.
Hunt and Hess g. I–III
g. I–IV astrocytoma
g. IV spondylolisthesis
MRI g.
Simpson G.
Spetzler-Martin g.
Gradenigo syndrome
gradient
g. amplifier
bipolar g.
g. coil
g. compensation
field g.
frequency-encoding g.
magnetic field g.
g. magnetic field
g. moment
g. moment nulling
net electrochemical potential g.
phase-encoding g.
pulsed g.

NOTES

G

gradient *(continued)*
readout g.
g. recalled echo
g. recalled echo technique
rephasing g.
rewinder g.
Ribot g.
slice-select encoding g.
g. slope
steep-dose g.
transmantle pressure g.
x g.
y g.
gradient-echo
g.-e. echo planar image
g.-e. magnetic resonance image
g.-e. MR image
g.-e. MR imaging
gradient-recalled
g.-r. acquisition in the steady state (GRASS)
g.-r. echo image
gradient-refocused
g.-r. imaging
g.-r. sequence
grading
De Monte g.
Fisher g.
Hirsch g.
Kernohan g.
Simpson g.
gradiometer
axial g.
Graefe
G. disease
G. sign
G. spot
graft
acellular human dermal g.
adipose g.
adrenal medulla g.
aortobifemoral bypass g.
autochthonous g.
autogenous bone g.
autologous fat g.
barrel staved g.
bone g.
bovine percardium dural g.
bypass g.
cable g.
carotid-vertebral vein bypass g.
circumferentially aortofemoral g.
clip g.
cranial bone g.
dural g.
fascicular g.
fat-patch g.
funicular g.
greater auricular nerve g.
Hemashield enhanced g.
human dural substitute g.
hydroxyapatite g.
interbody g.
interfascicular g.
intracranial-extracranial nerve g.
intracranial-intratemporal nerve g.
Keystone g.
g. material alternative
g. migration
nerve g.
petrous carotid-to-intradural carotid saphenous vein g.
posterior bone g.
posterolateral bone g.
radial artery g.
rib g.
roof-patch g.
saphenous vein bypass g.
saphenous vein patch g.
g. site
in situ tricortical iliac-crest block bone g.
skull bone g.
sleeve g.
split calvarial g.
split-thickness calvarial g.
strut g.
sural nerve bridge g.
sural nerve cable g.
Teflon tube g.
temporosuboccipital bone g.
tricortical iliac crest bone g.
Unilab Surgibone bovine bone g.
vascular patch g.
xenogeneic g.
grafting
allograft bone g.
g. anastomosis
autograft bone g.
bone g.
coronary artery bypass g.
fetal mesencephalic g.
fibular g.
hypophysial g.
posterolateral bone g.
strut g.
Grafton demineralized bone matrix
graft-versus-host disease (GVHD)
gram-negative
g.-n. bacillary meningitis
g.-n. bacillus
g.-n. endotoxin
Gram stain

grand
g. mal
g. mal epilepsy
g. mal seizure
grandmother cell
Granit loop
granular
g. cell myoblastoma
g. cell tumor
g. degeneration
g. ependymitis
g. layer
g. layer of cerebellar cortex
g. layer of cerebellum
g. layer of cerebral cortex
g. layer of retina
g. neuron
granulare
stratum g.
granularis
ependymitis g.
granulatio, pl. **granulationes**
granulationes arachnoideae
granulationes arachnoideales
granulation
arachnoid g.
arachnoidal g.
pacchionian g.
Virchow g.
granule
azurophilic g.
Birbeck g.
calcareous g.
g. cell
g. cell axon
g. cell proliferation
chromatic g.
chromophil g.
Crooke g.
lipofuscin g.
meningeal g.
Nissl g.
granulocyte
granulocyte-macrophage
g.-m. colony-stimulating factor
g.-m. colony-stimulating factor immunogene therapy (GM-CSF)
granulocytic
g. brain edema
g. sarcoma
granuloma
caseating g.
cholesterol g.
g. cryptococcal
eosinophilic g.
foreign body g.
Gagel g.
giant cell g.
intrasellar g.
lethal midline g.
parenchymal g.
petroclival cholesterol g.
granulomatosis
eosinophilic g.
Langerhans cell g.
lymphomatoid g.
Wegener g. (WG)
granulomatous
g. angiitis
g. angiitis of the central nervous system
g. angiitis of the CNS
g. arteritis
g. encephalitis
g. encephalomyelitis
g. hypophysitis
granulovacuolar degeneration
grape ending
graphanesthesia
graphesthesia
graphic
g. aphasia
g. impairment
g. violence
graphomotor
g. aphasia
g. control
g. skill
graphospasm
Grashey aphasia
grasp
g. channel
g. reflex
grasper
lion's claw g.
lion's paw g.
grasping reflex
GRASS
gradient-recalled acquisition in the steady state
2DFT G.

G

NOTES

GRASS *(continued)*
3DFT G.
sequential G.
Grasset
G. law
G. phenomenon
G. sign
Grasset-Bychowski sign
Grasset-Gaussel-Hoover sign
Grasset-Gaussel phenomenon
Grass stimulator S-44
gratifying work
grating
flicker frequency g.
sensorimotor g.
spatial frequency g.
Gratiolet
G. radiating fiber
G. radiation
gratitude
Graves
G. disease
G. ophthalmopathy
gravidarum
chorea g.
tetania g.
gravior
epilepsia g.
gravireceptors
gravis
adult-onset myasthenia g.
congenital myasthenia g.
juvenile myasthenia g.
myasthenia g. (MG)
neonatal myasthenia g.
neurasthenia g.
penicillamine-induced myasthenia g.
seronegative myasthenia g.
transient neonatal myasthenia g.
gravitational device
Gravol
gray (Gy)
g. baby syndrome
central g.
g. column
g. commissure
g. degeneration
dorsal central g.
g. fiber
g. layer of superior colliculus
g. matter (GM)
g. matter area
g. matter lactate
g. matter lactate level
g. matter region
g. matter tissue
periaqueductal central g.
periventricular g. (PVG)
g. ramus
g. substance
g. tuber
g. tubercle
G. type I, II synapse
g. wing
gray-matter necrosis
gray/white
g./w. matter difference
g./w. matter junction
great
g. anterior medullary artery
g. cerebral vein
g. cerebral vein of Galen
g. cerebral vein of Galen aneurysm
g. cistern
g. foramen
g. horizontal fissure
g. longitudinal fissure
g. toe reflex
g. transverse fissure of cerebrum
greater
g. auricular nerve graft
g. occipital nerve
g. rhomboid muscle
g. sciatic foramen
g. superficial petrosal nerve (GSPN)
Greenberg
G. retracting system
G. retractor
G. retractor frame
G. retractor set
Greenberg-Sugita
G.-S. retractor
G.-S. retractor grid
Greenberg-type bar
Greenfield
G. classification of spinocerebellar ataxia
G. disease
Greenwood bipolar and suction forceps
Greig
G. cephalopolysyndactyly
G. cephalopolysyndactyly syndrome
Grenoble stereotactic robot
GRH
gonadotropin-releasing hormone
grid
Greenberg-Sugita retractor g.
subdural g.
Griesinger sign
***GRIK1* gene**
grip
milkmaid's g.

pincer g.
syringe g.
grippe aurique
grip-strength test
grisea
commissura anterior g.
commissura posterior g.
substantia g.
griseae
columnae g.
griseofulvin peripheral neuropathy
griseum
indusium g.
groaning
nocturnal g.
Grocott stain
groove
anterior intermediate g.
anterolateral g.
anteromedian g.
arterial g.
frontal g.
meningioma of the olfactory g.
neural g.
occipital g.
olfactory g.
parasagittal g.
pontomedullary g.
posterior intermediate g.
posterolateral g.
retroolivary g.
sagittal g.
vascular g.
gross
g. medical error
G. Motor Function Measure (GMFM)
g. pathological feature
g. total resection
ground
g. bundle
g. electrode
group
g. A beta-hemolytic streptococcus
amygdala nucleus g.
g. analysis
AO g.
Brain Tumor Study G. (BTSG)
g. B streptococcus
buzz g.
galenic draining g.
glutethimide g.
neurogenic fiber type g.
osmophore g.
Parkinson Study G. (PSG)
pedunculopontine cholinergic g.
petrosal draining g.
Pittsburgh gamma knife g.
polyarteritis nodosa g.
primary g.
sapophore g.
Surgical Interbody Research G.
Swedish gamma knife g.
tentorial draining g.
transversospinalis muscle g.
UK Parkinson Disease Research G.
ventral respiratory g.
grouped discharge
grouping
clavus clinical g.
gastrointestinal symptom g.
pseudoneurological symptom g.
growing skull fracture
growth
g. arrest-specific gene
axonal g.
g. cone
g. factor inhibitor
g. fraction
g. hormone deficiency
g. hormone-producing adenoma
g. hormone-release inhibiting factor (GHRIF)
g. hormone-releasing hormone (GHRH)
g. hormone-secreting adenoma
meningioma g.
neurite g.
olfactory axonal g.
growth-associated protein
growth-hormone-secreting
g.-h.-s. pituitary
g.-h.-s. tumor
growth-inhibiting molecule
growth-promoting molecule
Gruber ligament
Gruca-Weiss spring
Gruenwald
G. ear forceps
G. neurosurgical rongeur
gryochrome

NOTES

GSA
general somatic afferent
***gsc* gene**
GSH
glutathione
GSHPx
glutathione persuades
GSNO
exogenous nitric oxide
GSPN
greater superficial petrosal nerve
GSR
galvanic skin reflex
galvanic skin resistance
galvanic skin response
GTC
generalized tonic-clonic
GTC convulsion
GTCS
generalized tonic-clonic seizure
GTO
Golgi tendon organ
GTP
guanosine triphosphate
Guam parkinsonism-dementia complex
guanethidine sulfate
guanfacine
guanidine
guanine/cytosine ratio
guanine nucleotide
guanophore
guanosine
g. diphosphate
g. monophosphate
g. triphosphate (GTP)
guanylate cyclase
guanylyl cyclase
guard
depth g.
Midas Rex bur g.
snore g.
UltraPower bur g.
guarded tripole
Gubler
G. hemiplegia
G. line
G. paralysis
G. syndrome
Gudden
G. atrophy
G. commissure
G. ganglion
G. tegmental nucleus
Guglielmi detachable coil (GDC)
guidance
axon g.
Brown-Roberts-Wells computerized tomography stereotactic g.
electrophysiological g.
fluoroscopic image g.
image g.
real-time g.
StealthStation system real-time g.
stereotactic g.
ultrasonographic g.
guide
Adson dural protector g.
AdTech electrode g.
AO stopped-drill g.
contoured anterior spinal plate drill g.
Cook stereotactic g.
Cushing saw g.
Davis saw g.
drill g.
Frazier dural g.
Ghajar g.
Gigli g.
Hall-Dundar drill g.
hydrophilic g.
medication g.
Navigus trajectory g.
NeuraGen nerve g.
nut alignment g.
stereotactic g.
g. wire
Yasargil ligature g.
guide-catheter
guidepin, guide pin
guidewire, guide wire
Choice PT g.
delivery g.
J-tipped g.
Platinum-Plus g.
Radifocus g.
Guillain-Barré
G.-B. polyneuritis
G.-B. postinfection peripheral neuropathy
G.-B. reflex
G.-B. syndrome
Guillain-Barré-Strohl syndrome
Guillain-Garcin syndrome
Guillain-Mollaret triangle
Guilland sign
Guinon disease
Guiot-Talairach construct
gullwing pattern
gumma
cerebral g.
gun
Omni clip g.

Gunn
Marcus G.
G. phenomenon
G. sign
G. syndrome
gustation
gustatoria
anosmia g.
gemma g.
gustatorium
organum g.
gustatorius
porus g.
gustatory
g. anesthesia
g. audition
g. aura
g. bud
g. cell
g. cortex
g. hallucination
g. hyperesthesia
g. lemniscus
g. nucleus
g. organ
g. pathway
g. pore
g. receiving area
g. receptor
g. sweating syndrome
gustatory-sudorific reflex
GUSTO-1
Global Utilization of Streptokinase and t-PA for Occluded Coronary Arteries
gustolacrimal reflex
gustometer
gustometry
gustus
organum g.
Guthrie test
gutter fracture
gutturotetany
Guyon canal
GVA
general visceral afferent
GVHD
graft-versus-host disease
Gy
gray
gynecophonous
gynergon
gynesic
gyral
g. atrophy
g. infarction
Gyralor superficial atrophy
gyrectomy
frontal g.
gyrencephalic
gyri (*pl. of* gyrus)
gyriform intracranial calcification
gyrochrome cell
gyromagnetic ratio
gyrometer
gyrosa
Gyroscan
gyrose
gyrospasm
gyrus, pl. **gyri**
angular g.
g. angularis
annectent g.
anterior central g.
anterior cingulate g.
anterior paracentral g.
anterior piriform g.
anterior transverse temporal g.
ascending frontal g.
ascending parietal g.
gyri breves insula
Broca g.
callosal g.
central g.
cerebral g.
gyri cerebri
gyri of cerebrum
cingulate g.
g. cinguli
contiguous supramarginal g.
deep transitional g.
dentate g.
g. dentatus
fasciolar g.
g. fasciolaris
first temporal g.
flattening of g.
fornicate g.
g. fornicatus
frontal g.
g. frontalis inferior
g. frontalis medialis
g. frontalis medius

G

NOTES

gyrus *(continued)*
g. frontalis superior
fusiform g.
g. fusiformis
g. geniculi
Heschl g.
hippocampal dentate g.
g. hippocampus
inferior frontal g.
inferior occipital g.
inferior parietal g.
inferior temporal g.
infracalcarine g.
insular g.
interlocking g.
intralimbic g.
isthmus of cingular g.
isthmus of cingulate g.
lamination of g.
lateral occipitotemporal g.
lateral olfactory g.
layer of dentate g.
lingual g.
g. lingualis
g. longus insula
marginal g.
medial frontal g.
medial occipitotemporal g.
medial olfactory g.
middle frontal g.
middle occipital g.
middle temporal g.
occipital g.
g. occipitotemporalis lateralis
g. occipitotemporalis medialis
g. olfactorius lateralis
g. olfactorius medialis
olfactory g.
gyri orbitales
orbital part of inferior frontal g.
paracentral g.
g. paracentralis
g. paracentralis anterior
g. paracentralis posterior
parahippocampal g.
g. parahippocampalis
paraterminal g.
g. paraterminalis
parietal g.
postcentral g.
g. postcentralis
posterior central g.
posterior cingulate g.
posterior fusiform g.
posterior paracentral g.
posterior transverse temporal g.
precentral g.
g. precentralis
preinsular g.
prepiriform g.
quadrate g.
g. rectus
Retzius g.
short insular g.
splenial g.
straight g.
subcallosal g.
g. subcallosus
subcollateral g.
superior frontal g.
superior occipital g.
superior parietal g.
superior temporal lobe g.
supracallosal g.
supramarginal g.
g. supramarginalis
tail of dentate g.
temporal g.
gyri temporales transversi
g. temporalis inferior
g. temporalis medius
g. temporalis superior
g. temporalis transversalis posterior
g. temporalis transversus anterior
g. temporalis transversus posterior habena
transitional g.
g. transitivi cerebri
transverse temporal g.
Turner marginal g.
uncal g.
uncinate g.
vein of olfactory g.

H
H field
H reflex
H response
H wave
H zone
H2
nuclei areae H, H1, H2
HAART
highly active antiretroviral therapy
habena, pl. **habenae**
gyrus temporalis transversus posterior h.
habenula, pl. **habenulae**
ganglion h.
nuclei habenulae
nucleus h.
habenulae perforatae
pineal h.
sulcus h.
trigone of h.
trigonum h.
habenular
h. body
h. commissure
h. nucleus
h. sulcus
h. trigone
habenularis
sulcus h.
habenularum
commissura h.
habenulointerpeduncularis
tractus h.
habenulointerpeduncular tract
habenulopeduncularis
tractus h.
habenulopeduncular tract
habenulothalamic tract
habit
h. chorea
h. cough
h. reversal training
h. spasm
h. tic
habitual seizure
habitus
h. apoplecticus
marfanoid h.
habromania
Hachinski
H. Ischemic Scale
H. ischemic score
hack
Hacker procedure
Haddad syndrome
Haeckel law
Haemophilus
H. aerophilus
H. influenzae
H. influenzae b
H. influenzae meningitis
H. parainfluenzae
Haenel symptom
Hageman factor
Hagen-Poiseuille law
Haglund disease
Hague Seizure Severity Scale
Hahn
H. echo
H. sign
Haid universal bone plate system
Haight-Finochietto rib spreader
Haight rib spreader
hair
auditory h.
h. cell
h. follicle
h. follicle receptor
Frey irritation h.
h. lead level
h. loss
olfactory h.
sensory h.
taste h.
von Frey h.
h. whorl pattern
hairline fracture
Hajdu-Cheney syndrome
Hajek
H. chisel
H. laminectomy punch
H. mallet
Hajek-Ballenger
H.-B. dissector
H.-B. septal elevator
Hajek-Koffler
H.-K. bone punch forceps
H.-K. laminectomy rongeur
H.-K. punch
Håkanson technique
Hakim
H. high-pressure valve
H. precision valve
H. programmable valve system
H. syndrome
Hakin-Cortis ventriculoperitoneal shunt

Hakuba
medial triangle of H.
Halcion
Haldol
half-and-half exposure
half base syndrome
half-Fourier imaging
half-life
drug h.-l.
half-NEX imaging
Halifax
H. clamp posterior cervical fixation
H. interlaminar clamp
H. interlaminar clamp system
Hall
H. neurosurgical craniotome
H. Osteon drill system kit
H. Osteon irrigation kit
H. Surgairtome II drill
H. UltraPower drill
H. Versipower drill
Hall-Dundar drill guide
Halle
H. bone curette
H. dura knife
H. nasal speculum
Haller
H. ansa
H. circle
H. line
H. unguis
halleri
circulus arteriosus h.
circulus venosus h.
Hallermann-Streiff syndrome
Hallervorden-Spatz
H.-S. disease
H.-S. syndrome
Hallervorden syndrome
Hallpike
H. maneuver
H. test
Hallpike-Bárány positioning maneuver
hallucal abnormality
hallucinated voice
hallucination
auditory h.
daytime h.
depressive auditory h.
depressive olfactory h.
depressive visual h.
drug-induced h.
fleeting auditory h.
fleeting visual h.
formed visual h.
gustatory h.
haptic h.
hypnagogic h.
hypnopompic h.
kaleidoscope h.
kinesthesia h.
lilliputian h.
nocturnal h.
nonpsychotic h.
olfactory h.
overt h.
palinoptic h.
running commentary h.
simple h.
sleep h.
speech h.
stump h.
tactile h.
third-person auditory h.
visual h.
hallucinative
hallucinatory
h. neuralgia
h. transient organic syndrome
hallucinogen
sedative h.
hallucinogenic hallucinosis
hallucinogen-induced
hallucinosis
hallucinogenic h.
peduncular h.
hallucinotic
halo
Ace low profile MR h.
Ace Mark III h.
h. apparatus
h. brace
Bremer h.
Brown-Roberts-Wells head ring h.
Houston h.
hypoechogenic peritumoral h.
h. phenomenon
Philadelphia h.
pulsating visual h.
h. retractor system
h. ring
Surgairtome II drill h.
h. vest
haloperidol condition
halo-ring adapter
Halotestin
halothane anesthesia
halo-vest immobilization
Halperon
Halstead modified technique
Halstead-Wepman Aphasia Screening Test

Halsted
H. artery forceps
H. mosquito forceps
HAMA
human antimouse antibody
hamartin
hamartoma
cortical h.
eccrine angiomatous h.
hypothalamic h.
subependymal h.
h. of the tuber cinereum
vascular h.
ventromedial hypothalamic h.
hamartomatosis
congenital h.
hamartomatous lipoma
hammer
Babinski percussion h.
Berliner percussion h.
Buck neurological h.
Buck percussion h.
Davis percussion h.
Dejerine-Davis percussion h.
Dejerine percussion h.
Epstein neurological h.
Küntscher h.
Monreal reflex h.
neurological h.
percussion h.
Rabiner neurological h.
slotted h.
Taylor percussion h.
Trömner percussion h.
Hammill Multiability Achievement Test
hammock bandage
Hammond disease
hamster cell
HAM/TSP
human T-cell lymphotropic virus type 1-associated myelopathy/tropical spastic paraparesis
hand
accoucheur's h.
all-median nerve h.
all-ulnar nerve h.
ape h.
h. ataxia
benediction h.
contralesional h.
dead h.
h. deformity
drop h.
H. Dynamometer Test
Gilliat-Summer nerve-damaged h.
h. grasp reflex
Marinesco succulent h.
mechanic's h.
h. nondominant
h. nondominant handedness
obstetric h.
obstetrical h.
h. palmar crease
phantom h.
preacher's h.
simian h.
striatal h.
H. Test, Revised 1983
upper h.
writing h.
handcuff neuropathy
handedness
hand nondominant h.
handgrip task
Handicapped
Developmental Assessment of the Severely H.
Handicaps
International Classification of Impairments, Disabilities and H. (ICIDH)
handle
bayonet h.
Cloward double-hinge cervical retractor h.
Hardy lateral knife h.
handpiece
CUSA system 200 straight autoclavable h.
Hand-Schüller-Christian disease
hand-shoulder syndrome
HANE
hereditary angioneurotic edema
hanging-drop equilibration
hangman's fracture
hangover
daytime sleep h.
Hanks buffered saline solution
Hannover
H. classification
H. system
Hansen disease

NOTES

H

haphalgesia
haplotype analysis
haptic hallucination
haptometer
hard
h. chancre
h. disk herniation
h. palate dissection
h. tissue replacement (HTR)
h. tissue replacement-malleable facial implant
h. tissue replacement-patient-matched (HTR-PMI)
h. tissue replacement-patient-matched implant
Harding W87 Test
hardware
TiMesh h.
Hardy
H. approach
H. attachment
H. bayonet dressing forceps
H. bivalve speculum
H. curette
H. dissector
H. lateral knife handle
H. lip retractor
H. microsurgical bayonet bipolar forceps
H. microsurgical enucleator
H. 5 mm mirror
H. pituitary spoon
H. 3-prong fork
H. sella punch forceps
H. sellar punch
H. suction tube
Hardy-Rand-Rittler plate
Hare Psychopathy Checklist: Screening Version
Harken rib spreader
harkoseride
Harmon cervical approach
harmonic
h. error field
h. function
harmonious interaction
Harm posterior cervical plate
Harms technique
HAROLD
hemispheric asymmetry reduction in older adults
HARP
Harvard Atherosclerosis Reversibility Project
Harriluque
H. sublaminar wiring modification
H. technique
Harrington
H. distraction
H. pedicle hook
H. rod
H. rod fixation
H. rod and hook system
H. rod instrumentation
H. rod instrumentation compression
H. rod instrumentation distraction outrigger device
H. rod instrumentation failure
H. rod instrumentation force application
H. scissors
H. spreader
Harris
H. migraine
H. syndrome
Harris-Smith cervical fusion
Hartel
H. technique
H. treatment
Harting body
Hartley-Krause operation
Hartnup disease
Hartshill
H. Ransford loop
H. rectangle
H. rectangle rod
Harvard Atherosclerosis Reversibility Project (HARP)
Hasegawa Dementia Scale
hatchet facies
Hausa Speaking Test
Hauser ambulation index
haut mal epilepsy
Haverfield-Scoville hemilaminectomy retractor
haversian canal
Hawthorn effect
Hayem encephalitis
Haynes brain cannula
HBMEC
human brain microvascular endothelial cell
HBO
hyperbaric oxygen
HBO therapy
HBr
citalopram HBr
galantamine HBr
hCG
human chorionic gonadotropin
HCG-secreting suprasellar immature teratoma

HCHWA-D
hereditary cerebral hemorrhage with amyloidosis-Dutch type
HCl
hydrochloride
buprenorphine HCl
chlorpromazine HCl
dexmethylphenidate HCl
imipramine HCl
lazabemide HCl
maprotiline HCl
methadone HCl
methamphetamine HCl
methylphenidate HCl
molindone HCl
naltrexone HCl
naratriptan HCl
nortriptyline HCl
tacrine HCl
tiagabine HCl
ziprasidone HCl
HCN-1 cell line
HCP
hypertrophic chromic pachymeningitis
HCT, Hct
hematocrit
HD
Hunting disorder
Huntington chorea
HDL
high-density lipoprotein
HDSA
Huntington Disease Society of America
HDT
head-down tilt
head
H. area
h. of caudate nucleus
h. cavity
h. circumference measurement
h. clamp
h. coil
h. computed tomography
h. erythromelalgia
h. fixation device
h. frame
h. injury
H. line
h. movement
h. nodding in spasmus nutans
h. position in intracranial pressure increase
h. ring
h. tetanus
h. tilt
h. trauma
h. trauma effect
whole h.
H. zone
headache
alarm-clock h.
analgesic rebound h.
basilar artery migraine h.
benign exertional h.
Bickerstaff migraine h.
bifrontal h.
bilious h.
bioccipital h.
bitemporal h.
blind h.
cataclysmic h.
catamenial migraine h.
cervicogenic h.
cheese reaction h.
chronic cluster h.
ciliary migraine h.
classic brain tumor h.
cluster h. (CH)
coital h.
cold stimulus h.
combination h.
cough h.
h. differential diagnosis
disabling h.
dull unremitting h.
episodic cluster h.
episodic tension-type h. (ETTH)
essential h.
evening h.
h. exacerbation
exertional h.
facioplegic migraine h.
featureless h.
fibrositic h.
frontal h.
generalized h.
giddy h.
helmet h.
hemiparesthetic migraine h.
high-altitude h.
histaminic h.

NOTES

H

headache *(continued)*
Horton h.
hot dog h.
hyperemic h.
hypertension-related h.
hyperventilation h.
hypnic h.
hypoxia-related h.
ice cream h.
ice-pick h.
idiopathic stabbing h.
h., insomnia, and depression (HID)
intraventricular h. (IVH)
ipsilateral h.
leakage h.
lower-half h.
matutinal h.
medication-induced h.
metabolic h.
migraine h.
migraine-like h.
mixed h.
monosodium glutamate-induced h.
morning h.
muscle contraction h.
nitrite h.
nodular h.
nonmigrainous vascular h.
nonpulsating h.
occipital h.
organic h.
paroxysmal migraine h.
pectoralgic migraine h.
periictal h.
h. phenotype
phobia-induced migraine h.
postconcussion h.
postictal migrainous h.
post-lumbar puncture h.
posttraumatic h.
preictal h.
premonitory h.
primary h.
psychogenic h.
pulsating h.
pyrexial h.
radiation-injury h.
rapid eye movement sleep-locked h.
recurring h.
reflex h.
REM sleep-locked h.
retinal migraine h.
seasonal migraine h.
secondary h.
sex h.
sick h.
sinus h.
sleep-related h.
spinal puncture h.
spondylotic h.
suboccipital h.
sudden-onset h.
suicide h.
swim-goggle h.
Symonds h.
symptomatic h.
syncopal migraine h.
h. syndrome
temporal h.
tension-type h.
tension-vascular h.
throbbing h.
thunderclap h.
toxic h.
traumatic h.
triptan rebound h.
unilateral migraine h.
vacuum h.
vascular h.
vasodilator h.
vasomotor h.
vestibular migraine h.
violent onset h.
weekend h.
whole cranial h.
Willis h.
Wolff h.

head-bobbing doll syndrome

head-down tilt (HDT)

head-dropping test

headframe
Kannon h.
Sugita h.
thousand-hands Kannon universal h.

headholder
Caspar h.
Gardner h.
integrated h.
Malcolm-Rand carbon-composite h.
Mayfield-Kees h.
Mayfield radiolucent h.
Mayfield skull-pin h.
pin h.
pinion h.
radiolucent cranial pin h.
Sugita h.
three-point h.

headlamp
Keeler video h.

headlight
high beam fiberoptic h.
LightWear h.
Orascoptic fiberoptic h.

Quadrilite 6000 fiberoptic h.
QuietLite Quadrilite 6000 fiberoptic h.
headrest
Brown-Roberts-Wells h.
Gardner-Wells h.
horseshoe h.
Light-Veley h.
Mayfield horseshoe h.
Mayfield-Kees h.
Mayfield radiolucent h.
multipurpose h.
pediatric h.
pin fixation h.
3-point h.
Reston foam-padded h.
Veley h.
headset
Instatrak h.
heads-up
h.-u. adjunctive endoscopy
h.-u. imaging system
head-to-head clinical trial
head-up tilt testing
health
bone h.
H. and Daily Living
heart
irritable h.
h. murmur
h. reflex
h. rhythm
heartbeat potential
heat
h. defense
h. effect
h. effector
h. exhaustion
h. hyperplasia
h. loss
h. shock protein
h. stress
heat-defense response
heating
eddy current h.
radiofrequency h.
heat-loss
h.-l. apparatus
h.-l. mechanism
h.-l. pathway
heat-regulating center
heavy
h. meromyosin
h. metal intoxication
h. metal neuropathy
h. particle radiotherapy
heavy-duty straight clip
heavy-metal neuritis
hebbian potentiation of synapse
hebetis
hecateromeric
hecatomeral cell
hecatomeric
hederiform ending
hedgehog gene
heel
h. tap
h. walking
heel-knee-shin test
heel-knee test
heel-tap
h.-t. reaction
h.-t. test
heel-to-knee-to-toe test
heel-to-shin test
Heidelberg concept
Heidenhain
H. disease
H. syndrome
H. type of spongiform encephalopathy
Heifetz
H. carotid occluder
H. clip
H. cranial perforator
H. cup serrated ring forceps
H. procedure
H. skull perforator
Heifetz-Weck clip
heightened sensory perception
height vertigo
Heilbronner
H. sign
H. thigh
Heine-Medin disease
Held
H. bundle
H. decussation
H. end bulb
helical
h. CT angiography
h. electrode

NOTES

helical-like filament
helices (*pl. of* helix)
helicopod gait
helicopodia
heliencephalitis
heliotrope rash
helix, pl. **helices**
helix-loop-helix (HLH)
h.-l.-h. response factor
helmet
collimator h.
cooling h.
h. headache
Sheffield collimator h.
Helmholtz coil
helminthic infection
Helweg bundle
Helwig tract
hemal gland
hemangioblastoma
benign capillary h.
spinal h.
third ventricular h.
hemangioendothelioma
epithelial h.
epithelioid h.
kaposiform h.
Masson vegetant intravascular h.
vertebral h.
hemangioma
h. of the brain
calvarial h.
capillary h.
cavernous h.
choroid plexus h.
dumbbell-shaped spinal cavernous h.
epidural cavernous h.
extraaxial cavernous h.
extradural h.
extramedullary h.
histiocytoid h.
infantile hemangioblastic h.
laryngeal h.
oral h.
pontomesencephalic cavernous h.
retropharyngeal h.
sacral h.
vertebral h.
hemangiomatosis
hemangiopericytoma
giant petroclival h.
meningeal h.
Hemashield enhanced graft
hematencephalon
hematocephaly
hematocrit (HCT, Hct)
hematoencephalic barrier
hematogenous cell infiltration
hematoma
acute subdural h.
balancing subdural h.
carotid plaque h.
cerebellar h.
chronic subdural h.
delayed traumatic intracerebral h. (DTICH)
dural h.
epidural h.
h. evacuation
evolving h.
extracerebral h.
extradural h.
facial h.
gelatinous h.
hemispheral h.
hypertensive h.
iatrogenic h.
infratemporal h.
interhemispheric h.
intracerebral h.
intracranial h.
intramural h.
intraparenchymal h.
intraventricular h.
isodense subdural h.
nasal septum h.
occipital h.
optic nerve sheath h.
parenchymatous h.
posterior fossa extradural h.
retromembranous h.
retropharyngeal h.
scalp h.
spinal epidural h. (SEH)
spontaneous spinal epidural h. (SSEH)
subdural h.
subgaleal h.
subperiosteal h.
sylvian h.
traumatic h.
Hematome system
hematomyelia
hematomyelopore
hematopoietic stem cell defect
hematoporphyrin derivative
hematorrhachis, hemorrhachis
h. externa
extradural h.
h. interna
subdural h.
hematoxylin
acid h.

Mayer h.
phosphotungstic acid h. (PTAH)
hematoxylin-eosin stain
heme
h. biosynthesis
h. synthesis
hemeralopia
hemiacrosomia
hemiageusia
hemiageustia
hemiakinesia
hemialgia
hemiamyosthenia
hemianalgesia
hemianesthesia
alternate h.
cerebral h.
crossed h.
h. cruciata
mesocephalic h.
pontile h.
spinal h.
hemianhidrosis
hemianopia, hemianopsia, hemiopia
altitudinal h.
bilateral homonymous h.
bitemporal h.
congruous h.
contralateral homonymous h.
dense h.
heteronymous h.
homonymous h.
ipsilateral h.
macular h.
macular-sparing h.
paracentral h.
partial h.
quandrantic h.
hemianopic scotoma
hemianosmia
hemiapraxia
hemiasomatognosia
hemiasynergia
hemiataxia
hemiathetosis
hemiatrophy
facial progressive h.
lingual h.
progressive lingual h.
hemiballism
hemiballismus
hemiballistic
hemibasal syndrome
hemicephalalgia
hemicerebrum
hemichorea
hemichorea-hemiballism syndrome
hemiconvulsion, hemiplegia, and epilepsy (HHE)
hemicord
hemicorporectomy
hemicorticectomy
cerebral h.
hemicrania
chronic paroxysmal h. (CHP, CPH)
h. continua
episodic paroxysmal h.
paroxysmal h.
hemicranial pain
hemicranicus
status h.
hemicraniectomy
hemicraniosis
hemicraniotomy
hemidecortication
cerebral h.
hemideficit
motor h.
sensible h.
hemidepersonalization
hemidysergia
hemidysesthesia
hemidystonia
hemiepilepsy
hemifacial
h. flushing
h. microsomia
h. spasm (HFS)
h. weakness
hemifield
contralesional h.
ipsilesional h.
h. loss
nasal h.
H. slide phenomenon
hemigeusia
hemihydranencephaly
hemihypalgesia
hemihyperesthesia
hemihyperkinesis
hemihypertonia
hemihypertrophied skull

NOTES

H

hemihypertrophy
hemihypesthesia
hemihypoesthesia
hemihypometria
hemihypotonia
hemilaminectomy
complete lateral h.
lumbar h.
partial h.
unilateral h.
hemilateral chorea
hemimegalencephaly
hemimicropsia
hemimyelomeningocele
hemineglect
h. syndrome
visuospatial h.
hemiopalgia
hemiopia (*var. of* hemianopia)
hemiparaplegia
hemiparesis
amobarbital-induced h.
ataxic h.
contralateral h.
dense h.
hemiparetic h.
herald h.
hypesthetic ataxic h.
ipsilateral h.
paradoxical ipsilateral h.
premature infant spastic h.
pure motor h.
residual h.
spastic h.
transient h.
hemiparesthesia
hemiparesthetic
h. migraine
h. migraine headache
hemiparetic hemiparesis
hemiparkinsonian stiffness
hemiplegia
acute acquired h.
acutely acquired h.
h. alternans
alternating hypoglossal h.
bilateral spastic h.
contralateral h.
crossed h.
h. cruciata
dense h.
double h.
facial h.
Gubler h.
hysterical h.
infantile h.
left h.
h. migraine
motor h.
pure motor h.
right h.
spastic h.
spinal h.
superior alternating h.
Wernicke-Mann spastic h.
hemiplegic
h. amyotrophy
h. gait
h. idiocy
h. migraine
h. rigidity
hemipontine syndrome
hemirachischisis
hemisection
spinal cord h.
hemisensory
h. disturbance
h. loss
h. syndrome
hemiseptum cerebri
hemisoma
hemisomatognosia
hemispasm
facial h.
hemispatial neglect
hemisphenoidotomy
hemispheral
h. hematoma
h. mass
hemisphere
cerebellar h.
h. of cerebellum
cerebral h.
commissure of cerebral h.
h. competition
dominant h.
face-dominant h.
face-nondominant h.
inferior surface of cerebellar h.
inferior vein of cerebellar h.
ipsilateral h.
medial surface of cerebral h.
mesial h.
nondominant h.
quadrate lobe of cerebral h.
h. sequence
h. stroke
superior surface of cerebellar h.
superior vein of cerebellar h.
superolateral face of cerebral h.
ventricle of cerebral h.
hemispherectomy

hemispheric
h. asymmetry reduction in older adults (HAROLD)
h. blood flow
h. cerebral dysgenesis
h. collapse
h. cross flow
h. disconnection syndrome
h. dynamic
h. gliosis
h. hippocampal cortex
h. infarction
hemispherical
h. contact probe
h. deafferentation
hemispherii
polus temporalis h.
hemispherotomy
transopercular h.
hemitetany
hemithermoanesthesia
hemitonia
hemitransfixion incision
hemitremor
hemivagotony
hemivertebra
hemizygosity
hemochromatosis
hemoclip
Samuels-Weck h.
hemodilution
isovolemic h.
prophylactic hypertensive hypervolemic h.
hemodynamic
cerebral h.
h. resuscitation
h. system
hemoflagellate
hemoglobin
h. glutamer-250[bovine] oxygen-based therapeutic system
h. H disease
h. SC disease
hemoglobinopathy
hemolysis
hemolytic uremia syndrome
hemolytic-uremic syndrome
hemoperfusion
hemophilia
Hemopure oxygen-based therapeutic system
hemorrhachis (*var. of* hematorrhachis)
hemorrhage
aneurysmal subarachnoid h.
apoplectic h.
arterial h.
artery of cerebral h.
brainstem h.
central nervous system h.
cerebellar h.
cerebral h.
cerebrovascular h.
choroid plexus h.
delayed traumatic intracerebral h.
Duret h.
eight-ball h.
epidural h.
extradural h.
flame-shaped h.
focus of h.
germinal matrix h.
Hunt and Hess grading scale for aneurysmal subarachnoid h.
hypertensive basal ganglia h.
hypotensive h.
Icelandic form of intracranial h.
intertrabecular h.
intracapsular h.
intracerebral h.
intracranial h.
intraocular h.
intraparenchymal h.
intraplaque h.
intratumor h.
intratumoral h.
intraventricular h.
Kistler classification of subarachnoid h.
lobar h.
mesencephalic h.
neonatal cerebral h.
neonatal intraventricular h.
nerve fiber layer h.
nonaneurysmal perimesencephalic subarachnoid h.
nondominant putaminal h.
parenchymal cerebral h.
parenchymatous h.
perianeurysmal h.
periaqueductal h.

NOTES

H

hemorrhage *(continued)*
perimesencephalic nonaneurysmal subarachnoid h.
periventricular intraventricular h. (PIH)
petechial h.
pontine h.
premature infant subarachnoid h.
primary pontine h.
primary subarachnoid supratentorial h.
putaminal h.
remote cerebellar h.
retinal h.
retrobulbar h.
slit h.
spinal cord h.
spinal epidural h.
spinal subarachnoid h.
spinal subdural h.
splinter h.
striate h.
subacute h.
subarachnoid h. (SAH)
subconjunctival h.
subcortical h.
subdural h.
subependymal h.
subgaleal h.
subhyaloid h.
subintimal h.
supratentorial subdural h.
syringomyelic h.
thalamic h.
thalamic-subthalamic h.
traumatic meningeal h.
traumatic subarachnoid h. (TSAH)
vitreous h.
hemorrhagic
h. contusion
h. dysangiogenesis
h. encephalopathy
h. fever
h. infarction
h. lesion
h. metastasis
h. necrosis
h. pachymeningitis
h. shearing injury
h. shock
h. softening
h. stroke
H. Stroke-Specific quality of life instrument (HSQuale)
h. transformation (HT)
hemorrhagica
encephalitis h.
hemorrheology
hemosiderin
h. deposition
h. reactional gliosis
h. ring
h. scar
hemosiderin-laden cell
hemosiderin-stained brain
hemosiderosis
cerebral h.
hemostasis
chemical h.
hemostasis-related protein
hemostat
Avitene microfibrillator collagen h.
h. awl
Crile h.
Surgicel fibrillator absorbable h.
hemostatic
h. forceps
h. plug formation
hemotympanum
Hemovac Hydrocoat drain
Hendler test
Henle
H. fiber layer
ligament of H.
H. membrane
H. nervous layer
H. rhomboid sinus
H. sheath
H. spine
Henoch chorea
Henoch-Schönlein purpura
Henry-Geist spinal fusion
henselae
Rochalimaea h.
Hensen
H. canal
H. cell
H. duct
H. node
heparin
low-molecular weight h.
h. sulfate
heparinization
heparinized
hepatic
h. apoprotein gene
h. coma
h. disease-associated neuropathy
h. encephalopathy
h. encephalopathy treatment
h. enzyme
h. injury
h. oxidative metabolism
h. porphyria

hepaticum
  coma h.
hepatis
  pars anterior faciei diaphragmatis h.
  pars posterior facies diaphragmatis h.
hepatocerebral
  h. degeneration
  h. disease
hepatocyte
  h. growth factor
  h. growth factor/scatter factor (HGF/SF)
hepatoiminodiacetic acid (HIDA)
hepatolenticular
  h. degeneration
  h. disease
hepatotoxicity
hepatropic virus
Heplock catheter
heptachlor
Heptalac
herald hemiparesis
Herbst
  H. appliance
  H. corpuscle
herculin
hereditaria
  adynamia episodica h.
hereditary
  h. angioneurotic edema (HANE)
  h. areflexic dystasia
  h. ataxic syndrome
  h. brachial plexus disorder
  h. branchial myoclonus
  h. cerebellar ataxia
  h. cerebellar ataxia of Marie
  h. cerebellar atrophy
  h. cerebral hemorrhage with amyloidosis-Dutch type (HCHWA-D)
  h. chin trembling
  h. coproporphyria
  h. dysphasic
  h. dysphasic dementia
  h. essential tremor
  h. hemorrhagic telangiectasia
  h. high-density lipoprotein deficiency
  h. hypertrophic neuropathy
  h. motor-sensory neuropathy (HMSN)
  h. myokymia
  h. neuropathic amyloidosis
  h. neuropathy with liability to pressure palsy (HNPP)
  h. neuropathy with susceptibility to pressure palsy
  h. nonprogressive chorea
  h. photomyoclonus
  h. posterior column ataxia
  h. radicular sensory neuropathy
  h. sensory and autonomic disorder
  h. sensory autonomic neuropathy, type 1–4 (HSAN-1–4)
  h. sensory motor neuropathy (HSMN)
  h. sensory neuropathy (HSN)
  h. sensory radicular neuropathy
  h. sensory radiculopathy
  h. spastic paraparesis (HSP)
  h. spastic paraplegia
  h. spinal ataxia
  h. spinocerebellar ataxia syndrome
  h. striatopallidal disease
heredoataxia
heredodegenerative
  h. disease
heredofamilial
  h. amyloidosis
  h. tremor
heredopathia atactica polyneuritiformis
heredotaxia
heregulin
Hering
  sinus nerve of H.
  H. sinus nerve
Hering-Breuer reflex
Hering-Traube wave
Hermann Brain Dominance Instrument
Hermetian symmetry
Hermetic
  H. external ventricular drainage system
  H. II drainage management system
  H. lumbar drainage system
hermeticism
hermsii
  Borrelia h.

NOTES

hernia
cerebral h.
meningeal h.
herniated
h. cervical disk
h. intervertebral disk
h. nucleus pulposus
herniation
brain h.
caudal transtentorial h.
central transtentorial h.
cerebellar tonsillar h.
h. of cerebellar tonsils
cerebral h.
cervical disk h.
cingulate h.
concentric h.
disk h.
extraforaminal lumbar disk h.
foramen magnum h.
foraminal h.
frank disk h.
hard disk h.
hippocampal h.
hippocampus h.
impending h.
incipient downward central brain h.
internal disk h.
intervertebral disk h.
intraspongy nuclear disk h.
lumbar disk h.
rostral transtentorial h.
soft disk h.
sphenoidal h.
spinal h.
subfalcial h.
subfalcine h.
subligamentous disk h.
h. syndrome
temporal lobe h.
tentorial h.
thoracic disk h.
tonsillar h.
transforaminal h.
transtentorial uncal h.
traumatic cervical disk h.
uncal transtentorial h.
herophili
torcular h.
herpes
geniculate h.
h. simplex
h. simplex virus (HSV)
h. simplex virus encephalitis (HSVE)
h. simplex virus genome
h. simplex virus type 1 (HSV-1)
h. simplex virus type 2 (HSV-2)
toxoplasmosis, other infections, rubella, cytomegalovirus infection, h.
h. zoster
h. zoster encephalitis
h. zoster neuritis
h. zoster ophthalmicus
h. zoster oticus
h. zoster virus infection
herpes/herpetic encephalitis
herpesvirus
h. encephalitis
human h. 6 (HHV6)
human herpesvirus-8/Kaposi sarcoma-associated h. (HHV-8/KSHV)
h. infection type 6, 7
Herpesvirus simiae
herpete
zoster sine h.
herpetic
h. meningoencephalitis
h. neuritis
Herring body
Herrmann
H. Brain Dominance Instrument, Revised
H. syndrome
Hers disease
Hertel
H. exophthalmometer
H. exophthalmometry examination
Heschl
H. convolution
H. gyrus
transverse temporal gyri of H.
Hess
H. screen test
trophotropic zone of H.
hetacillin
heteresthesia
heterochromatin
heterocyclic
heterodesmotic fiber
heterodimeric receptor
heteroganglionic
heterogeneity
allelic h.
clinical h.
etiological h.
genetic h.
locus h.
plaque h.
heterogeneous
h. condition
h. system disease

heterogenous disorder
heterogeny
heterogeusia
heterokinesia
heterokinesis
heterolalia
heterologous stimulus
heteromeral
heteromeric cell
heteromerous
heteromodal association cortex
heteromultimer
heteromultimeric complex
heteronuclear ribonucleic acid (hnRNA)
heteronymous
h. hemianopia
h. motoneuron
heteropathy
heterophasia
heterophemia, heterophemy
heteroplasm
heteropodal
heteropsia
diffuse h.
heteroreceptor
heterosexuality
heterosmia
heterosociality
heterosuggestibility
heterotonia
heterotonic
heterotopia
band h.
bilateral periventricular nodular h.
focal nodular h.
incomplete band h.
isolated periventricular nodular h.
neuronal h.
nodular h.
periventricular nodular h.
subcortical laminar h.
subependymal diffuse h.
heterotopic
h. gray matter
h. interstitial neuropathy of infancy
h. ossification
h. pain
heterotrimeric
heterotypic cortex
heterozygosity
heterozygote
Heubner
H. arteritis
artery of H.
H. disease
H. endarteritis
recurrent artery of H.
heutoscopy
Hewlett-Packard pressure monitor
Hexabrix
hexachlorophene toxicity
Hexadrol Phosphate
hexamethylmelamine
hexamethylpropyleneamineoxime
hexamethylpropyleneamine oxime (HMPAO)
hexapropymate
hexosaminidase
h. A
h. deficiency
hexose
Heyer-Pudenz valve
Heyer-Schulte
H.-S. antisiphon device
H.-S. bur hole valve
H.-S. neurosurgical shunt
H.-S. wound drain
HFF
high-frequency filter
HFF on electroencephalogram
HFPV
high-frequency percussive ventilation
HFS
hemifacial spasm
HGF/SF
hepatocyte growth factor/scatter factor
HHE
hemiconvulsion, hemiplegia, and epilepsy
H. syndrome
HHF35 muscle-specific actin tumor marker
HHV6
human herpesvirus 6
HHV-8/KSHV
human herpesvirus-8/Kaposi sarcoma-associated herpesvirus
HHV6-MS
human herpesvirus 6/multiple sclerosis
HHV6-specific
hiatus
h. semilunaris
tentorial h.

NOTES

H

Hibbs
H. spinal curette
H. spinal fusion gouge
Hibbs-Jones spinal fusion
Hibbs-Spratt spinal fusion curette
hiccup
endemic h.
idiopathic chronic h.
Hickman catheter
Hick syndrome
HID
headache, insomnia, and depression
HID syndrome
HIDA
hepatoiminodiacetic acid
technetium 99m HIDA
hidden observer phenomenon
hidradenoma
hidrocystoma
HIE
hypoxic ischemic encephalopathy
high
h. alpha coefficient
h. amplitude
h. animal protein
h. beam fiberoptic headlight
h. cervical spinal cord lesion
h. degree of competency
h. density area
h. energy X-ray beam
h. frequency deafness
h. linear filter
h. molecular weight cytokeratin tumor marker
h. muscular resistance bed
h. osmolar contrast medium
h. pontine lesion
h. potency neuroleptic
h. resolution chromosome analysis
h. sensitivity
h. sodium
h. steppage gait
h. utilizer
h. voltage slow and sharp activity
high-affinity binding site
high-air-loss bed
high-altitude headache
high-density
h.-d. lipoprotein (HDL)
h.-d. transient signal
high-dose dopaminergic agonist
high-energy
h.-e. brachytherapy
h.-e. cellular store
higher
h. center
h. cerebral dysfunction
h. cognitive function
h. neural function
h. order motion
high-filter frequency
high-force Sundt clip system
high-frequency
h.-f. activity
h.-f. filter (HFF)
h.-f. generator
h.-f. hearing impairment
h.-f. oscillation
h.-f. percussive ventilation (HFPV)
high-functioning patient
high-gain instability
high-grade
h.-g. glioma
h.-g. spondylolisthesis
h.-g. stenosis
high-intensity
h.-i. click stimulation
h.-i. lesion
h.-i. signal
high-lesion load
highly
h. active antiretroviral therapy (HAART)
h. selective vagotomy
h. unsaturated fatty acid (HUFA)
high-resolution
h.-r. brain SPECT
h.-r. brain SPECT system
h.-r. 3DFT MR imaging
h.-r. MRI
high-risk population
high-signal lesion
high-speed
h.-s. air drill
h.-s. microdrill
high-threshold mechanoreceptor
high-torque bur
High-Vision surgical telescope
high-voltage
h.-v. centrotemporal spike
h.-v. deflection
HI-induced brain damage
hila (*pl. of* hilum)
Hilal
H. coil
H. microcoil
hilar
h. adenopathy
h. cell
Hilger facial nerve stimulator
hillock
axon h.
facial h.

Hilton
H. law
H. method
hilum, pl. **hila**
h. of dentate nucleus
h. of inferior olivary nucleus
h. nuclei dentati
h. nuclei olivaris
h. nuclei olivaris caudalis
h. nuclei olivaris inferioris
h. of olivary nucleus
hilus of fascia dentata
H-imipramine binding
Hinck catheter
hindbrain
h. decompression
h. deformity
h. ischemia
h. vesicle
Hind III enzyme
hindlimb motor
***H. influenzae* type B meningitis**
hinged cast
hip
h. extensor gait
h. phenomenon
hip-flexion phenomenon
Hippel disease
Hippel-Lindau
H.-L. disease
von H.-L. (VHL)
hippocampal
h. activation
h. amnesia
h. commissure
h. complex
h. convolution
h. dentate gyrus
h. electroencephalogram
h. epilepsy
h. fissure
h. formation
h. formation atrophy
h. formation subdivision
h. herniation
h. infarction
h. monoamine concentration
h. neuronal loss
h. pyramidal cell loss
h. pyramidal neuron
h. raw volume
h. sclerosis
h. seizure discharge
h. slice
h. slice model of seizure
h. sprouting
h. sulcus
h. volume loss
h. volumetric loss
h. volumetry
h. vulnerability
hippocampal-amygdala complex
hippocampalis
formatio h.
sulcus h.
hippocampectomy
hippocampus, pl. **hippocampi**
alveus of h.
commissura h.
corpus fimbriatum h.
digitationes h.
fascia dentata h.
fimbria of h.
fissura h.
foot of h.
gyrus h.
h. herniation
layer of h.
h. major
mammalian h.
h. minor
minor h.
oriens layer of h.
pes h.
radiate layer of h.
rudimentum h.
h. sclerosis
strata h.
stratum lucidum h.
stratum moleculare h.
stratum oriens h.
stratum pyramidale h.
stratum radiatum h.
subiculum h.
sulcus h.
tenia h.
uncus gyri h.
Hippocratic aphorism
Hirano body
Hirsch
H. endonasal technique

NOTES

Hirsch *(continued)*
H. grading
H. hypophysis punch forceps
Hirschberg
H. reflex
H. sign
H. test
Hirschsprung disease
hirsutism
hirundinis
nidus h.
His
isthmus of H.
H. perivascular space
Histacryl Blue
histamine
h. cephalalgia
h. test in familial dysautonomia
histaminic
h. cephalalgia
h. headache
histidine metabolism disorder
histidinemia aminoaciduria
histidyl
histine
beta h.
histiocyte
epithelioid h.
histiocytoid hemangioma
histiocytoma
histiocytosis
diffuse cerebral h.
kerasin h.
sinus h.
histiocytosis X
Histoacryl
H. embolization
H. glue
histochemical study
histocompatability
histocompatibility
h. antigen
h. complex
histogram
peristimulus-time h. (PSTH)
histologic section
histology
posttraumatic brain h.
histolytica
Entamoeba h.
histomorphometric
histonectomy
histoneurology
histopathologic
histopathology
Histoplasma
H. capsulatum
H. infection
histoplasma
h. meningitis
h. polysaccharide antigen
histoplasmosis
disseminated central nervous system h.
disseminated CNS h.
historrhexis
history
neurologic-ophthalmologic h.
histotoxic hypoxia
Hitachi
H. scanning electron microscope
H. spectrophotometer
Hitch model
Hitzelberger sign
Hitzig girdle
HIV
human immunodeficiency virus
HIV encephalopathy
HIV myelopathy
HIV myopathy
HIV-1-envelope protein
HIV-associated dementia
Hivid
HIV-related
HIV-r. neuropathy
HIV-r. seizure
HIV-sensory neuropathy (HIV-SN)
HIV-SN
HIV-sensory neuropathy
HLA
human lymphocyte antigen
HLA class II
HLA DR15 (DR2) typing
HLA-Cw2
HLA-CW2 antigen
HLA-DQ6
HLA-DQA10102
HLA-DQAB10102
HLA-DQB10602
HLA-DR1
HLA-DR2 antigen
HLH
helix-loop-helix
HLH factor
HMPAO
hexamethylpropyleneamine oxime
hMSCs
human adult bone marrow mesenchymal stem cell
HMSN
hereditary motor-sensory neuropathy

HNK
human neonatal kidney
HNK cell
HNPP
hereditary neuropathy with liability to pressure palsy
hnRNA
heteronuclear ribonucleic acid
hNT neuron
Hoche
H. bundle
H. tract
Hochsinger
H. phenomenon
H. sign
HOCI
hypochlorous acid
hockey-stick dissector
Hodgkin
H. cycle
H. disease
H. lymphoma
Hodgkin-Huxley assumption
Hoehn
H. and Yahr Parkinson staging
H. and Yahr scale
H. and Yahr staging of Parkinson disease
Hoen
H. dural separator
H. intervertebral disk rongeur
H. lamina gouge
H. nerve hook
H. pituitary rongeur
H. ventricular needle
Hoffmann
H. and Mohr procedure
H. muscular atrophy
H. phenomenon
H. reflex
H. sign
Hoffmann-Werdnig syndrome
holder
Adson dural needle h.
Ayers needle h.
CBI stereotactic head h.
cordotomy hook h.
Crile needle h.
curved microneedle h.
Donaghy angled suture needle h.
endoscope h.
Holinger endarterectomy dissector h.
Jacobson needle h.
Malis needle h.
Micro-One needle h.
microsurgery needle h.
Micro-Two needle h.
needle h.
neurosurgical needle h.
Patil stereotactic head h.
ReFix stereotactic head h.
Sugita head h.
Texas Scottish Rite Hospital hook h.
Vari-Angle clip h.
Wangensteen needle h.
Webster needle h.
Yasargil needle h.
hole
bur h.
precoronal bur h.
h. preparation method
holiday
caffeine h.
Holinger endarterectomy dissector holder
holistic
h. approach
h. regimen
Hollander test
Hollenhorst plaque
Hollingshead-Redlich scale
Holmes
H. cerebellar degeneration disease
H. cortical cerebellar degeneration
H. phenomenon
H. sign
H. tremor
Holmes-Adie
H.-A. pupil
H.-A. syndrome
Holmes-Stewart phenomenon
holmium YAG laser
holocarboxylase
h. synthetase
h. synthetase deficiency
holocoenosis
holocord hydromyelia
holocrania
holography
digital h.

NOTES

H

holography *(continued)*
volumetric multiple exposure transmission h. (VMETH)
holohemispheric vasogenic edema
holophrastic
holoprosencephaly
alobar h.
holorachischisis
holotelencephaly
Holscher nerve root retractor
Holter
H. high-pressure valve
H. medium-pressure valve
H. monitor
H. monitor test
Holter-Hausner valve
Homans sign
Homén syndrome
homeodomain
h. factor
h. gene
h. protein
homeostasis
cellular ion h.
free radical h.
homeostatic balance
homeostenosis
Homer Wright rosette
HomeTrac
Saunders cervical H.
hominid
hominoid
homochronous
homocitrullinuria
homocysteine
h. acid
h. level
homocystinuria
adult-onset combined methylmalonic aciduria and h.
homodesmotic fiber
homofenazine
homogenate technique
homogeneity
field h.
spatial h.
homogeneous lesion
homogenous reinforcement
homoiopodal
homolateral
homolog
homologous
h. gene
h. stimulus
h. tetanus immune globulin (HTIG)
homomultimeric complex
homonomy
analysis of h.
homonymous
h. hemianopia
h. motoneuron
h. muscle
h. scintillating scotoma
homophone
homoplasmy
homotopic pain
homotypic cortex
homovanillic
h. acid (HVA)
h. acid concentration
h. acid test
homozygosity
homozygote
homozygous
dementia h.
h. state
homuncular organization phase reversal
homunculus
somatosensory h.
Honig
H. model
H. model of working memory
hood
dorsal aponeurotic expansion h.
H. masking technique
hook
Adson dissecting h.
Adson dural h.
Adson nerve h.
anatomic h.
André anatomical h.
ball-tip nerve h.
bifid h.
blunt nerve h.
Bobechko sliding barrel h.
calvarial h.
caudal h.
cautery h.
clawed pedicle h.
closed Cotrel-Dubousset h.
closed transverse process TSRH h.
Cloward cautery h.
Cloward dural h.
corkscrew dural h.
cranial Jacobs h.
Crile nerve h.
Culler h.
Cushing dural h.
Cushing gasserian ganglion h.
Cushing nerve h.
Dandy nerve h.
DePuy nerve h.
h. dislodgement

dissecting h.
downsized circular laminar h.
drop-entry (closed body) h.
dura h.
Fisch dural h.
Fisch micro h.
Frazier dural h.
Frazier nerve h.
ganglion h.
Harrington pedicle h.
Hoen nerve h.
h. hollow-ground connection design
intermediate C-D h.
Isola spinal implant system h.
Jannetta h.
Kennerdell-Maroon h.
Kilner h.
Krayenbuehl nerve h.
Lahey Clinic dural h.
Lahey Clinic nerve h.
laminar C-D h.
large ball nerve h.
Leatherman h.
Love nerve root h.
Lucae nerve h.
Malis nerve h.
Marino transsphenoidal h.
microball h.
Moe alar h.
Moe spinal h.
Moe square-ended h.
multispan fracture h.
Murphy ball h.
nerve h.
open C-D h.
pear-shaped nerve h.
pediatric C-D h.
pediatric TSRH h.
pedicle C-D h.
QPCA pear-shaped nerve h.
retractor handle Cloward dural h.
ribbed h.
Rosser crypt h.
Sachs dural h.
Scoville nerve root h.
Selverstone cordotomy h.
side-opening laminar h.
h. site
Smithwick button h.
Smithwick ganglion h.
Smithwick sympathectomy h.
Speare dural h.
square-ended h.
straight nerve h.
Strully dural h.
Texas Scottish Rite Hospital buttressed laminar h.
Texas Scottish Rite Hospital circular laminar h.
Texas Scottish Rite Hospital pedicle h.
Texas Scottish Rite Hospital trial h.
Toennis dural h.
top-entry (open body) h.
transection h.
transsphenoidal h.
TSRH buttressed laminar h.
TSRH circular laminar h.
TSRH pedicle h.
h. V-groove connection design
von Graefe strabismus h.
Weary nerve h.
Yasargil spring h.
Zielke bifid h.
Zimmer caudal h.

hookean body

hooked
h. bundle of Russell
h. fasciculus

hook-plate fixation

hook-to-screw L4-S1 compression construct

Hoover sign

Hopkins
H. II endoscope
H. Symptom Checklist–90 Total Score
H. syndrome

Hoppe-Goldflam disease

horizontal
h. cell of Cajal
h. cell of retina
h. conflict
h. eye movement
h. fissure of cerebellum
h. gaze
h. gaze palsy
h. gaze paresis
h. inhibition
h. pedicle diameter
h. vertigo

NOTES

horizontalis
fissura h.
hormonal
h. change
h. contraception
h. decline
h. difference
h. maturation
h. receptor
h. therapy
hormone
adrenocorticotropic h. (ACTH)
anterior pituitary h.
antidiuretic h. (ADH)
corticotropin-releasing h. (CRH)
ectopic h.
endogenous steroid h.
follicle-stimulating h. (FSH)
gonadotropin-releasing h. (GnRH, GRH)
growth hormone-releasing h. (GHRH)
hypothalamic regulating h.
luteinizing h. (LH)
luteinizing hormone-releasing h.
maternal thyroid h.
natriuretic h.
parathyroid h. (PTH)
peripheral steroid h.
prolactin-inhibiting h.
prolactin-releasing h. (PRH)
h. replacement
h. replacement therapy (HRT)
sex h.
steroid h.
supplemental steroid h.
syndrome of inappropriate secretion of antidiuretic h. (SIADH)
thyroid-stimulating h. (TSH)
thyrotropin-releasing h. (TRH)
horn
Ammon h.
anterior h.
apex of posterior h.
bulb of occipital h.
h. cell
cutaneous h.
dorsal h.
frontal h.
inferior h.
lateral ventricle occipital h.
lateral ventricle posterior h.
lateral ventricle temporal h.
occipital h.
posterior h.
spinal cord lateral h.
spinal cord ventral h.
temporal h.
tip of posterior h.
vein of posterior h.
ventral h.
Horner
H. ptosis
H. syndrome
Horner-Bernard syndrome
horse
charley h.
horseshoe
h. headrest
h. incision
horseshoe-shaped flap
Horsley
H. bone wax
H. dural separator
H. operation
H. rongeur
H. sign
Horsley-Clarke
H.-C. stereotactic apparatus
H.-C. stereotactic frame
Hortega
H. cell
H. neuroglia stain
Horton
H. disease
H. giant cell arteritis
H. headache
H. histamine cephalalgia
H. syndrome
hospital
Texas Scottish Rite H. (TSRH)
VA H.
hospital-acquired
h.-a. meningitis
h.-a. pneumonia
host
h. immune response
immunocompromised h.
hot
h. dog headache
h. knife
h. spot
h. water epilepsy
hot-spot phantom
Hounsfield unit (HU)
12-hour fasting lipid panel
hour-glass
h.-g. dressing
h.-g. tumor
House-Brackmann
H.-B. Facial Nerve Function Grading Scale
H.-B. Grading Scale
H.-B. Score

House-Fisch
H.-F. dural retractor
H.-F. dural spatula
housekeeping gene
Housepian
H. aneurysm clip
H. forceps
Houston halo
Howard spinal curette
Howmedica
H. Microfixation cranial plate
H. Microfixation System drill bit
H. Microfixation System plate cutter
H. Microfixation System plate-holding forceps
H. Microfixation System pliers
Hox gene
Ho:YAG laser
Hoyt-Spencer sign
H.P. Acthar Gel
hPVR
human poliovirus receptor
H1 receptor
H-reflex
357HR Magnum tablet
HRT
hormone replacement therapy
HSAN-1–4
hereditary sensory autonomic neuropathy, type 1–4
H-shaped microplate
HSMN
hereditary sensory motor neuropathy
HSN
hereditary sensory neuropathy
HSP
hereditary spastic paraparesis
HSQuale
Hemorrhagic Stroke-Specific quality of life instrument
HSV
herpes simplex virus
HSV encephalitis
HSV-1
herpes simplex virus type 1
HSV-2
herpes simplex virus type 2
HSVE
herpes simplex virus encephalitis
HT
hemorrhagic transformation
5-HT
5-hydroxytryptamine
5-HT agonist
5-HT receptor assay
5-HT releasing agent
5-HT reuptake inhibitor
5-HT1
serotonin 5-HT1
5HT1A antagonist
5-HT1 receptor
5-HT2 receptor
5-HT3 receptor
5-HT$_2$-D$_2$-antagonist
5HTIA receptor
HTIG
homologous tetanus immune globulin
HTLV
human T-cell leukemia virus
HTLV-associated myelopathy/tropical spastic paraparesis
HTLV-I associated myelopathy
5-HTP
5-hydroxytryptophan
HTR
hard tissue replacement
HTR polymer
5-HT$_{2C}$ receptor
HTR-MFI
H.-M. chin implant
H.-M. curved implant
H.-M. malar implant
H.-M. paranasal implant
H.-M. premaxillary implant
H.-M. ramus implant
H.-M. straight implant
HTR-PMI
hard tissue replacement-patient-matched
HTR-PMI implant
HU
Hounsfield unit
Hudson
H. brace
H. brace bur
H. cerebellar attachment
H. cranial drill set
H. cranial rongeur
H. drill
H. forceps
H. perforator

NOTES

HUFA
highly unsaturated fatty acid
huffer neuropathy
Hughes reflex
Hulka instrument
human
h. adult bone marrow mesenchymal stem cell (hMSCs)
h. antimouse antibody (HAMA)
h. botulism
h. brain microvascular endothelial cell (HBMEC)
h. chorionic gonadotropin (hCG)
h. chromosome 20
h. dural substitute
h. dural substitute graft
h. ecology
h. factor
h. herpesvirus 6 (HHV6)
h. herpesvirus-8/Kaposi sarcoma-associated herpesvirus (HHV-8/KSHV)
h. herpesvirus 6/multiple sclerosis (HHV6-MS)
h. immunodeficiency virus (HIV)
h. immunodeficiency virus infection
h. lymphocyte antigen (HLA)
h. neonatal kidney (HNK)
h. neonatal kidney cell
h. neurofilament light chain
h. poliovirus receptor (hPVR)
h. prion protein
h. Purkinje cell
h. relationship
h. strength
h. T-cell leukemia virus (HTLV)
h. T-cell lymphoma virus
h. T-cell lymphotropic virus
h. T-cell lymphotropic virus-associated myeloneuropathy
h. T-cell lymphotropic virus-associated myelopathy
h. T-cell lymphotropic virus type 1-associated myelopathy/tropical spastic paraparesis (HAM/TSP)
h. tetanus immune globulin
h. T-lymphotrophic virus-associated myelopathy
humanus
morsus h.
humeroperoneal muscular dystrophy
humoral
h. immune response
h. immune system
h. phototransduction
Humphrey visual field
Hunstad infusion needle
Hunt
H. angled serrated ring forceps
H. angled-tip forceps
H. atrophy
H. disease
H. grasping forceps
H. and Hess criteria
H. and Hess grade I–III
H. and Hess grading scale for aneurysmal subarachnoid hemorrhage
H. juvenile paralysis agitans
H. and Kosnik classification
H. neuralgia
H. paradoxical phenomenon
H. paradoxic phenomenon
H. syndrome
Hunt-Early technique
Hunter
H. canal
H. disease
H. dural separator
H. open cord tendon implant
H. operation
H. syndrome
hunterian
h. ligation
h. ligation of aneurysm
Hunter-McAlpine syndrome
Hunt-Hess
H.-H. aneurysm classification
H.-H. aneurysm grading system
H.-H. neurological classification
H.-H. subarachnoid hemorrhage scale
Hunting disorder (HD)
huntingtin protein
Huntington
H. chorea (HD)
H. disease
H. Disease Society of America (HDSA)
H. sign
Hunt-Kosnik classification of aneurysm
Hunt-Yasargil pituitary forceps
Hurd bone-cutting forceps
Hurler
H. disease
H. syndrome
Hurler-Scheie
H.-S. disease
H.-S. syndrome
Hurst disease
Hurteau skull plate anvil
Husk bone rongeur
Hutchinson
H. facies

H. mask
H. pupil
H. sign
H. type neuroblastoma
Hutchison
H. syndrome
H. triad in syphilis
HVA
homovanillic acid
HVA concentration
H-wave test
hyaline
h. arteriosclerosis
h. body of pituitary
h. degeneration
h. thickening
hyalin inclusion disease
hyalinization
Crooke h.
hyalophagia
hyaluronan
hyaluron-binding region
hyaluronic acid
hyaluronidase
hyatari
hybridization
fluorescence in situ h. (FISH)
Northern h.
in situ h.
suppression subtractive h. (SSH)
hybridoma
hydatid
cerebral h.
h. cyst
h. disease
Hydergine LC
hydralazine
h. hydrochloride
h. and hydrochlorothiazide
hydranencephaly
Hydrap-ES
hydrate
amyl h.
amylene h.
hydraulic-type
h.-t. disk prosthesis
h.-t. disk replacement
hydrazine toxicity
hydrencephalocele
hydrencephalomeningocele
hydrencephalus
hydrencephaly macrocephaly
hydride
butyl h.
hydroadipsia
hydrobromide
galantamine h.
hydrobulbia
hydrocarbon
aromatic h.
volatile h.
hydrocele spinalis
hydrocephalic
h. dementia
h. idiocy
h. periventricular radiolucency
hydrocephalocele
hydrocephaloid
hydrocephalus
acquired h.
acute h.
arrested h.
asymptomatic h.
bilateral h.
chronic communicating h.
cocktail chatter in h.
communicating h.
compensated h.
congenital h.
delayed h.
double compartment h.
external h.
h. ex vacuo
fetal h.
fulminant h.
idiopathic normal pressure h. (INPH)
infantile h.
internal h.
kaolin-induced h.
maximal h.
meningitic h.
multiloculated h.
neonatal h.
noncommunicating h.
normal-pressure h. (NPH)
normotensive h.
obstructing h.
obstructive h.
occult h.
otic h.
otitic h.

NOTES

hydrocephalus *(continued)*
h. oversecretion
posthemorrhagic h.
postinfectious h.
postmeningitic h.
posttraumatic h.
premature infant h.
primary h.
progressive h.
secondary h.
shunted h.
h. shunt procedure
subdural effusion with h.
symptomatic h.
tension h.
thrombotic h.
toxic h.
triventricular h.
uncompensated h.
unilateral h.
unshunted h.
vasospasm-related h.
X-linked h.
hydrocephaly
hydrochloride (HCl)
alphaprodine h.
amantadine h.
amitriptyline h.
aptiganel h.
azacyclonol h.
butaclamol h.
chlordiazepoxide h.
chlorpromazine h.
clonidine h.
cyclobenzaprine h.
cyproheptadine h.
dexclamol h.
dihydromorphinone h.
diphenhydramine h.
donepezil h.
dopamine h.
dothiepin h.
doxepin h.
doxorubicin h.
duloxetine h.
ethaverine h.
fluphenazine h.
hydralazine h.
hydromorphone h.
hydroxyzine h.
imafen h.
imipramine h.
isoetharine h.
meperidine h.
methadone h.
methylamphetamine h.
midodrine h.
naratriptan h.
nitrosourea h.
oxyphencyclimine h.
papaverine h.
perphenazine and amitriptyline h.
phencyclidine h.
procarbazine h.
promethazine h.
proparacaine h.
propranolol h.
ropinirole h.
sertraline h.
tiagabine h.
tizanidine h.
trifluoperazine h.
trihexyphenidyl h.
trimethobenzamide h.
tryptizol h.
venlafaxine h.
ziprasidone h.
hydrochlorothiazide
benazepril and h.
bupropion h.
hydralazine and h.
lisinopril and h.
methyldopa and h.
propranolol and h.
h. and spironolactone
h. and triamterene
hydrocortisone
Hydrocortone
H. Acetate
H. Phosphate
hydrodipsia
hydrodipsomania
HydroDIURIL
hydroencephalocele
hydroencephaly
Hydro-Ergoloid
hydrogel
copper sulfate h.
Hydrogel disk replacement
hydrogen ion concentration
hydrolase
dopamine beta h. (DPH)
epoxide h.
terminal h.
Hydrolene polymer
Hydroloid-G
hydroma
cystic h.
hydromania
hydromeningitis
hydromeningocele
hydromeningoencephalocele
hydromicrocephaly
hydromorphine

hydromorphone hydrochloride
hydromyelia
holocord h.
hydromyelocele
hydromyelomeningocele
hydronephrosis in spinal bifida cystica
Hydro-Par
hydroperoxide
phospholipid h.
4-hydroperoxycyclophosphamide
hydrophilic guide
hydrophilicity
hydrophobia
hydrophobic
h. ligand
h. tetanus
hydrophobicity algorithm
hydrophorograph
hydropneumatic massage
hydropneumogony
hydrops
endolymphatic h.
hypertensive meningeal h.
labyrinthine h.
hydrorachis
HydroStat IR
hydrosyringomyelia
hydroxide
magnesium aluminum h.
hydroxocobalamin
3-hydroxy-3-methyl-glutaric aciduria
hydroxyapatite
APS h.
h. graft
Interpore porus h.
hydroxybutyrate
beta h.
4-hydroxybutyric aciduria
hydroxychloroquine
hydroxycobalamin
17-hydroxycorticosteroid
6-hydroxydopamine (6-OHDA)
hydroxyethylmethacrylate
2-hydroxyethylmethacrylate
hydroxyethyl methacrylate polymerizing solution
2-hydroxyglutaric aciduria
5-hydroxyindoleacetic acid
3-hydroxyisobutyric aciduria
hydroxyisovaleric aminoaciduria
hydroxylase
tryptophan h.
tyrosine h.
hydroxylase-positive
tyrosine h.-p.
hydroxylation
hydroxyl radical
4-hydroxynonenal
hydroxyproline
hydroxyquinoline neurotoxicity
5-hydroxytryptamine (5-HT)
5-h. receptor assay
5-hydroxytryptophan (5-HTP)
hydroxyurea
hydroxyzine
h. hydrochloride
h. pamoate
hygroma
subdural h.
Hygroton
hyla
hylomania
hyoglossus muscle
hyoid
h. advancement
h. bone
h. suspension
hypalgesia, hypoalgesia
h. dolorosa
hypalgesic, hypalgetic
hypalgia
Hy-Pam
Hypaque
hypaxial
hypegiaphobia
hyperabduction syndrome
hyperactive
h. affect
h. sympathetic response
h. tendon reflex
hyperacusis, hyperacusia
hyperadrenalism
hyperadrenergic
h. response
h. state
hyperaesthetic
hyperageusia
hyperaldosteronism
hyperalgesia, hyperalgia
auditory h.
muscular h.

NOTES

hyperalgesic zone
hyperalgetic
hyperalgia (*var. of* hyperalgesia)
hyperalimentation
hyperammonemia
cerebroatrophic h.
valproate-associated h.
hyperamylasemia
hyperaphia
hyperaphic
hyperargininemia
hyperarousal
physiological h.
h. symptom
hyperbetaalaninemia aminoaciduria
hyperbilirubinemia
nonhemolytic h.
hyperbulia
hyperbulimia
hypercalcemia
neonatal h.
hypercalciuria
hypercapnia, hypercarbia
depressed ventilatory response to h.
hypercapnic responsiveness
hypercatabolism
hypercholesterolemia
familial h.
hypercinesis, hypercinesia
hyper-CKemia
idiopathic h.-C.
hypercoagulability
hypercoagulable state
hypercoagulation
hypercoenesthesia
hypercompensatory type
hypercortisolemia
hypercortisolism
hypercryalgesia
hypercryesthesia
hyperdopaminergic state
hyperdynamia
hyperdynamic
hyperemia
occlusive h.
relative h.
hyperemic
h. headache
h. response
hyperenergetic behavior
hypereosinophilic syndrome
hyperequilibrium
hyperergasia
hyperergia, hypergia
hyperergic encephalitis
hyperesthenia
hyperesthesia
auditory h.
cerebral h.
gustatory h.
muscular h.
h. olfactoria
olfactory h.
oneiric h.
h. optica
tactile h.
vaginal h.
hyperesthetic
hyperestrogenemia
hyperevolutism
hyperexcitability
neuronal h.
self-sustaining h.
hyperexcitation
neuron h.
hyperexplexia
hyperextension
intraoperative neck h.
hyperextension-hyperflexion injury
hyperfibrinolysis
hyperflexion
hyperfractionated
h. irradiation
h. radiotherapy
hyperfractionation
hyperfrontality
hyperfunction
adrenal cortical h.
hyperfusion
hypergammaglobulinemia
hypergamy
hyperganglionosis
hypergeusia
hypergia (*var. of* hyperergia)
hyperglycemia
ketotic h.
nonketotic h.
hyperglycinemia
nonketotic h.
hyperglycorrhachia
hyperhidrosis
palmar h.
sleep h.
hyperhomocysteinemia
hypericum perforatum
hyperinsulinemia
hyperinsulinism
hyperintense
h. hyperosmolality
h. lesion
hyperintensity
h. change
deep white matter h.

incidental punctate white matter h.
MRI signal h.
periventricular h.
punctate white matter h.
h. rating
h. severity
signal h.
subcortical h.
subcortical gray matter h.
white matter h.
hyperisotonia
hyperkalemia
hyperkalemic periodic paralysis
hyperkeratosis
hyperkinesis, hyperkinesia
h. sign
hyperkinetic
h. conduct disorder
h. dysarthria
h. encephalopathy
h. impulse disorder
h. motor disorder
h. reaction
h. syndrome
hyperkyphoscoliosis
neuropathic h.
hyperlaxity
joint h.
hyperlexia
hyperlipidemia
hyperlysinemia aminoaciduria
hyperlysinuria
hypermagnesemia
hypermetabolic
h. effect
h. tumor component
hypermetamorphosis
hypermethioninemia hyperornithinemia
hypermethylation
hypermetria
hypermimia
hypermotor seizure
hypermyelination
hypermyesthesia
hypermyotonia
hypernatremia
hypodipsic h.
hypernatremic encephalopathy
hypernephroma
hypernomic
hyperorality
hyperornithinemia
hypermethioninemia h.
hyperosmia
hyperosmolality
hyperintense h.
hyperosmolar
h. (hyperglycemic) nonketotic coma
h. hyperglycemic nonketotic syndrome
hyperosmolarity
hyperosmotic agent
hyperosphresia
hyperosphresis
hyperostosis
Caffey h.
diffuse idiopathic skeletal h. (DISH)
h. frontalis interna
hyperostotic
h. lesion
h. spondylosis
hyperoxaluria
hyperoxia
hyperpallesthesia
hyperparathyroidism
maternal h.
hyperpathia
hyperperfusion
h. syndrome
tissue h.
hyperphagia
hyperphenylalaninemia
hyperphosphatasia
hyperphosphorylated tau
hyperphrenic
hyperpipecolatemia
hyperpituitarism
hyperplasia
arachnoidal h.
congenital virilizing adrenal h.
fibromuscular h.
gingival h.
heat h.
multiglandular h.
papillary mucosal h.
somatotroph h.
static h.
vessel h.
hyperplastic-hypertrophic obesity
hyperplastic primary vitreous
hyperpolarization

NOTES

hyperpolarization-activated
h.-a. cationic current
h.-a. chloride current
hyperpolarize factor
hyperpolarizing current
hyperponesis
hyperponetic
hyperpragic
hyperpraxia
hyperprolactinemia
hyperprolinemia aminoaciduria
hyperpronation
hyperpyrexia
hyperreactive
hyperreflexia
asymmetric h.
autonomic h. (AH)
bilateral h.
detrusor h.
pathologic h.
spastic h.
unilateral h.
hyperresponsive
hypersalivation
hypersarcosinemia
hypersecretion
hypersecretory adenoma
hyperselaphesia
hypersensitivity
carotid sinus h.
denervation neuronal h.
h. vasculitis
hypersomnia
hypersomnic depression
hypersomnolence
central nervous system h.
idiopathic CNS h.
hypersomnolent
hyperstimulation
adrenergic h.
hypersympathicotonus
hypersynchronous
h. activity
h. discharge
h. electroencephalogram
hypersynchrony
hypnagogic h.
hypertarachia
hypertelorism
orbital h.
hypertension
benign intracranial h.
cerebral h.
idiopathic intracranial h. (IIH)
intracranial h.
malignant h.
neonatal h.
orthostatic h.
paroxysmal h.
postural h.
venous h.
hypertension-related headache
hypertensive
h. basal ganglia hemorrhage
h. dilation
h. encephalopathy
h. hematoma
h., hypervolemic, hemodilutional therapy
h. meningeal hydrops
h. pontine microhemorrhage
hyperthermalgesia
hyperthermesthesia
hyperthermia
malignant h.
microwave h.
rebound h.
hyperthermoesthesia
hyperthyroidism
apathetic h.
hyperthyroid neuropathy
hypertonia
sympathetic h.
treatment-emergent h.
hypertonic
h. absence
h. cerebral palsy
hypertonicity
hypertonus
hypertrichosis
hypertriglyceridemia
hypertrophic
h. arthritis
h. cervical
h. cervical pachymeningitis
h. chromic pachymeningitis (HCP)
h. cranial pachymeningitis
h. interstitial neuropathy
h. nodular gliosis
h. obesity
h. olivary degeneration
h. pachymeningitis dorsalis
hypertrophica
pachymeningitis cranialis h.
hypertrophied frenula syndrome
hypertrophy
facet h.
muscle h.
pons h.
pseudomuscular h.
uncovertebral joint h.
hypertropia
over-right h.
hypertryptophanemia

hyperuricemia
hypervalinemia
hypervascularity
intratumoral h.
hypervascularization
hyperventilation
h. activating technique
autonomic h.
h. headache
h. seizure
h. test
h. tetany
hypervigilance
hyperviscosity syndrome
hypervitaminosis A
hypervolemia
hypervolemic treatment
hypesthesia, hypoesthesia
brachiofacial cortical h.
contralateral tactical h.
olfactory h.
trigeminal h.
hypesthetic ataxic hemiparesis
hyphema
hypnagogic
h. hallucination
h. hypersynchrony
h. image
h. state
hypnalgia
hypnapagogic
hypnesthesia
hypnic
h. headache
h. jerk
hypnoanalytic
hypnocinematograph
hypnodrama
hypnogenesis
hypnogenic spot
hypnogogic
hypnoid
hypnoidal state
hypnolepsy
hypnomania
Hypnomidate
hypnopathy
hypnopedia
hypnophrenosis
hypnopompic
h. hallucination
h. image
hypnosis
hypnotic
h. action
h. activity
h. agent
h. drug
h. sedative
hypnotic-dependent sleep disorder
hypnotic-induced
hypnoticus
status h.
hypnotist
hypnotoid
hypoactive
h. affect
h. limbic structure
hypoactivity
glutamatergic h.
hypoacusis
hypoadrenalism
hypoaffective
hypoalgesia (*var. of* hypalgesia)
hypobetalipoproteinemia
hypoblast
hypobulia
hypocalcemia
neonatal h.
premature infant h.
hypocapnia
hypochlorous acid (HOCI)
hypochondria
hypochondriac
h. neurosis
h. paranoia
h. psychoneurotic reaction
hypochondriacal
monosymptomatic h.
h. reaction
hypochondrial reflex
hypochondroplasia
hypocomplementemic urticarial vasculitis
hypocondriaque
folie h.
hypocortisolemia
hypocretin
h. axon
h. neural pathway
hypocrisy

NOTES

H

hypocrite
hypocupremia
hypodensity
white matter h.
hypodepression
hypodipsic hypernatremia
hypoechogenic peritumoral halo
hypoequilibrium
hypoergic
hypoesthesia (*var. of* hypesthesia)
hypofibrinogenemia
hypofolatemia
hypofrontality
hypofunction
hypofunctionality
hypoganglionosis
hypogastric
h. ganglion
h. nerve
h. reflex
hypogastricus
nervus h.
plexus h.
hypogenetic corpus callosum
hypogeusesthesia
hypogeusia
hypoglossal
h. canal lesion
h. cranial nerve
h. eminence
h. nerve [CN XII]
h. nerve palsy
h. nerve paresis
h. nerve testing
h. neuralgia
h. neuropathy
h. nucleus
h. triangle
h. trigone
hypoglossale
trigonum h.
hypoglossal-facial nerve anastomosis
hypoglossalis
nucleus h.
hypoglossi
ansa h.
descendens h.
eminentia h.
nucleus nervi h.
nucleus prepositus h.
rami linguales nervi h.
trigonum nervi h.
tuberculum h.
hypoglosso
rami communicantes nervi lingualis cum nervo h.
hypoglossus
hypoglycemic
h. coma
h. encephalopathy
h. peripheral neuropathy
h. seizure
hypoglycorrhachia of cerebrospinal fluid
hypogonadism with anosmia
hypohypnotic
hypointensity
hypokalemia
thiazide-induced h.
hypokalemic
h. metabolic acidosis
h. periodic paralysis
hypokinetic
h. dysarthria
h. syndrome
hypokyphosis
right thoracic curve with h.
thoracic h.
hypolemmal
hypolipidemic
hypologia
hypomagnesemia
neonatal h.
hypomania
treatment-emergent h.
hypomanic quality
hypomelanosis of Ito
hypometabolism
parietooccipitotemporal h.
prefrontal h.
hypometamorphosis
hypometria
hypomimia
hypomotor seizure
hypomyelinating condition
hypomyelination
childhood ataxia with cerebral h.
hypomyelinogenesis
hyponatremia
hyponatremic encephalopathy
hyponoic
hypopallesthesia
hypoparathyroid
h. encephalopathy
h. tetany
hypoparathyroidism
hypoperfusion
biparietal h.
bitemporal h.
cerebellar h.
cerebral h.
delayed postischemic h.
mesial temporal h.
parietooccipital h.
posterior frontal h.

posterior parietal h.
h. syndrome
temporoparietal h.
hypophonia
hypophonic aphasia
hypophosphatemia
hypophrasia
hypophyseal (*var. of* hypophysial)
hypophysectomize
hypophysectomy
h. forceps
partial central h.
total h.
transethmosphenoidal h.
transsphenoidal h.
unilateral h.
hypophyseoportal system
hypophyseopriva
hypophyseoprivic
hypophyseos
infundibulum lobi posterioris h.
lobus anterior h.
lobus glandularis h.
lobus posterior h.
pars intermedia lobi anterioris h.
pars nervosa h.
pars pharyngea h.
hypophyseotropic
hypophysial, hypophyseal
h. aneurysm
h. cachexia
h. forceps
h. fossa
h. grafting
h. portal system
h. stalk
h. stalk
h. syndrome
hypophysiopriva
cachexia h.
hypophysioprivic
hypophysiosphenoidal syndrome
hypophysis
alpha cell of anterior lobe of h.
anterior lobe of h.
h. cerebri
chromophobe cells of anterior lobe of h.
distal part of anterior lobe of h.
glandular lobe of h.
infundibular part of anterior lobe of h.
neural lobe of h.
neural part of h.
pharyngeal h.
posterior lobe of h.
h. punch forceps
h. sicca
tentorium of h.
hypophysitis
giant cell granulomatous h.
granulomatous h.
lymphocytic h.
lymphoid h.
pseudotumoral lymphocytic h.
hypopituitarism
hypopituitary coma
hypoplasia
cerebellar h.
condylar h.
falx h.
optic nerve h.
pituitary h.
hypoponesis
hypopotentia
hypopraxia
hypopselaphesia
hyporeactive
hyporeflexia
multisegmental h.
radicular h.
hyposensitivity
hyposmia
hyposomnia
hyposomniac
hyposthenia
hypostheniant
hyposthenic
hyposympathicotonus
hypotaxia
hypotaxis
hypotelorism
hypotension
acute severe h.
idiopathic orthostatic h.
intracranial h. (IH)
neurogenic orthostatic h.
orthostatic h.
spontaneous intracranial h.
sympathotonic orthostatic h.

NOTES

hypotensive
h. hemorrhage
h. retinopathy
h. surgery
hypothalami
infundibulum h.
lamina terminalis h.
nucleus anterior h.
nucleus arcuatus h.
nucleus dorsalis h.
nucleus dorsomedialis h.
nucleus paraventricularis anterior h.
nucleus posterior h.
nucleus supraopticus h.
nucleus ventrolateralis h.
nucleus ventromedialis h.
hypothalamic
h. acromegaly
h. amenorrhea
h. area
h. astrocytoma
h. blood flow
h. dysfunction
h. dysregulation
h. glioma
h. glucocorticoid
h. hamartoma
h. hypophysial gonadal axis
h. infundibulum
h. lesion
h. nucleus
nucleus posterior h.
h. obesity
h. pacemaker cell
h. regulating hormone
h. regulatory input
h. savage syndrome
h. sulcus
h. thermostat
hypothalamicae
zona h.
hypothalamic/chiasmatic glioma
hypothalamicorum
rami nucleorum h.
hypothalamic-pituitary
h.-p. axis
h.-p. dysfunction
h.-p. system
hypothalamic-pituitary-adrenal axis
hypothalamic-pituitary-adrenocortical system
hypothalamic-releasing factor
hypothalamicus
ramus h.
sulcus h.
hypothalamocerebellar fiber
hypothalamohypophysial
h. portal system
h. tract
hypothalamohypophysialis
tractus h.
hypothalamospinal
h. fiber
h. tract
hypothalamospinales
fibrae h.
hypothalamotomy
hypothalamus
anterior h.
dorsomedial nucleus of h.
interstitial nuclei of anterior h.
lateral zone of h.
medial zone of h.
paraventricular nucleus of h.
posterior nucleus of h.
preoptic h.
supraoptic nucleus of h.
ventromedial nucleus of h.
zone of h.
Hypotherm Gel Kap
hypothermia
controlled h.
fatal h.
h. I-bolt
regional h.
hypothermic metabolic index
hypothesis, pl. **hypotheses**
alpha, beta, gamma h.
clonal evolution h.
congenital h.
dedifferentiation h.
degenerative h.
free radical h.
gate-control h.
jelly roll h.
lipid h.
misdifferentiation h.
mnemic h.
Penfield h.
upregulation/downregulation h.
hypothesis-driven
VOL-based h.-d.
hypothymic
hypothyroid
h. dwarfism
h. neuropathy
hypothyroidism
congenital h.
neonatal h.
premature infant h.
hypotonia
benign congenital h.
essential h.

focal neonatal h.
muscular h.
neonatal h.
nitrazepam-induced h.
hypotonic cerebral palsy
hypotonicity
hypotonus
hypotony
ocular h.
hypotropia
hypotube
nitinol h.
hypoventilation
h. coma
primary alveolar h.
hypovolemia
hypovolemic shock
hypoxanthine
h. guanine phosphoribosyltransferase
h. guanine phosphoribosyltransferase deficiency
hypoxemia
nocturnal h.
hypoxia
anemic h.
anoxic h.
cerebral h.
delayed coma after h.
histotoxic h.
hypoxic h.
ischemic h.
relative h.
short-term h.
stagnant h.
toxic h.
hypoxia-related headache
hypoxic
h. brain damage
h. cerebral vasodilatation
h. hypoxia
h. ischemia
h. ischemic encephalopathy (HIE)
h. ventilatory response
hypoxic-hypercarbic encephalopathy
hypoxic-ischemic
h.-i. brain
h.-i. brain damage
h.-i. injury
h.-i. insult
hypsarhythmia, hypsarrhythmia
hypsarrhythmic electroencephalographic pattern
hypsicephalic
hypsicephaly
hypsocephaly
hypsokinesis
Hyrtl
H. anastomosis
H. foramen
H. loop
hysteresis
hysterica
megalopia h.
suffocation h.
hysterical
h. amnesia
h. anesthesia
h. aphonia
h. ataxia
h. blindness
h. chorea
h. convulsion
h. dementia
h. depression
h. fugue state
h. gait
h. gait disorder
h. hearing impairment
h. hemiplegia
h. movement disorder
h. mutism
h. paralysis
h. polydipsia
h. pseudodementia
h. seizure
h. syncope
h. torticollis
h. tremor
h. visual loss
h. voices
hysteric coma-like state
hystericoneuralgic
hystericus
clavus h.
globus h.
hysterocatalepsy
hysteroepilepsy
hysteroepileptogenous point
hysterogenic
hysterogenous
hysteroid convulsion

NOTES

hysteromania

Hytrast

I
I band
I substance
IADL
instrumental activities of daily living
IADSA
intraarterial digital subtraction angiography
IAP
intermittent acute porphyria
iatrogenic
i. carotid-cavernous fistula
i. complication
i. discitis
i. disease
i. effect
i. elevatus
i. hematoma
i. instability
i. lumbar kyphosis
IBBB
intrablood-brain barrier
I-bolt
hypothermia I.-b.
Texas Scottish Rite Hospital I.-b.
I-boundary
Ibuprohm
Ibu-Tab
IC
illusionary contour
imprinting center
Codman IC
IC effect
ICA
internal carotid artery
ICA-occluded stable Xe/CT CBF study
ice
i. cream headache
i. pick-like pain
i. pick pain
ICEEG
intracranial electroencephalogram
Iceland disease
Icelandic form of intracranial hemorrhage
I-cell disease
ice-pick headache
ichthyotoxism
IC-IC
intracranial-intracranial
IC-IC bypass
ICIDH
International Classification of Impairments, Disabilities and Handicaps
I-complex
ICP
intracranial pressure
ICP Camino bolt
ICP catheter
ICP microsensor
ICP monitor
ICP wave form
ICP-T
intracranial pressure-temperature
ICP-T fiberoptic ICP intracranial temperature catheter
ICP-T fiberoptic ICP monitoring catheter
ictal
i. amnesia
i. automatism
i. cerebral perfusion pattern
i. confusional seizure
i. EEG pattern
i. epileptiform abnormality
i. epileptiform activity
i. epileptiform pattern
i. fear
i. focal epileptiform discharge
i. localization
i. onset zone
i. pattern on EEG
i. period
i. polygram
i. propagation
i. semiology
i. speech
i. vomiting
ictus
i. epilepticus
i. paralyticus
i. sanguinis
ICVM
intracranial vascular malformation
ID
index of difficulty
ida
tripa i.
idazoxan
IDEA
Individuals with Disabilities Education Act
idealizing transference
ideal spinal implant

ideational
i. agnosia
i. apraxia
ideatory apraxia
idebenone
idenenone
identical elements
identification process
identified trait
identity diffusion
ideokinetic apraxia
ideological orientation
ideomotion
ideomotor
i. apraxia
i. dyspraxia
ideoplastia
ideoplastic stage
ideovascular
IDET
intradiscal electrothermal therapy
IDET procedure
idiocy
amaurotic i.
athetosic i.
eclamptic i.
hemiplegic i.
hydrocephalic i.
mongolian i.
paraplegic i.
xerodermic i.
idiodynamic control
idiogamist
idiogenic osmoles
idioglossia
idioglottic
idiographic
idioimbecile
idiojunctional rhythm
idiolect
idiolog
idiomuscular
idiopathic
i. bilateral vestibulopathy
i. calcification
i. chronic hiccup
i. CNS hypersomnolence
i. facial nerve palsy
i. generalized epilepsy
i. generalized epilepsy syndrome
i. growth hormone deficiency
i. hyper-CKemia
i. hypertrophic cranial pachymeningitis
i. inflammatory myopathy (IIM)
i. intracranial hypertension (IIH)
i. intracranial pachymeningitis
i. meningitis
i. muscular atrophy
i. myelofibrosis (IMF)
i. normal pressure hydrocephalus (INPH)
i. orbital pseudotumor
i. orthostatic hypotension
i. Parkinson disease
i. Parsonage-Turner syndrome
i. partial epilepsy
i. peripheral neuropathy
i. plexus neuritis
i. polyneuropathy
i. recurring stupor
i. seizure
i. stabbing headache
i. thoracic scoliosis
i. thrombocytopenic purpura (ITP)
i. trigeminal neuralgia (ITN)
idiopathic/cryptogenic
idiopathy
idiophrenic
idioreflex
idiospasm
idiosyncrasia olfactoria
idiosyncratic
i. basis
i. intoxication
IDP
inflammatory demyelinating polyneuropathy
IDPL
injected dose per liter
iduronate sulfatase
IENF
intraepidermal nerve fiber
IFET
ischemic forearm exercise test
ifiasochism
verbal i.
IFN
interferon
IFN-B1a
Avonex
IFN-B1b
Betaferon
IFN-gamma
interferon-gamma
IGF
insulinlike growth factor
IgG
immunoglobulin G
Iggo receptor
IgM
immunoglobulin M
IgM antibody capture
IgM GM-1 antiganglioside antibody

IGMIT
image-guided minimally invasive therapy
IH
intracranial hypotension
IHS
International Headache Society
IHWOP
intracranial hypertension without papilledema
IIH
idiopathic intracranial hypertension
IIM
idiopathic inflammatory myopathy
Ikematsu
method of I.
I-labeled cocaine analog
ileocolic plexus
Iletin
Lente I. II
Protamine Zinc and I. I
Ilhéus encephalitis
iliac
i. artery injury
i. crest bone graft stabilization
i. crest resection
i. crest syndrome
i. fixation
i. post
i. screw
iliacus
plexus i.
iliocostal muscle
iliofemoral thrombosis
iliohypogastrici
ramus cutaneus anterior nervi i.
ramus cutaneus lateralis nervi i.
iliohypogastric nerve
iliohypogastricus
nervus i.
ilioinguinalis
nervus i.
ilioinguinal nerve
iliopsoas muscle
iliopubic nerve
iliopubicus
nervus i.
iliosacral
i. and iliac fixation construct
i. screw
Ilizarov corticotomy
IL-1
interleukin-1
illegal drug synthesis
illness
autoimmune i.
brain i.
comorbid i.
debilitating i.
dementing i.
fatigue of systemic i.
monophasic i.
neurological i.
objective severity of i.
outcome of i.
viral-mediated i.
illumination
Luxtec coaxial i.
illuminator
XL i.
illusion
auditory i.
i. des sosies
Kanizsa i.
i. of power
illusionary contour (IC)
illusory memory
imafen hydrochloride
image
accidental i.
i. acquisition time
angio i.
autoradiographic i.
axial magnetic resonance i.
axial spin-echo i.
B-mode i.
body i.
contrast-enhanced MR i.
coregistered i.
i. correlation
cross-sectional i.
dangerous i.
diffusion-weighted echo plantar i. (DW-EPI)
echo planar i.
i. foldover
i. formation principle
ghost i.
gradient-echo echo planar i.
gradient-echo magnetic resonance i.
gradient-echo MR i.
gradient-recalled echo i.

NOTES

image *(continued)*
i. guidance
i. guided solution
hypnagogic i.
hypnopompic i.
imperfect i.
incidental i.
in-phase i.
i. intensification
i. intensifier
long pulse repetition time/echo time i.
magnetic resonance i. (MRI)
midsagittal i.
motor i.
negative i.
i. neurosurgery
neutral i.
out-of-phase i.
PET i.
phantom i.
positive i.
proton-weighted i.
i. quality
raw speckled i.
reformatted i.
i. registration
sagittal spin-echo i.
sagittal T1-weighted SE i.
sagittal T1-weighted spin echo i.
sensory i.
short pulse repetition time/echo time i.
source i.
SPECT i.
spin-echo T1-weighted plan i.
stereotactic PET i.
tactile i.
thin-section i.
tilting of visual i.
T1-weighted magnetic resonance i.
T2-weighted magnetic resonance i.
T1-weighted MR i.
T2-weighted MR i.
T1-weighted spin-echo i.
T2-weighted spin-echo i.
T2-weighted turbo-gradient i.

ImageBox
MediLive I.

image-guided
i.-g. minimally invasive therapy (IGMIT)
i.-g. stereotactic brain biopsy

image-integrated surgery treatment planning

Imagent
I. BP
I. GI
I. LN
I. US

imager
CERESPECT brain i.
Magnes 2500 WH i.
1.5-T i.

imaging
BCI X9digitX Cardial I.
blood oxygen level-dependent functional magnetic resonance i. (BOLD f-MRI)
blood pool i.
brain i.
cerebrovascular magnetic resonance i.
chemical-shift i.
Chopper-Dixon hybrid i.
cine phase contrast magnetic resonance i.
color-flow i.
computerized infrared telethermographic i.
continuous-wave Doppler i.
contrast-enhanced MR i.
contrast enhancement i.
2DFT gradient-echo i.
3DFT gradient-echo MR i.
Diasonics magnetic resonance i.
diffuse tension i. (DTI)
diffusion-perfusion magnetic resonance i.
diffusion tension i.
diffusion tensor i. (DTI)
diffusion tensor magnetic resonance i. (diffusion tensor MRI)
diffusion-weighted i. (DWI)
diffusion-weighted magnetic resonance i.
digital vascular i. (DVI)
direct multiplanar i.
Dixon method opposed i.
Doppler i.
echo planar i.
fast i.
fat-suppression MR i.
FLAIR sequence magnetic resonance i.
flow-sensitive magnetic resonance i. (FS MRI)
flow-sensitive MR i.
fluid-attenuated inversion recovery sequence magnetic resonance i.
fluoroscopic i.
functional brain i.
functional magnetic resonance i. (f-MRI)

gadolinium-enhanced MR i.
Gd-DTPA-enhanced cranial MR i.
gradient-echo MR i.
gradient-refocused i.
half-Fourier i.
half-NEX i.
high-resolution 3DFT MR i.
intrinsic i.
line i.
Magnes magnetic source i.
magnetic resonance i. (MRI)
magnetic resonance perfusion i.
magnetic source i. (MSI)
i. method
i. modularity
MR volumetry i.
i. multiplanar
multiple line-scan i.
multiple plane i.
neurodiagnostic i.
neuroreceptor i.
neurovascular i.
nonproton magnetic resonance i.
nuclear i.
oblique sagittal gradient-echo MR i.
orthogonal polarized spectral i. (OPSI)
partial flip angle i.
partial Fourier i.
perfusion-weighted i.
phase-sensitive gradient-echo MR i.
planar spin i.
point i.
proton i.
pulsed Doppler i.
quantitative i.
radionuclide i.
rapid acquisition radiofrequency-echo steady state i.
real-time color Doppler i.
reproducible target i.
second harmonic i. (SHI)
sequential plane i.
sequential point i.
serial i.
short inversion recovery i.
simultaneous volume i.
spin-echo i.
spin-warp i.
structural magnetic resonance i.
i. study
subtraction i.
surface coil spectroscopic i.
surveillance i.
^{99m}Tc-HMPAO SPECT i.
Tc-99m HMPAO cerebral perfusion SPECT i.
three-dimensional fast low-angle shot i.
three-dimensional Fourier transform gradient-echo i.
time-variance i. (TVI)
transcranial real-time color Doppler i.
two-dimensional Fourier transform gradient-echo i.
two-dimensional proton echo-planar spectroscopic i.
in vivo i.

imbalance
acid-base i.
autonomic i.
calcium metabolism i.
dopamine-acetylcholine i.
electrolyte i.
magnesium i.
potassium i.
sodium i.
sympathetic i.
vasomotor i.

IMF
idiopathic myelofibrosis

imidazopyridine

iminoglycinuria

imipenem-cilastatin injection

imipramine
i. HCl
i. hydrochloride
i. neurotoxicity

imitative tetanus

Imitrex

immaturity
cognitive function i.

immediate
i. control
i. early gene
i. early gene cascade
i. posttraumatic automatism
i. posttraumatic convulsion

immigration
macrophage i.

NOTES

immitis
Coccidioides i.
immobile face
immobilization
halo-vest i.
i. method
postoperative i.
sternal occipital mandibular i.
sternooccipital-mandibular i. (SOMI)
Treponema pallidum i.
immobilizer
sternooccipitomanubrial i.
immortalized primary cell culture
immune
chorea i.
i. complex
i. dysregulation
i. mediated mechanism
i. response
i. system
immunity
cell-mediated i.
immunocompetent macrophage
immunocompromised host
immunocytochemical
i. analysis
i. assay
immunoelectrotransfer blot technique
immunofluorescence assay
immunoglobulin
i. G (IgG)
i. kappa light chain
i. M (IgM)
i. treatment
immunohistochemical
i. study
i. technique
immunohistochemistry
BrDu i.
Southwestern i.
immunologic
i. abnormality
i. aspect
i. dysfunction
i. nitric oxide synthase
immunological paralysis
immunology
multiple sclerosis i.
immunoperoxidase
i. method
i. procedure
i. staining
immunoreactive
plasma i. (PI-R)
immunostimulatory gene transfer
immunosuppressive
i. drug
i. effect
i. medication
i. therapy
immunotoxin
immunoturbidimetry analyzer
IMPA cephalometric measurement
impact
disruptive i.
pharmacologic i.
systemic i.
impactor
Cloward bone graft i.
vertebral body i.
impaired
Assessment for Persons Profoundly or Severely I.
i. attentional functioning
i. cerebral function
i. cognition
i. concentration
consciousness i.
i. control
i. drug metabolism
i. face recognition
i. limbic-diencephalic function
i. memory
i. migration of brain neuron
i. neuromuscular transmission
i. object recognition
i. vision
impairment
age-associated memory i.
age-related memory i.
anterior horn cell motor i.
autonomic i.
basic i.
category specific semantic i.
cerebral i.
Clinician Rated Overall Life I.
cognitive i.
communication i.
constructional i.
early speech i.
frontal lobe i.
functional/cognitive i.
functional hearing i.
gaze i.
general medical i.
global cognitive i.
global measure of i.
graphic i.
high-frequency hearing i.
hysterical hearing i.
initial spoken language i.
intellectual i.
level of i.
life i.

medical i.
memory i.
mental i.
mild cognitive i. (MCI)
motivation i.
motor i.
narrative speech perception i.
neurocognitive i.
nonlanguage cognitive i.
perceptual-motor ability i.
peripheral nerve level motor i.
phonologic assembly i.
preexisting cognitive i.
psychogenic hearing i.
psychomotor i.
i. Rating score
root level motor i.
saccade i.
semantic memory i.
sensory i.
severe i.
social i.
speech processing i.
spinal nerve level motor i.
spoken language i.
supranuclear vertical gaze i.
temporal lobe i.
transient cognitive i. (TCI)
upper motor neuron i.
vascular cognitive i.
verbal memory i.
visual memory i.
volitional i.

impar
ganglion i.
nervus i.

impedance
i. artifact
i. audiometry
electrode i.
i. method
middle ear i.
static acoustic i.

impediment
environmental i.

impending herniation

imperfect
i. image
i. image registration

imperfecta
dentinogenesis i.
osteogenesis i. (OI)

impersistence
motor i.

impingement
anterior cord i.
corpus callosal i.

implant
Activa Tremor Control System i.
Arenberg-Denver inner-ear valve i.
auditory brainstem i. (ABI)
broken existing i.
Ceratite ceramic i.
Christoferson disk bony i.
cochlear i.
custom i.
DTT i.
embryonic i.
epidural i.
epilepsy i.
i. fatigue
ferromagnetic i.
fetal dopaminergic tissue i.
fetal neural i.
Gliadel i.
hard tissue replacement-malleable facial i.
hard tissue replacement-patient-matched i.
HTR-MFI chin i.
HTR-MFI curved i.
HTR-MFI malar i.
HTR-MFI paranasal i.
HTR-MFI premaxillary i.
HTR-MFI ramus i.
HTR-MFI straight i.
HTR-PMI i.
Hunter open cord tendon i.
ideal spinal i.
iodine-125 i.
KLS-Martin i.
lumbar anterior-root stimulator i.
MacroSorb absorbable plate i.
metallic otologic i.
NeuroControl Freehand i.
nicardipine prolonged-release i.
Nucleus 24 multichannel auditory brainstem i.
otologic i.
patient-matched i.

NOTES

implant *(continued)*
- Polaris adjustable spinal cage i.
- i. removal
- Schwann-cell i.
- silicone i.
- i. survival rate
- tissue i.
- TSRH i.
- vagal nerve i.
- vagus stimulator i.
- Zielke VDS i.

implantation
- brachytherapy seed i.
- i. cone
- DBS electrode i.
- nerve i.
- screw i.
- subdural grid i.
- i. technique

implanted
- i. infusion pump
- i. polymer

implicit process

implosion therapy

impotentia generandi

impregnation
- Bodian silver i.

impressio
- i. petrosa pallii
- i. petrosa pallii incisura
- i. trigeminalis ossis temporalis
- i. trigemini ossis temporalis

impression
- basilar i.
- cervical spine basilar i.
- diagnostic i.

impressive aphasia

imprinting
- i. center (IC)
- i. center mutation analysis
- i. defect
- genomic i.

improper dose

improved
- i. communication skill
- Isollyl I.

improvement
- clinical i.
- cognitive i.
- life-changing i.
- spontaneous i.

impulse
- i. asynchrony
- forced i.
- nerve i.
- neural i.
- i. neurosis
- nociceptive i.

impulsive
- i. petit mal epilepsy
- i. spectrum

impulsive-aggressive trait

impulsivity
- counteracting i.
- lifetime i.

impunitive response

iMRI
- PoleStar N-10 i.

Imuran

imus
- nervus splanchnicus thoracicus i.

in
- in situ hybridization
- in situ photocoagulation
- in situ spinal fusion
- in situ tricortical iliac-crest block bone graft
- in toto
- in utero teratologic agent
- in vitro molecular study
- in vitro spectra
- in vivo benzodiazepine receptor binding
- in vivo brain functioning
- in vivo data
- in vivo ^{1}H magnetic resonance spectroscopy
- in vivo imaging
- in vivo optical spectroscopy (INVOS)
- in vivo situational exposure
- in vivo stereological assessment

inability to function independently

inactivation
- functional hippocampal i.

inactivator
- electrocerebral i.

inactivity
- behavioral i.
- electrocerebral i. (ECI)

inadequate
- i. impulse control
- i. stimulus
- i. therapy

inanimate learning device

inappropriate verbalizing

inattention
- sensory i.
- visual i.

inborn
- i. error of metabolism
- i. reflex

incapacitating drowsiness

incarceration
cauda equina i.
incendiare
monomanie i.
incentive system
incerta
zona i.
incidence
age-specific cumulative i.
myelopathy i.
nonunion i.
incidental
i. aneurysm
i. dual pathology
i. image
i. punctate white matter hyperintensity
incipient downward central brain herniation
incision
battledore i.
bifrontal i.
Brunner modified i.
Caldwell-Luc i.
circumscribing i.
coronal scalp i.
C-shaped i.
curved i.
deltoid-splitting i.
dural i.
elliptical i.
exploratory i.
eyebrow i.
hemitransfixion i.
horseshoe i.
Kocher collar i.
laterally convex dural i.
lateral rhinotomy i.
Lynch i.
Mayfield i.
midline i.
muscle-splitting i.
Naffziger straight midline i.
palatal mucosal i.
posterolateral costotransversectomy i.
right-sided submandibular transverse i.
S i.
scalp i.
skin i.
standard retroperitoneal flank i.
straight i.
tangential i.
transcortical i.
transverse i.
T-shaped i.
vertical midline i.
V-shaped i.
Weber-Fergusson i.
webspace i.
Y i.
incisional neuroma
incisive plexus
incisura, pl. **incisurae**
i. cerebelli anterior
i. cerebelli posterior
impressio petrosa pallii i.
i. jugularis ossis occipitalis
i. jugularis ossis temporalis
i. preoccipitalis
tentorial i.
i. tentorii
i. tentorii cerebelli
incisural
i. dissection
i. space
incisure
Lanterman i.
Lanterman-Schmidt i.
occipital bone jugular i.
preoccipital i.
Schmidt-Lanterman i.
temporal bone jugular i.
tentorial i.
i. of tentorium of cerebellum
inclusion
i. body
i. body encephalitis
i. body myopathy
i. cell disease
cytoplasmic i.
intracellular lipid i.
intraneuronal i.
i. lipoma
Pick i.
i. tumor
inclusion-body myositis
incogitant
incomplete
i. alexia
i. band heterotopia

NOTES

Indiana
I. tome carpal tunnel release system
I. type familial amyloid polyneuropathy
Indian variant lipofuscinosis
indicator
finger i.
sensor position i.
sleep position i. (SPI)
indices (*pl. of* index)
indicis
indicophose
indifference to pain syndrome
indifferent electrode
indigo carmine
indigotin disulfonate sodium
indirect
i. fracture
i. genetic transmission
i. mechanism
i. probe
i. reflex
i. striatopallidal pathway
indiscriminate lesion
indium-111
i. octreotide scintigraphy
indium cisternogram
indium-diethylene triamine pentaacetic acid study
Individuals with Disabilities Education Act (IDEA)
Indochron E-R capsule
indolamine function
indolaminergic pathway
indomethacin-responsive headache syndrome
induced
i. aphasia
i. factitious symptom
inducer
angiogenic i.
InDura intrathecal catheter and pump
indusium griseum
ineffective communication pattern
inequality
ventilation/perfusion i.
Inerpan flexible burn dressing
inertia
sleep i.
i. time
inescapable pain
inexact fiducial
inexorable decline
In-Exsufflator respiratory device
infancy
diencephalic syndrome of i.
familial autosomal recessive idiopathic myoclonic epilepsy of i.
heterotopic interstitial neuropathy of i.
melanotic neuroectodermal tumor of i. (MNTI)
spongy degeneration of i.
infant
traction response of i.
infantile
i. acid maltase deficiency
i. amnesia
i. beriberi
i. botulism
i. convulsion
i. diplegia
i. ganglioglioma
i. Gaucher disease
i. G_{M2} gangliosidosis
i. hemangioblastic hemangioma
i. hemiplegia
i. hydrocephalus
i. inflammatory multisystem disease
i. jerk myoclonus
i. lipofuscinosis
i. multisystem inflammatory disease
i. myofibrillar myopathy
i. myofibromatosis
i. neuroaxonal dystrophy
i. neuronal degeneration
i. neuropathy
i. progressive spinal muscular atrophy
i. Refsum disease
i. spasm
i. spastic paraplegia
i. subacute necrotizing encephalopathy
i. tetany
i. X-linked ataxia
i. X-linked deafness
infantilis
diataxia cerebralis i.

NOTES

infantilis *(continued)*
poliodystrophia cerebri progressiva i.
progressiva i.
Infant's
I. Feverall
I. Silapap
infarction, infarct
anterior communicating artery distribution i.
arteriolar i.
atherosclerotic i.
bicerebral i.
bilateral occipital i.
bilateral upper brain stem i.
borderzone i.
brain i.
brainstem i.
calcarine cortex i.
capsular i.
capsulocaudate i.
capsuloputaminal i.
capsuloputaminocaudate i.
cerebellar artery i.
cerebral artery i.
cerebrovascular i.
cortical i.
cryptogenic i.
cystic lacunar i.
i. dementia
dominant hemisphere i.
dorsopontomesencephalic lacunar i.
embolic i.
Freiberg so-called i.
frontal lobe i.
gyral i.
hemispheric i.
hemorrhagic i.
hippocampal i.
inferolateral i.
ischemic brainstem i.
ischemic cerebral i.
lacunar brain i.
large-artery i.
large-vessel i.
medium vessel i.
medullary i.
mesencephalic i.
midbrain i.
migraine-induced i.
migrainous i.
multiple cortical i.
myocardial i.
nonembolic i.
nonseptic embolic brain i.
occipital lobe i.
optic nerve i.
paramedian i.
parietooccipital i.
perinatal i.
photochemically-induced graded spinal cord i.
photothrombotic i.
pontine i.
posterior cerebral territory i.
putaminal i.
retinal i.
right frontoparietal i.
silent i.
small centrum ovale i.
small deep recent i.
small lacunar i.
small-penetrator i. (SPI)
small-vessel i.
spinal cord i.
striatocapsular i.
subcortical i.
subendocardial myocardial i.
temporal lobe i.
thalamic i.
thalamopeduncular i.
tuberothalamic i.
ventral pontine i.
vertebrobasilar i.
i. volume
watershed i.
white matter i.
infarctlike lesion
infection
Absidia i.
Acanthamoeba i.
amebic i.
arenavirus i.
bacterial i.
baculovirus i.
Campylobacter jejuni i.
Candida i.
central nervous system influenza virus i.
cerebral i.
cestode i.
chronic spinal epidural i.
chronic spinal intradural i.
closed disk space i.
clostridial i.
Coccidioides i.
congenital cytomegalovirus i.
congenital herpes simplex virus i.
Coxiella burnetii i.
cryptococcal i.
Cryptococcus i.
cryptogenic i.
cysticercal i.
disk space i.

enteric virus i.
enterovirus i.
epidural i.
extradural i.
extrameningeal tuberculous i.
fever caused by i. (FI)
focal i.
fungal i.
helminthic i.
herpesvirus i. type 6, 7
herpes zoster virus i.
Histoplasma i.
human immunodeficiency virus i.
intervertebral disk space i.
latent i.
Legionella pneumophila i.
lytic i.
meningeal i.
mosquito bite i.
Mucor i.
Mycobacterium tuberculosis i.
Mycoplasma i.
mycotic i.
myxovirus i.
Naegleria i.
nematode i.
neonatal enterovirus i.
neonatal herpes simplex virus i.
nervous system i.
nosocomial i.
odontogenic i.
ophthalmic zoster i.
opportunistic i.
orthomyxovirus i.
parainfluenza virus i.
paramyxovirus i.
parasitic i.
paraspinal i.
pediatric autoimmune neuropsychiatric diseases associated with streptococcal i. (PANDAS)
Phycomycetes rhizopus i.
poliomyelitis i.
poliovirus i.
postoperative i.
i. prevention
protozoan i.
retrovirus i.
rhabdovirus i.
Rhizopus i.
rickettsial i.
roseola i.
scalp i.
Shigella dysenteriae i.
slow-virus i.
spinal cord i.
spirochetal i.
streptococcal i.
togavirus i.
trematode i.
varicella zoster virus i.
ventriculostomy-related i.
viral i.
zoster virus i.

infection-related neuropathy

infectious
i. aneurysm
i. hepatitis peripheral neuropathy
i. mononucleosis
i. ophthalmoplegia
i. polyneuritis
i. polyneuritis syndrome
i. retinopathy

infectiva
polioencephalitis i.

inferior
i. anastomotic vein
i. anterocaudal cingulate cortex
i. aperture of axillary fossa
area vestibularis i.
i. basal vein
i. cerebellar artery
i. cerebellar peduncle
i. cerebral surface
i. cerebral vein
i. cervical ganglion
i. choroid plexus
i. choroid vein
colliculus i.
complexus olivaris i.
i. dental nerve
i. extradural approach
fasciculus longitudinalis i.
fasciculus occipitofrontalis i.
i. fovea
i. frontal convolution
i. frontal gyrus
i. frontal sulcus
i. ganglion of glossopharyngeal nerve
i. ganglion of vagus

NOTES

inferior *(continued)*
i. ganglion of vagus nerve
gyrus frontalis i.
gyrus temporalis i.
i. horn
i. horn of lateral ventricle
i. laryngeal nerve
lobulus parietalis i.
lobulus semilunaris i.
i. longitudinal fasciculus
i. longitudinal sinus
macula cribrosa i.
i. medullary velum
i. mesenteric ganglion
i. nasal colliculus
nervus cardiacus cervicalis i.
nervus cutaneous brachii lateralis i.
nervus gluteus i.
nervus laryngealis i.
nervus laryngeus i.
nevus alveolus i.
nucleus olivaris i.
nucleus salivarius i.
nucleus salivatorius i.
nucleus vestibularis i.
i. occipital gyrus
i. occipitofrontal fasciculus
oliva i.
i. olivary complex
i. olivary nucleus
i. olive
i. orbital fissure
i. orbitofrontal complex
i. parietal gyrus
i. parietal lobule
i. parietal region
i. part of vestibulocochlear nerve
pedunculus cerebellaris i.
pedunculus thalami i.
i. periventricular white matter
i. petrosal ganglion
i. petrosal sinus
plexus dentalis i.
plexus hypogastricus i.
plexus mesentericus i.
plexus rectalis i.
i. polioencephalitis
i. pontine syndrome
i. prefrontal cortex
i. quadrigeminal brachium
radiatio thalami i.
i. rectus muscle
i. root of ansa cervicalis
i. root of cervical loop
i. root of vestibulocochlear nerve
i. sagittal sinus
i. salivary nucleus
i. salivatory nucleus
i. semilunar lobule
sinus petrosus i.
sinus sagittalis i.
sulcus frontalis i.
sulcus temporalis i.
i. surface of cerebellar hemisphere
i. syndrome of red nucleus
tela choroidea i.
i. temporal convolution
i. temporal cortex
i. temporal gyrus
i. temporal sulcus
i. thalamic peduncle
i. thalamic radiation
i. thalamostriate vein
i. thyroid plexus
i. transvermian approach
i. vein of cerebellar hemisphere
i. vein of vermis
vena anastomotica i.
i. vena cava
vena choroidea i.
vena ventricularis i.
vena vermis i.
i. ventricular vein
i. vertebra
i. vestibular area
i. vestibular nucleus

inferiore
ramus communicans nervi laryngei superioris cum nervo laryngeo i.

inferiores
nervi anales i.
nervi clunium i.
nervi rectales i.
nuclei olivares i.
rami clunium i.
rami gluteales i.
venae cerebelli i.
venae cerebri i.
venae hemispherii cerebelli i.
venae thalamostriatae i.

inferioris
brachium colliculi i.
commissura colliculi i.
hilum nuclei olivaris i.
nuclei colliculi i.
nucleus linearis i.
nucleus reticularis intermedius pontis i.
pars opercularis gyri frontalis i.
pars orbitalis gyri frontalis i.
pars triangularis gyri frontalis i.
rami dentales inferiores plexus dentalis i.

rami gingivales inferiores plexus dentalis i.
vellus olivae i.

inferior-lateral endonasal transsphenoidal approach

inferius
brachium quadrigeminum i.
cornu i.
ganglion cervicale i.
ganglion mesentericum i.
velum medullare i.

inferofrontal fissure

inferolateral
i. infarction
i. pontine artery

inferolateralis
margo i.

infiltrating tumor

infiltration
hematogenous cell i.
paraneural i.
perineural i.

InFix interbody fusion system

inflammation
arterial i.
cartilage i.
ear cartilage i.
ischemic ocular i.
lipopolysaccharide-induced i.
neurogenic i. (NI)
spinal cord i.

inflammation-induced cell injury

inflammatory
i. cytokine
i. demyelinating disease
i. demyelinating neuropathy
i. demyelinating optic neuritis
i. demyelinating polyneuropathy (IDP)
i. demyelinating polyradiculoneuropathy
i. lesion
i. myopathy
i. response

inflow effect

influence
vestibulospinal i.

influenza
i. A antibody
i. A pandemic
i. virus myositis

influenzae
Haemophilus i.
Haemophilus i. b

influenzal encephalitis

information
afferent thermosensory i.
biochemical i.
release of i.
sensory i.
i. technology
thermosensory i.
i. underload
verbal i.

infracalcarine gyrus

infracerebral

infraclinoid aneurysm

infradian rhythm

infragranular
i. layer
i. region

infranuclear
i. lesion
i. paralysis
i. weakness

infraorbital
i. injection
i. nerve
i. plexus

infraorbitalis
nervus i.
rami labiales superiores nervi i.
rami nasales externi nervi i.
rami nasales interni nervi i.
rami palpebrales inferiores nervi i.

infrapiriform foramen

infrared
i. digitizer
i. light-reflecting sphere
i. thermography (IRT)

infraspinatus reflex

infraspinous fascia

infrastriate layer

infratemporal
i. approach
i. fossa (ITF)
i. fossa tumor
i. hematoma

infratentorial
i. arteriovenous malformation
i. compartment
i. lateral supracellular approach

NOTES

infratentorial *(continued)*
i. lesion
i. neoplastic syndrome
i. neurological tumor
i. region
i. structural syndrome
i. supracerebellar
i. venous drainage
infratentorial-Lindau tumor
infratrochlearis
nervus i.
rami palpebrales nervi i.
infratrochlear nerve
infundibula (*pl. of* infundibulum)
infundibular
i. body
i. dilatation
i. part
i. part of anterior lobe of hypophysis
i. recess
i. stalk
i. stem
infundibularis
nucleus i.
pars i.
recessus i.
infundibuli
recessus i.
infundibulohypophysitis
necrotizing i.
infundibuloma
infundibulotubular region
infundibulum, pl. **infundibula**
aditus ad i.
i. hypothalami
hypothalamic i.
iter ad i.
i. lobi posterioris hypophyseos
i. neurohypophyseos
Infusaid M400 constant flow pump
infusion
brain i.
brain-heart i. (BHI)
i. computed tomography
continuous extravascular i. (CEI)
continuous intrathecal baclofen i.
continuous intravenous i.
diastole-phased pulsatile i.
etomidate-propylene glycol i.
intraparenchymal i.
intraventricular i.
propofol i.
i. pump
Inge
I. cervical lamina spreader
I. laminectomy retractor
I. laminectomy spreader
Ingraham-Fowler tantalum clip
Ingraham skull punch forceps
ingravescent apoplexy
ingrowth
neuronal i.
inguinal
i. freckling
i. reflex
inhalation
CO_2 i.
oxygen i.
xenon i.
inherent contrast
inheritance
autosomal dominant i.
autosomal recessive i.
mendelian i.
inherited
i. ataxia
i. global neurodegenerative disorder
inhibited response
inhibition
collagenase i.
complement fixation i.
dopaminergic i.
GABAergic i.
$GABA_B$ receptor-mediated i.
GABAR-mediated i.
horizontal i.
mediated neuronal i.
paired-pulse i.
pervasive i.
Wedensky i.
inhibitor
acetyl cholinesterase i.
angiogenic i.
batimastat protease i.
calpain i.
carbonic anhydrase i.
caspase i.
catechol-methyl-transferase i.
catechol-*O*-methyltransferase i.
cholinesterase i.
COMT i.
converting enzyme i. (CEI)
COX-2 i.
cyclooxygenase i.
cysteine protease i.
cytokine i.
dopa decarboxylase i.
endothelial cell i.
epidermal growth factor-tyrosine kinase i. (EGPR-TKI)
excitatory amino acid receptor i.
excitotoxin i.

farnesyl transferase i.
growth factor i.
5-HT reuptake i.
marimastat protease i.
matrix metalloproteinase i.
metalloprotease i.
monoamine oxidase i. (MAOI)
monoamine oxidase-B i.
NOS i.
peptide i.
plasminogen activator i.
polyamine biosynthesis i.
protease i.
protein kinase C i.
reductase i.
selective norepinephrine reuptake i.
selective phosphodiesterase i.
selective serotonin reuptake i. (SSRI)
serotonin norepinephrine reuptake i.
signal transduction i.
Src i.
thromboxane synthase i.
tissue factor pathway i.
xanthine oxidase i.

inhibitory
i. amino acid
i. effect
i. fiber
i. ganglion
i. loop
i. nerve
i. neurotransmitter
i. postsynaptic current
i. postsynaptic potential (IPSP)
i. protein
i. regulatory input
i. synapse
i. transmitter
i. virus

inhomogeneity
field i.

iniencephaly

initial
i. segment
i. spoken language impairment
i. stage
i. stress reaction
i. upward deflection

initiative
Parkinson Research The Organized Genetic I. (PROGENI)

Inject-Ease

injected dose per liter (IDPL)

injection
Adlone I.
A-methaPred I.
AquaMEPHYTON I.
Ben-Allergin-50 I.
botulinum toxin i.
Calciferol I.
Calcimar I.
Campath subcu i.
Carnitor I.
Cibacalcin I.
conjunctival i.
Cytoxan I.
depMedalone I.
Depoject I.
Depo-Medrol I.
Depopred I.
D.H.E. 45 I.
Diazemuls I.
D-Med I.
Dopascan i.
Enlon I.
epidural steroid i.
etomidate i.
extradural i.
focal stereotactic i.
free-hand i.
imipenem-cilastatin i.
infraorbital i.
i. injury
intraarterial i.
intrahippocampal i.
intraneural phenol i.
intratumoral i.
intraventricular i.
Konakion I.
long-acting i.
Mestinon I.
Metastron I.
Miacalcin I.
M-Prednisol I.
Neosar I.
Osteocalcin I.
paramagnetic contrast i.
Regonol I.
Relefact TRH i.

NOTES

injection *(continued)*
retrobulbar i.
retrogasserian i.
Reversol I.
saline i.
Salmonine I.
stereotactic intracystic i.
sumatriptan succinate i.
Tensilon I.
THAM I.
THAM-E I.
Ureaphil I.

injured brain

injury
acceleration extension i.
accidental i.
acquired brain i. (ABI)
acute burst i.
acute central cervical spinal cord i.
avulsion i.
axonal shearing i.
axonotmetic i.
brachial plexus avulsion i.
brain i.
brainstem i. (BSI)
Brief Test of Head I.
burner i.
burst i.
cervical nerve root i.
cervical spine i.
chemical i.
chronic constrictive i. (CCI)
closed brain i. (CBI)
closed head i.
common iliac artery i.
contrecoup i.
crush i.
current of i.
diffuse axonal i. (DAI)
diffuse brain i.
diffuse white matter shearing i.
discoligamentous i.
diving spinal cord i.
electrical i.
endothelial i.
epileptogenic brain i.
Erb i.
Erb-Duchenne-Klumpke i.
excitotoxic neuronal cell i.
extension i.
extension-type cervical spine i.
flexion-distraction i.
flexion-extension i.
flexion-extension-mediated i.
fluid percussion head i.
focal cerebral head i.
Fränkel classification of spinal cord i.
global ischemic neuronal i.
head i.
hemorrhagic shearing i.
hepatic i.
hyperextension-hyperflexion i.
hypoxic-ischemic i.
iliac artery i.
inflammation-induced cell i.
injection i.
i. of intervertebral disk
ischemic i.
kainic acid-induced focal i.
laryngeal nerve i.
lightning i.
LSUMC classification of nerve i.
lumbar spine i.
lumbosacral spine plexus i.
middle column i.
mild head i.
minor head i. (MHI)
missile i.
multiple impact i.
neural i.
neuronal i.
nonmissile head i.
old nerve i.
open head i.
optic nerve i.
oxidative cellular i.
oxygen radical-induced cellular i.
parasympathetic nerve i.
past head i.
penetrating i.
perinatal obturator nerve i.
peripheral nerve i.
permanent i.
phrenic nerve i.
physical i.
i. potential
quadriplegic i.
radiation i.
radical induced brain i.
repetitive motion i. (RMI)
retraction i.
rotational i.
rotationally induced shear-strain i.
severe head i.
I. Severity Scale
shearing i.
skeletal muscle i.
soft tissue i.
i. spike
spinal cord i. (SCI)
sports-related spinal i.
stable cervical spine i.

stinger i.
suction i.
thoracic duct i.
thoracic spine i.
thoracolumbar spine flexion-distraction i.
three-column cervical spine i.
tracheal i.
transient plexus i.
traumatic brain i. (TBI)
two-column cervical spine i.
ureter i.
vascular i.
vena cava i.
vertebral artery i.
i. of war
whiplash i.
Wilbrand knee i.

injury-healing theory

in-line telesensor

innate reflex

inner

i. band of Baillarger
i. cone fiber
i. limiting layer
i. line of Baillarger
i. nuclear layer
i. plexiform layer
i. sheath of optic nerve
i. world

innervate

innervation

adrenergic i.
anomalous i.
i. apraxia
compensatory i.
reciprocal i.
rudimentary sympathetic i.

innervatory

i. apraxia
i. dyspraxia

innominata

substantia i.

innominate

i. angiogram
i. artery
i. substance
i. vein

Innovative Magnetic Resonance Imaging System

INO

internuclear ophthalmoplegia

inoculation

intracerebral i.

iNOS

isoform of NO synthase
stressed-induced iNOS

inositol

i. triphosphate
i. 1,4,5-triphosphate (IP_3)

inotropic component

INPH

idiopathic normal pressure hydrocephalus

in-phase image

input

afferent i.
arterial plasma i.
behavioral i.
cerebral sensory i.
cholinergic i.
cortical i.
emotional i.
hypothalamic regulatory i.
inhibitory regulatory i.
negativity of I. 1, 2
phonetic i.
positivity of I. 1, 2
regulatory i.
vestibulospinal i.

INR

international normalized ratio

insane

general paresis of the i.

insaniens

chorea i.

insecticide peripheral neuropathy

inserter, insertor

Texas Scottish Rite Hospital hook i.

insertion

C-D rod i.
i. equipment
oblique screw i.
pedicle screw i.
screw i.
sphenoidal electrode i.
Syracuse anterior I-plate i.

insertional activity

insertion/deletion polymorphism

insertor (*var. of* inserter)

inside-out signaling

NOTES

insomnia
altitude i.
chronic i.
conditioned i.
familial fatal i.
fatal familial i.
food allergy i.
long-term i.
nocturnal i.
posttraumatic i.
primary i.
psychophysiologic i.
psychophysiological i.
rebound i.
recurrent i.
short-term i.
sleep initiation i.
sleep maintenance i.
subjective i.
insomniac
insomnia-type
inspiratory
i. center
i. gasping
instability
atlantoaxial i.
autonomic i.
cervical spine atlantoaxial i.
emotional i.
endplate i.
fixation i.
high-gain i.
iatrogenic i.
lumbar spine i.
occipitoatlantoaxial i.
occipitocervical i.
phase i.
postural i.
sagittal plane i.
spinal i.
vasomotor i.
vertebral cervical i.
instantaneous axotomy
instant scan
Instat fibrin film
Instatrak
I. guidance system
I. headset
instillation procedure
instrument
Backlund stereotactic i.
20-channel Beckman EEG i.
Clarke stereotactic i.
Cloward i.
Craig vertebral body biopsy i.
digitized i.
Dwyer i.
Evershears surgical i.
Gamma knife i.
Hemorrhagic Stroke-Specific quality of life i. (HSQuale)
Hermann Brain Dominance I.
Hulka i.
interspinous segmental spinal i.
Kinetix i.
Kloehn craniofacial i.
Malis bipolar i.
micro-Doppler i.
Micro-Three microsurgery i.
i. migration
Millet neurological test i.
model TC2-64B pulsed-range gated Doppler i.
Nicolet Compass EMG i.
Nucleotome Endoflex i.
Nucleotome Flex II cannula i.
pencil-grip i.
personality disorder i.
pistol-grip i.
primer i.
pulsed-range gated Doppler i.
Radionics bipolar i.
rating i.
Richmond subarachnoid screw i.
Ruggles Surgical I.
solid-state i.
spark-gap i.
SpeedReducer i.
stereotactic i.
Ware i.
WHO i.
Yasargil i.
Yasargil-Aesculap i.
Zielke i.
instrumental
i. act
i. activities of daily living (IADL)
i. ADL
i. amusia
instrumentalism
instrumentation
anterior distraction i.
anterior-posterior fusion with segmental spinal i.
AO fixateur interne i.
AO notched i.
C-D i.
compression U-rod i.
Cotrel-Dubousset pedicle screw i.
Cotrel-Dubousset pedicular i.
Cotrel-Dubousset spinal i.
distraction i.
double Zielke i.
dynamic compression plate i.

Edwards i.
i. failure
Gellman i.
Harrington rod i.
interspinous segmental spinal i.
i. intervertebral
Jacobs locking hook spinal rod i.
Kambin i.
Kaneda anterior spinal i.
Louis i.
lumbar spine i.
lumbosacral spine transpedicular i.
Luque II segmental spinal i.
Luque semirigid segmental spinal i.
modular i.
Moss-Miami spinal i.
multiple hook assembly C-D i.
posterior cervical spinal i.
posterior distraction i.
posterior hook-rod spinal i.
rod-sleeve i.
sacral spine modular i.
sacral spine Universal i.
segmental spinal i.
spinal i.
Steffee i.
stereotactic i.
Texas Scottish Rite Hospital i.
transpedicular spinal i.
TSRH i.
universal i.
variable screw placement system i.
VSP plate i.
Zielke i.
Z-plate anterior thoracolumbar i.

insufficiency
adrenal i.
adrenocortical i.
anterior pituitary i.
aortic i.
convergence i.
divergence i.
mechanical i.
muscular i.
parathyroid i.
renal i.
respiratory i.
testicular i.
vertebrobasilar i.

insufficient sleep syndrome

insufflation
cranial i.

insula, pl. **insulae**
central sulcus of i.
circular sulcus of i.
gyri breves i.
gyrus longus i.
limen i.
lobus i.
long gyrus of the i.
i. operculum
i. of Reil
short gyrus of the i.
sulcus centralis i.
sulcus circularis i.
sulcus limitans of i.

insular
i. area
i. cistern
i. cortex
i. cortex tissue
i. epilepsy
i. gyrus
i. lobe
i. sclerosis
i. threshold
i. vein

insulares
venae i.

insularis
lobus i.
pars i.

insular-opercular syndrome

insulated electrode needle

insulin
i. coma treatment
i. effect
i. growth factor
i. hypoglycemia test
i. shock treatment

insulinlike growth factor (IGF)

insult
bihemispheral i.
CNS i.
excitoxic i.
hypoxic-ischemic i.
intraoperative neural i.
perinatal unilateral cerebral ischemic i.
putative i.

insult-induced neuronal damage

NOTES

intact
cognitively i.
i. spinous lamina
i. spinous process
integral
i. membrane glycoprotein
i. role
Integra Selector ultrasonic aspiration
integrated
i. ECT system
i. headholder
i. sideport access portal
integrative
i. approach
i. problem
integrity
electrophysiologic i.
physical i.
intellectual
i. ability
i. aphasia
i. aura
i. deficiency
i. exercise
i. function
i. function deficit
i. functioning
i. impairment
intense energy
intensification
image i.
intensifier
image i.
OEC-Diasonics mobile C-arm image i.
intensity
i. modulated radiation therapy
i. of trauma
intensive motor activity
Intensol
Diazepam I.
intention
motor i.
i. myoclonus
i. spasm
i. tremor
intent rating
intent-to-treat analysis
interacting cytokine
interaction
amygdala-prefrontal cortex-locus ceruleus i.
differential i.
dipole-dipole i.
electron-coupled nuclear spin-spin i.
glial neuronal i.
harmonious i.
neurochemical i.
pharmacodynamic i.
pharmacokinetic i.
physicochemical i.
i. process analysis
protein binding i.
proton-electron dipole-dipole i.
state-trait i.
treatment intensity-by-time i.
interactive
i. effect
i. voice response system
interannular segment
interarticularis
pars i.
interbody
i. fusion
i. graft
interbrain
intercalary neuron
intercalated nucleus
intercalation
intercalatus
nucleus i.
intercavernous sinus
intercellular
i. collagen
i. matrix
intercerebral
intercession
interclinoid
i. fold
i. ligament
intercolumnar tubercle
interconnected cerebral region
intercostal
i. artery
i. artery angiogram
i. muscle weakness
i. nerve
i. nerve nucleus
i. neuralgia
intercostales
nervi i.
intercostalis
rami mammarii laterales rami cutanei lateralis pectoralis nervi i.
rami mammarii mediales rami cutanei anterioris pectoralis nervi i.
ramus cutaneus anterior abdominalis nervi i.
ramus cutaneus anterior pectoralis nervi i.
ramus cutaneus lateralis abdominalis nervi i.

ramus cutaneus lateralis pectoralis nervi i.
intercostalium
rami musculares nervi nervorum i.
intercostobrachiales
nervi i.
intercostobrachial nerve
intercostohumeralis
intercrural
i. fissure
i. ganglion
i. space
interdigital
i. neuritis
i. transfer
interdural tumor
interear difference
interelectrode
interest
region of i. (ROI)
restricted i.
volume of i. (VOL)
voxel of i. (VOI)
interface
air-brain i.
long-term bone-instrumentation i.
motor i.
sensory i.
interfacet wiring and fusion
interfascial approach
interfascicular
i. fasciculus
i. graft
i. neuroglia
interfascicularis
fasciculus i. (FI)
interference
electromagnetic i. (EMI)
ipsilateral visuospatial i.
interferon (IFN)
alpha i.
i. beta-1a
i. beta-1b
i. flue-like
interferon-B
interferon-beta
i.-b. 1a
i.-b. 1b
interferon-gamma (IFN-gamma)
interfibrillary migration
interfissural
InterFix RP threaded spinal fusion cage device
interforniceal approach
interganglionic
intergemmal
intergyral
interhemicerebral
interhemispheric
i. cyst
i. fissure
i. hematoma
i. propagation time
i. synchrony
transcallosal i.
i. transcallosal-subchoroidal transvelum interpositum approach
interictal
i. behavior
i. behavior change
i. behavior syndrome
i. bisynchronous discharge
i. complex
i. EEG activity
i. electroencephalogram
i. epileptic personality
i. epileptiform abnormality
i. epileptiform activity
i. epileptiform spike
i. focal epileptiform discharge
i. generalized spike-and-wave discharge
i. pattern
i. period
i. phenomenon
i. physiologic dysfunction
i. sharp wave
i. spike discharge
interior band of Baillarger
interlaminar
i. clamp
i. decompression
interleukin
interleukin-1 (IL-l)
i. B-converting enzyme
interleukin-4
interleukin-5
interleukin-6
interleukin-7
interleukin-8
interleukin-9
interleukin-10

NOTES

interleukin-11
interleukin-12
interleukin-13
interlimb coordination
interlocking gyrus
interlocutor
intermanual conflict
intermaxillary fixation
intermedia
i. adenohypophyseos
area hypothalamica i.
columna i.
ganglia i.
massa i.
pars i.
regio hypothalamica i.
stria cochlearis i.
intermediae
nucleus dorsomedialis hypothalamicae i.
intermediary nerve
intermediate
i. acoustic stria
i. brain syndrome due to alcohol
i. C-D hook
i. cervical septum
i. column
i. column of spinal cord
i. ganglion
i. head fixator
i. hemispheric dynamic
i. hypothalamic area
i. hypothalamic region
i. layer
i. mass
i. nerve
i. part
i. part of adenohypophysis
i. spinal muscular atrophy
i. white layer of superior colliculus
i. zone
i. zone of spinal cord
intermedii
nervi supraclaviculares i.
rami temporales i.
intermediofacialis
nervus i.
intermediolateral
i. cell column
i. cell column of spinal cord
i. mesencephalic syndrome
i. nucleus
i. tract
intermediolateralis
nucleus i.
intermediomedialis
nucleus i.
ramus frontalis i.
intermediomedial nucleus
intermedium
septum cervicale i.
stratum griseum i.
stratum medullare i.
intermedius
nervus cutaneous dorsalis i.
nucleus linearis i.
nucleus ventralis i.
ventralis i.
intermeningeal
intermesentericus
plexus i.
intermittent
i. acute porphyria (IAP)
i. cramp
i. double-step gait
i. focal slowing
i. myoclonus epilepsy
i. neurogenic claudication
i. photic stimulation
i. rhythmic delta activity (IRDA)
i. tetanus
i. torticollis
intermodal competition
interna
capsula i.
globus pallidus i.
hematorrhachis i.
hyperostosis frontalis i.
lamina pyramidalis i.
mediodorsal globus pallidus i.
ophthalmoplegia i.
pachymeningitis i.
protuberantia occipitalis i.
tabula i.
internae
crus anterius capsulae i.
crus posterius capsulae i.
fibrae arcuatae i.
genu capsulae i.
pars cervicalis arteriae carotidis i.
pars lenticulothalamicus capsulae i.
pars retrolentiformis capsulae i.
pars sublentiformis capsulae i.
pars thalamolenticularis capsulae i.
rami cruris posterioris capsulae i.
rami genus capsulae i.
rami partis retrolentiformis capsulae i.
stria laminae granularis i.
stria laminae pyramidalis i.
venae cerebri i.

internal
i. architecture neuronal size
i. arcuate fiber
i. auditory canal
i. band of Baillarger
i. capsule
i. capsule anterior crus
i. capsule posterior crus
i. capsule syndrome
i. carotid angiogram
i. carotid artery (ICA)
i. carotid artery aneurysm
i. carotid artery balloon test occlusion
i. carotid balloon test
i. cerebral vein
i. circadian clock
i. corticotectal tract
i. decompression
i. disk herniation
i. fixation plate-screw system
i. fixation of spine
i. fixation spring
i. hydrocephalus
i. jugular vein
i. line of Baillarger
i. medullary lamina
i. meningitis
i. model
i. neurolysis
i. ophthalmoplegia
i. pillar cell
i. popliteal nerve
i. pulse generating unit
i. pyocephalus
i. representation
i. respiration
i. selection
i. sense
i. sheath of optic nerve
i. spinal fixation
I. State Scale
i. terminal filament
i. validity
i. vertebral venous plexus

internalis
globus pallidus i. (GPi)

international
I. Classification of Epilepsies and Epileptic Syndromes
I. Classification of Impairments, Disabilities and Handicaps (ICIDH)
I. Classification of Seizures
I. Cooperative Study on the Timing of Aneurysm Surgery
I. Headache Society (IHS)
Interpore Cross I.
I. League Against Epilepsy
i. normalized ratio (INR)
I. Study of Unruptured Intracranial Aneurysm (ISUIA)
I. 10–20 system of electrode placement
I. Working Formulation classification

interne
AO/ASIF fixateur i.
AO fixateur i.
construct AO fixateur i.
Dick AO fixateur i.
fixateur i.

interneuron
GABAergic cortical i.

interneuronal calcium modulation

interni
crista transversa meatus acustici i.
nervus musculi obturatorii i.

interno
ramus communicans nervi laryngei inferioris cum ramo laryngeo i.

internodal
i. distance
i. length
i. segment

internodale
segmentum i.

internode
Ranvier i.

internorum
stratum segmentorum externorum et i.

internuclearis
ophthalmoplegia i.

internuclear ophthalmoplegia (INO)

internucleosomal DNA fragmentation

internum
corpus geniculatum i.
filum terminale i.
stratum limitans i.

NOTES

internum *(continued)*
stratum nucleare i.
stratum plexiforme i.
internuncial
i. fiber
i. neuron
i. pathway
internus
globus pallidus i. (GPi)
nervus caroticus i.
nervus obturatorius i.
plexus caroticus i.
interoception
interoceptive
i. cue
i. nervous system
interoceptor
interofective system
interolivary
interoreceptive
interossei sign
interosseous branch of medial terminal branch of deep fibular nerve
interparietal sulcus
interpeak
i. delay
i. latency
interpedicular distance
interpeduncular
i. cistern
i. fossa
i. fossa lesion
i. ganglion
i. nucleus
i. space
i. trigone
interpeduncularis
cisterna i.
fossa i.
nucleus i.
substantia perforata i.
interpleural analgesia (IPA)
interpolation algorithm
Interpore
I. Cross International
I. porus hydroxyapatite
interposed nucleus
interpositi
cavum veli i.
interpositospinalis
tractus i.
interpositospinal tract
interpositum
velum i.
interpositus
nucleus i.
interpulse time
interradial plexus
interscalene triangle
interscapular reflex
intersegmental
i. aberration
i. covariation
i. fasciculus
i. fiber
i. reflex
intersemilunar fissure
intersemilunaris
fissura i.
interspace
ballooning of vertebral i.
cervical i.
i. collapse
lumbar i.
thoracic i.
interspike interval
interspinous
i. ligamentum
i. segmental spinal
i. segmental spinal instrument
i. segmental spinal instrumentation
i. segmental spinal instrumentation technique
interstimulus interval
interstitial
i. amygdaloid nucleus
i. brachytherapy
i. cell
i. hydrocephalic edema
i. neuritis
i. nuclei of anterior hypothalamus
i. nucleus of Cajal
i. nucleus of medial longitudinal fasciculus
i. polymyositis
i. radiation source
i. radiation therapy
i. radiotherapy
i. serotonin concentration
interstitialis
nucleus amygdalae i.
interstitiospinalis
tractus i.
interstitiospinal tract
interstriate layer
interthalamica
adhesio i.
interthalamic adhesion
interthalamicus
connexus i.
intertrabecular hemorrhage
intertrain interval
intertransverse process fusion
interuncal distance

intervaginal space of optic nerve
interval
atlantoaxial i.
interspike i.
interstimulus i.
intertrain i.
mean interpotential i. (MIPI)
time i.
intervention
biologic i.
clinical i.
cognitive i.
culture-specific i.
drug i.
early pharmacological i.
educational i.
experimental i.
exposure-based i.
free-hand ultrasound-guided i.
GAD-specific i.
pharmacologic i.
pharmacological i.
static i.
targeted i.
verbal i.
interventional neuroradiology
interventriculare
foramen i.
interventricular foramen
intervertebral
i. discitis
i. disk
i. disk compression
i. disk herniation
i. disk rupture
i. disk space infection
i. foramen
i. ganglion
instrumentation i.
i. osteochondrosis
i. punch
intervertebralis
annulus fibrous disci i.
calcinosis i.
nucleus pulposus disci i.
interview
I. Based Impression of Change
research i.
Zarit burden i.
intestinal
polyneuropathy, ophthalmoplegia, leukoencephalopathy, and i. (POLI)
i. trauma
intonation
voice i.
intoxicant
intoxicate
intoxication
aluminum i.
ammonia i.
anticonvulsant i.
bromide i.
Burundanga i.
fluoxetine i.
heavy metal i.
idiosyncratic i.
manganese i.
mercury i.
narcotic i.
pathologic i.
pathological i.
reversible i.
serum heavy metal i.
substance i.
thallium i.
water i.
intraabdominal
i. bleeding
i. neuroblastoma
intraaortic balloon pump
intraarachnoid
i. leptomeningeal malformation
i. neurovascular structure
intraarterial
i. Amytal testing
i. digital subtraction angiogram
i. digital subtraction angiography (IADSA)
i. drug delivery
i. flow
i. injection
intraaural attenuation
intraaxial
i. brain lesion
i. fiber
i. neoplasm
intrablood-brain barrier (IBBB)
intracanalicular lesion
intracapsular hemorrhage

intracarotid
i. amobarbital testing
i. marrow cell
i. sodium Amytal memory testing
intracavernous
i. carotid aneurysm
i. tumor
intracavitary irradiation
intracellular
i. calcium
i. calcium block
i. contribution
i. deoxyhemoglobin
i. energy metabolism
i. insoluble protein deposit
i. ion
i. lipid inclusion
i. metabolic pathway
i. metabolic process
i. second messenger
i. signal
intracephalic
intracerebellar
i. nucleus
intracerebral
i. aneurysm
i. arteriovenous malformation
i. depth electrode
i. depth electrode monitoring
i. ganglioma
i. hematoma
i. hemorrhage
i. Hodgkin lymphoma
i. hydatid cyst
i. inoculation
i. lesion
i. microdialysis
i. steal
intracerebroventricular administration of morphine
intracisternal
i. administration
i. fibrinolysis
i. puncture
intraclass correlation
intraconal mass
intracortical
i. axon
i. connection
i. inhibition and facilitation
i. transverse fiber
intracranial
i. aerocele
i. air
i. aneurysm
i. arachnoid cyst
i. arterial dolichoectasia
i. artery
i. astrocytoma
i. bleeding
i. brain volume
i. bruit
i. calcification
i. cavernous angioma
i. cholesteatoma
i. circulation
i. compliance
i. cryptococcosis
i. disease
i. electroencephalogram (ICEEG)
i. electroencephalography
i. epidural abscess
i. epidural pressure
i. ganglion
i. glioma
i. granulomatous arteritis
i. hematoma
i. hemorrhage
i. Hodgkin lymphoma
i. hypertension
i. hypertension without papilledema (IHWOP)
i. hypotension (IH)
intracranial to i.
i. mass lesion
i. meningioma
i. meningioma resection
i. MR angiography
i. navigation
i. neoplasm
i. neuroblastoma
i. occlusion
i. pachymeningitis
i. part of optic nerve
i. plasmacytoma
i. pneumatocele
i. pneumocele
i. pressure (ICP)
i. pressure catheter
i. pressure Express digital monitor
i. pressure increase
i. pressure microsensor
i. pressure-temperature (ICP-T)
i. raw volume
i. rhizotomy
i. sarcoidosis
i. schwannoma
i. seminoma
i. sinus thrombosis
i. steal phenomenon
i. steal syndrome
i. tuberculoma
i. tumor
i. vascular dissection

i. vascular malformation (ICVM, IVM)
i. venous malformation
i. venous sinus
intracranial-extracranial
i.-e. nerve graft
i.-e. transplantation
intracranial-intracranial (IC-IC)
i.-i. bypass
intracranial-intratemporal nerve graft
intracrine
intractable
i. grand mal epilepsy
i. pain
i. partial seizure
i. psychomotor epilepsy
intraculminalis
fissura i.
intraculminate fissure
intracutaneous
intracytoplasmic
intradermal angioma
intradiploic epidermoid cyst
intradiscal
i. electrothermal
i. electrothermal procedure
i. electrothermal therapy (IDET)
intradural
i. abscess
i. anastomosis
i. approach
i. arteriovenous fistula
i. dissection
i. draining vein
i. extramedullary mass lesion
i. inflammatory disease
i. lipoma
i. metastasis
i. phase
i. retractor
i. retromedullary arteriovenous fistula
i. segment
i. tumor
i. tumor surgery
intradural-extradural meningioma
intraepidermal
i. nerve fiber (IENF)
i. nerve fiber density
intrafascicular migration
intraforaminal approach
intrafusal fiber
intragemmal
intragracile sulcus
intragracilis
sulcus i.
intragyral
intrahippocampal
i. injection
i. microdialysis
intraictal physiologic dysfunction
intralabyrinthine schwannoma
intralamellaris
pachymeningitis i.
intralaminar nucleus
intralimbic gyrus
intraluminal thrombolysis
Intramedic PE-50 polyethylene tubing
intramedullary
i. ependymoma
i. epidermoid cyst
i. lymphoma
i. nail
i. spinal cord tumor
i. spinal lesion
i. toxoplasmosis
i. tractotomy
intrameningeal
intramodal target
intramolecular
i. dipole-dipole mechanism
i. relaxation
intramural
i. hematoma
i. plexus
intramuscular
i. absorption
i. administered drug
i. administration
i. neurolysis
intraneural
i. edema
i. ganglion cyst
i. neurofibrillary tangle
i. phenol injection
intraneuronal
i. fibrillary tangle
i. inclusion
i. inclusion disease
intranidal aneurysm
intransigent
intransitive limb

NOTES

intranuclear
- i. ophthalmoplegia
- i. receptor

intraocular
- i. hemorrhage
- i. neuritis
- i. pressure

intraocularis
- pars intralaminaris nervi optici i.
- pars prelaminaris nervi optici i.

intraoperative
- i. angiography
- i. balloon occlusion
- i. B-mode ultrasound
- i. cell saver
- i. cortical stimulation
- i. dural tear
- i. electrical cortical stimulation (IOECS)
- i. electrocorticography
- i. facial nerve monitoring
- i. lateral fluoroscopy
- i. microendoscopy
- i. MRI
- i. neck hyperextension
- i. neural insult
- i. neuromonitoring
- i. neurophysiological monitoring
- i. rupture
- i. stereotactic spatial localization
- i. ultrasonic probe
- i. x-ray

intraorbital
- i. arteriovenous malformation
- i. granular cell tumor
- i. lesion
- i. meningioma
- i. surgery

intraosseous
- i. meningioma
- i. schwannoma

intraparenchymal
- i. cyst
- i. drug delivery
- i. hematoma
- i. hemorrhage
- i. infusion
- i. mass
- i. meningioma
- i. periventricular echodensity

intraparietal
- i. sulcus
- i. sulcus of Turner

intraparietalis
- sulcus i.

intraparotideus
- plexus i.

intraperitoneal (IP)
- i. receptor

intrapial

intrapituitary cyst

intraplaque hemorrhage

intrapontine

intrapsychic
- i. change
- i. origin
- i. world

intrarachidian

Intrascan ultrasound

intrasegmental
- i. fiber
- i. reflex

intrasellar
- i. craniopharyngioma
- i. extension
- i. granuloma
- i. growth-hormone-secreting pituitary tumor
- i. lesion
- i. neuroadenohyphophyseal choristoma
- i. paraganglioma
- i. Rathke cleft cyst
- i. rhabdomyosarcoma

intrasinus transducer

intraspinal
- i. adenoma
- i. drug infusion system
- i. epidural pressure
- i. herniated disk
- i. lesion
- i. meningioma
- i. vascular malformation

intraspinous muscle

intraspongy nuclear disk herniation

intrasynaptic

intratentorial
- i. atrophy
- i. malformation
- i. supracerebellar approach

intraterritorial anastomosis

intratest scatter

intrathalamicae
- fibrae i.

intrathalamic fiber

intrathecal
- i. antibiotic
- i. drug therapy
- i. fluorescein
- i. IgG synthetic rate
- i. immunoglobulin synthesis
- i. morphine analgesia

i. morphinotherapy
i. neurolysis
i. octreotide
i. pain management
intrathoracic bleeding
intratumoral
i. arteriovenous shunt
i. chemotherapy
i. hemorrhage
i. hypervascularity
i. injection
intratumor hemorrhage
intrauterine shunt procedure
intravagal
i. glomus
i. paraganglioma
intravagale
glomus i.
intravascular
i. balloon occlusion
i. device
i. ligature
i. lymphoma
i. pressure
i. streaming
intravenous (IV, I.V.)
i. gamma globulin
i. immune globulin
i. immune globulin humoral therapy
i. immunoglobulin treatment
i. medication
i. oxygen-15 water bolus technique
i. regional anesthesia (IVRA)
i. regional sympathetic blockade
intraventricular (I-V)
i. catheter
i. drug delivery
i. endoscopy
i. headache (IVH)
i. hematoma
i. hemorrhage
i. infusion
i. injection
i. meningioma
i. septation
i. tumor
intravertebral
intravoxel phase dispersion
Intrel
I. II spinal cord stimulation system
I. II spinal cord stimulator
intrinsic
i. birefringence
i. brainstem tumor
i. capacity
i. cell suicide mechanism
i. damage
i. disease
i. factor deficiency
i. fiber
i. imaging
i. reflex
i. relationship
i. transverse connector
i. transverse connector role
intrinsic-negative runner
intrinsic-positive runner
introjective-projective cycle
intromittent organ
intron
Intropaque
Intropin
intrusive
i. memory
i. symptom
intubation
aqueductal i.
nasogastric i.
oral i.
intumescence
tympanic i.
intumescent
intumescentia
i. cervicalis
i. ganglioformis
i. lumbalis
i. lumbosacralis
i. tympanica
invagination
basilar i.
invasive
i. electroencephalographic monitoring
i. pituitary adenoma
i. tumor
Inventory-55
inventory
Behavior Change I.

NOTES

inventory *(continued)*
Bell Object Relations and Reality Testing I.
Brief Pain I.
Brief Symptom I.
Brigance Diagnostic Life Skills I.
Butcher Treatment Planning I.
Creative Behavior I.
Creative Styles I.
Daily Stress I.
DeLong Interest I.
Epilepsy Surgery I.-55
Johns Hopkins Functioning I.
Multidimensional Pain I.
Neuropsychiatric I.
Quality of Life I.
Quality of Life in Epilepsy-89 i.
Self-Description I.
sleep-awake activity i.
social stress and functionality i.
Talbieh Brief Distress I.
inverse
i. Anton syndrome
i. Argyll Robertson pupil
i. ocular bobbing
i. polymerase chain reaction-based detection of frataxin gene
i. square rule
i. treatment planning
inversed jaw-winking syndrome
inversion
i. recovery
i. time
inverted radial reflex
investigatory reflex
inveterate
involuntary
i. medication
i. movement
i. nervous system
i. repetitive movement disorder antineuronal antibody assay
i. time-out
involution
thymic i.
involutional
i. paranoid reaction
i. psychotic reaction
involvement
brain i.
bulbar i.
extraocular muscle i.
sarcoidosis neuromuscular i.
tumorous i.
INVOS
in vivo optical spectroscopy
INVOS 3100 cerebral oximeter monitoring system
INVOS transcranial cerebral oximeter
inward focus
iobenzamic acid
iobutoic acid
iocarmate meglumine
iocarmic acid
iocetamate
iodamic acid
iodamide
***Iodamoeba buetschlii* cerebral amebiasis**
iodatol
iodide
metocurine i.
radioactive i.
iodinated radiographic contrast
iodine
i. deficiency
isotopic i.
i. 131 MIBG
protein-bound i. (PBI)
iodine-125 implant
iodipamide
i. meglumine
i. methylglucamine
iodized oil
iodoalphionic acid
iodopyracet
iodoxamate
iodoxamic acid
iodoxyl
IOECS
intraoperative electrical cortical stimulation
ioglicate
ioglicic acid
ioglucol
ioglucomide
ioglunide
ioglycamic acid
ioglycamide
iogulamide
iohexol
i. CT ventriculogram
i. myelography
ion
argon i.
calcium i.
i. channel
i. channel disorder
i. flux
intracellular i.
positive i.
ionic stimulus

ionophore
calcium i.
ionophose
iopamidol contrast medium
iopanoate
iopanoic acid
iophendylate
iophenoxic acid
ioprocemic acid
iopromide
iopronic acid
iopydol
iopydone
iosefamate
iosefamic acid
ioseric acid
iosulamide
iosumetic acid
iotasul
ioteric acid
iothalamate
meglumine i.
iothalamic acid
I-o transforms
iotrol
iotroxamide
iotroxic acid
ioversol
Iowa Conners scale
ioxaglate
i. meglumine
i. sodium
ioxaglic acid
ioxithalamate
ioxithalamic acid
iozomic acid
IP
intraperitoneal
IP_3
inositol 1,4,5-triphosphate
IPA
interpleural analgesia
I-Paracaine
I-plate
Syracuse anterior I.-p.
ipodate acid
ipratropium bromide
ipsative score
ipsilateral
i. anosmia
i. approach
i. cerebellar ataxia
i. cerebellar sign
i. corticospinal tract sign
i. facial palsy
i. facial paralysis
i. facial paresis
i. gaze palsy
i. headache
i. hemianopia
i. hemiparesis
i. hemisphere
i. loss
i. mesial temporal sclerosis
i. mesial temporal structure
i. middle cerebral artery
i. monocular blindness
i. projection
i. reflex
i. somatosensory cortex
i. stroke
i. temporal cortex
i. tonic conjugate gaze
i. tonic deviation
i. tragus
i. transcallosal technique
i. vasogenic edema
i. visuospatial interference
ipsilesional hemifield
IPSP
inhibitory postsynaptic potential
I/Q imbalance ghost
IR
HydroStat IR
IRDA
intermittent rhythmic delta activity
IRDA on electroencephalogram
Iressa
iridis
rubeosis i.
Iriditope
iridium
iridium-192
iridocyclitis
iridoparalysis
iridoplegia
complete i.
reflex i.
sympathetic i.
iridotomy
argon laser i. (ALI)

NOTES

iris
i. Lisch nodule
i. neovascularization
i. stellate pattern
iritis
white i.
irkunii
iron
i. deficiency
i. ferrous sulfate
i. lung
i. metabolism
i. poisoning
i. replacement therapy
iron-ascorbate-DTPA
technetium 99m i.-a.-D.
iron-containing lesion
irradiation
conventional fractionated i.
convergent beam i.
excitatory i.
gamma i.
hyperfractionated i.
intracavitary i.
selective i.
stereotactic i.
whole brain i. (WBI)
irregular
i. nystagmus
i. sleep-wake pattern
Irrigant
Neosporin GU I.
irrigation bipolar system
irritability
mechanical i.
nervous i.
specific i.
irritable
i. heart
i. nociceptor
i. syndrome
irritation
meningeal i.
temperature i.
irritative
i. lesion
i. zone
IRT
infrared thermography
Isaacs-Mertens syndrome
Isaacs syndrome
ischemia
anoxic i.
brain i.
brainstem i.
cerebral i.
cerebrovascular i.
chronic ocular i.
cortical transient i.
focal artery i.
focal cerebral i.
global cerebral i.
hindbrain i.
hypoxic i.
ischemic i.
myoneural i.
nocturnal cardiac i.
posterior circulation i.
reversible i.
rostral brainstem i.
tourniquet i.
transient brain stem i.
vasomotor i.
vertebrobasilar i.
white matter i.
ischemia-induced elevation
ischemia-modifying factor
ischemic
i. anterior optic neuropathy
i. brain damage
i. brain edema
i. brainstem infarction
i. cascade
i. cerebral infarction
i. cerebrovascular disease
i. event
i. forearm exercise test (IFET)
i. hypoxia
i. injury
i. ischemia
i. lesion volume
i. lumbago
i. muscular atrophy
i. neuritis
i. neuron
i. neuronal cell death
i. ocular inflammation
i. pathology
i. penumbra
i. posterior optic neuropathy
i. preconditioning
i. stress
i. stroke
i. stroke pathophysiology
i. vascular dementia
i. white matter lesion
ischemic-hypoxic
i.-h. encephalopathy
i.-h. lesion
ischiadic
i. nerve
i. plexus
ischiadici
rami musculares nervi i.

ischiadicus
nervus i.
ischialgia
ischiodynia
ischioneuralgia
ischogyria
^{125}I seed
ISG
ISG viewing wand
ISG Wand navigation system
I-shaped scalp flap
Ishihara plate
island
i. of Calleja
neuroectodermal tumor pale i.
i. pedicle scalp flap
i. of Reil
syncytial i.
islet
Calleja i.
i. cell adenoma
***islet* gene**
Isle of Wight Study
ISO-30
isobutyl
isobutyl-2-cyanoacrylate
isocentric
i. linear accelerator
i. linear accelerator x-ray
isochromosome
isochronism
law of i.
isocoric pupil
isocortex
isodense
i. mass
i. subdural hematoma
isodisomy
isodose
i. curve
i. line
isoelectric
i. electroencephalogram
i. encephalogram
isoenergetic
isoenzyme
isoetharine hydrochloride
isoflavone
isoflurane anesthesia
isoform
brain i.
embryonic i.
four-repeat i.
i. of NO synthase (iNOS)
recombinant tau i.
three-repeat i.
isofrequency band
isointense lesion
Isola
I. spinal implant system
I. spinal implant system accessory
I. spinal implant system anchor
I. spinal implant system application
I. spinal implant system complication
I. spinal implant system component
I. spinal implant system design
I. spinal implant system dimension
I. spinal implant system eye rod
I. spinal implant system hook
I. spinal implant system iliac post
I. spinal implant system iliac screw
I. spinal implant system longitudinal member contouring
I. spinal implant system plate-rod combination
isolated
i. angiitis
i. angiitis of the central nervous system
i. gait ignition failure
i. periventricular nodular heterotopia
i. phobia
i. radial nerve palsy
isolation
anterior horn cell i.
fungus i.
mononuclear leukocyte i.
isolé
cerveau i.
encéphale i.
isoleucyl
Isollyl Improved
isomerase
glucosephosphate i.
isomeric function
isometheptene mucate
isometric tremor
isomorphous gliosis
Isonate

NOTES

isoniazid
i. neuropathy
i. polyneuropathy
i. therapy
isoniazid-induced pyridoxine deficiency
isonicotinic acid peripheral neuropathy
Isopap
Isopaque
isopotential
isoproterenol tilt table test
isosorbide dinitrate
isothiocyanate
allyl i.
isotope
i. cisternogram
i. cisternography
isotopic
i. cisternography
i. iodine
isotretinoin
isotropic
i. band
i. 3DFT
i. three-dimensional Fourier transform
isovaleric
i. acidemia aminoaciduria
i. aciduria
isovaleyl-CoA dehydrogenase
isovolemic hemodilution
isozyme
isthmi (*pl. of* isthmus)
isthmic spondylolisthesis
isthmoparalysis
isthmoplegia
isthmus, pl. **isthmi**
i. of cingular gyrus
i. of cingulate gyrus
ganglion i.
i. gyri cinguli
i. of gyrus cinguli
i. of gyrus fornicatus
i. of His
i. of limbic lobe
i. rhombencephali
rhombencephalic i.
ISUIA
International Study of Unruptured Intracranial Aneurysm
ITAC
T-cell alpha chemoattractant
itch-specific central neuron
ITC radiopaque balloon catheter
item-total correlation
iter
i. ad infundibulum
i. of Sylvius
i. a tertio ad quartum ventriculum
iterative discharge
ITF
infratemporal fossa
ithykyphosis, ithycyphosis
ithylordosis
IT-MS infusion therapy
ITN
idiopathic trigeminal neuralgia
Ito
hypomelanosis of I.
ITP
idiopathic thrombocytopenic purpura
itraconazole
Itrel
I. pulse generator
I. 3 Spinal Cord Stimulation System
I-V
intraventricular
IV, I.V.
intravenous
Campath IV
lamina IV
Ivalon
I. embolic sponge
I. foam
I. particle
I. wire coil
IVEC-10 neurotransmitter analyzer
IVH
intraventricular headache
IVM
intracranial vascular malformation
IVRA
intravenous regional anesthesia
Iwabuchi clip
IX
protoporphyrin IX
ixomyelitis

jabs and jolts syndrome
JACE-STIM electrotherapy stimulation device
jacket
Minerva j.
jackknife
j. attack
j. spasm
Jackson
J. epilepsy
J. law
J. rule
J. sign
J. spine table
J. vagoaccessory hypoglossal paralysis
jacksonian
j. epilepsy
j. march
j. seizure
Jackson-Pratt drain
Jackson-Weiss syndrome
Jacobs
J. locking hook spinal rod
J. locking hook spinal rod instrumentation
J. locking hook spinal rod instrumentation modification
J. locking hook spinal rod technique
Jacobson
J. endarterectomy spatula
J. microneurosurgical scissors
J. microprobe
J. microvascular knife
J. mosquito forceps
J. needle holder
J. nerve
J. plexus
J. probe
J. reflex
J. suture pusher
J. vessel knife
Jacobson-Potts vascular clamp
Jacod
J. syndrome
J. triad
Jaeger-Hamby procedure
Jahnke syndrome
jake paralysis
Jakob-Creutzfeldt disease
Jak-STAT mechanism
Jamaica
J. ginger poisoning
J. ginger polyneuritis
Jamaican
J. neuropathy
J. vomiting sickness
jamais vu aura
Jamestown
J. Canyon (JC)
J. Canyon virus (JCV)
Janet test
Jannetta
J. alligator forceps
J. aneurysm neck dissector
J. bayonet forceps
J. duckbill elevator
J. fork
J. hook
J. knife
J. microvascular decompression procedure
J. posterior fossa retractor
J. probe
Jannetta-Kurze dissecting scissors
Jansen
J. bone curette
J. mastoid retractor
J. monopolar forceps
J. rasp
J. rongeur
J. scalp retractor
Jansen-Middleton
J.-M. forceps
J.-M. rongeur
J.-M. scissors
Jansen-Wagner retractor
Jansky-Bielschowsky disease
Janz
J. juvenile myoclonic seizure
J. response
J. response on electroencephalogram
syndrome of J.
J. syndrome
Japanese
J. B encephalitis
J. encephalitis virus
J. Society of Sleep Research
J. suction tip
Japanese-type familial amyloid polyneuropathy
japonica
encephalitis j.
jararaca
Jarcho-Levin syndrome

Jarell forceps
jargon
j. aphasia
organ j.
Jarisch-Herxheimer
J.-H. fever
J.-H. fever reaction
Jarit
J. brain forceps
J. periosteal elevator
J. rotator
J. tendon-pulling forceps
Jarit-Kerrison laminectomy rongeur
Jarit-Liston bone rongeur
Jarit-Ruskin bone rongeur
Jarman Underprivileged Area
Jasco spectropolarimeter
jaundice
nuclear j.
jaunes
plaque j.
Javid
J. carotid clamp
J. shunt
jaw
j. claudication
j. jerk
j. winking
jaw-jerk reflex
jaw-winking
j.-w. phenomenon
j.-w. reflex
j.-w. syndrome
jaw-working reflex
JB
jugular bulb
JC
Jamestown Canyon
JC virus
JCV
Jamestown Canyon virus
JedMed TRI-GEM microscope
Jeep driver's disease
Jefferson
J. fracture
J. syndrome
jejuni
Campylobacter j.
jelly
j. nystagmus
j. roll hypothesis
Jendrassik maneuver
Jerald forceps
jerk
ankle j.
biceps j.
chin j.
crossed adductor j.
crossed knee j.
elbow j.
j. finger
flurry of myoclonic j.
forearm j.
hypnic j.
jaw j.
knee j.
leg j.
macro square-wave j.
myoclonic j.
nocturnal leg j.
nystagmoid j.
j. nystagmus
paretic j.
photomyoclonic j.
quadriceps j.
square-wave j.
supinator j.
tendon j.
triceps surae j.
jerking stiff-person syndrome
jerk-locked back-averaged recording
jerky nystagmus
Jervell-Lange-Nielsen syndrome
jessur
jet
j. lag phenomenon/syndrome
j. lag sleep disorder
jeweler's bipolar forceps
Jewett wave
jig
Ace Hershey halo j.
jinjinia bemar
jiryan
Joffroy
J. reflex
J. sign
Johanson-Blizzard syndrome
Johns Hopkins Functioning Inventory
Johnson brain tumor forceps
Johnston alopecia
joint
amp j.
apophysial j.
atlantoaxial j.
atlantooccipital j.
Charcot j.
facet j.
j. hyperlaxity
incudostapedial j.
neuropathic j.
radiohumeral j.
j. receptor
j. replacement
sacroiliac j.

j. sense
temporomandibular j.
zygapophyseal j.
joker dissector
Jolly
J. reaction
J. test
jolt
lancinating electric shocklike j.
Joplin neuroma
Joseph disease
Jostent graft stent
Joubert syndrome
journal
JPA
juvenile pilocytic astrocytoma
J receptor
J-sella deformity
J-tipped guidewire
juga cerebralia
jugular
j. bulb (JB)
j. bulb oxyhemoglobin saturation monitoring (SjO_2)
j. bulb venous oxygen saturation
j. chain lymph node
j. foramen
j. foramen mass
j. foramen muscle
j. foramen schwannoma
j. foramen syndrome
j. ganglion
j. glomus
j. nerve
j. sign
j. vein
j. vein dissection
jugulare
foramen j.
glomus j.
jugularis
nervus j.
jugulation
jugulocephalic vein
jugulosubclavian junction
jugulotympanicum
glomus j.
jumper
j. disease
j. disease of Maine
jumping Frenchmen of Maine disease
jumpy stump
junction
anterior cervical approach to cervicothoracic j.
cervicomedullary j.
cervicothoracic j.
craniocervical j.
craniovertebral j.
electrotonic j.
gap j.
gray/white matter j.
jugulosubclavian j.
liponeural j.
motor unit neuromuscular j.
myoneural j.
neuromuscular j.
parietotemporooccipital j.
pontomedullary j.
pontomesencephalic j.
posterior craniocervical j.
postsynaptic neuromuscular j.
sylvian/rolandic j.
temporoparietal j. (TPJ)
thoracolumbar j.
junctional
j. dilation
j. kyphosis
j. scotoma of Traquair
junctural feature
Junin virus
juramentado
jurisprudential teaching model
Juster reflex
justification
neurobiological j.
juvenile
j. absence epilepsy
j. absence seizure
j. amyotrophy
j. angiofibroma
j. arteriovenous malformation
j. cerebellar astrocytoma
j. chorea
j. dermatomyositis
j. fibromatosis
j. justice system
j. myasthenia gravis
j. myoclonic epilepsy
j. myxedema
j. neuronal ceroid lipofuscinosis

NOTES

juvenile *(continued)*
j. nonneuropathic Niemann-Pick disease
j. papillomatosis
j. parkinsonism
j. pilocytic astrocytoma (JPA)
j. rheumatoid arthritis
j. spinal muscular atrophy
j. violence
juvenilis
dementia paralytica j.
juxtaarticular cyst
juxtacortical
j. chondroma
j. sarcoma
juxtallocortex
juxtamembrane
juxtapapillary uveitis
juxtapulmonary receptor
juxtarestiform body
juxtarestiforme
corpus j.

K
potassium
K complex
K index
K+
K+ Care
K+ Care Effervescent
K-2000 surgical saw blade
Kadian sustained-release morphine capsule
Kaes
K. feltwork
line of K.
K. line
K. stria
Kaes-Bechterew
band of K.-B.
K.-B. layer
K.-B. stria
Kahn syndrome
kainate receptor
kainic
k. acid
k. acid-induced focal injury
Kaiser-Meyer-Olkin measure
kaleidoscope hallucination
Kales
criteria of Rechtschaffen and K.
kallikrein gene
Kallmann syndrome
Kaltostat dressing
Kambin instrumentation
Kanavel approach
Kandel stereotactic apparatus
Kaneda
K. anterior spinal instrumentation
K. anterior spinal/scoliosis system
K. anterior spinal system
K. anterior spine stabilizing device
K. SR spinal system
Kanizsa illusion
Kannon headframe
Kaochlor-Eff
Kaochlor SF
kaolin clotting time
kaolin-induced hydrocephalus
Kaon
Kap
Hypotherm Gel K.
Kaplan agnesis
Kaplan-Meier
K.-M. survival analysis
K.-M. survival curve
kaposiform hemangioendothelioma
Kaposi sarcoma
kappa
k. light chain
k. opiate receptor
k. wave
Kapseals
Dilantin K.
Karlin microknife
Karnofsky
K. Performance Scale
K. performance score (KPS)
K. rating scale
Kartagener syndrome
karyochrome cell
Kasabach-Merritt syndrome
Katayama fever
Kato
technique of Miyazaki and K.
Katz ADL Index
Katzmann Orientation-Memory-Concentration questionnaire
Katzman test
kava
k. extract
kava k.
kavain
kavalactones
kavapyrones
Kawasaki disease
Kawase
K. anterior petrosectomy
K. triangle
Kayser-Fleischer
K.-F. corneal ring
K-Centrum anterior spinal fixation system
***KCNQ2* gene**
***KCNQ3* gene**
33-kDa antigen
56kD protein
Keane Mobility bed
Kearns-Sayre
K.-S. disease
K.-S. syndrome
Kearns-Sayre-Shy (KSS)
Keeler
K. Galilean loupe
K. panoramic loupe
K. video headlamp
Keen
K. operation
K. point

Keep · kinase

Keep
K. Alert capsule
K. GOing caplet
Kehrer reflex
keirospasm
Keitel index
K-Electrolyte Effervescent
Kelly-Goerss COMPASS stereotactic system
Kelly stereotactic system
Kelvin body
Kennedy
K. disease
K. disease test
K. syndrome
Kennedy-Fischbeck disease
Kennerdell-Maroon
K.-M. dissector
K.-M. elevator
K.-M. hook
K.-M. orbital retractor
K.-M. technique
Kenney Self-Care Questionnaire
Kenny ADL index
Kerandel symptom
kerasin histiocytosis
keratan sulfate
keratitis
neuroparalytic k.
neurotrophic k.
k. paralytica
keratoacanthoma
keratoconjunctivitis sicca
keratocyst
keratoderma blennorrhagicum
keratopathy
band k.
exposure k.
keratosis
k. obturans
seborrheic k.
keratotic lesion
keraunoneurosis
Kerlix dressing
kernicterus
neonatal k.
premature infant k.
Kernig
K. sign
K. test
Kernohan
K. classification of brain tumor
K. grading
K. notch
K. notch phenomenon
K. notch syndrome
K. sign
K. system
K. system of glioma classification
Kerns-Sayre syndrome
Kerr
K. clip
K. sign
Kerrison
K. bone punch
K. bone punch kinesthesiometer
K. microronguer
K. rongeur
Keryx Biopharmaceuticals
Kestenbaum procedure
ketamine
NMDA antagonist k.
ketanserin
ketoacid accumulation
ketoaciduria
branched-chain k.
ketorolac tromethamine
ketotic
k. glycine
k. hyperglycemia
Kety-Schmidt method
Key elevator
keyhole
k. craniotomy
k. laminectomy
k. surgery
transsylvian k.
Key-Retzius
foramen of K.-R.
Keystone graft
K-Gen Effervescent
kidney
human neonatal k. (HNK)
Kiel classification
Kienböck phenomenon
killer
natural k. (NK)
Killian
K. gouge
K. operation
K. septum speculum
Kilner hook
Kiloh-Nevin
K.-N. ocular form or progressive muscular dystrophy
K.-N. ocular myopathy
K.-N. syndrome
KinAir bed
kinanesthesia
kinase
calcium-calmodulin k. II
c-jun N-Terminal k.
creatine k. (CK)
DNA protein k.

focal adhesion k. (FAK)
mitogen-activated protein k.
phosphoglycerate k.
phosphorylase k.
protein k.
protein k. C (PKC)
seine k.
serum creatinine k.
threonine k.
tyrosine k.
kindled seizure
kindling
amygdala k.
delay of k.
k. process
Kindt carotid clamp
kinematic
forelimb k.
kinematograph
kinesia paradoxica
kinesigenic
k. ataxia
k. attack
k. chorea
k. choreoathetosis
kinesioneurosis
kinesipathy
kinesthesia hallucination
kinesthesiometer
Kerrison bone punch k.
kinesthesis
kinesthetic
k. aura
k. sense
kinetic
k. ataxia
k. cervical spine
k. drive
k. model
k. modeling
k. perimetry
k. strabismus
k. tremor
kinetics
cellular k.
first-order elimination k.
zero-order elimination k.
Kinetix instrument
King
K. type I–V curve
K. type II, V scoliosis
K. type IV curve posterior correction
kink
cervicomedullary k.
kinky-hair disease
Kinnier-Wilson disease
kinocilium
Kinsbourne syndrome
Kirby-Bauer disk diffusion method
Kirschner
K. pin
K. wire
K. wire placement
Kisch reflex
Kistler
K. classification of subarachnoid hemorrhage
K. subarachnoid hemorrhage classification
kit
Ceretec imaging k.
ELISA Quantikine k.
Hall Osteon drill system k.
Hall Osteon irrigation k.
KLS-Martin modular neuro k.
KTP dual disk k.
Laitinen high-precision stereotactic-assisted radiation therapy k.
Laitinen percutaneous tumor biopsy k.
Laserscope discography k.
Micro E irrigation k.
Micro 100 irrigation k.
Ototome irrigation k.
PainBuster infusion pump management k.
Radiofocus introducer B k.
Shiley distention k.
START k.
stereotactic-assisted radiation therapy k.
TANGENT posterior impacted instrument k.
Vectastain ABC k.
Klaus height index
Klearway oral appliance
K-Lease
Klebsiella pneumoniae **meningitis**
kleeblattschädel
Kleine-Levin syndrome
Kleist sign

NOTES

Klippel disease
Klippel-Feil
K.-F. deformity
K.-F. syndrome
Klippel-Trenaunay syndrome
Klippel-Trenaunay-Weber syndrome
Klippel-Weil sign
Kloehn craniofacial instrument
Klonopin
Klorvess Effervescent
Klotrix
KLS-Martin
KLS-M. center-drive screw
KLS-M. implant
KLS-M. modular neuro kit
Klumpke
K. palsy
K. paralysis
Klumpke-Dejerine
K.-D. paralysis
K.-D. syndrome
Klüver
method of K.
Klüver-Barrera Luxol fast blue stain
Klüver-Bucy syndrome
K-Lyte/Cl
K-Lyte Effervescent
KM universal battery charger
knee
k. jerk
k. phenomenon
k. reflex
Wilbrand k.
knee-chest position
knee-jerk reflex
knife
Adson dural k.
Adson right-angle k.
angular k.
arachnoid k.
Bucy cordotomy k.
canal k.
clasp k.
Cottle k.
Crile gasserian ganglion k.
Cushing dural hook k.
diamond k.
discission k.
electric k.
Frazier cordotomy k.
Frazier pituitary k.
Freer-Swanson ganglion k.
gamma k.
Halle dura k.
hot k.
Jacobson microvascular k.
Jacobson vessel k.
Jannetta k.
Leksell gamma k.
Leksell Model C gamma k.
model U gamma k.
Olivecrona trigeminal k.
photon k.
platelet-shaped k.
Rayport dural dissector and k.
201-source cobalt-60 gamma k.
Stecher arachnoid k.
Toennis dura k.
Weary cordotomy k.
X K.
Yasargil arachnoid k.
Yasargil microvascular k.
Knight forceps
Knighton hemilaminectomy retractor
knismogenic
knob
olfactory k.
synaptic k.
Knodt rod
K-Norm
knuckle
cervical aortic k.
k. under
Koala Pad graphics tablet
Kobayashi retractor
Kocher
K. clamp
K. collar incision
K. dissector
K. point
K. reflex
Kocher-Debré-Semelaigne syndrome
Kocher-Lovelace clamp
Koenen tumor
Koerber-Salus-Elschnig syndrome
Koerte-Ballance operation
Koerte procedure
Kohlmeier-Degos syndrome
Kohnstamm phenomenon
Kojewnikoff epilepsy
kok disease
kola
gotu k.
Kölliker-Fuse nucleus
Kölliker reticulum
Kolyum
Komai stereotactic head frame
Komet
K. K-2000 surgical saw blade
K. K-wire/Steinman pin and delivery tray system
K. medical battery tester
K. Medical/Brasseler USA XK-95 high-speed drill system

K. medical replacement batteries
K. XK-95
K. XK-95 high-speed surgical drill system
Konakion Injection
koniocortex
auditory k.
Kontrast U
konzo disease
Korsakoff (K's)
K. amnesia
K. syndrome
korsakoffian amnesia
Körte-Balance operation
Kostuik
K. rod
K. screw
Kostuik-Harrington
K.-H. device
K.-H. distraction system
Kozhevnikov
K. epilepsy
K. spring-summer encephalitis
KPS
Karnofsky performance score
Krabbe
K. Arnold-Chiari malformation
K. diffuse sclerosis
K. disease
K. leukodystrophy
K. syndrome
Krabbe-Weber-Dimitri disease
Kraepelina paranoia
Kraepelin-Morel disease
Kraepelin schema
Krause
K. corpuscle
K. denervation
K. end bulb
K. operation
K. respiratory bundle
K. terminal bulb
Krayenbuehl nerve hook
Krimsky test
Kronecker
K. aneurysm needle
K. center
***krox* gene**
Kruskal-Wallis
K.-W. H test
K.-W. test
K's
Korsakoff
K's disease
K's syndrome
k-space reordered by inversion time at each slice position
KSS
Kearns-Sayre-Shy
KTP/532 surgical laser
KTP dual disk kit
kubisagari, kubisagaru
Kufs disease
Kugelberg-Welander
K.-W. disease
K.-W. juvenile spinal muscle atrophy
K.-W. syndrome
Kühne
K. phenomenon
K. spindle
K. terminal plate
Kuhnt intermediary tissue
Kümmell spondylitis
Kundalini yoga
Küntscher
K. hammer
K. nail
Kurtzke
K. Expanded Disability Status Scale
K. multiple sclerosis disability scale
K. score
Kurze
K. dissection scissors
K. suction-irrigator
Kussmaul
K. aphasia
K. coma
K. paralysis
Kussmaul-Landry paralysis
Kveim test
K-wire placement
kymatism
kymoparalytica
myohypertrophia k.
kynurenic acid
kynurenine aminotransferase
Kyoto Multi-Institutional Study Group Pediatric Neurology
kyphoplasty

NOTES

kyphoscoliosis
- neurofibromatosis k.
- k. secondary to neurofibromatosis
- severe k.
- thoracolumbar k.

kyphosis
- acute angular k.
- k. brace
- Cobb method of measuring k.
- congenital k.
- k. correction
- k. creation
- iatrogenic lumbar k.
- junctional k.
- lumbar k.
- postlaminectomy k.
- posttraumatic k.
- right thoracic curve with junctional k.
- Scheuermann k.
- thoracic k.
- thoracolumbar k.

kyphotic
- k. deformity
- k. deformity pathomechanics

KyphX inflatable bone tamp

L4-5 disk disease
L5-S1 disk disease
LA
leukoariosis
Inderal L.
Labbé
L. neurocirculatory syndrome
vein of L.
L. vein
labeling
l. index
photoaffinity l.
terminal deoxynucleotide transferase-mediated nick end l. (TUNEL)
labia (*pl. of* labium)
labial
l. dysarthria
l. nerve
l. paralysis
labiochorea
labioglossolaryngeal
l. palsy
l. paralysis
labioglossomandibular approach
labioglossopharyngeal
l. paralysis
labiomandibular
l. approach
l. glossotomy
labium, pl. **labia**
l. cerebri
laboratory
basement l.
l. study
Venereal Disease Research L. (VDRL)
labyrinth
vestibular l.
labyrinthectomy
unit l. (UL)
labyrinthine
l. aplasia
l. apoplexy
l. concussion syndrome
l. disease
l. disorder
l. fistula test
l. hydrops
l. righting reflex
l. torticollis
l. vertigo
labyrinthitis
laceration
brain l.
cerebral l.
scalp l.
lacerum
foramen l.
L-acetylcarnitine
lack
l. of clear-cut cerebral dominance
l. of efficacy
energy l.
lacrimal
l. duct
l. gland
l. gland dysfunction
l. nerve
l. reflex
lacrimalis
nervus l.
pars orbitalis glandulae l.
lacrimogustatory reflex
La Crosse encephalitis
lactate
brain l.
calcium l.
l. dehydrogenase
global brain l.
gray matter l.
regional brain l.
Ringer l.
sodium l.
white matter l.
lactation
lactic
l. acidosis
l. acid production in perinatal asphyxia
l. acid serum level
lactoferrin
lactose metabolism
lactosuria
lactotroph cell
lactotrophic
Lactrodectus mactans
lacuna, pl. **lacunae**
cerebral l.
l. cerebri
lateral l.
lacunae laterales
lacunae lateralis
parasinusoidal l.
lacunaire
état l.
lacunar
l. amnesia
l. brain infarction

lacunar *(continued)*
l. state
l. stroke
l. stroke manifestation
l. syndrome
lacunaris
status l.
lacunar-molecular layer
lacune
lacunosum
stratum moleculare et substratum l.
lacunosus
status l.
Ladd fiberoptic system
laeso
vertigo ab stomacho l.
Lafora
L. body
L. body disease
L. familial myoclonic epilepsy
laforin
lagophthalmos
Lahey
L. Clinic dural hook
L. Clinic nerve hook
L. score
Laitinen
L. high-precision stereotactic-assisted radiation therapy kit
L. percutaneous tumor biopsy kit
L. stereoadapter
L. stereoguide 2000 arc-centered stereotactic frame
L. stereotactic head frame
L. stereotactic system
lake
lateral l.
venous l.
Lake-Cavanaugh disease
lalognosis
laloplegia
L-alpha-acetylmethadiol 3
Lamaze technique
lambda
l. light chain
l. wave
lambdoid
l. activity
l. craniosynostosis
l. plagiocephaly
l. synostosis
lambdoidal suture
Lambert-Eaton
L.-E. myasthenic syndrome (LEMS)
L.-E. syndrome (LES)
Lambert syndrome
lamella, pl. **lamellae**
basal l.
triangular l.
vitreous l.
lamellar sheath
lamellated corpuscle
lamellosa
corpuscula l.
lamellosum
corpusculum l.
Lamictal
lamina, pl. **laminae**
l. I
l. IV
l. V
l. VI
l. affixa
l. alaris
laminae albae cerebelli
l. arcus vertebrae
basal l.
l. basalis
l. basalis choroideae
basilar l.
l. basilaris cochlea
l. of the cerebral cortex
l. choroidea
l. choroidea epithelialis
l. cinerea
l. cribrosa
l. dorsalis
epithelial l.
external medullary l.
intact spinous l.
internal medullary l.
laminae medullares cerebelli
laminae medullares thalami
l. medullaris
l. medullaris lateralis
l. medullaris lateralis corporis striati
l. medullaris medialis
l. medullaris medialis corporis striati
l. medullaris medialis nuclei lentiformis
l. medullaris thalami externa
l. of mesencephalic tectum
l. molecularis
l. molecularis corticis cerebri
l. multiformis
periclaustral l.
l. plexiformis corticis cerebri
l. pyramidalis externa
l. pyramidalis ganglionaris
l. pyramidalis interna
l. quadrigemina
quadrigeminal l.

Rexed l.
l. of Rexed
rostral l.
l. rostralis
l. septi pellucidi
l. of septum pellucidum
spinal l.
spinal l. II
laminae spinalis
l. spinalis II
l. spreader
l. supraneuroporica
l. tectalis mesencephali
l. tecti
l. tecti mesencephali
l. terminalis (LT)
l. terminalis cerebri
l. terminalis of cerebrum
l. terminalis hypothalami
l. ventralis
l. of vertebral arch
l. vitrea

lamin a/c gene (LMNA)

laminaplasty
Tsuji l.

laminar
l. C-D hook
l. cortex posterior aspect
l. cortical necrosis
l. cortical sclerosis

laminated cortex

lamination of gyrus

laminectomized spine

laminectomy
Beckman-Eaton l.
Beckman-Weitlaner l.
cervical spine l.
decompressive l.
Gill l.
Girdlestone l.
keyhole l.
multilevel l.
osteoplastic l.
4-place l.
l. punch forceps
l. roll
single-level decompressive l.

laminin

laminoforaminotomy

laminoplasty
distraction l.
en bloc l.
open door l.
spinous process-splitting l.
l. with extended foraminoplasty for cervical myelopathy

laminotomy
microendoscopic l.
microscopic l. (ML)
unilateral l.

Lamitrode lead

lamivudine
zidovudine and l.

lamotrigine

Lance-Adams syndrome

lancinating
l. electric shocklike jolt
l. pain

lancisi
striae l.

Lancisi longitudinal nerve

Lanci stria

Landau
L. reflex
L. syndrome

Landau-Kleffner syndrome

landmark
glabella-inion line l.
pedicle l.
surface l.

Landolt
L. pituitary speculum
L. spreader

Landouzy-Dejerine
L.-D. atrophy
L.-D. disease
L.-D. muscular dystrophy

Landouzy dystrophy

Landouzy-Grasset law

Landry
L. paralysis
L. syndrome

Landry-Guillain-Barré-Strohl syndrome

Landry-Guillain-Barré syndrome

Langenbeck periosteal elevator

Langer-Giedion syndrome

Langerhans
L. cell
L. cell granulomatosis

Langley nerve

language
l. alteration

NOTES

language *(continued)*
l. area
l. associated cortex
l. disturbance
l. lateralization
l. manipulation
l. therapy
l. zone
lanreotide
Lanterman
L. cleft
L. incisure
L. segment
Lanterman-Schmidt incisure
lanthanide
Lapidus bed
Laplacian montage on electroencephalogram
Lapras catheter
lapse
memory l.
lapsus lingua
large
l. ball nerve hook
l. polymorphic ganglion cell
l. vessel vasculitis
large-artery infarction
large-egress cannula
large-vessel infarction
Larmor
L. equation
L. frequency
L. precession
Larodopa
Lars Frisén
laryngeal
l. atresia
l. chorea
l. crisis
l. dysarthria
l. epilepsy
l. hemangioma
l. nerve
l. nerve injury
l. syncope
l. vertigo
laryngectomy
laryngismus
laryngoparalysis
laryngoplegia
laryngospasm
laryngospastic reflex
Lasègue
L. disease
L. sign
L. syndrome
L. syndrome I, II
L. test
laser
argon l.
l. beam
carbon dioxide l.
Cavitron l.
l. disk decompression (LDD)
l. Doppler flowmeter (LDF)
l. Doppler flowmetry
l. Doppler spectroscopy
l. Doppler velocimetry
holmium YAG l.
Ho:YAG l.
KTP/532 surgical l.
Nd:YAG l.
l. nucleotomy
orthogonal l.
l. photocoagulation (LPC)
l. scanning microscope (LSM)
Sharplan l.
l. speckle
l. speckle pattern
l. surgery
Surgica K6 l.
l. uvulopalatoplasty (LUPP)
VersaPulse holmium l.
laser-assisted
l.-a. palatoplasty
l.-a. spinal endoscopy
l.-a. uvulopalatoplasty (LAUP)
Laserflo Doppler probe
Laserflow
L. blood perfusion monitor
L. BPM^2 real time cerebral perfusion monitor
laser-nephelometric assay for betaB-TP
Laserscope discography kit
Lassa fever virus
lata
Tutoplast fascia l.
Latarjet nerve
late
l. after depolarization
l. distal hereditary myopathy
l. epilepsy
l. infantile lipofuscinosis
l. luteal phase of menstrual cycle
l. Lyme neuroborreliosis
l. seizure
l. whiplash syndrome
late-life
l.-l. dementia
l.-l. migraine accompaniment
latency
blink reflex l.
distal motor l.

l. distal motor
increased rapid eye movement l.
interpeak l.
mean sleep l.
l. proximal
REM l.
residual l.
sensory l.
sleep l.
terminal l.
l. of tibialis anterior activation

latency-evoked potential

latent

l. epilepsy
l. infection
l. period
l. reflex
l. tetany
l. zone

late-onset

l.-o. ataxia
l.-o. category
l.-o. Werdnig-Hoffmann disease

late-phase long-term potentiation (L-LTP)

lateral

l. amygdaloid nucleus
l. aperture
l. aperture of fourth ventricle
l. aperture of the fourth ventricle
l. atrial vein
l. central tegmental field
l. cerebellar region
l. cerebellomedullary cistern
l. cerebral fissure
l. cerebral fossa
l. cerebral sulcus
l. cervical nucleus
l. column
l. column of spinal cord
l. corticospinal tract
l. cuneate nucleus
l. direct vein
L. Dominance Examination
l. dorsal tegmentum
l. dorsal tegmentum nucleus
l. extracavitary approach
l. extracavity approach
l. fasciculus proprius
l. femoral cutaneous nerve
l. fillet
l. foramina of Luschka
l. fossa of brain
l. funiculus
l. funiculus of spinal cord
l. gaze
l. gaze nystagmus
l. gaze palsy
l. geniculate body
l. geniculate nucleus (LGN)
l. ground bundle
l. habenular nucleus
l. hemispheric dynamic
l. hypothalamic area
l. hypothalamic region
l. inferior pontine syndrome
l. intermediate substance
l. intradural approach
l. lacuna
l. lake
l. lemniscus
l. lemniscus trigone
l. line organ
l. listhesis
l. longitudinal stria
l. medullary lamina of corpus striatum
l. medullary lamina of lentiform nucleus
l. medullary syndrome
l. midpontine syndrome
l. neocortex
l. nucleus of mammillary body
l. nucleus of medulla oblongata
l. nucleus of thalamus
l. nucleus of trapezoid body
l. occipital artery
l. occipital sulcus
l. occipitotemporal gyrus
l. olfactory gyrus
l. olfactory stria
l. olfactory tract
l. orbitofrontal circuit
l. orbitofrontal cortex
l. parabrachial nucleus
l. pericuneate nucleus
l. periventricular white matter
l. posterior choroidal
l. posterior choroidal artery
l. posterior nucleus
l. preoptic nucleus
l. projection

L

NOTES

lateral *(continued)*
l. proprius bundle
l. pterygoid nerve
l. pulvinar nucleus
l. pyramidal fasciculus
l. pyramidal tract
l. rachiotomy
l. raphespinal tract
l. recess of fourth ventricle
l. recess stenosis
l. rectus muscle
l. rectus palsy
l. recumbent position
l. reticular nucleus
l. reticulospinal tract
l. rhinotomy
l. rhinotomy incision
l. roentgenogram
l. root of median nerve
l. root of optic tract
l. rostral supplementary motor area
l. rotation
l. sellar compartment
l. semicircular canal (LSC)
l. septal nucleus
l. sinus
l. sinus thrombosis
l. skull base
l. spinal sclerosis
l. spinothalamic tract
l. superior olivary nucleus
l. superior pontine syndrome
l. tarsorrhaphy
l. temporal epileptogenic lesion
l. temporal resection
l. terminal branch of deep fibular nerve
l. thalamic peduncle
l. thoracic meningocele
l. tuberal nucleus
l. vein of lateral ventricle
l. ventricle floor
l. ventricle occipital horn
l. ventricle posterior horn
l. ventricle temporal horn
l. vertigo
l. vestibular nucleus
l. vestibulospinal tract
l. zone
l. zone of hypothalamus

laterale
cornu l.
corpus geniculatum l.

laterales
lacunae l.
nervi supraclaviculares l.
nuclei tuberales l.
rami medullares l.
ramus choroidei posteriores l.
venae directae l.

lateralis
area hypothalamica l.
arteria occipitalis l.
arteria orbitofrontalis l.
bulbus cornus occipitalis ventriculi l.
bulbus cornus posterioris ventriculi l.
cisterna cerebellomedullaris l.
cisterna fossae l.
cisterna sulci l.
columna l.
cornu anterius ventriculi l.
cornu frontale ventriculi l.
cornu inferius ventriculi l.
cornu occipitale ventriculi l.
cornu posterius ventriculi l.
cornu temporale ventriculi l.
ductus semicircularis l.
fasciculus corticospinalis l.
fasciculus proprius l.
fasciculus pyramidalis l.
fissura cerebri l.
funiculus l.
globus pallidus l.
gyrus occipitotemporalis l.
gyrus olfactorius l.
lacunae l.
lamina medullaris l.
lemniscus l.
nervi digitales plantares communes nervi plantaris l.
nervi digitales plantares proprii nervi plantaris l.
nervus ampullaris l.
nervus cutaneous dorsalis l.
nervus cutaneous femoralis l.
nervus cutaneous femoris l.
nervus cutaneous surae l.
nervus cutaneus antebrachii l.
nervus pectoralis l.
nervus plantaris l.
nervus pterygoideus l.
nuclei lemnisci l.
nucleus amygdalae l.
nucleus centralis l.
nucleus cervicalis l.
nucleus corporis geniculati l.
nucleus corporis mammillaris l.
nucleus dorsalis corporis geniculati l.
nucleus geniculatus l.
nucleus habenularis l.
nucleus lemnisci l.

nucleus mamillaris l.
nucleus olivaris superior l.
nucleus parabrachialis l.
nucleus paragigantocellular l.
nucleus pericuneatus l.
nucleus preopticus l.
nucleus septalis l.
nucleus tractus olfactorii l.
nucleus ventralis l.
nucleus ventralis corporis geniculati l.
nucleus ventralis corporis geniculi l.
nucleus vestibularis l.
pars centralis ventriculi l.
pars dorsalis corporis geniculati l.
pars ventralis corporis geniculati l.
pedunculus thalami l.
plexus choroideus ventriculi l.
rami corporis geniculati l.
ramus choroidei ventriculi l.
ramus profundus nervi plantaris l.
ramus superficialis nervi plantaris l.
regio hypothalamica l.
stria longitudinalis l.
stria olfactoria l.
substantia intermedia centralis et l.
sulcus occipitalis l.
tela choroidea ventriculi l.
tractus corticospinalis l.
tractus pyramidalis l.
tractus raphespinalis l.
tractus spinothalamicus l.
tractus vestibulospinalis l.
trigonum collaterale ventriculi l.
trigonum lemnisci l.
vena atrii l.
vena lateralis ventriculi l.
vena medialis ventriculi l.
vena recessus l.
ventralis posterior l.
ventriculus l.
zona l.

laterality
crossed l.

lateralization
fetal planum temporal l.
language l.

lateralized
l. activity
l. artifact
l. brain language system

laterally convex dural incision

lateral-onset temporal lobe epilepsy

lateriflora
Scutellaria l.

later-life depression

laterodorsal tegmental nucleus

lateropulsion
l. of body movement
l. of eye movement

latex
l. agglutination
l. balloon
l. particle agglutination test

latex-covered pledget

lathyrism

Latin American Sleep Society

latissimus dorsi muscle

lattice
l. degeneration
l. field

latticed layer

laughing
l. seizure
l. sickness

laughter reflex

Laumonier ganglion

LAUP
laser-assisted uvulopalatoplasty

Laurence-Biedl syndrome

Laurence-Moon-Bardet-Biedl syndrome

Laurence-Moon-Biedl syndrome

Laurence-Moon syndrome

Lausanne stereotactic robot

law
l.'s of association
autonomic affective l.
l. of average localization
Bastian l.
Bastian-Bruns l.
Bell l.
Bell-Magendie l.
Bernoulli l.
Boltzmann distribution l.
Bowditch l.
Broadbent l.
l. of denervation
Flatau l.
Flouren l.
Gerhardt-Semon l.

NOTES

law *(continued)*
Grasset l.
Haeckel l.
Hagen-Poiseuille l.
Hilton l.
l. of isochronism
Jackson l.
Landouzy-Grasset l.
Leyden l.
Magendie l.
Müller l.
Poiseuille l.
l. of referred pain
restraint l.
Ribot l.
Ritter l.
Rosenbach l.
Semon l.
Sherrington l.
L. of Specific Nerve Energy
Stokes l.
l. of thirds
three strikes l.
van der Kolk l.
wallerian l.

Lawford syndrome

layer
bacillary l.
l. of Bechterew
Bekhterev l.
l. of cerebellar cortex
l. of cerebral cortex
claustral l.
l. of dentate gyrus
dysfibrous l.
ependymal l.
epithelial choroid l.
external granular l.
fillet l.
fusiform l.
ganglionic l.
granular l.
Henle fiber l.
Henle nervous l.
l. of hippocampus
infragranular l.
infrastriate l.
inner limiting l.
inner nuclear l.
inner plexiform l.
intermediate l.
interstriate l.
Kaes-Bechterew l.
lacunar-molecular l.
latticed l.
magnocellular l.
mantle l.
marginal l.
Meynert l.
mitral cell l.
molecular l.
multiform l.
l. of nerve fiber
neuroepithelial l.
olfactory nerve l.
optic l.
oriens l.
outer limiting l.
outer nuclear l. (ONL)
outer plexiform l.
peripapillary nerve fiber l.
piriform neuron l.
l. of piriform neuron
plexiform l.
polymorphous l.
Purkinje cell l.
pyramidal cell l.
radiant l.
l. of rods and cones
rostral l.
spindle-celled l.
stria of internal granular l.
stria of internal pyramidal l.
stria internal pyramidal l.
stria of molecular l.
subcallosal l.
superior colliculus l.
suprastriate l.
ventricular l.
Waldeyer zonal l.
zonular l.

lazabemide HCl

lazaroid

Lazarus effect

L-baclofen

LBE
line bisection error

LBP
low back pain

LC
locus coeruleus
Hydergine LC

LCBF
local cerebral blood flow

LCMV
lymphocytic choriomeningitis virus

LDA
low-density area

LDD
laser disk decompression
L. delivery system
L. procedure

LDF
laser Doppler flowmeter
lumbodorsal fascia
LDL
low-density lipoprotein
L-dopa
on-off effect of L.-d.
L.-d. stimulation test
L-dopa/benserazide
lead
colic l.
deep brain l.
dual octapolar l.
dual quadrapolar l.
EEG with NP l.
l. encephalitis
l. encephalopathy
eye l.
frontopolar l.
Lamitrode l.
model 300 NCP bipolar l.
NCP l.
l. neuropathy
octapolar l.
l. palsy
l. paralysis
l. poisoning
lead-pipe rigidity
leak
anastomotic l.
cerebrospinal fluid l.
leaky l.
sentinel l.
leakage
cerebrospinal fluid l.
chylous l.
l. headache
leaky leak
Leão spreading depression
least-square residual
Leatherman hook
Leber
L. congenital amaurosis
L. disease
L. hereditary optic atrophy
LED
light-emitting diode
LED probe
Lee
L. disk prosthesis
L. ganglion
Leeds Anxiety Scale
LeFort
L. classification
L. fracture
L. osteotomy
left
l. atrial myxoma
l. bundle branch block
l. common carotid artery
extension, sidebent right, rotated l. (ESRRL)
l. frontal lobe
l. hemiplegia
l. hemisphere damage (LHD)
l. hemisphere dominance
l. planum temporal
l. thoracolumbar major curve pattern
l. ventricle
l. ventricular function
l. visuospatial neglect
left-bearing nystagmus
left-right asymmetry
left/right hemisphere dominance
left-sided
l.-s. apraxia
l.-s. thoracotomy
left-to-right shunt
leftward saccade
leg
champagne-bottle l.
l. jerk
l. pain
l. phenomenon
restless l.'s
l. sign
legasthenia
Legend high speed pneumatic system
Legendre
L. function
L. sign
Legg disease
***Legionella pneumophila* infection**
leg-raising test
leiasthenia
Leibinger
L. 3-D plate
L. microplate
L. Micro Plus plate
L. Micro Plus screw

NOTES

Leibinger *(continued)*
L. Micro System cranial fixation plate
L. Micro System drill bit
L. Micro System plate cutter
L. Micro System plate-holding forceps
L. Micro System pliers
L. titanium mini-Würzburg implant system
Leica vibrating knife microtome
Leichtenstern
L. encephalitis
L. phenomenon
L. sign
Leiden factor V
Leigh
L. disease
L. necrotizing encephalopathy
L. subacute necrotizing encephalomyelitis
L. syndrome
leiodystonia
leiomyoma
extraspinal l.
leiomyosarcoma
disseminated l.
Leksell
L. adapter to Mayfield device
L. apparatus
L. arc
L. gamma knife
L. gamma knife target series
L. GammaPlan computerized program
L. Micro-Stereotactic system
L. Model C gamma knife
L. Model G stereotactic frame
L. posteroventral pallidotomy
L. rongeur
L. selector
L. stereotactic gamma unit
L. stereotactic gamma unit lens
L. SurgiPlan computerized program
L. technique
Leksell-Elekta stereotactic frame
Lemieux-Neemeh syndrome
Lemmon sternal spreader
lemniscal
l. fiber
l. pathway
l. system
l. trigone
lemniscorum
decussatio l.
lemniscus, pl. **lemnisci**
acoustic l.
auditory l.
decussation of medial l.
gustatory l.
lateral l.
l. lateralis
medial l.
l. medialis
nucleus of lateral l.
spinal l.
l. spinalis
stratum interolivare l.
trigeminal l.
l. trigeminalis
trigone of lateral l.
trigonum l.
LEMS
Lambert-Eaton myasthenic syndrome
length
age-dependent l.
chord l.
crown-heel l. (CH)
crown-rump l.
internodal l.
pedicle screw chord l.
pedicle screw path l.
pulse l.
lengthening
distal catheter l.
l. reaction
Lenhossék process
Lenke
L. classification of adolescent idiopathic scoliosis
L. scoring system
Lennert lymphoma
Lennox-Gastaut
L.-G. pattern
L.-G. syndrome
Lennox syndrome
lens
crossed l.
Leksell stereotactic gamma unit l.
275mm objective l.
nucleus of l.
Lente Iletin II
lenticula, pl. **lenticulae**
lenticular
l. ansa
l. aphasia
l. fasciculus
l. ganglion
l. loop
l. nucleus
l. progressive degeneration
lenticularis
ansa l.
dystonia l.

fasciculus l.
nucleus of the ansa l.
nucleus ansae l.
lenticulooptic
lenticulostriate
l. artery (LSA)
lenticulothalamic
lentiformis
capsulae nuclei l.
discus l.
lamina medullaris medialis nuclei l.
nucleus l.
lentiform nucleus
lentiginosis
centrofacial l.
lentis
ectopia l.
nucleus l.
lentiviral vector
leonine facial feature
leontiasis ossea
Leopard syndrome
Leponex
leprae
Mycobacterium l.
leprosy
anesthetic l.
articular l.
dry l.
mutilating l.
l. peripheral neuropathy
trophoneurotic l.
leprous
l. neuropathy
l. polyneuritis
leptin
l. level
l. secretion
l. signal
leptomeningeal
l. anastomosis
l. capillary-venous angiomatosis
l. carcinoma
l. carcinomatosis
l. cyst
l. enhancement postcontrast administration
l. fibrosis
l. gliomatosis
l. metastasis
l. neoplastic disease
l. tumor
l. venous angioma
leptomeningeal/wedge cortical biopsy
leptomeninges
leptomeningeum
spatium l.
leptomeningioma
leptomeningitis
basilar l.
sarcomatous l.
leptomeningopathy
leptomeninx
leptomyelolipoma
Leptomyxid
leptospirosis
l. lymphocytic meningitis
Leriche
L. operation
L. sympathectomy
L. syndrome
Leri sign
LeRoy-Raney scalp clip
LeRoy scalp clip-applying forceps
LES
Lambert-Eaton syndrome
Lesch-Nyhan
L.-N. disease
L.-N. syndrome
Leser-Trélat sign
lesion
acute cerebellar hemispheric l.
afferent digital l.
afferent nerve l.
angiocentric immunoproliferative l.
anterior parietal l.
anterochiasmatic l.
atrophic l.
auricular l.
axonal l.
basal ganglionic l.
biparietal l.
brachial plexus l.
brain l.
brainstem l.
bubbly bone l.
callosal l.
cavernous sinus l.
central l.
centrotemporoparietal l.
cerebral l.
cerebrovascular l.

NOTES

lesion *(continued)*
cervical cord l.
chiasmal l.
chiasmatic l.
circumscribed l.
compressive mass l.
compressive trigeminal nerve l.
conus medullaris l.
cortical l.
corticospinal pathway l.
cyclops l.
deep white matter l. (DWML)
demyelinating trigeminal nerve l.
destructive stereotactic l.
diencephalic l.
diffuse pontine l.
discharging l.
discoid skin l.
dominant hemisphere l.
dorsal root entry zone l.
dumbbell l.
Duret l.
entry zone l.
epicortical l.
epileptogenic structural l.
epileptogenic temporal l.
excitatory l.
extraaxial l.
extraconal l.
extracranial mass l.
extramesial temporal l.
fimbria-fornix l.
focal l.
frank l.
frontal lobe l.
frontal white matter l.
l. generation
hemorrhagic l.
high cervical spinal cord l.
high-intensity l.
high pontine l.
high-signal l.
homogeneous l.
hyperintense l.
hyperostotic l.
hypoglossal canal l.
hypothalamic l.
indiscriminate l.
infarctlike l.
inflammatory l.
infranuclear l.
infratentorial l.
interpeduncular fossa l.
intraaxial brain l.
intracanalicular l.
intracerebral l.
intracranial mass l.
intradural extramedullary mass l.
intramedullary spinal l.
intraorbital l.
intrasellar l.
intraspinal l.
iron-containing l.
irritative l.
ischemic-hypoxic l.
ischemic white matter l.
isointense l.
keratotic l.
lateral temporal epileptogenic l.
leukoencephalopathic l.
l. load
low-density l.
lower motor neuron l.
mass l.
Meckel cave l.
median nerve l.
mesial temporal epileptogenic l.
metabolic l.
metameric l.
microscopic l.
midbrain l.
midline developmental l.
mucous membrane l.
multiple focal l.
nail l.
nasal l.
neoplastic l.
neurofibrillary l.
neurogenic l.
nondominant hemisphere l.
nonmeningiomatous malignant l.
nucleus basalis l.
occipital l.
ocular l.
optic nerve l.
oral herpes l.
orbitomedial/cingulate l.
pallidal l.
paraorbital l.
parasagittal l.
parasellar l.
parietal cortex l.
parietal lobe l.
parietooccipital l.
peripheral nerve l.
peripheral oculomotor l.
periventricular hyperintense l.
periventricular white matter l.
Perthes-Bankart l.
petroclival l.
phrenic nerve l.
pigment epithelial l.
pituitary stalk l.
pontine l.

posterior column l.
posterior compartment l.
posterior fossa l.
posterior language area l.
posttraumatic frontal l.
prepontine l.
pretectal l.
pseudocystic hypodense l.
pseudomedial longitudinal fasciculus l.
pyramidal tract l.
radiofrequency l.
regurgitant l.
retrobulbar l.
retrochiasmal l.
retrochiasmatic l.
retrocochlear l.
ring-wall l.
root entry-zone l.
rotationally induced shear-strain l.
sciatic nerve l.
senile leukoencephalopathic l.
single enhancing CT l.
skip l.
space-occupying brain l.
spinal l.
striatal l.
structural brain l.
subcortical l.
subtentorial l.
supranuclear l.
suprasellar l.
supratentorial structural l.
synchronous l.
tectal l.
thalamic l.
transverse cord l.
ulnar nerve l.
underlying mass l.
underlying structural l.
upper motor neuron l.
well-defined focal brain l.
white matter l. (WML)

lesionectomy
computer-assisted volumetric stereotactic l.
stereotactic l.

lesion-induced cortical plasticity

lesioning
dorsal root entry zone l.
DREZ l.
nucleus caudalis-nucleus solitarius DREZ l.
radiofrequency l.
thermal l.
trigeminal nucleus caudalis l.

lesser superficial petrosal nerve (LSPN)

LET
linear energy transfer

lethal midline granuloma

lethargica
encephalitis l.

lethargy

lethica
aphasia l.

letter
l. blindness
l. fluency test

Letterer-Siwe disease

leucine
l. degradation
l. serum level
l. zipper family
l. zipper gene

leucotomy

leucovorin

leukemia
central nervous system l.
l. inhibitory factor (LIF)
periventricular l.
l. therapy affecting cognitive function

Leukeran

leukoaraiosis

leukoariosis (LA)

leukocyte
cerebrospinal fluid l.
eosinophilic l.
polymorphonuclear l. (PML)
l. scintigraphy
tumor-infiltrating l. (TIL)

leukocytoclastic vasculitis

leukocytosis
emotional l.

leukodystrophia cerebri progressiva

leukodystrophy
adrenal l.
Canavan l.
globoid cell l.
Krabbe l.
metachromatic l.
metachromic l.

L

NOTES

leukodystrophy *(continued)*
Pelizaeus-Merzbacher l.
spongiform l.
spongy degeneration l.
sudanophilic l.
l. with diffuse Rosenthal fiber formation
leukoencephalitis
acute epidemic l.
acute necrotizing hemorrhagic l.
necrotizing hemorrhagic l.
l. periaxialis concentrica
postinfectious l.
postvaccinial l.
sclerosing l.
subacute sclerosing l.
van Bogaert sclerosing l.
viral l.
leukoencephalopathic lesion
leukoencephalopathy
cerebral autosomal dominant arteriopathy with subcortical infarcts and l. (CADASIL)
cerebral autosomal recessive arteriopathy with subcortical infarcts and l. (CARASIL)
diffuse necrotizing l.
metachromatic l.
multifocal l.
necrotizing l.
polycystic lipomembranous osteodysplasia with sclerosing l. (PLOSL)
progressive multifocal l. (PML)
l. radiation
subacute sclerosing l.
subcortical l.
leukoencephaly
focal pontine l.
progressive necrotizing l.
leukokoria
leukomalacia
cystic periventricular l.
periventricular l. (PVL)
premature infant periventricular l.
leukomyelitis
necrotizing hemorrhage l.
leukomyelopathy
leukopenia
transient l.
leukopoiesis
leukotome
leukotomy
bimedial frontal l.
limbic l.
prefrontal l.
transorbital l.
ventromedial frontal l.
leukotriene
leuprolide acetate
LEV
levetiracetam
levallorphan tartrate
levator
l. ani nerve
l. palpebrae muscle
l. scapulae
level
l. of abstraction
l. of activity
agitation l.
air-fluid l.
l. of alertness
ammonia blood l.
bilirubin serum l.
blood alcohol l. (BAL)
carnitine serum l.
cerebrospinal fluid ferritin l.
ceruloplasmin serum l.
cholesterol serum l.
circulating leptin l.
l. of cognitive function
l. of consciousness
cortisol l.
creatinine kinase serum l.
criterion l.
l. of depression
l. of disruption
dissociation l.
effective l.
E-selectin l.
estrogen l.
expression l.
flucytosine blood l.
l. of functioning
L. of Functioning Scale
glucose blood l.
gray matter lactate l.
hair lead l.
homocysteine l.
l. of impairment
lactic acid serum l.
leptin l.
leucine serum l.
linear interpolation l.
lipid serum l.
liver enzyme serum l.
low energy l.
lower circulating estrogen l.
meningioma prostaglandin l.
mental l.
molecular l.
muscle enzyme serum l.

neural noise l.
neural pathway l.
orotic acid urine l.
oxalic acid urine l.
pathological l.
perceptual l.
performance l.
phenylalanine serum l.
phosphocreatinine l.
phytanic acid l.
pipecolic acid l.
plasma homocysteine l.
plasma leptin l.
posttest l.
primitive emotional l.
progesterone l.
proline urine l.
l. of psychological pain
red cell folic acid l.
serum ammonia l.
serum androgen l.
serum caffeine l.
serum folic acid l.
spinal l.
symptom l.
thyroid-stimulating hormone l.
urea blood l.
uric acid l.
vertebral l.
vitamin B12 l.
white matter lactate l.
zinc protoporphyrin l.

level-dependent
level-of-care criterion
levetiracetam (LEV)
Levine-Critchley syndrome
Levin thermocouple cordotomy electrode
levo-alpha-acetylmethadol
levocarnitine
levodopa
l. and carbidopa
l. ethylester
levodopa/carbidopa
levodopa-induced dyskinesia
levonorgestrel
levopromazine
Levoxine
Lévy-Roussy syndrome
Lewis blood group activity
Lewy
L. body
L. body dementia
L. body disease
Lexapro
lexical
l. access
l. agraphia
l. process
lexical-syntactic deficit
lexipafant
Lex-Ton spinal frame
Leyden
L. ataxia
L. law
L. neuritis
Leyden-Möbius
L.-M. muscular dystrophy
L.-M. syndrome
Leydig
L. neuron
L. tumor cell
Leyla
L. brain retractor
L. self-retaining tractor bar
L. self-retaining tractor bar lift
LFF
low-frequency filter
LFF on electroencephalogram
LGG
low-grade glioma
LGMD2B
limb girdle muscular dystrophy type 2B
LGN
lateral geniculate nucleus
LH
luteinizing hormone
LHD
left hemisphere damage
Lhermitte
L. phenomenon
L. sign
Lhermitte-Duclos disease
liberae
terminationes nervorum l.
Librium
Lichtheim
L. aphasia
L. disease
L. plaque
L. sign
L. syndrome

NOTES

licorice
deglycyrrhizinated l.
licostinel
Licox partial pressure of oxygen measuring computer
Liddell-Sherrington reflex
Liddle
L. dexamethasone suppression test
L. psychomotor poverty
lid nystagmus
lidocaine
l. test
l. transdermal patch
Lidoderm
LidodexNS
lidofenin
technetium 99m l.
Liebowitz Social Anxiety Scale
lienalis
plexus l.
lienal plexus
Liepmann apraxia
LIF
leukemia inhibitory factor
life
l. impairment
L. Satisfaction Index
L. Skills Profile
L. Skills Profile index
l. span
L. Span Study
l. stressor
life-changing improvement
lifetime impulsivity
life-year
quality-adjusted l.-y. (QUALY)
Li-Fraumeni syndrome
lift
Leyla self-retaining tractor bar l.
pneumatic chair l.
lifter
Yasargil tissue l.
Ligaclip
L. applier
L. clip
Ethicon L.
ligament
alar l.
anterior longitudinal l.
atlantoepistrophic l.
axial-occipital l.
coccygeal l.
costotransverse l.
costovertebral l.
cruciate l.
dentate l.
denticulate l.
fracture-dislocation with anterior l.
Gruber l.
l. of Henle
interclinoid l.
longitudinal l.
mamilloaccessory l. (MAL)
occipital-atlas-axis l.
ossification of the posterior longitudinal l. (OPLL)
petrosphenoidal l.
posterior longitudinal l.
Struthers l.
transverse atlantal l.
yellow l.
ligamentectomy
bilateral l.
ligamentum, pl. **ligamenta**
l. denticulatum
l. flavum
interspinous l.
ligand
l. concentration
hydrophobic l.
l. occupation
putative endogenous l.
receptor l.
l. selection
ligand-gated ion channel
ligase
ubiquitin protein l.
ligation
hunterian l.
ligature
intravascular l.
light
l. chain paraprotein
l. exposure
glare of l.
l. meromyosin
l. microscopy study
l. sleep
light-emitting diode (LED)
lightheaded
lightning
l. attacks in infantile spasm
l. injury
light-prompted button task
Light-Veley headrest
LightWare micro retractor
LightWear headlight
lignoceroyl coenzyme A synthase deficiency
Lilienthal rib spreader
Liliequist
membrane of L.
lilliputian hallucination

limb
afferent l.
l.'s of bony semicircular canal
branch to internal capsule, posterior l.
branch to internal capsule, retrolentiform l.
efferent l.
l. girdle muscular dystrophy type 2B (LGMD2B)
intransitive l.
l. movement disorder
l. muscle
l. myokymia
phantom l.
l. psychogenic disorder
l. weakness
limb-girdle muscular dystrophy
limb-girdle-trunk paresis
limbic
l. activation
l. brain region
l. circuitry
l. cortex
l. dopamine receptor
l. effect
l. encephalitis
l. leukotomy
l. lobe
l. neuronal firing rate
l. system
l. system pathway
l. system structure
limbic-related region
limbicus
lobus l.
Limbitrol
limb-kinetic
l.-k. apraxia
l.-k. dyspraxia
limbus vertebra
limen, pl. **limina**
l. insula
l. to twoness
***LIM* gene**
LIM-HD
LIM-homeodomain
LIM-homeodomain (LIM-HD)
limina (*pl. of* limen)
liminal stimulus
liminometer
limit
extreme narrowing l.
limitans
glia l.
sulcus l.
limitation
conceptual l.
empirical l.
receiver l.
limited
l. effect
l. symptom attack
limiting
l. sulcus
l. sulcus of fourth ventricle
l. sulcus of Reil
l. sulcus of rhomboid fossa
limit-setting sleep disorder
***LIM*-kinase gene**
limp
antalgic l.
l. wristed
Limulus
L. amebocyte lysate assay
limulus lysate assay of cerebrospinal fluid
LINAC
linear accelerator
Boston LINAC
LINAC radiosurgery
LINAC radiosurgery system
LINAC-based radiosurgical system
Lindamood Auditory Conceptualization
Lindau
L. disease
L. tumor
Lindau-von Hippel disease
Linder
L. sign
L. test
Lindermann bur
Linde XeScan
line
AC-PC l.
anterior commissure-posterior commissure l.
l. artifact
Baillarger l.
basal l.
l. of Bechterew
bimastoid l.

NOTES

line *(continued)*
l. bisection error (LBE)
cell l.
central sacral l.
Chamberlain palatooccipital l.
Chaussier l.
choroid l.
clivus canal l.
digastric l.
Donaldson l.
Fishgold l.
foramen magnum l.
l. frequency noise dot
Garrett orientation l.
l. of Gennari
Gennari l.
glabella-inion l.
Gubler l.
Haller l.
HCN-1 cell l.
Head l.
l. imaging
isodose l.
l. of Kaes
Kaes l.
linear regression l.
logarithmic regression l.
Lorentzian l.
M l.
major dense l.
major period l.
McGregor basal l.
McRae foramen magnum l.
Mees l.
midpoint to meatal l.
neural cell l.
Obersteiner-Redlich l.
occipital l.
palatooccipital l.
period l.
posterior canal l.
radiosignal l.
recruitment l.
rolandic l.
l. scanning
SH-SY5Y cell l.
simian l.
soft l.
spinolamellar l.
spinous interlaminar l.
sylvian l.
tender l.
Ullmann l.
Voigt l.
Wackenheim clivus canal l.
l. width

linear
l. accelerator (LINAC)
l. accelerator radiosurgery
l. accelerator system
l. chromosome
l. craniectomy
l. energy transfer (LET)
l. interpolation level
l. least-square regression analysis
l. nucleus
l. perspective
l. rate-response function
l. regression analysis
l. regression line
l. scale
l. skull fracture

line-derived
glial cell l.-d.

lingering fear

lingua, pl. **linguae**
l. cerebelli
l. franca
lapsus l.
nucleus fibrosus l.
septum l.
tremor l.

linguadental

lingual
l. airway dysfunction
l. corpuscle
l. gyrus
l. hemiatrophy
l. muscle
l. nerve
l. paralysis
l. plexus
l. septum
l. trophoneurosis
l. vein

lingual-facial-buccal dyskinesia

lingualis
gyrus l.
nervus l.
rami fauciales nervi l.
rami isthmi faucium nervi l.
rami linguales nervi l.

lingualplasty

lingula, pl. **lingulae**
l. cerebelli
l. of cerebellum
vincula l.

lingular

linguofacial vein

Link
L. SB Charité disk
L. SB Charité disk prosthesis

linkage
l. analysis
l. object
rod l.
lion's
l. claw grasper
l. paw grasper
Lioresal
liothyronine sodium
lip
l. reflex
l. smacking automatism
lipase
acid l.
lipectomy
lipedematous alopecia
lipid
l. bilayer
cell membrane l.
l. hypothesis
l. metabolic disorder
l. metabolism disorder
l. myopathy
l. peroxidation
l. recycling
serum l.
l. serum level
l. storage disorder
lipid-containing vesicle
lipid-laden stromal cell
lipidosis, pl. **lipidoses**
cerebral l.
cerebroside l.
familial neurovisceral l.
galactosylceramide l.
ganglioside l.
neuronal l.
sphingomyelin l.
sulfatide l.
lipid-protein bilayer
Lipiodol
lipodermatosis
lipodystrophy
lipofuscin granule
lipofuscinosis
adult l.
ceroid l.
Finnish variant of neuronal ceroid l.
l. granular osmiophilic deposit
Indian variant l.
infantile l.
juvenile neuronal ceroid l.
late infantile l.
neuronal ceroid l.
lipogranulomatosis
Farber l.
lipohyalinosis
lipohyalinotic
lipoid metabolism
lipoidosis
cerebroside l.
lipolysis
membrane l.
lipolytic enzyme
lipoma
epidermoid l.
hamartomatous l.
inclusion l.
intradural l.
quadrigeminal cistern l.
spinal l.
subarachnoid l.
subcutaneous l.
tectal l.
lipomatosis
epidural l.
lipomeningocele
lipomyelocele
lipomyelomeningocele
lipomyeloschisis
liponeural junction
lipophilic
l. chloroethylnitrosourea
l. compound
l. morpholinoanthracycline
lipophilin
lipopolysaccharide
lipopolysaccharide-induced inflammation
lipoprotein
high-density l. (HDL)
low-density l. (LDL)
l. metabolic disorder
l. receptor-related
liposarcoma
liposomal
liposome
cytarabine l.
Lipoxide
lipoxygenase pathway
Liqui-Char

NOTES

liquid
L. Embolic System
ethylene vinyl alcohol copolymer l.
liquor cerebrospinalis
***LIS1* gene**
Lisch nodule
lisinopril and hydrochlorothiazide
LISREL 8 program
Lissauer
L. bundle
L. column
column of Spitzka and L.
L. fasciculus
L. marginal zone
L. paralysis
L. tract
L. tract of spinal cord
lissencephalia
lissencephalic syndrome
lissencephaly
l. syndrome
Walker l.
X-linked l.
Listeria
L. monocytogenes
L. monocytogenes meningitis
listhesis
lateral l.
lisuride
liter
injected dose per l. (IDPL)
literacy deficiency
literal
l. agraphia
l. paraphasia
literalis
dysarthria l.
lithium
l. carbonate
l. dose
l. treatment
Litmosoides carinii
Little disease
livedo reticularis
liver
l. damage
l. encephalopathy
l. enzyme serum level
l. flap
l. function test
l. phosphorylase
l. span
l. transplantation
Livierato sign
living
activities of daily l. (ADL)
Communication Activities of Daily L.
Communicative Abilities in Daily L.
l. death
Health and Daily L.
instrumental activities of daily l. (IADL)
Reintegration to Normal L. (RNL)
tasks of independent l.
L-LTP
late-phase long-term potentiation
LM
lower motoneuron
lower motor
LMN
lower motor neuron
LMNA
lamin a/c gene
LN
Imagent LN
load
axial l.
high-lesion l.
lesion l.
sensory l.
loading
axial l.
Edwards modular system dynamic l.
salient l.
l. strategy
lobar
l. atrophy
l. division
l. dysfunction
l. hemorrhage
l. sclerosis
lobata
Pueraria l.
lobe
burst temporal l.
cerebral l.
l. of cerebrum
cuneiform l.
falciform l.
flocculonodular l.
frontal l.
insular l.
isthmus of limbic l.
left frontal l.
limbic l.
medial temporal l.
mesial aspect of temporal l.
mesial part of frontal l.
mesiobasal temporal l.
mesiotemporal l.

neural l.
occipital l.
olfactory l.
optic l.
parietal l.
piriform l.
prefrontal l.
quadrate l.
right frontal l.
semilunar l.
Spigelius l.
temporal l.
uncus of temporal l.
vagal l.
visceral l.

lobectomy
anterior temporal l.
anteromesial temporal l.
Falconer l.
nondominant temporal l.
occipital l.
temporal l.

lobi (*pl. of* lobus)

lobotomy
frontal l.
prefrontal l.
radical prefrontal l.
transorbital l.

Lobstein ganglion

lobule
ala of central l.
ansiform l.
anterior lunate l.
anterior paracentral l.
biventer l.
biventral l.
central l.
flocculonodular l.
gracile l.
inferior parietal l.
inferior semilunar l.
myxoid l.
paracentral l.
paramedian l.
parietal l.
posterior lunate l.
quadrangular l.
quadrate l.
semilunar l.
simple l.
slender l.
superior parietal l. (SPL)
superior semilunar l.
wing of central l.

lobulet, lobulette

lobulus, pl. **lobuli**
l. biventer
l. biventralis
l. centralis corporis cerebelli
l. clivi
l. culminis
l. cuneiformis
l. folii
l. fusiformis
l. gracilis
l. paracentralis
l. paramedianus
l. paramedianus cerebelli
l. parietalis inferior
l. parietalis superior
l. quadrangularis
l. quadrangularis anterior cerebelli
l. quadrangularis posterior cerebelli
l. quadratus
lobuli semilunares
l. semilunaris caudalis
l. semilunaris inferior
l. semilunaris rostralis
l. semilunaris superior
l. simplex
l. simplex cerebelli

lobus, pl. **lobi**
l. anterior hypophyseos
lobi cerebri
l. clivi
l. falciformis
l. flocculonodularis
l. frontalis
l. frontalis cerebri
l. glandularis hypophyseos
l. insula
l. insularis
l. limbicus
l. nervosus
l. nervosus neurohypophyseos
l. occipitalis
l. occipitalis cerebri
l. parietalis
l. parietalis cerebri
l. posterior cerebelli
l. posterior hypophyseos
l. rostralis cerebelli

L

NOTES

lobus *(continued)*
l. temporalis
l. vagi
local
l. anesthesia
l. cerebral blood flow (LCBF)
l. circuit theory
l. diagnostic block
l. epilepsy
l. excitatory state
l. field distortion
l. lymph node
l. reduction in amplitude
l. reflex
l. sign
l. syncope
l. tetanus
l. tic
l. vasoconstrictive action
localization
l. agnosia
autoradiographic l.
cerebral l.
2D graphic l.
dipole l.
frame fixation-scanner assisted target l.
ictal l.
intraoperative stereotactic spatial l.
law of average l.
manual target l.
pedicle l.
pneumotaxic l.
scanner assisted target l.
spatial l.
stereotactic l.
stereotactic anatomic target l.
subcellular l.
target l.
ultrasonographic l.
x-ray l.
localization-related
l.-r. epilepsy
l.-r. seizure
localized
l. amnesia
l. electroencephalographic seizure pattern
l. evoked potential
l. magnetic resonance
l. pruritus
l. restorative central nervous system gene therapy
localizer
Flashpoint 5000 3-D l.
Mayfield fiducial l.
Risser l.
Suetens-Gybels-Vandermeulen angiographic l.
ultrasonic l.
location
brain l.
cervical sympathetic chain l.
pedicle l.
locative
entity l.
locator
Gill Thomas l.
loci (*pl. of* locus)
lock
l. finger
l. spasm
locked facet
locked-in syndrome
locoism
locomotion
brachial l.
locomotor ataxia
loco weed
loculation syndrome
loculus, pl. **loculi**
meningeal l.
locus, pl. **loci**
l. caeruleus
l. cerulean
l. cinereus
l. coeruleus (LC)
l. coeruleus region
l. ferrugineus
l. heterogeneity
l. niger
l. perforatus anticus
l. perforatus posticus
quantitative trait l. (QTL)
Loewenthal
L. bundle
L. tract
loflazepate
ethyl l.
log
sleep l.
logagnosia
logagraphia
logamnesia
logaphasia
logarithmic regression line
logarithm of the odds score
logasthenia
logical memory subtest score
logistic regression equation
logomachy
logopathy
logoplegia
Logor

logospasm
LOH10
loss of heterozygosity chromosome 10
Lombard voice-reflex test
lomustine (CCNU)
long
l. association fiber
L. Beach stereotactic robot
l. gyrus of the insula
l. pulse repetition time/echo time image
l. pulse repetition time/long echo time
l. pulse repetition time/long echo time spin-echo
l. root of ciliary ganglion
l. segment spinal fusion
l. sleep (LS)
l. sleeper
l. thoracic nerve
l. thoracic palsy
long-acting
l.-a. injectable medication
l.-a. injection
longae
fibrae associationes l.
long-chain fatty acid
longi
nervi ciliares l.
longitudinal
l. assessment
l. cerebral fissure
l. experimental study design
l. expert evaluation using all available data
l. fissure of cerebrum
l. ligament
l. ligament rupture
l. magnetization
l. medial bundle
l. member to anchor connector
l. pontine bundle
l. pontine fasciculus
l. pontine fiber
l. relaxation
l. scan
l. sinus thrombus
l. spinal bar
longitudinales
fibrae pontis l.
long-lasting drug effect
long-standing corticosteroid administration
longstanding symptom
long-stay ward
long-term
l.-t. associative memory
l.-t. bone-instrumentation interface
l.-t. course
l.-t. declarative memory
l.-t. effectiveness
l.-t. effects of trauma
l.-t. insomnia
l.-t. naturalistic study
l.-t. storage of memory
l.-t. vasomotor tone renin
longus
l. capitis muscle
l. cervicis colli muscle
nervus thoracicus l.
loop
Blair-Ivy l.
corticobasal ganglia-cortical parallel l.
corticobasal ganglionic-thalamocortical l.
gamma l.
Granit l.
Hartshill Ransford l.
l. of hypoglossal nerve
Hyrtl l.
inferior root of cervical l.
inhibitory l.
lenticular l.
Meyer l.
Meyer-Archambault l.
neuronal feedback l.
neuronal feed-forward l.
pallidostriatal feedback l.
peduncular l.
Ransford l.
l. of spinal nerve
subclavian l.
superior root of cervical l.
l. synapse
unipolar cutting l.
vascular l.
Vieussens l.
Lophophora williamsii
Lopressor
lorazepam

NOTES

lordosis
l. creation
lumbar spine l.
l. preservation
thoracic spine l.
Lorentzian line
Lorenz
L. cranial plate
L. cranial screw
L. Neuro/skull base titanium osteosynthesis system
L. titanium screws and plate
Lorenzo oil
Lorfan
losigamone
loss
allelic l.
amygdala volumetric l.
axonal l.
blood l.
bone l.
cell l.
central sensory l.
color vision l.
complete visual l.
l. of consciousness
contralateral l.
cortical sensory l.
Dejerine onion peel sensory l.
dense sensory l.
dissociated sensory l.
l. of energy metabolism
functional l.
gag reflex l.
gaze-evoked visual l.
glucocorticoid-induced bone l.
hair l.
heat l.
hemifield l.
hemisensory l.
l. of heterozygosity chromosome 10 (LOH10)
hippocampal neuronal l.
hippocampal pyramidal cell l.
hippocampal volume l.
hippocampal volumetric l.
hysterical visual l.
l. of independence
ipsilateral l.
lumbar lordosis iatrogenic l.
mechanical visual l.
l. of memory
natural hearing l.
neuronal l.
nonspecific neuronal l.
partial visual l.
peripheral sensory l.
permanent visual l.
primary afferent l.
progressive visual l.
l. of response
retrocochlear hearing l.
saddle-area sensory l.
l. of sensitivity
sensory l.
signal l.
stocking-glove sensory l.
surgical hearing l.
synapse l.
topographic memory l.
transient monocular visual l.
unilateral visual l.
visual acuity l.
volumetric l.
weight l.
loss-of-resistance technique
Lotronex
lotus neuropathy
Lou Gehrig disease
Louis-Bar syndrome
Louis instrumentation
lounging position
loupe
binocular l.
Keeler Galilean l.
Keeler panoramic l.
l. magnification
loup-garou
Love
L. nerve root hook
L. nerve root retractor
L. pituitary rongeur
Love-Adson wire tightener
Love-Gruenwald
L.-G. cranial rongeur
L.-G. disk rongeur
L.-G. intervertebral disk forceps
L.-G. pituitary forceps
L.-G. pituitary rongeur
Love-Kerrison
L.-K. laminectomy rongeur
L.-K. rongeur forceps
Lovén reflex
low
l. alpha coefficient
l. anger threshold
l. back pain (LBP)
l. back pain psychogenic disorder
l. back syndrome
l. blood gas partition
l. bone mass
l. calcium
l. cervical approach
l. delirium

l. EMG tone
l. energy level
l. linear frequency
l. lumbar spine fracture
l. molecular weight cytokeratin
l. penetrance-high frequency gene
l. physical activity
l. potassium
L. Profile valve
l. serum albumin
l. single thoracic curve
l. tension glaucoma
l. threshold of competency
l. voltage EEG

low-air-loss bed
low-amplitude activity
low-degree astrocytoma
low-density
l.-d. area (LDA)
l.-d. lesion
l.-d. lipoprotein (LDL)
l.-d. lipoprotein receptor

low-dose
l.-d. dopaminergic agonist
l.-d. estrogen replacement
l.-d. strategy

Löwenberg
L. canal
L. scala

low-energy gamma radiation
lower
l. abdominal periosteal reflex
l. basilar aneurysm
l. cervical spine
l. cervical spine fusion
l. cervical spine posterior stabilization
l. cervical spine procedure
l. circulating estrogen level
l. clivus
l. hook trial
l. limb dysmetria
l. lumbar spine
l. motoneuron (LM)
l. motor (LM)
l. motor neuron (LMN)
l. motor neuron disease
l. motor neuron dysarthria
l. motor neuron dysfunction
l. motor neuron lesion
l. motor neuron paralysis
l. motor neuron syndrome
l. pons
l. posterior lumbar spine and sacrum surgery
l. radicular syndrome
l. thoracic pedicle
l. thoracic spine

lower-half headache
lowest saturation of oxygen
Lowe syndrome
low-filter frequency
low-frequency
l.-f. activity
l.-f. filter (LFF)

low-grade
l.-g. astrocytoma
l.-g. glioma (LGG)

low-key response
low-melt temperature agarose
low-molecular weight heparin
low-pass filter
Lowry-MacLean syndrome
low-tension glaucoma
low-threshold
l.-t. mechanoreceptive (LTM)
l.-t. mechanoreceptor

low-voltage
l.-v. activity
l.-v. calibration

loxapine
loxia
Loxitane C
Lozol
LP
lumbar puncture

LPC
laser photocoagulation

LS
long sleep
Micro-K LS

LSA
lenticulostriate artery

LSC
lateral semicircular canal

L-shaped
L.-s. aneurysm clip
L.-s. microplate

LSI
lumbar spine index

LSM
laser scanning microscope

NOTES

LSM-GB200 confocal laser scanning microscope
LSPN
lesser superficial petrosal nerve
LSUMC
LSUMC classification of motor and sensory function
LSUMC classification of nerve injury
LT
lamina terminalis
LTM
low-threshold mechanoreceptive
L-triiodothyronine
L-tryptophan
L-type calcium channel
LU26-054
lubeluzole
Lucae
L. bone mallet
L. nerve hook
Lucas and Drucker Motor Index
Luc ethmoid forceps
Luciani triad
lucidum
septum l.
Lückenschädel
lucubrate
Ludiomil
ludotherapy
Ludwig
depressor nerve of L.
L. ganglion
L. nerve
Luer-Lok stopcock
luetic
l. aneurysm
l. meningitis
Luft disease
Luhr
L. Microfixation cranial plate
L. Microfixation System drill bit
L. Microfixation System pliers
L. micro plate
L. microplate
L. mini plate
L. pan plate
lumbago
ischemic l.
lumbales
nervi splanchnici l.
lumbalia
ganglia l.
segmentum l. 1–5
lumbalis
cisterna l.
intumescentia l.
plexus l.
rami musculares plexus l.
ramus lateralis rami posterioris nervi l.
ramus medialis rami posterioris nervi l.
segmentum medullae spinalis l.
lumbalium
rami anteriores nervorum l.
rami dorsales nervorum l.
rami posteriores nervorum l.
rami ventrales nervorum l.
lumbar
l. anterior-root stimulator implant
l. arachnoid peritoneal shunt
l. artery
l. catheter
l. cistern
cisterna l.
l. curve
l. discectomy
l. disk disease
l. disk herniation
l. disk rupture
l. drain
l. drainage
l. enlargement of spinal cord
l. epidural steroid
l. facet disease
l. flat back syndrome
l. ganglion
l. hemilaminectomy
L. I/F CAGE
l. interbody fusion
l. interspace
l. kyphosis
l. lordosis iatrogenic loss
l. lordosis preservation
l. meningocele
l. myelography
l. nerve
l. part of diaphragm
l. part of spinal cord
l. pedicle fixation
l. pedicle marker
l. pedicle screw
l. periosteal turnover flap
l. plexopathy
l. plexus
l. port
l. puncture (LP)
l. puncture needle
l. puncture pain
l. reflex
l. rheumatism
l. scoliosis
l. spinal stenosis

l. spine biopsy
l. spine burst fracture
l. spine decompression
l. spine index (LSI)
l. spine injury
l. spine instability
l. spine instrumentation
l. spine kyphotic deformity
l. spine lordosis
l. spine model
l. spine pedicle diameter
l. spine rotational stability
l. spine segmental fixation
l. spine stabilization
l. spine transpedicular fixation
l. spine trauma
l. spine vertebral osteosynthesis
l. spondylosis
l. sympathectomy
l. synovial cyst
l. theco-peritoneal shunt syndrome
l. tumor
l. vertebra

lumbares
nervi splanchnici l.

lumbaria
segmentum l.

lumbaris
plexus l.

lumbarization

lumbar-peritoneal
l.-p. shunt
l.-p. shunting

lumboaortic intermesenteric plexus

lumbo-atrial shunt

lumbodorsal fascia (LDF)

lumboinguinalis
nervus l.

lumboinguinal nerve

lumboperitoneal shunt

lumbosacral
l. corset
l. enlargement
l. enlargement of spinal cord
l. fusion
l. junction bone density
l. junction cortical thickness
l. junction fracture
l. meningocele
l. myelomeningocele
l. plexus neuritis
l. radiculopathy
l. spine plexus injury
l. spine transpedicular instrumentation
l. trunk
l. vertebra

lumbosacralis
intumescentia l.
plexus l.
truncus l.

luminal
l. occlusion
l. perfusate

Lumsden
L. center
pneumotaxic center of L.

lunate
l. fissure
l. sulcus

lunatus
sulcus l.

Lundborg myoclonic epilepsy

lung
iron l.
trench l.

lupinosis

LUPP
laser uvulopalatoplasty

Lupron

lupus
l. anticoagulant
l. cerebritis
l. erythematosus
l. erythematosus cell
l. erythematosus peripheral neuropathy

Luque
L. II segmental spinal instrumentation
L. instrumentation concave technique
L. instrumentation convex technique
L. loop fixation
L. rectangle
L. ring
L. rod
L. rod migration
L. semirigid segmental spinal instrumentation
L. sublaminar wiring technique
L. wire

NOTES

Luque-Galveston
L.-G. fixation
L.-G. post
Luschka
foramen of L.
lateral foramina of L.
L. nerve
Lust
L. phenomenon
L. reflex
L. sign
lusterless eye
lutea
macula l.
luteae
fovea centralis maculae l.
luteal phase progesterone
luteinizing
l. hormone (LH)
l. hormone-releasing hormone
luteum
corpus l.
punctum l.
Luvox
luxation
rotatory l.
Luxtec
L. coaxial illumination
L. illuminated surgical telescope
luxury
l. perfusion
l. perfusion syndrome
Luys
L. body
centre médian de L.
nucleus of L.
luysii
corpus l.
Lyell syndrome
Lyme
L. borreliosis
L. disease
L. encephalopathy
L. neuroborreliosis
L. neuropathy
lymphadenopathy
lymphangioma
lymphoblastoid
lymphocyte
CD4 l.
cytotoxic l.
peripheral blood l.
tumor-infiltrating l. (TIL)
lymphocyte:PMN ratio in cerebrospinal fluid
lymphocytic
l. adenohypophysitis
l. choriomeningitis
l. choriomeningitis virus (LCMV)
l. choriomeningitis virus encephalitis
l. hypophysitis
l. meningitis
l. pleocytosis
l. pleocytosis-depressed glucose in cerebrospinal fluid
lymphocytopenia
lymphocytosis
atypical l.
lymphoepithelial parotid tumor
lymphoepithelioma
lymphogranuloma venereum encephalitis
lymphoid hypophysitis
lymphokine
lymphokine-activated killer cell
lymphoma
angiotropic l.
central nervous system l.
centroblastic B-cell l.
cerebral l.
CNS l.
Hodgkin l.
intracerebral Hodgkin l.
intracranial Hodgkin l.
intramedullary l.
intravascular l.
Lennert l.
malignant l.
meningeal l.
non-Hodgkin l. (NHL)
primary brain l.
primary central nervous system l. (PCNSL)
primary CNS l.
primary intramedullary l.
primary leptomeningeal l.
primary nervous system l.
solitary extranodal l.
lymphomagenesis
lymphomatoid granulomatosis
lymphomatosum
cystadenoma l.
lymphomatous
l. meningitis
l. tumor
lymphopathy
ataxic l.
lymphoproliferative disorder
lymphotoxin
Lynch incision
Lyodura
Lyodura-associated Creutzfeldt-Jakob disease
lyophilized cadaveric dura

lypressin
lyra davidis
lysergic acid diethylamide and strychnine
lysine metabolism disorder
lysolecithin patching
lysosomal
  l. enzymatic activity
  l. storage disease
  l. storage disorder
lytic infection
Lytico-Bodig disease

NOTES

L

M
M line
M response
M segment
M vector
M wave
M1
M1 agonist
M1 segment aneurysm
M2
M2 artery segment
M2 branch
M2 segment of right middle cerebral artery
99m
CEA-Tc 99m
Pertscan 99m
M-2 anterior plate system
MAC
minimal alveolar concentration
MAC EIA
MacCarty forceps
MacDonald dissector
MacDougall diet for multiple sclerosis
Macewen
M. sign
M. symptom
Machado-Joseph disease
Machiafava-Bignami disease
machine
Accuray Neurotron 1000 m.
m. artifact
Burdick Eclipse ECG m.
TECA-TD20 EMG m.
Machover
mAChR
muscarinic acetylcholine receptor
Mach 16 Select wire
Machupo virus
Mackenzie syndrome
macrencephaly, macrencephalia
macro
m. square-wave jerk
m. stimulation
macroadenoma
enclosed m.
pituitary m.
macroaneurysm
macrocephalic, macrocephalous
macrocephaly, macrocephalia
hydrencephaly m.
m. with somatic and genital growth delay
macrocheilia
macrocrania
macrocranium
macrocryoglobulinemia peripheral neuropathy
macro-eCVR-FV circulation
macroelectrical stimulation
macroelectrode technique
macroencephalia
macroencephalon
macroencephaly
macroglia cell
macroglobulinemia
m. peripheral neuropathy
Waldenstrom m.
m. of Waldenstrom
macroglossia
macrognathia
macrogyria
macroinstrument
macromolecule
cellular m.
myelin m.
macrophage
activated m.
m. immigration
immunocompetent m.
perivascular m.
macrophage-derived cell
macrophthalmos
MacroPore sheet
macropsia
macroscopic
m. dysgenesis
m. magnetization moment
m. magnetization vector
MacroSorb absorbable plate implant
macrostereognosia
Macrotec
mactans
Lactrodectus m.
macula, pl. **maculae**
m. communicans
m. cribrosa
maculae cribrosae
m. cribrosa inferior
m. cribrosa media
m. cribrosa quarta
m. cribrosa superior
m. densa
m. lutea
neuroepithelium of m.
m. retinae
m. sacculi
m. utriculi

M

macular
m. fasciculus
m. hemianopia
m. sparing
macularis
fasciculus m.
macular-sparing hemianopia
maculocerebral
maculoneural bundle
maculopapular rash
madazolam
Mad Hatter syndrome
M-ADL
morphine-Adcon-L
M-ADL paste
madness
myxedema m.
madreporic coral
madurae
Actinomadura m.
Maffucci syndrome
MAG
myelin-associated glycoprotein
MAG3
Technescan M.
magaldrate
3M Agee carpal tunnel release system
Magellan electromagnetic navigation system
Magendie
foramen of M.
M. law
median foramen of M.
M. space
Magendie-Hertwig
M.-H. sign
M.-H. syndrome
Magerl
M. hook-plate system
method of M.
M. plate-screw system
M. posterior C1-C2 screw fixation
magic
M. B1 balloon
m. bone
M. microcatheter
m. thinking
M. Wallstent
MAGIC syndrome
magna
arteria radicularis m.
chorda m.
chorea m.
cisterna m.
mega cisterna m.
radicularis m.
vena cerebri m.
Magnacal
magnae
cisterna venae m.
Magnan
M. sign
M. trombone movement
Magnes
M. magnetic source imaging
M. 2500 WH imager
magnesium
m. aluminum hydroxide
m. balance
m. carbonate
m. chloride
m. deficiency infantile tremor syndrome
m. gluconate
m. hydroxide suspension
m. imbalance
m. oxide
m. salicylate
m. sulfate
MAGNES MEG system
magnet
Alnico Magneprobe m.
cobalt samarium m.
C-shaped resistive m.
field m.
main field m.
m. mode
open m.
permanent m.
PoleStar m.
m. quench
m. reaction
m. reflex
resistive m.
m. shielding
superconducting m.
0.5-T superconducting m.
magnetic
m. apraxia
m. dipole
m. disk
m. field
m. field gradient
m. field vector
m. moment
m. resonance (MR)
m. resonance angiogram
m. resonance angiography (MRA)
m. resonance image (MRI)
m. resonance imaging (MRI)
m. resonance marker
m. resonance neurography (MRN)
m. resonance perfusion imaging
m. resonance signal

m. resonance spectroscopy (MRS)
m. resonance tomography (MRT)
m. resonance venography (MRV)
m. seizure therapy
m. shielded cabin
somatosensory evoked m.
m. source imaging (MSI)
m. stimulator
m. susceptibility
m. susceptibility artifact

magnetization
longitudinal m.
spatial modulation of m. (SPAMM)
spin m.
transverse m.

magnetization-prepared rapid acquisition gradient echo sequence (MPRAGE)

magnetoelectric stimulation

magnetoelectrophysiology

magnetoencephalogram (M-EEG, MEG)

magnetoencephalograph

magnetoencephalography (MEG)

magnetohydrodynamic effect

Magnetom
M. Open scanner
M. SP 4000 1.5-Tesla system
M. Vision scanner

magnetometer
8-channel whole-head m.

magnetometry
synthetic aperture m. (SAM)

magnetophosphene

Magnevist

magni
ramus posterior nervi auricularis m.

magnification
loupe m.

magnitude
perturbation m.

magnocell

magnocellular
m. basal forebrain
m. deficit
m. dysfunction
m. layer
m. neuron
m. pathway
m. reticular nucleus
m. visual system

magnocellularia
strata m.

magnocellularis
nucleus medialis m.
nucleus reticularis m.

magnum
M. 800 bed
foramen m.

magnus
M. and de Kleijn neck reflex
nervus auricularis m.
nucleus raphes m.
m. raphe nucleus

Magonate

Magstim
M. 200
M. 200 stimulator

maidenhair tree

main
m. cuneate nucleus
m. d'accoucheur
m. effect
m. en griffe deformity
m. en singe
m. field
m. field magnet
m. sensory nucleus of the trigeminus
m. succulente

Maine
jumper disease of M.

maintenance
m. medication
m. of wakefulness test (MWT)

maitre de plaiser

major
m. break
chorea m.
m. dense line
epilepsia m.
m. epilepsy
m. forceps
m. form
hippocampus m.
m. histocompatibility complex (MHC)
m. life stress
m. motor aphasia
m. motor seizure
nervus occipitalis m.
nervus palatinus m.
nervus petrosus m.
nervus splanchnicus thoracicus m.

NOTES

M

major *(continued)*
m. period line
m. psychiatric syndrome
m. risk period
m. solution
majoris
rami nasales posteriores inferiores nervi palatini m.
sulcus nervi petrosi m.
makros
MAL
mamilloaccessory ligament
mal
m. d'orient
grand m.
petit m.
pyknoleptic petit m.
malabsorption
fat m.
m. syndrome peripheral neuropathy
vitamin D m.
Malacarne
M. pyramid
M. space
malacia traumatica
maladaptive
m. coping
m. mechanism
m. pattern
m. pattern of motivation
maladie
m. des tics
m. du doute
malaise
postexertional m.
malalignment
ocular m.
malar eminence
malaria
cerebellar m.
cerebral m.
therapeutic m.
malate
almotriptan m.
Malcolm-Rand carbon-composite headholder
maleate
chlorpheniramine m.
fluvoxamine m.
methysergide m.
perhexiline m.
prochlorperazine m.
timolol m.
trimipramine m.
malevolent thought system
malfeasance
malformation
angiographically occult intracranial vascular m. (AOIVM)
angiographically visualized vascular m. (AVVM)
Arnold-Chiari m.
arteriovenous m. (AVM)
auditory arteriovenous m.
bone occipital m.
brain arteriovenous m. (BAVM)
brainstem cavernous m.
cavernous m. (CM)
central nervous system m.
cerebral venous m. (CVM)
cerebrovascular m.
Chiari m. (I–IV)
congenital m.
cortical m.
craniofacial m.
cryptic arteriovenous m.
cryptic cerebrovascular m.
cryptic vascular m.
Dandy-Walker m.
developmental m.
dural arteriovenous m.
familial arteriovenous m.
flocculonodular arteriovenous m.
Galen vein m.
glomus arteriovenous m.
infratentorial arteriovenous m.
intraarachnoid leptomeningeal m.
intracerebral arteriovenous m.
intracranial vascular m. (ICVM, IVM)
intracranial venous m.
intraorbital arteriovenous m.
intraspinal vascular m.
intratentorial m.
juvenile arteriovenous m.
Krabbe Arnold-Chiari m.
medial hemispheric arteriovenous m.
obliterated arteriovenous m.
occipital m.
occult cerebrovascular m. (OCVM)
Osler-Weber-Rendu arteriovenous m.
pial arteriovenous m.
punctate cavernous m.
radiculomeningeal spinal vascular m.
Spetzler-Martin classification of arteriovenous m.
spinal cord arteriovenous m.
split-cord m.
structural m.
supratentorial arteriovenous m.
thalamocaudate arteriovenous m.

vascular m.
vein of Galen m.
venous m.
Wyburn-Mason arteriovenous m.

Malibu orthosis

malignancy
anterior skull base m.
nasopharyngeal m.
skull-base m.

malignant
m. astrocytoma
m. atrophic papulosis
m. eccrine poroma
m. endovascular papillary angioendothelioma
m. external otitis
m. familial myoclonic epilepsy
m. fibrohistiocytoma
m. germ cell tumor
m. glioma
m. hypertension
m. hyperthermia
m. lymphoma
m. meningioma
m. neuroleptic syndrome
m. phenotype
m. purpura
m. stupor
m. teratoma

mali-mali

Malis
M. angled bayonet forceps
M. bipolar cautery scissors
M. bipolar instrument
M. bipolar microcoagulator
M. brain retractor
M. CMC-II bipolar coagulator
M. CMC-III electrosurgical system
M. curette
M. dissector
M. electrocoagulation unit
M. elevator
M. irrigating bipolar CMC-III
M. irrigation forceps
M. jeweler's bipolar forceps
M. ligature passer
M. needle holder
M. nerve hook
M. neurological scissors
M. solid state coagulator
M. vessel supporter

Malis-Jensen microbipolar forceps

malleable
m. endoscope
m. microsurgical suction device
m. multipore suction tube

malleatory
m. chorea
m. spasm

mallet
Hajek m.
Lucae bone m.

malnutrition infantile tremor syndrome

malocclusion

malternative drink

malum vertebrale suboccipitale

mamillare
corpus m.

mamillaris
nuclei corporis m.
pedunculus corporis m.

mamillary, mammillary
m. body
m. body volume
m. region

mamilloaccessory
m. ligament (MAL)
m. notch
m. ridge

mamillopeduncular tract

mamillotegmental
m. fasciculus
m. tract

mamillotegmentalis
fasciculus m.

mamillothalamic
m. fasciculus
m. tract

mamillothalamicus
fasciculus m.

mammalian
m. cell
m. hippocampus
m. olfactory system
m. vomeronasal system

mammary
m. body
m. neuralgia

mammillary (*var. of* mamillary)

mammillotegmental fasciculus

mammillothalamic fasciculus

mammosomatotroph cell adenoma

NOTES

management
intrathecal pain m.
nonpharmacologic behavior m.
seizure m.
Manchester and Oxford Universities Scale for the Psychopathological Assessment of Dementia (MOUSEPAD)
mandibular
m. advancing device
m. condylectomy
m. fixation
m. nerve
m. notch electrode
m. osteotomy
m. reflex
m. repositioner
m. retraction
m. swing technique
mandibularis
nervus m.
ramus meningeus nervi m.
mandibulofacial dysostosis
mandibulotomy
mandrel, mandril
steam-shaping m.
maneuver
Adson modified m.
Allen m.
Bárány m.
Bielschowsky m.
Buzzard m.
Dandy m.
Dix-Hallpike m.
doll's eye m.
Gowers m.
Hallpike m.
Hallpike-Bárány positioning m.
Jendrassik m.
nasal airflow-inducing m. (NAIM)
passive-aggressive m.
Phalen m.
Schreiber m.
Spurling m.
Valsalva m.
manganese
m. chloride
m. intoxication
m. toxicity
m. toxin
manic
m. patient
m. stare
m. syndrome
manie
m. de perfection
m. de rumination
manifest
m. symptom
m. tetany
manifesta
spina bifida m.
manifestation
behavioral m.
characteristic m.
clinical m.
m. of depression
lacunar stroke m.
neurobehavioral m.
neuroimaging m.
neurotic m.
psychophysiologic m.
m. of resistance
somatic neurologic m.
m. of violence
man-in-a-barrel syndrome
manipulation
cranial nerve m.
language m.
m. stage
syntactic m.
manipulator
Mehrkoordinaten m. (MKM)
manner
allosteric m.
psychical m.
mannitol
m. in intracranial pressure increase
mannitol-induced cerebral vasodilatation
Mannkopf sign
mannose in mucolipidosis
mannose-terminated-glucocerebrosidase
mannosidase
mannosidosis
alpha m.
beta m.
Mann-Whitney test
MANOVA
multiple analysis of variance
mansoni
Schistosoma m.
mantle
brain m.
cerebral m.
m. layer
m. sclerosis
Mantoux interdermal tuberculin skin test
manual
M. of Internal Fixation
m. target localization
m. vernier scale
manubrium
MAO-A gene polymorphism

MAOI
monoamine oxidase inhibitor
MAO spectrophotometric assay
MAP
mitogen-activated protein
map
brain electrical activity m.
phase-contrast m.
retinotopic m.
somatosensory m.
statistical parametric m. (SPM)
Z score m.
maple
maplike skull
mapped epilepsy syndrome
mapping
behavior m.
brain electrical activity m.
brainstem diencephalic m.
cortical m.
electrical stimulation m.
electrophysiological m.
genetic m.
phase m.
radiotherapy brain m.
somatosensory m.
spatiotemporal brain m.
speech and motor m.
stimulation m.
Talairach whole-brain m.
two-dimensional m.
maprotiline HCl
marantic
m. thrombosis
m. thrombus
marasmic
m. thrombosis
m. thrombus
marbled appearance of basal ganglion
Marcaine
Marcé study
march
jacksonian m.
Marchac forehead template
Marchant zone
marche a petits plantar aspect
Marchi
M. ball
M. degeneration
M. globule
M. reaction
M. tract
Marchiafava-Bignami
M.-B. aminoaciduria
M.-B. disease
M.-B. syndrome
Marconi Medical Systems console
Marcus
M. grading scale for avascular necrosis
M. Gunn
M. Gunn phenomenon
M. Gunn pupil
M. Gunn syndrome
marfanoid
m. craniosynostosis syndrome
m. habitus
Marfan syndrome
margaritoma
margaroid tumor
margin
dural m.
marginal
m. branch of cingulate sulcus
m. fasciculus
m. gyrus
m. layer
m. sinus
m. zone
marginalis
fasciculus m.
ramus m.
sinus m.
sulcus m.
marginally therapeutic dose
marginis
cornu inferius m.
margo
m. inferior cerebri
m. inferolateralis
m. inferolateralis hemispherii cerebri
m. inferomedialis hemispherii cerebri
m. medialis cerebri
m. superomedialis
m. superomedialis cerebri
Margrel transfacetal screw technique
Marie
M. ataxia
hereditary cerebellar ataxia of M.

NOTES

Marie *(continued)*
M. quadrilateral sign
M. quadrilateral space
Marie-Foix-Alajouanine
M.-F.-A. cerebellar atrophy
M.-F.-A. disease
Marie-Foix sign
Marie-Strümpell
M.-S. disease
M.-S. encephalitis
Marie-Tooth disease
marimastat
M. BB5416
M. protease inhibitor
Marin Amat syndrome
Marinesco
M. sign
M. succulent hand
Marinesco-Garland syndrome
Marinesco-Radovici reflex
Marinesco-Sjögren syndrome
Marino
M. transsphenoidal curette
M. transsphenoidal dissector
M. transsphenoidal enucleator
M. transsphenoidal hook
Marinol
mariposia
marked motor agitation
marker
biochemical phenotypic m.
biochemical tumor m.
biologic m.
cerebral fluid m.
m. chromosome
desmin tumor m.
discoid m.
DNA m.
epithelial membrane antigen tumor m.
factor VIII antigen tumor m.
fiducial m.
glial-specific m.
HHF35 muscle-specific actin tumor m.
high molecular weight cytokeratin tumor m.
lumbar pedicle m.
magnetic resonance m.
metallic skin m.
pedicle m.
phenotypic m.
roentgenographic opaque m.
Schwann cell m.
serum m.
S-100 tumor m.
surface fiducial m.
thoracic pedicle m.
tumor m.
vimentin tumor m.
m. X syndrome
Markham-Meyerding hemilaminectomy retractor
Markov decision analysis model
Marlex
marmoratus
status m.
Maroon-Jannetta dissector
Maroteaux-Lamy
M.-L. disease
M.-L. syndrome
Marpres
marrow
bone m.
vertebral m.
Marsden and Harrison criteria
marsupial notch
Martin-Bell syndrome
Martin-Gruber anastomosis
Martin nerve root retractor
Martinotti cell
Maryland
M. coma scale
M. tissue grasping forceps
M. type familial amyloid polyneuropathy
Masini sign
mask
m. facies
Hutchinson m.
Parkinson m.
Parrot m.
tabetic m.
masked
m. epilepsy
m. facies
masking
metacontrast m.
m. pain
white noise m.
masklike
m. face
m. facies
mass
m. action theory
black m.
cerebellar m.
m. doubling time
m. effect
external auditory canal m.
fat-free m.
free-fat m. (FFM)
hemispheral m.
intermediate m.

intraconal m.
intraparenchymal m.
isodense m.
jugular foramen m.
m. lesion
low bone m.
m. media
muscle m.
parameningeal m.
parasagittal intracranial m.
parasellar m.
peak bone m.
petrous apex m.
pineal region m.
m. reflex
serpiginous m.
m. spectrometer
suprasellar m.
supratentorial m.
thermogenic tissue m.
tigroid m.
vascular intratympanic m.
massage
carotid sinus m.
digital temple m.
hydropneumatic m.
nerve-point m.
m. treatment
massager
Cryocup ice m.
massa intermedia
masseter
m. reflex
m. strength
masseteric nerve
massetericus
nervus m.
massive spasm
Masson
M. trichrome stain
M. vegetant intravascular hemangioendothelioma
Masson-Fontana stain
MAST
minimal access spinal technology
master gland
mastication disorder
masticatoria
monoplegia m.
masticatorius
nucleus m.
masticatory
m. attack
m. diplegia
m. nucleus
m. spasm
mastocytosis
systemic m.
mastoid
m. air cell
m. antrum
m. complex
m. process
m. retractor
Matas
M. operation
M. test
M. treatment
matchbox sign
matching
prototype m.
m. and tuning network
mater
cranial arachnoid m.
cranial pia m.
dura m.
pia m.
sinus of dura m.
spinal arachnoid m.
spinal pia m.
transverse sinus of dura m.
venous sinus of dura m.
material
alloplastic m.
ballistic m.
Biocoral graft m.
Elgiloy clip m.
Glasflex m.
MP-35 clip m.
NeuroCell-HD porcine fetal neural m.
NeuroCell-PD porcine fetal neural m.
neutral m.
nonferrous m.
Phynox cobalt alloy clip m.
precollagenous filamentous m.
verbal m.
maternal
m. competency
m. deprivation syndrome
m. dysfunction

NOTES

maternal · maximum

maternal *(continued)*
m. hyperparathyroidism
m. thyroid hormone
mathematical optimization and logical dimensioning for radiotherapy
***math* gene**
Matricaria recutita
matris
sinus transversus durae m.
matrix
m. adhesion
DuraGen dural graft m.
extracellular m. (ECM)
germinal m.
Grafton demineralized bone m.
intercellular m.
m. metalloproteinase (MMP)
m. metalloproteinase inhibitor
m. molecule
parenchymal m.
m. protein
rigid body transformation m.
matter
anisotropy of white m.
cortical gray m.
deep white m.
gray m. (GM)
heterotopic gray m.
inferior periventricular white m.
lateral periventricular white m.
medial periventricular white m.
occipital gray m. (Occip GM)
occipital white m.
parahippocampal white m.
periaqueductal gray m.
periventricular gray m.
periventricular white m.
pontine gray m.
sclerosis of white m.
subcortical gray m.
superior periventricular white m.
white m.
mattress
Akros extended care m.
Akros pressure m.
eggcrate m.
Matulane
maturation
glial cell m.
hormonal m.
neocortex m.
neuroblast m.
Pandy m.
maturational change
maturity
cognitive m.
motor m.
matutinal
m. epilepsy
m. headache
Mauthner
M. cell
M. fiber
M. membrane
M. sheath
Maxalt
Maxenon 300 watt xenon light source
Maxicamera
Gamma M.
Maxidone
maxillaris
nervus m.
rami alveolares superiores anteriores nervi m.
rami alveolares superiores posteriores nervi m.
rami nasales posteriores superiores laterales nervi m.
rami nasales posteriores superiores mediales nervi m.
rami orbitales nervi m.
ramus alveolaris superior medius nervi m.
ramus meningeus nervi m.
maxillary
m. antrum
m. artery
m. nerve
m. osteotomy
m. plexus
m. sinus
m. vein
maxillofacial
m. fracture
m. plating system
m. trauma
maxillomandibular artery
Maxillume 250 watt quartz halogen light source
Maxima II TENS unit
maximal
m. effect
m. electroshock-induced seizure
m. electroshock seizure (MES)
m. hydrocephalus
m. plasma concentration
m. stimulus
m. voluntary contraction
maximum
full width at half m. (FWHM)
full-width half m.
m. intensity pixel reconstruction
m. intensity projection
m. intent rating

m. lethality rating
m. saccade peak velocity
m. tolerable amount
m. tolerated dose
m. voluntary contraction (MVC)

maximus gait
Maxwell pair
Mayberg limbic-cortical dysregulation model
Mayer
M. hematoxylin
M. reflex

Mayer-Gross closing-in phenomenon
Mayerson sign
Mayfield
M. aneurysm clip
M. brain spatula
M. disposable skull pin
M. fiducial localizer
M. fixation frame
M. head clamp
M. headrest system
M. horseshoe headrest
M. incision
M. miniature clip applier
M. neurosurgical skill clamp
M. pinion
M. radiolucent base unit
M. radiolucent headholder
M. radiolucent headrest
M. rongeur
M. skull cap pin
M. skull-pin headholder
M. spinal curette
M. surgical system
M. temporary aneurysm clip applier
M. tongs

Mayfield/ACCISS stereotactic device
Mayfield-Kees
M.-K. headholder
M.-K. headrest
M.-K. skull fixation apparatus
M.-K. table attachment

Mayo
M. Alzheimer Disease Center/Alzheimer Disease Patient Registry
M. Asymptomatic Carotid Endarterectomy Study
M. block anesthesia
M. Clinic stereotactic robot
M. scissors

May-White syndrome
Mazzoni corpuscle
MBP
myelin basic protein

MBP-reactive T cell
MCA
middle cerebral artery

McArdle disease
MCAT
middle cerebral artery thrombosis

McCain
M. TMJ cannula
M. TMJ trocar

McCarthy reflex
McCormac reflex
MCD
medullary collecting duct
medullary cystic disease

McDowell Impairment Index
McFadden cross-legged clip
McFadden-Kees clip
McGill
M. forceps
M. Pain Questionnaire

McGregor basal line
McGuire screw system
M-channel
m-chlorophenylpiperazine
MCI
mild cognitive impairment

McKenzie
M. brain clip forceps
M. clip-applying forceps
M. clip-bending forceps
M. clip-introducing forceps
M. enlarging bur
M. hemostasis clip
M. perforating twist drill
M. reservoir
M. silver clip

McLain-Weinstein classification of spinal tumors
McLeod syndrome
McLone and Knepper etiological theory
McRae foramen magnum line
MCTD
mixed connective tissue disease

m-current

NOTES

MCV
motor conduction velocity
MD
mitochondrial disease
movement duration
MDAS
Memorial Delirium Assessment Scale
MDM2
murine double minute 2
MDM2 gene
MDMA
methylenedioxymethamphetamine
mean
m. alpha frequency
m. arterial blood pressure
m. consecutive difference
m. corpuscular volume
m. interpotential interval (MIPI)
m. intracranial raw volume
m. normalized whole brain volume
m. sleep latency
m. sorted difference
standard error of the m. (SEM)
m. total weighted sum score
m. weighted score
measles
m. encephalitis
m. panencephalitis
m. peripheral neuropathy
m., rubella and zoster (MRZ)
measure
m. of balance
baseline m.
behavioral assessment m.
Bench Mark M.'s
cognitive m.
course of illness m.
diagnostic m.
dissociation m.
Functional Independence M.
functioning m.
m. of general cognitive functioning
global m.
Gross Motor Function M. (GMFM)
Kaiser-Meyer-Olkin m.
neglect m.
neurocognitive m.
neuropsychologic m.
number-recency m.
objective m.
outcome m.
overall cognitive m.
phenomenological m.
pretreatment m.
quality of life m.
quantitative m.
repeated m. (rm)
Schütz M.'s
sensitive m.
state-dependent m.
Surrogate Outcome M.
symptom m.
therapeutic m.
measured stress
measurement
blood flow m.
cephalometric m.
m. effect
endoesophageal pressure m.
m. error
head circumference m.
IMPA cephalometric m.
M-mode electrocardiographic m.
premature infant head circumference m.
quality-of-life m.
reference m.
Schober m.
xenon CT m.
measurement/monitoring
nasal pressure m.
meatus
external acoustic m.
mebendazole
mechanical
m. anosmia
m. insufficiency
m. irritability
m. nociceptor
m. plate design
m. ventilation
m. vertigo
m. visual loss
mechanical-type disk prosthesis
mechanicoreceptor
mechanics
quantum m.
spinal m.
mechanic's hand
mechanism
airstream m.
analogous brain m.
arousal m.
association m.
basic brain m.
brain metabolic m.
caspase-independent m.
causal m.
causative m.
clamping m.
cognitive m.
m. of correction
disengagement m.
dissociable m.

emotional m.
endogenous brain m.
free radical scavenging m.
fundamental neural m.
gating m.
genomic m.
glutamergic m.
heat-loss m.
immune mediated m.
indirect m.
intramolecular dipole-dipole m.
intrinsic cell suicide m.
Jak-STAT m.
maladaptive m.
metabolic m.
mote-beam m.
neural m.
neurobiological m.
neuronal m.
one-way flow m.
osmotic m.
paracrine m.
perceptual/cognitive m.
pharmacological m.
plastic compensatory m.
postsynaptic compensatory m.
primary m.
relapse m.
rotating m.
spring m.
sunburst m.
thermogenic m.
vasculitic m.
mechanoceptor
mechanoporation
mechanoreceptive
low-threshold m. (LTM)
mechanoreceptor
cutaneous m.
m. fiber
high-threshold m.
low-threshold m.
pacinian m.
Ruffini m.
mechanoreflex
mechanosensory
Meckel
M. cave
M. cave lesion
M. ganglion
M. lesser ganglion
M. space
M. sphenopalatine ganglionectomy
Meckel-Gruber syndrome
meckelii
cavum m.
MeCP2 gene
Medarsed
MED^next bone dissecting system
Medelec five-channel neurophysiological device
media (*pl. of* medium)
mediae
pars sphenoidalis arteriae cerebralis m.
medial
m. accessory olivary nucleus
m. amygdaloid nucleus
m. atrial vein
m. branch C2
m. central nucleus of thalamus
m. central tegmental field
m. cerebral surface
m. dorsal nucleus of thalamus
m. eminence
m. eminence of rhomboid
m. epicondylectomy
m. extradural approach
m. fillet
m. forebrain bundle
m. frontal cortex
m. frontal gyrus
m. frontal lobe syndrome
m. geniculate body
m. geniculate nucleus (MGN)
m. habenular nucleus
m. hemispheric arteriovenous malformation
m. hemispheric dynamic
m. inferior pontine syndrome
m. lemniscus
m. longitudinal bundle
m. longitudinal fasciculus (MLF)
m. longitudinal stria
m. magnocellular nucleus
m. medullary lamina of corpus striatum
m. medullary lamina of lentiform nucleus
m. medullary syndrome
m. nucleus of thalamus
m. nucleus of trapezoid body

NOTES

medial *(continued)*
m. occipital artery
m. occipitotemporal gyrus
m. olfactory gyrus
m. olfactory stria
m. operculum
m. orbitofrontal cortex
m. parabrachial nucleus
m. pericuneate nucleus
m. periventricular white matter
m. plantar nerve
m. posterior choroidal
m. prefrontal cortex (mPFC)
m. preoptic area
m. preoptic nucleus
m. rectus muscle
m. reticulospinal tract
m. root of median nerve
root of olfactory tract, lateral and m.
m. root of optic tract
m. rostral supplementary motor area
m. septal nucleus
m. striate artery
m. sulcus of crus cerebri
m. superior olivary nucleus
m. superior temporal
m. surface of cerebral hemisphere
m. temporal cortex
m. temporal lobe
m. temporal lobe epilepsy
m. temporal memory system
m. temporal structure
m. terminal branch of deep fibular nerve
m. terminal nucleus (MTN)
m. triangle of Hakuba
m. vein of lateral ventricle
m. ventral nucleus
ventral posterior m. (VPM)
m. vestibular nucleus
m. vestibulospinal tract
m. zone
m. zone of hypothalamus

mediale
corpus geniculatum m.

mediales
decussatio lemnisci m.
nervi supraclaviculares m.
nuclei geniculati m.
rami clunium m.
rami gluteales m.
rami medullares m.
ramus choroidei posteriores m.

medialis
arteria occipitalis m.
arteria orbitofrontalis m.
eminentia m.
fasciculus longitudinalis m.
globus pallidus m.
gyrus frontalis m.
gyrus occipitotemporalis m.
gyrus olfactorius m.
lamina medullaris m.
lemniscus m.
nervi digitales dorsales hallucis lateralis et digit secundi m.
nervi digitales plantares communes nervi plantaris m.
nervi digitales plantares proprii nervi plantaris m.
nervus cutaneous antebrachii m.
nervus cutaneous brachii m.
nervus cutaneous dorsalis m.
nervus cutaneous surae m.
nervus pectoralis m.
nervus plantaris m.
nervus pterygoideus m.
nuclei corporis geniculati m.
nucleus amygdalae basalis m.
nucleus campi m.
nucleus corporis geniculati m.
nucleus corporis mammillaris m.
nucleus dorsalis corporis geniculati m.
nucleus habenularis m.
nucleus interstitiales fasciculi longitudinalis m.
nucleus mamillaris m.
nucleus olivaris accessorius m.
nucleus olivaris superior m.
nucleus parabrachialis m.
nucleus pericuneatus m.
nucleus preopticus m.
nucleus septalis m.
nucleus ventralis corporis geniculati m.
nucleus vestibularis m.
pars dorsalis corporis geniculati m.
pars ventralis corporis geniculati m.
ramus anterior nervi cutanei antebrachii m.
ramus posterior nervi cutanei antebrachii m.
stria longitudinalis m.
stria olfactoria m.
tractus vestibulospinalis m.
vena atrii m.
zona m.

median
m. aperture
m. aperture of fourth ventricle
m. cleft face syndrome

m. corpectomy
m. eminence
m. face syndrome
m. foramen of Magendie
m. frontal sulcus
m. longitudinal fasciculus
m. mixed nerve action potential
m. nerve
m. nerve entrapment
m. nerve lesion
m. nerve trauma
m. preoptic nucleus
m. raphe of medulla oblongata
m. raphe nucleus
m. raphe of pons
m. sternotomy brachial plexopathy
m. sulcus of fourth ventricle

mediana
eminentia m.

mediani
nervi digitales palmares communes nervi m.
nervi digitales palmares proprii nervi m.
radix lateralis nervi m.
radix medialis nervi m.
rami musculares nervi m.
ramus palmaris nervi m.

medianum
centrum m.

medianus
nervus m.
nucleus preopticus m.
nucleus raphes m.

mediated neuronal inhibition

medical
m. comorbidity
m. effect
m. impairment
M. Research Council (MRC)
M. Research Council scale for strength testing
m. taper schedule
m. utilization
m. value system

medically
m. intractable partial epilepsy
m. refractory partial seizure

medical/neurological disorder

medication
adjunctive m.
anticholinergic m.
antiretroviral m.
antiseizure m.
antiviral m.
continuous maintenance m.
dopaminergic m.
m. dosage
ergot-derived m.
forced m.
m. guide
immunosuppressive m.
intravenous m.
involuntary m.
long-acting injectable m.
maintenance m.
neuroleptic m.
peripherally acting anticholinergic m.
prophylactic m.
psychiatric m.
psychotropic m.
m. reduction
m. refractoriness
m. regimen
m. side effect
m. stigma
m. tapering
m. taper schedule
vasodilating antihypertensive m.
weight-neutral psychotic m.

medication-induced
m.-i. depressive syndrome
m.-i. headache
m.-i. movement disorder
m.-i. REM sleep suppression

medication-related side effect

medicine
American Academy of Sleep M.
Band-Aid m.
complementary m.
constitutional m.
electrodiagnostic m.
evidence-based m.
Western m.

Medicus bed

Mediflow pillow

Medihaler ergotamine

medii
nervi clunium m.

MediLive ImageBox

Medin disease

M

NOTES

mediodorsal
m. globus pallidus interna
m. nucleus
mediodorsalis
nucleus m.
mediopubic reflex
medioventralis
nucleus m.
Medisorb drug delivery system
MediSpacer
Airlife M.
meditation-based stress reduction
Mediterranean myoclonus
medium, pl. **media**
arteria cerebri media
cella media
contrast media
culture m.
Dulbecco modified Eagle m.
Eagle minimum essential m.
ganglion cervicale m.
high osmolar contrast m.
iopamidol contrast m.
macula cribrosa media
mass media
otitis media
scala media
stratum griseum m.
m. vessel infarction
media violence
violent media
^{133}XeSPECT contrast m.
medius
gyrus frontalis m.
gyrus temporalis m.
nervus cardiacus cervicalis m.
nervus meningeus m.
pedunculus cerebellaris m.
plexus rectalis m.
sulcus frontalis m.
sulcus temporalis m.
MedNext high-speed drill
Medos-Hakim valve
Medos valve
Medpacific LD 5000 Laser-Doppler perfusion monitor
Medrad infusion pump
Medrol Dosepak
medronate
technetium 99m m.
medroxyprogesterone acetate
MED system
Medtronic
M. Midas Rex Legend system
M. 3470 pulse generator
M. Sofamor Danek
M. SynchroMed implantable pump
M. Xtrel neurostimulator
medulla, pl. **medullae**
m. oblongata
m. oblongata lateral funiculus
m. oblongata reticular formation
posterior pyramid of the m.
pyramid of m.
rostral ventrolateral m.
m. spinalis
ventrolateral surface of the m.
medullar
medullare
centrum m.
medullares
striae m.
medullaris
conus m.
lamina m.
stria m.
substantia m.
tethered conus m.
tubus m.
medullary
m. artery
m. artery of brain
m. body of cerebellum
m. body of vermis
m. center
m. chemoreceptor
m. collecting duct (MCD)
m. cone
m. cystic disease (MCD)
m. fold
m. glioma
m. infarction
m. inhibitory region
m. inhibitory zone
m. lamina of thalamus
m. layer of thalamus
m. plate
m. protrusion
m. pyramidotomy
m. raphe
m. raphe nucleus
m. reticulospinal tract
m. segment
m. sheath
m. sign
m. solitary tract
m. striae of fourth ventricle
m. stria of thalamus
m. substance
m. syndrome
m. taenia of thalamus
m. tenia
m. tractotomy

m. tube
m. tumor
medullated nerve fiber
medullation
medullectomy
medullitis
medulloblastoma
desmoplastic m.
familial m.
melanotic m.
vermian m.
medullocell
medulloepithelioma
medullomyoblastoma
medullopontine sulcus
medullovasculosa
area m.
zona m.
M-EEG
magnetoencephalogram
MEEP
miniature end-plate potential
Mees line
mefenamic acid
Mefoxin
MEG
magnetoencephalogram
magnetoencephalography
M. head-based coordinate system
M. sensor
M. sensorimotor mapping coordinate
mega
m. cisterna magna
M. Tilt and Turn bed
Mega-Air bed
megacephalia
megacephalic
megacephalous
megacephaly
megadolichobasilar anomaly
megadolichovertebrobasilar anomaly
megalencephalon
megalencephaly
unilateral m.
megalgia
megalocephaly, megalocephalia
megaloencephalic
megaloencephalon
megaloencephaly
megalopapilla
megalopia hysterica
meglumine
diatrizoate m.
iocarmate m.
iodipamide m.
m. iothalamate
ioxaglate m.
m. metrizoate
Mehrkoordinaten manipulator (MKM)
Meige
M. disease
M. syndrome
Meissner
M. corpuscle
M. ganglion
M. plexus
melancholia agitata
melancholic type
melancholium
omego m.
melanin pigment
melanocyte
melanocyte-inhibiting factor
melanocytoma
meningeal m.
melanophore
melanophorin
melanosis
neurocutaneous m.
melanotic
m. medulloblastoma
m. neuroectodermal tumor
m. neuroectodermal tumor of infancy (MNTI)
melanotropin-releasing factor (MRF)
melarsoprol
MELAS
mitochondrial encephalomyopathy with lactic acidosis and strokelike episodes
mitochondrial myopathy, encephalopathy, lactic acidosis, strokelike episodes
M. syndrome
melatonin-replacement therapy
melatonin test
Melissa officinalis
melitensis
Brucella m.
Melkersson-Rosenthal syndrome
Melkersson syndrome
Mellaril
mellituria

Melmon and Rosen classification
Melnick-Fraser syndrome
melphalan
Melzack and Wall gate theory
memantine
membrana, pl. **membranae**
m. basilaris
m. cerebri
m. limitans gliae
m. versicolor
membranacea
crura m.
membrane
arachnoid m.
m. attack complex
basement m.
basilar m.
brain synaptic m.
branch of auriculotemporal nerve to tympanic m.
m. capacitance
caroticooculomotor m.
choroid m.
diencephalic m.
m. excitability
Fielding m.
glial limiting m.
Henle m.
m. ion channel
m. of Liliequist
m. lipolysis
Mauthner m.
mesencephalic m.
neuronal m.
nitrocellulose m.
m. phenotype
m. phosphatidylserine exposure
pial-glial m.
postsynaptic m.
m. potential
Preclude spinal m.
presynaptic m.
sarcolemma m.
Schwann m.
spiral m.
synaptic m.
vestibular m.
vitreous m.
membrane-anchored aspartyl protease
membrane-associated protein
membrane-bound glycoprotein
membranectomy
membranous cochlea
memento mori
MEM-4104K
Neuropak Four EMG/Evoked Response Measuring System Model M.
memoration
amnesic m.
Memorial
M. Delirium Assessment Scale (MDAS)
M. Symptom Assessment Scale
memory
accuracy of m.
anterograde m.
Bower model of mood-congruent m.
m. consolidation
declarative m.
m. deterioration
m. disturbance
m. dysfunction
episodic m.
euthymic m.
event m.
factual m.
m. function
m. function deficit
Honig model of working m.
illusory m.
impaired m.
m. impairment
m. index
intrusive m.
m. lapse
long-term associative m.
long-term declarative m.
long-term storage of m.
loss of m.
nonautobiographical m.
nondeclarative m.
nonverbal m.
m. organization
m. paradigm
m. performance
m. process
m. processing
prospective m.
recall m.
recent m.
recognition m.
recovered m.
remote m.
m. retrieval strategy
retrograde m.
Ribot law of m.
secondary verbal m.
selective m.
semantic m.

senile m.
short-term declarative m.
short-term visual m.
spatial m.
superior long-term m.
m. system
tapping m.
m. task
top-down organization of m.
m. trace
verbal episodic m.
veridical m.
visual episodic m.
visuospatial m.
working m.
memory-continuous performance
memory-guided saccade
Memotherm stent
MEMS
microelectromechanical system
MEN
multiple endocrine neoplasia
MEN II, III
MEN-1–3
multiple endocrine neoplasia, type 1–3
Mendel
M. dorsal foot reflex
M. instep reflex
Mendel-Bechterew reflex
Mendel-Bekhterev sign
mendelian inheritance
mendicancy
pathological m.
Menezes
method of M.
Mengo encephalitis
Ménière
M. disease
M. syndrome
meningeal
m. angiomatosis
m. anthrax
m. artery
m. biopsy
m. carcinoma
m. carcinomatosis
m. diverticula
m. fibrosis
m. filament
m. gliomatosis
m. granule
m. hemangiopericytoma
m. hernia
m. infection
m. irritation
m. loculus
m. lymphoma
m. melanocytoma
m. nerve
m. neurosarcoidosis
m. neurosyphilis
m. pachymeningitis
m. pathogen
m. plexus
m. sign
m. syphilis
m. tumor
m. vein
méningéale
tache m.
meningematoma
meningeocortical
meningeorrhaphy
meninges (*pl. of* meninx)
meningeus
plexus m.
meninghematoma
meningioangiomatosis
meningioma
anaplastic m.
angioblastic m.
angioplastic m.
angle m.
atypical m.
benign m.
bifrontal malignant m.
cavernous sinus m.
clinoidal m.
clival m.
clivus m.
complex m.
convexity m.
craniospinal m.
cutaneous m.
cystic intraparenchymal m.
dermal m.
endotheliomatous m.
en plaque m.
epidural m.
extracranial m.
extradural m.
falcotentorial m.

NOTES

M

meningioma *(continued)*
falx m.
fibroblastic m.
m. formation
frontal convexity m.
m. growth
intracranial m.
intradural-extradural m.
intraorbital m.
intraosseous m.
intraparenchymal m.
intraspinal m.
intraventricular m.
malignant m.
meningothelial m.
metastasizing m.
olfactory groove m.
m. of the olfactory groove
optic nerve sheath m.
papillary m.
parasagittal m.
parasellar tentorial m.
parietal m.
perioptic m.
peritorcular m.
petroclinoclival m.
petroclival m.
petroclivotentorial m.
pineal m.
posterior fossa m.
m. prostaglandin level
psammomatous m.
m. resection
secretory m.
sphenoid ridge m.
sphenoid wing m.
sphenoorbital m.
spinocranial m.
subdural m.
subfrontal m.
suprasellar m.
supratentorial m. (STM)
syncytial m.
tentorial apex m.
tentorial leaf m.
thoracic m.
torcular m.
transitional m.
tuberculum sella m.
tuberculum sellae m.

meningioma-associated cerebral edema

meningiomatosis

meningiorrhaphy

meningis

meningism

meningitic
m. hydrocephalus
m. neurosyphilis
m. streak

meningitidis
Neisseria m.

meningitis, pl. **meningitides**
Acanthamoeba m.
actinomycosis lymphocytic m.
acute cerebrospinal m. (ACM)
acute purulent m.
aseptic uremic m.
Bacilles anthracis m.
bacterial m.
basilar m.
benign lymphocytic m.
beta hemolytic streptococcus m.
blastomyocotic m.
candidal m.
carcinomatous m.
cerebrospinal m.
chemical aseptic m.
Citrobacter m.
CMV m.
coccidioidal m.
community-acquired bacterial m.
coxsackievirus m.
cryptococcal m.
cytomegalovirus m.
echovirus m.
enterovirus m.
eosinophilic m.
epidemic cerebrospinal m.
epidural m.
external m.
fungal m.
gram-negative bacillary m.
Haemophilus influenzae m.
H. influenzae type B m.
histoplasma m.
hospital-acquired m.
idiopathic m.
m. inflammatory response
internal m.
Klebsiella pneumoniae m.
leptospirosis lymphocytic m.
Listeria monocytogenes m.
luetic m.
lymphocytic m.
lymphomatous m.
meningococcal m.
Mima polymorpha m.
Mollaret m.
mumps m.
Naegleria m.
Neisseria meningitidis m.
neonatal m.
neoplastic m.
occlusive m.

ornithosis lymphocytic m.
m. ossificans
otitic m.
paragonimiasis lymphocytic m.
pneumococcal m.
premature infant m.
Proteus m.
purulent m.
pyogenic m.
septic m.
serosa m.
m. serosa circumscripta
serous m.
m. serous spinalis
sinogenic m.
spinal m.
staphylococcal m.
sterile m.
streptococcal m.
subacute m.
sympathetic m.
m. sympathica
tubercular m.
tuberculosis m.
tuberculous m.
viral m.

meningoarteritis

meningocele
lateral thoracic m.
lumbar m.
lumbosacral m.
sacral m.
spinal m.
spurious m.
traumatic m.

meningocephalitis

meningocerebral cicatrix

meningocerebritis

meningococcal
m. endotoxin
m. meningitis

meningococcemia
acute fulminating m.

meningocortical

meningocyte

meningoencephalitis
acute primary hemorrhagic m.
amebic m.
arbovirus m.
aseptic m. (AME)
bacterial m.
biundulant m.
chronic progressive syphilitic m.
eosinophilic m.
herpetic m.
mumps m.
murine typhus m.
nonvasculitic autoimmune inflammatory m.
primary amebic m.
Rocky Mountain spotted fever m.
sterile m.
syphilitic m.
toxoplasmic m.

meningoencephalocele
basal m.
ethmoidal m.
sphenoethmoidal m.
sphenoorbital m.
sphenopharyngeal m.
transsphenoidal m.

meningoencephalomyelitis

meningoencephalomyelopathy

meningoencephalopathy

meningofibrobplastoma

meningogenic

meningohydroencephalocele

meningohypophyseal
m. branch
m. trunk

meningoma

meningomyelitis
syphilitic m.

meningomyelocele

meningomyeloencephalitis

meningopathy

meningopolyneuritis
tick-borne m.

meningorachidian vein

meningoradicular

meningoradiculitis

meningorhachidian, meningorrhachidian

meningorrhagia

meningorrhea

meningothelial
m. appearance
m. arachnoid cell
m. meningioma

meningothelioma

meningotyphoid fever

NOTES

meningovascular
m. neurosyphilis
m. syphilis
meningovasculitis
syphilitic m.
meninigitis
Pasteurella m.
meninx, pl. **meninges**
basilar meninges
m. fibrosa
m. primitiva
primitive m.
m. serosa
m. tenuis
vascular m.
m. vasculosa
meniscus, pl. **menisci**
tactile m.
m. tactus
menkeiti
Menkes
M. disease
M. kinky hair syndrome
menstrual
m. cycle
m. epilepsy
m. migraine
mental
m. agraphia
m. alertness
M. Alternation Test
m. arousal
m. claudication
m. data
m. flexibility
m. impairment
m. level
m. model
m. nerve
m. phenomenon
m. retardation
m. speed
m. status change
m. workload
mentalis
nervus m.
rami gingivales nervi m.
rami labiales nervi m.
rami mentales nervi m.
mentally competent
mentation
slowed m.
menu
registration m.
Menzel
M. ataxia
M. olivopontocerebellar atrophy
M. olivopontocerebellar degeneration
MEP
motor evoked potential
multimodality evoked potential
meperidine
m. analog
m. hydrochloride
m. and promethazine
Mephyton Oral
meprobamate
MEQ
Morningness-Eveningness Questionnaire
meralgia paresthetica
mercuralis
erethism m.
mercurial tremor
mercury
m. intoxication
m. peripheral neuropathy
m. poisoning
m. toxicity
m. toxin
Meretoja syndrome
Meretoja-type familial amyloid polyneuropathy
meridian
extraordinary m. (EM)
Merkel
M. corpuscle
M. tactile cell
M. tactile disk
Merocel tampon
merocoxalgia
meromyosin
heavy m.
light m.
merorachischisis, merorrhachischisis
merosin deficiency
merosin-positive congenital muscular dystrophy
merosmia
MERRF
myoclonus epilepsy with ragged red fiber
MERRF syndrome
MERRLA
myoclonus epilepsy with ragged red fibers-lactic acidosis
MERRLA syndrome
Mersiline tape
Mersilk black silk suture
mertiatide
technetium 99m m.
merycism
Merzbacher-Pelizaeus disease

MES
maximal electroshock seizure
MES test
mesaxon
mescal button
mesem
per m.
mesencephali
apertura aqueductus m.
aqueductus m.
fibrae corticonucleares m.
formatio reticularis tegmenti m.
lamina tectalis m.
lamina tecti m.
nuclei reticulares m.
sulcus lateralis m.
tectum m.
tegmentum m.
mesencephalic
m. cistern
m. corticonuclear fiber
m. flexure
m. hemorrhage
m. infarction
m. membrane
m. neuron
m. nucleus
m. nucleus of trigeminal nerve
m. nucleus of the trigeminus
m. premotor structure
m. reticular formation
m. sign
m. tegmentum
m. tissue
m. tractotomy
m. tract of trigeminal nerve
m. transition area
m. transplant
m. vein
mesencephalicae
venae m.
mesencephalicum
tectum m.
tegmentum m.
mesencephalicus
nucleus cuneiformis m.
mesencephalitis
mesencephalohypophyseal
mesencephalon
m. aqueduct
oculomotor sulcus of m.
m. reticular formation
reticular nuclei of m.
ventral m.
mesencephalooculofacial angiomatosis
mesencephalotomy
mesenchymal drift
mesenchyme
paraxial m.
mesenrhomboencephalitis
mesenteric vasculitis
mesh
Dumbach cranial titanium m.
polylactic acid m.
tantalum m.
Teflon m.
mesial
m. aspect of temporal lobe
m. cerebral structure
m. epileptogenic cortex
m. hemisphere
m. part of frontal lobe
m. prefrontal cortical area
m. surface
m. temporal epileptogenic lesion
m. temporal hypoperfusion
m. temporal sclerosis
mesial-frontal cortex
mesiobasal
m. limbic epilepsy
m. temporal lobe
mesiotemporal lobe
mesoblastic sensibility
mesocephalic hemianesthesia
mesocortex
mesocortical
m. dopamine pathway
m. dopaminergic system
mesocorticolimbic dopaminergic abnormality
mesoderm
mesoglia
mesoglial cell
mesolimbic
m. dopamine pathway
m. dopamine system
m. selectivity
mesolobus
mesomorphic
mesoneuritis
nodular m.
mesorhachischisis

NOTES

mesoridazine
mesostriatal system abnormality
mesothelioma
fibrous m.
messenger
eukaryotic m.
intracellular second m.
m. ribonucleic acid
Mestinon
M. Injection
M. Syrup
M. Timespan
mesulergin
mesylate
benztropine m.
bromocriptine m.
dihydroergotamine m.
doxazosin m.
pergolide m.
rasagiline m.
reboxetine m.
traxoprodil m.
ziprasidone m.
metabolic
m. abnormality
m. acidosis
m. activation
m. activity
m. alkalosis
m. capability
m. change
m. coma
m. conversion
m. derangement
m. difference
m. disorder
m. disorder screening
m. effect
m. encephalitis
m. encephalopathy
m. headache
m. increase
m. lesion
m. mechanism
m. pathway
m. process
m. rate
m. response
metabolism
abnormal m.
albumin m.
alcohol m.
arachidonic acid m.
m. at rest
brain glucose m.
caffeine m.
carbohydrate m.
carnitine muscle m.
cerebellar m.
cholesterol m.
cortical m.
cytochrome P450 m.
dopamine m.
drug m.
energy m.
frontal m.
glial m.
global m.
glucose m.
glutamate m.
hepatic oxidative m.
impaired drug m.
inborn error of m.
intracellular energy m.
iron m.
lactose m.
lipoid m.
loss of energy m.
metal m.
methadone m.
neuronal m.
nitrogen m.
nucleic acid m.
parallel pathways of m.
phosphate m.
phytol m.
porphyrin m.
prefrontal m.
psychotropic m.
purine m.
regional brain glucose m.
regional glucose m.
striatal m.
striatus-orbitofrontal m.
temporal lobe m.
metabolite
active m.
bupropion m.
phosphoinositol m.
toxic m.
metabotropic
m. glutamate
m. glutamate receptor (mGluR1)
metacarpohypothenar reflex
metacarpothenar reflex
metachromatic
m. leukodystrophy
m. leukodystrophy neuropathy
m. leukoencephalopathy
metachromic leukodystrophy
metachronous neoplasm
metacognitive capacity
metacontrast masking

Metadate
M. CD
M. CD extended-release capsule
metaiodobenzyl-guanidine (MIBG)
metal
m. electrode
m. failure
m. fatigue
m. metabolic disorder
m. metabolism
m. neuropathy
m. object
m. plate
metallic
m. cranioplasty
m. foreign body
m. otologic implant
m. skin marker
m. toxin
m. tremor
metalloendoprotease
metalloprotease inhibitor
metalloproteinase
matrix m. (MMP)
tissue inhibitor of m. (TIMP)
metal-produced neuropathy
metamemory
metameric
m. lesion
m. nervous system
m. syndrome
metamorphopsia
metamorphose
metanalysis
metaraminol bitartrate
metastasis, pl. **metastases**
brain m.
calvarial m.
cerebral m.
choroidal m.
distant m.
drop m.
dural m.
extradural spinal m.
hemorrhagic m.
intradural m.
leptomeningeal m.
miliary brain m.
ocular m.
retrobulbar orbital m.
spinal m.
subarachnoid space m.
metastasizing meningioma
metastatic
m. brain tumor
m. disease
m. tumor removal
Metastron Injection
metatarsalgia
Morton m.
metatarsal reflex
metathalamus
metencephalic
metencephalon
metencephalospinal
metenkephalin
meter
BioTrainer exercise m.
clip force m.
methacrylate
dimethylaminoethyl m.
methadone
m. HCl
m. hydrochloride
m. metabolism
methamphetamine HCl
methanol poisoning
methantheline
methazolamide
methcathinone
methemoglobin
methexenyl
methicillin-resistant staphylococci
methiodal
methionine
methocarbamol
method
Anel m.
Antyllus m.
assessment m.
avidin-biotin-complex-peroxidase m.
brain electrical activity m. (BEAM)
brain imaging m.
Brasdor m.
bundle-nailing m.
Cavalieri direct estimator m.
clinical m.
cognitive m.
Coleman m.
Cooper m.
correlation m.

NOTES

M

method *(continued)*
Deaver m.
diagnostic m.
m. of Dickman
Dickson m.
dose reduction m.
Fairbanks m.
FDG m.
Flesh-Kincaid m.
Fujita m.
m. of Glees
Hilton m.
hole preparation m.
m. of Ikematsu
imaging m.
immobilization m.
immunoperoxidase m.
impedance m.
Kety-Schmidt m.
Kirby-Bauer disk diffusion m.
m. of Klüver
m. of Magerl
m. of Menezes
Moore m.
Pavlov m.
phase-contrast m.
Purmann m.
Q-sort m.
rating m.
reduction m.
Scarpa m.
Seldinger m.
Simmons m.
steady-state m.
m. of successive approximation
Taylor series linearization m.
Thane m.
Turnbull m.
Wardrop m.
Westergren m.
Winston-Lutz m.
Wintrobe m.
Xe clearance m.
xenon m.
zeta m.
methodical chorea
methotrexate
m. poisoning
m. sodium
methsuximide
methyl
m. alcohol peripheral neuropathy
m. alcohol poisoning
m. alcohol toxicity
m. alcohol toxin
m. dopa
methylamphetamine hydrochloride
methylcarbamic
methyl-CpG-binding protein
3-methylcrontyonyl-CoA carboxylase
***N*-methyl-D-aspartate**
N-m.-D.-a. receptor
N-m.-D.-a. receptor antagonist
methyldopa and hydrochlorothiazide
methylene
m. blue
m. tetrahydrofolate reductase defect
methylenedioxymethamphetamine (MDMA)
m. and phencyclidine
methylglucamine
iodipamide m.
3-methylglutaconic aciduria
methylglyoxal bis(guanylhydrazone)
methylmalonic
m. acidemia
m. aciduria
m. aminoaciduria
methylmalonyl-CoA
methylmalonyl-CoA mutase
methylmethacrylate
m. block
m. cranioplastic plug
m. cranioplasty
m. spacer
methylphenidate
m. administration
m. HCl
m. HCl extended-release capsule
methylphenidate-induced change
1-methyl-4-phenyl-1,2,3,6-tetrahydropyridine
methylprednisolone
m. acetate
m. and sodium succinate
methylxanthine-induced postural tremor
MethyPatch
methysergide maleate
metocurine iodide
metolazone
metopic
m. craniectomy
m. suture
m. synostosis
metopoplasty
metoprolol tartrate
Metrazol
metrizamide
m. contrast study
m. myelography
metrizamide-enhanced CT
metrizamide-filled balloon
metrizoate
meglumine m.

metrizoic acid
metronidazole
METRx system
metyrapone test
Metzenbaum scissors
mevalonate kinase deficiency
mevalonic aciduria
mevinolin
Mexate-AQ
mexiletine
Meyer
M. loop
M. sublaminar wiring technique
Meyer-Archambault loop
Meyerding
M. laminectomy blade
M. laminectomy retractor
Meyerding-Scoville blade
Meynert
basal nucleus of M.
M. commissure
M. fasciculus
fasciculus of M.
M. fountain decussation
M. layer
nucleus basalis of M.
retroflex bundle of M.
M. retroflex bundle
M. solitary cell
M. tract
MFD
monorhythmic frontal delta
M. activity
M. Test
M. waves on electroencephalogram
MFMN
multifocal motor neuropathy
MFS
Miller-Fisher syndrome
MG
myasthenia gravis
MGBG
mitoguazone
mGluR1
metabotropic glutamate receptor
MGN
medial geniculate nucleus
MHC
major histocompatibility complex
MHI
minor head injury
Miacalcin
M. Injection
M. Nasal Spray
Miami
M. Acute Care cervical collar
M. J collar
mianserin
MIBG
metaiodobenzyl-guanidine
iodine 131 MIBG
micans
degeneratio m.
mication
mice
CRF knockout m.
Michele vertebral body trephine
Michel scalp clip
Michotte visual stimulus
micrencephalous
micrencephaly, micrencephalia
Micrins microsurgical suture
Micro
M. E irrigation kit
M. 100 irrigation kit
M. link fiber
M. Plus screw
microabscess
candidal m.
microadenoma
cystic m.
pituitary m.
microadenomectomy
selective m.
microaerophilic streptococci
Micro-Aire blade
microaneurysm
microangiogenesis
microangiopathy
mineralizing m.
microarray
microartery forceps
microball hook
microbipolar forceps
microbore Tygon tube
microcatheter
Excel double-tipped m.
Magic m.
Prowler-14 m.
Prowler double-tipped m.
Rapid Transit m.
m. system

NOTES

microcatheter *(continued)*
Tracker Excel m.
variable stiffness m.
microcephaly
encephaloclastic m.
schizencephalic m.
MicroChoice electric powered surgical system
microcirculation
nerve root m.
microcirculatory
m. perfusion
m. red cell flux
microclip
Yasargil m.
microcoagulator
Malis bipolar m.
microcoil
endothelin-1 platinum-Dacron m.
Hilal m.
platinum m.
platinum-Dacron m.
Microcomputer Imaging Device/M2
microconnector
titanium m.
microcosm
microcoulomb
microcrania
microcup forceps
microcurette, microcuret
Rhoton m.
Yasargil m.
microcyst
microdactyly
microdialysis
intracerebral m.
intrahippocampal m.
microdipole
microdiscectomy, microdiskectomy
microdissector
Rhoton m.
Yasargil m.
micro-Doppler instrument
microdrill
high-speed m.
system high-speed m.
microdysgenesia
cortical m.
microdysgenesis
micro-eCVR-FV circulation
microelectrode recording
microelectroencephalography
microelectromechanical system (MEMS)
microembolic signal
microembolism
cerebral m.
silent m.
microencephaly
microendoscopic
m. discectomy system
m. foraminotomy
m. laminotomy
microendoscopy
intraoperative m.
MicroFET2 muscle test
microfibrillar collagen
microfilament
microforceps
Yasargil m.
microglia cell
microgliacyte
microglial
m. cluster
m. nodular encephalitis
microglioma
microgliomatosis
microgliosis
microglobulin
$beta_2$ m.
micrognathia
Robin sequence m.
micrograph
electron m.
micrographia
micrography
MicroGuide microelectrode recording system
microguidewire
FasDasher-14 m.
Transcend m.
microgyria
perisylvian m.
microgyrus
microhemagglutination-*T. pallidum* test
microhemorrhage
hypertensive pontine m.
microhook
Rhoton m.
microinfarction
microinjection
Micro-K
M.-K. 10 Extencaps
M.-K. LS
microknife
Karlin m.
microlumbar discectomy
microMax drill system
micromesh
titanium m.
MicroNeedle
Colorado M.
microneurography
microneurosurgery
microneurovascular anastomosis

Micro-One needle holder
microoperative
m. procedure
m. treatment
Micropaque
microphthalmos
micropituicyte
micropituitary rongeur
microplate
C-shaped m.
H-shaped m.
Leibinger m.
L-shaped m.
Luhr m.
Storz Microsystem m.
Synthes Microsystem m.
Micro-Plus titanium plating system
microporosity
microprobe
Jacobson m.
microprolactinoma
micropsia
micropsychotic dimension
microptic
microrasp
Yasargil m.
microretractor
flexible arm m.
microronguer
Kerrison m.
microsaccadic flutter
microsatellite
microsaw
oscillating m.
Zimmer m.
microscissors
curved conventional m.
straight m.
Yasargil m.
microscope
Elekta Robotic Surgical M.
Hitachi scanning electron m.
JedMed TRI-GEM m.
laser scanning m. (LSM)
LSM-GB200 confocal laser scanning m.
MKM m.
Moller MMS-900 m.
Nikon Labophot-2 m.
Omni 2 m.
operating m. VM 900
operative m.
OPMI surgical m.
Philips 400 transmission electron m.
pneumatic m.
robotic m.
surgical m.
SurgiScope robotic m.
VARIMIC 900 m.
Vario m.
Zeiss Axiovert m.
Zeiss-Contraves operating m.
Zeiss MKM m.
Zeiss operating m.
Zeiss OpMi CS-NC2 surgical m.
Zeiss OPMI Neuro/NC4 surgical m.
zoom m.
microscopic
m. endoscopy surgery
m. foraminotomy
m. laminotomy (ML)
m. lesion
m. neurosurgery
m. neurosurgery endoscopic-assisted
m. polyangiitis
microscopy
electron m.
scanning electron m.
transillumination m.
MicroSeal adapter
microseme
microsensor
ICP m.
intracranial pressure m.
microsleep
microsmatic
microsmic
Micro-Softplate
micro-Soft Stream sidehole infusion catheter
microsomal isoenzyme metabolism profile
microsomia
hemifacial m.
MicroSpan Capnometer 8800
microsphere
degradable starch m.'s (DSM)
microstaple
Barouk m.
microstomia

NOTES

Microsulfon
microsurgery
m. discectomy
endoscope-controlled m.
m. forceps
frameless stereotactic m.
Möller m.
m. needle holder
microsurgical
m. discectomy (MSD)
m. DREZotomy
m. neck clipping
m. procedure
m. thoracoscopic vertebrectomy
microsuture
microsystem
micro-thin plastic fiber
Micro-Three microsurgery instrument
microtome
Leica vibrating knife m.
microtopography
Microtrast
microtubule
cytoplasmic m.
microtubule-associated protein
microtubule-binding
m.-b. domain
m.-b. repeat
Micro-Two
M.-T. forceps
M.-T. needle holder
M.-T. scissors
Micro-Vac suction catheter
microvascular
m. anastomosis
m. clip
m. compression syndrome
m. decompression (MVD)
m. forceps
m. pressure (MVP)
Microvena retrieval device
microvesicular steatosis
microvolt (μV)
microwave hyperthermia
Microzide
Micro-Z neuromuscular stimulator
micturition
m. center
m. reflex
m. syncope
MID
multiinfarct dementia
Midamor
Midas
M. Rex bur guard
M. Rex craniotome
M. Rex craniotomy saw
M. Rex drill
M. Rex instrumentation system
M. Rex power system
midazolam
midbrain
aqueduct of m.
m. deafness
m. infarction
m. lesion
opening of aqueduct of m.
m. reticular formation
rostral m.
tectum of m.
tegmentum of m.
m. tegmentum
m. vesicle
midcervical flexion myelopathy
middle
m. cerebellar peduncle
m. cerebral artery (MCA)
m. cerebral artery occlusion
m. cerebral artery thrombosis (MCAT)
m. cervical ganglion
m. column injury
m. cranial fossa
m. cranial fossa approach
m. cranial fossa cyst
m. ear impedance
m. fossa craniotomy approach
m. fossa exposure
m. fossa floor/petrous dissection
m. fossa transtentorial translabyrinthine approach
m. frontal convolution
m. frontal gyrus
m. frontal sulcus
m. glial cell line-derived neurotrophic factor
m. gray layer of superior colliculus
m. hemorrhoidal plexus
m. lobe of cerebellum
m. meningeal artery (MMA)
m. occipital gyrus
m. posterior temporobasal vein
m. radicular syndrome
m. temporal convolution
m. temporal focal spike
m. temporal gyrus
m. temporal sulcus
midface
m. degloving
m. degloving technique
m. hypoplasia syndrome
m. retrusion
midget bipolar cell

midlife cardiovascular risk factor
midline
m. developmental lesion
m. exposure
m. fusion defect
m. incision
m. myelotomy
m. shift
m. spinal approach
m. syndrome
m. tumor
midodrine hydrochloride
midpoint to meatal line
midpontine syndrome
midsagittal
m. diameter
m. image
m. section
midtegmentum
midtemporal seizure
Mierzejewski effect
Miethke dual-switch valve
mieux
faute de m.
Mifeprex
mifepristone
migraine
abdominal m.
acephalgic m.
acute confusional m.
affective prodrome of m.
autosomal dominant m.
basilar artery m.
Bickerstaff m.
Brobdingnagian disorder of visual perception in m.
catamenial m.
catastrophic m.
ciliary m.
classic m.
common m.
complicated m.
confusional m.
m. equivalent
facial m.
facioplegic m.
familial hemiplegic m. (FHM)
fulgurating m.
Harris m.
m. headache
hemiparesthetic m.
hemiplegia m.
hemiplegic m.
menstrual m.
migraine sans m.
neurologic m.
ophthalmic m.
ophthalmoplegic m.
paroxysmal m.
pectoralgic m.
retinal m.
seasonal m.
syncopal m.
unilateral m.
m. variant
m. vasospasm
vestibular m.
m. with aura
m. without aura (MwoA)
migraine-induced
m.-i. infarction
m.-i. stroke
migraine-like headache
migraine-neuralgia analgesic
migraineur
depressed m.
epileptic m.
migrainosus
status m.
migrainous
m. aura
m. cranial neuralgia
m. infarction
m. symptom
Migranal
migrans
erythema chronicum m.
visceral larva m.
migration
m. abnormality
electrode m.
graft m.
instrument m.
interfibrillary m.
intrafascicular m.
Luque rod m.
neuroblast m.
neuroepithelial cell m.
neuronal m.
perifascicular m.
rod m.

M

NOTES

migration *(continued)*
transendothelial m.
vertical m.
migratory
m. arthralgia
m. cell
Mikaelsson catheter
Mikulicz operation
mild
m. cognitive impairment (MCI)
m. dementia
m. head injury
m. mental retardation
m. subsyndromal symptom
Miles punch biopsy forceps
miliary
m. aneurysm
m. brain metastasis
m. pulmonary tuberculosis
military neurosurgery
milk-ejection reflex
milkmaid's grip
Millard-Gubler syndrome
Mille
M. Pattes screw
M. Pattes technique
Miller-Dieker syndrome
Miller-Fisher
M.-F. syndrome (MFS)
M.-F. test
M.-F. variant of Guillain-Barré syndrome
Milles syndrome
Millet neurological test instrument
Milligan dissector
Millipore
M. filter
M. suture
Mills dressing
milrinone
Miltex rib spreader
Milton disease
Miltown
Milwaukee brace
Mima polymorpha meningitis
mimetic
m. chorea
m. convulsion
m. muscle
m. paralysis
mimic
m. convulsion
m. spasm
m. tic
mimicry
molecular m.
Minamata disease
mind
m. blindness
m. power
mind/body dualism
mineralizing microangiopathy
Minerin
miner's
m. cramp
m. nystagmus
Minerva
M. jacket
M. vest
mini
m. applier
M. Orbita plate
M. Würzburg implant system
M. Würzburg screw
miniature end-plate potential (MEEP)
minicore-multicore myopathy
minicore myopathy
minimal
m. access spinal technology (MAST)
m. alveolar concentration (MAC)
m. brain dysfunction
m. lethal dose (MLD)
minimalist surgical strategy
minimally conscious state
Minimax 200 watt light source
minimizing stimulation
minimum
m. duration
m. effective concentration
m. incision surgery
m. intensity projection
mini-open
m.-o. approach
m.-o. technique
miniplate
m. strut
titanium m.
minisomotic infusion pump
mini-Sugita clip
Minnesota Regional Sleep Disorders Center
minor
chorea m.
M. disease
epilepsia m.
m. forceps
m. form
m. head injury (MHI)
hippocampus m.
m. hippocampus
m. motor seizure
nervus occipitalis m.
nervus petrosus m.

nervus splanchnicus thoracicus m.
M. sign
minores
nervi palatini m.
minoris
ramus renalis nervi splanchnici m.
sulcus nervi petrosi m.
minorum
rami tonsillares nervorum palatinorum m.
minute
murine double m. 2 (MDM2)
m. object
miosis
paralytic m.
spastic m.
MIPI
mean interpotential interval
Mira
M. cautery
M. Mark III cranial drill
M. Mark III cranial drill set
M. Mark V craniotome
M. Mark V craniotome set
mirabile
rete m.
MIRAGE study
Mirapex
mirror
Hardy 5 mm m.
m. of Wernicke
mirror-writing
miryachit, myriachit
misconception
sleep-state m.
misdifferentiation hypothesis
misdirection phenomenon
misery perfusion
Mishler valve
Miskimon cerebellar retractor
mismatch negativity
misonidazole
misoprostol
misregistration
flow m.
oblique flow m.
missense mutation
missile
m. effect
m. injury
Mistichelli crossing
mitamachen
Mitchell disease
mitgehen
Mithracin
mitior
epilepsia m.
mitochondria
fatty acid transport into m.
mitochondrial
m. condensation
m. cytopathy
m. defect
m. deoxyribonucleic acid analysis
m. disease (MD)
m. DNA
m. encephalomyopathy with lactic acidosis and strokelike episodes (MELAS)
m. encephalomyopathy with sensorimotor polyneuropathy
m. encephalopathy
m. free radical generation
m. metabolic disorder
m. myopathy
m. myopathy, encephalopathy, lactic acidosis, strokelike episodes (MELAS)
m. neurogastrointestinal encephalomyopathy
m. neurogastrointestinal encephalopathy (MNGIE)
m. neuropathy
Mitofsky-Aaksberg random digit dialing procedure
mitogen
mitogen-activated
m.-a. protein (MAP)
m.-a. protein kinase
mitoguazone (MGBG)
mitosis
neural tube formation m.
mitotane
mitotic
m. segregation
m. spindle apparatus
mitoxantrone
mitral
m. cell
m. cell layer
m. valve prolapse

NOTES

mixed
m. anxiety-depression
m. aphasia
m. bipolar state
m. cerebral dominance
m. connective tissue disease (MCTD)
m. form cerebral palsy
m. frequency EEG
m. germ cell tumor
m. glioma
m. growth hormone-prolactin cell adenoma
m. headache
m. nerve
m. paralysis
m. pineal tumor
m. receptive/expressive language disorder
m. spasm
m. up
mixed-type
m.-t. epilepsy
m.-t. psychopathic personality
mixoscopia
Mixter ventricular needle
mixture
epinephrine-anesthetic m.
thrombogenic ferrous m.
mixtus
nervus m.
Miyoshi myopathy (MM)
Mizuho
M. aneurysm sizer-dissector
M. surgical Doppler
MKM
Mehrkoordinaten manipulator
MKM fiducial
MKM microscope
MKM stereotactic image-guided system
MKM workstation
ML
microscopic laminotomy
ML4
mucolipidosis type IV
MLD
minimal lethal dose
MLF
medial longitudinal fasciculus
MM
Miyoshi myopathy
MMA
middle meningeal artery
275mm objective lens
M-mode electrocardiographic measurement
MMP
matrix metalloproteinase
MMS-900
MMS-900 balancing tool
MMS-900 microscope balancer
M'Naghten test
MNC
mononuclear cell
MND
motor neuron disease
mneme
mnemic, mnemenic
m. hypothesis
m. theory
mnemism
theory of m.
m. theory
mnemonics
MNGIE
mitochondrial neurogastrointestinal encephalopathy
MNSC
motor nerve conduction study
MNTI
melanotic neuroectodermal tumor of infancy
Moban
mobile spasm
Möbius
M. disease
M. syndrome
modafinil
modal dose
mode
magnet m.
normal m.
quiet wakefulness m.
syntaxic m.
transcranial Doppler B m.
model
affective schematic mental m.
affect-related schematic mental m.
affect trauma m.
Baddeley m.
biomedical m.
corpectomy m.
developmental-vulnerability m.
Hitch m.
Honig m.
internal m.
jurisprudential teaching m.
kinetic m.
lumbar spine m.
Markov decision analysis m.
Mayberg limbic-cortical dysregulation m.
mental m.

multimodal treatment m.
m. 300 NCP bipolar lead
nonaffective schematic mental m.
m. 100 pulse generator
m. 101 pulse generator
schematic mental m.
standard kinetic m.
subcortical dysfunction m.
m. TC2-64B pulsed-range gated Doppler instrument
treatment m.
m. U gamma knife
vitro matrigel m.

modeling
forward m.
kinetic m.

modification
body m.
C-D screw m.
Harriluque sublaminar wiring m.
Jacobs locking hook spinal rod instrumentation m.
posttranslational m.
m. or Woodson

modified
M. Autonomic Perception Questionnaire
m. Fischer classification
m. Gilsbach technique
m. Harrington rod
m. McGill Pain Questionnaire
M. Rankin Scale
m. Robert Jones dressing
m. Simpson-Angus Rating Scale
m. Stroop effect

modifier
biologic response m.

modular instrumentation

modularity
imaging m.

modulation
dopaminergic m.
interneuronal calcium m.
pain m.

modulator
circadian m.
selective estrogen receptor m. (SERM)

module
CUSA electrosurgical m.
Nd:YAG m.

Modulock posterior spinal fixation

Moduretic

Moe
M. alar hook
M. rod
M. spinal hook
M. square-ended hook
M. system

Moersch-Woltmann syndrome

mofetil
mycophenolate m.

MOG
myelin oligodendrocyte glycoprotein

mogiarthria

mogigraphia

mogilalia

mogiphonia

moiety
reelin m.

Moire topographic scoliosis assessment

molar behavior

molded vacuum pillow

molecular
m. approach
m. behavior
m. diagnostic technique
m. dualism
m. genetics
m. layer
m. layer of cerebellar cortex
m. layer of cerebellum
m. layer of cerebral cortex
m. layer of olfactory bulb
m. layer of retina
m. layer stria
m. level
m. mimicry
m. neurosurgery
m. plexus

molecular-based conceptual therapy

moleculare
stratum m.

molecularis
lamina m.
stria laminae m.

molecule
Abeta m.
adhesion m.
cell adhesion m. (CAM)
endothelial adhesion m.
feel-good m.

NOTES

molecule *(continued)*
glucose transporter m.
growth-inhibiting m.
growth-promoting m.
matrix m.
nerve-cell adhesion m.
neural-cell adhesion m. (NCAM)
second-messenger m.
Molie capsule
molimen climactericum virile
molindone HCl
Mollaret meningitis
Möller microsurgery
Moller MMS-900 microscope
mollis
chorea m.
molluscum fibrosum
molybdenum cofactor deficiency
moment
gradient m.
macroscopic magnetization m.
magnetic m.
three-point bending m.
momentum
angular m.
Monakow
M. bundle
fasciculus aberrans of M.
M. fiber
M. nucleus
M. syndrome
M. tract
Monarch spinal system
monathetosis
monaxonic
Mondini syndrome
Mondonesi reflex
MO needle
monesthetic
mongolian idiocy
monitor
bispectral EEG m.
Camino fiberoptic ICP m.
Camino OLM ICP m.
canopy ventilation m.
Cardiocap II pressure m.
4-channel Transcranial Doppler m.
Cortexplorer cerebral blood flow m.
Datex infrared CO_2 m.
Doppler ultrasound m.
electronic m.
Hewlett-Packard pressure m.
Holter m.
ICP m.
intracranial pressure Express digital m.
Laserflow blood perfusion m.
Laserflow BPM^2 real time cerebral perfusion m.
Medpacific LD 5000 Laser-Doppler perfusion m.
Moor MBF3D m.
Nerve Integrity M. 2
Nicolet Nerve Integrity M. (NIM-2)
Palmar cutaneous temperature m.
SentiLite EEG m.
SentiLite neurological m.
Sentinel-4 neurological m.
Steritek ICP mini m.
monitor-2
Xomed nerve integrity m.
Xomed-Treace nerve integrity m.
monitoring
anesthetic m.
bedside multimodality m.
brain electrical activity m. (BEAM)
cardiac m.
clinical m.
closed circuit television m.
continuous video-EEG m. (CCTV-EEG)
cranial nerve m.
diagnostic m.
Doppler precordial end-tidal carbon dioxide m.
ECoG m.
electronic m.
end-tidal carbon dioxide m.
end-tidal nitrogen m.
esophageal pH m.
esophageal pressure m.
fetal heart rate m.
F-wave m.
intracerebral depth electrode m.
intraoperative facial nerve m.
intraoperative neurophysiological m.
invasive electroencephalographic m.
jugular bulb oxyhemoglobin saturation m. (SjO_2)
neurophysiological m.
m. probe
real-time m.
scalp EEG m.
screw position perioperative m.
seizure m.
somatosensory evoked potential m.
spinal cord function intraoperative m.
subdural ICP m.
m. technique
transcutaneous carbon dioxide m.
transcutaneous oxygen m.

video-EEG m.
video electroencephalographic m.
visual-function m.

monoamine
m. oxidase-B inhibitor
m. oxidase inhibitor (MAOI)
m. oxidase inhibitor-serotonergic agent

monoaminergic
m. fiber
m. pathway
m. system

monobactam
monobloc advancement
monoblock
butterfly-shaped m.

monobloc-type appliance
monochorea
monoclonal
m. antibody
m. antiglial fibrillary acidic protein
m. gammopathy

monocular
m. blindness
m. heads-up display imaging system

monocystic craniopharyngioma
monocyte
monocytogenes
Listeria m.

monofilament
von Frey m.

monoganglial
monogenetic disorder
Mono-Gesic
monogynous
monolayer
endothelial m.

monolithic adult block
monomanie
m. du vol
m. erotique
m. incendiare

monomelic
m. amyotrophy
m. muscular atrophy
m. paresis

monomer
acrylamide m.

monomorphic activity
monomyoplegia
mononeural
mononeuralgia
mononeuric
mononeuritis multiplex
mononeuropathy
entrapment m.
multifocal m.
multiple m.
m. multiplex
phrenic m.

mononuclear
m. cell (MNC)
m. leukocyte isolation
m. pleocytosis
m. pleocytosis of cerebrospinal fluid

mononucleosis
infectious m.
m. peripheral neuropathy

mononucleotide
flavin m. (FMN)

monoparesis
monoparesthesia
monophagic
monophasia
monophasic
m. action potential
m. illness
m. wave
m. waveform

monophosphate
adenosine 3′,5′-cyclic m. (cAMP)
cyclic adenosine m.
guanosine m.

Monoplace hyperbaric chamber
monoplegia
crural m.
m. masticatoria
spastic m.

monoplegic
monopolar
m. cathodal stimulator
m. cautery
m. electrocautery
m. needle electrode
m. stimulating electrode
m. tissue forceps

monoportal ventriculoscopy
monorail aspiration catheter
monorhythmic
m. frontal delta (MFD)

NOTES

monorhythmic *(continued)*
m. frontal delta activity
m. sinusoidal delta activity
monosodium
m. glutamate
m. glutamate-induced headache
m. glutamate poisoning
monosomy
chromosome (9_p) m.
monospasm
monosymptomatic hypochondriacal
monosynaptic
m. connection
m. reflex arc
m. reflex discharge
m. segmental reflex response
m. stretch reflex
monotheism
monotherapy
cabergoline m.
pramipexole m.
ropinirole m.
topiramate m.
monotreme
Monreal reflex hammer
Monro
M. aqueduct
M. fissure
foramen of M.
foramina of M.
M. sulcus
Monro-Kel Roussy-Lévy hereditary areflexic dystasia
montage
bipolar m.
reference m.
transverse bipolar m.
monticulus, pl. **monticuli**
m. cerebelli
clivus m.
mood
m. disturbance
m. elevation
m. regulator
m. spectrum disorder
m. stabilization
m. state
mood-stabilizing agent
Mooney face
moon facies
Moore method
Moor MBF3D monitor
mooseri
Rochalimaea m.
Morand spur
morbilliform rash
morcellation
morcellement
morcellize
Morel-Kraepelin disease
Morgagni
M. disease
M. syndrome
M. tubercle
Morgagni-Adams-Stokes syndrome
Morganella morganii
Morgan-Russell scale
mori
memento m.
Morley peritoneocutaneous reflex
morning
m. glory syndrome
m. headache
Morningness-Eveningness Questionnaire (MEQ)
Moro reflex
morphine
intracerebroventricular administration of m.
morphine-Adcon-L (M-ADL)
morphine-naloxone test
morphinotherapy
intrathecal m.
morpholinoanthracycline
lipophilic m.
morphologic
m. change
m. study
morphological
m. deformation
m. difference
morphology
cerebrovascular m.
neuronal m.
qualitative m.
quantitative m.
morphometric
m. abnormality
m. technique
morphometry
m. analysis
brain m.
pedicle m.
voxel-based m.
morphosynthesis
Morquio
M. disease
M. syndrome
M. syndrome type A, B
Morscher
M. anterior cervical plate
M. titanium cervical plate
Morse sternal spreader
morsus humanus

mort douce
Morton
M. disease
M. foot
M. metatarsalgia
M. neuralgia
M. neuroma
Morvan
M. chorea
M. disease
M. syndrome
MOSP
myelin/oligodendrocyte-specific protein
mosquito
m. bite infection
m. clamp
m. forceps
Moss-Harms basket
Moss-Miami
M.-M. polyaxial screw
M.-M. spinal instrumentation
M.-M. spinal system
mossy
m. cell
m. fiber
m. fiber sprouting
mote-beam mechanism
moth-eaten alopecia
Mother Jones dressing
motility
m. adhesion
extraocular m.
ocular m.
motion
active integral range of m. (AIROM)
m. artifact
brownian m.
coherent m.
m. concentration
higher order m.
m. picture violence
m. segment
m. sense
m. sickness
spinal range of m. (SROM)
motivation
characteristic pattern of m.
m. factor
m. impairment
maladaptive pattern of m.
motivational
m. enhancement therapy
m. process
motivational/behavioral factor
motive
abundancy m.
effectance m.
motiveless resistance
motoceptor
motoneuron
alpha m.
beta m.
gamma m.
heteronymous m.
homonymous m.
lower m. (LM)
peripheral m.
upper m.
motor
m. abnormality
m. activity
m. agraphia
m. alexia
m. amusia
m. aphasia
m. apraxia
m. ataxia
m. aura
m. cell
m. conduction
m. conduction block
m. conduction velocity (MCV)
m. control
m. cortex
m. dapsone neuropathy
m. decussation
m. deficit
m. development examination
m. endplate
m. evoked potential (MEP)
m. fiber
m. finding
m. fluctuation
forelimb m.
m. function
m. hemideficit
m. hemiplegia
hindlimb m.
m. image
m. impairment
m. impersistence

M

NOTES

motor *(continued)*
m. intention
m. interface
m. jacksonian attack
latency distal m.
lower m. (LM)
m. maturity
m. neglect
m. nerve conduction study (MNSC)
m. nerve terminal
m. neuron
m. neuron disease (MND)
m. neuron disorder
m. neuron paralysis
m. neuron senescence
m. nucleus
m. nucleus of facial nerve
m. nucleus of trigeminal nerve
m. nucleus of trigeminus
m. overflow
m. paradigm
m. pathways disease
m. phenomenon
m. point
m. point block
m. psychogenic disorder
m. region
m. response
m. restlessness
m. retardation
m. retardation developmental delay disorder
m. root of ciliary ganglion
m. root of mandibular nerve
m. root of spinal nerve
m. root of submandibular nerve
m. root of trigeminal nerve
m. seizure
m. sign
m. slowing
m. speech area
m. speech center
m. strength
m. strip
m. subtype
m. system
m. system disease
m. system syndrome
m. task
m. thalamus
m. threshold
m. tract
m. unit (MU)
m. unit action potential (MUAP)
m. unit axon
m. unit discharge
m. unit muscle
m. unit neuromuscular junction
m. unit potential (MUP)
m. unit potential amplitude potential
m. zone

motori

motoria
decussatio m.
radix m.

motoric
m. abnormality
m. phenomenon
m. region
m. slowing

motorically

motoricity

motorius
nervus m.

motorneuronal pool inhibitory neuron

motor-verbal

motrice
tache m.

Motricity Index

Mount
M. laminectomy rongeur
M. syndrome

Mount-Reback syndrome

MOUSEPAD
Manchester and Oxford Universities Scale for the Psychopathological Assessment of Dementia

mouth
downturned corners of the m.
m. occlusion pressure
tapir m.

movement
m. artifact
associated m.
bizarre asynchronous m.
choreic m.
choreiform m.
cocaine-induced choreoathetoid m.
conjugate contraversive eye m.
conjugated eye m.
coreoathetoid m.
decomposition of m.
discordance of m.
m. disorder
m. duration (MD)
dysconjugate m.
dystonic m.
extraocular m. (EOM)
fast saccadic eye m.
fluidity of m.
head m.
horizontal eye m.

involuntary m.
lateropulsion of body m.
lateropulsion of eye m.
Magnan trombone m.
neurobiotactic m.
nonrapid eye m. (NREM)
paradoxical abdominal m.
passive m.
peak-dose choreoathetoid dyskinetic m.
periodic leg m.
periodic limb m. (PLM)
psychotropic m.
pursuit eye m.
quasi-purposeful m.
rapid alternating m.
rapid eye m. (REM)
reaching-grasping m.
reflex m.
repetitive m.
rhythmic m.
saccadic pursuit eye m.
m. sense
sequential opposition finger m.
skilled finger m.
sleep-onset rapid eye m.
slow lateral eye m.
slow rolling eye m.
smooth pursuit eye m.
stereotyped m.
stereotypic m.
tardive m.
transitive limb m.
vergence m.
vertical eye m.

M-oxy

moyamoya
m. collateral enlargement
m. disease
m. syndrome

Moynihan forceps

Mozart effect

MP-35 clip material

mPFC
medial prefrontal cortex

MPM I multi-parameter monitoring system

MPPP
multidisciplinary pilot project program

MPRAGE
magnetization-prepared rapid acquisition gradient echo sequence

M-Prednisol Injection

MPTP-induced parkinsonism

MR
magnetic resonance
MR angiogram
gadolinium diethylenetriamine pentaacetic acid-enhanced MR
MR imaging with gadolinium enhancement
MR spectroscopy
surface coil MR
MR volumetry imaging

MRA
magnetic resonance angiography
CE MRA
contrast-enhanced MR angiography

MRC
Medical Research Council
MRC scale for strength testing

MRF
melanotropin-releasing factor

MRI
magnetic resonance image
magnetic resonance imaging
brain MRI
MRI compatibility
contrast-enhanced MRI
diffusion tensor MRI
diffusion tensor magnetic resonance imaging
FS MRI
flow-sensitive magnetic resonance imaging
gadolinium-enhanced MRI
MRI grade
high-resolution MRI
intraoperative MRI
nonproton MRI
open clam-shell MRI
MRI scan
MRI signal hyperintensity
structural MRI
MRI volumetry
whole-spine MRI

MRI-based brain anatomy

MRN
magnetic resonance neurography

M

NOTES

MRS
magnetic resonance spectroscopy
multivoxel MRS
MRT
magnetic resonance tomography
MRV
magnetic resonance venography
MRZ
measles, rubella and zoster
MRZ reaction
MS
multiple sclerosis
MS etiopathogenesis
MS pathway
Rebif MS
MSA
multisystem atrophy
MSD
microsurgical discectomy
MSI
magnetic source imaging
MSLT
multiple sleep latency test
MSLT with electroencephalogram
MST
multiple subpial transection
99mTc
technetium 99m, or 99mTc
^{99}mTc-HMPAO
MTC Ventcontrol ventricular catheter
MTD
multiple tic disorder
mtDNA depletion syndrome
MTN
medial terminal nucleus
MTS
MTS electrohydraulic piston
MU
motor unit
mu
m. opiate receptor
m. rhythm
m. wave
MUAP
motor unit action potential
MUAP on electromyogram
mucate
isometheptene m.
Much-Holzmann reaction
mucin-secreting adenocarcinoma
mucocele
clival m.
erosive sphenoid m.
m. formation
paranasal m.
sphenoid m.
mucocutaneous lymph node syndrome
mucolipidosis
mannose in m.
m. type IV (ML4)
mucopolysaccharide
mucopolysaccharidosis I–VI
mucopyocele
m. of the clivus
nasal sinus m.
Mucor
Mucoraceae
***Mucor* infection**
mucormycosis
Mucosil
mucosulfatidosis
mucous
m. membrane lesion
m. retention cyst
Muir
tract of Bruce and M.
mulberry-like nodule
Mulholland and Gunn criteria
Mullan
M. percutaneous trigeminal ganglion microcompression set
M. triangle
M. wire
Müller
M. fiber
M. ganglion
M. glial
M. law
M. muscle
M. radial cell
M. trigone
mullerian duct aplasia, renal aplasia, cervicothoracic somite dysplasia (MURCS)
Müller-König
M.-K. procedure
M.-K. transposition
multiarc LINAC radiosurgery
Multichannel ABI
multicomponent
m. program
multicore
m. disease
m. myopathy
multicystic
m. encephalomalacia
m. encephalopathy
multidetermined behavior
multidimensional
m. assessment
m. assessment of outcome
m. family therapy
m. Fourier transform

m. framework
M. Pain Inventory
multidisciplinary pilot project program (MPPP)
MultiDop XS system
multienzyme
pyruvate dehydrogenase m.
multifacet circumplex
multifaceted nature
multifactorial
m. etiology
m. event
multifocal
m. acquired motor axonopathy
m. fibrosclerosis
m. glioma
m. leukoencephalopathy
m. mononeuropathy
m. motor neuropathy (MFMN)
m. myoclonus
m. paroxysm
m. placoid pigment epitheliopathy
m. subcortical demyelination
multiform
m. layer
m. layer of cerebral cortex
multiforme
erythema m.
giant cell glioblastoma m.
glioblastoma m. (GBM)
stratum m.
multiforme-like
erythema m.-l.
multiformis
lamina m.
multifrequency transcranial Doppler
multiganglionic
multiglandular hyperplasia
multihandicapped
multiinfarct
m. dementia (MID)
m. progressive supranuclear palsy
Multi-Institutional Research in Alzheimer Genetic Epidemiology
multilead electrode
multileaf collimator
multilevel laminectomy
multilobar resection
multiloculated hydrocephalus
multimodal
m. association cortex
m. code
m. therapeutic approach
m. therapy
m. treatment model
multimodality
m. evoked potential (MEP)
m. image coregistration
Multiplace chamber
multiplanar
imaging m.
multiple
m. analysis of variance (MANOVA)
m. association
m. buccal frenulum
m. carboxylase deficiency
m. congenital anomaly
m. cortical infarction
m. discharge
m. endocrine neoplasia (MEN)
m. endocrine neoplasia, type 1–3 (MEN-1–3)
m. focal lesion
m. hook assembly
m. hook assembly C-D instrumentation
m. impact injury
m. intracranial aneurysm
m. line-scan imaging
m. medically unexplained symptom
m. mononeuropathy
m. mucosal neuroma syndrome
m. myeloma
m. myeloma peripheral neuropathy
m. neuritis
m. neuroma
m. operations syndrome
m. plane imaging
m. sclerosis (MS)
m. sclerosis ataxia
m. sclerosis chronic progressive pattern
m. sclerosis dementia
m. sclerosis immunology
m. sclerosis pathophysiology
m. sclerosis plaque
m. sclerosis relapse
m. sclerosis-type organic
m. sclerosis variant
m. sensitive point
m. sleep latency test (MSLT)

NOTES

multiple *(continued)*
m. spike population
m. subpial transection (MST)
m. synostosis
m. system atrophy
m. targeting
m. tic disorder (MTD)
m. victimization
multiple-choice testing
multiple-dose regimen
multiple-episode patient
multiple-point sacral fixation
multiple-tracer approach
multiplex
arthrogryposis congenita m.
diabetic mononeuritis m.
mononeuritis m.
mononeuropathy m.
myoclonus m.
paramyoclonus m.
multipolar
m. cell
m. neuron
multipolarity
multipore suction tip
multipotential cell
multipurpose headrest
multisegmental hyporeflexia
multisomatoform disorder
multispan fracture hook
multispeaker phonetic noise
Multispect 3 camera
multistate
multisynaptic
multisystem
m. atrophy (MSA)
m. therapy
multisystemic
m. therapy
m. therapy approach
multivariate technique
multivoxel
m. MRS
m. technique
multocida
Pasteurella m.
mumbling automatism
mumps
m. encephalitis
m. facial nerve palsy
m. meningitis
m. meningoencephalitis
m. peripheral neuropathy
m. vaccination complication
MUP
motor unit potential
mural thrombus
muramyl peptide
MURCS
mullerian duct aplasia, renal aplasia, cervicothoracic somite dysplasia
MURCS syndrome
murine
m. double minute 2 (MDM2)
m. typhus
m. typhus meningoencephalitis
murmur
brain m.
heart m.
Murphy
M. ball hook
M. rake retractor
MurphyScope neurologic device
Murray
M. Valley disease
M. Valley encephalitis
Musashi-1
muscarine poisoning
muscarinic
m. acetylcholine receptor (mAChR)
m. cholinergic blockade
m. side effect
muscimol
muscle
m. absence
m. activity
agonist m.
antagonist m.
anterior scalene m.
anterior serratus m.
m. atonia
m. atrophy
m. biopsy
branch of glossopharyngeal nerve to stylopharyngeus m.
cervicis m.
m. contraction headache
m. cramp
cranial m.
m. denervation
depressor anguli oris m.
digastric m.
m. dissection
distal m.
m. endplate
m. enzyme serum level
m. examination
external intercostal m.
m. fascicle
m. fiber
m. fiber action potential
m. fiber type disproportion
m. fibrosis
m. filter

flexor carpi radialis m.
Gantzer m.
greater rhomboid m.
homonymous m.
hyoglossus m.
m. hypertrophy
iliocostal m.
iliopsoas m.
inferior rectus m.
m. inflammatory disorder
intraspinous m.
jugular foramen m.
lateral rectus m.
latissimus dorsi m.
levator palpebrae m.
limb m.
lingual m.
longus capitis m.
longus cervicis colli m.
m. mass
medial rectus m.
mimetic m.
motor unit m.
Müller m.
m. myotonic disorder
nuchal m.
ocular m.
omohyoid m.
orbicularis orbis m.
orbicularis oris m.
orbicular oculi m.
m. pain
palatoglossus m.
palatopharyngeus m.
paraspinal m.
pectoralis major m.
m. periodic paralysis
pharyngeal constrictor m.
m. phosphorylase
platysma m.
m. pseudohypertrophy
psoas m.
m. psychogenic disorder
m. receptor
rectus lateralis abducens oculomotor m.
m. relaxant
m. rigidity
Rouget m.
sacrospinalis m.
scalenus anticus m.
m. sense
skeletal m.
smooth m.
somatic m.
m. spasm
m. spindle
sternocleidomastoid m.
sternohyoid m.
sternomastoid m.
sternothyroid m.
strap m.
m. strength
m. stretch reflex
striated m.
styloglossus m.
stylohyoid m.
stylopharyngeus m.
superior rectus m.
temporalis m.
teres major m.
m. tone
m. tone inhibitor system
trapezius m.
vascular smooth m.
m. wasting

muscle-eye-brain disease
muscle-fascia-Gelfoam combination
muscle-paretic nystagmus
muscle-relaxing effect
muscle-splitting incision
musculaire
folie m.
muscular
m. anesthesia
m. atrophy
m. branch of deep fibular nerve
m. dystrophy
facioscapulohumeral m.
m. hyperalgesia
m. hyperesthesia
m. hypotonia
m. insufficiency
m. pseudohypertrophy
m. reflex
m. sense
m. trophoneurosis
muscularis
ramus m.
musculature
axial m.
bulbar m.

M

NOTES

musculocutanei
rami musculares nervi m.
musculocutaneous nerve
musculocutaneus
nervus m.
musculorum
m. deformans
dystonia m.
musculoskeletal
m. deformity
m. psychogenic disorder
musculospiral
m. nerve
m. paralysis
musical
m. agraphia
m. alexia
musician's cramp
musicogenic epilepsy
Mussen frame
mussitans
delirium m.
mussitation
Mustargen
mutant
presenilin m.
mutase
methylmalonyl-CoA m.
phosphoglycerate m.
mutation
deletion m.
missense m.
point m.
single point m.
tandem double m.
tumor suppressor gene m.
UBE3A m.
mutilating
m. acropathy
m. leprosy
mutism
akinetic m.
apathetic akinetic m.
cerebellar m.
elective m.
hysterical m.
pure word m.
voluntary m.
muttering delirium
MVC
maximum voluntary contraction
MVD
microvascular decompression
MVP
microvascular pressure
MwoA
migraine without aura
MWT
maintenance of wakefulness test
myalgia cruris epidemica
myalgic asthenia
myasthenia
m. gravis (MG)
m. gravis evaluation
m. snarl
myasthenic
m. crisis
m. facies
m. ptosis
m. reaction
m. syndrome
myatonia, myatony
mycetism cerebralis
mycetismus
mycobacteria
mycobacterial
Mycobacterium
M. leprae
M. tuberculosis
M. tuberculosis infection
mycophenolate mofetil
Mycoplasma
Mycoplasma arthritidis
Mycoplasma infection
Mycoplasma pneumoniae encephalitis
mycosis
mycotic
m. infection
m. intracranial aneurysm
mydriasis
alternating m.
paralytic m.
spasmodic m.
spastic m.
springing m.
mydriatic rigidity
myelalgia
myelapoplexy
myelatelia
myelauxe
myelencephalic vein
myelencephalitis
myelencephalon
myelic
myelin
m. basic protein (MBP)
m. basic protein deficiency
m. body
m. breakdown
m. degradation
m. figure
m. macromolecule

m. oligodendrocyte glycoprotein (MOG)
oral bovine m.
m. ovoid
peripheral nerve m.
m. sheath
m. tissue stain

myelin-associated glycoprotein (MAG)

myelinated
m. axon
m. nerve
m. nerve fiber
m. nerve fiber function

myelinating phenotype

myelination
m. of axon
central nervous system m.
peripheral nerve m.

myelinic neuroma

myelinization

myelinoclasis
acute perivascular m.
postinfection perivascular m.

myelinoclastic
m. diffuse cerebral sclerosis
m. disease

myelinogenesis

myelinogenetic

myelinogeny

myelin/oligodendrocyte glycoprotein

myelin/oligodendrocyte-specific protein (MOSP)

myelinolysis
central pontine m.

myelinopathy

myelinotoxic

myelinotoxicity

myelin-producing cell

myelitic

myelitis
acute necrotizing m.
acute transverse m.
ascending m.
bulbar m.
complete transverse m.
concussion m.
demyelinated m.
Foix-Alajouanine m.
funicular m.
neurooptic m.
periependymal m.
postinfectious m.
postvaccinal m.
subacute necrotizing m.
syphilitic m.
systemic m.
transverse m.
m. vaccinia
viral m.

myeloarchitectonics

myeloarchitecture

myelocele

myeloclast

myelocyst

myelocystic

myelocystocele
terminal m.

myelocystomeningocele

myelocyte

myelodiastasis

myelodysplasia

myelodysplastic

myeloencephalic

myeloencephalitis
eosinophilic m.

myelofibrosis
idiopathic m. (IMF)
m. osteosclerosis

myelofugal

myelogenesis

myelogenic

myelogenous

myelogeny

myelogram

myelography
cervical m.
computed tomographic metrizamide m.
computer-assisted m. (CAM)
delayed computed tomographic m.
iohexol m.
lumbar m.
metrizamide m.
spinal evaluation m.
water-soluble contrast m.

myeloid elastase

myelolysis

myeloma
multiple m.
osteosclerotic m.

myeloma-associated neuropathy

M

NOTES

myelomalacia
angiodysgenetic m.
cystic m.
myelomenia
myelomeningitis
myelomeningocele
lumbosacral m.
spina bifida m.
myeloneuritis
myeloneuropathy
cassava plant tropical m.
human T-cell lymphotropic virus-associated m.
tropical m.
myeloparalysis
myelopathic muscular atrophy
myelopathy
acute partial m.
acute transverse m.
AIDS-associated vacuolar m.
AIDS-related m.
carcinomatous m.
cervical spondylosis without m.
cervical spondylotic m.
chronic progressive m.
compressive m.
diabetic m.
HIV m.
HTLV-I associated m.
human T-cell lymphotropic virus-associated m.
human T-lymphotrophic virus-associated m.
m. incidence
laminoplasty with extended foraminoplasty for cervical m.
midcervical flexion m.
necrotizing m.
paracarcinomatous m.
paraneoplastic m.
radiation m.
reducing body m.
spondylotic m.
subacute necrotic m.
subacute necrotizing m.
m. syndrome
systemic m.
transverse m.
traumatic m.
tropical spastic paraparesis/HTLV-I associated m.
vacuolar m.
vascular m.
myeloperoxidase
myelopetal
myelophthisic
myelophthisis
myeloplegia
myelopore
myeloproliferative disorder
myeloradiculitis
myeloradiculodysplasia
myeloradiculopathy
myeloradiculopolyneuronitis
myelorrhagia
myelorrhaphy
myeloschisis
myelosclerosis
myelosis
funicular m.
myelosyphilis
myelosyringosis
myelotome
myelotomography
myelotomy
Bischof m.
commissural m.
extralemniscal m.
midline m.
T m.
myenteric plexus
myentericus
plexus (nervosus) m.
Myer fiber
Myers model of perinatal asphyxia
Myerson sign
myesthesia
mylohyoideus
nervus m.
mylohyoid nerve
Myloral
myoadenylate
m. deaminase
m. deaminase deficiency
myoblastoma
granular cell m.
Myobloc
myobradia
myocardial infarction
myocelialgia
myoclonia
eyelid m.
fibrillary m.
myoclonic
m. absence
m. astatic epilepsy
m. dystonia
m. encephalopathy
m. encephalopathy syndrome
m. epilepsy of adolescence
m. epilepsy with ragged red fiber
m. epilepsy with ragged red fiber myopathy

m. epilepsy with ragged red fiber syndrome
m. jerk
m. opsoclonus
M. SE
myoclonica
dyssynergia cerebellaris m.
myoclonic-astatic petit mal seizure
myoclonus
Baltic m.
benign infantile m.
benign neonatal sleep m.
cortical m.
m. epilepsy
m. epilepsy with ragged red fiber (MERRF)
m. epilepsy with ragged red fibers-lactic acidosis (MERRLA)
epileptic negative m.
essential m.
fragmentary m.
hereditary branchial m.
infantile jerk m.
intention m.
Mediterranean m.
multifocal m.
m. multiplex
nocturnal m.
nonepileptic m.
ocular m.
oculopalatal m.
palatal m.
palatoocular m.
paraneoplastic opsoclonus m.
postanoxic m.
postencephalitic m.
posthypoxic m.
preictal m.
propriospinal m.
m. reticular reflex
sleep m.
spinal segmental m.
stimulus sensitive m.
tardive m.
m. tardive
myocutaneous flap
Myodil
myodynia
myodystonia
myodystony
myodystrophy, myodystrophia
myoedema
myoesthesis, myoesthesia
myofascial
m. pain
m. syndrome
myofibril
myofibrillar infantile myopathy
myofibrillary disarray
myofibroblast
myofibromatosis
infantile m.
myogenic
m. motor evoked potential
m. paralysis
m. tonus
myoglobinuria
drug-induced m.
exercise-induced m.
myogram
myography
myohypertrophia kymoparalytica
myoinositol
myokymia
eyelid m.
facial m.
generalized m.
hereditary m.
limb m.
myokymia-cramp syndrome
myokymic discharge
myomedulloblastoma
myonecrotic myopathy
myoneural
m. ischemia
m. junction
myoneuralgia
postural m.
myoneurasthenia
myoneurogastrointestinal encephalopathy
myoneuroma
myopalmus
myoparalysis
myoparesis
myopathic
m. atrophy
m. carnitine deficiency
m. facies
m. gait
m. spasm
myopathy
acute steroid quadriplegic m.

NOTES

M

myopathy *(continued)*
alcoholic m.
bland m.
centronuclear m.
congenital m.
critical illness m.
desmin storage m.
distal m.
HIV m.
idiopathic inflammatory m. (IIM)
inclusion body m.
infantile myofibrillar m.
inflammatory m.
Kiloh-Nevin ocular m.
late distal hereditary m.
lipid m.
minicore m.
minicore-multicore m.
mitochondrial m.
Miyoshi m. (MM)
multicore m.
myoclonic epilepsy with ragged red fiber m.
myofibrillar infantile m.
myonecrotic m.
myotubular m.
nemaline m.
nondystrophin m.
polysaccharide storage m.
proximal myotonic m. (PROMM)
quadriceps m.
sarcotubular m.
thyrotoxic m.
trilaminar m.
tubular aggregate m.
Welander distal m.
Xp21 m.
Z-band in nemaline m.
myophosphorylase deficiency
myopia
axial m.
myopsychic
myopsychopathy
myopsychosis
myorelaxant activity
myorhythmia
oculomasticatory m.
myosalgia
myoschwannoma
Myoscint
myoseism
myosin filament
myositis
cancer-associated m.
cervical tension m.
childhood m.
eosinophilic m.
inclusion-body m.
influenza virus m.
orbital m.
m. ossificans
myospasm, myospasmus
cervical m.
myospasmia
myotatic
m. contraction
m. contracture
m. reflex
myotome
myotomy
genioglossus advancement-hyoid m.
myotone
myotonia
m. acquisita
m. atrophica
Becker m.
chondrodystrophic m.
m. chondrodystrophic
m. congenita
m. dystrophica
m. neonatorum
potassium-aggravated m. (PAM)
myotonic
m. afterdischarge
m. discharge
m. dystrophy gene
m. facies
m. muscular dystrophy
m. potential
m. pupil
m. response
myotonica
dystrophia m.
myotonoid
myotonus
myotony
myotubular myopathy
myriachit (*var. of* miryachit)
myristic acid
Mysoline
Mytelase
M. Caplet
M. chloride
myxedema
m. coma
m. depression
juvenile m.
m. madness
m. peripheral neuropathy
myxoglioma
myxoid lobule
myxoma
atrial m.
left atrial m.

myxomatous
m. cell
m. thickening

myxoneuroma
myxopapillary ependymoma
myxovirus infection

NOTES

NAA
National Aphasia Association
NABTC
North American Brain Tumor Consortium
nabumetone
***N*-acetylaspartic acid**
***N*-acetylglucosamine-6-sulfate sulfatase**
***N*-acetylglutamate deficiency**
***N*-acetylneuraminic acid**
nAChR
nicotinic acetylcholine receptor
NADPH
nicotinamide adenine dinucleotide phosphate
NADPH-diaphorase
Naegleria
N. fowleri
N. infection
N. meningitis
nafate
Nafcil
Naffziger
N. straight midline incision
N. syndrome
N. test
Naftidrofuryl
Nageotte
N. bracelet
N. cell
Nager Miller syndrome
nail
intramedullary n.
Küntscher n.
n. lesion
NAIM
nasal airflow-inducing maneuver
NAIP
neuronal apoptosis inhibitory protein
naked axon
naked-eye direct vision surgery
naltrexone HCl
Nam
nicotinamide
naming
category-specific n.
nandrolone decanoate
nap
diurnal n.
napping
daytime n.
napsylate
Naqua
naratriptan
n. HCl
n. hydrochloride
narcissistic
n. character structure
n. feature
narcohypnia
narcolepsy
N. Network
non-REM n.
narcoleptic
n. tetrad
n. triad
narcoplexy
narcosis
CO_2 n.
nitrogen n.
narcotic intoxication
Nardil
NARP
neuropathy, ataxia, retinitis pigmentosa
narrative
n. data
n. speech
n. speech perception
n. speech perception impairment
narrow
n. AO dynamic compression plate
n. bipole
n. tripole
narrow-bite bone rongeur
narrowing
degenerative n.
nasal
n. airflow-inducing maneuver (NAIM)
n. cavity
n. chondritis
n. continuous positive airway pressure
n. CPAP
n. ganglion
n. glioma
n. hemifield
n. lesion
n. mucosal sac
n. pressure measurement/monitoring
n. reflex
n. septum hematoma
n. sinus
n. sinus mucopyocele
n. surgery
nasal-temporal asymmetry

N

nascentium
trismus n.
nascent motor unit potential
NASCET
North American Symptomatic Carotid Endarterectomy Trial
NASCIS
National Acute Spinal Cord Injury Studies
Nashold
N. biopsy needle
N. TC electrode
nasion
nasociliari
ramus communicans cum nervo n.
nasociliaris
n. nerve
nervus n.
radix n.
nasociliary
n. nerve
n. neuralgia
n. root
nasoethmoidal encephalocele
nasofrontal encephalocele
nasofrontalis
fonticulus n.
nasogastric
n. intubation
n. tube
nasomental reflex
nasoorbital encephalocele
nasopalatine
n. nerve
n. plexus
nasopalatinus
nervus n.
nasopharyngeal
n. angiofibroma
n. blastomycosis
n. cooling
n. electrode
n. electrode placement (PG)
n. malignancy
n. mucus retention cyst
nasopharyngolaryngoscopy
nasopharyngoscopy
nasopharynx
Nasu-Hakola disease
Natecor
National
N. Acute Spinal Cord Injury Studies (NASCIS)
N. Aphasia Association (NAA)
N. Comorbidity Study
N. Death Index
N. Institute of Neurological and Communicative Disorders and Stroke (NINCDS-ADRDA)
N. Institute of Neurological Disorders and Stroke (NINDS)
N. Institutes of Health Stroke Scale (NIHSS)
N. Mental Health Association (NMHA)
N. Rehabilitation Association
N. Society for Epilepsy (NSE)
N. Spine Network (NSN)
N. Treatment Improvement Evaluation Study
natriuresis
natriuretic hormone
natural
n. chemotherapy agent
n. hearing loss
n. killer (NK)
n. killer cell
n. progesterone
naturalistic
n. design
n. followup study
nature
multifaceted n.
subcortical n.
Naturetin
nausea anesthesia
nauseous
navicular abdomen
navigation
Cybon surgical n.
intracranial n.
navigator
Operating Arm stereotactic n.
Zeiss STN surgical tool n.
Navigus
N. cranial base and cap
N. trajectory guide
Navy neurologic screening examination
N-butyl
N-b. cyanoacrylate
N-b. 2-cyanoacrylate with lipiodol adhesive agent
NC
neurogenic claudication
NCA
nuclear cerebral angiography
NCAM
neural-cell adhesion molecule
NCC
neurocysticercosis
NCP
NeuroCybernetic prosthesis
NCP lead

NCP programming wand
NCP System
NCS
nerve conduction study
NCV
nerve conduction velocity
1505 NDSB occlusion balloon catheter
Nd:YAG
neodymium:yttrium-aluminum-garnet
Nd:YAG laser
Nd:YAG module
NE
neurologic examination
near
n. reflex spasm
n. syncope
near-infrared spectroscopy (NIRS)
nebulin
NEC
neuroendocrine carcinoma
neck
n. of aneurysm
n. circumference
n. pain
potato tumor of n.
n. righting reflex
n. sign
n. stiffness
n. stimulation
n. tonic reflex
transverse nerve of the n.
n. weakness
wry n.
neck-tongue syndrome
necrencephalus
necrolysis
epidermal n.
toxic epidermal n. (TEN)
necrosis
acute tubular n.
aseptic n.
caseous n.
cell n.
cerebral radiation n.
coagulative n.
cystic medial n.
gray-matter n.
hemorrhagic n.
laminar cortical n.
Marcus grading scale for avascular n.
occlusal n.
pituitary n.
postpartum n.
pressure n.
radiation n.
tubular n.
tumor n.
vasculitic n.
necrotizing
n. angiitis
n. encephalitis
n. encephalomyelitis
n. encephalomyelopathy
n. encephalopathy
n. granulomatous systemic arteritis
n. hemorrhage leukomyelitis
n. hemorrhagic leukoencephalitis
n. infundibulohypophysitis
n. leukoencephalopathy
n. myelopathy
n. vasculitis
NEE
needle electrode examination
needle
Adson n.
aneurysm n.
angled n.
n. aspiration
atraumatic Sprotte n.
Backlund biopsy n.
Bier lumbar puncture n.
brain biopsy n.
butterfly n.
Colorado MicroDissection n.
Cone ventricular n.
Cournand arteriogram n.
Cournand-Grino arteriogram n.
Cushing ventricular n.
Dandy ventricular n.
D'Errico ventricular n.
n. dissector
n. electrode
n. electrode examination (NEE)
n. electromyographic
n. electromyography
n. EMG
epidural n.
Espocan combined spinal/epidural n.
Frazier ventricular n.
Hoen ventricular n.
n. holder

N

NOTES

needle *(continued)*
Hunstad infusion n.
insulated electrode n.
Kronecker aneurysm n.
lumbar puncture n.
Mixter ventricular n.
MO n.
Nashold biopsy n.
neurography n.
Pace ventricular n.
Poppen ventricular n.
Quincke spinal n.
R-K n.
Scoville ventricular n.
Sedan-Nashold n.
Shaw aneurysm n.
Sheldon-Spatz vertebral arteriogram n.
Smiley-Williams arteriogram n.
spinal n.
Sprotte epidural n.
Sprotte spinal n.
straight n.
Thermistor n.
titanium alloy n.
n. trephination system
Tuohy n.
ventricular n.
ventriculostomy n.
Whitacre spinal n.
needle-in-the-eye syndrome
needle-nose rongeur
NEEG
normal electroencephalogram
neencephalon
nefazodone
Neftel disease
negative
n. afterpotential
n. aspiration
n. change
n. dromotropism
n. feedback
n. image
n. immunosuppressive effect
n. myoclonic seizure
n. myoclonus state
n. picture-caption pair
n. priming effect
n. priming task
negatively
n. bathmotropic
n. correlated region
negative-pressure ventilation
negativity
early right-anterior n.
n. of Input 1, 2
mismatch n.
phonological mismatch n. (PMN)
right anterior-temporal n.
visual mismatch n. (VMMN)
neglect
emotional n.
hemispatial n.
left visuospatial n.
n. measure
motor n.
thalamic n.
visuospatial n.
Negri body
Negri-Jacod syndrome
Negro
N. phenomenon
N. sign
Neisseria
N. meningitidis
N. meningitidis meningitis
Nélaton syndrome
nelfinavir
Nelson
N. rib spreader
N. syndrome
N. tumor
nemaline myopathy
nematode infection
Nembutal Sodium
nemonapride
Neo-Calglucon
neocerebellum
neocinetic
Neo-Cobefrin
Carbocaine with N.-C.
neocortex
lateral n.
n. maturation
neocortical
n. association area
n. coverage
n. epilepsy
n. region
NeoDerm dressing
neodymium:yttrium-aluminum-garnet (Nd:YAG)
neoencephalon
neoendorphin
neoformans
Cryptococcus n.
Neo-Iopax
neokinetic
neolalia
neolalism
neologism
neomycin

neonatal
n. abstinence syndrome
n. adrenoleukodystrophy
n. alloimmune thrombocytopenia
n. apoplexy
n. asphyxia
n. breath-holding spell
n. cerebral hemorrhage
n. drug addiction seizure
n. enterovirus infection
n. extracorporal membrane oxygenation
n. hemorrhagic disease
n. herpes simplex virus infection
n. hydrocephalus
n. hypercalcemia
n. hypertension
n. hypocalcemia
n. hypoglycemic seizure
n. hypomagnesemia
n. hypothyroidism
n. hypotonia
n. intraventricular hemorrhage
n. kernicterus
n. language development
n. meningitis
n. myasthenia gravis
n. opiate withdrawal
n. poliomyelitis
n. polycythemia
n. tetanus
n. tetany
n. tyrosinemia aminoaciduria
n. withdrawal syndrome

neonate asphyxia
neonatorum
encephalitis n.
myotonia n.
tetania n.
tetanus n.
trismus n.

neopallium
Neopap
neoplasia
adenohypophyseal n.
multiple endocrine n. (MEN)
multiple endocrine n., type 1–3 (MEN-1–3)
prostatic intraepithelial n. (PIN)

neoplasm
cranial nerve n.
de novo metachronous n.
extensive n.
frontal n.
intraaxial n.
intracranial n.
metachronous n.
pearly n.
pineal parenchymal n.
spinal cord n.
temporal horn n.
trochlear nerve n.

neoplastic
n. aneurysm
n. angioendotheliomatosis
n. arachnoiditis
n. lesion
n. meningitis

neopterin
serum n.

Neosar Injection
neospinothalmic tract
Neosporin GU Irrigant
neostigmine test
neostriatum
Neo-Synephrine
neothalamus
neovascularization
iris n.
subretinal n.

nepenthic
nephelometric assay
nephralgic crisis
nephritis
shunt n.

Nephro-Calci
nephrosis
nephrotopic
nephrotoxicity
Néri sign
Nernst equation
nerve
abdominopelvic splanchnic n.
abducens n.
abducent n. [CN VI]
accelerator n.
accessory n. [CN XI]
accessory phrenic n.
accommodation of n.
accompanying vein of hypoglossal n.
acoustic n.

NOTES

N

nerve *(continued)*
n. action potential
afferent digital n.
alveolar n.
ampullar n.
anal n.
Andersch n.
anococcygeal n.
anomalous nonrecurrent right inferior laryngeal n.
antebrachial cutaneous n.
anterior abdominal cutaneous branch of intercostal n.
anterior ampullary n.
anterior antebrachial n.
anterior auricular n.
anterior branch of axillary n.
anterior branch of thoracic n.
anterior cutaneous branch of femoral n.
anterior cutaneous branch of iliohypogastric n.
anterior cutaneous branch of intercostal n.
anterior ethmoidal n.
anterior femoral cutaneous n.
anterior interosseous n.
anterior pectoral cutaneous branch of intercostal n.
anterior pulmonary branch of vagus n.
anterior ramus of cervical n.
anterior ramus of lumbar n.
anterior ramus of sacral n.
anterior ramus of spinal n.
anterior ramus of thoracic n.
anterior root of spinal n.
anterior superior alveolar branches of infraorbital n.
aortic n.
area of facial n.
Arnold n.
articular branch of deep fibular n.
auditory n.
augmentor n.
auricular branch of vagus n.
auriculotemporal n.
autonomic n.
axillary n.
baroreceptor n.
Bell n.
n. biopsy
Bock n.
brachial cutaneous n.
buccal n.
buccinator n.
cardiac n.
caroticotympanic n.
carotid branch of glossopharyngeal n. [CN IX]
carotid sinus n.
cavernosal n.
cavernous n.
celiac n.
n. cell
n. cell body
n. center
centrifugal n.
centripetal n.
cerebral n.
cervical n.
chorda tympani n.
ciliary n.
circumflex n.
cluneal n.
coccygeal n.
cochlear part of vestibulocochlear n.
cochlear root of eighth n.
cochlear root of vestibulocochlear n.
common fibular n.
common peroneal n.
communicating branch of anterior interosseous nerve with ulnar n.
communicating branch of auriculotemporal nerve with facial n.
communicating branch of chorda tympani with lingual n.
communicating branch of facial nerve with glossopharyngeal n.
communicating branch of lacrimal nerve with zygomatic n.
communicating branch of lingual nerve with hypoglossal n.
communicating branch of median nerve with ulnar n.
communicating branch of otic ganglion to auriculotemporal n.
communicating branch of otic ganglion with medial pterygoid n.
communicating branch of radial nerve with ulnar n.
communicating branch of spinal n.
communicating branch of superficial radial nerve with ulnar n.
communicating branch of tympanic plexus with auricular branch of vagus n.
communicating branch with nasociliary n.
n. compression
n. compression syndrome

n. conduction study (NCS)
n. conduction velocity (NCV)
n. conduction velocity study
Cotunnius n.
cranial n.
crural interosseus n.
cubital n.
cutaneous n.
Cyon n.
n. deafness
n. decompression
decussation of trochlear n.
dental n.
descending tract of trigeminal n.
diaphragmatic n.
digastric n.
digital n.
n. discontinuity
dorsal root of spinal n.
dorsal scapular n.
efferent n.
eighth cranial n. [CN VIII]
eleventh cranial n. [CN XI]
encephalic n.
n. ending
n. entrapment
n. entrapment neuralgia
esodic n.
ethmoidal n.
excitor n.
excitoreflex n.
exodic n.
external popliteal n.
external sheath of optic n.
facial n. [CN VII]
n. fascicle
femoral cutaneous n.
fenestrated oculomotor n.
n. fiber
n. fiber layer hemorrhage
n. fibril
fibrous sheath of optic n.
fibular n.
n. field
fifth cranial n. [CN V]
first cranial n. [CN I]
fourth cervical n. (C4)
fourth cranial n. [CN IV]
frontal n.
furcal n.
fusimotor n.
Galen n.
gangliated n.
n. ganglion
ganglion of facial n.
ganglionic layer of optic n.
ganglionic stratum of optic n.
ganglion of intermediate n.
Gaskell n.
gastric n.
geniculum of facial n.
genitofemoral n.
genu of the facial n.
glossopharyngeal cranial n. [CN IX]
gluteal n.
n. graft
greater occipital n.
greater superficial petrosal n. (GSPN)
n. growth factor (NGF)
n. growth factor antiserum
Hering sinus n.
n. hook
hypogastric n.
hypoglossal n. [CN XII]
hypoglossal cranial n.
iliohypogastric n.
ilioinguinal n.
iliopubic n.
n. implantation
n. impulse
inferior dental n.
inferior ganglion of glossopharyngeal n.
inferior ganglion of vagus n.
inferior laryngeal n.
inferior part of vestibulocochlear n.
inferior root of vestibulocochlear n.
infraorbital n.
infratrochlear n.
inhibitory n.
inner sheath of optic n.
N. Integrity Monitor 2
intercostal n.
intercostobrachial n.
intermediary n.
intermediate n.
internal popliteal n.
internal sheath of optic n.

NOTES

nerve *(continued)*
interosseous branch of medial terminal branch of deep fibular n.
intervaginal space of optic n.
intracranial part of optic n.
ischiadic n.
Jacobson n.
jugular n.
labial n.
lacrimal n.
Lancisi longitudinal n.
Langley n.
laryngeal n.
Latarjet n.
lateral femoral cutaneous n.
lateral pterygoid n.
lateral root of median n.
lateral terminal branch of deep fibular n.
lesser superficial petrosal n. (LSPN)
levator ani n.
lingual n.
long thoracic n.
loop of hypoglossal n.
loop of spinal n.
Ludwig n.
lumbar n.
lumboinguinal n.
Luschka n.
mandibular n.
masseteric n.
maxillary n.
medial plantar n.
medial root of median n.
medial terminal branch of deep fibular n.
median n.
meningeal n.
mental n.
mesencephalic nucleus of trigeminal n.
mesencephalic tract of trigeminal n.
mixed n.
motor nucleus of facial n.
motor nucleus of trigeminal n.
motor root of mandibular n.
motor root of spinal n.
motor root of submandibular n.
motor root of trigeminal n.
muscular branch of deep fibular n.
musculocutaneous n.
musculospiral n.
myelinated n.
mylohyoid n.
nasociliaris n.
nasociliary n.
nasopalatine n.
ninth cranial n. [CN IX]
nucleus of abducent n.
nucleus of accessory n.
nucleus of acoustic n.
nucleus of cranial n.
nucleus of hypoglossal n.
nucleus of oculomotor n.
nucleus of phrenic n.
nucleus of pudendal n.
nucleus of trigeminal n.
nucleus of trochlear n.
nucleus of vagus n.
obturator n.
occipital n.
oculomotor n. [CN III]
olfactory cranial n.
ophthalmic recurrent n.
optic n. [CN II]
outer sheath of optic n.
n. pain
palatine n.
n. palsy
n. papilla
parasympathetic n.
parotid n.
pathetic n.
pectineus n.
pectoral n.
perforating cutaneous n.
perineal n.
peripheral n.
perivascular n.
peroneal n.
petrosal n.
pharyngeal plexus of vagus n.
phrenic n.
phrenicoabdominal n.
pilomotor n.
piriform n.
plantar n.
n. plexus
plexus of spinal n.
pneumogastric n.
popliteal n.
posterior branch of axillary n.
posterior communicating n.
posterior interosseous n.
posterior nucleus of oculomotor n.
posterior nucleus of vagus n.
posterior pulmonary branch of vagus n.
posterior root of spinal n.
posterior tibial n.
presacral n.
pressor n.

pressoreceptor n.
principal sensory nucleus of trigeminal n.
pterygoid canal n.
pterygopalatine n.
pudendal n.
quadratus femoris n.
radial n.
rectal n.
recurrent laryngeal n. (RLN)
recurrent meningeal n.
n. regrowth
n. root
n. root avulsion
n. root block
n. root edema
n. root embarrassment
root of facial n.
n. root microcirculation
n. root retractor
n. root sheath effacement
root of trigeminal n.
saccular n.
sacral n.
saphenous n.
sartorius n.
scapular n.
Scarpa n.
sciatic n.
scrotal n.
second cervical n.
second cranial n. [CN II]
secretomotor n.
secretory n.
sensory ganglion of cranial n.
sensory ganglion of encephalic n.
sensory root of mandibular n.
sensory root of spinal n.
sensory root of trigeminal n.
seventh cranial n. [CN VII]
n. sheath
n. sheath tumor
sinuvertebral n.
sixth cranial n. [CN VI]
small sciatic n.
n. of smell
somatic n.
spermatic n.
sphenopalatine n.
sphincter ani n.
spinal nucleus of accessory n.
spinal nucleus of trigeminal n.
spinal tract of trigeminal n.
splanchnic n.
stapedial n.
stapedius n.
statoacoustic n.
n. stimulator
n. stroma
n. stump
stylohyoid n.
stylopharyngeal n.
subclavian n.
subclavius n.
subcostal n.
sublingual n.
submaxillary n.
suboccipital n.
subscapular n.
sudomotor n.
sulcus of the oculomotor n.
superficial petrosal n.
superior ganglion of glossopharyngeal n.
superior ganglion of vagus n.
superior laryngeal n. (SLN)
superior part of vestibulocochlear n.
superior root of vestibulocochlear n.
supraclavicular n.
supraorbital n.
suprascapular n.
supratrochlear n.
sural cutaneous n.
sural sensory n.
n. suture
sympathetic n.
temporal n.
tensor tympani n.
tensor veli palatini n.
tenth cranial n. [CN X]
tentorial n.
terminal n.
third cranial n. [CN III]
thoracic splanchnic n.
thoracodorsal n.
tibial n.
Tiedemann n.
tonsillar n.
n. tract
trifacial n.

N

NOTES

nerve *(continued)*
trigeminal cranial n.
trigone of auditory n.
trigone of hypoglossal n.
trigone of vagus n.
trochlear n. [CN IV]
trochlear cranial n.
tympanic n.
ulnar n.
unmyelinated n.
utricular n.
utriculoampullarly n.
vagal part of accessory n.
vaginal n.
vagus cranial n.
vagus cranial n. [CN X]
Valentin n.
vascular circle of optic n.
vasoconstrictor n.
vasodilator n.
vasomotor n.
vasosensory n.
ventral branch of thoracic n.
ventral medial nuclei of oculomotor n.
ventral ramus of thoracic n.
ventral root of spinal n.
vertebral n.
vestibular part of vestibulocochlear n.
vestibular root of vestibulocochlear n.
vestibulocochlear n. [CN VIII]
vidian n.
visceral nuclei of oculomotor n.
Willis n.
Wrisberg n.
n. of Wrisberg
zygomatic n.
zygomaticofacial branch of zygomatic n.
zygomaticotemporal branch of zygomatic n.

nerve-action current

nerve-cell adhesion molecule

nerveless

nerve-point massage

nervi (*pl. of* nervus)

nervimotility

nervimotion

nervimotor

nervimuscular

nervine

nervomuscular

nervorum
ansae n.
nervus n.

nervosa
anorexia n.
foramina n.
pars n.

nervosi
pars cranialis partis parasympathici divisionis autonomici systematis n.
pars parasympathetica divisionis autonomici systematis n.
pars peripherica systematis n.
pars sympathica divisionis autonomici systematis n.

nervosum
systema n.
Willis centrum n.

nervosus
lobus n.
plexus n.
status n.

nervous
n. asthenopia
n. bladder
n. chill
n. consumption
n. discharge
n. distribution
n. fatigability
n. irritability
n. system
n. system infection
n. system structure
n. tissue

nervus, pl. **nervi**
n. abducens [CN VI]
n. acusticus
n. acusticus [CN VIII]
nervi alveolares superiores
n. ampullaris anterior
n. ampullaris lateralis
n. ampullaris posterior
nervi anales inferiores
n. anococcygeus
n. articularis
nervi auriculares anteriores
n. auricularis magnus
n. auricularis posterior
n. auriculotemporalis
n. autonomicus
n. axillaris
n. buccalis
n. canalis pterygoidei
nervi cardiaci thoracici
n. cardiacus cervicalis inferior
n. cardiacus cervicalis medius
n. cardiacus cervicalis superior
nervi carotici externi
nervi caroticotympanici

n. caroticus internus
nervi cavernosi clitoridis
nervi cavernosi penis
nervi cervicales
nervi ciliares breves
nervi ciliares longi
nervi clunium inferiores
nervi clunium medii
nervi clunium superiores
n. coccygeus
n. cochlearis
nervi craniales
n. cutaneous antebrachii medialis
n. cutaneous antebrachii posterior
n. cutaneous brachii lateralis inferior
n. cutaneous brachii lateralis superior
n. cutaneous brachii medialis
n. cutaneous brachii posterior
n. cutaneous dorsalis intermedius
n. cutaneous dorsalis lateralis
n. cutaneous dorsalis medialis
n. cutaneous femoralis lateralis
n. cutaneous femoralis posterior
n. cutaneous femoris lateralis
n. cutaneous femoris posterior
n. cutaneous perforans
n. cutaneous surae lateralis
n. cutaneous surae medialis
n. cutaneus
n. cutaneus antebrachii lateralis
nervi digitales dorsales hallucis lateralis et digit secundi medialis
nervi digitales dorsales nervi radialis
nervi digitales dorsales nervi ulnaris
nervi digitales dorsales pedis
nervi digitales palmares communes nervi mediani
nervi digitales palmares communes nervi ulnaris
nervi digitales palmares proprii nervi mediani
nervi digitales palmares proprii nervi ulnaris
nervi digitales plantares communes nervi plantaris lateralis
nervi digitales plantares communes nervi plantaris medialis
nervi digitales plantares proprii nervi plantaris lateralis
nervi digitales plantares proprii nervi plantaris medialis
n. dorsalis clitoridis
n. dorsalis penis
n. dorsalis scapulae
nervi encephalici
nervi erigentes
n. ethmoidalis anterior
n. ethmoidalis posterior
n. facialis [CN VII]
n. femoralis
n. fibularis communis
n. fibularis profundus
n. fibularis superficialis
n. frontalis
n. glossopharyngeus [CN IX]
n. gluteus inferior
n. gluteus superior
n. hypogastricus
n. iliohypogastricus
n. ilioinguinalis
n. iliopubicus
n. impar
n. infraorbitalis
n. infratrochlearis
nervi intercostales
nervi intercostobrachiales
n. intermediofacialis
n. intermedius neuralgia
n. interosseus antebrachii anterior
n. interosseus antebrachii posterior
n. interosseus cruris
n. ischiadicus
n. jugularis
nervi labiales anteriores
nervi labiales posteriores
n. lacrimalis
n. laryngealis inferior
n. laryngealis recurrens
n. laryngealis superior
n. laryngeus inferior
n. laryngeus recurrens
n. laryngeus superior
n. lingualis
n. lumboinguinalis
n. mandibularis
n. massetericus
n. maxillaris
n. meatus acustici externi

NOTES

nervus *(continued)*
n. medianus
n. meningeus medius
n. mentalis
n. mixtus
n. motorius
n. musculi obturatorii interni
n. musculi piriformis
n. musculi quadrati femoris
n. musculi tensoris tympani
n. musculi tensoris veli palatini
n. musculocutaneus
n. mylohyoideus
n. nasociliaris
n. nasopalatinus
n. nervorum
n. obturatorius
n. obturatorius accessorius
n. obturatorius internus
n. occipitalis major
n. occipitalis minor
n. occipitalis tertius
n. octavus [CN VIII]
n. oculomotorius [CN III]
nervi olfactorii
n. olfactorius [CN I]
n. ophthalmicus
n. opticus [CN II]
nervi palatini
nervi palatini minores
n. palatinus major
n. pectoralis lateralis
n. pectoralis medialis
nervi peroneales
n. peroneus profundus
n. peroneus profundus accessorius
n. peroneus superficialis
n. petrosus major
n. petrosus minor
n. petrosus profundus
n. pharyngeus
nervi phrenici accessorii
n. phrenicus
n. plantaris lateralis
n. plantaris medialis
n. presacralis
n. pterygoideus lateralis
n. pterygoideus medialis
nervi pterygopalatini
n. pudendus
n. quadratus femoris
n. radialis
nervi rectales inferiores
n. saccularis
nervi sacrales et nervus coccygeus
n. saphenus
n. sciaticus
nervi scrotales anteriores
nervi scrotales posteriores
n. sensorius
n. spermaticus externus
nervi spinales
n. spinosus
nervi splanchnici lumbales
nervi splanchnici lumbares
nervi splanchnici pelvici
nervi splanchnici sacrales
n. splanchnicus thoracicus imus
n. splanchnicus thoracicus major
n. splanchnicus thoracicus minor
n. stapedius
n. statoacusticus [CN VIII]
n. subclavius
n. sublingualis
n. suboccipitalis
nervi subscapulares
nervi supraclaviculares
nervi supraclaviculares intermedii
nervi supraclaviculares laterales
nervi supraclaviculares mediales
nervi supraclaviculares posteriores
n. supraorbitalis
n. suprascapularis
n. supratrochlearis
n. suralis
nervi temporales profundi
n. terminalis
n. thoracicus longus
n. thoracodorsalis
n. tibialis
n. transversus cervicalis
n. transversus colli
n. trigeminalis
n. trigeminus [CN V]
n. trochlearis [CN IV]
n. tympanicus
n. ulnaris
n. utricularis
n. utriculoampullaris
nervi vaginales
nervi vasorum
n. vestibulocochlearis [CN VIII]
n. visceralis
n. zygomaticus

nesidioblastosis

nest
choristoma n.

nestin

net
n. electrochemical potential gradient
Neuro n.

netilmicin

netrin

network
matching and tuning n.
Narcolepsy N.
National Spine N. (NSN)
neural n.
neurofibrillar n.
prefrontal-insular cerebellar n.
thalamocortical n.
wide area n.
Neucalm
Neuhauser syndrome
neuradynamia
NeuraGen nerve guide
neuragmia
neural
n. activation
n. arc
n. arch resection
n. axis
n. canal
n. capacity
n. cell line
n. crest
n. crest cell
n. crest precursor
n. crest syndrome
n. crest tumor localization study
n. cyst
n. cytoarchitecture
n. darwinism
n. deafness
n. discharge
n. dissector
n. ectoderm
n. fold
n. foramen
n. foramen remodeling
n. function
n. ganglion
n. groove
n. growth factor
n. hamster cell
n. imaging study
n. impulse
n. injury
n. layer of retina
n. lobe
n. lobe of hypophysis
n. lobe of neurohypophysis
n. lobe of pituitary gland
n. mechanism
n. migration disorder
n. network
n. noise level
n. part of hypophysis
n. pathway
n. pathway level
n. placode
n. plasticity
n. plate
n. plate formation
n. progenitor cell
n. prosthesis
n. regeneration
n. segment
n. stalk
n. stem cell
n. structure
n. substrate
n. system
n. transplantation
n. tube
n. tube closure
n. tube defect (NTD)
n. tube development disorder
n. tube floor plate cell
n. tube formation mitosis
neural-cell adhesion molecule (NCAM)
neuralgia
abdominal n.
atypical facial n.
atypical trigeminal n.
chronic migrainous n.
ciliary n.
cranial n.
delayed-onset postherpetic n.
epileptiform n.
facial n.
n. facialis vera
Fothergill n.
geniculate n.
glossopharyngeal n. (GPN)
hallucinatory n.
Hunt n.
hypoglossal n.
idiopathic trigeminal n. (ITN)
intercostal n.
mammary n.
migrainous cranial n.
Morton n.
nasociliary n.
nerve entrapment n.

N

NOTES

neuralgia *(continued)*
nervus intermedius n.
occipital n.
otic n.
paratrigeminal n.
periodic migrainous n.
peripheral n.
petrosal n.
postherpetic n. (PHN)
posttraumatic n.
pterygopalatine n.
Raeder paratrigeminal n.
red n.
reminiscent n.
sciatic n.
Sluder n.
sphenopalatine n.
stump n.
suboccipital n.
supraorbital n.
symptomatic n.
Trélate-Charlin n.
trifacial n.
trifocal n.
trigeminal n. (TN)
trigger point n.
vagoglossopharyngeal n.
Vail n.
vidian n.
neuralgic
n. amyotrophy
n. pain syndrome
neuralgiform
neurally mediated syncope
neuramebimeter
neuraminidase deficiency
neuranagenesis
neurapophysis
neurapraxia
peripheral nerve n.
neurarchy
neurasthenia
angioparalytic n.
angiopathic n.
gastric n.
n. gravis
n. praecox
primary n.
pulsating n.
sexual n.
traumatic n.
neurasthenic
n. personality
n. psychoneurosis reaction
neuraxial
neuraxis staging
neuraxon, neuraxone
neure
neurectasia
neurectasis
neurectasy
neurectomy, neuroectomy
Cotte presacral n.
obturator n.
occipital n.
presacral n.
retrogasserian n.
Sonneberg n.
vestibular n.
neurectopia
neurectopy
neureglin (NRG)
Neurelan
neurepithelial
neurepithelium
neurergic
neurexcitotoxicity
neurexeresis
neuriatria, neuriatry
neurilemma, neurolemma
n. cell
neurilemmitis
neurilemoma
acoustic n.
Antoni type A, B n.
neurility
neurimotility
neurimotor
neurinoma
acoustic n.
dumbbell-shaped n.
trigeminal nerve n.
neurite
dystrophic n.
n. extension
n. growth
n. outgrowth
n. overgrowth
neuritic
n. cytoskeletal abnormality
n. muscular atrophy
n. plaque
neuriticum
atrophoderma n.
neuritis, pl. **neuritides**
adventitial n.
ascending n.
axial n.
brachial plexus n.
central n.
descending n.
Eichhorst n.
eighth nerve herpetic n.
endemic n.

fallopian n.
Gombault n.
heavy-metal n.
herpes zoster n.
herpetic n.
idiopathic plexus n.
inflammatory demyelinating optic n.
interdigital n.
interstitial n.
intraocular n.
ischemic n.
Leyden n.
lumbosacral plexus n.
multiple n.
occipital n.
optic n.
orbital optic n.
n. ossificans
parenchymatous n.
periaxial n.
postocular optic n.
radiation n.
radicular n.
relapsing hypertrophic n.
retrobulbar optic n.
sciatic n.
segmental n.
serum n.
shoulder-girdle n.
suboccipital n.
syphilitic n.
toxic n.
traction n.
traumatic n.
unilateral optic n.
vestibular n.

neuro
n. convex transducer
N. net
N. N-50 lesion generator
n. trend probe

neuroacanthocytosis
neuroactive amino acid
neuroadenolysis
neuro-AIDS
neuroallergy
neuroamebiasis
neuroanastomosis
autogenous cable graft interposition VII-VII n.

neuroanatomic
n. circuit
n. connection
n. pathway

neuroanatomical
neuroanatomy of aging
neuroanesthesia
neuroarthropathy
atrophic n.

neuroastrocytoma
neuroaugmentation
neuroaugmentive
NeuroAvitene applicator
neuroaxonal dystrophy
neurobehavioral
n. consequence
n. feature
n. manifestation
n. sequela
n. symptom

neuro-Behçet disease
neurobiological
n. cause
n. factor
n. justification
n. mechanism
n. perspective

neurobiologist
neurobiology of early childhood development
neurobiotactic movement
neurobiotaxis
neuroblast
n. maturation
n. migration
n. redundancy
sympathetic n.

neuroblastoma
cerebral n.
dumbbell n.
dumbbell-type n.
Hutchinson type n.
intraabdominal n.
intracranial n.
occipital n.
olfactory n.
Pepper n.

Neurobloc
neuroborreliosis
late Lyme n.
Lyme n.

NOTES

N

neurocan
neurocardiac
neurocardiogenic syncope
neurocele
NeuroCell
NeuroCell-HD
N.-HD neural cell transplant product
N.-HD porcine fetal neural material
NeuroCell-PD
N.-PD porcine fetal neural material
N.-PD porcine neural cell transplant product
neuroceptor
neurochemical
n. change
n. disequilibrium
n. effect
n. interaction
n. pathway
n. transmission
neurochemistry
neurochitin
neurochorioretinitis
neurochoroiditis
neurocirculatory
n. asthenia
n. disorder
neurocladism
neurocognitive
n. alteration
n. impairment
n. index
n. measure
n. process
neurocommunication
NeuroControl Freehand implant
neurocranial granulomatous arteritis
neurocristopathy
neurocutaneous
n. angiomatosis
n. melanosis
n. syndrome
NeuroCybernetic
N. prosthesis (NCP)
N. Prosthesis System (NPS)
neurocysticercosis (NCC)
neurocyte
neurocytolysis
neurocytoma
central n.
neurodegeneration
glutamate receptor-mediated n.
neurodegenerative
n. disease
n. disorder
neurodendrite
neurodendron
neurodermal sinus
neurodiagnostic
n. imaging
n. procedure
neurodissector
Penfield n.
NeuroDrape surgical drape
neurodynia
neuroectoderm
neuroectodermal
n. tumor
n. tumor desmoplastic variant
n. tumor pale island
neuroectodermatosis
neuroectomy (*var. of* neurectomy)
neuroeffector
neuroelectricity
neuroembryology
neuroencephalomyelopathy
neuroendocrine
n. carcinoma (NEC)
n. index
n. test
n. transducer
n. transducer cell
n. tumor localization study
neuroendocrinology
neuroendoscope
Neuroview n.
neuroendoscopic third ventriculostomy
neuroendoscopy
computer-assisted n.
neuroenteric cyst
neuroepithelial
n. cell
n. cell migration
n. cell proliferation
n. cyst
n. layer
n. layer of retina
n. tumor
neuroepithelioma
neuroepithelium
n. of ampullary crest
n. cristae ampullaris
n. of macula
neuroexcitatory state
neurofiber
afferent n.
association n.
autonomic n.
commissural n.
efferent n.
postganglionic n.
preganglionic n.
projection n.

somatic n.
tangential n.
visceral n.
neurofibra, pl. **neurofibrae**
neurofibrae afferentes
n. associationis
neurofibrae autonomicae
n. commissuralis
neurofibrae efferentes
neurofibrae postganglionares
neurofibrae postganglionicae
neurofibrae pregangionares
neurofibrae preganglionicae
n. projectionis
neurofibrae somaticae
neurofibrae tangentiales
neurofibrae viscerales
neurofibrarum
stratum n.
neurofibril
neurofibrilla
neurofibrillar
n. network
neurofibrillary
n. degeneration
n. lesion
n. tangle
n. tangle score
neurofibrillatory
neurofibroma
aryepiglottic fold n.
dumbbell n.
nonplexiform cutaneous n.
orbital n.
plexiform n.
solitary n.
spinal n.
neurofibromatosis
n. 1 (NF-1)
n. 2 (NF-2)
abortive n.
central type n.
cutaneous n.
incomplete n.
n. kyphoscoliosis
kyphoscoliosis secondary to n.
peripheral n.
segmental n.
n. type 1, 2
von Recklinghausen n.
neurofibromin
neurofibrosarcoma
neurofilament expression
neurogangliitis
neuroganglion
neurogenetic
neurogenic
n. arthropathy
n. atrophy
n. bladder
n. claudication (NC)
n. disorder
n. dysphagia
n. fiber type group
n. fracture
n. inflammation (NI)
n. lesion
n. motor evoked potential
n. orthostatic hypotension
n. process
n. pulmonary edema (NPE)
n. tonus
n. torticollis
n. ulcer
neurogenous
neurogerontology
neuroglia
n. cell
interfascicular n.
peripheral n.
neurogliacyte
neuroglial, neurogliar
n. fiber
neurogliocyte
neurogliocytoma
neuroglioma ganglionare
neuroglioma ganglionare
neurogliomatosis
neuroglycopenia
neurogram
neurography
magnetic resonance n. (MRN)
n. needle
Neuroguard transcranial Doppler
neurohemal
neurohistology
neurohormonal
neurohormone
NeuroHub
neurohumor
neurohumoralism
neurohumoral transmission

NOTES

neurohypophysectomy
neurohypophyseos
infundibulum n.
lobus nervosus n.
pars nervosa n.
neurohypophysial
neurohypophysis
neural lobe of n.
neuroid
neuroimaging
n. approach
n. assessment
functional n.
n. manifestation
structural n.
n. study
three-dimensional n.
neuroimmunology
neuroimmunomodulatory
Neuroinformatics
Office of N. (ONI)
neurokeratin
neurokinin
neurolemma (*var. of* neurilemma)
neurolemmal sheath cell
neuroleptanalgesia
neuroleptic
n. adjunct
n. bioavailability
conventional n.
n. dosage
n. dose
n. dosing
n. drug
n. exposure
high potency n.
n. malignant syndrome (NMS)
n. medication
n. sensitivity
traditional n.
typical n.
neuroleptic-free patient
neuroleptic-induced
neuroleptic-naive patient
neurolinguist
neurolinguistic programming
neurolinguistics
NeuroLink II EEG data acquisition system
Neurolite
neurologic
n. company
n. complication
n. diagnosis
n. disease
n. disorder
n. dysregulation
n. evaluation
n. event
n. examination (NE)
n. feature
n. migraine
n. rehabilitation
n. sign
n. symptom
n. syndrome
neurological
n. deficit
n. hammer
n. illness
neurologic-ophthalmologic history
neurologist
neurology
American Board of Psychiatry and N. (ABPN)
clinical n.
environmental n.
geriatric n.
Kyoto Multi-Institutional Study Group Pediatric N.
psychiatry and n.
restorative n.
neurolues
neurolymph
neurolymphomatosis
neurolysis
alcohol n.
chemical n.
internal n.
intramuscular n.
intrathecal n.
phenol n.
trigeminal n.
neurolytic block
neuroma
acoustic n.
amputation n.
n. cutis
extracanicular acoustic n.
extrapineal pinealoma false n.
facial n.
false n.
fibrillary n.
gasserian ganglion n.
incisional n.
Joplin n.
Morton n.
multiple n.
myelinic n.
neuromata n.
nevoid n.
peripheral nerve n.
plexiform n.
posttraumatic n.

stump n.
n. telangiectodes
traumatic n.
trigeminal n.
true n.
Verneuil n.
neuromagnetic response
neuromagnetometer
whole-head n.
neuromalacia
neuromalakia
neuromata neuroma
NeuroMate robotic technology
neuromatosa
elephantiasis n.
neuromatosis
neuromechanism
neuromediator
Neuromed Octrode implantable device
Neuromeet nerve approximator
neuromeningeal
neuromere
neurometabolic disorder
Neurometer CPT/C for nerve evaluation
neuromodulation
neuromodulator
neuromonitoring
intraoperative n.
neuromuscular
n. atrophy
n. blockade
n. blocking agent
n. condition
n. disease
n. electrical stimulation
n. junction
n. junction disorder
n. junction transmission
n. scoliosis
n. scoliosis orthotic treatment
n. spindle (NMS)
neuromusculoskeletal syndrome
neuromyal
neuromyasthenia
epidemic n.
neuromyelitis optica
neuromyic
neuromyopathy
carcinomatous n.
neuromyositis
neuromyotonia
neuromyotonic discharge
neuron
abnormal epileptic n.
afferent n.
alpha motor n.
aspiny n.
autonomic motor n.
bipolar n.
brainstem n.
canonical n.
central respiratory n.
cerebellar granule n.
cholinergic n.
cold-sensitive n.
collateral sprouting n.
cortical pyramidal n.
corticobulbar motor n.
corticospinal motor n.
dopaminergic n.
dorsal horn n.
dorsal spinocerebellar tract n.
dystrophic n.
epileptic n.
excitatory pyramidal n.
fetal brain transitory n.
first-order n.
GABAergic n.
gamma motor n.
ganglionic motor n.
giant n.
glutamate-containing n.
glutamatergic n.
Golgi type I, II n.
granular n.
hippocampal pyramidal n.
hNT n.
n. hyperexcitation
impaired migration of brain n.
intercalary n.
internuncial n.
ischemic n.
itch-specific central n.
layer of piriform n.
Leydig n.
lower motor n. (LMN)
magnocellular n.
mesencephalic n.
motor n.
motorneuronal pool inhibitory n.
multipolar n.
noradrenergic n.

NOTES

N

neuron *(continued)*
olfactory sensory n. (OSN)
pedunculopontine n.
peripheral sensory n.
phrenic motor n.
piriform n.
polymorphic n.
postganglionic motor n.
postsynaptic n.
preganglionic motor n.
premotor n.
presynaptic n.
primary afferent n.
primary sensory n.
projection n.
pseudounipolar n.
Purkinje n.
pyramidal n.
redundant n.
sacral dorsal commissural n.
secondary sensory n.
second-order n.
sensory n.
somatic motor n.
somesthetic n.
spiny n.
stellate n.
striatal n.
thalamic reticular n.
n. theory
n. threshold
unipolar n.
upper motor n. (UMN)
visceral motor n.
vomeronasal sensory n. (VSN)
warm-sensitive n.

neuronal
n. achromasia
n. activation
n. adhesion
n. aggregate
n. apoptosis inhibitory protein (NAIP)
n. cell apoptosis
n. ceroid lipofuscinosis
n. ceroid lipofuscinosis curvilinear body
n. cytoplasm
n. damage
n. death
n. degeneration
n. differentiation
n. element firing
n. excitability
n. feedback loop
n. feed-forward loop
n. function
n. heterotopia
n. hyperexcitability
n. ingrowth
n. injury
n. lipidosis
n. loss
n. lysosomal storage disorder
n. mechanism
n. membrane
n. metabolism
n. migraine disorder
n. migration
n. migration abnormality
n. migration disorder
n. morphology
n. NAHPH-diaphorase/NOS expression
n. nitric oxide synthase (nNOS)
n. pathology
n. plasticity
n. precursor
n. process
n. pruning
n. regeneration
n. reuptake
n. shrinkage
n. signal
n. size
n. somata
n. specificity
n. spike activity
n. sprouting
n. stabilizing agent
n. structure
n. subpopulation
n. tumor
n. viability

neuronavigation
frameless and armless stereotactic n.

neuronavigator
three-dimensional digitizer n.

neuronavigator-guided brain surgery

neurone

neuronitis
vestibular n.

neuronopathy
sensory n.
X-linked recessive bulbospinal n.

neuronophage

neuronophagia

neuronophagy

neuronotropic

neuron-specific
n.-s. cytoskeletal protein
n.-s. enolase (NSE)

Neurontin

neuronyxis
neurooncologic disease
neurooncology
neuroophthalmic disorder
neuroophthalmology
neurooptic myelitis
neurootology
neuropacemaker
Neuropak
N. Four EMG/Evoked Response Measuring System Model MEM-4104K
N. 8 system
neuropapillitis
neuroparalysis
neuroparalytic
n. keratitis
n. ophthalmia
neuropath
neuropathic
n. arthritis
n. arthropathy
n. atrophy
n. hyperkyphoscoliosis
n. joint
n. pain
neuropathogenesis
neuropathogenicity
neuropathologic examination
neuropathology
Alzheimer disease n.
neuropathy
acquired demyelinative n.
acromegalic n.
acrylamide peripheral n.
acute axonal motor n.
acute ischemic brachial n.
acute motor-sensory axonal sensory n.
acute sensory-motor axonal n.
AIDS n.
alcoholic peripheral n.
alcohol-induced peripheral n.
alkaloid n.
amyloid n.
amyloidosis peripheral n.
anterior ischemic optic n. (AION)
anterograde fast component n.
arsenic peripheral n.
asymmetric motor n.
n., ataxia, retinitis pigmentosa (NARP)
auditory n.
autonomic n.
autosympathectomy secondary to n.
avitaminosis B_{12} peripheral n.
axonal n.
bacterial peripheral n.
barbiturate peripheral n.
Bassen-Kornzweig peripheral n.
botulism peripheral n.
brachial plexus n.
brucellosis peripheral n.
bulbar hereditary motor n.
B vitamin deficiency n.
carcinoma peripheral n.
carcinomatous n.
chronic hepatic failure peripheral n.
chronic inflammatory demyelinating sensorimotor n.
compression n.
compressive n.
congenital hypomyelination n.
congenital sensory n.
cranial n.
Cuban epidemic n.
dapsone n.
Dejerine-Sottas peripheral n.
demyelinating n.
Denis Browne n.
Denny-Brown sensory radicular n.
diabetic n.
dinitrophenol peripheral n.
diphtheria peripheral n.
diphtheritic n.
distal symmetric axonal sensorimotor n.
dying-back n.
emetine peripheral n.
entrapment n.
ethyl alcohol peripheral n.
facial n.
familial amyloid n.
femoral n.
focal n.
giant axonal n.
glossopharyngeal n.
gold peripheral n.
griseofulvin peripheral n.
Guillain-Barré postinfection peripheral n.

NOTES

neuropathy *(continued)*
handcuff n.
heavy metal n.
hepatic disease-associated n.
hereditary hypertrophic n.
hereditary motor-sensory n. (HMSN)
hereditary radicular sensory n.
hereditary sensory n. (HSN)
hereditary sensory autonomic n., type 1–4 (HSAN-1–4)
hereditary sensory motor n. (HSMN)
hereditary sensory radicular n.
HIV-related n.
HIV-sensory n. (HIV-SN)
huffer n.
hyperthyroid n.
hypertrophic interstitial n.
hypoglossal n.
hypoglycemic peripheral n.
hypothyroid n.
idiopathic peripheral n.
infantile n.
infection-related n.
infectious hepatitis peripheral n.
inflammatory demyelinating n.
insecticide peripheral n.
ischemic anterior optic n.
ischemic posterior optic n.
isoniazid n.
isonicotinic acid peripheral n.
Jamaican n.
lead n.
leprosy peripheral n.
leprous n.
lotus n.
lupus erythematosus peripheral n.
Lyme n.
macrocryoglobulinemia peripheral n.
macroglobulinemia peripheral n.
malabsorption syndrome peripheral n.
measles peripheral n.
mercury peripheral n.
metachromatic leukodystrophy n.
metal n.
metal-produced n.
methyl alcohol peripheral n.
mitochondrial n.
mononucleosis peripheral n.
motor dapsone n.
multifocal motor n. (MFMN)
multiple myeloma peripheral n.
mumps peripheral n.
myeloma-associated n.
myxedema peripheral n.
nitrofurantoin n.
nonprogressive n.
nutritional n.
occupational n.
oculomotor n.
onion bulb n.
optic n.
pantothenic acid deficiency peripheral n.
paraneoplastic n.
paraproteinemic n.
periaxial n.
peripheral n.
peroneal entrapment n.
phrenic n.
polyarteritis nodosa peripheral n.
porphyria peripheral n.
porphyric n.
pressure n.
progressive hypertrophic interstitial n.
pure sensory n.
radiation n.
radicular n.
Refsum peripheral n.
relapsing n.
retrograde fast component n.
rheumatoid n.
sacral plexus n.
sarcoid n.
sarcoidosis peripheral n.
segmental n.
senile n.
sensorimotor peripheral n.
sensory n.
sensory-motor-autonomic n.
serum sickness peripheral n.
Shy-Drager n.
slow component n.
small-fiber n. (SFN)
sprue peripheral n.
steroid-sensitive n.
subacute demyelinating n.
subacute myelooptic n. (SMON)
subclinical n.
sulfonamide peripheral n.
suprascapular n.
symmetrical diffuse n.
symmetric distal n.
Tangier peripheral n.
thallium peripheral n.
therapeutic agent-related n.
TOCP n.
    triorthocresyl phosphate neuropathy
tomaculous n.
toxic n.

traumatic n.
tricresyl phosphate peripheral n.
trigeminal n.
triorthocresyl phosphate n. (TOCP neuropathy)
tropical ataxic n. (TAN)
tuberculosis peripheral n.
typhoid peripheral n.
ulnar n.
uremia peripheral n.
uremic n.
vaccination peripheral n.
vagus n.
vasculitic n.
vestibulocochlear n.
vincristine peripheral n.
vitamin B_{12} n.
Wegener granulomatosis-associated n.
Whipple disease peripheral n.

neuropeptide
n. change
n. gene
plasma n. Y
n. Y (NPY)

neuropharmacology
functional n.

neurophilic

neurophthalmology

neurophysins

neurophysiological
n. monitoring
n. phenotypic factor

neurophysiology

neuropil, neuropile
n. thread

neuroplasm

neuroplasmic

neuroplasticity

neuroplastic response

neuroplasty
epidural n.

neuroplegic

neuroplexus

neuropodia

neuropodion

neuropodium

neuropore
anterior n.
caudal n.
posterior n.
rostral n.

neuropraxia

Neuroprobe

neuroprogenitor cell

neuroprosthesis

neuroprotection

neuroprotective effect

neuroprotein

neuropsychiatric
n. condition
n. disorder
n. drug
n. feature
N. Inventory
N. Inventory/nursing home version
n. systemic lupus erythematosus

neuropsychiatrist
American College of N.'s

neuropsychiatry
Schedules for Clinical Assessment in N.

neuropsychologic
n. area
n. characteristic
n. deficit
n. disorder
n. domain
n. functioning
n. measure
n. performance
n. test
n. testing

neuropsychologically relevant task

neuropsychological profile

neuropsychologist

neuropsychology
clinical n.
cognitive n.

neuropsychopathic

neuropsychopathy

neuroradiology
interventional n.
pediatric n.

neuroreceptor imaging

neurorecidive

neurorecurrence

neuroregeneration

neuroregulator

neurorehabilitation

neurorelapse

NOTES

neuroretinal angiomatosis
neuroretinitis
neurorrhaphy
epineurial n.
neurosarcocleisis
neurosarcoidosis
meningeal n.
neurosarcoma
NEURO-SAT frameless isocentric stereotactic system
neuroschisis
neuroschwannoma
neuroscience
behavioral n.
cognitive n.
en N.
psychotherapeutic n.
neuroscientist
clinical n.
neurosecretion
neurosecretory
n. cell
n. substance
neurosegmental
neurosensory
neuroses (*pl. of* neurosis)
neuroshunting
Neurosign 100 constant current stimulator
neurosis, pl. **neuroses**
accident n.
acute posttraumatic n.
hypochondriac n.
impulse n.
obsessional n.
postconcussion n.
posttraumatic n.
situation n.
situational n.
n. tarda
torsion n.
traumatic n.
neuroskeletal
neurosome
neurosonology
neurospasm
neurosplanchnic
neurospongioma
neurospongium
Neurostation One
Neurostat-Mark
Westco N.-M. II
neurostatus
neurosteroid
neurosthenia
neurostimulation
neurostimulator
Medtronic Xtrel n.
Synergy Versitrel n.
neurosurgeon
AANS/CNS Joint Committee of Military N.'s
neurosurgery
functional n.
image n.
microscopic n.
military n.
molecular n.
stereotactic n.
neurosurgical
N. Cervical Spine Scale
n. needle holder
n. procedure
n. stereotactic robot
neurosuture
neurosyphilis
asymptomatic n.
cerebrovascular n.
congenital n.
meningeal n.
meningitic n.
meningovascular n.
ophthalmic n.
parenchymatous n.
paretic n.
tabetic n.
neurotabes
Dejerine peripheral n.
neurotaxis
neurotendinous
n. organ
n. spindle
neurotensin
neuroterminal
neurothekeoma
neurothele
neurotherapeutics
neurotherapy
neurothlipsia, neurothlipsis
neurotic
n. anxiety state
n. depressive state
n. factor
n. manifestation
neurotica
alopecia n.
neuroticism
neurotization
neurotize
neurotmesis
neurotology
neurotome

neurotomy
radiofrequency n.
retrogasserian n.
Spiller-Frazier n.
neurotonic congestion
neurotony
neurotoxic
neurotoxicity
additive n.
antibiotic n.
antihistamine n.
beta-lactam antibiotic n.
boric acid n.
codeine n.
dextroamphetamine n.
diphenoxylate n.
dopamine n.
dose-dependent n.
ferrous sulfate n.
FK-506 n.
glutamate n.
hydroxyquinoline n.
imipramine n.
nitric oxide-mediated n.
piperazine n.
neurotoxin
neurotransmission
adrenergic n.
cholinergic n.
dopamine n.
dysregulated n.
glutamatergic n.
neurotransmitter
adrenergic n.
amino acid n.
excitatory n.
false n.
inhibitory n.
n. metabolic enzyme
n. release
n. transporter
n. vessel docking
neurotransplantation
neurotrauma
NeuroTrek microelectrode recording system
Neurotrend
N. continuous multiparameter system
N. sensor
neurotripsy
neurotrophic
n. atrophy
n. factor
n. factor expression
n. keratitis
n. ulcer
neurotrophin
neurotrophy
neurotropic
n. effect
n. virus
neurotropism
neurotropy
neurotrosis
neurotubule
neurovaricosis
neurovaricosity
neurovascular
n. flap
n. imaging
n. tree
neurovegetative
Neuroview
N. integrated visualization system
N. neuroendoscope
neurovirology
neurovirulence
neurovirulent
neurovisceral
neuroviscerolipidosis
familial n.
Neurturin
neururgic
Neutraceuticals
third-generation N.
neutral
n. image
n. material
neutralization
anterior n.
Neutra-Phos
Neutra-Phos-K
neutropenia
neutropenic
never-medicated patient
Nevin-Jones subacute spongiform encephalopathy
nevirapine
nevoid
n. amentia

NOTES

nevoid *(continued)*
n. basal cell carcinoma syndrome
n. neuroma
nevra
névropathique
famille n.
nevus alveolus inferior
new
n. variant Creutzfeldt-Jakob disease
N. York Longitudinal Study
N. York University Parkinson's Disease Scale
newborn drug withdrawal
Newcastle
N. classification
N. disease virus
newer-generation device
newly emergent categorical change
Newman-Keuls Test
new-onset seizure
Newport collar
newtonian body
NF-1
neurofibromatosis 1
NF-2
neurofibromatosis 2
NGF
nerve growth factor
NHL
non-Hodgkin lymphoma
NI
neurogenic inflammation
nicardipine prolonged-release implant
NicErase-SL
Nichrome cylindrical electrode
Nicola
N. forceps
N. pituitary rongeur
N. rasp
N. scissors
Nicolau septineuritis
Nicolet
N. Compass EMG instrument
N. Nerve Integrity Monitor (NIM-2)
N. Pathfinder I
N. Pathfinder I recording device
N. Viking II electrophysiologic system
nicotinamide (Nam)
n. adenine dinucleotide phosphate (NADPH)
nicotine-induced seizure
nicotinic acetylcholine receptor (nAChR)
Nicotrol NS
nictitans
spasmus n.
nictitate
nictitating spasm
nictitation
nidulans
Aspergillus n.
nidus
n. avis
n. definition
n. hirundinis
n. obliteration
Niemann disease
Niemann-Pick
N.-P. disease (NPD)
N.-P. disease, type A, B, C
niente
dolce far n.
nifedipine
nifurtimox
niger
Aspergillus n.
locus n.
nucleus n.
night
n. pain
n. palsy
nighttime awakening
nigra
fetal substantia n.
substantia n. (SN)
nigrae
pars compacta substantiae n.
pars reticularis substantiae n.
rami substantiae n.
nigral TH-positve cell
nigropallidal
nigrostriatal
n. dopaminergic system
n. dopamine system
n. pathway
n. tract
nigrostriate
n. fiber
n. tract
nigrum
tapetum n.
NIHSS
National Institutes of Health Stroke Scale
Nijmegen breakage syndrome
Nikon Labophot-2 microscope
NIM-2
Nicolet Nerve Integrity Monitor
nimodipine
Nimotop capsule
nimustine
NINCDS-ADRDA
National Institute of Neurological and Communicative Disorders and Stroke

NINDS
National Institute of Neurological Disorders and Stroke
Nintendo epilepsy
ninth cranial nerve [CN IX]
niobium-titanium
Niopam
Nipah virus encephalitis
Nipride
NIR Royal Advanced stent
NIRS
near-infrared spectroscopy
Nishioka system
Nishizaki-Wakabayashi suction tube
Nissl
N. body
N. degeneration
N. granule
N. substance
nitinol hypotube
Nitoman
nitrate
butyl n.
gallium n.
nitrazepam
nitrazepam-induced hypotonia
nitric
n. acid
n. oxide
n. oxide-mediated neurotoxicity
n. oxide synthase (NOS)
nitrite
amyl n.
n. headache
nitrocellulose membrane
nitrofurantoin
n. neuropathy
n. polyneuropathy
nitrogen
blood urea n. (BUN)
n. metabolism
n. narcosis
n. wasting
nitroprusside
sodium n. (SNP)
nitrosourea hydrochloride
nitrous oxide
nizofenone
NK
natural killer
***nkx* gene**
NLS
nonlinear least square
NMDA
N. antagonist ketamine
N. receptor
N. receptor antagonist
N-methyl-4-phenyl-1,2,3,6-tetrahydropyridine
***N*-methylspiroperidol**
NMHA
National Mental Health Association
NMR
nuclear magnetic resonance
NMS
neuroleptic malignant syndrome
neuromuscular spindle
nNOS
neuronal nitric oxide synthase
No. 2
Barbidonna N.
Nocardia
N. asteroides
N. farcinica
N. nova
nocardial brain abscess
nocardiosis
central nervous system n. (CNS nocardiosis)
cerebral n.
CNS n.
central nervous system nocardiosis
nociception
nociceptive
n. impulse
n. pain
n. reflex
n. stimulation
nociceptor
n. activation
angry backfiring C n. (ABC syndrome)
C-fiber n.
cutaneous n.
irritable n.
mechanical n.
polymodal n.
primary afferent n.
nocifensor
n. reflex
nociinfluence
nociperception

NOTES

N

nocturna
chorea n.
nocturnal
n. agitation
n. awakening
n. cardiac ischemia
n. confusion
n. confusional episode
n. dyspnea
n. eating syndrome
n. enuresis
n. epilepsy
n. groaning
n. hallucination
n. hypotensive episode
n. hypoxemia
n. insomnia
n. leg cramp
n. leg jerk
n. myoclonus
n. oxygen saturation
n. pain
n. paroxysmal dystonia
n. polysomnography
n. restlessness
n. seizure
n. sleep
n. spell
n. stridor
n. vertigo
n. vocalization
n. wandering
nodding spasm
node
accessory nerve lymph n.
Babès n.
flocculonodular n.
Hensen n.
jugular chain lymph n.
local lymph n.
primitive n.
n. of Ranvier
Ranvier n.
Schmorl n.
vital n.
nodosa
periarteritis n.
polyarteritis n.
trichorrhexis n.
nodose ganglion
nodular
n. enhancement
n. headache
n. heterotopia
n. induration of temporal artery
n. mesoneuritis
n. panencephalitis
nodule
Babès n.
glial n.
iris Lisch n.
Lisch n.
mulberry-like n.
Schmorl n.
n. of vermis
nodulus, pl. **noduli**
n. cerebelli
vermal n.
n. vermis
noetic
noeud vital
noggin **gene**
NO-induced DNA degradation
noire
bete n.
noise
acoustic n.
n. condition
diagnostic n.
gaussian n.
multispeaker phonetic n.
phonetic n.
n. reduction device
noli me tangere
Nolvadex
Nomad-LE EMG
nominal
n. aphasia
n. standard dose
nonacoustic schwannoma
nonadapting receptor
nonaffective schematic mental model
non-Alzheimer frontal lobe type dementia
nonamphetamine
central nervous system stimulant, n.
nonanaplastic oligodendroglioma
nonaneurysmal perimesencephalic subarachnoid hemorrhage
non-aplastic glioma
nonautobiographical memory
nonaxial
nonbiological artifact
noncephalic electrode
noncerebral activity
nonchromaffin paraganglioma
noncommunicating hydrocephalus
noncontained disk
nonconvulsive
n. seizure
n. status epilepticus
nondampened waveform
nondecalcified trabecula

nondeclarative memory
nondepolarizing
nondepressed skull fracture
nondetachable
n. endovascular balloon
n. occlusive balloon
n. silicone balloon catheter
nondominant
hand n.
n. hemisphere
n. hemisphere lesion
n. putaminal hemorrhage
n. temporal lobectomy
nondystrophin myopathy
noneloquent area
nonembolic infarction
nonencapsulated
n. nerve ending
n. nerve glomerulus
nonenteric cyst
nonepileptic
n. event
n. myoclonic contraction
n. myoclonus
n. seizure
nonepileptiform activity
nonferromagnetic clip
nonferrous material
nonfluent aphasia
nonfocal elevation
non-fragilis
Bacteroides n.-f.
nonfunctional and repetitive motor behavior
nonfunctioning adenoma
nongerminoma malignant germ cell tumor
nonhemolytic hyperbilirubinemia
non-Hodgkin lymphoma (NHL)
nonhomonymous field defect
noninvasive
n. brain imaging study
n. carotid baroceptor stimulation
n. positive pressure ventilation
nonionic contrast agent
nonketotic
n. glycine
n. hyperglycemia
n. hyperglycemic hyperosmolar coma
n. hyperglycinemia
nonlacunar syndrome
nonlanguage cognitive impairment
nonlesional cortical resection
nonlinear
n. developmental curve
n. least square (NLS)
n. rate-response function
nonmedullated fiber
nonmeningiomatous malignant lesion
nonmicrosurgical procedure
nonmigrainous vascular headache
nonmissile head injury
nonmyelinated
nonneoplastic disease
non-neural cell
nonneuropathic
nonolfactory cortex
nonorganic aphonia
nonparalytic poliomyelitis
nonparetic eye performance
non-paretic eye valid reaction time
nonpathological dissociation
nonpenetrating trauma
nonphantom study
nonpharmacologic behavior management
nonphysiologic artifact
nonplexiform cutaneous neurofibroma
nonprogressive
n. myoclonus condition
n. neuropathy
nonproton
n. magnetic resonance imaging
n. MRI
nonpsychotic
n. Alzheimer patient
n. hallucination
n. posttraumatic brain syndrome
n. severity psychoorganic syndrome
nonpulsating headache
nonrandom rating
nonrapid
n. eye movement (NREM)
n. eye movement sleep
nonreference recording
non-REM
n.-R. narcolepsy
n.-R. sleep
nonrheumatic atrial fibrillation
nonselective expression of transgene
nonseptic embolic brain infarction
nonshivering thermogenesis

NOTES

nonsignificant protective effect
nonspastic paraparesis
nonspecific
n. encephalomyeloneuropathy
n. neuronal loss
n. neurotic factor
n. response rate
n. stimulation
n. system
nonstereotactic PET
nonsynaptic transmission
nontoxic gene expression
nonturbulence subscale
nontyphoidal salmonellosis
nonunion
n. incidence
n. rate
nonvasculitic autoimmune inflammatory meningoencephalitis
nonverbal
n. abstractive ability
n. cue
n. memory
n. synthesizing ability
n. tactile attention task
nonviral infectious disease
Noonan syndrome
noradrenergic
n. effect
n. neuron
n. system function
Norco
Norcuron
Nordstadt classification
no-reflow phenomenon
norepinephrine
peripheral n.
n. toxicity
Norland digital oscilloscope
normal
n. circuitry
n. electroencephalogram (NEEG)
n. heat defense
n. mode
n. perfusion pressure breakthrough (NPPB)
n. resting potential
n. thermogenesis
normal-frequency band
normalization principle
normalized whole brain volume
normal-pressure hydrocephalus (NPH)
Norman-Roberts syndrome
Norman-Wood syndrome
normative aspect
normocapnia
normokalemic periodic paralysis
normotensive hydrocephalus
normotonic
normoxic diffusion
norm violator
Norpace
Norpramin
Norrie disease
North
N. American Brain Tumor Consortium (NABTC)
N. American Spine Society Questionnaire
N. American Symptomatic Carotid Endarterectomy Trial (NASCET)
Northern
N. blot analysis
N. epilepsy with mental retardation
N. hybridization
N. Manhattan Stroke Study
northern
Northwick Park Index of Independence in ADL index
nortriptyline HCl
NOS
nitric oxide synthase
N. inhibitor
nose-bridge-lid reflex
nosecone
CEM handswitching n.
nose-eye reflex
nose spray test
nosocomial infection
nosotropic
notanencephalia
notch
anterior cerebellar n.
n. filter
Kernohan n.
mamilloaccessory n.
marsupial n.
posterior cerebellar n.
preoccipital n.
semilunar n.
n. of tentorium
notched appearance of spike-wave discharge
***notch* gene**
notencephalocele
Nothnagel syndrome
notochord
notochordoma
Nottingham Health Profiles
nova
Nocardia n.
Novalis shaped beam surgery
Novantrone

novel
n. memory task
n. recall task
n. stimulus
n. task performance
novo
de n.
Novo-10a CBF measuring device
Novodorm
Novopaque
Novus
N. hydrocephalic valve
N. mini valve
noxious agent
NPD
Niemann-Pick disease
NPE
neurogenic pulmonary edema
NPH
normal-pressure hydrocephalus
NPPB
normal perfusion pressure breakthrough
NPS
NeuroCybernetic Prosthesis System
NPY
neuropeptide Y
N_1 receptor
N_2 receptor
NREM
nonrapid eye movement
NRG
neureglin
NS2000 bipolar generator system
NSE
National Society for Epilepsy
neuron-specific enolase
NSN
National Spine Network
NT2 cell
NTD
neural tube defect
N-terminal signal
N-terminus
nuchal
n. dystonia
n. muscle
n. rigidity
nuchocephalic reflex
nuclear
n. agenesis
n. aplasia
n. bag
n. bag fiber
n. cerebral angiography (NCA)
n. chain
n. chain fiber
n. depression
n. envelope
n. imaging
n. jaundice
n. layer of cerebellum
n. layer of retina
n. magnetic relaxation dispersion
n. magnetic resonance (NMR)
n. magnetization vector
n. MR scan
n. ophthalmoplegia
n. psuedoinclusion
n. receptor
n. relaxation
n. signal
n. spin
n. spin quantum number
nuclei (*pl. of* nucleus)
nucleic acid metabolism
nucleocortical fiber
nucleofugal
nucleolus
subthalamic n. (STN)
nucleolysis
percutaneous laser n.
nucleon
nucleopetal
Nucleopore filter
nucleoside adenosine
nucleotide
guanine n.
Nucleotome
N. aspiration probe
N. Endoflex instrument
N. Flex II cannula instrument
N. Flex II flexible cutting probe
N. procedure
nucleotomy
laser n.
nucleus, pl. **nuclei**
abducens n.
n. of abducent nerve
nuclei accessorii nevi oculomotorii
nuclei accessorii tractus optici
n. accessorius columnae anterioris medullae spinalis

NOTES

nucleus *(continued)*
accessory basal amygdaloid n.
accessory cuneate n.
n. of accessory nerve
accessory oculomotor n.
accessory olivary n.
n. accumbens
n. accumbens septi
acoustic n.
n. of acoustic nerve
n. acusticus
aerosolized droplet n.
n. alae cinereae
almond n.
ambiguous n.
n. ambiguus
ambiguus n.
n. amygdalae
n. amygdalae basalis medialis
n. amygdalae centralis
n. amygdalae corticalis
n. amygdalae interstitialis
n. amygdalae lateralis
amygdaloid n.
n. ansae lenticularis
n. of the ansa lenticularis
anterior n.
n. anterior corporis trapezoidei
anterior dorsal n.
nuclei anteriores thalami
anterior extremity of caudate n.
n. anterior hypothalami
anterior hypothalamic n.
anterior interpositus n.
anterior olfactory n.
anterior periventricular n.
n. anterodorsalis
n. anterodorsalis thalami
anterodorsal thalamic n.
n. anteroinferior thalami
n. anterolateralis
n. anterolateralis medullae spinalis
n. anteromedialis
n. anteromedialis nervi oculomotorii
n. anteromedialis thalami
anteromedial thalamic n.
n. anterosuperior thalami
n. anteroventralis
n. anteroventralis thalami
anteroventral thalamic n.
arcuate n.
nuclei arcuati
n. arcuatus
n. arcuatus hypothalami
n. arcuatus of intermediate hypothalamic area
n. arcuatus medullae oblongatae
n. arcuatus of medulla oblongata
n. arcuatus thalami
nuclei areae H, H1, H2
auditory n.
autonomic oculomotor n.
autonomic visceral motor n.
basal n.
nuclei basales
n. basalis of Ganser
n. basalis lesion
n. basalis of Meynert
basolateral amygdaloid n.
basomedial amygdaloid n.
Bechterew n.
Blumenau n.
body of caudate n.
branchiomotor n.
bulbar n.
Burdach n.
caeruleun n.
n. of Cajal
n. campi dorsalis
n. campi medialis
nuclei campi perizonalis
n. campi ventralis
nuclei camporum perizonalium
catecholaminergic n.
nuclei of caudal colliculus
n. caudalis centralis
n. caudalis-nucleus solitarius DREZ lesioning
caudal olivary n.
caudal pontine reticular n.
caudate n.
n. caudatus
central amygdaloid n.
central caudate n.
n. centralis lateralis
n. centralis lateralis thalami
n. centralis medialis thalami
n. centralis medullae spinalis
n. centralis superior raphes
n. centralis tegmenti superior
centromedian thalamic n.
n. centromedianus
n. centromedianus thalami
cerebellar n.
nuclei cerebellares
nuclei cerebelli
n. ceruleus
cervical n.
n. cervicalis lateralis
Clarke n.
cochlear n.
nuclei cochleares
n. cochlearis anterior
n. cochlearis posterior

n. coeruleus
nuclei colliculi caudalis
nuclei colliculi inferioris
n. commissurae posterioris
n. commissuralis nevi vagi
n. commissuralis rhomboidalis
n. corporis geniculati lateralis
n. corporis geniculati medialis
nuclei corporis geniculati medialis
nuclei corporis mamillaris
n. corporis mammillaris lateralis
n. corporis mammillaris medialis
cortical amygdaloid n.
cranial motor n.
n. of cranial nerve
cranial olivary n.
cuneate n.
n. of cuneate fasciculus
n. cuneatus
n. cuneatus accessorius
n. cuneatus pars centralis
n. cuneatus pars rostralis
n. cuneatus tubercle
cuneiform n.
n. cuneiformis
n. cuneiformis mesencephalicus
n. of Darkschewitsch
deep cerebellar n.
Deiters n.
dentate n.
n. dentatus
n. dentatus cerebelli
depigmentation of noradrenergic brainstem n.
dorsal accessory olivary n.
dorsal cochlear n.
nuclei dorsales thalami
n. of dorsal field
n. dorsalis of Clarke
n. dorsalis corporis geniculati lateralis
n. dorsalis corporis geniculati medialis
n. dorsalis corporis trapezoidei
n. dorsalis hypothalami
n. dorsalis lateralis thalami
n. dorsalis nervi oculomotorii
n. dorsalis nervi vagi
n. dorsalis raphe
dorsal lateral geniculate n.
dorsal premammillary n.
dorsal raphe n.
dorsal septal n.
dorsal thoracic n.
dorsal vagal n.
dorsolateral n.
n. dorsolateralis medullae spinalis
dorsomedial hypothalamic n.
n. dorsomedialis hypothalami
n. dorsomedialis hypothalamicae intermediae
n. dorsomedialis medullae spinalis
Edinger n.
Edinger-Westphal n.
electrical stimulation of centromedian thalamic n.
emboliform n.
n. emboliformis
endolemniscal n.
n. endolemniscalis
endopeduncular n.
n. endopeduncularis
external cuneate n.
extrajunctional n.
extrapyramidal n.
n. facialis
facial motor n.
n. fasciculi gracilis
fastigial n.
n. fastigiatus
n. fastigii
n. fibrosus lingua
filiform n.
n. filiformis
force n.
n. funiculi cuneati
n. funiculi gracilis
n. gelatinosus
gelatinous n.
geniculate n.
nuclei geniculati mediales
n. geniculatus lateralis
geniculatus lateralis n.
n. gigantocellularis medullae oblongatae
globose n.
n. globosus
n. of Goll
Goll column n.
gracile n.
n. gracilis tubercle
Gudden tegmental n.

NOTES

nucleus *(continued)*
gustatory n.
n. habenula
nuclei habenulae
habenular n.
n. habenularis lateralis
n. habenularis medialis
head of caudate n.
hilum of dentate n.
hilum of inferior olivary n.
hilum of olivary n.
hypoglossal n.
n. hypoglossalis
n. of hypoglossal nerve
hypothalamic n.
n. hypothalamicus anterior
n. hypothalamicus dorsalis
n. hypothalamicus dorsomedialis
n. hypothalamicus posterior
n. hypothalamicus ventrolateralis
n. hypothalamicus ventromedialis
nuclei of inferior colliculus
n. inferior nervi trigeminalis
inferior olivary n.
inferior salivary n.
inferior salivatory n.
inferior syndrome of red n.
inferior vestibular n.
n. infundibularis
intercalated n.
n. intercalatus
intercostal nerve n.
intermediolateral n.
n. intermediolateralis
intermediomedial n.
n. intermediomedialis
n. intermediomedialis medullae spinalis
interpeduncular n.
n. interpeduncularis
interposed n.
n. interpositus
n. interpositus anterior
n. interpositus posterior
interstitial amygdaloid n.
n. interstitiales fasciculi longitudinalis medialis
nuclei interstitiales hypothalami anterioris
intracerebellar n.
intralaminar n.
nuclei intralaminares thalami
Kölliker-Fuse n.
lateral amygdaloid n.
lateral cervical n.
lateral cuneate n.
lateral dorsal tegmentum n.
lateral geniculate n. (LGN)
n. of lateral geniculate body
lateral habenular n.
n. lateralis cerebelli
n. lateralis corporis trapezoidei
n. lateralis dorsalis thalami
n. lateralis medullae oblongatae
n. lateralis posterior
n. of lateral lemniscus
lateral medullary lamina of lentiform n.
n. of lateral olfactory stria
n. of the lateral olfactory tract
lateral parabrachial n.
lateral pericuneate n.
lateral posterior n.
lateral preoptic n.
lateral pulvinar n.
lateral reticular n.
lateral septal n.
lateral superior olivary n.
lateral tuberal n.
lateral vestibular n.
laterodorsal tegmental n.
n. lemnisci lateralis
nuclei lemnisci lateralis
n. of lens
lenticular n.
lentiform n.
n. lentiformis
n. lentis
linear n.
n. linearis inferioris
n. linearis intermedius
n. linearis superior
n. of Luys
magnocellular reticular n.
magnus raphe n.
main cuneate n.
n. mamillaris lateralis
n. mamillaris medialis
n. of mamillary body
n. masticatorius
masticatory n.
medial accessory olivary n.
medial amygdaloid n.
nuclei mediales thalami
n. of medial field
medial geniculate n. (MGN)
n. of medial geniculate body
medial habenular n.
n. medialis centralis thalami
n. medialis cerebelli
n. medialis corporis trapezoidei
n. medialis magnocellularis
n. medialis magnocellularis corporis geniculati

medial magnocellular n.
medial medullary lamina of lentiform n.
medial parabrachial n.
medial pericuneate n.
medial preoptic n.
medial septal n.
medial superior olivary n.
medial terminal n. (MTN)
medial ventral n.
medial vestibular n.
median preoptic n.
median raphe n.
mediodorsal n.
n. mediodorsalis
n. medioventralis
medullary raphe n.
mesencephalic n.
n. mesencephalicus nervi trigemini
n. mesencephalicus trigeminalis
Monakow n.
motor n.
n. motorius nervi trigemini
n. motorius trigeminalis
N. 24 multichannel auditory brainstem implant
n. nervi abducentis
nuclei nervi cochlearis
n. nervi cranialis
n. nervi facialis
n. nervi glossopharyngei
n. nervi hypoglossi
n. nervi oculomotorii
n. nervi phrenici
n. nervi pudendi
nuclei nervi trigeminalis
nuclei nervi trigemini
n. nervi trochlearis
nuclei nervi vagi
nuclei nervi vestibulocochlearis
nuclei nervorum cranialium
n. niger
obscurus raphe n.
oculomotor n.
nuclei oculomotorii accessorii
nuclei oculomotorii autonomici
n. oculomotorius
n. of oculomotor nerve
n. olfactorius anterior
nuclei olivares caudales
nuclei olivares inferiores
n. olivaris
n. olivaris accessorius dorsalis
n. olivaris accessorius medialis
n. olivaris accessorius posterior
n. olivaris cranialis
n. olivaris inferior
n. olivaris principalis
n. olivaris rostralis
n. olivaris superior
n. olivaris superior lateralis
n. olivaris superior medialis
olivary n.
Onuf n.
Onufrowicz n.
oral pontine reticular n.
nuclei of origin
nuclei originis
n. originis
oval hyperchromatic n.
pallidal raphe n.
n. pallidus raphes
parabigeminal n.
n. parabigeminalis
parabrachial n.
nuclei parabrachiales
n. parabrachialis lateralis
n. parabrachialis medialis
n. paracentralis thalami
parafascicular n.
n. parafascicularis thalami
n. paragigantocellular lateralis
paralemniscal n.
n. paralemniscalis
paramedial reticular n.
paramedian n.
n. paramedianus dorsalis
n. paramedianus posterior
paranigral n.
n. paranigralis
parapeduncular n.
n. parapeduncularis
n. parasolitarius
nuclei parasympathici sacrales
n. parataenialis thalami
paraventricular n.
nuclei paraventriculares thalami
n. paraventricularis
n. paraventricularis anterior hypothalami
n. paraventricularis posterior thalami
pars magnocellularis n.

NOTES

nucleus *(continued)*
pedunculopontine tegmental n.
n. pericuneatus lateralis
n. pericuneatus medialis
perifornical n.
n. perifornicalis
perihypoglossal n.
nuclei perihypoglossales
nuclei periolivares
periolivary n.
peripeduncular n.
n. peripeduncularis
peritrigeminal n.
n. peritrigeminalis
n. periventricularis posterior
n. periventricularis ventralis
periventricular preoptic n.
n. of perizonal field
Perlia n.
phrenic motor n.
n. of phrenic nerve
n. phrenicus columnae anterioris medullae spinalis
pontine raphe n.
pontine reticular n.
n. pontinus nervi trigeminalis
n. pontis raphes
pontobulbar n.
n. pontobulbaris
postbulbar motor n.
posterior accessory olivary n.
n. of posterior commissure
nuclei posteriores thalami
n. posterior hypothalami
n. posterior hypothalamic
posterior hypothalamic n.
posterior interpositus n.
n. posterior nervi vagi
posterior periventricular n.
posterior raphe n.
n. posterior raphes
posterior thoracic n.
posterolateral n.
n. posterolateralis medullae spinalis
posteromedial n.
n. posteromedialis medullae spinales
precommissural septal n.
pregeniculate n.
n. pregeniculatus
n. premammillaris dorsalis
n. premammillaris ventralis
preoptic n.
n. preopticus lateralis
n. preopticus medialis
n. preopticus medianus
n. preopticus periventricularis
n. prepositus hypoglossi
prerubral n.
n. of prerubral field
pretectal n.
nuclei pretectales
n. principalis nervi trigemini
principal olivary n.
n. proprius
prosthetic disk n. (PDN)
n. of pudendal nerve
n. pulposus
n. pulposus disci intervertebralis
pulvinar n.
nuclei pulvinares
nuclei pulvinares thalami
pyknotic n.
n. pyramidalis
raphe n.
n. raphes magnus
n. raphes medianus
n. raphes obscurus
n. raphes pallidus
n. raphes pontis
n. raphes posterior
red n.
reticular n.
n. reticulares medullae oblongatae
nuclei reticulares mesencephali
nuclei reticulares pontis
nuclei reticulares raphes
n. reticularis intermedius gigantocellularis
n. reticularis intermedius medullae oblongatae
n. reticularis intermedius pontis inferioris
n. reticularis intermedius pontis superioris
n. reticularis lateralis medullae oblongatae
n. reticularis magnocellularis
n. reticularis paragigantocellularis
n. reticularis paramedianus
n. reticularis paramedianus precerebelli
n. reticularis parvocellularis
n. reticularis pontis caudalis
n. reticularis pontis oralis
n. reticularis pontis rostralis
n. reticularis tegmentalis pontinus
n. reticularis tegmenti pontis
n. reticularis thalami
n. reticularis trigeminalis pedunculopontinus
n. reticulatus thalami
reticulotegmental n.
n. retroambiguus
retrodorsal n.

n. retrodorsolateralis medullae spinale
retrofacial n.
n. retrofacialis
retroposterior lateral n.
retroposterolateralis n.
n. retroposterolateralis medulla spinalis
n. reuniens
rhombencephalic gustatory n.
rhomboid n.
n. robustus archistriatalis
Roller n.
roof n.
rostral interstitial n.
rostral olivary n.
n. ruber
sacral dorsal commissural n. (SDCN)
sacral parasympathetic n.
n. saguli
sagulum n.
n. salivarius inferior
n. salivarius superior
salivary n.
n. salivatorius inferior
n. salivatorius superior
salivatory n.
Schwalbe n.
Schwann n.
secondary sensory n.
n. semilunaris
n. sensorius inferior nervi trigeminalis
n. sensorius principalis nervi trigemini
n. sensorius superior nervi trigemini
sensory n.
septal n.
n. septalis lateralis
n. septalis medialis
n. septalis precommissuralis
septofimbrial n.
Siemerling n.
sole n.
nuclei solitarii
n. solitarius
n. of solitary tract
somatic motor n.
somesthetic relay n.
special visceral efferent n.
special visceral motor n.
spherical n.
n. spinalis nervi accessorii
n. spinalis nervi trigemini
spinal trigeminal n.
Spitzka n.
Staderini n.
Stilling n.
n. striae terminalis
striate n.
subcaeruleus n.
n. subceruleus
subcortical limbic n.
subcuneiform n.
n. subcuneiformis
subhypoglossal n.
n. subhypoglossalis
sublingual n.
subparabrachial n.
n. subparabrachialis
subthalamic n. (STN)
n. subthalamicus
superior central raphe n.
superior central tegmental n.
superior olivary n.
superior salivary n.
superior salivatory n.
superior vestibular n.
suprachiasmatic n.
n. suprachiasmaticus
supralemniscal n.
n. supralemniscalis
n. supramammillaris
supramammillary n.
supraoptic n.
n. supraopticus
n. supraopticus hypothalami
tail of caudate n.
tectal n.
n. tecti
nuclei tegmentales anteriores
n. tegmentalis pedunculopontinus
n. tegmentalis posterolateralis
tegmental pedunculopontine reticular n.
nuclei tegmenti
n. tegmenti pontis caudalis
n. tegmenti pontis oralis
terminal n.
nuclei terminales

NOTES

N

nucleus *(continued)*
nuclei terminationis
n. terminationis
thalamic gustatory n.
thoracic n.
n. thoracicus
n. thoracicus dorsalis
n. thoracicus posterior
n. tractus mesencephalici nervi trigeminalis
n. tractus mesencephali nervi trigemini
n. tractus olfactorii lateralis
nuclei tractus solitarii
n. tractus solitarii
n. tractus spinalis nervi trigemini
n. of trapezoid body
triangular n.
n. triangularis
nuclei triangularis septi
triangular septal n.
trigeminal mesencephalic n.
trigeminal motor n.
n. of trigeminal nerve
trochlear n.
n. of trochlear nerve
tuberal n.
nuclei tuberales
nuclei tuberales laterales
tubercle of cuneate n.
n. tuberomammillaris
tuberomammillary n.
n. vagalis dorsalis
n. of vagus nerve
vein of caudate n.
ventral anterior n.
nuclei ventrales laterales thalami
nuclei ventrales mediales thalami
nuclei ventrales thalami
n. of ventral field
ventral intermediate n. (VIM)
ventral intermediate thalamic n.
n. ventralis
n. ventralis anterior
n. ventralis anterior thalami
n. ventralis corporis geniculati lateralis
n. ventralis corporis geniculati medialis
n. ventralis corporis geniculi lateralis
n. ventralis corporis trapezoidei
n. ventralis intermedius
n. ventralis intermedius thalami
n. ventralis lateralis
n. ventralis posterior intermedius thalami
n. ventralis posterior thalami
n. ventralis posterolateralis
n. ventralis posterolateralis thalami
n. ventralis posteromedialis
n. ventralis posteromedialis thalami
ventral lateral geniculate n.
ventral posterior n.
ventral posteroinferior n.
ventral posterolateral n.
ventral posteromedial n.
ventral premammillary n.
ventral principal n.
ventral tier thalamic n.
ventrobasal n.
nuclei ventrobasales
ventrocaudal n.
n. ventro-intermedius
ventrolateral n.
n. ventrolateralis hypothalami
n. ventrolateralis medullae spinalis
ventromedial n.
ventromedial hypothalamic n.
n. ventromedialis hypothalami
n. ventromedialis medullae spinalis
vestibular n.
nuclei vestibulares
n. vestibularis caudalis
n. vestibularis inferior
n. vestibularis lateralis
n. vestibularis medialis
n. vestibularis rostralis
n. vestibularis superior
vestibulocochlear n.
nuclei viscerales nervi oculomotorii
Voit n.
Westphal n.

NuLev
null-cell adenoma
null-condition detection threshold
***null* gene**
nulling
gradient moment n.
null position nystagmus
numb
n. cheek syndrome
n. chin syndrome
number
n. of excitation
nuclear spin quantum n.
quantum n.
Reynolds n.
wave n.
number-recency measure
***numb* gene**
numbing symptom
numbness
emotional n.

facial n.
periodic hemilingual n.
waking n.
Nurolon suture
Nurrl protein
nursing home placement
nut alignment guide
nutans
chorea n.
epilepsia n.
head nodding in spasmus n.
spasmus n.
nutation
nutatory
nuthkavihak
nutraceutical
n. data
n. product
nutrient vessel
nutrition
parenteral n.
total parenteral n. (TPN)
nutritional
n. change
n. neuropathy
n. polyneuropathy
n. status
n. type cerebellar atrophy
nyctalgia
Nyegaard
Nymox urinary test
Nyquist
N. frequency
N. sampling criteria
Nyssen-van Bogaert syndrome
nystagmoid jerk
nystagmus
abduction n.
acquired n.
alternating n.
apogeotropic n.
asymmetric n.
bow-tie n.
Bruns n.
caloric n.
central n.
cerebellar n.
circular n.
coarse n.
congenital n.
conjugate n.
contralateral monocular n.
convergence-evoked n.
convergence-retraction n.
diagonal n.
dissociated n.
downbeat n.
down-moving optokinetic n.
drug-induced n.
dysjunctive n.
elliptical n.
end-gaze physiologic n.
end-point n.
n. examination
fine rapid n.
first-degree n.
fixation n.
gaze-evoked n.
gaze-paretic n.
irregular n.
jelly n.
jerk n.
jerky n.
lateral gaze n.
left-bearing n.
lid n.
miner's n.
muscle-paretic n.
null position n.
oblique n.
ocular bobbing n.
ocular dysmetria n.
ocular flutter n.
oculomasticatory myorrhythmia n.
opsoclonus n.
optokinetic n. (OKN)
palatal n.
paretic n.
paroxysmal positional n.
party n.
pendular n.
periodic alternating n. (PAN)
peripheral n.
phasic n.
positional n.
postrotational n.
railway n.
rapid n.
rebound n.
refractory convergence n.
resilient n.
retraction n.

NOTES

nystagmus *(continued)*
retraction-convergence n.
n. retractorius
reversed optokinetic n.
right-bearing n.
rotary n.
rotatory n.
second-degree n.
seesaw n. (SSN)
sensory-deprivation n.
spasmus mutans n.
spontaneous n.
third-degree continuous spontaneous n.
torsional n.
toxic n.
transient n.
true n.
unidirectional n.
upbeating n.
vertical n.
vestibular end-organ n.
voluntary n.

nystagmus-myoclonus

OAA
oxaloacetate
OBAS
Oregon Brain Aging Study
OBD
organic brain disease
obdormition
Obersteiner-Redlich
O.-R. line
O.-R. zone
Oberto mouth prop
obesity
hyperplastic-hypertrophic o.
hypertrophic o.
hypothalamic o.
o. hypoventilation syndrome
obex
O. plugging
object
o. agnosia
o. blindness
functional o.
linkage o.
metal o.
minute o.
pointed o.
primary o.
objective
o. assessment
o. measure
o. motor score
o. pulsatile tinnitus
o. sensation
o. severity
o. severity of illness
o. trauma characteristic
o. vertigo
objectivism
objectivity
oblique
o. bundle of pons
o. flow misregistration
o. gastric fiber
o. nystagmus
o. pontine fasciculus
o. sagittal gradient-echo MR imaging
o. screw insertion
o. transcorporeal approach
obliquus reflex
obliterans
thromboangiitis o.
obliterated
o. arteriovenous malformation
o. basal cistern
obliteration
cortical o.
nidus o.
transcatheter o.
obliterative
o. arachnoiditis
o. arteritis
oblongata
anterior column of medulla o.
anterior median fissure of medulla o.
dorsal median fissure of medulla o.
gigantocellular nucleus of medulla o.
gracile fasciculus of medulla o.
lateral nucleus of medulla o.
median raphe of medulla o.
medulla o.
nucleus arcuatus of medulla o.
posterior median fissure of medulla o.
posterior median sulcus of medulla o.
pyramid of medulla o.
raphe mediana medullae o.
raphe medullae o.
reticular nuclei of medulla o.
sensory decussation of medulla o.
vein of medulla o.
ventral median fissure of medulla o.
oblongatae
fasciculus gracilis medullae o.
fissura mediana anterior medullae o.
fissura mediana ventralis medullae o.
foramen caecum medullae o.
foramen cecum medullae o.
formatio reticularis medullae o.
funiculus lateralis medullae o.
funiculus posterior medullae o.
nucleus arcuatus medullae o.
nucleus gigantocellularis medullae o.
nucleus lateralis medullae o.
nucleus reticulares medullae o.
nucleus reticularis intermedius medullae o.

oblongatae *(continued)*
nucleus reticularis lateralis medullae o.
pyramis medullae o.
raphe medullae o.
sulcus anterolateralis medullae o.
sulcus dorsolateralis medullae o.
sulcus medianus dorsalis medullae o.
sulcus medianus posterior medullae o.
sulcus posterolateralis medullae o.
sulcus ventrolateralis medullae o.
tractus solitarius medullae o.
venae medullae o.
oblongatal
OBS
organic brain syndrome
obscurus
nucleus raphes o.
o. raphe nucleus
obsessional
o. compulsive inventory alpha
o. neurosis
o. Q factor
o. reaction
o. thinking
obstacle sense
obstetric
o. hand
o. palsy
o. paralysis
obstetrical
o. hand
o. paralysis
obstructing hydrocephalus
obstruction
cranial venous o.
incomplete upper airway o.
retinal venous o.
retina venous o.
upper airway o.
venous outflow o.
venular o.
obstructive
o. hydrocephalus
o. sleep apnea-hypopnea (OSAH)
o. sleep apnea-hypopnea syndrome (OSAHS)
o. sleep apnea syndrome (OSAS)
OBT
Olivier-Bertrand-Tipal
OBT stereotactic frame
obtained finding
obturans
keratosis o.
obturator
o. nerve
o. neurectomy
obturatorii
rami musculares rami anterioris nervi o.
rami musculares rami posterioris nervi o.
ramus anterior nervi o.
ramus cutaneus lateralis pectoralis nervi o.
ramus posterior nervi o.
obturatorius
nervus o.
Occip GM
occipital
o. alpha
o. artery
o. association
o. association cortical area
o. bone
o. bone jugular incisure
o. bossing
o. cortex
o. cortex damage
o. cortex tissue
o. cortical dysplasia of Taylor
o. corticectomy
o. dominant intermittent rhythmic delta activity
o. encephalocele
o. eye field
o. forceps
o. glioblastoma
o. gray matter (Occip GM)
o. groove
o. gyrus
o. headache
o. hematoma
o. horn
o. interhemispheric approach
o. intermittent rhythmic delta activity (OIRDA)
o. lesion
o. line
o. lobe
o. lobe of cerebrum
o. lobectomy
o. lobe epilepsy
o. lobe infarction
o. lobe seizure
o. lobe tumor
o. malformation
o. nerve
o. neuralgia
o. neurectomy
o. neuritis

o. neuroblastoma
o. operculum
o. pain
o. part of corpus callosum
o. plexus
o. pole
o. pole of cerebrum
o. resection
o. sinus
o. stripe
o. transtentorial
o. white matter
occipital-atlas-axis ligament
occipitalis
arteria o.
forceps o.
incisura jugularis ossis o.
lobus o.
polus o.
processus intrajugularis ossis o.
processus jugularis ossis o.
sinus o.
stria o.
occipital-supracerebellar
occipitoatlantoaxial
o. complex
o. fusion
o. instability
occipitocervical
o. arthrodesis
o. fixation
o. fusion
o. instability
o. stabilization
occipitocollicular tract
occipitofrontal fasciculus
occipitofrontalis
fasciculus o.
occipitomastoid suture
occipitonuchal region
occipitoparietal artery occlusion
occipitopontile tract
occipitopontinae
fibrae o.
occipitopontine
o. fiber
o. tract
occipitopontinus
tractus o.
occipito-subtemporal approach
occipitotectal
o. fiber
o. tract
occipitotectales
fibrae o.
occipitotemporal
o. convolution
o. cortex
o. sulcus
occipitotemporalis
ramus o.
sulcus o.
occipitothalamic radiation
occiput
flat o.
occluded sinus
occluder
Heifetz carotid o.
occlusal necrosis
occlusion
aneurysm o.
aqueductal o.
o. balloon catheter with silicone balloon
balloon test o.
branch artery o.
carotid artery o. (CAO)
chronic o.
o. coil
distal o.
dural sinus o.
endovascular balloon o.
internal carotid artery balloon test o.
intracranial o.
intraoperative balloon o.
intravascular balloon o.
luminal o.
middle cerebral artery o.
occipitoparietal artery o.
posterotemporal artery o.
pre-Rolandic artery o.
proximal balloon o.
retina arterial o.
retinal arterial o.
retinal artery o.
sinovenous o.
sinus o.
superior sagittal sinus o.
Test balloon o.
thrombotic o.

NOTES

occlusion *(continued)*
transtorcular o.
transverse sinus o.
vascular o.
ventral spinal artery o.
ventricular catheter o.
vertebral artery o.
occlusion/stenosis
occlusive
o. cerebrovascular disease
o. hyperemia
o. meningitis
occulomotor pathway
occult
o. cerebrovascular malformation (OCVM)
o. frontal focus
o. hydrocephalus
o. spinal dysraphism
occulta
spina bifida o.
occultum
cranium bifidum o.
occupancy
D_2 o.
preferential o.
receptor o.
occupation
ligand o.
occupational
o. neuropathy
o. neurotic disorder
o. spasm
o. therapy
ochronosis
octapeptide
cholecystokinin o. (CCK-8)
octapolar lead
octavi
pars cochlearis nevi o.
pars vestibularis nervi o.
octavus
nervus o. [CN VIII]
octopus visual field analyzer
OctreoScan scanner
octreotide
intrathecal o.
ocular
o. alignment
o. bobbing
o. bobbing nystagmus
o. cup
o. deviation
o. dipping
o. dyskinesia
o. dysmetria
o. dysmetria nystagmus
o. flutter
o. flutter nystagmus
o. hypotony
o. ischemic syndrome
o. lesion
o. malalignment
o. metastasis
o. motility
o. motility examination
o. motor apraxia
o. motor ataxia
o. motor disturbance
o. motor syndrome
o. muscle
o. myoclonus
o. pain
o. paralysis
o. photoreceptor
o. pneumoplethysmography
o. pseudomyasthenia
o. pulse
o. tilt reaction
o. torticollis
o. vertigo
o. vesicle
oculi
pars orbitalis musculi orbicularis o.
tapetum o.
Oculinum
oculoauricular reflex
oculocephalic
o. reflex
o. test
oculocephalogyric
o. crisis
o. reflex
oculocerebrorenal syndrome
oculocerebrovasculometry
oculocraniosomatic disease
oculoencephalic angiomatosis
oculogastrointestinal muscular dystrophy
oculographic artifact
oculogyric crisis
oculomasticatory
o. myorhythmia
o. myorrhythmia nystagmus
oculomotor
o. abnormality
o. nerve [CN III]
o. nerve examination
o. nerve paralysis
o. nerve paresis
o. neuropathy
o. nuclear complex
o. nucleus
o. nucleus raphes
o. ptosis

o. reflex
o. response
o. root of ciliary ganglion
o. sulcus
o. sulcus of mesencephalon
o. system
o. trigone
oculomotorii
nuclei accessorii nevi o.
nuclei viscerales nervi o.
nucleus anteromedialis nervi o.
nucleus dorsalis nervi o.
nucleus nervi o.
ramus inferior nervi o.
ramus superior nervi o.
sulcus nervi o.
oculomotorius
nervus o. [CN III]
nucleus o.
sulcus o.
oculopalatal myoclonus
oculopharyngeal
o. muscular dystrophy (OPMD)
o. syndrome
oculoplethysmography
oculorespiratory reflex
oculospinal
oculosympathetic
o. dysfunction
o. ptosis
oculovestibular reflex
OCVM
occult cerebrovascular malformation
odaxesmus
Odense Pharmacoepidemiological Database (OPED)
Oden syndrome
ODI
oxygen desaturation index
ODN
oligodeoxynucleotide
odogenesis
odonterism
odontoblast
odontogenic infection
odontoid
o. dysplasia
o. fracture
o. fracture internal fixation
o. fracture stabilization
o. process
o. process osteosynthesis
o. process resection
odontoideum
os o.
odontoneuralgia
odorant receptor (OR)
OEC-Diasonics mobile C-arm image intensifier
Oenothera biennis
oesophagealis
plexus o.
oesophageus
plexus o.
Office of Neuroinformatics (ONI)
officinalis
Melissa o.
off-period dystonia
offset frequency
Ogura operation
6-OHDA
6-hydroxydopamine
ohm
OI
osteogenesis imperfecta
oil
brominized o.
ethiodized o.
evening primrose o. (EPO)
iodized o.
Lorenzo o.
OIRDA
occipital intermittent rhythmic delta activity
OIRDA on electroencephalogram
Ojemann cortical stimulator
okadaic acid
OKAN
optokinetic afternystagmus
Oklahoma tick fever virus
OKN
optokinetic nystagmus
OKS
optokinetic stimulation
OKT3
OKT3 monoclonal antibody
OKT3 uremic
olanzapine
olanzapine-associated DKA
OLC
oligodendrocyte-like cell

NOTES

old
o. nerve injury
oldest o.
Oldberg
O. brain retractor
O. dissector
O. intervertebral disk rongeur
O. pituitary forceps
O. pituitary rongeur
oldest old
old-old patient
old-sergeant syndrome
olecranon reflex
olfactant
olfaction
olfactology
olfactometer
olfactometry
olfactoria
fila o.
hyperesthesia o.
idiosyncrasia o.
olfactoriae
striae o.
olfactorii
nervi o.
vena gyri o.
olfactorium
organum o.
trigonum o.
tuberculum o.
olfactorius
bulbus o.
nervus o. [CN I]
sulcus o.
tractus o.
olfactory
o. amnesia
o. anesthesia
o. area
o. aura
o. axonal growth
o. brain
o. bulb
o. bundle
o. coefficient
o. cortex
o. cranial nerve
o. deficit
o. epithelium
o. esthesioneuroblastoma
o. filum
o. glomerulus
o. groove
o. groove meningioma
o. gyrus
o. hair
o. hallucination
o. hyperesthesia
o. hypesthesia
o. knob
o. lobe
o. nerve examination
o. nerve layer
o. neuroblastoma
o. organ
o. pathway
o. peduncle
o. pyramid
o. receptor
o. receptor cell
o. rod
o. root
o. sensory neuron (OSN)
o. sheathing cell
o. stria
o. sulcus
o. system
o. tract
o. trigone
o. tubercle
o. vestibule
olfactus
organum o.
oligemia
oligemic
oligoastrocytoma
oligoblast
oligoclonal band
oligodendria
oligodendroblast
oligodendroblastoma
oligodendrocyte
o. lineage cell
o. progenitor (OP)
o. progenitor recruitment
oligodendrocyte-like cell (OLC)
oligodendroglia cell
oligodendroglioma
anaplastic o.
nonanaplastic o.
pleomorphic o.
supratentorial o.
oligodeoxynucleotide (ODN)
oligoglia
oligonucleotide
antisense o.
oligopeptidase
brain prolyl o.
prolyl o.
oligosaccharide chain
oligosynaptic
Oliphant

olisbos
oliva, pl. **olivae**
o. inferior
siliqua olivae
o. superior
olivare
amiculum o.
corpus o.
olivaris
hilum nuclei o.
nucleus o.
olivarum
commissura o.
olivary
o. body
o. degeneration
o. eminence
o. nucleus
olive
accessory o.
inferior o.
superior o.
Olivecrona
O. aneurysm clamp
O. brain spatula
O. clip
O. clip applier
O. dura dissector
O. dura scissors
O. rasp
O. rongeur
O. trigeminal knife
O. trigeminal scissors
O. wire saw
Olivecrona-Gigli saw
Olivecrona-Toennis clip-applying forceps
Olivier-Bertrand-Talairach stereotactic head frame
Olivier-Bertrand-Tipal (OBT)
O.-B.-T. frame
olivifugal
olivipetal
olivocerebellar
o. fiber
o. tract
olivocerebellaris
tractus o.
olivocochlear
o. bundle
o. bundle of Rasmussen
o. tract
olivocochlearis
tractus o.
olivopontocerebellar
o. atrophy
o. degeneration
olivospinal
o. fiber
o. tract
olivospinales
fibrae o.
Ollier disease
Olmsted County Study
3-O-MD
3-O-methyldopa
omego melancholium
Omersch-Woltman syndrome
3-O-methyldopa (3-O-MD)
Ommaya
O. reservoir
O. ventriculoperitoneal shunt
Omni
O. clip gun
O. 2 microscope
Omnipaque
omnipresent dysphoria
Omniscan
Omni-Vent
omohyoid muscle
omphalocele-exstrophy-imperforate anus-spinal defects complex
OMS
opsoclonus-myoclonus syndrome
oncocytoma
oncogene
ras o.
oncolytic virus
oncoprotein
c-erbB-2-encoded o.
OncoRad OV103
OncoScint
O. CR/OV
O. OV103
O. PR
OncoTrac
Oncovin
ondansetron
Ondine curse
one
Neurostation O.
one-and-a-half syndrome

NOTES

oneiric, oniric
o. hyperesthesia
oneirique
delire o.
oneiroid
oneironanalysis
one-sided chorea
one-way flow mechanism
ongoing
o. cognitive process
o. neuroleptic treatment
ONI
Office of Neuroinformatics
onion
o. bulb change
o. bulb formation
o. bulb neuropathy
onion-skin distribution
oniric (*var. of* oneiric)
ONL
outer nuclear layer
on-off
o.-o. effect of L-dopa
o.-o. flushing reservoir
o.-o. motor fluctuation
o.-o. phenomenon
on-period dystonia
ONSD
optic nerve sheath decompression
onset
wake after sleep o. (WASO)
ontogenic process
ontogeny
Onuf nucleus
Onufrowicz nucleus
ONYX-015 virus
Onyx liquid embolic agent
oophagia
Oort
bundle of O.
OP
oligodendrocyte progenitor
opalgia
Opalski cell
OPED
Odense Pharmacoepidemiological Database
open
o. angiography
o. C-D hook
o. clam-shell MRI
o. cordotomy
o. door laminoplasty
o. exit foramen
o. head injury
o. loop reflex
o. magnet
o. skull fracture
o. stereotactic craniotomy
opening
o. of aqueduct of midbrain
o. of cerebral aqueduct
o. pressure
open-label trial
open-mouthed anteroposterior tomogram
operant
tact o.
operating
O. Arm stereotactic navigator
o. microscope VM 900
operation
aneurysmal clipping o.
Ball o.
Brooks-Gallie cervical o.
Brooks-Jenkins cervical o.
cingulate o.
Cloward o.
concrete o.
Cotte o.
Dana o.
Dandy o.
decompression o.
floating-forehead o.
Frazier-Spiller o.
Gardner o.
Hartley-Krause o.
Horsley o.
Hunter o.
Keen o.
Killian o.
Koerte-Ballance o.
Körte-Balance o.
Krause o.
Leriche o.
Matas o.
Mikulicz o.
Ogura o.
Schloffer o.
Smith-Robinson o.
stereotactic o.
Stoffel o.
Stookey-Scarff o.
synchrocyclotron o.
tongue-in-groove o.
Torkildsen o.
O. Versus Aspirin study
operative
o. microscope
o. trajectory
o. wedge frame
opercula (*pl. of* operculum)
opercular
o. cortex

o. epilepsy
o. part
opercularis
pars o.
operculi
operculum, pl. **opercula**
frontal o.
o. frontale
frontoparietal o.
o. frontoparietale
insula o.
medial o.
occipital o.
parietal o.
o. parietale
sylvian o.
temporal o.
o. temporale
O-PET technique
OPG
osteoprotegerin
ophiophobia
ophresiophobia
ophryosis
ophthalmencephalon
ophthalmia
neuroparalytic o.
ophthalmic
o. artery
o. artery aneurysm
o. disorder
o. migraine
o. neurosyphilis
o. plexus
o. recurrent nerve
o. segment
o. segment aneurysm
o. system
o. vein
o. vesicle
zoster o.
o. zoster
o. zoster infection
ophthalmica
vesicula o.
zona o.
ophthalmici
ramus meningeus recurrens nervi o.
ramus tentorii nervi o.
ophthalmicus
caliculus o.
herpes zoster o.
nervus o.
ophthalmodynamometer
Bailliart o.
compression o.
ophthalmodynamometry
suction o.
ophthalmologic examination
ophthalmoneuritis
ophthalmoneuromyelitis
ophthalmoparesis
progressive external o.
ophthalmopathy
Graves o.
ophthalmoplegia
chronic progressive external o. (CPEO)
o. externa
fascicular o.
infectious o.
o. interna
internal o.
internuclear o. (INO)
o. internuclearis
intranuclear o.
nuclear o.
orbital o.
o. and paralysis
Parinaud o.
o. partialis
o. plus
o. progressiva
progressive external o. (PEO)
pseudointernuclear o.
supranuclear o.
o. totalis
ophthalmoplegic migraine
ophthalmoplethysmography
ophthalmoscopy
opiate receptor
opioid
o. peptide
o. peptide in seizure
o. poisoning
o. precursor protein
opioid-dependent patient
opiophagorum
tremor o.
opisthion
opisthoporeia
opisthotonic

NOTES

opisthotonoid
opisthotonos, opisthotonus
o. position
OPLL
ossification of the posterior longitudinal ligament
OPMD
oculopharyngeal muscular dystrophy
OPMI
OPMI microscopic drape
OPMI surgical microscope
OPMI Vario/NC 33 system
Oppenheim
O. disease
O. reflex
O. sign
O. syndrome
opportunistic infection
opprobrium
OPSI
orthogonal polarized spectral imaging
opsialgia
OpSite dressing
opsoclonia
opsoclonus
myoclonic o.
o. nystagmus
opsoclonus-myoclonus syndrome (OMS)
OPTAx system
optic
o. agnosia
o. aphasia
o. ataxia
o. canal
o. chiasm
o. chiasmal syndrome
o. chiasm compression
o. chiasm tumor
o. cup
o. decussation
o. disk
o. disk edema with a macular star
o. disk pallor
o. disk swelling
o. fissure
o. layer
o. lobe
o. nerve astrocytoma
o. nerve atrophy
o. nerve [CN II]
o. nerve examination
o. nerve glioma
o. nerve hypoplasia
o. nerve infarction
o. nerve injury
o. nerve lesion
o. nerve sheath decompression (ONSD)
o. nerve sheath hematoma
o. nerve sheath meningioma
o. neuritis
o. neuropathy
o. part of retina
o. pathway glioma
o. pathway tumor
o. radiation
o. recess
o. tectum
o. thalamus
o. tract
o. tract compression
o. tract syndrome
o. vesicle
optica
hyperesthesia o.
neuromyelitis o.
radiatio o.
optical
o. alexia
o. densitometry
o. device
o. digitizer
o. image guided surgery system with dynamic referencing
o. righting reflex
o. shingle
o. system
optici
circulus vasculosus nervi o.
nuclei accessorii tractus o.
pars canalis nervi o.
pars intracanalicularis nervi o.
pars intracranialis nervi o.
pars intraocularis nervi o.
pars orbitalis nervi o.
radix lateralis tractus o.
radix medialis tractus o.
rami tractus o.
stratum ganglionare nervi o.
vaginae nervi o.
vagina externa nervi o.
vagina interna nervi o.
opticocarotid triangle
opticocerebral syndrome
opticochiasmatic cistern
opticociliary
opticofacial reflex
opticokinetic (*var. of* optokinetic)
opticopyramidal syndrome
opticostriate region
opticum
brachium o.

chiasma o.
stratum o.
opticus
nervus o. [CN II]
recessus o.
tractus o.
optimal
o. group size
o. treatment strategy
Optiray
optochiasmic
optokinetic, opticokinetic
o. afternystagmus (OKAN)
o. disorder
o. nystagmus (OKN)
o. reflex dysfunction
o. stimulation (OKS)
Optotrak motion and position measurement system
OR
odorant receptor
Orabilex
Oragrafin
oral
o. administered drug
o. administration
o. alimentary automatism
o. antiviral agent
o. appliance
o. appliance therapy
o. apraxia
o. atresia
o. bovine myelin
Calciferol O.
o. cavity
o. contraceptive-induced chorea
o. corticosteroid
Cytoxan O.
Dormarex O.
o. dose
Drisdol O.
o. dyskinesia
o. hemangioma
o. herpes lesion
o. intubation
Mephyton O.
o. pontine reticular nucleus
o. progesterone
o. retraction
o. supplementation
o. ulceration
VitaCarn O.
oral-biting period
oral-buccal-lingual dyskinesia
oral-facial-digital syndrome
oralis
nucleus reticularis pontis o.
nucleus tegmenti pontis o.
Oramorph
Orap
Orascoptic
O. fiberoptic headlight
O. loupe extension
Oravue
Orbeli effect
orbicularis
o. oculi reflex
o. orbis muscle
o. oris muscle
o. pupillary reflex
sign of the o.
o. sign
orbicular oculi muscle
Orbis-Sigma cerebrospinal fluid shunt valve
orbital
o. apex syndrome
o. blood flow
o. cephalocele
o. chemosis
o. decompression
o. disease
o. dystopia
o. encephalocele
o. floor fracture
o. floor syndrome
o. granulocytic sarcoma
o. hypertelorism
o. myositis
o. neurofibroma
o. ophthalmoplegia
o. optic neuritis
o. part
o. part of inferior frontal gyrus
o. plate
o. prefrontal cortex
o. pseudotumor
o. region
o. solitary fibrous tumor
o. sulcus
o. varix

NOTES

orbital *(continued)*
o. vein
o. venous approach
o. zygomatic craniotomy
orbitales
gyri o.
sulci o.
orbitalis
pars o.
orbitofrontal
o. activity
o. approach
o. area
o. cortex
o. epilepsy
o. syndrome
orbitomedial/cingulate lesion
orbitopathy
thyroid o.
orbitotomy
orbitozygomatic
o. mandibular osteotomy
o. temporopolar approach
orbivirus
Oregon Brain Aging Study (OBAS)
organ
annulospiral o.
auditory o.
Bidder o.
circumventricular o.
Corti o.
effector o.
encapsulated end o.
end o.
Golgi tendon o. (GTO)
gustatory o.
intromittent o.
o. jargon
lateral line o.
neurotendinous o.
olfactory o.
parapineal o.
parietal o.
reinnervation of target o.
Ruffini o.
sense o.
sensory o.
o. of smell
o. of special sense
spiral o.
statoacoustic o.
subcommissural o.
subfornical o.
tactile o.
o. of taste
terminal o.
o. of touch
o. transplantation
vestibular o.
vestibulocochlear o.
o. of vision
visual o.
vomeronasal o.
o. of Zuckerkandl
organa (*pl. of* organum)
organelle
cellular o.
cytoplasmic o.
organic
o. acidemia
o. aciduria
o. affective syndrome
o. amnesia
o. amnestic syndrome
o. anxiety disorder
o. brain disease (OBD)
o. brain disorder
o. brain syndrome (OBS)
o. contracture
o. delusional disorder
o. delusional syndrome
o. drivenness
o. dysfunction
o. etiology
o. hallucinosis syndrome
o. headache
o. mental disorder
o. mental syndrome
o. mood disorder
o. mood syndrome
multiple sclerosis-type o.
o. pain
o. personality disorder
o. psychiatric disorder
o. solvent
o. vertigo
organism
causative o.
cryptococcal o.
o. embolus
organismic
organism-specific antibody index
organization
cortical o.
memory o.
World Health O. (WHO)
organizer
o. gene
Spemann o.
organoleptic
organophosphate pesticide poisoning
organophosphorus insecticide poisoning
organum, pl. **organa**
o. auditus

o. gustatorium
o. gustus
o. olfactorium
o. olfactus
organa sensoria
organa sensuum
o. spirale
o. subcommissurale
o. subfornicale
o. tactus
o. vasculosum
o. vasculosum laminae terminalis
o. vasculosum of lamina terminalis
o. vestibulocochleare
o. visus

Orgaran
Orgogozo score for neurological deficit
oriens
o. layer
o. layer of hippocampus
stratum o.

orientation
body spatial o.
coronal o.
ideological o.
reverse o.
sagittal o.
theoretical o.
transverse o.
whole focus o.

oriented
alert and o. (AAO)
o. and alert
o. in all spheres
awake, alert, and o.

orienting
o. reflex
o. response

origin
anomalous o.
apparent o.
deep o.
ectal o.
ental o.
intrapsychic o.
nuclei of o.
psychodynamic o.
psychogenic o.
real o.
Schwann cell o.
superficial o.
o. of violence

originis
nuclei o.
nucleus o.

Orinase
ORION anterior cervical plate
ornithine
o. decarboxylase
o. transcarbamoylase
o. transcarbamylase
o. transcarbamylase deficiency (OTCD)

ornithine-ketoacid
o.-k. aminotransferase
o.-k. aminotransferase deficiency

ornithinemia
ornithosis lymphocytic meningitis
orolingual-buccal dyskinesia
oromandibular dystonia
oromotor dyspraxia
oropharyngeal
o. airway space
o. dystonia
o. reflex

orotic acid urine level
Orozco cervical plate
orphan
enteric cytopathic human o. (ECHO)
o. train

orphenadrine
Orpington Prognosis Scale
Orthawear antiembolism stockings
orthochorea
orthodox sleep
orthodromic
orthodromically
Orthofix Cervical-Stim stimulator
orthogenics
orthognathic
orthogonal
o. angiography
o. combination
o. depression factor
o. film
o. laser
o. polarized spectral imaging (OPSI)
o. square Helmholtz coil
o. x-ray

NOTES

orthograde degeneration
orthographic process
orthomyxovirus infection
orthosis, pl. **orthoses**
cervicothoracic o.
CranioCap custom-made cranial o.
Flex Foam o.
Malibu o.
postoperative lumbosacral o.
thoracolumbar standing o.
thoracolumbosacral o.
orthostatic
o. edema
o. epileptoid
o. fluctuation
o. hypertension
o. hypotension
o. stability
o. syncope
o. tremor
orthosympathetic
orthotonos, orthotonus
o. position
orthriogenesis
os
os odontoideum
os priapi
OSAH
obstructive sleep apnea-hypopnea
OSAHS
obstructive sleep apnea-hypopnea syndrome
Osaka telesensor
OSAS
obstructive sleep apnea syndrome
Osborn band
Os-Cal 500
oscillating microsaw
oscillation
high-frequency o.
oscillatory brain activity
oscillopsia
oscilloscope
Norland digital o.
Tektronix 2214 o.
OSI modular table system
Osler-Rendu-Weber syndrome
Osler-Weber-Rendu arteriovenous malformation
osmatic
osmesis
osmesthesia
osmicate
osmics
osmoceptor
osmoles
idiogenic o.
osmology
osmophobia
osmophore group
osmoreceptor
osmosis
osmotherapy
osmotic
o. demyelination
o. demyelination syndrome
o. mechanism
OSN
olfactory sensory neuron
osphresiology
osphretic
OssaTron device
ossea
crura o.
leontiasis o.
ossicle
Tutoplast auditory o.
ossificans
fibrodysplasia o.
meningitis o.
myositis o.
neuritis o.
ossification
heterotopic o.
o. of the posterior longitudinal ligament (OPLL)
ossifying
o. arachnoiditis
o. fibroma
osteitis deformans
osteoblastoma
Osteocalcin Injection
osteochondroma
osteochondrosis
intervertebral o.
osteoclastic
osteodiastasis
osteogenesis imperfecta (OI)
osteogenic sarcoma
osteoid osteoma
osteolysis
osteoma
choroidal o.
osteoid o.
osteomalacia
Osteomed
osteomyelitis
cranial o.
pyogenic o.
spinal o.
osteonecrosis
syphilitic o.
osteopathic scoliosis

osteopetrosis
cranial o.
osteophyte formation
osteoplastic
o. bone flap
o. craniotomy
o. laminectomy
osteoporosis
o. circumscripta
o. circumscripta cranii
disuse o.
glucocorticoid-induced o.
posttraumatic o.
steroid-induced o.
o. with vertebral collapse and neurologic deficit
osteoporotic spine
osteoprotegerin (OPG)
osteoradionecrosis
osteosarcoma
osteosclerosis
myelofibrosis o.
osteosclerotic myeloma
OsteoSet
osteosynthesis
anterior column o.
cranial o.
facial o.
lumbar spine vertebral o.
odontoid process o.
plate-screw o.
posterior column o.
thoracic spine vertebral o.
thoracolumbar spine vertebral o.
vertebral o.
wire o.
osteotome
Cherry o.
Cloward spinal fusion o.
osteotomy
craniofacial o.
ethmoidal o.
frontonasomaxillary o.
frontoorbital o.
glabellar exposure o.
LeFort o.
mandibular o.
maxillary o.
orbitozygomatic mandibular o.
Tessier o.
ostium tympanicum tubae auditivae
OSV II Smart Valve system
Oswestry
O. Low Back Pain Disability Questionnaire
O. score
otalgia
geniculate o.
tabetic o.
OTCD
ornithine transcarbamylase deficiency
otic
o. abscess
o. capsule
o. ganglion
o. hydrocephalus
o. neuralgia
otici
radix parasympathica ganglii o.
radix sensoria ganglii o.
oticum
ganglion o.
rami ganglionares nervi maxillaris ad ganglion o.
oticus
herpes zoster o.
otitic
o. abscess
o. hydrocephalus
o. meningitis
otitis
malignant external o.
o. media
otocerebritis
otoconial plug
otocyst
otoencephalitis
otoganglion
otogeny
otologic implant
otoneuralgia
otoneurology
otorhinorrhea
otorrhea
cerebrospinal fluid o.
otosclerosis
Ototome irrigation kit
ototoxic
ototoxicity
***otx* gene**
Ouchterlony double diffusion technique

outcome
o. assessment
global o.
o. of illness
o. measure
multidimensional assessment of o.
overall management o.
premature infant neurodevelopmental o.
primary efficacy o.
psychosocial symptom o.
seizure-free o.
o. study
therapeutic o.
treatment o.
outer
o. band of Baillarger
o. cone fiber
o. limiting layer
o. line of Baillarger
o. mesaxon of the myelin sheath
o. nuclear layer (ONL)
o. plexiform layer
o. sheath of optic nerve
outgrowth
chemoattractant axonal o.
neurite o.
outlet
o. syndrome
thoracic o.
out-of-phase
o.-o.-p. image
o.-o.-p. waveform
output
cortical motor o.
sympathetic o.
outside-in signaling
outward focus
OV103
OncoRad O.
OncoScint O.
ovabain-like compound
oval
o. area of Flechsig
o. corpuscle
o. fasciculus
o. hyperchromatic nucleus
ovale
centrum o.
foramen o.
patent foramen o.
white matter of the centrum o.
ovalis
fossa o.
ovarian
o. androgen secretion
o. function
overabstract speech
overall
o. cognitive functioning
o. cognitive measure
o. disability
o. management outcome
o. risk index
o. survival
overconcern with sleep
overdrainage syndrome
overflow
motor o.
receiver o.
overfocusing disorder
overgrowth
neurite o.
overhang
bony o.
overlapping agitation
overlap syndrome in polymyositis
overload
receiver o.
sensory o.
overrepresented
over-right hypertropia
oversecretion
hydrocephalus o.
overshooting
saccadic o.
overt
o. agitation
o. hallucination
o. weeping
Overtime tablet
overuse phenomenon
OVM
postirradiation O.
ovoid
myelin o.
Owen gauze dressing
Owsley acid
oxacillin
oxalate
escitalopram o.
o. pryoantimonate technique
oxalic acid urine level
oxaloacetate (OAA)
oxandrole
oxazepam
OXC
oxcarbazepine
oxcarbazepine (OXC)
oxidant
endogenous o.
oxidase
cytochrome c o.
xanthine o.

oxidation
alpha-ketoglutarate o.
fatty acid o.
pyruvate o.
o. state
oxidative
o. cellular injury
o. degeneration
o. phosphorylation
o. stress
o. stress signaling
oxide
exogenous nitric o. (GSNO)
magnesium o.
nitric o.
nitrous o.
superparamagnetic iron o.
oxidized
o. cotton
o. regenerated cellulose
oxidronate
technetium 99m o.
oxime
hexamethylpropyleneamine o. (HMPAO)
^{99m}Tc-hexamethylpropyleneamine o.
oximeter
INVOS transcranial cerebral o.
pulse o.
Somanetics INVOS 3100 cerebral o.
oximetry
continuous venous o.
pulse o.
oxolinic acid
oxoprolinuria
oxyacoia
oxyaphia
oxybarbiturate
oxybutynin chloride
Oxycel
oxycellulose
oxycephalia
oxycephalic
oxycephalous
oxycephaly
oxychlorosene
oxyecoia
oxyesthesia
oxygen
cerebral metabolic rate of o. ($CMRO_2$)
o. desaturation index (ODI)
o. extraction fraction (EOF)
o. free radical
hyperbaric o. (HBO)
o. inhalation
partial venous gas tension of o.
o. radical attack
o. radical-induced cellular injury
regional cerebral metabolic rate of o.
saturation of o. (SaO2)
o. tension
o. therapy
oxygenation
cerebral hemodynamics and o.
extracorporeal membrane o.
neonatal extracorporal membrane o.
oxygeusia
oxylate
sodium o.
oxymetazoline nasal spray
oxyosmia
oxyosphresia
oxyphenbutazone
oxyphencyclimine hydrochloride
oxytocin

NOTES

1p
chromosome 1p
6p
chromosome 6p
p170 glycoprotein
P3 probe
p53 gene
PA
plasminogen activator
presenilin
tissue-type PA
urokinase-type PA
Pabenol
pacchionian
p. body
p. corpuscle
p. foramen
p. gland
p. granulation
Pacchioni foramen
Paced Auditory Serial Addition Test
pacemaker
circadian p.
Pace ventricular needle
Pachon test
pachydermatocele
pachygyria
pachyleptomeningitis
pachymeninges
pachymeningitis
p. cranialis hypertrophica
p. externa
hemorrhagic p.
hypertrophic cervical p.
hypertrophic chromic p. (HCP)
hypertrophic cranial p.
idiopathic hypertrophic cranial p.
idiopathic intracranial p.
p. interna
intracranial p.
p. intralamellaris
meningeal p.
purulent p.
pyogenic p.
spinal p.
syphilitic cerebral hypertrophic p.
pachymeningopathy
pachymeninx
pacinian
p. corpuscle
p. mechanoreceptor
Pacini corpuscle
packer
Woodson dura p.
packing
Avitene p.
endosaccular p.
Vaseline gauze p.
paclitaxel
PAD
primary afferent depolarization
pad
cotton p.
Gelfoam p.
parapharyngeal fat p.
pharyngeal fat p.
paddies
cotton p.
Padgett baseline pinch gauge
PAE
pediatric and adolescent epilepsy
PAF
platelet-activating factor
Paget disease
paidology
pain
p. asymbolia
atypical facial p.
back p.
bone p.
brain central p.
causalgic p.
central post-stroke p.
chronic intractable p.
core p.
deafferentation p.
deliberate infliction of p.
dermatome p.
diabetic neuropathy neuralgia p.
p. disorder
effected p.
end-zone p.
extraterritorial spontaneous p.
eye p.
facial p.
faciocephalic p.
functional p.
gate control theory of p.
girdle p.
Goody's Body P.
hemicranial p.
heterotopic p.
homotopic p.
ice pick p.
ice pick-like p.
inescapable p.
p. intensity threshold
intractable p.

pain *(continued)*
lancinating p.
law of referred p.
leg p.
level of psychological p.
low back p. (LBP)
lumbar puncture p.
masking p.
p. modulation
muscle p.
myofascial p.
neck p.
nerve p.
neuropathic p.
night p.
nociceptive p.
nocturnal p.
occipital p.
ocular p.
organic p.
paroxysmal evoked p.
P. Patient Profile
P. Perception Profile
peripheral deafferentation p.
phantom limb p.
phantom tooth p.
physical p.
posttraumatic p.
psychogenic chest p.
psychogenic pelvic p.
psychogenic precordial p.
radicular distribution of p.
p. reaction
recurrent p.
referred p.
rest p.
retroorbital p.
root p.
sciatic p.
p. sense
short-lasting unilateral neuralgiform p.
skin graft harvesting p.
somatic p.
somatoform p.
spinal cord p.
p. spot
tabetic p.
tactile p.
p. and temperature pathway
terebrating p.
thalamic p.
p. threshold reduction
p. transduction
unilateral p.
venipuncture p.
visceral p.
viscerogenic referred p.

PainBuster infusion pump management kit
Paine retinaculatome
painful
p. anesthesia
p. leg and moving fingers syndrome
p. leg and moving toes syndrome
p. paraplegia

painless aura
pain-sensitive vessel
pair
coherent negative picture-caption p.
coherent positive picture-caption p.
control picture-caption p.
Maxwell p.
negative picture-caption p.
picture-caption p.
positive picture-caption p.
reference picture-caption p.

paired
p. electrode recording
p. gene
p. helical filament

paired-pulse inhibition
palatal
p. lift prosthesis
p. mucosal eruption
p. mucosal incision
p. myoclonus
p. nystagmus
p. paresis
p. reflex
p. split
p. surgery
p. syndrome

palatine nerve
palatini
nervi p.
nervus musculi tensoris veli p.
tensor veli p.

palatinum
velum p.

palatoglossus muscle
palatooccipital line
palatoocular myoclonus
palatopharyngeal
p. flap
p. paralysis of Avellis

palatopharyngeus muscle
palatopharyngoplasty
palatoplasty
laser-assisted p.
radiofrequency p.

palatoplegia

paleencephalon
paleocerebellar
paleocerebellum
paleocortex
paleokinetic
paleologic thinking
paleophrenia
paleopsychic
paleostriatal syndrome
paleostriatum
paleothalamus
paligraphia
palikinesia, palicinesia
palilalia
palilexia
palilogia
palindrome
palindromic encephalopathy
palingnosticum
  delirium p.
palinlexia
palinopia
palinopsia
palinoptic hallucination
palinphrasia, paliphrasia
pallanesthesia
pallesthesia
pallesthetic sensibility
pallidal
  p. atrophy
  p. degeneration
  p. lesion
  p. raphe nucleus
  p. syndrome
pallidectomy
pallidi
  rami globi p.
pallidoamygdalotomy
pallidoansection
pallidoansotomy
pallidofugal
pallidostriatal feedback loop
pallidotomy
  Leksell posteroventral p.
  posteroventral p.
  stereotactic p.
  ventroposterior medial p.
  ventroposterolateral p.
  VPL p.
pallidum
  dorsal p.
  p. dorsale
  p. I, II
  posteroventral sensorimotor p.
  Treponema p.
  ventral p.
  p. ventrale
pallidus
  globus p.
  nucleus raphes p.
  ventral globus p.
pallii
  impressio petrosa p.
Pallister-Hall syndrome
Pallister-Killian syndrome
pallium
  petrosal impression of the p.
pallor
  optic disk p.
palmar
  p. crease
  P. cutaneous temperature monitor
  p. hyperhidrosis
  p. reflex
Palmaz-Schatz stent
Palmaz stent
palm-chin reflex
palmi
palmic
palmitate
palmitic acid
palmitoyl acyl-CoA
palmitoylation
palmitoyltransferase
  carnitine p.
palmodic
palmomental
  p. reflex
  p. test
palmus
palpatometry
palsy
  abducens nerve p.
  American Academy of Cerebral P.
  ataxic cerebral p.
  atonic cerebral p.
  backpack p.
  Bell p.
  bilateral gaze p.
  birth p.
  brachial birth p.
  bridegroom's p.

NOTES

P

palsy *(continued)*
bulbar p.
cerebellar cerebral p.
cerebral p.
choreoathetoid cerebral p.
craft p.
cranial nerve p.
creeping p.
crutch p.
Dejerine-Klumpke p.
diabetic oculomotor p.
diabetic third nerve p.
double elevator p.
dystonic cerebral p.
Erb p.
Erb-Duchenne p.
extraocular muscle p.
extrapyramidal cerebral p.
facial p.
feeding difficulties in cerebral p.
Féréol-Graux p.
fourth nerve p.
gaze p.
hereditary neuropathy with liability to pressure p. (HNPP)
hereditary neuropathy with susceptibility to pressure p.
horizontal gaze p.
hypertonic cerebral p.
hypoglossal nerve p.
hypotonic cerebral p.
idiopathic facial nerve p.
ipsilateral facial p.
ipsilateral gaze p.
isolated radial nerve p.
Klumpke p.
labioglossolaryngeal p.
lateral gaze p.
lateral rectus p.
lead p.
long thoracic p.
mixed form cerebral p.
multiinfarct progressive supranuclear p.
mumps facial nerve p.
nerve p.
night p.
obstetric p.
peripheral nerve pressure p.
peripheral occulomotor p.
peroneal nerve p.
persistent facial p.
postganglionic oculosympathetic p.
posticus p.
pressure p.
progressive infantile bulbar p.
progressive supranuclear p. (PSP)
pseudoabducens p.
pseudobulbar p.
pure athetoid p.
pure spastic p.
pyramidal cerebral p.
right sixth nerve p.
saccadic p.
Saturday night p.
scrivener's p.
seventh nerve p.
shaking p.
sixth cranial nerve p.
spastic bulbar p.
spastic cerebral p.
spinal accessory p.
stimulation program in cerebral p.
supranuclear gaze p.
Tapia vagohypoglossal p.
tardy median p.
tardy ulnar nerve p.
third nerve p.
trembling p.
trochlear nerve p.
vertical gaze p.
wasting p.

PAM
potassium-aggravated myotonia

pamabrom

pamidronate

pamoate
hydroxyzine p.

PAN
periodic alternating nystagmus

panacea

Panama cut

panasthenia

panautonomic

pancerebellar ataxia

panchreston

Pancoast
P. syndrome
P. tumor

pancreatic
p. carcinoma
p. encephalopathy

pancreaticus
plexus p.

pancreatitis

pancuronium bromide

pancytopenia

PANDAS
pediatric autoimmune neuropsychiatric diseases associated with streptococcal infection
pediatric autoimmune neuropsychiatric disorder associated with streptococci

pandemic
p. epidemiology
influenza A p.
pandiculation
Pandy maturation
pandysautonomia
acute p.
panel
Flushmesh p.
12-hour fasting lipid p.
panencephalitis
measles p.
nodular p.
Pette-Döring p.
progressive rubella p.
rubella p.
sclerosing p.
subacute sclerosing p. (SSPE)
panesthesia
panesthetic
Panevril
pang
brow p.
P. type agenesis
panhypopituitarism
panicogenic effect
Panlor
panneuritis endemica
panneurosis
panodic
panplegia
pan-potency
Pansch fissure
PANSS
Positive and Negative Syndrome Scale
PANSS-EC
Positive and Negative Syndrome Scale-Component Excited
pansynostosis
pantalgia
pantanencephalia
pantanencephaly
panthodic
panting center
Pantopaque
Pantopon
pantothenic acid deficiency peripheral neuropathy
PAP
positive airway pressure
bilevel PAP (BiPAP)
papaverine hydrochloride
papaverine-soaked Gelfoam
paper stop artifact
Papez
P. circle
P. circuit
papilla, pl. **papillae**
acoustic p.
nerve p.
papillary
p. meningioma
p. mucosal hyperplasia
papilledema
axoplasmic flow and p.
intracranial hypertension without p. (IHWOP)
papilliferous cystoma
papillitis
papilloma, pl. **papillomata**
choroid plexus p.
papillomatosis
juvenile p.
papillomatous
cystic p.
papillophlebitis
papovavirus
PAPS
3′-phosphoadenosine 5′-phosphosulfate
papulosis
malignant atrophic p.
paraanalgesia
paraanesthesia
paraballism
parabigeminalis
nucleus p.
parabigeminal nucleus
parabrachiales
nuclei p.
parabrachial nucleus
paracarcinomatous
p. encephalomyelopathy
p. myelopathy
paracenesthesia
paracentesis
paracentral
p. fissure
p. gyrus
p. hemianopia
p. lobule
p. nucleus of thalamus

NOTES

P

paracentral *(continued)*
p. scotoma
p. sulcus
paracentralis
gyrus p.
lobulus p.
sulcus p.
paracerebellar
paracetamol
parachiasmal epidermoid tumor
parachlorophenylalanine
parachute
p. reflex
p. response
paracinesia (*var. of* parakinesia)
paracinesis
paraclinoid internal carotid artery aneurysm
Paracoccidioides brasiliensis
paracousis (*var. of* paracusis)
paracrine mechanism
paracusia
paracusis, paracousis
paradigm
complex p.
double step p.
event-related innocuous somatosensory stimulation p.
gap p.
memory p.
motor p.
positive-going p.
risk p.
stimuli p.
task p.
three-stimulus p.
paradigmatic
paradox
calcium p.
pH p.
paradoxica
kinesia p.
paradoxical
p. abdominal movement
p. air embolism
p. cerebral embolism
p. cold response
p. combination
p. contraction
p. depression
p. diaphragm phenomenon
p. effect
p. extensor reflex
p. flexor reflex
p. ipsilateral hemiparesis
p. patellar reflex
p. phenomenon of dystonia
p. pupil
p. pupillary phenomenon
p. pupillary reflex
p. sleep
p. stimulation
p. triceps reflex
paraepilepsy
paraequilibrium
paraesthesia
parafalcine region
parafalx
parafascicular nucleus
paraffin
p. embedding
Tissuewax p.
paraflocculus
ventral p.
p. ventralis
parafollicular cell
paraganglioma
intrasellar p.
intravagal p.
nonchromaffin p.
parageusia
parageusic
paragigantocellularis
nucleus reticularis p.
paragloboside
sulfated glucuronyl p. (SGPG)
sulfate-3-glucuronyl p.
sulfate-3-glucuronyllactosaminyl p.
sulfoglucuronyl lactosaminyl p.
paragonimiasis lymphocytic meningitis
paragrammatism
paragraphia
parahaemolyticus
Vibrio p.
parahippocampal
p. activation
p. gyrus
p. white matter
parahippocampalis
gyrus p.
uncus gyri p.
parahippochampus
parahypophysis
parainfluenzae
Haemophilus p.
parainfluenza virus infection
paraisopropyliminodiacetic acid (PIPIDA)
parakinesia, paracinesia
parakinesis
parakinetic
paralalia
paraldehyde
paralemniscalis
nucleus p.

paralemniscal nucleus
paraleprosis
paralexia
paralexic
paralgesia
paralgesic
paralgia
paralimbic
- p. cortex
- p. region

paralinguistic feature
parallel
- p. fiber
- p. pathways of metabolism
- p. subsystem

paralog
paralogical thinking
paralogism
paralogistic
paralogy
paralysis, pl. **paralyses**
- abducens nerve p.
- acute ascending p.
- acute atrophic p.
- p. agitans
- ascending p.
- Avellis p.
- backpack p.
- Benedikt ipsilateral oculomotor p.
- Brown-Séquard p.
- bulbar p.
- central p.
- chronic basal meningitis with cranial nerve p.
- compression p.
- conjugate p.
- contralateral facial p.
- crossed p.
- crutch p.
- Cruveilhier p.
- decubitus p.
- deglutition p.
- Dejerine-Klumpke p.
- diphtheritic p.
- Duchenne p.
- Duchenne-Erb p.
- Erb-Duchenne p.
- Erb spinal p.
- extraocular p.
- facial nerve p.
- familial hypokalemic periodic p.
- faucial p.
- flaccid p.
- gaze p.
- generalized p.
- ginger p.
- global p.
- glossolabiolaryngeal p.
- glossolabiopharyngeal p.
- glossopalatolabial p.
- glossopharyngeal nerve p.
- glossopharyngeolabial p.
- Gubler p.
- hyperkalemic periodic p.
- hypokalemic periodic p.
- hysterical p.
- immunological p.
- infranuclear p.
- ipsilateral facial p.
- Jackson vagoaccessory hypoglossal p.
- jake p.
- Klumpke p.
- Klumpke-Dejerine p.
- Kussmaul p.
- Kussmaul-Landry p.
- labial p.
- labioglossolaryngeal p.
- labioglossopharyngeal p.
- Landry p.
- lead p.
- lingual p.
- Lissauer p.
- lower motor neuron p.
- mimetic p.
- mixed p.
- motor neuron p.
- muscle periodic p.
- musculospiral p.
- myogenic p.
- normokalemic periodic p.
- obstetric p.
- obstetrical p.
- ocular p.
- oculomotor nerve p.
- ophthalmoplegia and p.
- periodic p.
- peripheral facial p.
- peroneal p.
- phonetic p.
- phrenic nerve p.
- physiologic sleep p.

NOTES

paralysis *(continued)*
postdiphtheritic p.
postepileptic p.
posthemiplegic p.
posticus p.
Pott p.
predominantly predormital sleep p.
pressure p.
progressive bulbar p.
pseudobulbar p.
pseudohypertrophic muscular p.
radial p.
Ramsay Hunt p.
rectus p.
reflex p.
Remak p.
residual p.
rucksack p.
saccade p.
sensory p.
Simmer p.
sleep p.
sodium-responsive periodic p.
spastic spinal p.
spinal p.
spinomuscular p.
supranuclear p.
tegmental mesencephalic p.
thyrotoxic periodic p. (TPP)
tick p.
Todd postepileptic p.
transient flaccid p.
trigeminal p.
trochlear nerve p.
upper motor neuron p.
vasomotor p.
vocal cord p.
vocal fold p.
waking p.
wasting p.
Zenker p.
paralytic ileus
paralytic
p. chorea
p. dementia
p. miosis
p. mydriasis
p. poliomyelitis
p. pontine exotropia
p. psychosomatic disorder
p. scoliosis
p. stroke
paralytica
aphonia p.
dementia p.
keratitis p.
paralyticus
ictus p.
paralytique
folie p.
paralytogenic
paralyzant
paralyzing
p. depression
p. vertigo
paramagnetic
p. contrast
p. contrast enhancement
p. contrast injection
p. relaxation
paramedial reticular nucleus
paramedian
p. durotomy
p. infarction
p. lobule
p. mesencephalic syndrome
p. nucleus
p. pontine reticular formation (PPRF)
p. region
p. thalamopeduncular artery
p. thalamus
p. triangle
paramedianus
lobulus p.
nucleus reticularis p.
parameningeal mass
parameter
aberrant laboratory p.
pharmacokinetic p.
psychiatric p.
stimulation p.
suprasegmental p.
treatment intensity p.
paramethoxyamphetamine
parametrismus
paramimia
paramusia
paramyoclonus multiplex
paramyotonia
ataxic p.
p. congenita
congenital p.
symptomatic p.
paramyotonus
paramyxovirus infection
paranalgesia
paranasal
p. mucocele
p. sinus
p. sinus tumor
paraneoplastic
cerebellar degeneration p.

p. cerebellar degeneration
p. cerebral degeneration
p. encephalomyelitis
p. encephalomyelopathy
p. myelopathy
p. neurological disease
p. neurologic disease
p. neurologic disorder
p. neurologic syndrome
p. neuropathy
p. opsoclonus myoclonus
p. pain syndrome
p. polyneuropathy
p. syndrome

paranesthesia
paraneural infiltration
paraneurone
paranigralis
nucleus p.
paranigral nucleus
paranodal region
paranoia
hypochondriac p.
Kraepelina p.
Seglas-type p.
paranoic
reformatory p.
paranoid
p. involutional reaction
p. state
p. thinking
p. type
paranoides
paranoid-type
p.-t. arteriosclerotic
p.-t. arteriosclerotic dementia
p.-t. presenile dementia
p.-t. psycho-organic syndrome
p.-t. senile dementia
paranormal capacity
paranuclear
paraolfactorii
sulci p.
paraolfactory cortical area
paraorbital lesion
paraosmia
paraparesia
paraparesis
acute-onset p.
chronic p.
hereditary spastic p. (HSP)
HTLV-associated myelopathy/tropical spastic p.
human T-cell lymphotropic virus type 1-associated myelopathy/tropical spastic p. (HAM/TSP)
nonspastic p.
spastic p.
tropical spastic p.
X-linked spastic p.
paraparetic
parapeduncularis
nucleus p.
parapeduncular nucleus
parapharyngeal
p. fat pad
p. wall
paraphasia, paraphrasia
central p.
literal p.
phonemic p.
thematic p.
paraphasic
paraphia
paraphilia
troilism p.
paraphrasia (*var. of* paraphasia)
paraphrenic
paraphronia
paraphysial, paraphyseal
p. body
p. cyst
paraphysis, pl. **paraphyses**
parapineal organ
paraplectic
paraplegia
American Spinal Injury Association/International Medical Society of P. (ASIA/IMSOP)
ataxic p.
congenital spastic p.
p. dolorosa
Erb syphilitic spastic p.
p. in extension
familial spastic p.
p. in flexion
hereditary spastic p.
infantile spastic p.
painful p.
peripheral p.
postoperative p.

NOTES

paraplegia *(continued)*
Pott p.
senile p.
spastic p.
superior p.
syphilitic p.
tetanoid p.
toxic p.
tropical spastic p.
paraplegic
p. idiocy
p. spasm
p. spastic gait
paraplegiform
paraplegin
parapoplexy
parapraxia
parapraxis, pl. **parapraxes**
paraprotein
light chain p.
paraproteinemia
paraproteinemic neuropathy
parapsia
parapsis
parareflexia
pararmusia
parasagittal
p. falx
p. groove
p. intracranial mass
p. lesion
p. meningioma
p. section
parasellar
p. cistern
p. dysgerminoma
p. lesion
p. mass
p. region
p. tentorial meningioma
p. tumor
parasinoidal
p. sinus
p. space
parasinusoidal lacuna
parasitic
p. brain abscess
p. infection
parasolitarius
nucleus p.
parasomnia
parasomniac
parasomnias
parasomnia-type
paraspecific stimulation
paraspinal
p. infection
p. muscle
p. rod application
Parastep I System
parastriate
p. area
p. cortex
parasubiculum
parasympathetic
p. nerve
p. nerve injury
p. nervous system
p. part
p. root of ciliary ganglion
p. root of otic ganglion
p. root of pterygopalatine ganglion
p. root of sublingual ganglion
p. root of submandibular ganglion
parasympathica
pars p.
parasympathotonia
parataxic
paraterminal
p. body
p. gyrus
paraterminale
corpus p.
paraterminalis
gyrus p.
parathyreopriva
tetania p.
parathyroid
p. gland
p. hormone (PTH)
p. hormonelike protein (PLP)
p. insufficiency
p. tetany
parathyroprival tetany
paratonia progressiva
paratonic rigidity
Paratrend 7 sensor
paratrigeminal
p. neuralgia
p. syndrome
paratriptan
paratype
paraventricular
p. cyst
p. fiber
p. nucleus
p. nucleus of hypothalamus
paraventriculares
fibrae p.
paraventricularis
nucleus p.
paraventriculohypophysiales
fibrae p.

paraventriculohypophysialis
tractus p.
paraventriculohypophysial tract
paravertebral
p. ganglion
p. venous plexus
paraxial mesenchyme
paraxon
parchment crackling
parectropia
parencephalia
parencephalitis
parencephalocele
parencephalous
parenchyma
brain p.
parenchymal
p. bacillary peliosis
p. cerebral hemorrhage
p. granuloma
p. matrix
parenchymatous
p. atrophy
p. cell of corpus pineale
p. cerebellar degeneration
p. hematoma
p. hemorrhage
p. neuritis
p. neurosyphilis
p. syphilis
parent artery
parenteral
p. alimentation
p. formula
p. nutrition
paresis
abducens nerve p.
accessory nerve p.
bibrachial p.
canal p.
central facial p.
cerebral gaze p.
congenital suprabulbar p.
crural p.
distal motor p.
downward gaze p.
elevation p.
extraocular muscle p.
flaccid p.
gaze p.
general p.
horizontal gaze p.
hypoglossal nerve p.
ipsilateral facial p.
limb-girdle-trunk p.
monomelic p.
oculomotor nerve p.
palatal p.
postictal p.
progressive extraocular p.
pseudoabducens nerve p.
spastic p.
trochlear nerve p.
upward gaze p.
vertical gaze p.
watershed area p.
zoster p.
paresthesia
Berger p.
Bernhardt p.
transient facial p.
paresthetica
brachialgia statica p.
cheiralgia p.
gonyalgia p.
meralgia p.
paresthetic pseudopolycythemia
paretic
p. agraphia
p. analgesia
p. dementia
p. eye
p. jerk
p. neurosyphilis
p. nystagmus
Pargonimus westermani
pargyline
paries, gen. **parietis**, pl. **parietes**
p. vestibularis ductus cochlearis
parietal
p. body
p. cell vagotomy
p. cortex
p. cortex damage
p. cortex lesion
p. corticectomy
p. craniotomy
p. encephalocele
p. foramen
p. gyrus
p. lobe
p. lobe of cerebrum

NOTES

parietal · parotid

parietal *(continued)*
p. lobe epilepsy
p. lobe lesion
p. lobe syndrome
p. lobe tumor
p. lobule
p. meningioma
p. neocortical association area
p. operculum
p. organ
p. pathology
p. plane
p. tissue
p. vein
parietale
operculum p.
parietales
venae p.
parietalis
lobus p.
parietes (*pl. of* paries)
parietis (*gen. of* paries)
parietooccipital
p. craniotomy
p. fissure
p. hypoperfusion
p. infarction
p. lesion
p. sulcus
parietooccipitalis
parietooccipitalis
arcus p.
arteriae p.
fissura p.
ramus p.
sulcus p.
parietooccipitotemporal hypometabolism
parietopontinae
fibrae p.
parietopontine
p. fiber
p. tract
parietopontinus
tractus p.
parietosquamous suture
parietotemporal area
parietotemporooccipital junction
parietotemporopontinae
fibrae p.
parietotemporopontine fiber
Parinaud
P. ophthalmoplegia
P. sign
P. syndrome
park bench position
Parkes Weber syndrome
Parkin
P. protein
wild-type P.
Parkinson
de-novo P.
P. disease
P. disease and lateral sclerosis-dementia complex
P. Disease Quality of Life Scale (PDQUALIF)
P. Disease Questionnaire (PDQ-39)
P. facies
P. mask
P. Research The Organized Genetic Initiative (PROGENI)
P. Research The Organized Genetic Initiative study
P. sign
P. Study Group (PSG)
P. triangle
parkinsonian
p. crisis
p. dysarthria
p. gait
p. postmenopausal women
p. symptom
p. syndrome
parkinsonism
amyotrophy p.
autosomal recessive juvenile p. (AR-JP)
deprenyl and tocopherol antioxidative therapy of p. (DATATOP)
juvenile p.
MPTP-induced p.
postencephalitic p.
p. tremor
vascular p.
parkinsonism-dementia
Parkinson-plus syndrome
Parlodel
Parnate
parolfactoria
area p.
parolfactory
p. area
p. sulcus
parolivary body
paroniria salax
paronymous
parosmia
parotid
p. dissection
p. duct
p. nerve

p. plexus
p. tumor
parotideus
plexus p.
parotitis
paroxysm
childhood epilepsy with occipital p.
multifocal p.
paroxysmal
p. alpha activity
p. atrial fibrillation
p. bursting
p. cerebral dysrhythmia
p. convulsion
dyskinesia p.
p. epileptiform discharge
p. evoked pain
p. exertional dyskinesia
p. hemicrania
p. hypertension
p. kinesigenic choreoathetosis
p. kinesigenic dyskinesia
p. migraine
p. migraine headache
p. nocturnal dystonia
p. nonkinesigenic dyskinesia (PNKD)
p. positional nystagmus
p. sleep
p. sleep disorder
p. torticollis
p. vertigo
Parrot
P. disease
P. mask
P. sign
Parry-Romberg
P.-R. disease
P.-R. syndrome
pars
p. abdominalis autonomica
p. abdominalis systematis
p. anterior
p. anterior commissurae anterioris
p. anterior commissurae rostralis
p. anterior faciei diaphragmatis hepatis
p. anterior facies diaphragmatis
p. anterior fornicis vaginae
p. anterior fornix vaginae
p. anterior lobuli quadrangularis anterioris
p. anterior pedunculi cerebri
p. anterior pontis
p. autonomica systematis nervosi peripherici
p. basilaris pontis
p. basolateralis corporis amygdaloidei
p. canalis nervi optici
p. caudalis
p. caudalis nervi vestibularis
p. centralis ventriculi lateralis
p. cervicalis arteriae carotidis internae
p. cervicalis ductus thoracici
p. cervicalis esophagi
p. cervicalis medullae spinalis
p. coccygea medullae spinalis
p. cochlearis
p. cochlearis nervi vestibulocochlearis
p. cochlearis nevi octavi
p. compacta
p. compacta substantiae nigrae
p. corticalis
p. corticomedialis corporis amygdaloidei
p. cranialis partis parasympathici divisionis autonomici systematis nervosi
p. cupularis
p. cupularis recessus epitympanici
p. distalis
p. distalis adenohypophyseos
p. dorsalis corporis geniculati lateralis
p. dorsalis corporis geniculati medialis
p. dorsalis diencephali
p. dorsalis lobuli qudrangularis anterioris
p. dorsalis pedunculi cerebri
p. dorsalis pontis
p. duralis fili terminalis
p. flaccida
p. frontalis corporis callosi
p. inferior alae lobuli centralis
p. inferior nervi vestibularis
p. inferoposterior lobuli quadrangularis

NOTES

P

pars *(continued)*
p. infraclavicularis plexus brachialis
p. infundibularis
p. insularis
p. interarticularis
p. intermedia
p. intermedia adenohypophyseos
p. intermedia commissura bulborum
p. intermedia lobi anterioris hypophyseos
p. intracanalicularis nervi optici
p. intracranialis nervi optici
p. intralaminaris nervi optici intraocularis
p. intraocularis nervi optici
p. lateralis nuclei accumbentis
p. lenticulothalamicus capsulae internae
p. lumbalis diaphragmatis
p. lumbalis medullae spinalis
p. magnocellularis nucleus
p. medialis nuclei accumbentis
p. nervosa
p. nervosa hypophyseos
p. nervosa neurohypophyseos
p. occipitalis corporis callosi
p. olfactoria corporis amygdaloidei
p. opercularis
p. opercularis gyri frontalis inferioris
p. optica retinae
p. orbitalis
p. orbitalis glandulae lacrimalis
p. orbitalis gyri frontalis inferioris
p. orbitalis musculi orbicularis oculi
p. orbitalis nervi optici
p. orbitalis ossis frontalis
p. parasympathetica divisionis autonomici systematis nervosi
p. parasympathica
p. parasympathica divisionis automaticae systematis nervosi peripherici
p. parvocellularis nuclei rubri
p. pelvica autonomica
p. pelvica partis parasympatheticae systematis nervosi autonomici
p. pelvica systematis autonomici
p. peripherica
p. peripherica systematis nervosi
p. pharyngea hypophyseos
p. pialis fili terminalis
p. plana
p. plicata
p. posterior commissurae anterioris
p. posterior commissurae rostralis
p. posterior facies diaphragmatis hepatis
p. posterior fornix vaginae
p. posterior lobuli quadrangularis anterioris
p. postlaminalis nervi optici vaginae
p. precommunicalis arteriae cerebri anterioris
p. prelaminaris nervi optici intraocularis
p. reticularis substantiae nigrae
p. reticulata
p. retrolentiformis capsulae internae
p. retrolentiformis cruris posterior
p. rostralis nervi vestibularis
p. sacralis medullae spinalis
p. sellaris
p. sphenoidalis arteriae cerebralis mediae
p. spinalis nervi accessorii
p. sublentiformis capsulae internae
p. sublentiformis cruris posterioris
p. superior ali lobuli centralis
p. superior nervi vestibularis
p. supraclavicularis plexus brachialis
p. sympathica
p. sympathica divisionis autonomici systematis nervosi
p. tensa
p. thalamolenticularis capsulae internae
p. thoracica aortae
p. thoracica autonomica
p. thoracica ductus thoracici
p. thoracica esophagi
p. thoracica medullae spinalis
p. thoracica systematis autonomici
p. triangularis
p. triangularis gyri frontalis inferioris
p. tuberalis
p. vagalis
p. vagalis nervi accessorii
p. vascularis
p. vasculosa
p. ventralis corporis geniculati lateralis
p. ventralis corporis geniculati medialis
p. ventralis diencephali
p. ventralis lobuli quadrangularis anterioris
p. ventralis pedunculi cerebri
p. ventralis pontis
p. vertebralis
p. vestibularis nervi octavi

p. vestibularis nervi vestibulocochlearis
Parsidol
Parsitan
Parsonage-Aldren-Turner syndrome
Parsonage-Turner
P.-T. disease
P.-T. syndrome
part
autonomic p.
cupular p.
cupulate p.
infundibular p.
intermediate p.
opercular p.
orbital p.
parasympathetic p.
sympathetic p.
triangular p.
vertebral p.
parthenium
Tanacetum p.
partial
p. agenesis
p. arterial gas tension of carbon dioxide
p. central hypophysectomy
p. complex epilepsy
p. complex seizure
p. disability
p. facetectomy
p. flip angle imaging
p. Fourier imaging
p. hemianopia
p. hemilaminectomy
p. homonymous field defect
p. labyrinthectomy petrous apicectomy approach
p. nominal aphasia
p. oxygen pressure of brain tissue ($PbrO_2$)
p. pressure
p. saturation
p. temporal lobe epilepsy
p. thromboplastin time (PTT)
p. venous gas tension of oxygen
p. visual loss
partialis
ophthalmoplegia p.
rachischisis p.
partial-onset seizure
partial-thickness craniectomy
particle
p. beam
p. beam radiosurgery
p. domain
electron transport p. (ETP)
Ivalon p.
polyvinyl alcohol p.
proteinaceous infectious p.
signal recognition p. (SRP)
viral p.
particulate embolization
partition
brain-blood p.
low blood gas p.
party nystagmus
parvalbumin (PV)
parvocellularia
strata p.
parvocellularis
nucleus reticularis p.
PAS
periodic acid-Schiff
PAS-positive circular body
PASS
Postural Assessment Scale for Stroke Patients
passage
adiabatic fast p.
bouton en p.
wire p.
passer
Malis ligature p.
passive
p. extension
p. flexion
p. movement
p. tremor
passive-aggressive
p.-a. feature
p.-a. maneuver
paste
M-ADL p.
Pasteurella
P. meninigitis
P. multocida
past head injury
Patau syndrome
patch
acetylsalicylic acid p.
Dura-Guard dural repair p.

NOTES

patch *(continued)*
lidocaine transdermal p.
selegiline p.
shagreen p.
striosome p.
Tissue-Guard bovine pericardial p.
transdermal p.
patch-clamp
whole-cell p.-c.
patched gene
patching
lysolecithin p.
patchy retrograde amnesia
patellar
p. clonus
p. plexus
p. tendon reflex
patelloadductor reflex
patellometer
patency
valve p.
patent foramen ovale
pathema
pathematic aphasia
pathergy phenomenon
pathetic nerve
pathfinder
Nicolet P. I
pathogen
meningeal p.
p. of violence
pathogenesis
biologic p.
poliomyelitis p.
pathogenic
p. dystonia
p. factor
pathognomonic sign
pathologic
p. hyperreflexia
p. intoxication
p. spondylolisthesis
p. spontaneous activity
pathological
p. change
p. communication
p. dissociation
p. drowsiness
p. feature
p. finding
p. grief reaction
p. intoxication
p. level
p. mendicancy
p. mood state
p. personality
p. response
p. sleepiness
p. study
pathology
anatomic p.
borderline p.
cerebrovascular p.
cognitive p.
cortical p.
deep white matter p.
dental p.
Down syndrome p.
dual p.
incidental dual p.
ischemic p.
neuronal p.
parietal p.
personality p.
phenotype p.
secondary dual p.
subcortical p.
synuclein p.
true dual p.
white matter p.
pathomechanics
kyphotic deformity p.
spinal fusion p.
pathophysiologic
p. factor
p. process
pathophysiological
p. basis
p. cascade
p. role
pathophysiology
p. of delirium
ischemic stroke p.
multiple sclerosis p.
tremor p.
pathway
abducens p.
accessory conduction p. (ACP)
afferent p.
amygdalofugal p.
auditory p.
basal forebrain cholinergic p.
basic brain p.
biochemical p.
brain dopaminergic p.
catabolic p.
catecholaminergic p.
central auditory p.
cerebellar p.
cerebrospinal fluid p.
corticobulbar p.
corticofugal p.
corticospinal motor p.
CSF outflow p.

dentatoolivary p.
descending motor p.
dopamine p.
dopaminergic tuberoinfundibular p.
dorsal column sensory p.
efferent p.
extrapyramidal p.
extrathalamic p.
final common p.
frontopontocerebellar p.
frontostriatal p.
geniculocortical p.
glutamatergic p.
gustatory p.
heat-loss p.
hypocretin neural p.
indirect striatopallidal p.
indolaminergic p.
internuncial p.
intracellular metabolic p.
lemniscal p.
limbic system p.
lipoxygenase p.
magnocellular p.
mesocortical dopamine p.
mesolimbic dopamine p.
metabolic p.
monoaminergic p.
MS p.
neural p.
neuroanatomic p.
neurochemical p.
nigrostriatal p.
occulomotor p.
olfactory p.
pain and temperature p.
pentose phosphate p. (PPP)
peptidergic p.
perforant p.
perforating p.
pilomotor p.
pontine cholinergic p.
pyramidal p.
ras signaling p.
reticulocortical p.
reticulothalamocortical p.
retinal p.
retrochiasmal visual p.
sensory p.
serotonergic p.
signal transduction p.
stretch reflex p.
synaptic p.
thalamocortical p.
trigeminovascular p.
tuberoinfundibular p.
ubiquitin p.
vasoconstrictor p.
ventral amygdalofugal p.
visceromotor p.
visual p.

patient

adult scoliosis p.
akinetic p.
amnesic p.
p. autonomy
bipolar p.
borderline p.
catatonic p.
delirious p.
demented p.
dementia p.
disruptive psychotic p.
dissociative p.
dysphoric p.
first-episode p.
full-dose-treated p.
high-functioning p.
manic p.
multiple-episode p.
neuroleptic-free p.
neuroleptic-naive p.
never-medicated p.
nonpsychotic Alzheimer p.
old-old p.
opioid-dependent p.
peregrinating p.
p. placement criterion
p. positioning
Postural Assessment Scale for Stroke P.'s (PASS)
psychotic Alzheimer p.
rapid metabolizer p.
slow metabolizer p.
sudden and unexplained death in epilepsy p. (SUDEP)
suicidal depressed p.
symptomatic p.
treatment-intolerant p.
unipolar p.
variable screw placement system-plated p.

NOTES

patient-centered approach
patient-controlled analgesia (PCA)
patient-matched
hard tissue replacement-p.-m. (HTR-PMI)
p.-m. implant
Patil
P. stereotactic head frame
P. stereotactic head holder
P. stereotactic system II
Patrick
P. sign
P. test
pattern
aberrant gamma burst p.
alpha p.
anomalous parental vocal p.
Antoni p. (type A & B)
beaten copper p.
p. of care
catamenial seizure p.
change in sleep p.
chicken-wire vascular p.
chronic p.
convergence-divergence p.
dermatoglyphic p.
desynchronized discharge p.
discharge p.
double major curve p.
Down syndrome dermatoglyphic p.
EEG alpha p.
electroencephalogram burst suppression p.
electroencephalographic p.
electromyographic incomplete interference p.
p. of expression
field p.
fixed-action p.
p. generator
glycosylation p.
gullwing p.
hair whorl p.
hypsarrhythmic electroencephalographic p.
ictal cerebral perfusion p.
ictal EEG p.
ictal epileptiform p.
ineffective communication p.
interictal p.
iris stellate p.
irregular sleep-wake p.
laser speckle p.
left thoracolumbar major curve p.
Lennox-Gastaut p.
localized electroencephalographic seizure p.
maladaptive p.
multiple sclerosis chronic progressive p.
polygenic-threshold p.
radiofrequency homogeneity p.
recruitment p.
repeating p.
p. of repetitive behavior
right thoracic left lumbar curve p.
right thoracic minor curve p.
seizure p.
speech p.
spike-and-wave p.
storiform p.
syndromal p.
syndromic p.
temporal p.
type II curve p.
whorling p.
patterned
p. alopecia
p. stimulus
pattern-induced epilepsy
patterning synaptic connection
pattern-reversal stimulus
pattern-sensitive epilepsy
patting automatism
patty
polyclot p.
pauciimmune necrotizing vasculitis
paucisynaptic
Pauli exclusion principle
Paulus trocar
pause
apneic p.
respiratory p.
Pausinystalia yohimbe
pauvre
paving stone degeneration
Pavlov method
pavor incubus
Pavulon
***pax* gene**
Paxil
Paykel classification
Payne syndrome
PBD
peroxisome biogenesis disorder
PBI
protein-bound iodine
PBMC
peripheral blood mononuclear cell
$PbrO_2$
partial oxygen pressure of brain tissue
$PbrO_2$ monitoring probe
PBS
phosphate-buffered saline

PC12 cell
PC-2048B positron emission tomograph
PCA
patient-controlled analgesia
DAT for PCA
PCD
programmed cell death
PCMRA
phase contrast magnetic resonance angiography
PCNSL
primary central nervous system lymphoma
PCO_2
PComA
posterior communicating artery
PCP
posterior clinoid process
PCR
polymerase chain reaction
false-negative PCR
frataxin gene PCR
X25 PCR
PCV
procarbazine, lomustine (CCNU), vincristine
PCV chemotherapy
PD
phenyldichloroarsine
cyclothymic PD
PD Quality of Life Scale (PDQUALIF)
PDA
polymorphic delta activity
PDA on electroencephalogram
PDGF
platelet-derived growth factor
PDH
pyruvate dehydrogenase
PDH complex
PDM
Bontril PDM
PDN
prosthetic disk nucleus
PDN device
PDN prosthetic disk
PDQ-39
Parkinson Disease Questionnaire
PDQUALIF
Parkinson Disease Quality of Life Scale
PD Quality of Life Scale
PE
plasma exchange
PEA
percentage of error in amplitude
PEAK
PEAK polyaxial anterior cervical fixation system
peak
p. absorption spike
p. behavioral effect
p. bone mass
Bragg ionization p.
p. expiratory flow rate
p. score
peak-dose
p.-d. choreoathetoid dyskinetic movement
p.-d. dyskinesia
peak-to-peak amplitude
Péan
P. clamp
P. forceps
peapod intervertebral disk forceps
pear bur
pearl-and-string sign
pearl-chain appearance
pearl tumor
pearly
p. neoplasm
p. tumor
pear-shaped nerve hook
Pearson
P. correlation coefficient pedantic
P. syndrome
pectineus nerve
pectoral
p. nerve
p. reflex
pectoralgia
pectoralgic
p. migraine
p. migraine headache
pectoralis major muscle
pectoris
Prinzmetal vasospastic angina p.
pectus renalis
pedal system
pedantic
Pearson correlation coefficient p.
pediatric
p. and adolescent epilepsy (PAE)

NOTES

pediatric *(continued)*
p. autoimmune neuropsychiatric diseases associated with streptococcal infection (PANDAS)
p. autoimmune neuropsychiatric disorder associated with streptococci (PANDAS)
p. brain stem glioma
p. C-D hook
p. Cotrel-Dubousset rod
p. headrest
p. moyamoya disease
p. neuroradiology
p. polypharmacy
p. supratentorial hemispheric tumor
p. TSRH hook
p. Wada testing
pedication
pedicle
p. anatomy
p. axis angle
p. C-D hook
p. cortex disruption
p. diameter
p. dimension
p. entrance point
p. evaluation
p. landmark
p. localization
p. location
lower thoracic p.
p. marker
p. morphometry
rigid p.
p. screw
p. screw breakage
p. screw chord length
p. screw construct
p. screw construct peg
p. screw hardware prominence
p. screw insertion
p. screw linkage design
p. screw path length
p. screw plating
p. screw pullout strength
p. screw-rod fixation
p. sounding probe
thoracic p.
pedicled pericranial flap
pedicular fixation
pedi-gravity assisted valve
pedionalgia
pedioneuralgia
pedis
nervi digitales dorsales p.
peduncle
caudal cerebellar p. (CCP)
cerebellar p.
cerebral p.
p. of corpus callosum
cranial cerebellar p.
decussation of superior cerebellar p.
p. of flocculus
inferior cerebellar p.
inferior thalamic p.
lateral thalamic p.
p. of mamillary body
middle cerebellar p.
olfactory p.
pineal p.
pontine cerebellar p.
rostral cerebellar p.
superior cerebellar p.
thalamic p.
ventral thalamic p.
peduncular
p. ansa
p. hallucinosis
p. loop
peduncularis ansa p.
p. vein
pedunculares
rami p.
venae p.
peduncularis
ansa p.
p. ansa peduncular
pedunculi (*pl. of* pedunculus)
p. cerebellares
p. cerebelli
pedunculomamillaris
fasciculus p.
pedunculomammillary fasciculus
pedunculopontine
p. cholinergic group
p. neuron
p. tegmental nucleus
p. tegmentum
pedunculopontinus
nucleus reticularis trigeminalis p.
nucleus tegmentalis p.
pedunculotomy
pedunculus, pl. **pedunculi**
basis p.
p. cerebellaris caudalis
p. cerebellaris inferior
p. cerebellaris medius
p. cerebellaris pontinus
p. cerebellaris superior
p. cerebralis
p. cerebri
p. corporis callosi
p. corporis mamillaris

p. corpus pinealis
p. flocculus
pes p.
p. of pineal body
p. thalami inferior
p. thalami lateralis
p. thalami ventralis

PEEP
positive end-expiratory pressure

Peet splanchnic resection

peg
fibular p.
pedicle screw construct p.

Peganone

Peiper-Beyer laminectomy rongeur

pejoration

peliosis
parenchymal bacillary p.

Pelizaeus-Merzbacher
P.-M. disease
P.-M. leukodystrophy
P.-M. sclerosis

pellagra
Casal necklace appearance in p.
p. dementia

pellicle

pellucidi
cavitas septi p.
cavum septi p.
lamina septi p.
vena anterior septi p.
vena posterior septi p.

pellucidum
anterior vein of septum p.
cavity of septum p.
cavum septum p.
lamina of septum p.
posterior vein of septum p.
septum p.
vein of septum p.

pelopsia

Pelorus
P. stereotactic frame
P. surgical system

pelvic
p. fixation
p. ganglion
p. plexus

pelvica
ganglia p.

pelvici
nervi splanchnici p.

pelvicorum
radix parasympathica gangliorum p.

pelvicus
plexus p.

pelvina
ganglia p.
plexus p.

pelvis
crossed reflex of p.

pelvofemoral muscular dystrophy

PemADD
PemADD CT

PEMF
pulsed electromagnetic field

pemoline

Pena-Shokeir syndrome

pencil-grip instrument

Pende sign

pendetide
satumomab p.

Pendred syndrome

pendular nystagmus

pendulum of diagnosis

penetrating
p. injury
p. trauma

penetration
anterior cortex p.
antibiotic p.
vertebral body anterior cortex p.

Penfield
P. dissector
P. hypothesis
P. neurodissector

penicillamine

penicillamine-induced myasthenia gravis

Penicillium

penile reflex

penis
nervi cavernosi p.
nervus dorsalis p.
p. reflex

penitence

penitentiare
folie p.

Penn cube function formula

pentaacetate
gadolinium diethylenetriamine p.

pentastarch

NOTES

P

pentobarbital
p. coma
p. in status epilepticus
pentose phosphate pathway (PPP)
pentoxifylline
pentylenetetrazol
penumbra
ischemic p.
penumbral region
PEO
progressive external ophthalmoplegia
Pepper
P. neuroblastoma
P. syndrome
P. tumor
peptic
peptide
Abeta p.
alpha beta p.
amyloid beta p.
atrial natriuretic p. (ANP)
brain natriuretic p.
calcitonin gene-related p. (CGRP)
p. cotransmitter
C-type natriuretic p.
p. inhibitor
muramyl p.
opioid p.
vasoactive intestinal p.
peptidergic
p. fiber
p. pathway
percentage of error in amplitude (PEA)
percentile
percept analysis
perception
altered spatial p.
altered time p.
p. analysis
auditory p.
complex visual p.
endopsychic p.
figure-ground p.
heightened sensory p.
narrative speech p.
spatial p.
speech p.
perceptorium
perceptual
p. aspect
p. disturbance
p. emotive stimulus
p. error
p. filtering
p. level
p. motor skill
p. process
perceptual/cognitive mechanism
perceptual-identification test
perceptual-motor ability impairment
perchlorate extract
Perclose closure device
percussion
distal tingling on p. (DTP)
p. hammer
percutaneous
p. balloon commissurotomy
p. cabling
p. cordotomy
p. discoscope
p. electrode array
p. endoscopic recanalization
p. epidural electrode
p. glycerol rhizolysis
p. intraarterial embolization
p. laser nucleolysis
p. radiofrequency gangliolysis
p. radiofrequency retrogasserian rhizotomy (PRFR)
p. radiofrequency rhizolysis
p. radiofrequency sympathectomy
p. retrogasserian glycerol chemoneurolysis
p. retrogasserian glycerol rhizolysis (PRGR)
p. retrogasserian glycerol rhizotomy
p. spinal endoscope
p. stimulation
p. thecoperitoneal shunt
p. thermocoagulation
p. transvenous coil embolization
p. trigeminal nerve compression
peregrinating patient
perencephaly
perescutes
persecuteurs p.
Perez reflex
perfection
manie de p.
perfluorocarbon
perfluorooctyl bromide
perforans
nervus cutaneous p.
perforant pathway
perforatae
habenulae p.
perforated space
perforating
p. bur
p. cutaneous nerve
p. pathway
perforation
esophageal p.
vascular p.

perforator
Acra-Cut cranial p.
Aesculap skull p.
cranial p.
Cushing cranial p.
Heifetz cranial p.
Heifetz skull p.
Hudson p.
powered automatic skull p.
Raney p.
perforatum
hypericum p.
performance
cognitive p.
p. level
memory p.
memory-continuous p.
neuropsychologic p.
nonparetic eye p.
novel task p.
P. Oriented Balance and Mobility Assessment
recall p.
P. Scale Scores
task p.
Taylor Complex Figure task p.
vocational p.
work p.
Perf-Plate cranial plate
perfusate
p. drip
luminal p.
perfusion
cerebral p.
critical p.
p. deficit
luxury p.
microcirculatory p.
misery p.
transcardiac p.
perfusion-weighted imaging
pergolide mesylate
perhexiline maleate
periamygdaloid
p. area
p. cortex
perianal reflex
perianeurysmal hemorrhage
periapical abscess
periaqueductal
p. central gray
p. glioma
p. gray matter
p. gray substance
p. hemorrhage
periaqueductalis
substantia grisea p.
periarterial
p. plexus of choroid artery
p. sympathectomy
periarterialis
plexus p.
periarteritis nodosa
periaxial
p. neuritis
p. neuropathy
periaxialis
encephalitis p.
periaxonal
pericallosa
cisterna p.
pericallosal
p. azygos artery
p. cistern
pericapillary encephalorrhagia
pericardial reflex
pericaryon
pericentromeric region of chromosome 16q
periclaustral lamina
pericorpuscular synapse
pericranial temporalis flap
pericranii
sinus p.
pericranitis
pericranium
pericyte edema generation
pericytosis
peridendritic
peridural
peridurale
spatium p.
periencephalitis
periendoneurium
periependymal myelitis
perifascicular
p. atrophy
p. migration
perifocal edema
periforaminal

NOTES

P

perifornical
p. area
p. nucleus
perifornicalis
nucleus p.
perigangliitis
periganglionic
perigemmal
periglial
periglomerular cell
perihematomal
perihypoglossal
p. nuclear complex
p. nucleus
perihypoglossales
nuclei p.
periictal headache
periinsular
perikarya
perikaryon
perilesional inhibitory cortex
perilocus ceruleus
perilymphatic
p. duct
p. fistula
perilymphaticus
ductus p.
perilymph fistula (PLF)
perimedullary venous system
perimeningitis
perimenstrual progesterone withdrawal
perimesencephalic
p. cistern
p. nonaneurysmal subarachnoid hemorrhage
perimetry
Goldman p.
kinetic p.
perimyelitis
perimysium
perinatal
p. anoxia
p. asphyxia
p. clavicle fracture
p. craniocerebral trauma
p. development
p. humerus fracture
p. infarction
p. obturator nerve injury
p. unilateral cerebral ischemic insult
perineal
p. nerve
p. post
perineural
p. anesthesia
p. fibroblastoma
p. infiltration
perineuria
perineurial cyst
perineuritic
perineuritis
perineurium
perineuronal
p. end foot
p. space
perinuclear
period
absolute refractory p.
amblyogenic p.
apneustic p.
cluster p.
ictal p.
interictal p.
latent p.
p. lateralized epileptiform discharge
p. line
major risk p.
oral-biting p.
readout p.
relative refractory p.
sensorimotor p.
silent p.
sleep onset p. (SOP)
treatment p.
periodic
p. acid-Schiff (PAS)
p. acid-Schiff-hematoxylin stain
p. alternating gaze
p. alternating nystagmus (PAN)
p. edema
p. hemilingual numbness
p. lateralizing epileptiform discharge (PLED)
p. leg movement
p. limb movement (PLM)
p. limb movement disorder (PLMD)
p. limb movement during sleep (PLMS)
p. limb movement of sleep (PLMS)
p. migrainous neuralgia
p. paralysis
p. sharp wave complex
p. vestibular ataxia (PVA)
periolivares
nuclei p.
periolivary nucleus
perioperative
p. anoxia
p. cisternography

p. complication
p. reduction
perioptic
p. meningioma
p. subarachnoid space
periorbita
periorbital ecchymosis
periosteal
p. elevator
p. reflex
periostitis interna cranii
peripachymeningitis
peripapillary nerve fiber layer
peripapullar astrocyte
peripatetic
peripeduncularis
nucleus p.
peripeduncular nucleus
peripheral
p. antimuscarinic side effect
p. aromatization
p. avulsion
p. benzodiazepine receptor
p. blood lymphocyte
p. blood mononuclear cell (PBMC)
p. catecholamine
p. catecholamine receptor
p. chemoreceptor
p. cholinergic activity
p. deafferentation pain
p. dysarthria
p. electromyographic activity
p. facial paralysis
p. glioma
p. motoneuron
p. myelin protein 22
p. nerve
p. nerve axotomy
p. nerve disease
p. nerve entrapment syndrome
p. nerve fascicle
p. nerve injury
p. nerve lesion
p. nerve level motor impairment
p. nerve myelin
p. nerve myelination
p. nerve neurapraxia
p. nerve neuroma
p. nerve pressure palsy
p. nerve regeneration
p. nerve regeneration conduit
p. nerve sheath tumor
p. nerve trauma
p. nervous system (PNS)
p. nervous system disorder
p. neuralgia
p. neuroectodermal tumor
p. neurofibromatosis
p. neuroglia
p. neuropathic pain syndrome
p. neuropathy
p. nociceptor activation
p. nociceptor sensitization
p. norepinephrine
p. nystagmus
p. occulomotor palsy
p. oculomotor lesion
p. paraplegia
p. part of nervous system
p. sensory loss
p. sensory neuron
p. steroid hormone
p. tabes
p. tissue
p. trigeminal nerve branch
p. vascular disease
p. vasomotor disturbance
p. vertigo
p. vestibular system
peripherally
p. acting anticholinergic medication
p. inserted central catheter (PICC)
peripheraphose
peripherica
pars p.
peripherici
divisio autonomica systematis nervosi p.
pars autonomica systematis nervosi p.
pars parasympathica divisionis automaticae systematis nervosi p.
periphericum
systema nervosum p.
peripherophose
periphery dose
periphlebitis retinae
perirolandic parietal cortex
perispondylitis
perissodactylous
peristimulus-time histogram (PSTH)

NOTES

peristriate
p. area
p. cortex
perisylvian
p. cortex
p. microgyria
p. region
perithelial small cell sarcoma
peritoneal
p. catheter
subdural p.
peritoneum
peritorcular meningioma
peritraumatic predictor
peritrigeminalis
nucleus p.
peritrigeminal nucleus
Peritrode
peritumoral
p. band
p. brain edema
periungual fibroma
perivascular
p. change
p. cuff
p. cuffing
p. end foot
p. foot
p. gliosis
p. macrophage
p. mononuclear cell
p. nerve
p. nerve-ending stimulation
p. sheath
p. space
periventricular
p. disease
p. fiber
p. gray (PVG)
p. gray matter
p. gray matter area
p. gray region
p. gray substance
p. hyperintense lesion
p. hyperintensity
p. intraventricular hemorrhage (PIH)
p. leukemia
p. leukomalacia (PVL)
p. nodular heterotopia
p. preoptic nucleus
p. radiolucency
p. white matter
p. white matter lesion
p. zone
periventriculares
fibrae p.
periventricularis
nucleus preopticus p.
zona p.
perizonalis
nuclei campi p.
perizonalium
nuclei camporum p.
Perkin-Elmer
Applied Biosystems P.-E.
perlée
tumeur p.
Perlia
convergence nucleus of P.
P. nucleus
Perls stain
permanent
p. cranial nerve deficit
p. injury
p. magnet
p. section
p. sympathectomy
p. vegetative state
p. visual loss
Permax
per mesem
permissive
p. hypothesis of affective
p. substrate
Perneczky-designed microscope-assisting endoscope
perocephalic edema
peroneal
p. entrapment neuropathy
p. muscular atrophy
p. nerve
p. nerve palsy
p. paralysis
p. phenomenon
p. sign
p. somatosensory evoked potential
peroneales
nervi p.
peroxidase
glutathione p.
peroxidation
lipid p.
peroxisomal
p. disease
p. metabolic disorder
peroxisome biogenesis disorder (PBD)
peroxynitrite anion
perpendicular fasciculus
perpetrator of violence
perphenazine and amitriptyline hydrochloride
perplexing behavior

Perroncito
P. apparatus
P. spiral
persecuteurs perescutes
persenilin gene
perseverative agraphia
persistence
cerebral artery fetal p.
persistent
p. clonus
p. facial palsy
p. primitive carotid-basilar artery anastomosis
p. rumination
p. tremor
p. trigeminal artery anastomosis
p. vegetative state (PVS)
personality
abnormal p.
p. abnormality
amoral p.
brooding p.
p. change
p. dimension
p. disorder instrument
interictal epileptic p.
mixed-type psychopathic p.
neurasthenic p.
pathological p.
p. pathology
p. theory
von Zerssen circumplex model of premorbid p.
Personnel Identification Card (PIC)
perspective
behavioral p.
biologic p.
developmental p.
linear p.
neurobiological p.
psychoanalytic p.
psychosocial p.
religious p.
symptomatic p.
perspective-taking skill
perspiration artifact
persuades
glutathione p. (GSHPx)
Perthes-Bankart lesion
Pertofrane
Pertscan 99m
perturbation
p. magnitude
torque-pulse p.
pertussis-toxin-catalyzed ADP-ribosylation
pertussis vaccination encephalopathy
pervasive
p. developmental disorder
p. inhibition
pes
p. anserinus
p. cavus deformity
p. cavus in Friedreich ataxia
p. hippocampus
p. pedunculus
PET
positive emission tomography
positron emission tomography
PET image
nonstereotactic PET
PET scan
PET technique
petechia, pl. **petechiae**
petechial hemorrhage
PET-FDG
positron emission tomography-fluorodeoxyglucose
PET-guided stereotactic biopsy
pethidine
petit
p. mal
p. mal epilepsy
p. mal seizure
p. mal variant
Petit syndrome
petroclinoclival meningioma
petroclinoid fold
petroclival
p. cholesterol granuloma
p. lesion
p. meningioma
p. tumor
petroclivotentorial meningioma
petrooccipitalis
fissura p.
petrosa
vena p.
petrosal
p. approach
p. draining group
p. ganglion

NOTES

petrosal *(continued)*
p. impression of the pallium
p. nerve
p. neuralgia
p. sinus
p. sinus sampling
petrosectomy
Kawase anterior p.
petrositis
petrosphenoidal ligament
petrosphenoid syndrome
petrosquamosal sinus
petrosquamous
p. sinus
p. suture
petrous
p. apex
p. apex mass
p. bone
p. carotid artery
p. carotid-to-intradural carotid saphenous vein graft
p. ganglion
p. ridge chemodectoma
petrousitis
Pette-Döring
P.-D. disease
P.-D. panencephalitis
Peyronie disease
Peyton brain spatula
PF
Fiorgen P.
Pfeiffer syndrome
Pfuhl sign
PG
nasopharyngeal electrode placement
PGD
phosphogluconate dehydrogenase
P-glycoprotein
PGR
psychogalvanic response
phacoma, phakoma
phacomatosis, phakomatosis
phagocytosis
phakoma (*var. of* phacoma)
phalangeal cell
Phalen
P. maneuver
P. sign
P. test
phantom
p. absence seizure
p. arm
p. base
Compass stereotactic p.
gelatin p.
p. hand
hot-spot p.
p. image
p. limb
p. limb pain
Plexiglas p.
sensory p.
p. shock syndrome
three-dimensional SPECT p.
p. tooth pain
phantosmia
PHA-P
phytohemagglutinin-A-P
pharmacodynamic interaction
pharmacogenomics
pharmacokinetic
p. interaction
p. parameter
protein binding p.
pharmacologic
p. agent
p. factor
p. impact
p. intervention
p. sensitivity
pharmacological
p. agent
p. antagonism
p. approach
p. armamentarium
p. blockade
p. difference
p. intervention
p. mechanism
p. predictor
p. property
p. stimulus
Pharmacopeia
pharmacoresistent epilepsy
pharmacotherapy
conventional p.
p. regimen
pharyngeal
p. airway
p. anesthesia
p. cleft
p. constrictor muscle
p. fat pad
p. hypophysis
p. plexus of vagus nerve
p. pouch
p. reflex
p. tissue
p. tubercle
p. wall
p. weakness
pharyngeus
nervus p.

pharyngismus
pharyngoplegia
pharyngospasm
pharyngotympanic cephalalgia
phase
absolute construction of p.
p. angle
ascension p.
p. cancellation
p. coherence
p. contrast magnetic resonance angiography (PCMRA)
p. cycling
delayed sleep p.
p. encoding
extradural p.
p. instability
intradural p.
p. mapping
p. position
postambivalent p.
recovery p.
reference p.
relaxation p.
p. reversal
p. reversal potential
rising p.
p. shift
tonic p.
transverse magnetization p.
treatment p.
vector p.
walking swing p.
phase-contrast
p.-c. map
p.-c. method
p.-c. technique
phased-array
p.-a. coil
p.-a. color-flow ultrasound system
phase-dependent
phase-encoding
p.-e. direction
p.-e. gradient
phase-sensitive
p.-s. detector
p.-s. gradient-echo MR imaging
phase-shift effect
phasic
p. alertness
p. nystagmus
p. reflex
p. twitching
phencyclidine
p. and amphetamine/methamphetamine
p. delirium
p. hydrochloride
methylenedioxymethamphetamine and p.
p. thiophene
phenelzine
phenobarbital
ephedrine, theophylline, p.
very high dose p.
phenobutiodil
phenol
p. motor point block
p. neurolysis
phenolphthalein
phenolsulfonphthalein (PSP)
phenomena (*pl. of* phenomenon)
phenomenalistic causality
phenomenological
p. characteristic
p. measure
phenomenology
clinical p.
delirium p.
phenomenon, pl. **phenomena**
alien limb p.
arm p.
Babinski p.
baked brain p.
Bell p.
bilateral motor p.
breakthrough p.
centralization p.
cervicolumbar p.
cheek p.
clasp-knife p.
clinical p.
cogwheel p.
crossed phrenic p.
Cushing p.
Dandy-Walker p.
Dejerine hand p.
Dejerine-Lichtheim p.
doll's eyes p.
doll's head p.
Doppelganger p.
Duckworth p.

NOTES

phenomenon *(continued)*
Erben p.
escape p.
facialis p.
Fere p.
finger p.
freezing p.
Galassi pupillary p.
Gibbs p.
Gowers p.
Grasset p.
Grasset-Gaussel p.
Gunn p.
halo p.
Hemifield slide p.
hidden observer p.
hip p.
hip-flexion p.
Hochsinger p.
Hoffmann p.
Holmes p.
Holmes-Stewart p.
Hunt paradoxic p.
Hunt paradoxical p.
interictal p.
intracranial steal p.
jaw-winking p.
Kernohan notch p.
Kienböck p.
knee p.
Kohnstamm p.
Kühne p.
leg p.
Leichtenstern p.
Lhermitte p.
Lust p.
Marcus Gunn p.
Mayer-Gross closing-in p.
mental p.
misdirection p.
motor p.
motoric p.
Negro p.
no-reflow p.
on-off p.
overuse p.
paradoxical diaphragm p.
paradoxical pupillary p.
pathergy p.
peroneal p.
Philippe-Gombault p.
polyspike-spike wave p.
Pool p.
psychomotor p.
psychotic-like p.
Pulfrich p.
Queckenstedt p.
radial p.
Raynaud p.
rebound p.
release p.
Riddoch p.
Ritter-Rollet p.
Rust p.
Schiff-Sherrington p.
Schlesinger p.
Schramm p.
Schüller p.
seizurelike p.
Sherrington p.
soft psychotic-like p.
Souques p.
springlike p.
staircase p.
steal p.
Strümpell p.
tibial p.
toe p.
tongue p.
transient visual p.
Trousseau p.
Uhthoff p.
vacuum p.
visual p.
warmup p.
wearing-off p.
Wedensky p.
Wernicke hemianopic pupillary p.
Westphal p.
Westphal-Piltz p.
Wever-Bray p.

phenomenon/syndrome
Fregoli p.
jet lag p.

phenothiazine toxic effect

phenotype
alcohol-related p.
clinical p.
DMD p.
headache p.
malignant p.
membrane p.
myelinating p.
p. pathology

phenotypic
p. expression
p. factor
p. marker
p. study

phenoxybenzamine

phentermine

phenylalanine
p. hydroxylase deficiency

p. hydroxylase therapy in phenylketonuria
p. serum level
phenylalaninemia
phenylalkylamine
3-phenylaminoalanine
phenylbutazone
phenylbutyrate
phenyldichloroarsine (PD)
phenylketonuria (PKU)
p. genetic factor
phenylalanine hydroxylase therapy in p.
p. treatment
phenylpiperazine
phenylpiperidine
phenylpropranolamine
phenylpropylamine
phenyl-*t*-butyl-nitrone
Phenytek
phenytoin-induced
p.-i. chorea
p.-i. choreoathetosis
phenytoin interaction with other drug
pheochromocytoma and neuroblastoma localization study
pheromonal
pheromone
Philadelphia
P. collar
P. halo
Philippe-Gombault phenomenon
Philippe triangle
Philippson reflex
Philips
P. Gyroscan S5, S15
P. linear accelerator
P. Tomoscan
P. 400 transmission electron microscope
Philly bolt
Phineas Gage syndrome
phi rhythm
phlebitis
sinus p.
phlebography
phlegmatic
PHN
postherpetic neuralgia
phobia
blood/injection p.
generalized social p.
isolated p.
p. reaction
universal p.
phobia-induced migraine headache
phobic reaction
Phoenix
P. ancillary valve
P. Anti-Blok ventricular catheter
P. cranial drill
P. cruciform valve
P. fifth ventricle system
pholcodine
phonatory spasm
phonemic paraphasia
phonetic
p. input
p. noise
p. paralysis
phonic spasm
phonoangiography
quantitative spectral p.
Phono-Graphix program
phonologic
p. assembly impairment
p. syntactic syndrome
phonological
p. agraphia
p. mismatch negativity (PMN)
p. process
phonomyoclonus
phonomyography
phonoreceptor
phoria
phose
phosis
phosphacan
phosphatase
alkaline p.
pyruvate dehydrogenase p.
tyrosine p.
phosphate
dibasic calcium p.
disopyramide p.
Hexadrol P.
Hydrocortone P.
p. metabolism
nicotinamide adenine dinucleotide p. (NADPH)

NOTES

phosphate *(continued)*
potassium phosphate and sodium p.
sodium p.
phosphate-buffered saline (PBS)
phosphate-regulating gene with homologies to endopeptidases on the X-chromosome
phosphate-wasting syndrome
phosphatidylinositol
phosphatidylserine (PO)
phosphene
3′-phosphoadenosine 5′-phosphosulfate (PAPS)
phosphocreatine
phosphocreatinine
frontal p.
p. level
phosphofructokinase
p. transferase deficiency
phosphogluconate dehydrogenase (PGD)
phosphoglycerate
p. kinase
p. kinase deficiency
p. mutase
p. mutase deficiency
phosphoinositol metabolite
phosphokinase
creatine p.
phospholipid hydroperoxide
phospholipid-related signal transduction
phosphoribosyl pyrophosphate synthetase superactivity
phosphoribosyltransferase
hypoxanthine guanine p.
phosphorus
p. nuclear magnetic resonance spectroscopy
serum p.
phosphorus-31
phosphorylase
p. deficiency
p. kinase
liver p.
muscle p.
phosphorylate tau protein
phosphorylation
oxidative p.
posttranslation p.
protein tyrosine p.
tau p.
5′-phosphosulfate
adenosine 5′-p. (APS)
3′-phosphoadenosine 5′-p. (PAPS)
phosphotungstic acid hematoxylin (PTAH)
photalgia
photesthesia
photic
p. afterdischarge
p. driving
p. stimulation
p. stimulation activating technique
p. stimulus
photic-induced epileptiform activity
photic-sneeze reflex
photism
photoaffinity labeling
Photoarticulation Test
photochemically-induced graded spinal cord infarction
photocoagulation
laser p. (LPC)
in situ p.
photoconvulsive
photodynamic therapy
photodynia
photodysphoria
photoesthetic
photofrin porfimer sodium
photogenic epilepsy
photometrazol
photomicrograph
photomicroscope
Zeiss IIIRS p.
photomyoclonic jerk
photomyoclonus
hereditary p.
photon
p. beam radiosurgery
p. knife
P. Radiosurgery System
p. ray
photonic radiosurgical system
photoparoxysmal response (PPR)
photophobia
photophobic
photopsia
photoptarmosis
photoradiation therapy
photoreceptor
ocular p.
photosensitivity
photosensitizer
photothrombosis
arterial p.
photothrombotic infarction
phototransduction
humoral p.
pH paradox
phrenalgia
phrenectomy
phrenemphraxis
phrenic
p. ganglion

p. mononeuropathy
p. motor neuron
p. motor nucleus
p. nerve
p. nerve conduction time
p. nerve injury
p. nerve lesion
p. nerve paralysis
p. neuropathy
p. nucleus of anterior column of spinal cord
p. plexus

phrenica
ganglia p.

phrenicectomy

phrenici
nucleus nervi p.
rami phrenicoabdominales nervi p.
ramus pericardiacus nervi p.

phreniclasia

phreniclasis

phrenicoabdominal nerve

phrenicoexeresis

phreniconeurectomy

phrenicotomy

phrenicotripsy

phrenicus
nervus p.

phrenoglottic

phrenologist

phrenology

phrenoplegia

phrenospasm

phrenotropic

phrictopathic

phthisica
spes p.

phthisis bulbus

PHY
physostigmine

***Phycomycetes rhizopus* infection**

phylogenetic predecessor

phylogeny

Phynox cobalt alloy clip material

physaliphora
ecchordosis p.

physaliphore

physaliphorous cell

physical
p. activity
p. attack
p. comorbid disorder
p. danger
p. disturbance
p. exercise
p. functioning
p. injury
p. integrity
p. pain
p. restraints
p. skill
p. therapy
p. withdrawal

Physicians' Global Rating Scale

physicochemical
p. interaction
p. principle

physiognomic

physiologic
p. epilepsy
p. sleep paralysis
p. slowing
p. tetanus
p. tremor
p. zero

physiological
p. antagonism
p. arousal
p. artifact
p. component
p. drive
p. hyperarousal
p. reflex

physiology
respiratory p.
p. of women

physiopsychic

physiotherapy

physocephaly

physostigmine (PHY)

phytanic acid level

phytohemagglutinin-A-P (PHA-P)

phytol metabolism

phytonadione

pi
p. procedure
p. rhythm

pia
p. mater
p. mater cranialis
p. mater encephali
p. mater spinalis

NOTES

pia-arachnoid cell
piagetian theory of moral reasoning development
pial
p. arteriovenous malformation
p. artery
p. cortical vessel
p. funnel
p. part of filum terminale
p. terminal filament
p. tissue
piale
filum terminale p.
pial-glial membrane
pianist's cramp
piarachnitis
piarachnoid
PIC
Personnel Identification Card
PICA
posterior inferior cerebellar artery
posterior inferior communicating artery
PICA aneurysm
PICA index
PICC
peripherally inserted central catheter
Pick
P. atrophy
P. body
P. bundle
P. cell
P. disease
P. inclusion
P. syndrome
Picker scanner
Picornaviridae
picornavirus
pictorial aphasia
picture
Allen p.
Blacky p.
p. in picture technique
picture-caption pair
pieds terminaux
piesesthesia, piezesthesia
piesimeter, piezometer
piety
filial p.
piezesthesia (*var. of* piesesthesia)
piezoelectric potential
piezometer (*var. of* piesimeter)
piezoresistive transducer
piezosensor
PIF
prolactin-inhibiting factor
pigment
acute posterior multifocal placoid p.
p. epithelial lesion
p. gene
melanin p.
pigmentary retinopathy
pigmented
p. layer of retina
p. villonodular synovitis (PVS)
pigmenti
incontinentia p.
pigmentosa
neuropathy, ataxia, retinitis p. (NARP)
retinitis p.
pigmentosum
xeroderma p.
PIH
periventricular intraventricular hemorrhage
pili torti
pillar
p. cell
p. cell of Corti
Corti p.
p. of fornix
pillar-and-post microsurgical retractor
pillow
Mediflow p.
molded vacuum p.
pill-rolling tremor
pilocytic juvenile astrocytoma
piloid
p. astrocytoma
p. gliosis
pilojection
pilomatrixoma
pilomotor
p. fiber
p. nerve
p. pathway
p. reflex
pilomyxoid astrocytoma
pilonidal sinus
pilot program
Piltz sign
pimethixene
pimozide
PIN
prostatic intraepithelial neoplasia
PIN entrapment
pin
AO guide p.
p. fixation headrest
p. headholder
Kirschner p.

Mayfield disposable skull p.
Mayfield skull cap p.
p. sensation
Steinmann p.
Synthes guide p.
torlone fixation p.
pincer grip
pinch
digital p.
pindolol
pineal
p. body
p. cell
p. cell tumor
p. cyst
p. germinoma
p. gland
p. habenula
p. meningioma
p. parenchymal neoplasm
p. parenchymal tumor
p. peduncle
p. recess
p. region
p. regional choriocarcinoma
p. region mass
p. region teratoma
p. region tumor
p. stalk
p. ventricle
pineale
chief cell of corpus p.
corpus p.
parenchymatous cell of corpus p.
pinealectomy
pinealis
glandula p.
pedunculus corpus p.
recessus p.
pinealoblastoma
pinealocyte
pinealocytoma
pinealoma
ectopic p.
extrapineal p.
pinealopathy
pineoblastoma
pineocytoma
ping-pong
p.-p. appearance
p.-p. fracture
p.-p. gaze
pinion
p. headholder
Mayfield p.
pink collar worker
pinocytosis
pinocytotic vesicle
pins-and-needles sensation
pinwheel
Safe-T-Wheel p.
Piotrowski sign
pipecolic acid level
piperazine neurotoxicity
piperidine
piperidyl
pipe stemming of ankle-brachial index
PIPIDA
paraisopropyliminodiacetic acid
technetium 99m P.
pipoglutamic aciduria
pipradrol
PI-R
plasma immunoreactive
piracetam
piribedil
piriform
p. area
p. cortex
p. lobe
p. nerve
p. neuron
p. neuron layer
piriformis
nervus musculi p.
p. syndrome
piriformium
stratum neuronorum p.
pirisudanol
pirlindole
Pisces electrode
Pisces-Quad electrode
pistol-grip instrument
piston
MTS electrohydraulic p.
Pitanguy
P. oval skin resection
P. plastic surgery
pitch contour
Pitt-Rogers-Dank syndrome

NOTES

Pittsburgh
P. gamma knife group
P. Sleep Quality Index
pituicyte
pituicytoma
pituitaria
glandula p.
pituitary
p. abscess
p. adamantinoma
p. adenoma
p. adiposity
p. ameloblastoma
p. apoplexy
p. autoimmunity
p. basophilia
cachexia p.
p. cachexia
p. curette
p. dwarfism
p. dysfunction
p. dystopia
p. forceps
p. gland
growth-hormone-secreting p.
hyaline body of p.
p. hypoplasia
p. macroadenoma
p. microadenoma
p. necrosis
p. portal system
p. prolactin release
p. replacement therapy
p. spoon
p. stalk
p. stalk lesion
p. stalk section
p. tumor
***pitx* gene**
PIVKA
protein induced by vitamin K absence
pivotal role
PKC
protein kinase C
PKU
phenylketonuria
placebo-controlled
p.-c. drug study
p.-c. trial
placebo response rate
4-place laminectomy
placement
bone graft p.
carotid artery angioplasty and stent p.
clip p.
endosaccular coil p.
International 10–20 system of electrode p.
Kirschner wire p.
K-wire p.
nasopharyngeal electrode p. (PG)
nursing home p.
plate p.
posterolateral bone graft p.
rod p.
sacral screw p.
subdural electrode p.
therapeutic school p.
therapeutic vocational p.
variable screw p.
placode
neural p.
placoid pigment epitheliopathy
PLACS
protease-linked activation cloning system
plagiocephaly
lambdoid p.
plain
Citanest P.
p. forceps
p. radiography
p. tomography
p. x-ray
plaiser
maitre de p.
plana
pars p.
planar
p. reconstruction
p. spin imaging
P. Stereotaxic Atlas of the Human Brain
plane
Aeby p.
arachnoid p.
coronal insonation p.
frontal p.
frontoparallel p.
parietal p.
sagittal p.
sensitive p.
subplatysmal p.
superior temporal p.
vertical p.
planning
comprehensive treatment p.
conceptual p.
image-integrated surgery treatment p.
inverse treatment p.
preoperative p.
spatial p.
planotopokinesia

plantalgia
plantar
p. muscle reflex
p. nerve
planum
fetal p.
p. polare
p. sphenoidale
p. temporale
p. temporale asymmetry
plaque
Abeta-centered neuritic p.
AMY p.
argyrophil p.
atherosclerotic p.
cortical neuritic p.
fibromyelinic p.
fibrous p.
p. heterogeneity
Hollenhorst p.
p. jaunes
Lichtheim p.
multiple sclerosis p.
neuritic p.
Redlich-Fisher miliary p.
p. reduction assay
sclérose en p.
sclerotic p.
senile p.
p. shadow
tuberculoma en p.
plasma
delta-function arterial p.
p. dopamine beta-hydroxylase
p. elastase
p. exchange (PE)
p. factor
p. fatty acid
p. fibrinolytic enzyme system
p. glutamate concentration
p. homocysteine level
p. immunoreactive (PI-R)
p. leptin level
p. membrane dopamine transporter
p. neuropeptide Y
p. protein
p. thromboplastin
plasmacytoma
intracranial p.
primary intracranial p.
plasmapheresis
Plasmatein
plasmatofibrous astrocyte
plasmin-antiplasmin complex
plasminogen
p. activator (PA)
p. activator inhibitor
Plasmodium falciparum
plastic
p. collar
p. compensatory mechanism
p. reorganization
p. scalp clip
plastic-covered hydrogel disk
plasticity
axonal p.
cortical p.
dendritic p.
experience-induced cortical p.
lesion-induced cortical p.
neural p.
neuronal p.
somatosensory p.
synapse p.
synaptic p.
Plastizote cervical collar
plasty
aqueductal p.
plate
alar p.
American Optical Hardy-Rand-Rittler color p.
AO dynamic compression p.
AO reconstruction p.
ASIF broad dynamic compression bone p.
ASIF T p.
basal p.
bone p.
broad AO dynamic compression p.
butterfly-shaped monobloc vertebral p.
cartilage p.
cartilaginous end p.
Caspar anterior cervical p.
Caspar trapezoidal p.
cervical p.
commissural p.
contoured anterior spinal p.
cortical p.
cranial bone fixation p.
craniocervical p.

NOTES

plate *(continued)*
cranioplasty p.
cribriform p.
3D titanium mini bone p.
end p.
E-Z Flap cranial bone p.
p. fixation
floor p.
Hardy-Rand-Rittler p.
Harm posterior cervical p.
Howmedica Microfixation cranial p.
Ishihara p.
Kühne terminal p.
Leibinger 3-D p.
Leibinger Micro Plus p.
Leibinger Micro System cranial fixation p.
Lorenz cranial p.
Lorenz titanium screws and p.
Luhr micro p.
Luhr Microfixation cranial p.
Luhr mini p.
Luhr pan p.
medullary p.
metal p.
Mini Orbita p.
Morscher anterior cervical p.
Morscher titanium cervical p.
narrow AO dynamic compression p.
neural p.
orbital p.
ORION anterior cervical p.
Orozco cervical p.
Perf-Plate cranial p.
p. placement
prochordal p.
Profile anterior spinal p.
Profil-O-Plastic p.
quadrigeminal p.
roof p.
round hole p.
Roy-Camille p.
skull p.
sole p.
spinous process p.
stainless steel preformed skull p.
Steffee p.
Storz Microsystems cranial fixation p.
symmetrical sacral p.
symmetrical thoracic vertebral p.
Synthes cervical p.
Synthes Microsystem cranial fixation p.
tantalum preformed skull p.
tectal p.
terminal p.
thoracolumbosacral p.
titanium p.
TSRH p.
vascular foot p.
vertebral p.
Vitallium p.
wing p.

platelet
p. count
p. glycoprotein Ia/IIa deficiency
p. glycoprotein IIb/IIIa
p. thromboxane release

platelet-activating factor (PAF)

platelet-derived growth factor (PDGF)

platelet-fibrin embolus

platelet-shaped knife

plate-screw
p.-s. fixation
p.-s. osteosynthesis

plate-spacer washer

platform
positioning p.
StealthStation treatment guidance p.

plating
anterior spinal p.
Caspar p.
pedicle screw p.
posterior spinal p.
Steffee p.

Platinol

platinum
p. coil
p. microcoil
p. ring

platinum-based drug

platinum-Dacron microcoil

Platinum-Plus guidewire

platybasia

platysmal reflex

platysma muscle

Plavix

PLED
periodic lateralizing epileptiform discharge
synchronous bilateral PLED

pledget
cotton p.
cottonoid p.
Gelfoam p.
latex-covered p.

pleiotrophin

pleocytosis
cerebrospinal fluid p.
p. of cerebrospinal fluid
lymphocytic p.
mononuclear p.

pleomorphic
- p. adenoma
- p. oligodendroglioma
- p. xanthoastrocytoma (PXA)

Pletal
plethysmograph
plethysmography
- air p.
- venous occlusion p. (*pl. of* VOP)

pleura
pleurodynia
pleurothotonos, pleurothotonus
pleusirs
- folie à p.

plexectomy
plexiform
- p. layer
- p. layer of cerebral cortex
- p. layer of retina
- p. neurofibroma
- p. neuroma

plexiformis
- stria laminae p.

Plexiglas phantom
plexitis
- brachial p.

plexopathy
- brachial p.
- lumbar p.
- median sternotomy brachial p.
- radiation p.
- radiation-induced p.
- sacral p.

plexus
- abdominal aortic p.
- anterior cerebral artery p.
- anular p.
- p. aorticus abdominalis
- p. aorticus thoracalis
- p. aorticus thoracicus
- ascending pharyngeal p.
- Auerbach p.
- autonomic p.
- p. autonomici
- p. autonomicus
- Batson p.
- brachial p.
- p. brachialis
- cardiac p.
- p. cardiacus
- p. caroticus communis
- p. caroticus externus
- p. caroticus internus
- carotid p.
- cavernous p.
- celiac p.
- cervical p.
- p. cervicalis
- choroid p.
- p. of choroid artery
- p. choroideus
- p. choroideus ventriculi lateralis
- p. choroideus ventriculi quarti
- p. choroideus ventriculi tertii
- ciliary ganglionic p.
- coccygeal p.
- p. coccygeus
- p. coeliacus
- common carotid nervous p.
- communicating branch of facial nerve with tympanic p.
- communicating branch of intermediate nerve with tympanic p.
- crural p.
- Cruveilhier p.
- p. deferentialis
- p. dentalis inferior
- p. dentalis superior
- diaphragmatic p.
- p. of ductus deferens
- p. entericus
- epidural venous p.
- epigastric p.
- Erb-Duchenne-Klumpke injury to brachial p.
- esophageal p.
- p. esophagealis
- p. esophageus
- Exner p.
- external maxillary p.
- external vertebral venous p.
- facial p.
- p. femoralis
- ganglia of autonomic p.
- gastric coronary p.
- p. gastrici
- gastroepiploic p.
- p. hypogastricus
- p. hypogastricus inferior
- p. hypogastricus superior
- ileocolic p.

NOTES

plexus *(continued)*
p. iliacus
incisive p.
inferior choroid p.
inferior thyroid p.
infraorbital p.
p. intermesentericus
internal vertebral venous p.
interradial p.
intramural p.
p. intraparotideus
ischiadic p.
Jacobson p.
lienal p.
p. lienalis
lingual p.
p. lumbalis
lumbar p.
p. lumbaris
lumboaortic intermesenteric p.
p. lumbosacralis
maxillary p.
p. of medial cerebral artery
Meissner p.
meningeal p.
p. meningeus
p. mesentericus inferior
p. mesentericus superior
middle hemorrhoidal p.
molecular p.
myenteric p.
nasopalatine p.
nerve p.
p. nervorum spinalium
p. nervosus
p. nervosus celiacus
p. (nervosus) myentericus
p. (nervosus) submucosus
occipital p.
p. oesophagealis
p. oesophageus
ophthalmic p.
p. pancreaticus
paravertebral venous p.
parotid p.
p. parotideus
patellar p.
pelvic p.
p. pelvicus
p. pelvina
p. periarterialis
p. pharyngeus nervi vagi
phrenic p.
popliteal p.
posterior auricular p.
prevertebral p.
prostatic p.
p. prostaticus
pterygoid p.
p. pulmonalis
p. rectalis inferior
p. rectalis medius
p. rectalis superior
sacral p.
p. sacralis
sagittal p.
Santorini p.
sciatic p.
solar p.
spermatic p.
spinal nerve p.
p. of spinal nerve
p. splenicus
p. subclavius
subdermal p.
submucous intestinal p.
subsartorial p.
p. subserosus
subtrapezius p.
superficial temporal p.
superior hemorrhoidal p.
superior thyroid p.
supraradial p.
p. suprarenalis
sympathetic p.
tentorial p.
thoracic aortic p.
tonsillar p.
p. tympanicus
p. uretericus
p. uterovaginalis
vaginal p.
vascular p.
p. vascularis
venous p.
vertebral p.
p. vertebralis
vesical p.
p. vesicale
p. vesicalis
vidian p.
visceral p.
p. visceralis

PLF
perilymph fistula

plica choroidea

plicata
pars p.

pliers
Howmedica Microfixation System p.
Leibinger Micro System p.
Luhr Microfixation System p.

PLIF
posterior lumbar interbody fusion
PLM
periodic limb movement
PLMD
periodic limb movement disorder
PLMS
periodic limb movement during sleep
periodic limb movement of sleep
PLMS index
PLOSL
polycystic lipomembranous osteodysplasia with sclerosing leukoencephalopathy
plot
funnel p.
PLP
parathyroid hormonelike protein
plug
methylmethacrylate cranioplastic p.
otoconial p.
soaked fat p.
soaked muscle p.
plugging
Obex p.
plumbism
plumula
plus
APAP P.
generalized epilepsy with febrile seizures p. (GEFS+)
ophthalmoplegia p.
Siemens Somatom P.
PME
progressive myoclonus epilepsy
PML
polymorphonuclear leukocyte
progressive multifocal leukoencephalopathy
PMN
phonological mismatch negativity
***PMP-22* gene**
PMR
polymyalgia rheumatica
PNET
primitive neuroectodermal tumor
pneumatic
p. chair lift
p. microscope
pneumatocele
p. cranii
extracranial p.
intracranial p.
pneumatocephalus
pneumatorrhachis (*var. of* pneumorrhachis)
pneumatosis
epidural p.
pneumobulbar
pneumocele
extracranial p.
intracranial p.
pneumocephalus
epidural p.
tension p.
pneumococcal
p. meningitis
p. pneumonia
pneumocrania
pneumocranium
Pneumocystis carinii
pneumoencephalocele
pneumoencephalogram
pneumoencephalography
pneumoencephalos
pneumogastric nerve
pneumogram
pneumograph
pneumonia
hospital-acquired p.
pneumococcal p.
pneumoniae
cephalosporin-resistant *Staphylococcus p.*
drug-resistant Streptococcus p. (DRSP)
Staphylococcus p.
Streptococcus p.
pneumoorbitography
pneumoplethysmography
ocular p.
pneumorrhachis, pneumatorrhachis
pneumosinus dilatans
pneumotachogram
pneumotachograph
pneumotachometer
pneumotaxic
p. center
p. center of Lumsden
p. localization
pneumotonometry
pneumoventricle

NOTES

P

pneumoventriculi
PNF
proprioceptive neuromuscular facilitation
PNF exercise
PNKD
paroxysmal nonkinesigenic dyskinesia
PNS
peripheral nervous system
PO
phosphatidylserine
pococurante
podismus
podospasm
podospasmus
POEMS
polyneuropathy, organomegaly, endocrinopathy, monoclonal gammopathy, skin changes
P. syndrome
poikilothermia
point
anchoring p.
anterior commissure-posterior commissure reference p.
apophysary p.
apophysial p.
Baker p.
Barker p.
Crutchfield drill p.
entry p.
Erb p.
extra p. (Ex)
hysteroepileptogenous p.
p. imaging
Keen p.
Kocher p.
motor p.
multiple sensitive p.
p. mutation
pedicle entrance p.
powered automatic stopping drill p.
pressure p.
pressure-arresting p.
pressure-exciting p.
retromandibular tender p.
sacral brim target p.
p. scanning
self-stopping drill p.
sensitive p.
supraclavicular p.
supraorbital p.
sylvian p.
tender p.
time p.
trigger p.
Trousseau p.
Valleix p.
Vogt p.
Vogt-Hueter p.
Ziemssen motor p.
pointed
p. awl
p. object
pointes
torsades de p.
3-point headrest
pointing test
point-resolved spectroscopy (PRESS)
7-point scale
poise
Poiseuille
P. equation
P. law
poisoning
alcoholic p.
arsenic p.
barbiturate p.
carbon monoxide p.
carbon tetrachloride p.
cholinesterase inhibitory p.
curare p.
cyanide p.
ethylene glycol p.
iron p.
Jamaica ginger p.
lead p.
mercury p.
methanol p.
methotrexate p.
methyl alcohol p.
monosodium glutamate p.
muscarine p.
opioid p.
organophosphate pesticide p.
organophosphorus insecticide p.
pyrimethamine p.
thallium p.
valproic acid p.
poker spine
Poland syndrome
polar
p. artery
p. coordinate system
p. spongioblastoma
p. sulcus
polare
planum p.
spongioblastoma p.
Polaris
P. adjustable spinal cage implant
P. camera system
P. position tracker

polarity
dynamic p.
reverse p.
Polar-Mate coagulator
polarographic
pole
frontal p.
occipital p.
temporal p.
PoleStar
P. magnet
P. N-10 iMRI
POLI
polyneuropathy, ophthalmoplegia, leukoencephalopathy, and intestinal
poliencephalitis
poliencephalomyelitis
polio
French p.
polioclastic
poliodystrophia
p. cerebri
p. cerebri progressiva infantilis
poliodystrophy
cerebral p.
progressive cerebral p.
progressive infantile p.
polioencephalitis
p. infectiva
inferior p.
superior hemorrhagic p.
polioencephalomeningomyelitis
polioencephalomyelitis
polioencephalopathy
polioencephalotropic
poliomyelencephalitis
poliomyelitis
abortive p.
acute anterior p.
acute bulbar p.
acute lateral p.
acute paralytic p.
anterior p.
ascending p.
bulbar p.
cerebral p.
chronic anterior p.
endemic p.
epidemic p.
p. infection
neonatal p.
nonparalytic p.
paralytic p.
p. pathogenesis
postinoculation p.
postvaccinal p.
spinal paralytic p.
p. treatment
poliomyelitis-induced respiratory failure
poliomyeloencephalitis
poliomyelopathy
poliovirus infection
polus
p. frontalis
p. frontalis hemispherii cerebri
p. occipitalis
p. occipitalis hemispherii cerebri
p. temporalis
p. temporalis cerebri
p. temporalis hemispherii
polyacrylamide
sodium dodecyl sulfate p. (SDS-PAGE)
polyamine biosynthesis inhibitor
polyangiitis
microscopic p.
polyanhydride
p. biodegradable polymer wafer
p. poly[bis(carboxyphenoxy-propane)-sebacic acid]
polyanhydroglucuronic acid
polyarteritis
p. nodosa
p. nodosa group
p. nodosa peripheral neuropathy
polyaxial screw
polyaxonic
polychondritis
relapsing p.
Polycillin-N
polycinematosomnography
Polycitra-K
polyclonal antibody
polyclonia
polyclot patty
polycystic
p. lipomembranous osteodysplasia with sclerosing leukoencephalopathy (PLOSL)
p. ovary syndrome

NOTES

polycythemia
neonatal p.
p. vera
polydipsia
hysterical p.
polyene thread
polyesthesia
polyethylene
p. intravenous catheter
p. sleeve
p. terephthalate fabric
polyganglionic
polygenic-threshold pattern
polyglot
polyglucosan storage disease
polyglutamine
p. disease
p. stretching
polygram
ictal p.
polygyria
polyhydramnios
polyhydroxyethylmethacrylate
polylactic
p. acid
p. acid mesh
polyleptic
polymacrogyria
polymer
cellulose acetate p.
p. drug delivery
p. encapsulation
HTR p.
Hydrolene p.
implanted p.
polymerase
p. chain reaction (PCR)
p. chain reaction technique
polymerization
polymethylmethacrylate
polymicrogyria
polyminimyoclonus
polymodal nociceptor
polymorphic
p. delta activity (PDA)
p. epilepsy of childhood
p. neuron
polymorphism
insertion/deletion p.
MAO-A gene p.
restriction fragment length p. (RFLP)
sequence p.
polymorphonuclear leukocyte (PML)
polymorphous layer
polymyalgia
p. arteritica
p. rheumatica (PMR)
polymyoclonus
dentatorubral cerebellar atrophy with p.
polymyositis
interstitial p.
overlap syndrome in p.
polymyositis/dermatomyositis
polymyxin
polyneural
polyneuralgia
polyneuric
polyneuritic
polyneuritiformis
heredopathia atactica p.
polyneuritis
acute febrile p.
acute idiopathic p.
acute infective p.
acute postinfective p.
anemic p.
chronic familial p.
cranial p.
erythredema p.
Guillain-Barré p.
infectious p.
Jamaica ginger p.
leprous p.
postinfectious p.
polyneuromyositis
polyneuronitis
polyneuropathy
acute inflammatory p.
acute painful p.
acute postinfectious p.
alcoholic p.
amyloid p.
anemic p.
arsenic p.
arsenical p.
autoimmune demyelinating p. (AIDP)
axonal p.
axon loss p.
buckthorn p.
carcinomatous p.
chronic inflammatory demyelinating p. (CIDP)
chronic relapsing p.
critical illness p.
demyelinating p.
diabetic sensorimotor p.
diphtheric p.
distal sensory p. (DSP)
distal symmetric p.

dying-back p.
dysimmune p.
familial amyloidotic p.
Finnish type familial amyloid p.
gait disorder, autoantibody, late-age onset, p.
generalized p.
gestational p.
idiopathic p.
Indiana type familial amyloid p.
inflammatory demyelinating p. (IDP)
isoniazid p.
Japanese-type familial amyloid p.
Maryland type familial amyloid p.
Meretoja-type familial amyloid p.
mitochondrial encephalomyopathy with sensorimotor p.
nitrofurantoin p.
nutritional p.
p., ophthalmoplegia, leukoencephalopathy, and intestinal (POLI)
p., organomegaly, endocrinopathy, monoclonal gammopathy, skin changes (POEMS)
p., organomegaly, endocrinopathy, myeloma, and skin change
paraneoplastic p.
porphyric p.
Portuguese type familial amyloid p.
recurrent p.
Rukavina-type familial amyloid p.
sarcoid p.
segmental demyelinating p.
sensorimotor axonal p.
subacute p.
symmetric p.
symmetrical sensory p.
thallium p.
uremic p.
Van Allen type familial amyloid p.

polyomavirus
polyopia
polyp
antrochoanal p.
polypectomy
polypeptide
calcitonin gene-related p.
p. hormone gene
vasoactive intestinal p. (VIP)
polypeptidorrhachia
polypharmacy
pediatric p.
rational p.
polyphasic motor unit
polyplegia
polypneic center
polypropylene suture
poly-Q-tract
polyradiculitis
polyradiculomyelitis
CMV p.
cytomegalovirus p. (CMV-PRAM)
polyradiculomyopathy
polyradiculoneuritis
acute idiopathic demyelinating p. (AIDP)
polyradiculoneuropathy
acute inflammatory demyelinating p.
chronic inflammatory demyelinating p. (CIDP)
chronic relapsing p.
demyelinating p.
inflammatory demyelinating p.
polyradiculopathy
acute inflammatory demyelinating p.
chronic inflammatory demyelinating p.
diabetic p.
polyrhythmic activity
polysaccharide storage myopathy
polysensitivity
polysensory
polyserositis
polysomnogram
polysomnograph (PSG)
polysomnographic
p. abnormality
p. study
polysomnography
Atlas of p.
full-night p.
nocturnal p.
polyspike-and-wave discharge
polyspike-spike wave phenomenon
polyspike-wave complex
polysynaptic discharge
polytetrafluoroethylene
expanded p. (ePTFE)

NOTES

P

polytherapy
rational p.
p. regimen
polytomography
polyvinyl
p. acetate emulsion
p. alcohol
p. alcohol foam
p. alcohol particle
polyvinylpyrrolidone (PVP)
polyvitamin
Pompe
P. disease
P. disease, type 2
pond fracture
ponesiatrics
ponograph
pons, pl. **pontes**
anterior part of p.
basilar part of p.
p. cerebelli
dorsal part of p.
p. et cerebellum
p. hypertrophy
lower p.
median raphe of p.
oblique bundle of p.
raphe of p.
p. reticular formation
reticular nuclei of p.
tegmentum of p.
transverse fiber of p.
upper p.
p. varolii
vein of p.
ventral part of p.
pontem
rami ad p.
ponticulus promontorii
pontile
p. apoplexy
p. hemianesthesia
pontina
raphe mediana p.
pontine
p. angioma
p. angle
p. angle tumor
p. apoplexy
p. artery
p. cerebellar peduncle
p. cholinergic pathway
p. cistern
p. corticonuclear fiber
p. flexure
p. glioma
p. gray matter
p. hemorrhage
p. hydatid cyst
p. infarction
p. lateral gaze center
p. lesion
p. paramedian reticular formation
p. parareticular formation
p. raphe nucleus
p. reticular nucleus
p. sign
p. syndrome
p. tegmentum
p. tractotomy
p. vein
pontinus
nucleus reticularis tegmentalis p.
pedunculus cerebellaris p.
pontis
basis p.
brachium p.
cisterna p.
fasciculi longitudinales p.
fasciculus obliquus p.
fibrae corticonucleares p.
formatio reticularis tegmenti p.
nuclei reticulares p.
nucleus raphes p.
nucleus reticularis tegmenti p.
pars anterior p.
pars basilaris p.
pars dorsalis p.
pars ventralis p.
raphe p.
sulcus basilaris p.
taenia p.
tegmentum p.
venae p.
pontobulbar
p. body
p. nucleus
p. sulcus
pontobulbare
corpus p.
pontobulbaris
nucleus p.
pontobulbia
pontocerebellar
p. fiber
p. recess
p. trigone
pontocerebellare
trigonum p.
pontocerebellares
fibrae p.
pontocerebellaris
angulus p.
cisterna p.

pontocerebellum
pontogeniculooccipital spike-inhibiting activity
pontomedullary
p. epidermoid cyst
p. groove
p. junction
p. separation
p. sulcus
pontomesencephalic
p. cavernous hemangioma
p. junction
p. vein
pontomesencephalica
vena p.
pontopeduncular sulculus
pontoreticulospinalis
tractus p.
pontoreticulospinal tract
pontosubicular degeneration
Pool phenomenon
Pool-Schlesinger sign
popliteal
p. artery
p. nerve
p. plexus
Poppen
P. intervertebral disk laminectomy rongeur
P. ventricular needle
Poppen-Blalock carotid clamp
Poppen-Gelpi laminectomy retractor
population
high-risk p.
multiple spike p.
p. stratification
target p.
Porch Index of Communicative Ability
porcine
p. cell transplantation
p. dopaminergic cell
pore
gustatory p.
taste p.
porencephalia (*var. of* porencephaly)
porencephalic, porencephalous
p. cyst
porencephalitis
porencephaly, porencephalia
congenital p.
encephaloclastic p.
schizencephalic p.
pornerastic
porocarcinoma
poroma
malignant eccrine p.
porosis, pl. **poroses**
cerebral p.
porphobilinogen
p. deaminase
urinary p.
porphyria
acute intermittent p.
delta-aminolevulinate dehydratase p.
hepatic p.
intermittent acute p. (IAP)
p. peripheral neuropathy
p. synthesizing enzyme
variegate p.
porphyric
p. neuropathy
p. polyneuropathy
porphyrin
p. compound
p. metabolism
port
lumbar p.
p. wine stain
porta, pl. **portae**
portal
integrated sideport access p.
p. systemic encephalopathy
porte manteau procedure
Porteus
portmanteau word
Portnoy
P. DPV device
P. ventricular cannula
P. ventricular catheter
portosystemic shunt
Portuguese-Azorean disease
Portuguese type familial amyloid polyneuropathy
porus
p. acusticus
p. gustatorius
position
p. agnosia
angular p.
p. of attack
brow-down p.

NOTES

position *(continued)*
decubitus p.
emprosthotonos p.
fetal p.
knee-chest p.
k-space reordered by inversion time at each slice p.
lateral recumbent p.
lounging p.
opisthotonos p.
orthotonos p.
park bench p.
phase p.
prone p.
reverse Trendelenburg p.
semi-Fowler p.
p. sense
sitting p.
supine p.
translational p.
Trendelenburg p.
tuck p.
positional
p. nystagmus
p. therapy
p. vertigo
p. vertigo of Bárány
positioning
patient p.
p. platform
proper neck p.
position-specific tremor
positive
p. ability
p. afterpotential
p. airway pressure (PAP)
P. Attention Behavior
p. dromotropism
p. effect
p. emission tomography (PET)
p. end-expiratory pressure (PEEP)
p. feedback
p. image
p. ion
P. and Negative Stroke Scale
P. and Negative Syndrome Scale (PANSS)
P. and Negative Syndrome Scale-Component Excited (PANSS-EC)
p. occipital sharp transient
p. occipital sharp transients of sleep (POSTS)
p. picture-caption pair
p. result
p. score
p. sharp wave
p. symptom
p. symptom dimension
positive airway pressure (PAP)
positive-going paradigm
positively
p. bathmotropic
p. correlated region
positivity of Input 1, 2
positron
p. emission tomography (PET)
p. emission tomography-fluorodeoxyglucose (PET-FDG)
p. emission tomography technique
p. emission tomography with [^{18}F]-labeled
post
p. baseline visit
Caspar retraction p.
p. hoc analysis
p. hoc stimulation
p. hoc stratification
p. hoc test
p. hoc testing
iliac p.
Isola spinal implant system iliac p.
Luque-Galveston p.
perineal p.
p. recovery
p. stroke depression
p. TIA depression
postactivation
p. depression
p. exhaustion
p. facilitation
postadrenalectomy syndrome
postambivalence
postambivalent
p. phase
p. phase stage
postanoxic
p. coma
p. dystonia
p. encephalopathy
p. myoclonus
postapoplectic epilepsy
postbasic stare
postbulbar motor nucleus
postcardiotomy
postcentral
p. area
p. fissure
p. gyrus
p. resection
p. sulcus
postcentralis
gyrus p.
sulcus p.

postchiasmic eminence
postclival
p. fissure
p. sulcus
postcommissurales
fibrae p.
postcommissural fiber
postconcussion
p. amnesia
p. headache
p. neurosis
p. syndrome
postconcussive amnesia
postcontusional brain syndrome
postcontusion syndrome encephalopathy
postdiphtheritic paralysis
post-ECT
postelectroconvulsive
postembolization angiogram
postencephalitic
p. behavior syndrome
p. myoclonus
p. parkinsonism
postepileptic paralysis
posterior
p. accessory olivary nucleus
p. acoustic stria
p. alexia
p. aphasia
area hypothalamica p.
arteria cerebelli inferior p.
arteria cerebri p.
arteria choroidea p.
arteria spinalis p.
arteria temporalis p.
p. atlantoaxial arthrodesis
p. auricular plexus
p. beaten copper appearance
p. bone graft
p. branch of axillary nerve
p. callosal vein
p. callosotomy
p. canal line
p. central convolution
p. central gyrus
p. cerebellar artery
p. cerebellar notch
cerebellomedullaris p.
p. cerebellomedullary cistern
p. cerebral artery
p. cerebral commissure
p. cerebral territory infarction
p. cervical fixation
p. cervical spinal instrumentation
p. cervical spine surgery
p. choroidal artery
p. cingulate
p. cingulate gyrus
p. cingulate region
p. circle of Willis
p. circulation ischemia
cisterna cerebellomedullaris p.
p. clinoid process (PCP)
columna p.
p. column cordotomy
p. column lesion
p. column osteosynthesis
p. column of spinal cord
p. column syndrome
commissura alba p.
commissura grisea p.
p. communicating artery (PComA)
p. communicating nerve
p. compartment lesion
p. construct
p. cord syndrome
p. cranial fossa
p. craniocervical junction
p. decompression
decussatio tegmentalis p.
p. distraction instrumentation
p. dominant activity
ductus semicircularis p.
p. ecchymosis
p. external arcuate fiber
fasciculus longitudinalis p.
p. fasciculus proprius
p. fixation system biomechanics
forceps p.
p. fossa aneurysm
p. fossa approach
p. fossa-atrial shunt
p. fossa craniotomy
p. fossa dural arteriovenous fistula
p. fossa extradural hematoma
p. fossa lesion
p. fossa meningioma
p. fossa syndrome
p. fossa tumor
p. frontal hypoperfusion
p. funiculus
p. fusiform gyrus

NOTES

posterior *(continued)*
p. gray commissure
gyrus paracentralis p.
gyrus temporalis transversalis p.
p. hippocampal activation
p. hook-rod spinal instrumentation
p. horn
p. hypothalamic area
p. hypothalamic nucleus
p. hypothalamic region
incisura cerebelli p.
p. inferior cerebellar artery (PICA)
p. inferior cerebellar artery syndrome
p. inferior communicating artery (PICA)
p. inferior communicating artery aneurysm
p. interbody lumbar spinal fusion
p. intercavernous sinus
p. intermediate groove
p. intermediate sulcus
p. interosseous nerve
p. interpositus nucleus
p. interspinous wiring
p. joint syndrome
p. lacerate foramen
p. language area lesion
p. language cortex
p. leukoencephalopathy syndrome
p. limb of internal capsule
p. lobe of cerebellum
p. lobe of hypophysis
p. lobe of pituitary gland
p. longitudinal bundle
p. longitudinal ligament
p. lower cervical spine stabilization
p. lower cervical spine surgery
p. lumbar interbody fusion (PLIF)
p. lumbar interbody fusion surgery
p. lumbar spine and sacrum surgery
p. lunate lobule
p. marginal vein
p. medial nucleus of thalamus
p. median fissure
p. median fissure of medulla oblongata
p. median fissure of spinal cord
p. median sulcus of medulla oblongata
p. median sulcus of spinal cord
p. medullary velum
nervus ampullaris p.
nervus auricularis p.
nervus cutaneous antebrachii p.
nervus cutaneous brachii p.
nervus cutaneous femoralis p.
nervus cutaneous femoris p.
nervus ethmoidalis p.
nervus interosseus antebrachii p.
p. neuropore
p. notch of cerebellum
p. nuclear complex of the thalamus
nucleus cochlearis p.
nucleus hypothalamicus p.
p. nucleus of hypothalamus
nucleus interpositus p.
nucleus lateralis p.
p. nucleus of oculomotor nerve
nucleus olivaris accessorius p.
nucleus paramedianus p.
nucleus periventricularis p.
nucleus raphes p.
nucleus thoracicus p.
p. nucleus of vagus nerve
p. occipitocervical approach
p. paracentral gyrus
p. parietal cortex (PPC)
p. parietal hypoperfusion
p. parolfactory sulcus
pars retrolentiformis cruris p.
p. peduncle of thalamus
p. perforated substance
p. pericallosal vein
p. periventricular nucleus
p. pillar of fornix
p. pituitary fossa
p. pituitary gland ectopia
posterioris apex cornus p.
p. primary ramus
p. pulmonary branch of vagus nerve
p. pyramid of the medulla
p. quadrigeminal body
p. rachischisis
radiatio thalami p.
radiatio thalamica p.
radix p.
p. raphe nucleus
p. recess
p. recess of interpeduncular fossa
recessus p.
regio hypothalamica p.
p. rhizotomy
p. rhythm
p. rod system
p. root
p. root of ansa cervicalis
p. root ganglion
p. root of spinal nerve
p. segmental fixation
p. semicircular canal (PSC)

sinus intercavernosus p.
spina bifida p.
p. spinal artery
p. spinal cord syndrome
p. spinal fusion
p. spinal plating
p. spinal sclerosis
p. spinocerebellar tract
stria cochlearis p.
substantia perforata p.
sulcus intermedius p.
sulcus lateralis p.
sulcus parolfactorius p.
p. superior fissure
p. surgical exposure of sacrum and coccyx
p. tegmental decussation
p. temporobasal vein
p. thalamic radiation
p. thalamic tubercle
p. thoracic nucleus
p. tibial nerve
p. tibial nerve-evoked potential
tractus spinocerebellaris p.
tractus trigeminothalamicus p.
p. transverse temporal gyrus
p. trigeminothalamic tract
p. truncal vagotomy
truncus vagalis p.
p. upper cervical spine surgery
p. vagal trunk
p. vein of corpus callosum
p. vein of septum pellucidum
vena septi pellucidi p.
ventralis oralis p.
p. vermis syndrome
p. vomer

posteriores
fibrae arcuatae externae p.
nervi labiales p.
nervi scrotales p.
nervi supraclaviculares p.
rami temporales p.

posteriori
a p.

posterioris
apex cornus p.
p. apex cornus posterior
bulbus cornus p.
cervix columnae p.
nucleus commissurae p.
pars sublentiformis cruris p.
rami gastrici posteriores trunci vagalis p.
rami perineales nervi cutanei femoris p.
ramus occipitalis nervi auricularis p.
vena cornus p.

posterior-lateral lumbar spinal fusion

posterius
cornu p.
corpus quadrigeminum p.
foramen caecum p.

posteroinferior
p. cerebellar artery
ventral p. (VPI)

posterolateral
p. approach
p. bone graft
p. bone grafting
p. bone graft placement
p. costotransversectomy
p. costotransversectomy incision
p. costotransversectomy technique
p. fissure
p. groove
p. lumbosacral fusion
p. nucleus
p. sclerosis
p. spinal artery
p. sulcus
p. tract
ventral p. (VPL)

posterolateralis
fissura p.
nucleus tegmentalis p.
nucleus ventralis p.
sulcus p.
tractus p.

posteromedialis
nucleus ventralis p.
ramus frontalis p.
ventralis p.

posteromedial nucleus

posteromedian column of spinal cord

posteroparietal

posterotemporal
p. artery occlusion

posteroventral
p. pallidotomy
p. sensorimotor pallidum

NOTES

postexertional malaise
postfundibular eminence
postganglionares
neurofibrae p.
postganglionic
p. efferent
p. motor neuron
p. nerve fiber
p. neurofiber
p. oculosympathetic palsy
postganglionicae
neurofibrae p.
posthemiplegic
p. athetosis
p. chorea
p. paralysis
posthemorrhagic hydrocephalus
postherpetic
p. neuralgia (PHN)
p. neuralgia prophylaxis
posthippocampal fissure
posthypnotic amnesia
posthypophysectomy traction syndrome
posthypoxic myoclonus
postictal
p. blood flow switch
p. cognitive dysfunction
p. migrainous headache
p. paresis
p. slowing
p. suppression
posticus
locus perforatus p.
p. palsy
p. paralysis
tetanus p.
postinduction
p. caudate
p. occipital cortex
postinfection
p. encephalomyelopathy
p. perivascular myelinoclasis
postinfectious
p. disseminated encephalomyelitis
p. hydrocephalus
p. leukoencephalitis
p. myelitis
p. polyneuritis
postinfective encephalitis
postinoculation poliomyelitis
postirradiation OVM
postischemic seizure
postjunctional
postlaminectomy
p.-l. kyphosis
p.-l. syndrome
p.-l. two-level spondylolisthesis
postleucotomy syndrome
postlingual fissure
postlobotomy syndrome
post-lumbar puncture headache
postlumbar puncture syndrome
postlunate fissure
postmalaria neurologic syndrome
postmeningitic hydrocephalus
postmenopausal seizure
postmortem
p. brain tissue
p. data
p. finding
p. spinal cord
p. study
p. technique
post-movement beta desynchronization
postneuritic atrophy
postnodular sulcus
postocular optic neuritis
postoperative
p. angiogram
p. arachnoiditis
p. bracing
p. care
p. confusion
p. corticosteroid
p. extubation
p. immobilization
p. infection
p. lumbosacral orthosis
p. paraplegia
p. regimen
p. skull defect
p. tetany
postparainfectious encephalomyelitis
postparalytic
postpartum
p. necrosis
p. pituitary necrosis syndrome
p. syndrome
postpolio
p. sequela
p. syndrome
postpoliomyelitis syndrome
postprandial
postpsychotic
postpuberty
postpubescence
postpump seizure
postpyramidal
p. fissure
p. sulcus
postpyramidalis
fissura p.
postradiation fibrosis
postrape syndrome

postrema
area p.
p. area posttraumatic
postrhinal fissure
postrolandic
p. area
postrotational nystagmus
POSTS
positive occipital sharp transients of sleep
POSTS on electroencephalogram
postspell symptom
postspike facilitation
poststress ankle/arm Doppler index
postsylvian
postsynaptic
p. compensatory mechanism
p. cortical neuronal potential
p. enhancement
p. excitation
p. fold
p. 5-HT2 receptor
p. 5-HT3 receptor
p. membrane
p. neuromuscular junction
p. neuron
p. stimulation
posttest level
posttetanic
p. exhaustion
p. facilitation
p. potentiation (PTP)
posttorque pulse
posttorture syndrome
posttranslational modification
posttranslation phosphorylation
posttraumatic
p. amnesia
p. amnestic syndrome
p. apoplexy
p. apoplexy of Bollinger
p. brain histology
p. brain syndrome
p. delirium
p. dementia
p. epilepsy
p. epileptiform activity
p. frontal lesion
p. headache
p. hydrocephalus
p. insomnia
p. intradiploic pseudomeningocele
p. kyphosis
p. leptomeningeal cyst
p. neck syndrome
p. neuralgia
p. neuroma
p. neurosis
p. osteoporosis
p. pain
p. pain syndrome
postrema area p.
p. spinal deformity
p. stress symptom
p. symptom formation
p. vertigo
postural
P. Assessment Scale for Stroke Patients (PASS)
p. hypertension
p. instability
p. myoneuralgia
p. orthostatic tachycardia syndrome
p. reaction
p. reflex
p. syncope
p. tremor
p. unsteadiness
p. vertigo
posture
p. agnosia
p. examination
p. reflex abnormality
p. sense
posturing
axial p.
bizarre p.
decerebrate p.
decorticate p.
unilateral dystonic p.
posturography
postvaccinal
p. encephalitis
p. encephalomyelitis
p. encephalomyelopathy
p. encephalopathy
p. myelitis
p. poliomyelitis
postvaccinial leukoencephalitis
potassium (K)
p. acetate
p. acetate, potassium bicarbonate, and potassium citrate

NOTES

potassium *(continued)*
p. bicarbonate
p. bicarbonate and potassium chloride, effervescent
p. bicarbonate, potassium chloride, and potassium citrate
p. bicarbonate and potassium citrate, effervescent
p. bromide
p. channel
p. channel gene
p. chloride
p. chloride and potassium gluconate
p. citrate and citric acid
p. citrate and potassium gluconate
p. imbalance
low p.
p. phosphate and sodium phosphate
p. salicylate
serum p.
potassium-aggravated myotonia (PAM)
potatorum
tremor p.
potato tumor of neck
potency
antidopaminergic p.
potential
abuse p.
acoustic evoked p.
action p.
auditory compound actional p.
auditory evoked p.
biphasic action p.
bizarre high-frequency p.
brain p.
brainstem auditory evoked p. (BAEP)
brainstem evoked p.
cerebral p.
cochlear microphonic p.
compound motor action p. (CMAP)
compound muscle action p. (CMAP)
compound nerve action p. (CNAP)
p. correlation
cortical somatosensory evoked p.
p. cumulative trauma disorder
demarcation p.
dermatosensory evoked p.
direct auditory compound actional p.
direct cortical stimulation and somatosensory evoked p. (SSEP)
electrical evoked p.
electromyographic p.
endplate p. (EPP)
equal p.
event-related p.
evoked p. (EP)
excitatory postsynaptic p. (EPSP, ESEP)
extracellular action p.
extrapyramidal symptom p.
extreme somatosensory evoked p.
fasciculation p.
fibrillation p.
generator p.
giant motor unit action p.
glossokinetic p.
heartbeat p.
inhibitory postsynaptic p. (IPSP)
injury p.
latency-evoked p.
localized evoked p.
median mixed nerve action p.
membrane p.
miniature end-plate p. (MEEP)
monophasic action p.
motor evoked p. (MEP)
motor unit p. (MUP)
motor unit action p. (MUAP)
motor unit potential amplitude p.
multimodality evoked p. (MEP)
muscle fiber action p.
myogenic motor evoked p.
myotonic p.
nascent motor unit p.
nerve action p.
neurogenic motor evoked p.
normal resting p.
peroneal somatosensory evoked p.
phase reversal p.
piezoelectric p.
posterior tibial nerve-evoked p.
postsynaptic cortical neuronal p.
p. predisposing factor
pretreatment binding p.
prothrombotic p.
pudendal somatosensory evoked p.
receptor p.
resting membrane p.
rhythmic repetitive muscle p.
satellite p.
scalp electrical p.
sensory compound action p.
sensory evoked p. (SEP)
sensory nerve action p. (SNAP)
serrated action p.
small motor unit p.
somatosensory evoked p. (SSEP)
spike p.
spinal sensory evoked p.
steady-state visual evoked p.

suicide p.
p. suicide victim
sural sensory p.
transcranial motor evoked p. (TeMEP)
transmembrane p. (TMP)
trigeminal evoked p. (TEP)
unpatterned flash visual evoked p.
visual evoked p. (VEP)
visual evoked cortical p.
weight gain p.

potentiation
late-phase long-term p. (L-LTP)
posttetanic p. (PTP)
short-term p. (STP)

potentiometer
angle position p.

Pott
P. abscess
P. disease
P. paralysis
P. paraplegia
P. puffy tumor

Potter syndrome

Potzl syndrome

pouch
Blake p.
pharyngeal p.
Rathke p.
spinal extradural arachnoid p.

Pourfour du Petit syndrome

pouting reflex

poverty
Liddle psychomotor p.
p. of speech

povidone-iodine
aqueous p.-i.

Powassan
P. encephalitis
P. virus

powder
antibiotic p.
Avitene p.

power
p. amplifier
combined predictive p.
p. drill
p. dynamic
endocratic p.
global field p. (GFP)
illusion of p.
mind p.
predictive p.
processing p.
p. router
p. spectral analysis

powered
p. automatic skull perforator
p. automatic stopping drill
p. automatic stopping drill point

PPA
primary progressive aphasia

PPC
posterior parietal cortex

PPP
pentose phosphate pathway

PPPMA
progressive postpolio muscle atrophy

PPR
photoparoxysmal response

PPRF
paramedian pontine reticular formation

PPT
preprotachykinin

PQ calcium channel

PR
OncoScint PR

practiced task

Prader-Willi syndrome

praecox
dementia p.
neurasthenia p.

pragmatagnosia

pragmatamnesia

pramipexole
p. dihydrochloride
p. monotherapy
p. study

prandic epilepsy

praxis
visual constructional p.

praziquantel

preacher's hand

prealbumin protein

preamplifier
epoxy-mounted p.

preataxic

precapillary end foot

Precedex

precentral
p. area
p. cerebellar vein

NOTES

P

precentral *(continued)*
p. fissure
p. gyrus
p. sulcus
precentralis
fissura p.
gyrus p.
sulcus p.
precerebelli
nucleus reticularis paramedianus p.
precession
fast imaging with steady p. (FISP)
Larmor p.
steady-state free p.
precessional frequency
prechiasmatic sulcus
prechiasmaticus
sulcus p.
prechiasmatis
sulcus p.
precipitating stimulus
preclinical stage
preclival
p. fissure
p. sulcus
Preclude
P. dura substitute prosthesis
P. spinal membrane
precognition
precollagenous filamentous material
precoma
precommissural
p. bundle
p. septal area
p. septal nucleus
p. septum
precommissurales
fibrae p.
precommissuralis
nucleus septalis p.
preconditioning
ischemic p.
preconsciousness
precontoured unit rod
preconvulsive
precoronal bur hole
precueing
auditory spatial p.
preculminalis
fissura p.
preculminate fissure
precuneal fissure
precunealis
arteria p.
precuneate
precuneus
precursor
neural crest p.
neuronal p.
p. sign to rupture of aneurysm
precursory symptom
predatory violence
predecessor
phylogenetic p.
predementia
predictive
p. characteristic
p. factor
p. power
p. property
p. relationship
predictor
peritraumatic p.
pharmacological p.
symptom-related p.
predisposition
fundamental p.
predominantly predormital sleep paralysis
predormital
predormitum
predorsal bundle
preexcision spike
preexisting
p. cognitive impairment
p. dementia
p. representation
preference
gaze p.
preferential
p. anosmia
p. occupancy
prefixation
prefixed chiasm
prefrontal
p. cortex
p. cortex activation
p. cortex of the brain
p. cortical area
p. cortical volume
p. flow
p. hypometabolism
p. leukotomy
p. lobe
p. lobotomy
p. metabolism
p. region
p. vein
prefrontales
venae p.
prefrontal-insular cerebellar network
pregabalin

pregangionares
neurofibrae p.
preganglionic
p. autonomic fiber
p. efferent
p. motor neuron
p. nerve fiber
p. neurofiber
preganglionicae
neurofibrae p.
pregeniculate nucleus
pregeniculatus
nucleus p.
prehemiplegic chorea
preictal
p. headache
p. myoclonus
preinduction
p. occipital cortex
p. thickness
preinsular gyrus
preischemic blood glucose
preketamine
prelemniscal radiation (RAPRL)
preliminary analysis
prelipid substance
prematura
alopecia p.
premature
p. closure
p. confrontation
p. discharge
p. infant bowing reflex
p. infant head circumference measurement
p. infant hydrocephalus
p. infant hypocalcemia
p. infant hypothyroidism
p. infant kernicterus
p. infant meningitis
p. infant neurodevelopmental outcome
p. infant periventricular leukomalacia
p. infant pontosubicular degeneration
p. infant seizure
p. infant spastic hemiparesis
p. infant subarachnoid hemorrhage
p. infant tyrosinemia
premedullary
p. arteriovenous fistular
p. cistern
premenstrual dysphoria
PremiCron nonabsorbable suture
Premier anterior cervical plate system
premonitory
p. headache
p. stage
p. symptom
premorbid
p. ability
p. cognition
p. dementia
p. functioning
p. personality trait
p. trauma
premotor
p. area
p. cortex
p. neuron
p. syndrome
prenodular fissure
preoccipital
p. incisure
p. notch
preoccipitalis
incisura p.
preoperative
p. angiogram
p. angiography
p. evaluation
p. planning
p. preparation
p. sedation
p. tomography
preoptic
p. area
p. hypothalamus
p. nucleus
p. recess
p. region
preoptica
area p.
preparalytic
preparation
facet joint p.
preoperative p.
rod contour p.
wire contour p.

NOTES

prepiriform
p. cortex
p. gyrus
prepontine
p. cistern
p. lesion
p. region
preprotachykinin (PPT)
prepyramidal
p. fissure
p. sulcus
p. tract
prepyramidalis
fissura p.
pre-Rolandic artery occlusion
prerolandic sulcus
prerubral
p. field
p. nucleus
prerupture of aneurysm
presacral
p. nerve
p. neurectomy
p. sympathectomy
presacralis
nervus p.
presaturation pulse
presbyacusis, presbycusis
presenile dementia
presenilin (PA)
p. 1 (PS1)
p. 2 (PS2)
p. gene
p. mutant
preservation
carotid p.
lordosis p.
lumbar lordosis p.
p. technique
zone of partial p.
preservative-free normal saline
preserved conduction velocity
presigmoid approach
PRESS
point-resolved spectroscopy
press
environmental p.
pressor
p. fiber
p. nerve
pressoreceptive
pressoreceptor
p. nerve
p. reflex
p. system
pressosensitive
pressure
p. algometer
p. anesthesia
p. autoregulation
p. autoregulatory status
bilevel positive airway p. (BiPAP)
carbon dioxide arterial p.
central venous p.
cerebral perfusion p.
cerebrospinal fluid p.
closure p.
colloid oncotic p.
p. cone
continuous positive airway p. (CPAP)
cranial perfusion p.
diastolic blood p.
p. distension technique
feeding mean arterial p. (FMAP)
p. gauge
increased intracranial p.
intracranial p. (ICP)
intracranial epidural p.
intraocular p.
intraspinal epidural p.
intravascular p.
mean arterial blood p.
microvascular p. (MVP)
mouth occlusion p.
nasal continuous positive airway p.
p. necrosis
p. neuropathy
opening p.
p. palsy
p. paralysis
partial p.
p. point
positive airway p. (PAP)
positive end-expiratory p. (PEEP)
pulmonary capillary wedge p.
raised intracranial p.
p. receptor
regional cerebral perfusion p. (rCPP)
p. sense
p. of speech
supraglottic p.
tentorial p.
transdiaphragmatic p.
transducer-measured intracranial venous p.
pressure-arresting point
pressure-exciting point
pressure-gradient change
pressure-volume index
Preston ligamentum flavum forceps
prestriate area

presubiculum
presumptive basis
presurgical assessment
presylvian fissure
presynaptic
p. congenital myasthenic syndrome
p. membrane
p. membrane protein
p. nerve ending
p. neuron
p. stimulation
subsensitization of p.
p. terminal
presyncope
pretectal
p. area
p. lesion
p. nucleus
p. region
p. syndrome
pretectales
nuclei p.
pretectalis
area p.
pretectoolivares
fibrae p.
pretectoolivary fiber
pretectum
prethymectomy
pretraumatic
p. amnesia
p. risk factor
p. vulnerability
pretreatment
p. binding potential
p. measure
prevention
infection p.
rod rotation p.
preverbal attentional processing
prevertebral
p. ganglion
p. plexus
Prévost sign
PRF
prolactin-releasing factor
PRFR
percutaneous radiofrequency retrogasserian rhizotomy
PRGR
percutaneous retrogasserian glycerol rhizolysis
PRH
prolactin-releasing hormone
priapi
os p.
primary
p. active compound
p. afferent depolarization (PAD)
p. afferent loss
p. afferent neuron
p. afferent nociceptor
p. alveolar hypoventilation
p. amebic meningoencephalitis
p. amenorrhea
p. aminoaciduria
p. angiitis
p. angiitis of the central nervous system
p. angiitis of the CNS
p. antiphospholipid antibody syndrome
p. auditory cortex
p. axotomy
p. brain lymphoma
p. brain tumor
p. brain vesicle
p. central nervous system lymphoma (PCNSL)
p. clip
p. CNS lymphoma
p. drive
p. dystonia
p. effect
p. efficacy outcome
p. ending
p. end-to-end anastomosis
p. enduring negative symptom
p. enuresis
p. epidural cyst
p. fibromyalgia syndrome
p. fissure of cerebellum
p. generalized epilepsy
p. generalized seizure
p. group
p. headache
p. hydrocephalus
p. idiopathic seizure
p. insomnia
p. intracranial plasmacytoma

NOTES

primary *(continued)*
p. intramedullary lymphoma
p. lateral sclerosis
p. leptomeningeal lymphoma
p. mechanism
p. motor area
p. nervous system lymphoma
p. neurasthenia
p. neuroectodermal tumor
p. neuronal cell
p. neuronal degeneration
p. nonenduring negative symptom
p. object
p. optic atrophy
p. orthostatic tremor
p. pharmacological approach
p. pontine hemorrhage
p. process
p. progressive amyotrophy
p. progressive aphasia (PPA)
p. progressive cerebellar degeneration
p. receiving area
p. receptive area
p. rhinencephalic psychomotor epilepsy
p. risk factor
p. senile dementia
p. sensation
p. sensorimotor cortex
p. sensory cortex
p. sensory neuron
p. shock
p. Sjögren syndrome
p. somatic problem
p. somatomotor area
p. somatosensory area
p. somatosensory cortex
p. subarachnoid supratentorial hemorrhage
p. synaptic cleft
p. thought disorder
p. trunk syndrome
p. vertigo
p. victim
p. visual area
p. visual cortex
p. vitreous

primary/secondary distinction
primate dorsal stream
primates motor cortex
primer instrument
primidone
priming dose
primitiva
meninx p.

primitive
p. emotional level
p. lamina terminalis
p. maxillary vein
p. meninx
p. neuroectodermal tumor (PNET)
p. neuroepithelial tumor
p. node
p. otic artery
p. streak
p. trigeminal artery
p. trigeminal artery variant

primordial inferior hypophysial artery
principal
p. olivary nucleus
p. sensory nucleus of trigeminal nerve
p. sensory nucleus of the trigeminus

principal-components analysis
principalis
nucleus olivaris p.

principle
Bolam P.
image formation p.
normalization p.
Pauli exclusion p.
physicochemical p.
Tarasoff p.
wellness p.

Pringle disease
prinomastat
Prinzmetal vasospastic angina pectoris
Priodax
prion
p. analog
p. disease
p. protein (PrP)

prism
Fresnel paste-on p.

PRL
prolactin

proaccelerin
proapoptotic
proband
p. condition
p. status

PROBE
PRO-ton Brain exam

probe
bipolar cautery p.
Bipolar Circumactive P. (BICAP)
Bunnell dissecting p.
Bunnell forwarding p.
Dandy p.
Doppler p.
electromagnetic flow p.

electromagnetic focusing field p.
extended sector ultrasonic p.
fluoroptic thermometry p.
gearshift p.
hemispherical contact p.
indirect p.
intraoperative ultrasonic p.
Jacobson p.
Jannetta p.
Laserflo Doppler p.
LED p.
monitoring p.
neuro trend p.
Nucleotome aspiration p.
Nucleotome Flex II flexible cutting p.
P3 p.
$PbrO_2$ monitoring p.
pedicle sounding p.
right-angle blunt p.
SpineStat p.
TCD p.
Transonics flow p.
ultrasonic p.
Vasamedics laser Doppler flow p.
virtual p.

problem
conceptual p.
core p.
Daily Record of Severity of P.'s
fundamental conceptual p.
integrative p.
primary somatic p.
sleep p.
somatic p.
subtle memory p.

Probst bundle

Procanbid

procarbazine
p. hydrochloride
p., lomustine (CCNU), vincristine (PCV)

Procedure-200
Shedler-Western Assessment P.

procedure
ablative central neurosurgical p.
activation p.
Albee shelf p.
analysis p.
anterior stabilization p.
assessment p.
Bonferroni-Dunn p.
Buschke Free and Cued Selective Reminding P.
Caldwell-Luc p.
carotid ablative p.
carotid Amytal p.
cervical spine stabilization p.
clinical p.
Cloward p.
cloze p.
coiling p.
Colonna shelf p.
debulking p.
demyelinating p.
Dewar posterior cervical fixation p.
DREZ p.
EDAS p.
EEG activating p.
egg-shelling p.
electrophysiological p.
extracranial-to-intracranial bypass p.
fetal shunt p.
genioglossus advancement p.
Gill p.
Hacker p.
Heifetz p.
Hoffmann and Mohr p.
hydrocephalus shunt p.
IDET p.
immunoperoxidase p.
instillation p.
intradiscal electrothermal p.
intrauterine shunt p.
Jaeger-Hamby p.
Jannetta microvascular decompression p.
Kestenbaum p.
Koerte p.
LDD p.
lower cervical spine p.
microoperative p.
microsurgical p.
Mitofsky-Aaksberg random digit dialing p.
Müller-König p.
neurodiagnostic p.
neurosurgical p.
nonmicrosurgical p.
Nucleotome p.
pi p.
porte manteau p.

NOTES

procedure *(continued)*
prototype matching p.
psychophysical p.
Q-sort p.
radiosurgical lesioning p.
rating p.
retrogasserian p.
Scaramella p.
single bur hole p.
Smith-Robinson p.
standard rating p.
surgical p.
SWAP p.
SWAP-200 assessment p.
transnasal septal displacement p.
two-stage p.
upper cervical spine p.
ventriculovascular shunt p.
Wada p.

Proceed hemostatic agent

procerus sign

process
absent spinous p.
active pathophysiologic p.
affective p.
age-related deterioration p.
age-related developmental p.
anterior clinoid p.
apical p.
autoimmune p.
axonal p.
brain p.
central timing p.
clinoid p.
common central p.
continuous inflammatory p.
declarative memory p.
deficient spinous p.
Deiters p.
dendritic p.
deterioration p.
developmental p.
diagnostic p.
emotional memory p.
environmental p.
escalative p.
executive p.
fundamental cognitive p.
GFAP-stained p.
identification p.
implicit p.
intact spinous p.
intracellular metabolic p.
kindling p.
Lenhossék p.
lexical p.
mastoid p.
memory p.
metabolic p.
motivational p.
neurocognitive p.
neurogenic p.
neuronal p.
odontoid p.
ongoing cognitive p.
ontogenic p.
orthographic p.
pathophysiologic p.
perceptual p.
phonological p.
posterior clinoid p. (PCP)
primary p.
secondary p.
semantic p.
sensory p.
spinous p.
stress-illness p.
sublexical p.
sucker p.
uncinate p.
viscerosensory p.
withdrawal p.

processing
affective p.
affect-related p.
altered tau p.
p. area
beta-amyloid p.
cell p.
declarative emotional memory p.
emotional information p.
emotional memory p.
memory p.
p. power
preverbal attentional p.
receptive language p.
signal p.
speech p.
speed of p.
tau p.
temporal p.
p. time
visual motor p.
word p.

processus
p. intrajugularis ossis occipitalis
p. intrajugularis ossis temporalis
p. jugularis ossis occipitalis

prochlorperazine maleate

prochordal plate

procoagulant
endothelial cell-derived p.

proconvulsant effect

proctalgia fugax

proctoparalysis
proctoplegia
proctospasm
procursiva
  aura p.
procursive
  p. chorea
  p. epilepsy
procyclidine
prodromal psychotic symptom
prodrome
  dementia p.
  epileptic p.
product
  gene p.
  NeuroCell-HD neural cell transplant p.
  NeuroCell-PD porcine neural cell transplant p.
  nutraceutical p.
  Valleylab neurosurgical p.
  Vertigraft allograft p.
production
  adrenal androgen p.
  eicosanoid p.
  emotion p.
  endolymph p.
  word p.
prodynorphin
proencephalon
proenkephalin
Proetz test
Pro-Fast
  P.-F. HS capsule
  P.-F. SR capsule
profile
  P. anterior plate system
  P. anterior spinal plate
  Aphasia Diagnostic P.'s
  Communication Skills P.
  conversion V p.
  demyelinative spinal fluid p.
  Derogatis Stress P.
  diagnostic p.
  Emory Functional Ambulation P.
  eye-motor-verbal p.
  Functional Limitation P. (FLP)
  Life Skills P.
  microsomal isoenzyme metabolism p.
  P. of Mood States, Vigor
  neuropsychological p.
  Nottingham Health P.'s
  Pain Patient P.
  Pain Perception P.
  Q-score p.
  risk-benefit p.
  Sickness Impact P. (SIP)
  symptom p.
  therapeutic p.
  velocity p.
  P. VS
profiling
  facial p.
Profil-O-Plastic plate
profunda
  cisterna intercruralis p.
  vena cerebri media p.
profundae
  fibrae pontis p.
  venae cerebri p.
profundi
  nervi temporales p.
  rami musculares nervi fibularis p.
  rami musculares nervi peronei p.
profundum
  stratum album p.
  stratum griseum p.
  stratum medullare p.
profundus
  nervus fibularis p.
  nervus peroneus p.
  nervus petrosus p.
PROGENI
 Parkinson Research The Organized Genetic Initiative
  PROGENI study
progenitor
  p. cell
  oligodendrocyte p. (OP)
  temperature-sensitive neural p.
progestational activity
progesterone
  p. effect
  p. level
  luteal phase p.
  natural p.
  oral p.
  p. receptor
  p. secretion
  synthetic p.
progestin

NOTES

P

prognostic
P. Scale
p. status
Prograf
program
cerebral palsy infant stimulation p.
clinical intervention p.
coercion p.
FEAR p.
Leksell GammaPlan computerized p.
Leksell SurgiPlan computerized p.
LISREL 8 p.
multicomponent p.
multidisciplinary pilot project p. (MPPP)
Phono-Graphix p.
pilot p.
research p.
standard bone algorithm p.
treatment p.
UPBEAT p.
programmable
p. pulse generator
p. valve
programmed cell death (PCD)
programming
neurolinguistic p.
P. Wand
progressing stroke
progression
backward p.
clinical p.
cross-legged p.
dementia p.
symptom p.
progression-free survival
progressiva
dementia paratonia p.
dysbasia lordotica p.
dyssynergia cerebellaris p.
dystonia deformans p.
dystrophia musculorum p.
p. infantilis
leukodystrophia cerebri p.
ophthalmoplegia p.
paratonia p.
progressive
p. bulbar palsy of childhood
p. bulbar paralysis
p. bulbar paralysis of childhood
p. cerebellar tremor
p. cerebral
p. cerebral poliodystrophy
p. circumscribed cerebral atrophy
p. degenerative subcortical encephalopathy
P. Deterioration Scale
p. dialysis encephalopathy
p. dysarthria
p. epilepsy with mental retardation
p. epileptogenesis
p. external ophthalmoparesis
p. external ophthalmoplegia (PEO)
p. extraocular paresis
p. familial myoclonic epilepsy
p. flaccid quadriparesis
p. hydrocephalus
p. hypertrophic interstitial neuropathy
p. infantile bulbar palsy
p. infantile poliodystrophy
p. infantile spinal muscular atrophy
p. leptomeningeal fibrosis
p. lingual hemiatrophy
p. multifocal leukoencephalopathy (PML)
p. multifocal leuko-J encephalopathy
p. muscular dystrophy
p. myoclonic epilepsy
p. myoclonus epilepsy (PME)
p. necrotizing leukoencephaly
p. neuromuscular atrophy
p. neuropathic muscle atrophy
p. nonfluent aphasia
p. nuclear amyotrophy
p. posthemorrhagic ventriculomegaly
p. postpolio muscle atrophy (PPPMA)
p. rubella panencephalitis
p. spinal amyotrophy
p. spinal muscular atrophy
p. spongiform encephalopathy
p. subcortical encephalopathy
p. subcortical gliosis
p. supranuclear palsy (PSP)
p. systemic sclerosis
p. torsion spasm
p. traumatic encephalopathy
p. ventricular dilation
p. visual loss
ProHance
project
Harvard Atherosclerosis Reversibility P. (HARP)
projection
anteroposterior p.
p. area
axial p.
Caldwell p.
cerebrocerebellar p.
dopamine p.
dopaminergic p.

feedback p.
feedforward p.
p. fiber
filtered-back p.
ipsilateral p.
lateral p.
maximum intensity p.
minimum intensity p.
p. neurofiber
p. neuron
retrospective p.
sagittal p.
p. system
thalamocortical p.

projectionis
neurofibra p.

projective test

prolactin (PRL)
p. elevation
p. release
p. response
serum p.

prolactin-inhibiting
p.-i. factor (PIF)
p.-i. hormone

prolactinoma

prolactin-producing adenoma

prolactin-releasing
p.-r. factor (PRF)
p.-r. hormone (PRH)

prolactin-secreting
p.-s. pituitary adenoma
p.-s. pituitary tumor

prolapse
disk p.
mitral valve p.

proliferation
cell p.
control cell p.
dendrite p.
fibroblastic p.
granule cell p.
neuroepithelial cell p.
smooth muscle p.

proliferative malignant glial cell

proline urine level

Prolixin

Prolo function-economic rating scale

Proloid

prolongation
pulse repetition time p.

prolonged
p. exposure
p. nocturnal sleep
p. sedation

Prolopa

prolyl oligopeptidase

promethazine
p. hydrochloride
meperidine and p.

prominence
pedicle screw hardware p.

prominent phobic anxiety component

Prominol

PROMM
proximal myotonic myopathy

promontorii
ponticulus p.
subiculum p.

promoter
endogenous chromosomal p.

pronation sign

pronator
p. reflex
p. teres syndrome

prone
p. position
p. to relapse
p. straight leg raising test

pronuclei

proopiomelanocortin

ProOsteon 200R and 500R

prop
Oberto mouth p.

propagation
p. of activity
ictal p.

propallylonal

propantheline

proparacaine hydrochloride

Propavan

propentofylline

proper
p. fasciculus
p. neck positioning

properdin

property
affective p.
androgenic p.
anxiolytic p.
pharmacological p.
predictive p.

NOTES

property *(continued)*
receptor-binding p.
reinforcing p.
sedative p.
shape p.
thermoregulatory p.
thermosensory p.
prophylactic
p. anticonvulsant therapy
p. hypertensive hypervolemic hemodilution
p. medication
prophylaxis
anaphylactic shock p.
anticonvulsant p.
antimicrobial p.
postherpetic neuralgia p.
stroke p.
Propionibacterium acnes
propionic
p. acidemia
p. aciduria
propionyl-CoA carboxylase
Proplast
proplexus
propofol infusion
proportional sensitivity
proposagnosia
propranolamine
propranolol
p. hydrochloride
p. and hydrochlorothiazide
propria
dura p.
proprii
fasciculi p.
proprioception deficit
proprioceptive
p. nervous system
p. neuromuscular facilitation (PNF)
p. reflex
p. sense
p. sensibility
p. sensory deficit
p. vertigo
proprioceptor
propriospinal
p. myoclonus
p. system
proprius
anterior fasciculus p.
fasciculus anterior p.
fasciculus lateralis p.
lateral fasciculus p.
nucleus p.
posterior fasciculus p.
proptosis
propulsive gait
propylene glycol toxicity
propyliodone
prosencephalon
prosocele
prosocoele
Prosom
prosopagnosia
prosopalgia
prosopodiplegia
prosoponeuralgia
prosopoplegia
prosopospasm
prospective
p. experimental study design
p. memory
prostacyclin
prostaglandin
Prostaphlin
prostate-specific antigen (PSA)
prostatic
p. intraepithelial neoplasia (PIN)
p. plexus
prostaticus
plexus p.
prosthesis
AcroFlex disk p.
acrylic p.
articulating disk p.
auditory p.
ball-type disk p.
Bristol disk p.
Bryan cervical disk p.
Charité disk p.
composite disk p.
Cummins disk p.
elastic-type disk p.
hydraulic-type disk p.
Lee disk p.
Link SB Charité disk p.
mechanical-type disk p.
neural p.
NeuroCybernetic p. (NCP)
palatal lift p.
Preclude dura substitute p.
sacral segmental nerve stimulation implantable neural p.
spinal disk p.
prosthetic
p. disc nucleus device
p. disk nucleus (PDN)
p. heart valve
Prostigmin test
Protamine Zinc and Iletin I
protease
cysteine p.
p. inhibitor

membrane-anchored aspartyl p.
serine p.

protease-linked activation cloning system (PLACS)

protection
airway p.
cerebral p.

protective
p. effect
p. laryngeal reflex

protector
Adson dural p.

protein
p. 2
Abeta p.
acetylcholine-binding p.
alpha-synuclein p.
Alzheimer precursor p. (APP)
amyloid precursor p. (APP)
antiapoptotic p.
antiglial fibrillary acidic p.
argyrophil organizer region p.
B amyloid p.
basement membrane p.
Bence Jones p.
beta amyloid p.
betaB-Trace p. (beta-B-TP)
bifunctional p.
p. binding
p. binding interaction
p. binding pharmacokinetic
bone morphogenetic p. (BMP)
bone morphogenic p. (BMP)
brain-enriched hyaluronan binding p.
cAMP receptor p. (CRP)
cAMP response element binding p.
cellular prion p. (PrP^c)
cerebrospinal fluid p.
p. concentration
connexin 32 p.
C-reactive p.
CREB binding p.
p. C, S deficiency
cyclin-dependent kinase inhibitory p.
cytoskeletal p.
dynein p.
p. electrophoresis
encephalitogenic p.
estrogen-related p.
extracellular matrix p.
extracellular signal-regulated p.
FAK p.
FOS p.
G p.
gamma carboxylated p.
glial fibrillary acidic p. (GFAP)
growth-associated p.
heat shock p.
hemostasis-related p.
high animal p.
HIV-1-envelope p.
homeodomain p.
human prion p.
huntingtin p.
p. induced by vitamin K absence (PIVKA)
inhibitory p.
56 kD p.
p. kinase
p. kinase C (PKC)
p. kinase C inhibitor
matrix p.
membrane-associated p.
methyl-CpG-binding p.
microtubule-associated p.
mitogen-activated p. (MAP)
monoclonal antiglial fibrillary acidic p.
myelin basic p. (MBP)
myelin/oligodendrocyte-specific p. (MOSP)
neuronal apoptosis inhibitory p. (NAIP)
neuron-specific cytoskeletal p.
Nurrl p.
opioid precursor p.
parathyroid hormonelike p. (PLP)
Parkin p.
peripheral myelin p. 22
phosphorylate tau p.
plasma p.
prealbumin p.
presynaptic membrane p.
prion p. (PrP)
proteoglycan p.
proteolipid p.
ras p.
reelin p.
S-100 p.
S-100beta p.

NOTES

P

protein *(continued)*
p. S deficiency
serum p.
synaptosome associated p.
p. synthesis
tau p.
transthyretin p.
p. tyrosine phosphorylation
voltage-sensitive p.
p. zero
proteinaceous infectious particle
proteinase
aspartic p.
cysteine p.
serine p.
protein-bound iodine (PBI)
proteoglycan
aggrecan p.
biglycan p.
brevican p.
chondroitin sulfate p.
disk matrix p.
extracellular matrix p.
p. protein
versican p.
proteolipid protein
proteolysis
proteolytic fragment
proteomic
proteosome
extracellular p.
***Proteus* meningitis**
Proteus syndrome
prothrombin time (PT)
prothrombotic potential
protirelin
protocol
Computer-Aided Neurovascular Analysis and Simulation p. (CANVAS)
Dana-Farber Cancer Institute p.
Dysphagia Evaluation P.
fractionation p.
Gliadel wafer treatment p.
surveillance p.
treatment p.
Wada p.
proton
p. beam
p. beam radiation
p. density
p. density weighting
p. imaging
p. magnetic resonance spectroscopy
p. nuclear magnetic resonance spectroscopy
p. relaxation time
p. spectrum
PRO-ton Brain exam (PROBE)
proton-electron dipole-dipole interaction
proton-weighted image
Protopam
protopathic sensibility
protoplasmaticum
astrocytoma p.
protoplasmic
p. astrocyte
p. astrocytoma
protoporphyria
erythrocyte p.
protoporphyrin IX
protospasm
prototaxic
prototype
p. matching
p. matching procedure
protozoan infection
protracta
catatonia p.
protriptyline
protruded disk
protrusio defect
protrusion
disk p.
medullary p.
pseudopodial p.
protuberans
dermatofibrosarcoma p.
protuberantia occipitalis interna
Providence scoliosis system
Provigil
provocative testing
prowazekii
Rochalimaea p.
Prowler
P. double-tipped microcatheter
P. Plus catheter
Prowler-14 microcatheter
proximal
p. axonopathy
p. balloon occlusion
p. carotid ring
p. clipping
latency p.
p. myotonic myopathy (PROMM)
p. segment retraction
proximoataxia
Prozac Weekly
Prozine
PrP
prion protein
PrP^c
cellular prion protein

PrP-C (normal form)
***PrP* gene**
PrP-Sc (abnormal form)
Pruitt-Inahara shunt
pruning
neuronal p.
pruritus
localized p.
p. vulvae
PS1
presenilin 1
PS2
presenilin 2
PSA
prostate-specific antigen
psalteria (*pl. of* psalterium)
psalterial
psalterii
cavum p.
psalterium, pl. **psalteria**
psammocarcinoma
psammoma
p. body
Virchow p.
psammomatoid ossifying fibroma
psammomatous meningioma
psammous
PSC
posterior semicircular canal
P segment
pselaphesia, pselaphesis
pseudagraphia
Pseudallescheria boydii
pseudaphia
pseudarthrosis
documented p.
failed back syndrome with documented p.
p. rate
p. repair
pseudesthesia, pseudoesthesia
pseudoabducens
p. nerve paresis
p. palsy
pseudoagrammatism
pseudoagraphia
pseudoaneurysm
pseudoapoplexy
pseudoapraxia
pseudo-Argyll Robertson pupil
pseudoarthritis
pseudoataxia
pseudoathetosis
pseudoauthenticity
pseudo-battered child syndrome
pseudobulbar
p. palsy
p. paralysis
p. speech
pseudocele
pseudocephalocele
pseudocholinesterase
pseudochorea
pseudochromesthesia
pseudoclonus
pseudocoma
pseudocyesis
pseudocyst
secreting glial p.
pseudocystic hypodense lesion
pseudodebility
pseudodementia
p. of depression
depressive p.
hysterical p.
pseudoephedrine
pseudoepileptic seizure
pseudoepileptiform activity
pseudoesthesia (*var. of* pseudesthesia)
pseudofracture
pseudoganglion
Bochdalek p.
Cloquet p.
Valentin p.
pseudogene
pseudogeusesthesia
pseudogeusia
pseudo-Graefe sign
pseudo-Hurler
p.-H. disease
p.-H. syndrome
pseudohydrocephaly
pseudohypertrophic
p. muscular atrophy
p. muscular dystrophy
p. muscular paralysis
pseudohypertrophy
muscle p.
muscular p.
pseudohypnotics
pseudohypoparathyroidism
pseudoinclusion

NOTES

pseudointernuclear ophthalmoplegia
pseudoirreversible mechanism of action
pseudologia
pseudolumen
pseudomalignancy
pseudomedial longitudinal fasciculus lesion
pseudomemory
pseudomeningitis
pseudomeningocele
posttraumatic intradiploic p.
traumatic p.
Pseudomonaceae
Pseudomonas
P. aeruginosa
P. exotoxin
pseudomotivation
pseudomotor cerebri
pseudomuscular hypertrophy
pseudomyasthenia
ocular p.
pseudomyotonia
Debré-Sémélaigne p.
p. disease
pseudoneoplasm
pseudoneurological symptom grouping
pseudoneuroma
pseudoneuronophagia
pseudonomania
pseudonymity
pseudonymous
pseudoobstruction
pseudopalisading astrocytoma
pseudopapilledema
pseudoparalysis
arthritic general p.
congenital atonic p.
pseudoparaplegia
Basedow p.
pseudoparesis
pseudophotesthesia
pseudoplegia
pseudopodial protrusion
pseudopolycythemia
paresthetic p.
pseudopsammoma body
pseudopseudohypoparathyroidism
pseudoptosis
pseudopuberty
pseudorandom
pseudoreminiscence
pseudorosette
pseudosauthenticity
pseudosclerosis
Westphal p.
Westphal-Strümpell p.
pseudoseizure
pseudosplenium
pseudotabes
diabetic p.
pupillotonic p.
pseudotail
pseudotetanus
pseudotrismus
pseudotrisomy 13 syndrome
pseudotumor
p. cerebri
idiopathic orbital p.
orbital p.
pseudotumoral lymphocytic hypophysitis
pseudounipolar
p. ganglion cell
p. neuron
pseudoventricle
pseudovertigo
pseudovomiting
pseudo-Wernicke syndrome
pseudoxanthoma elasticum
pseudo-Zellweger syndrome
PSG
Parkinson Study Group
polysomnograph
Albert Grass Heritage PSG
psittacosis encephalitis
PS Medical Flow Control valve
psoas
p. abscess
p. muscle
psoriasis spondylitica
psoriatic arthritis
PSP
phenolsulfonphthalein
progressive supranuclear palsy
PSTH
peristimulus-time histogram
psuedoinclusion
nuclear p.
psuedoperiodic discharge
psychiatric
p. effect
p. medication
p. parameter
p. syndrome
psychiatry
American Association for Geriatric P. (AAGP)
Association of Directors of Medical Student Education in P. (ADMSEP)
p. and neurology
psychic
p. blindness
p. seizure

p. tic
p. wound
psychical
p. aura
p. manner
psychoactive chemical
psychoanalytic perspective
psychocardiac reflex
psychodynamic
p. effect
p. origin
psychoepileptic episode
psychogalvanic
p. reaction
p. reflex
p. reflex/response
p. response (PGR)
psychogenic
p. amnesia
p. chest pain
p. duodenal ulcer
p. dystonia
p. effort syndrome
p. epilepsy
p. fatigability
p. gastric ulcer
p. headache
p. hearing impairment
p. learning disorder
p. limb disorder
p. motor disorder
p. muscle disorder
p. musculoskeletal disorder
p. neurocirculatory disorder
p. nonepileptic seizure
p. obsessional disorder
p. origin
p. pain disorder
p. pelvic pain
p. peptic ulcer
p. precordial pain
p. respiratory disorder
p. rheumatic disorder
p. sexual disorder
p. skin disorder
p. sleep disorder
p. stomach disorder
p. torticollis
p. tremor
p. vertigo
psychological
p. consequence
p. construct
p. effect
p. response
p. state
p. strength
p. symptom
p. trauma
p. weakness
psychological/physiological arousal
psychologic test
psychometric
p. advantage
p. validity
psychomotor
p. abnormality
p. attack
p. behavioral disturbance
p. delay
p. epilepsy
p. impairment
p. phenomenon
p. retardation
p. seizure
p. slowing
p. speed
p. status
p. stress reaction
p. stupor
p. swelling
psychoneurotic depressive reaction
psychoorganic syndrome
psychopathic trait
psychopathologic accompaniment
psychopathology rating scale
psychopharmacologic agent
psychophysical procedure
psychophysiologic
p. insomnia
p. manifestation
psychophysiological insomnia
psychosensory aphasia
psychosine accumulation
psychosocial
p. function
p. perspective
p. symptom outcome
psychostimulant
p. drug
p. effect

NOTES

psychotherapeutic
p. approach
p. neuroscience
p. therapy
psychotic
p. Alzheimer patient
p. brain syndrome
p. choreoathetosis
p. depressive reaction
p. relapse
psychotic-like phenomenon
psychotomimetic agent
psychotropic
p. agent
p. medication
p. metabolism
p. movement
psychovisual therapy
psychroalgia
psychroesthesia
psychrophobia
PT
prothrombin time
PTAH
phosphotungstic acid hematoxylin
***ptc* gene**
8pter-23
chromosome 8pter-23
pterion
pterional
p. approach
p. craniotomy
pterygoid
p. canal nerve
p. fossa
p. plexus
pterygoidei
nervus canalis p.
pterygomaxillary suture
pterygopalatine
p. fossa
p. ganglion
p. nerve
p. neuralgia
pterygopalatini
nervi p.
radix intermedia ganglii p.
radix parasympathica ganglii p.
radix sensoria ganglii p.
radix sympathica ganglii p.
rami orbitales ganglii p.
ramus pharyngeus ganglii p.
pterygopalatinum
ganglion p.
rami ganglionares nervi maxillaris ad ganglion p.
PTH
parathyroid hormone
ptosed
ptosis, pl. **ptoses**
cerebral p.
eyelid p.
Horner p.
myasthenic p.
oculomotor p.
oculosympathetic p.
p. sympathetica
ptotic
PTP
posttetanic potentiation
PTS-Ultrason
PTT
partial thromboplastin time
pudendal
p. nerve
p. SEP
p. somatosensory evoked potential
pudendi
nucleus nervi p.
pudendus
nervus p.
Pudenz
P. shunt
P. valve
P. ventricular catheter
Pudenz-Heyer-Schulte valve
Pudenz-Heyer shunt system
Pueraria lobata
puer eternus
puerperal eclampsia
pugilistica
dementia p.
Puka
Pulfrich phenomenon
pullout
screw p.
p. strength
pull test
Pulmonair 40 bed
pulmonale
glomus p.
pulmonalis
plexus p.
rami pulmonales plexus p.
pulmonary
p. arteriovenous shunt
p. capillary wedge pressure
p. edema
p. embolism
p. encephalopathy
p. glomus
p. tuberculosis
pulmonocoronary reflex

pulp
vertebral p.
pulposus
herniated nucleus p.
nucleus p.
Pulsar infusion pump
pulsatile tinnitus
pulsatility
Gosling p.
p. index
pulsating
p. electromagnetic field
p. headache
p. neurasthenia
p. visual halo
pulsation
p. artifact
carotid p.
pulse
entoptic p.
p. flip angle
p. generator
p. length
ocular p.
p. oximeter
p. oximetry
posttorque p.
presaturation p.
radiofrequency p.
p. rate
p. repetition time
p. repetition time prolongation
RF p.
p. sequence
p. synchronous sound
p. timing diagram
p. transit time
p. wave artifact
p. wave Doppler
p. width
pulsed
p. Doppler
p. Doppler imaging
p. electromagnetic field (PEMF)
p. fluorography
p. gradient
pulsed-field gel electrophoresis
pulsed-range gated Doppler instrument
pulse-gated cine phase contrast sequence
pulseless disease
pulvinar
p. nucleus
p. nucleus of thalamus
p. thalami
pulvinares
nuclei p.
pulvinotomy
pump
Cordis Secor implantable p.
drug infusion p.
implanted infusion p.
InDura intrathecal catheter and p.
Infusaid M400 constant flow p.
infusion p.
intraaortic balloon p.
Medrad infusion p.
Medtronic SynchroMed implantable p.
minisomotic infusion p.
Pulsar infusion p.
Shiley-Infusaid p.
SynchroMed model 8611H prototype implantable p.
volumetric infusion p.
punch
bone p.
Cone skull p.
disk p.
dural p.
Fehling TOP ejector p.
Ferris Smith-Kerrison p.
Hajek-Koffler p.
Hajek laminectomy p.
Hardy sellar p.
intervertebral p.
Kerrison bone p.
Raney laminectomy p.
p. rongeur
Roton sellar p.
sellar p.
skull p.
punch-drunk syndrome
puncta (*pl. of* punctum)
punctata
rhizomelic chondrodysplasia p.
punctate
p. cavernous malformation
p. white matter hyperintensity
punctual stimulation
punctum, gen. **puncti**, pl. **puncta**
p. dolorosum

NOTES

punctum *(continued)*
p. luteum
p. vasculosum
puncture
Bernard p.
brain p.
cisternal p.
cranial p.
intracisternal p.
lumbar p. (LP)
Quincke p.
spinal p.
stereotactic p.
sternal p.
thecal p.
ventricle p.
ventricular p.
Puno-Winter-Byrd (PWB)
P.-W.-B. system
pupil
absent p.
Adie-Holmes p.
Adie tonic p.
Argyll Robertson p.
blown p.
Bumke p.
consensual response p.
corn-picker's p.
dilated poorly reactive p.
enlarged p.
fixed p.
Holmes-Adie p.
Hutchinson p.
inverse Argyll Robertson p.
isocoric p.
p. light-near dissociation
Marcus Gunn p.
myotonic p.
paradoxical p.
pseudo-Argyll Robertson p.
p. reactivity
rigid p.
Robertson p.
p. size disparity
tonic p.
tonically dilated p.
pupillary
p. abnormality
p. light reflex
p. light response
p. reactivity
pupillary-skin reflex
pupillatonia
pupillometry
pupillomotor
pupilloplegia
pupillotonic pseudotabes
purchase
bony p.
pure
p. absence
p. agraphia
p. alexia
p. aphasia
p. athetoid palsy
p. autonomic failure
p. depression
p. hemisensory stroke
p. limb apraxia
p. motor hemiparesis
p. motor hemiplegia
p. sensory neuropathy
p. sensory stroke
p. spastic palsy
p. tone discrimination
p. word deafness
p. word mutism
pure-tone
p.-t. audiometry
p.-t. average
purine
p. metabolic disorder
p. metabolism
p. nucleotide phosphorylase deficiency
Purkinje
P. cell
P. cell degeneration
P. cell layer
P. corpuscle
P. neuron
Purmann method
Puros Accugraft allograft
purpura
brain p.
Henoch-Schönlein p.
idiopathic thrombocytopenic p. (ITP)
malignant p.
thrombotic thrombocytopenic p.
purpurea
Claviceps p.
pursuit
p. defect
p. eye movement
saccadic p.
smooth p.
p. system
purulent
p. encephalitis
p. meningitis
p. pachymeningitis
pusher
Jacobson suture p.

putamen
ventral p.
putaminal
p. hemorrhage
p. infarction
putative
p. effect
p. endogenous ligand
p. insult
putatively poor-prognosis deficit syndrome
Putnam-Dana syndrome
putty
Bishop p.
Puusepp reflex
PV
parvalbumin
PV foam
PV positive cell
PVA
periodic vestibular ataxia
PVG
periventricular gray
PVL
periventricular leukomalacia
PVP
polyvinylpyrrolidone
PVS
persistent vegetative state
pigmented villonodular synovitis
PWB
Puno-Winter-Byrd
PXA
pleomorphic xanthoastrocytoma
pyelography
pyencephalus
pyknoepilepsy
pyknolepsy
pyknoleptic petit mal
pyknomorphic
pyknomorphous
pyknotic nucleus
pyla
pylar
pyocephalus
circumscribed p.
external p.
internal p.
pyogenes
Streptococcus p.
pyogenic
p. brain abscess
p. discitis
p. meningitis
p. osteomyelitis
p. pachymeningitis
pyogenica
encephalitis p.
pyramid
anterior p.
cerebellar p.
decussation of p.
Malacarne p.
p. of medulla
p. of medulla oblongata
olfactory p.
P. Scale
p. sign
syndrome of the p.
p. of tympanum
p. of vermis
pyramidal
p. cell
p. cell layer
p. cerebral palsy
p. decussation
p. eminence
p. fiber
p. neuron
p. pathway
p. radiation
p. system
p. tract
p. tract disease
p. tract lesion
p. tractotomy
p. tract sign
p. trocar
pyramidale
stratum p.
pyramidales
fibrae p.
pyramidalis
eminentia p.
nucleus p.
radiatio p.
tractus p.
pyramidis, pl. **pyramides**
fasciculus circumolivaris p.

NOTES

P

pyramidotomy
medullary p.
spinal p.
pyramidum
decussatio p.
pyramis
p. bulbus
p. of cerebellum
p. medullae oblongatae
p. tympani
p. vermis
pyranocarboxylic acid class
pyrazinamide
pyrazolopyrimidine
pyrexial headache
pyridostigmine bromide
pyridoxine deficiency
pyridoxine-deficiency seizure
pyriform
p. area
p. cortex
p. softening
pyrimethamine
p. poisoning
p. sulfadoxine
pyrimidine metabolic disorder
pyrogen
endogenous p. (EP)
pyromaniac
pyrophosphate
technetium 99m p.
technetium stannous p.
pyruvate
p. carboxylase
p. carboxylase deficiency
p. dehydrogenase (PDH)
p. dehydrogenase complex
p. dehydrogenase multienzyme
p. dehydrogenase phosphatase
p. kinase deficiency
p. oxidation
pyschasthenia
pyschoplegia
Pythium

Q
Q factor
Q fever
Q score
Q test
2q
chromosome 2q
2q21-33
chromosome 2q21-33
2q24
chromosome 2q24
6q24
chromosome 6q24
8q
chromosome 8q
8q13-21
chromosome 8q13-21
8q24
chromosome 8q24
10q22-24
chromosome 10q22-24
15q14
chromosome 15q14
15q24
chromosome 15q24
16q
chromosome 16q
pericentromeric region of chromosome 16q
19q11-13
chromosome 19q11-13
19q13.3
chromosome 19q13.3
20q
chromosome 20q
20q13.2
chromosome 20q13.2
20q13.3
chromosome 20q13.3
21q22.1
chromosome 21q22.1
21q22.3
chromosome 21q22.3
15q11-13 region
15q11-q13 deletion
QALE
quality-adjusted life expectancy
QEEG
quantitative electroencephalogram
QNP
quinpirole
QPCA pear-shaped nerve hook
Q-SART
Quantitative Sudomotor Axon Reflex test
Quantitative Sudomotor Axon Reflex Test
Q-score profile
Q-sit
Q-sort
Q.-s. method
Q.-s. procedure
Q.-s. technique
QST
quantitative sensory test
terminal QST
QTL
quantitative trait locus
Quad electrode
Quadramet
quadrangularis
lobulus q.
pars inferoposterior lobuli q.
quadrangular lobule
quadrantanopia
quadrantanopsia
upper homonymous q.
quadrate
q. gyrus
q. lobe
q. lobe of cerebral hemisphere
q. lobule
quadrature
q. detector
q. head coil
quadratus
q. femoris nerve
lobulus q.
quadriceps
q. gait
q. jerk
q. muscle biopsy
q. myopathy
q. reflex
quadrigemina
corpora q.
lamina q.
quadrigeminal
q. arachnoid cyst
q. body
q. cistern
q. cistern lipoma
q. lamina
q. plate
quadrigeminalis
cisterna q.
quadrigeminum
Quadrilite 6000 fiberoptic headlight

quadriparesis
progressive flaccid q.
spastic q.
quadriplegia
spastic q.
static spastic q.
quadriplegic injury
quadrupedal extensor reflex
quadruple sectoranopia
qualitative morphology
quality
compulsive q.
Q. of Crisis Support scale
q. factor
hypomanic q.
image q.
Q. of Life in Epilepsy-89 inventory
Q. of Life Inventory
q. of life measure
Q. of Life Scale
sleep q.
quality-adjusted
q.-a. life expectancy (QALE)
q.-a. life-year (QUALY)
quality-of-life measurement
QUALY
quality-adjusted life-year
quandrantic hemianopia
quantal release deficiency
quantification
color velocity imaging q.
quantitative
q. data
q. EEG analysis
q. electroencephalogram (QEEG)
q. imaging
q. measure
q. morphology
q. morphometric technique
q. motor unit potential analysis
q. receptor autoradiography
Q. Scoring System
q. sensory test (QST)
q. spectral phonoangiography
Q. Sudomotor Axon Reflex Test (Q-SART)
q. trait locus (QTL)
quantum
q. mechanics
q. number
quarta
crista q.
macula cribrosa q.
quarti
apertura lateralis ventriculi q.
apertura mediana ventriculi q.
foramen lateralis ventriculi q.
plexus choroideus ventriculi q.
ramus choroidei ventriculi q.
ramus choroideus ventriculi q.
recessus lateralis ventriculi q.
striae medullares ventriculi q.
sulcus limitans ventriculi q.
sulcus medianus ventriculi q.
taenia ventriculi q.
tegmen ventriculi q.
tela choroidea ventriculi q.
tenia ventriculi q.
ventriculi q.
quartus
ventriculus q.
Quartzo device
quasi-purposeful movement
quavering voice
quazepam
Queckenstedt
Q. phenomenon
Q. sign
Q. test
Queckenstedt-Stookey test
quench
magnet q.
questionnaire
Abbreviated Life Event Q.
Ages and Stages Q.'s
Cognitive Failures Q.
Communications Profile Q.
Community College Student Experiences Q. (CCSEQ)
Cree Q.
Edinburgh Q.
Frankfurt Complaint Q.
Katzmann Orientation-Memory-Concentration q.
Kenney Self-Care Q.
McGill Pain Q.
Modified Autonomic Perception Q.
modified McGill Pain Q.
Morningness-Eveningness Q. (MEQ)
North American Spine Society Q.
Oswestry Low Back Pain Disability Q.
Parkinson Disease Q. (PDQ-39)
Roland-Morris disability q.
Short-Form McGill Pain Q. (SF-MPQ)
Stanford Acute Stress Reaction Q.
St. George Anxiety Q.
quetiapine fumarate
Quick
Q. Connect twist drill
Q. Neurological Screening Test

QuickAnchor
  Resolve Q.
Quickcap electrode cap
QuietLite Quadrilite 6000 fiberoptic headlight
quiet wakefulness mode
quinacrine fluorescent banding
Quincke
  Q. disease
  Q. edema
  Q. puncture
  Q. spinal needle
quinidine
quinine ascorbate
quinolinate
quinolinic acid
quinolone
quinpirole (QNP)
quintana
  Rochalimaea q.
quintus
  ventriculus q.
quinuclidinyl benzilate
quiritarian epilepsy
quisqualic acid
quoque
  tu q.
quotient
  Ayala q.
  Brain-Age Q.

NOTES

500R
ProOsteon 200R and 500R
RA
robustus archistriatalis
RAATE
Recovery Attitude and Treatment Evaluator
RAATE score
RAB
remote afterloading brachytherapy
rabic tubercle
rabies virus
Rabiner neurological hammer
Rabot disease
raccoon eye
racetrack Microtron MM50 accelerator
rachial
rachicentesis
rachidial
rachidian
rachigraph
rachilysis
rachiocentesis
rachiochysis
rachiometer
rachiomyelitis
rachiopathy
rachioplegia
rachioscoliosis
rachiotome, rachitome
rachiotomy, rachitomy
lateral r.
rachischisis
r. partialis
posterior r.
r. totalis
rachitome (*var. of* rachiotome)
Racz Tun-L-Kath catheter
radial
r. artery
r. artery graft
r. glia
r. glial cell
r. nerve
r. nerve trauma
r. paralysis
r. phenomenon
r. reflex
radialis
flexor carpi r. (FCR)
nervi digitales dorsales nervi r.
nervus r.
rami musculares nervi r.
ramus communicans ulnaris nervi r.
ramus profundus nervi r.
ramus superficialis nervi r.
r. sign
radiant layer
radiata
corona r.
radiate
r. crown
r. layer of hippocampus
radiatio, pl. **radiationes**
r. acustica
r. corporis callosi
r. inferior thalami
r. optica
r. pyramidalis
r. thalami anterior
r. thalamica posterior
r. thalami centralis
r. thalami inferior
r. thalami posterior
radiation
acoustic r.
r. angiopathy
anterior thalamic r.
auditory r.
r. beam
beta-emitting r.
Bragg peak r.
central thalamic r.
r. of corpus callosum
r. effect
electromagnetic r.
r. exposure
fibrosis r.
focal r.
geniculocalcarine r.
Gratiolet r.
inferior thalamic r.
r. injury
leukoencephalopathy r.
low-energy gamma r.
r. myelopathy
r. necrosis
r. neuritis
r. neuropathy
occipitothalamic r.
optic r.
r. plexopathy
posterior thalamic r.
prelemniscal r. (RAPRL)
proton beam r.
pyramidal r.
r. retinopathy
single-fraction r.

R

radiation *(continued)*
stereotactic gamma r.
tegmental r.
temporal lobe r.
thalamic r.
thalamostriate r.
thalamotemporal r.
r. therapy
r. vasculitis
r. vasculopathy
Wernicke r.
radiation-induced
r.-i. glioma
r.-i. plexopathy
r.-i. vasculopathy
radiation-injury headache
radiatum
stratum r.
radical
r. decompressive craniotomy
diflavin free r.
free r.
r. fringe
hydroxyl r.
r. induced brain injury
oxygen free r.
r. prefrontal lobotomy
superoxide anion r.
radices (*pl. of* radix)
radicis
radicotomy
radiculalgia
radicular
r. cyst
r. distribution of pain
r. fiber
r. filum
r. hyporeflexia
r. motor deficit
r. neuritis
r. neuropathy
r. syndrome
r. vein
radicularia
fila r.
radicularis magna
radiculectomy
radiculitis
acute brachial r.
radiculoganglionitis
radiculomedullary
r. fistula
r. syndrome
radiculomeningeal spinal vascular malformation
radiculomeningomyelitis
radiculomyelopathy
radiculoneuritis
radiculoneuropathy
radiculopathy
cervical r.
diabetic thoracic r.
hereditary sensory r.
lumbosacral r.
spondylotic caudal r.
radiculospinal artery
Radifocus guidewire
radioactive
r. count
r. iodide
r. tracer
r. yttrium (^{90}Y)
r. yttrium seed
radiobicipital reflex
radiocapitellar joint ganglion
radioencephalogram
radioencephalography
radiofluoroscopy
televised r.
Radiofocus introducer B kit
radiofrequency (RF)
r. eddy current
r. electromagnetic field
r. generator
r. head coil
r. heating
r. homogeneity pattern
r. lesion
r. lesioning
r. needle electrode system
r. neurotomy
r. palatoplasty
r. pulse
r. rhizotomy
r. spoiling
r. thermocoagulation
r. thoracic sympathectomy
r. transmitter
R. Triage System (RAFTS)
radiofrequency-induced echo
radiograph
Waters view r.
radiography
digital r. (DR)
plain r.
radiohumeral joint
radioimmunoassay
radioimmunoprecipitation (RIP)
radioimmunotherapy
radioisotope
r. cisternogram
r. cisternography
r. scan
r. uptake

radiolabeled neurotrophic factor
radiolabeling
radiologic abnormality
radiological pressure-volume index
radiolucency
hydrocephalic periventricular r.
periventricular r.
radiolucent
r. cranial pin headholder
r. operating room table extension
radionecrosis
radioneuritis
Radionics
R. bipolar coagulation unit
R. bipolar instrument
R. CRW stereotactic head frame
R. RF lesion generator
radionucleotide (RN)
r. scanning
radionuclide
r. bone scan
r. cisternography
r. imaging
r. study
radiopaque fiducial
radioperiosteal reflex
radiopharmaceutical
radioreceptor
radiosensitizer
radiosignal line
radiosurgery
advanced design LINAC r.
arteriovenous malformation r.
Bragg peak r.
charged particle r.
cranial r.
extracranial r.
gamma knife r. (GKRS)
LINAC r.
linear accelerator r.
multiarc LINAC r.
particle beam r.
photon beam r.
repeat r.
stereotactic r. (SRS)
trunnion-guided r.
radiosurgical lesioning procedure
radiotherapy
r. brain mapping
external beam r. (EBRT)
fractionated r.
heavy particle r.
hyperfractionated r.
interstitial r.
mathematical optimization and logical dimensioning for r.
stereotactic linear accelerator r.
radiotracer
radius of angulation
radix, pl. **radices**
r. anterior
r. anterior ansae cervicalis
r. anterior nervi spinalis
r. brevis ganglii ciliaris
r. cochlearis
r. cochlearis nervi vestibulocochlearis
radices craniales
r. cranialis nervi accessorii
r. dorsalis
r. dorsalis nervi spinalis
r. inferior ansae cervicalis
r. inferior nervi vestibulocochlearis
r. intermedia ganglii pterygopalatini
r. lateralis nervi mediani
r. lateralis tractus optici
r. longa ganglii ciliaris
r. medialis nervi mediani
r. medialis tractus optici
r. motoria
r. motoria nervi spinalis
r. nasociliaris
r. nasociliaris ganglii ciliaris
r. nervi facialis
radices nervi trigemini
r. oculomotoria ganglii ciliaris
r. parasympathica ganglii ciliaris
r. parasympathica ganglii otici
r. parasympathica ganglii pterygopalatini
r. parasympathica ganglii sublingualis
r. parasympathica ganglii submandibularis
r. parasympathica gangliorum pelvicorum
radices plexus brachialis
r. posterior
r. posterior ansae cervicalis
r. posterior nervi spinalis
r. sensoria ganglii otici
r. sensoria ganglii pterygopalatini

radix *(continued)*
r. sensoria ganglii submandibularis
r. sensoria nervi spinalis
r. sensoria nervi trigemini
radices spinales
r. spinalis nervi accessorii
r. superior ansae cervicalis
r. superior nervi vestibulocochlearis
r. sympathica ganglii ciliaris
r. sympathica ganglii pterygopalatini
r. ventralis
r. ventralis nervi spinalis
r. vestibularis
r. vestibularis nervi vestibulocochlearis
Radovici sign
Raeder
R. paratrigeminal neuralgia
R. paratrigeminal syndrome
RAFTS
Radiofrequency Triage System
ragged red fiber (RRF)
Ragin' Cajun disease
RAI
respiratory arousal index
railway nystagmus
Raimondi
R. infant scalp hemostatic forceps
R. low pressure shunt
R. peritoneal catheter
R. spring catheter
R. ventricular catheter
Rainin clip-bending spatula
raised intracranial pressure
raisonnante
folie r.
raloxifene
Rambaud syndrome
rami (*pl. of* ramus)
ramicotomy
ramisection
ramitis
ramp stimulation
Ramsay
R. Hunt paralysis
R. Hunt syndrome, type I, II
R. Hunt type of inherited dentatorubral degeneration
ramus, pl. **rami**
rami ad pontem
r. albus nevi spinalis
rami alveolares superiores anteriores nervi maxillaris
rami alveolares superiores posteriores nervi maxillaris
r. alveolaris superior medius nervi maxillaris
rami anteriores nervorum cervicalium
rami anteriores nervorum lumbalium
rami anteriores nervorum sacralium
rami anteriores nervorum thoracicorum
r. anterior nervi auricularis
r. anterior nervi coccygei
r. anterior nervi cutanei antebrachii medialis
r. anterior nervi obturatorii
r. anterior nervi spinalis
r. anterior sulci lateralis cerebri
r. articularis
r. articularis nervi vagi
r. ascendens sulci lateralis cerebri
r. autonomicus
rami bronchiales anteriores nervi vagi
rami bronchiales nervi vagi
rami bronchiales posteriores nervi vagi
rami buccales nervi facialis
rami calcanei laterales nervi suralis
rami calcanei mediales nervi tibialis
rami cardiaci cervicales inferiores nervi vagi
rami cardiaci cervicales superiores nervi vagi
rami cardiaci thoracici
rami cardiaci thoracici nervi vagi
rami caudae nuclei caudati
rami celiaci nervi vagi
rami centrales anteromediales
r. cervicalis nervi facialis
r. chiasmaticus
rami choroidei
r. choroidei posteriores laterales
r. choroidei posteriores mediales
r. choroidei ventriculi lateralis
r. choroidei ventriculi quarti
r. choroidei ventriculi tertii
r. choroideus ventriculi quarti
r. cingularis
rami clivales
rami clunium inferiores
rami clunium mediales
rami clunium superiores
r. colli nervi facialis
r. communicans
r. communicans albus nervi spinalis
r. communicans cochlearis nervi vestibularis
r. communicans cum nervo glossopharyngeo

r. communicans cum nervo nasociliari
r. communicans fibularis nervi fibularis communis
r. communicans griseus nervi spinalis
r. communicans nervi facialis cum nervo glossopharyngeo
r. communicans nervi glossopharyngei cum chorda tympani
r. communicans nervi glossopharyngei cum nervo auriculotemporali
r. communicans nervi glossopharyngei ramo auriculari nervi vagi
r. communicans nervi glossopharyngei ramo meningeo nervi vagi
r. communicans nervi intermedii cum nervo vagi
r. communicans nervi intermedii cum plexu tympanico
r. communicans nervi lacrimalis cum nervo zygomatico
r. communicans nervi laryngei inferioris cum ramo laryngeo interno
r. communicans nervi laryngei superioris cum nervo laryngeo inferiore
r. communicans nervi lingualis cum chorda tympani
r. communicans nervi mediani com nervo ulnari
r. communicans nervi nasociliaris cum ganglio ciliari
r. communicans nervi vagi cum nervo glossopharyngeo
r. communicans peroneus nervi peronei communis
r. communicans ulnaris nervi radialis
rami communicantes
rami communicantes nervi auriculotemporalis cum nervi faciali
rami communicantes nervi lingualis cum nervo hypoglosso
rami communicantes nervorum spinalium
rami corporis amygdaloidei
r. corporis callosi dorsalis
rami corporis geniculati lateralis
rami cruris posterioris capsulae internae
rami cutanei anteriores nervi femoralis
rami cutanei cruris medialis nervi sapheni
r. cutaneus
r. cutaneus anterior abdominalis nervi intercostalis
r. cutaneus anterior nervi iliohypogastrici
r. cutaneus anterior pectoralis nervi intercostalis
r. cutaneus lateralis abdominalis nervi intercostalis
r. cutaneus lateralis nervi iliohypogastrici
r. cutaneus lateralis pectoralis nervi intercostalis
r. cutaneus lateralis pectoralis nervi obturatorii
rami dentales inferiores plexus dentalis inferioris
rami dentales superiores plexus dentalis superiores
r. digastricus nervi facialis
dorsal r.
rami dorsales nervorum cervicalium
rami dorsales nervorum lumbalium
rami dorsales nervorum sacralium
rami dorsales nervorum thoracicorum
r. dorsalis nervi coccygei
r. dorsalis nervi spinalis
r. dorsalis nervi ulnaris
rami esophagei nervi laryngei recurrentis
r. externus nervi accessorii
r. externus nervi laryngei superioris
rami fauciales nervi lingualis
r. femoralis nervi genitofemoralis
r. frontalis anteromedialis
r. frontalis intermediomedialis
r. frontalis posteromedialis
rami ganglionares nervi lingualis ad ganglion submandibulare

NOTES

ramus *(continued)*
rami ganglionares nervi maxillaris ad ganglion oticum
rami ganglionares nervi maxillaris ad ganglion pterygopalatinum
rami gastrici anteriores trunci vagalis anterioris
rami gastrici nervi vagi
rami gastrici posteriores trunci vagalis posterioris
r. genitalis nervi genitofemoralis
rami genus capsulae internae
rami gingivales inferiores plexus dentalis inferioris
rami gingivales nervi mentalis
rami gingivales superiores plexus dentalis superioris
rami glandulares ganglii submandibularis
rami globi pallidi
rami gluteales inferiores
rami gluteales mediales
rami gluteales superiores
gray r.
r. griseus nervi spinalis
rami hepatici trunci vagalis anterioris
r. hypothalamicus
rami inferiores nervi transversi colli
r. inferior nervi oculomotorii
r. infrapatellaris nervi sapheni
rami interganglionares trunci sympathici
r. internus nervi accessorii
r. internus nervi laryngei superioris
rami isthmi faucium nervi lingualis
rami labiales nervi mentalis
rami labiales superiores nervi infraorbitalis
rami laryngopharyngei ganglii cervicalis superioris
r. lateralis nervi supraorbitalis
r. lateralis rami posterioris nervi cervicalis
r. lateralis rami posterioris nervi lumbalis
r. lateralis rami posterioris nervi sacralis
r. lateralis rami posterioris nervi thoracici
rami linguales nervi glossopharyngei
rami linguales nervi hypoglossi
rami linguales nervi lingualis
r. lingualis nervi facialis
rami mammarii laterales rami cutanei lateralis pectoralis nervi intercostalis
rami mammarii mediales rami cutanei anterioris pectoralis nervi intercostalis
r. marginalis
r. marginalis mandibularis nervi facialis
r. medialis nervi supraorbitalis
r. medialis rami posterioris nervi cervicalis
r. medialis rami posterioris nervi lumbalis
r. medialis rami posterioris nervi sacralis
r. medialis rami posterioris nervi thoracici
rami medullares laterales
rami medullares mediales
r. membranae tympani nervi auriculotemporalis
r. meningeus nervi mandibularis
r. meningeus nervi maxillaris
r. meningeus nervi spinalis
r. meningeus nervi vagi
r. meningeus recurrens nervi ophthalmici
rami mentales nervi mentalis
rami musculares nervi femoralis
rami musculares nervi fibularis profundi
rami musculares nervi ischiadici
rami musculares nervi mediani
rami musculares nervi musculocutanei
rami musculares nervi nervorum intercostalium
rami musculares nervi peronei profundi
rami musculares nervi peronei superficialis
rami musculares nervi radialis
rami musculares nervi tibialis
rami musculares nervi ulnaris
rami musculares plexus lumbalis
rami musculares rami anterioris nervi obturatorii
rami musculares rami externi nervi accessorii
rami musculares rami posterioris nervi obturatorii
r. muscularis
r. musculi stylopharyngei nervi glossopharyngei
rami nasales externi nervi infraorbitalis

rami nasales interni laterales nervi ethmoidalis anterioris
rami nasales interni mediales nervi ethmoidalis anterioris
rami nasales interni nervi infraorbitalis
rami nasales nervi ethmoidalis anterioris
rami nasales posteriores inferiores nervi palatini majoris
rami nasales posteriores superiores laterales nervi maxillaris
rami nasales posteriores superiores mediales nervi maxillaris
r. nasalis externus nervi ethmoidalis anterioris
r. nervi oculomotorii ganglii ad ciliare
rami nucleorum hypothalamicorum
r. occipitalis nervi auricularis posterioris
r. occipitotemporalis
rami oesophageales gangliorum thoracicorum
rami oesophagei nervi laryngei recurrentis
rami orbitales ganglii pterygopalatini
rami orbitales nervi maxillaris
r. palmaris nervi mediani
r. palmaris nervi ulnaris
rami palpebrales inferiores nervi infraorbitalis
rami palpebrales nervi infratrochlearis
r. parietooccipitalis
rami parotidei nervi auriculotemporalis
rami partis retrolentiformis capsulae internae
rami pedunculares
r. pericardiacus nervi phrenici
rami perineales nervi cutanei femoris posterioris
rami pharyngeal nervi glossopharyngei
rami pharyngei nervi laryngei recurrentis
r. pharyngeus ganglii pterygopalatini
r. pharyngeus nervi vagi
rami phrenicoabdominales nervi phrenici
rami posteriores nervorum cervicalium
rami posteriores nervorum lumbalium
rami posteriores nervorum sacralium
rami posteriores nervorum thoracicorum
r. posterior nervi auricularis magni
r. posterior nervi coccygei
r. posterior nervi cutanei antebrachii medialis
r. posterior nervi obturatorii
r. posterior nervi spinalis
posterior primary r.
r. posterior sulci lateralis cerebri
r. profundus nervi plantaris lateralis
r. profundus nervi radialis
r. profundus nervi ulnaris
rami pulmonales plexus pulmonalis
rami pulmonales thoracici gangliorum thoracicorum
r. recurrens nervi spinalis
rami renales nervi vagi
rami renales plexus coeliaci
r. renalis nervi splanchnici minoris
r. sinus carotici
r. sinus carotici nervi glossopharyngei
r. stylohyoideus nervi facialis
rami substantiae nigrae
r. superficialis nervi plantaris lateralis
r. superficialis nervi radialis
r. superficialis nervi ulnaris
rami superiores nervi transversi colli
r. superior nervi oculomotorii
r. sympathicus ad ganglion submandibulare
r. sympathicus ganglii ciliaris
rami temporales anteriores
rami temporales intermedii
rami temporales posteriores
rami temporales superficiales nervi auriculotemporalis
r. tentorii nervi ophthalmici
rami thalamici
r. thalamicus
r. thyrohyoideus ansae cervicalis

NOTES

ramus *(continued)*
r. tonsillae cerebellae
rami tonsillares nervi glossopharyngei
rami tonsillares nervorum palatinorum minorum
rami tracheales nervi laryngei recurrentis
rami tracheales nervi recurrentis
rami tractus optici
r. tubalis plexus tympanici
r. tubarius plexus tympanici
rami tuberis cinerei
ventral r.
rami ventrales nervorum cervicalium
rami ventrales nervorum lumbalium
rami ventrales nervorum sacralium
rami ventrales nervorum thoracicorum
r. ventralis nervi coccygei
r. ventralis nervi spinalis
r. visceralis
white r.
rami zygomatici nervi facialis
r. zygomaticofacialis nervi zygomatici
r. zygomaticotemporalis nervi zygomatici

Rand
R. Functional Limitations Battery
R. Physical Capacities Battery

random
r. digital dialing
r. urine testing
r. wave

randomized
r. clinical trial
r. controlled trial
R. Trial of Tirilazad Mesylate in Patients With Acute Stroke (RANTTAS)

Raney
R. coagulating forceps
R. laminectomy punch
R. laminectomy rongeur
R. perforator
R. rongeur forceps
R. scalp clip
R. scalp clip applier
R. scalp clip-applying forceps
R. stirrup-loop curette

range
alpha frequency r.
dose r.
extreme r.
frequency r.
significant r.
subclinical r.
therapeutic r.

ranine

ranitidine

Ransford loop

RANTES
regulated on activation, normal T-cell expressed, and secreted

RANTTAS
Randomized Trial of Tirilazad Mesylate in Patients With Acute Stroke
RANTTAS study

Ranvier
R. cross
R. internode
node of R.
R. node
R. segment
R. tactile disk

rapamycin

RAPD
relative afferent pupillary defect

raphe
r. corporis callosi
dorsal r.
r. mediana medullae oblongata
r. mediana pontina
r. medullae oblongata
r. medullae oblongatae
medullary r.
r. nuclei region
r. nucleus
nucleus dorsalis r.
r. of pons
r. pontis
serotonergic dorsal r.
Stilling r.

raphes
nuclei reticulares r.
nucleus centralis superior r.
nucleus pallidus r.
nucleus pontis r.
nucleus posterior r.
oculomotor nucleus r.

raphespinal fiber

rapid
r. acquisition radiofrequency-echo steady state imaging
r. alternating movement
r. eye movement (REM)
r. eye movement deprivation
r. eye movement onset blinking
r. eye movement sleep
r. eye movement sleep behavior
r. eye movement sleep-locked headache

r. fluctuating course
r. metabolizer patient
r. nystagmus
r. plasma reagin (RPR)
r. spin echo (RSE)
r. time-zone change syndrome
R. Transit catheter
R. Transit microcatheter
rapidly adaptic receptor
Rapidpoint Access/Rapidpoint Coag
RAPRL
prelemniscal radiation
raptus
status r.
rarefaction
r. stimulation
r. stimulus
RAS
reticular activating system
ras
r. protein
r. signaling pathway
rasagiline mesylate
rash
bull's eye r.
butterfly r.
heliotrope r.
maculopapular r.
morbilliform r.
scarlatiniform r.
target r.
Rasmussen
bundle of R.
R. chronic focal encephalitis
R. nerve fiber
olivocochlear bundle of R.
R. olivocochlear bundle
R. syndrome
ras **oncogene**
rasp
Jansen r.
Nicola r.
Olivecrona r.
Yasargil r.
raspatory
rate
alternate motion r. (AMR)
cerebral metabolic r.
clearance r.
compliance r.
decline r.
erythrocyte sedimentation r. (ESR)
exacerbation r.
false-positive r.
fusion nonunion r.
implant survival r.
intrathecal IgG synthetic r.
limbic neuronal firing r.
metabolic r.
nonspecific response r.
nonunion r.
peak expiratory flow r.
placebo response r.
pseudarthrosis r.
pulse r.
r. of recovery
r. of recovery at discharge
relapse r.
specific absorption r.
r. of speech
transverse relaxation r.
treatment completion r.
treatment response r.
T2 relaxation r.
vertebral osteosynthesis fusion r.
rate-limiting enzyme
Rathke
R. cleft cyst
R. pouch
R. pouch cyst
R. pouch tumor
rating
baseline r.
Clinical Dementia R. (CDR)
clinician r.
dimensional r.
hyperintensity r.
r. instrument
intent r.
maximum intent r.
maximum lethality r.
r. method
nonrandom r.
r. procedure
ratio
absolute terminal innervation r.
bicaudate r.
CD4/CD8 r.
choline:*N*-acetyl-aspartate r.
Cho:NAA r.
contrast-to-noise r. (CNR)
Cre + Cho r.

NOTES

ratio *(continued)*
CSF-to serum glucose r.
distribution volume r. (DVR)
embolus-to-blood r.
estrogen-to-progesterone r.
Evans r.
functional terminal innervation r.
guanine/cytosine r.
gyromagnetic r.
international normalized r. (INR)
risk r.
risk-benefit r.
signal-to-noise r. (SNR)
T r.
^{99m}Tc HMPAO T/C r.
Torg r.
tumor:cerebellum r.
tumor:healthy tissue r.
rational
r. polypharmacy
r. polytherapy
r. problem solving
Ratliff avascular necrosis classification
raw
r. Q score
r. speckled image
r. volume
ray
R. brain spatula
R. brain spatula spoon
gamma r.
photon r.
R. pituitary curette
R. RRE-TM thermistor electrode
R. TFC
R. threaded fusion cage
Raybar 75
Raymond
R. apoplexy
R. syndrome
Raymond-Cestan syndrome
Raynaud
R. disease
R. phenomenon
R. syndrome
Rayport
R. dural dissector and knife
R. dural and knife dissector
Ray-Tec sponge
ray-tracing reconstruction
Rayvist
RBD
REM sleep behavior disorder
RBE
relative biologic effectiveness
RBS
right brain stroke
RC
real contour
rCBF
regional cerebral blood flow
rCBV
relative cerebral blood volume
rCPP
regional cerebral perfusion pressure
RDD
Rosai-Dorfman disease
RDI
respiratory disturbance index
reaching-grasping movement
reaction
abnormal r.
acute dystonic r. (ADR)
acute organic r.
affective r.
agitated r.
allergic r.
amplification r.
anaphylactoid r.
arousal r.
Arthus r.
aseptic meningeal r.
Asian alcohol flush r.
astrocytic r.
autoimmune r.
axon r.
axonal r.
Bekhterev r.
chronic paranoid r.
compulsive r.
consciousness stress r.
contrast dye r.
conversion r.
r. of degeneration
delayed hypersensitivity r.
depressive psychoneurotic r.
depressive psychotic r.
depressive situational r.
dissociative psychoneurotic r.
doll's eye r.
drug r.
dystonic r.
echo r.
exogenous r.
Fenton r.
galvanic skin r.
gemistocytic r.
glial r.
heel-tap r.
hyperkinetic r.
hypochondriacal r.
hypochondriac psychoneurotic r.
initial stress r.
involutional paranoid r.

involutional psychotic r.
Jarisch-Herxheimer fever r.
Jolly r.
lengthening r.
R. Level Scale
magnet r.
Marchi r.
MRZ r.
Much-Holzmann r.
myasthenic r.
neurasthenic psychoneurosis r.
obsessional r.
ocular tilt r.
pain r.
paranoid involutional r.
pathological grief r.
phobia r.
phobic r.
polymerase chain r. (PCR)
postural r.
psychogalvanic r.
psychomotor stress r.
psychoneurotic depressive r.
psychotic depressive r.
retrograde axon r.
reverse transcriptase polymerase chain r. (RT-PCR)
situational stress r.
sleeplessness associated with acute emotional conflicts or r.
sleeplessness associated with intermittent emotional conflicts or r.
startle r.
stress r.
tendon r.
r. time
Wernicke r.

reaction/response
startle r.

reactivation
varicella-zoster virus r.
VZV r.

reactive
r. astrocyte
r. cell
r. gliosis
r. oxygen species (ROS)
r. seizure

reactivity
emotional r.
pupil r.
pupillary r.

readout
r. delay
r. gradient
r. period

reagin
rapid plasma r. (RPR)

real
r. contour (RC)
r. origin

reality
r. distortion
r. therapy

real-life stimulus

real-time
r.-t. color Doppler imaging
r.-t. guidance
r.-t. monitoring

reaming awl

reanimation
facial r.

Rebif MS

rebleed
aneurysmal r.

rebleeding of aneurysm

rebound
r. effect
r. hyperthermia
r. insomnia
r. nystagmus
r. phenomenon
REM r.
r. suppression

reboxetine mesylate

recalcitrant

recall
event r.
r. failure
r. memory
r. performance
recognition versus r.
remote r.

recall-accuracy
code substitution-immediate r.-a.

recalled-delay

recanalization
angiographic r.
percutaneous endoscopic r.
TCD r.

NOTES

receiver
r. bandwidth
r. coil
r. limitation
r. operating characteristic (ROC)
r. overflow
r. overload
r. saturation
recency effect
recent memory
receptive
r. aphasia
r. area
r. dysphagia
r. dysprosody
r. language processing
receptoma
receptor
A1 adenosine r.
acetylcholine r. (AChR)
ACH r.
activated estrogen r.
adenosine r.
adrenergic r.
r. affinity
AI adenosine r. (AIAR)
alpha-adrenergic r.
alpha-2 adrenergic r.
AMPA r.
androgen r.
benzodiazepine postsynaptic r.
calcitonin receptor-like r. (CRLR)
catecholamine r.
central benzodiazepine r.
cerebral acetylcholine nicotinic r.
chemosensory r.
cold r.
contact r.
cutaneous r.
D2 r.
D3 r.
r. density
r. dimerization
dopamine D_2 r.
epidermal growth factor r. (EGFR)
epsilon opiate r.
estrogen r.
excitatory amino acid r.
extrasynaptic r.
fibroblast growth factor r. 2 (FGFR2)
GABA r.
$GABA_A$ r. (GABAR)
$GABA_B$ r.
glutamate r.
glutamate r. 1 (GluR1)
G-protein-coupled r. (GPCR)
gustatory r.
H1 r.
hair follicle r.
heterodimeric r.
hormonal r.
5-HT1 r.
5-HT2 r.
5-HT3 r.
5-HT_{2C} r.
5HTIA r.
human poliovirus r. (hPVR)
Iggo r.
intranuclear r.
intraperitoneal r.
J r.
joint r.
juxtapulmonary r.
kainate r.
kappa opiate r.
r. ligand
limbic dopamine r.
low-density lipoprotein r.
metabotropic glutamate r. (mGluR1)
N-methyl-D-aspartate r.
mu opiate r.
muscarinic acetylcholine r. (mAChR)
muscle r.
N_1 r.
N_2 r.
nicotinic acetylcholine r. (nAChR)
NMDA r.
nonadapting r.
nuclear r.
r. occupancy
odorant r. (OR)
olfactory r.
opiate r.
peripheral benzodiazepine r.
peripheral catecholamine r.
postsynaptic 5-HT2 r.
postsynaptic 5-HT3 r.
r. potential
pressure r.
progesterone r.
r. protein tyrosine phosphatase zeta/beta (RPTP zeta/beta)
rapidly adaptic r.
retroviral CB r.
sensory neuron-specific G protein-coupled r. (SNSRs)
serotonin 5-HT_2 r.
signal transducing r.
slowly adaptic r.
stretch r.
striatal r.
r. subunit

tactile r.
thermal r.
touch r.
Trk r.
tumor necrosis factor r. (TNFR)
tyrosine-kinase r.
r. up-regulation
urokinase plasminogen activator r.
vanilloid VR1 r. (VR1)
very low-density lipoprotein r.
viral r.
warmth r.

receptor-binding property

receptor-mediated current

receptor-related
lipoprotein r.-r.

recess
anterior r.
cerebellopontine r.
chiasmatic r.
cochlear r.
cupular part of epitympanic r.
frontoethmoidal r.
infundibular r.
optic r.
pineal r.
pontocerebellar r.
posterior r.
preoptic r.
Reichert cochlear r.
sphenoethmoidal r.
supraoptic r.
suprapineal r.
Tarin r.
triangular r.

recessive dystonia musculorum deformans

recessus
r. anterior
r. cochlearis
r. infundibularis
r. infundibuli
r. lateralis ventriculi quarti
r. opticus
r. pinealis
r. posterior
r. supraopticus
r. suprapinealis
r. triangularis

Rechtschaffen
criteria of R.

recipiomotor

reciprocal
r. circuitry
r. connection
r. innervation

Recklinghausen disease

recognition
impaired face r.
impaired object r.
r. memory
R. Memory Test (RMT)
r. test
r. time
r. versus recall

recombinant
r. DNA technique
r. human tumor necrosis factor-alpha
r. tau isoform
r. tissue plasminogen activator (RTPA)

reconnaissance
fausse r.

reconstruction
craniofacial r.
maximum intensity pixel r.
planar r.
ray-tracing r.
split bone graft r.
surface r.
three-dimensional r.

record
Candidate Profile R.
r. electrode

Recorder
SnoreSat Sleep R.

recording
ambulatory EEG r.
concurrent video-EEG r.
continuous electromyographic r.
continuous on-line r.
deep brain microelectrode r.
depth r.
r. electrode
jerk-locked back-averaged r.
microelectrode r.
nonreference r.
paired electrode r.
videocassette r.
whole-cell r.

recovered memory

NOTES

recovery
R. Attitude and Treatment Evaluator (RAATE)
fluid-attenuated inversion r. (FLAIR)
full interepisode r.
inversion r.
r. phase
post r.
rate of r.
saturation r.
short-tau inversion r.
short TI inversion r. (STIR)
short time inversion r.
r. of vision
recruiting response
recruitment
r. line
oligodendrocyte progenitor r.
r. pattern
recta
vasa r.
rectal nerve
rectangle
Hartshill r.
Luque r.
rectangular
r. awl
r. brain spatula
rectocardiac reflex
rectolaryngeal reflex
rectus
gyrus r.
r. lateralis abducens oculomotor muscle
r. paralysis
sinus r.
recurrence
seizure r.
recurrens
arteria r.
nervus laryngealis r.
nervus laryngeus r.
recurrent
r. artery of Heubner
r. course
r. encephalopathy
r. enteric cyst
r. insomnia
r. laryngeal nerve (RLN)
r. meningeal nerve
r. mood disorder
r. pain
r. panic attack
r. perforating artery
r. polyneuropathy
r. tumor
recurrentis
rami esophagei nervi laryngei r.
rami oesophagei nervi laryngei r.
rami pharyngei nervi laryngei r.
rami tracheales nervi r.
rami tracheales nervi laryngei r.
recurring
r. headache
r. symptom
recutita
Matricaria r.
recycling
lipid r.
red
r. cell folic acid level
r. eye
r. man syndrome
r. neck syndrome
r. neuralgia
r. nucleus
r. softening
redifferentiation
Redlich-Fisher miliary plaque
Red-O-Pack drain
redox factor-1
reducer
Cloward cervical dislocation r.
reducing body myelopathy
reductase
aldose r.
dihydropteridine r.
r. inhibitor
reduction
r. of amplitude
CBF r.
contrast sensitivity r.
cumulative medication r.
dose r.
r. fixation
fracture r.
fracture-dislocation r.
r. glossectomy
medication r.
meditation-based stress r.
r. method
pain threshold r.
perioperative r.
ritual r.
smoking-related r.
spondylolisthesis r.
r. stabilization
swan-neck deformity r.
symptom r.
r. technique
reductionism
biologic r.

redundancy
neuroblast r.
synapse r.
redundant neuron
reelin
r. gene
r. immunoreactive band
r. moiety
r. protein
reference
r. electrode
r. measurement
r. montage
r. phase
r. picture-caption pair
referencing
dynamic r.
optical image guided surgery system with dynamic r.
referential
referred
r. pain
r. sensation
ReFix
R. noninvasive fixation
R. stereotactic head fixator
R. stereotactic head holder
reflectance spectrophotometry
reflect edema
reflectometry
reflex
abdominal r.
abdominocardiac r.
abnormal nocturnal respiratory r.
Abrams heart r.
Achilles r.
acoustic r.
acousticopalpebral r. (APR)
acquired r.
acromial r.
r. action
adductor foot r.
adductor thigh r.
allied r.
anal r.
ankle r.
r. anosmia
antagonistic r.
anticus r.
antigravity r.
aponeurotic r.
r. arc
asymmetric tonic neck r.
attenuation r.
attitudinal r.
auditooculogyric r.
auditory oculogyric r.
auriculopalpebral r.
auropalpebral r.
axon r.
Babinski r.
back of foot r.
Barkman r.
basal joint r.
Bechterew-Mendel r.
behavior r.
Bekhterev deep r.
Bekhterev-Mendel r.
Benedek r.
Bezold-Jarisch r.
biceps femoris r.
Bing r.
bladder r.
blepharocardiac r.
blink r.
body righting r.
bone r.
bowing r.
brachioradial r.
brachioradialis r.
brain r.
bregmocardiac r.
Brissaud r.
Brudzinski r.
bulbocavernosus r.
bulbomimic r.
bulbospongiosus r.
carotid sinus r.
cephalopalpebral r.
cervicocollic r.
C-fiber r.
Chaddock r.
chain r.
r. change
chin r.
Chodzko r.
ciliospinal r.
r. circuit
clasp-knife r.
closed loop r.
cochleoorbicular r.
cochleopalpebral r.

R

NOTES

reflex *(continued)*
cochleopupillary r.
cochleostapedial r.
concealed r.
conditioned r. (CR)
contralateral r.
r. control
convulsive r.
coordinated r.
corneal r.
corneomandibular r.
corneomental r.
corneopterygoid r.
costal arch r.
costopectoral r.
cough r.
cranial r.
craniocardiac r.
cremasteric r.
crossed adductor r.
crossed extension r.
crossed knee r.
crossed spinoadductor r.
cry r.
cuboidodigital r.
Cushing r.
cutaneous pupil r.
dartos r.
darwinian r.
deep abdominal r.
deep tendon r. (DTR)
defense r.
deglutition r.
Dejerine r.
delayed r.
depressor r.
detrusor r.
diffused r.
digital r.
r. disorder
diving r.
doll's eye r.
dorsal r.
dorsum pedis r.
elbow r.
enterogastric r.
epigastric r.
r. epilepsy
Erben r.
erector spinae r.
erector-spinal r.
Escherich r.
esophagosalivary r.
external auditory meatus r.
external oblique r.
eye-closure r.
facial r.
faucial r.
femoral r.
femoroabdominal r.
finger-thumb r.
flexor r.
foot r.
forced grasping r.
front-tap r.
gag r.
Galant r.
galvanic skin r. (GSR)
gastrocolic r.
gastroileac r.
Geigel r.
Gifford r.
gill withdrawal r.
glabellar r.
gluteal r.
Golda r.
Golgi r.
Gordon r.
grasp r.
grasping r.
great toe r.
Guillain-Barré r.
gustatory-sudorific r.
gustolacrimal r.
H r.
hand grasp r.
r. headache
heart r.
Hering-Breuer r.
Hirschberg r.
Hoffmann r.
Hughes r.
hyperactive tendon r.
hypochondrial r.
hypogastric r.
inborn r.
indirect r.
infraspinatus r.
inguinal r.
innate r.
interscapular r.
intersegmental r.
intrasegmental r.
intrinsic r.
inverted radial r.
investigatory r.
ipsilateral r.
r. iridoplegia
Jacobson r.
jaw-jerk r.
jaw-winking r.
jaw-working r.
Joffroy r.
Juster r.

Kehrer r.
Kisch r.
knee r.
knee-jerk r.
Kocher r.
labyrinthine righting r.
lacrimal r.
lacrimogustatory r.
Landau r.
laryngospastic r.
latent r.
laughter r.
Liddell-Sherrington r.
lip r.
local r.
Lovén r.
lower abdominal periosteal r.
lumbar r.
Lust r.
magnet r.
Magnus and de Kleijn neck r.
mandibular r.
Marinesco-Radovici r.
mass r.
masseter r.
Mayer r.
McCarthy r.
McCormac r.
mediopubic r.
Mendel-Bechterew r.
Mendel dorsal foot r.
Mendel instep r.
metacarpohypothenar r.
metacarpothenar r.
metatarsal r.
micturition r.
milk-ejection r.
Mondonesi r.
monosynaptic stretch r.
Morley peritoneocutaneous r.
Moro r.
r. movement
muscle stretch r.
muscular r.
myoclonus reticular r.
myotatic r.
nasal r.
nasomental r.
neck righting r.
neck tonic r.
r. neurogenic bladder
r. neurologic activity
nociceptive r.
nocifensor r.
nose-bridge-lid r.
nose-eye r.
nuchocephalic r.
obliquus r.
oculoauricular r.
oculocephalic r.
oculocephalogyric r.
oculomotor r.
oculorespiratory r.
oculovestibular r.
olecranon r.
open loop r.
Oppenheim r.
optical righting r.
opticofacial r.
orbicularis oculi r.
orbicularis pupillary r.
orienting r.
oropharyngeal r.
palatal r.
palmar r.
palm-chin r.
palmomental r.
parachute r.
paradoxical extensor r.
paradoxical flexor r.
paradoxical patellar r.
paradoxical pupillary r.
paradoxical triceps r.
r. paralysis
patellar tendon r.
patelloadductor r.
pectoral r.
penile r.
penis r.
Perez r.
perianal r.
pericardial r.
periosteal r.
pharyngeal r.
phasic r.
Philippson r.
photic-sneeze r.
physiological r.
pilomotor r.
plantar muscle r.
platysmal r.
postural r.

NOTES

reflex *(continued)*
pouting r.
premature infant bowing r.
pressoreceptor r.
pronator r.
proprioceptive r.
protective laryngeal r.
psychocardiac r.
psychogalvanic r.
pulmonocoronary r.
pupillary light r.
pupillary-skin r.
Puusepp r.
quadriceps r.
quadrupedal extensor r.
radial r.
radiobicipital r.
radioperiosteal r.
rectocardiac r.
rectolaryngeal r.
regional r.
Remak r.
respiratory r.
Riddoch mass r.
righting r.
Roger r.
rooting r.
Rossolimo r.
Ruggeri r.
Saenger r.
scapular r.
scapulohumeral r.
scapuloperiosteal r.
Schäffer r.
scratch r.
segmental medullary r.
semimembranosus r.
semitendinosus r.
r. sensation
sexual r.
simple r.
sinus r.
skin r.
skin-muscle r.
skin-pupillary r.
snapping r.
Snellen r.
snout r.
sole tap r.
somatointestinal r.
r. spasm
spinal monosynaptic r.
spinoadductor r.
stapes r.
Starling r.
startle r.
static r.
statokinetic r.
statotonic r.
sternobrachial r.
sternutatory r.
Stookey r.
stretch r.
Strümpell r.
styloradial r.
suck r.
superficial r.
supination r.
supinator longus r.
supraorbital r.
suprapatellar r.
suprapubic r.
supraumbilical r.
swallowing r.
r. sympathetic dystrophy (RSD)
r. sympathetic dystrophy syndrome (RSDS)
synchronous r.
r. syncope
tarsophalangeal r.
tendo Achillis r.
tendon r.
testicular compression r.
r. testing
r. therapy
Throckmorton r.
thumb r.
tibioadductor r.
toe r.
tonic r.
trace conditioned r.
trained r.
triceps surae r.
trigeminofacial r.
trochanter r.
Trömner r.
ulnar r.
unconditional r.
unconditioned r.
upper abdominal periosteal r.
upper airway r.
urinary r.
utricular r.
vagus r.
vasopressor r.
venorespiratory r.
vesical r.
vestibular r.
vestibuloocular r. (VOR)
vestibulospinal r.
virile r.
visceral r.
viscerogenic r.
visceromotor r.

viscerosensory r.
visual orbicularis r.
vomiting r.
Weingrow r.
Westphal pupillary r.
wink r.
withdrawal r.
wrist clonus r.
zygomatic r.
reflexogenic
r. syncope
r. zone
reflexogenous
reflexograph
reflexology
reflexometer
reflexophil
reflexophile
reflexotherapy
reflex/response
psychogalvanic r.
reflux
vesicoureteral r.
reformatory paranoic
reformatted image
reformulation
sequential diagrammatic r.
refractoriness
medication r.
refractory
r. convergence nystagmus
r. erectile dysfunction
r. localization-related seizure
r. partial epilepsy
r. state
r. status epilepticus
Refsum
R. disease
R. peripheral neuropathy
R. syndrome
regenerate nerve sprouting
regeneration
aberrant r.
axon r.
axonal r.
cranial nerve r.
neural r.
neuronal r.
peripheral nerve r.
regimen
drug r.
holistic r.
medication r.
multiple-dose r.
pharmacotherapy r.
polytherapy r.
postoperative r.
steady-state r.
treatment r.
regio
r. hypothalamica anterior
r. hypothalamica dorsalis
r. hypothalamica intermedia
r. hypothalamica lateralis
r. hypothalamica posterior
region
anterior head r.
anterior hypothalamic r.
anterior insula r.
auditory r.
basal forebrain r.
bridge r.
Broca r.
carboxyl-terminal r.
central gray matter r.
cerebellar r.
cerebral r.
circumscribed r.
cortical gray r.
craniocervical r.
deep white matter r.
dopamine-innervated limbic r.
dorsal anterior cingulate r.
dorsal hypothalamic r.
dorsal limbic r.
dorsal neocortical r.
dorsolateral r.
extrapolar r.
frontal brain r.
germ cell tumor with synchronous lesions in pineal and suprasellar r.
gray matter r.
hyaluron-binding r.
inferior parietal r.
infragranular r.
infratentorial r.
infundibulotubular r.
interconnected cerebral r.
r. of interest (ROI)
intermediate hypothalamic r.
lateral cerebellar r.

NOTES

region *(continued)*
- lateral hypothalamic r.
- limbic brain r.
- limbic-related r.
- locus coeruleus r.
- mamillary r.
- medullary inhibitory r.
- motor r.
- motoric r.
- negatively correlated r.
- neocortical r.
- occipitonuchal r.
- opticostriate r.
- orbital r.
- parafalcine r.
- paralimbic r.
- paramedian r.
- paranodal r.
- parasellar r.
- penumbral r.
- perisylvian r.
- periventricular gray r.
- pineal r.
- positively correlated r.
- posterior cingulate r.
- posterior hypothalamic r.
- prefrontal r.
- preoptic r.
- prepontine r.
- pretectal r.
- 15q11-13 r.
- raphe nuclei r.
- rolandic r.
- sellar r.
- sensory r.
- septal r.
- silver-staining nucleolar organizer r. (AgNOR)
- speech perception r.
- subcortical gray r.
- subgenual cingulate r.
- subicular r.
- supraoptic r.
- suprasellar r.
- temporal speech r.
- temporomesial r.
- terminal r.
- thalamic r.
- transentorhinal r.
- ventral paralimbic r.
- visual r.
- watershed r.
- Wernicke r.
- white matter r.

regional
- r. brain glucose metabolism
- r. brain lactate
- r. brain parenchymal volume
- r. cerebral blood flow (rCBF)
- r. cerebral blood flow scintigraphy
- r. cerebral metabolic rate of oxygen
- r. cerebral perfusion pressure (rCPP)
- r. distribution
- r. glucose metabolism
- r. glucose metabolism at rest
- r. hypothermia
- r. oxygen extraction fraction
- r. oxygen saturation (rSO_2)
- r. reflex

registration
- r. error
- image r.
- imperfect image r.
- r. menu
- segmental r.
- subvoxel r.
- surface vessel r.

registry
- Acoustic Neuroma R.
- Alzheimer Disease Patient R. (ADPR)
- Brain Tumor R.
- Mayo Alzheimer Disease Center/Alzheimer Disease Patient R.
- Rush Alzheimer R.

Regitine

Regonol Injection

regressive electric shock therapy (REST)

regrowth
- axon r.
- nerve r.

regular
- r. eating schedule
- r. sleeping schedule
- r. waking schedule

regulated on activation, normal T-cell expressed, and secreted (RANTES)

regulation
- cerebrovascular r.
- emotional r.
- top-down r.
- volume r.
- weight r.

regulator
- mood r.
- suction Regugauge r.

regulatory
- r. center
- r. input
- r. role

Regulus frameless stereotactic system
regurgitant lesion
rehabilitation
aquatic r.
neurologic r.
Rehbein rib spreader
Reichert
R. cochlear recess
R. stereotaxy system
R. substance
substantia innominata of R.
Reichert-Mundinger
R.-M. apparatus
R.-M. stereotactic head frame
R.-M. syndrome
R.-M. technique
Reichert-Mundinger-Fischer stereotactic head frame
Reid baseline
Reil
R. ansa
R. band
circular sulcus of R.
insula of R.
island of R.
limiting sulcus of R.
R. ribbon
substantia innominata of R.
R. sulcus
taeniola corporis callosi of R.
threshold of island of R.
R. triangle
R. trigone
Reilly body
reinforcement
drug r.
homogenous r.
Teflon mesh r.
reinforcing
r. agent
r. drug response
r. effect
r. property
r. stimulus
reinnervated
r. fiber
r. motor unit
reinnervation
r. of target organ
Reintegration
R. to Normal Living (RNL)
R. to Normal Living Index
Reissner fiber
Reitan-Klove Sensory Perceptual Evaluation/Examination
Reiter syndrome
relapse
r. mechanism
multiple sclerosis r.
prone to r.
psychotic r.
r. rate
relapse-prevention
relapsing
r. fever
r. hypertrophic neuritis
r. neuropathy
r. polychondritis
relapsing-remitting (RR)
r.-r. multiple sclerosis (RRMS)
relation
afferent r.
dose-response r.
efferent r.
relational
r. alliance
r. efficacy
r. threshold
relationship
attachment r.
brain-behavior r.
complainant-listener r.
complex r.
counterintuitive r.
dose-response r.
forced r.
genetic r.
human r.
intrinsic r.
predictive r.
r. tool
relative
r. afferent pupillary defect (RAPD)
r. band amplitude
r. biological effectiveness
r. biologic effectiveness (RBE)
r. cerebral blood volume (rCBV)
r. hyperemia
r. hypoxia

NOTES

relative *(continued)*
r. optical density (ROD)
r. refractory period
relaxant
muscle r.
relaxation
applied r.
r. constant
dipole-dipole r.
intramolecular r.
longitudinal r.
nuclear r.
paramagnetic r.
r. phase
r. rate enhancement
r. response
spin-lattice r.
spin-spin r.
state of mindful r.
stress r.
T1 r.
T2 r.
r. theory
r. time
transverse r.
relaxation/tension
relay
spinothalamic r.
thalamic r.
thalamocortical r.
release
dopamine r.
r. of information
neurotransmitter r.
r. phenomenon
pituitary prolactin r.
platelet thromboxane r.
prolactin r.
sustained r. (SR)
voltage-dependent neurotransmitter r.
Relefact TRH injection
relevance
clinical r.
reliability
split-half r.
religious
r. difference
r. dynamic
r. perspective
***reln* gene**
Relpax
Relton-Hall frame
REM
rapid eye movement
REM deprivation
REM latency
REM onset blinking
REM rebound
REM sleep behavior disorder (RBD)
REM sleep-locked headache
REM sleep-related disorder
remacemide
Remak
R. fiber
R. ganglion
R. paralysis
R. reflex
R. sign
R. symptom
Remeron SolTab
Remind Cap
reminiscent
r. aura
r. neuralgia
Reminyl
remission
full r.
remodeled forehead
remodeling
bone r.
craniofacial r.
neural foramen r.
remote
r. afterloading brachytherapy (RAB)
r. cerebellar hemorrhage
r. memory
r. recall
r. symptomatic seizure
removal
Arana-Iniquez intracranial cyst r.
Dowling intracranial cyst r.
implant r.
metastatic tumor r.
rib r.
transsphenoidal r.
remoxipride
REM-sleep behavior
remyelinate
remyelination
renal
r. dysfunction
r. function
r. ganglion
r. insufficiency
renalia
ganglia r.
renalis
pectus r.
Renaut body
Rendu-Osler angiomatosis
Rendu-Osler-Weber disease
renifleur

renin
long-term vasomotor tone r.
renin-angiotensin
renitent
Renografin
Renografin-60
Renografin-76
Reno-M
Reno-M-30
Reno-M-60
Reno-M-Dip
Renovist II
Renovue
Renshaw cell
ReoPro
reorganization
cortical r.
plastic r.
somatotopographic r.
repair
cranial nerve r.
Gardner meningocele r.
pseudarthrosis r.
rod fracture r.
reparative response
repeat
microtubule-binding r.
r. radiosurgery
trinucleotide r.
variable number tandem r. (VNTR)
repeated
r. FID
r. measure (rm)
repeating pattern
repetition time
repetitive
r. discharge
r. motion injury (RMI)
r. motion syndrome (RMS)
r. movement
r. nerve stimulation
r. rumination
r. temporalis muscle temperature
r. transcranial magnetic stimulation (rTMS)
r. violence
r. watching
rephasing
even-echo r.
r. gradient
replacement
Bristol disk r.
disk r.
elastic-type disk r.
facet r.
hard tissue r. (HTR)
hormone r.
hydraulic-type disk r.
Hydrogel disk r.
joint r.
low-dose estrogen r.
spinal disk r.
tile plate facet r.
valve r.
repolarization
repositioner
mandibular r.
representation
Cartesian coordinate r.
internal r.
preexisting r.
spherical coordinate r.
representational
abstract versus r.
reprocessing
eye movement desensitization and r. (EMDR)
reproducible target imaging
repulsive axon guidance signal
Requip
requirement
energy r.
rerupture of aneurysm
Rescriptor
rescue
autologous bone marrow r.
bone marrow r.
research
Australian Council for Education R.
biologic r.
construct r.
cross-sectional r.
empirical r.
epidemiological r.
European Society for Sleep R.
r. interview
Japanese Society of Sleep R.
r. program
taxonomic r.
twin r.

NOTES

resection
anterior craniofacial r.
anteromedial temporal lobe r.
Badgley iliac wing r.
caudal lamina r.
condyle r.
cortical r.
craniofacial r.
dorsolateral r.
electroencephalography-guided cortical r.
en bloc r.
extralesional hippocampal r.
extratemporal r.
gross total r.
iliac crest r.
intracranial meningioma r.
lateral temporal r.
meningioma r.
multilobar r.
neural arch r.
nonlesional cortical r.
occipital r.
odontoid process r.
Peet splanchnic r.
Pitanguy oval skin r.
r. of pituitary tumor, transfacial approach
postcentral r.
seizure foci r.
surgical r.
temporal r.
transcranial r.
transoral odontoid r.
transthoracic vertebral body r.
tumor r.
vertebral r.
volumetric r.
resective epilepsy surgery
reserve
cross-flow r.
reservoir
Accu-Flo CSF r.
Braden flushing r.
McKenzie r.
Ommaya r.
on-off flushing r.
retromastoid Ommaya r.
Rickham r.
Salmon Rickham ventriculostomy r.
side-port flat-bottomed Ommaya r.
r. sign
suboccipital Ommaya r.
ventricular catheter r.
ventricular Ommaya r.
residual
r. aura
r. autoparalytic syndrome
r. dense nasal defect
r. hemiparesis
r. latency
least-square r.
r. negative symptom
r. paralysis
r. positive symptom
r. vertigo
resilient nystagmus
resin
Spurr epoxy r.
resistance
estimated cerebrovascular r.
galvanic skin r. (GSR)
manifestation of r.
motiveless r.
upper airway r.
r. vessel
resistant
r. epilepsy
treatment r.
resistive magnet
resolution threshold
Resolve QuickAnchor
resolving ischemic neurologic deficit (RIND)
resonance
fast-scan magnetic r.
localized magnetic r.
magnetic r. (MR)
nuclear magnetic r. (NMR)
stochastic r.
resonant frequency
resonator
birdcage r.
respiration
ataxic r.
Biot r.
Cheyne-Stokes r.
corneal r.
diffusion r.
electrophrenic r.
internal r.
tissue r.
respirator
r. brain
Drinker tank r.
respiratory
r. acidosis
r. alkalosis
r. anosmia
r. arousal index (RAI)
r. ataxia
r. center
r. chain
r. chain complex I deficiency

r. disorder
r. disturbance index (RDI)
r. effort-related arousal
r. embarrassment
r. event arousal
r. insufficiency
r. pause
r. physiology
r. reflex
r. system

respiratory-related arousal

respite care

respondent condition

response

abnormal muscle r.
achromatic r.
acute genomic r.
acute nociceptive r.
adverse autonomic r.
A-fiber evoked r.
agitation r.
alpha r.
AMPA receptor-mediated r.
amperometric r.
amygdala r.
angiogenic r.
antidromic r.
antiparkinsonian r.
auditory brainstem r. (ABR)
auditory brainstem-evoked r. (ABR)
auditory evoked r.
auditory visual-evoked r.
automated brainstem auditory evoked r. (ABaer)
automatic auditory brainstem r.
average evoked r.
axon r.
biphasic locomotor r.
blink r.
Bobath r.
brain metabolic r.
brainstem auditory evoked r. (BAER)
brainstem evoked r.
bulldog r.
buttress r.
caffeine r.
C-fiber evoked r.
chronic r.
cingulate r.
clasp-knife r.
clinical r.
conditioned drug r.
consistent r.
coping r.
Cushing r.
decremental r.
decrementing r.
discrete emotional r.
dissociative r.
dorsal horn neuronal r.
dysregulated stress r.
electromyographic r.
evoked cortical r.
exaggerated r.
extensor plantar r.
extensor toe r.
eye-blink r.
F r.
fabulized r.
fastigial pressor r.
fetal r.
galvanic skin r. (GSR)
r. generalization general learning ability
genital r.
glutamatergic r.
H r.
heat-defense r.
host immune r.
humoral immune r.
hyperactive sympathetic r.
hyperadrenergic r.
hyperemic r.
hypoxic ventilatory r.
immune r.
impunitive r.
inconsistent r.
incremental r.
inflammatory r.
inhibited r.
Janz r.
loss of r.
low-key r.
M r.
meningitis inflammatory r.
metabolic r.
monosynaptic segmental reflex r.
motor r.
myotonic r.
neuromagnetic r.
neuroplastic r.

NOTES

response *(continued)*
oculomotor r.
orienting r.
parachute r.
paradoxical cold r.
pathological r.
photoparoxysmal r. (PPR)
r. processing time
prolactin r.
psychogalvanic r. (PGR)
psychological r.
pupillary light r.
recruiting r.
reinforcing drug r.
relaxation r.
reparative r.
reward-irrelevant r.
segmentary r.
skin conductance r.
somatosensory evoked r. (SER)
sonomotor r.
spatial r.
spinally elicited peripheral nerve r. (SEPNR)
steady-state r. (SSR)
stepping r.
supramaximal r.
sympathetic skin r.
sympathoadrenomedullary r.
syntagmatic r.
thalamic r.
therapeutic r.
thermoeffector r.
thermoregulatory r.
theta r.
tissue-type metabolic r.
unconditioned r.
visual evoked r. (VER)

response-produced cue

responsiveness
absence of emotional r.
hypercapnic r.

REST
regressive electric shock therapy
REST condition

rest
aneurysmal r.
metabolism at r.
r. pain
regional glucose metabolism at r.
r. tremor

Restcue bed

restiform
r. body
r. eminence

restiforme
corpus r.

restiformis
eminentia r.

resting
r. ankle/arm Doppler index
r. anterior cingulate flow
r. membrane potential
r. PET study
r. state
r. T cell
r. tone
r. tremor

restless
r. legs
r. legs syndrome (RLS)
r. leg syndrome

restlessness
motor r.
nocturnal r.

Reston
R. dressing
R. foam-padded headrest

restorative neurology

Restoril

restraint
r. law
physical r.

restricted
r. focus
r. interest

restricting
cognitive r.

restriction
r. endonuclease
r. fragment length polymorphism (RFLP)
gown r.
r. of inward gaze

restrictive criterion

result
anomalous r.
biometric r.
concordant r.
positive r.

Resume electrode

resuscitation
hemodynamic r.

retainer
tongue r.

retardata
ejaculatio r.

retardation
fetal growth r.
mental r.
mild mental r.
motor r.
Northern epilepsy with mental r.
progressive epilepsy with mental r.

psychomotor r.
Spastic Paraplegia, Ataxia, Mental R. (SPAR)

retarded
TMR Performance Profile for the Severely and Moderately R.

rete
carotid r.
r. mirabile
r. mirabile caroticum

retention
brain r.
fluid r.
sodium-water r.

reticula (*pl. of* reticulum)

reticular
r. activating system (RAS)
r. formation
r. nuclei of the brainstem
r. nuclei of medulla oblongata
r. nuclei of mesencephalon
r. nuclei of pons
r. nucleus
r. nucleus of thalamus
r. substance

reticularis
formatio r.
livedo r.
substantia r.

reticulata
pars r.
substantia nigra pars r. (sNr)

reticulocerebellar tract

reticulocortical pathway

reticulocytosis
cerebroside r.

reticulospinalis
tractus r.

reticulospinal tract

reticulotegmental nucleus

reticulothalamocortical pathway

reticulotomy

reticulum, pl. **reticula**
r. cell sarcoma
endoplasmic r.
Kölliker r.
sarcoplasmic r.
smooth endoplasmic r.
r. stain

retifism

retigabine

retina
r. arterial occlusion
blood and thunder r.
cerebral layer of r.
cone cell of r.
external nuclear layer of r.
ganglion cell of r.
ganglionic cell layer of r.
ganglionic layer of r.
granular layer of r.
horizontal cell of r.
molecular layer of r.
neural layer of r.
neuroepithelial layer of r.
nuclear layer of r.
optic part of r.
pigmented layer of r.
plexiform layer of r.
rod cell of r.
sustentacular fiber of r.
r. venous obstruction

retinaculatome
Paine r.

retinae
fovea centralis r.
macula r.
pars optica r.
periphlebitis r.
strata nuclearia externa et interna r.
stratum cerebrale r.
stratum ganglionare r.
stratum moleculare r.
stratum neuroepitheliale r.
stratum nucleare externum et internum r.
stratum nucleare internum r.
stratum pigmenti r.
stratum plexiforme externum et internum r.

retinal
r. angioma
r. arterial occlusion
r. artery occlusion
r. cone
r. cyst
r. degeneration
r. detachment
r. embolism
r. ganglion cell (RGC)
r. hemorrhage

NOTES

retinal *(continued)*
r. infarction
r. migraine
r. migraine headache
r. pathway
r. pigment epitheliopathy
r. pigment epithelium
r. stroke
r. vasculitis
r. venous obstruction
retinitis pigmentosa
retinoblastoma
ectopic intracranial r.
r. gene
retinocerebral angiomatosis
retinocochleocerebral arteriolopathy
retinofugal target
retinoic acid
retinoid
retinoneuropathy
toxic r.
retinopathy
arterial-occlusive r.
hypotensive r.
infectious r.
pigmentary r.
radiation r.
stasis r.
venous stasis r.
retinothalamic projection fiber
retinotopic map
retioculopituicyte
retracting suture
retraction
brain r.
cerebellar r.
r. injury
mandibular r.
r. nystagmus
oral r.
proximal segment r.
sigmoid sinus r.
soft palate r.
temporal lobe r.
retraction-convergence nystagmus
retraction-induced cerebral damage
retractor
Adson-Anderson cerebellar r.
Adson hemilaminectomy r.
Anderson-Adson scalp r.
angled nerve root r.
Apfelbaum r.
Army-Navy r.
Badgley laminectomy r.
Ballantine hemilaminectomy r.
Beckman r.
Beckman-Eaton laminectomy r.
Beckman-Weitlaner laminectomy r.
r. blade
Bookwalter r.
brain r.
Budde halo ring r.
Burford r.
Campbell nerve root r.
Caspar cervical r.
cerebellar r.
Cherry brain r.
Cherry laminectomy r.
Cloward blade r.
Cloward brain r.
Cloward cervical r.
Cloward-Cushing vein r.
Cloward dural r.
Cloward-Hoen laminectomy r.
Cloward lumbar lamina r.
Cloward nerve root r.
Cloward skin r.
Cloward small cervical r.
Cloward tissue r.
collapsible tissue r.
Cone laminectomy r.
Cone scalp r.
Cottle-Neivert r.
Crile r.
Crockard r.
Cushing bivalve r.
Cushing decompressive r.
Cushing nerve r.
Cushing subtemporal r.
Cushing vein r.
Davis brain r.
Davis scalp r.
Deaver r.
deep r.
D'Errico-Adson r.
D'Errico nerve root r.
double fishhook r.
Downing r.
dural r.
Enker brain r.
fan r.
Farley r.
Finochietto r.
flexible arm r.
Frazier laminectomy r.
Frazier lighted brain r.
French brain r.
Gelpi r.
Glaser automatic laminectomy r.
Goulet r.
Greenberg r.
Greenberg-Sugita r.
r. handle Cloward dural hook
Hardy lip r.

Haverfield-Scoville hemilaminectomy r.
Holscher nerve root r.
House-Fisch dural r.
Inge laminectomy r.
intradural r.
Jannetta posterior fossa r.
Jansen mastoid r.
Jansen scalp r.
Jansen-Wagner r.
Kennerdell-Maroon orbital r.
Knighton hemilaminectomy r.
Kobayashi r.
Leyla brain r.
LightWare micro r.
Love nerve root r.
Malis brain r.
Markham-Meyerding hemilaminectomy r.
Martin nerve root r.
mastoid r.
Meyerding laminectomy r.
Miskimon cerebellar r.
Murphy rake r.
nerve root r.
Oldberg brain r.
pillar-and-post microsurgical r.
Poppen-Gelpi laminectomy r.
Roos brachial plexus root r.
Schwartz laminectomy r.
Scoville cervical disk r.
Scoville-Haverfield hemilaminectomy r.
Scoville hemilaminectomy r.
Scoville nerve root r.
Scoville-Richter laminectomy r.
self-retaining brain r.
Senn r.
Sheldon hemilaminectomy r.
single hook r.
Smith nerve root suction r.
Spurling nerve root r.
stereotactic r.
Stuck laminectomy r.
Sugita r.
Taylor r.
Teflon-coated brain r.
Temple-Fay laminectomy r.
Tew cranial spinal r.
titanium wound r.
Tuffier laminectomy r.
Tuffier-Raney r.
Valin hemilaminectomy r.
Weary nerve root r.
Weitlaner r.
Weitlaner-Beckman r.
Wiltse-Gelpi r.
Yasargil r.
Yasargil-Leyla brain r.

retractorius
nystagmus r.

retraining
breathing r.

retrieval
word r.

retroactive amnesia

retroambiguus
nucleus r.

retroauricular edema

retrobulbar
r. hemorrhage
r. injection
r. lesion
r. optic neuritis
r. orbital metastasis

retrobulbaris
tractus r.

retrochiasmal
r. lesion
r. visual pathway

retrochiasmatic
r. area
r. lesion

retrochiasmatica
area r.

retrocochlear
r. deafness
r. hearing loss
r. lesion

retrocollic spasm

retrocollis dystonia

retrocursive absence

retrodorsal nucleus

retrofacialis
nucleus r.

retrofacial nucleus

retroflex
r. bundle of Meynert
r. fasciculus

retroflexus
fasciculus r.

NOTES

retrogasserian
r. anhydrous glycerol injection therapy
r. injection
r. neurectomy
r. neurotomy
r. procedure
r. rhizotomy
retrognathia
retrognathism
retrograde
r. axon reaction
r. blood flow
r. chromatolysis
r. degeneration
r. fast component neuropathy
r. memory
r. transport
retrography
retrogressive differentiation
retrolabyrinthine-presigmoid approach
retrolabyrinthine-transsigmoid approach
retrolental fibroplasia
retrolenticular
r. limb of internal capsule
r. part of internal capsule
retrolentiform limb of internal capsule
retrolingual
retrolisthesis
retromandibular tender point
retromastoid
r. approach
r. craniotomy
r. Ommaya reservoir
r. suboccipital craniectomy
retromembranous hematoma
retroocular
retroolivaris
area r.
sulcus r.
retroolivary
r. area
r. groove
retroorbital pain
retroparotid space syndrome
retroperitoneal
r. approach
r. fibrosis
retropharyngeal
r. abscess
r. approach
r. hemangioma
r. hematoma
r. space
retroposterior lateral nucleus
retroposterolateralis nucleus
retropulsed bone excision
retropulsion
retrosigmoid
r. approach
r. craniectomy
retrospection
retrospective
r. experimental study design
r. projection
retrotarsal fold
retrothalamica
cisterna r.
retrotonsillar fissure
retrovesical center
retroviral CB receptor
retrovirus infection
retrusion
midface r.
Rett syndrome
Retzius
R. fiber
R. foramen
foramen of Key and R.
R. gyrus
sheath of Key and R.
reuniens
canaliculus r.
canalis r.
ductus r.
nucleus r.
reuptake
r. blockade
neuronal r.
revascularization
brain r.
cerebral r.
reverberating circuit
reversal
deficit r.
homuncular organization phase r.
phase r.
reverse
r. analgesia
r. causality
r. learning function
r. ocular bobbing
r. orientation
r. polarity
r. transcriptase polymerase chain reaction (RT-PCR)
r. Trendelenburg position
reverse-angled curette
reversed optokinetic nystagmus
reversible
r. C-arm
r. cognitive impairment of depression
r. decortication

dementia r.
r. intoxication
r. ischemia
r. ischemic neurological deficit
r. ischemic neurologic defect
r. ischemic neurologic deficit (RIND)
r. ischemic neurologic disability (RIND)
r. motor neuron disease
r. posterior leukoencephalopathy syndrome (RPLS)
r. shock

Reversol Injection
ReVia
Revilliod sign
revindication
Revised
Bracken Basic Concept Scale, R.
Brigance Diagnostic Comprehensive Inventory of Basic Skills, R.
Clymer-Barrett Readiness Test, R.
Comprehensive Identification Process, R.
Continuous Visual Memory Test, R.
Derogatis Affects Balance Scale, R.
Herrmann Brain Dominance Instrument, R.
R. Physical Anhedonia Scale
R. Trauma Score

revision
Fast Health Knowledge Test, 1986 R.
UltraPower r.

revolving door syndrome
reward
r. circuitry
r. system

reward-irrelevant response
rewinder gradient
Rexed
lamina of R.
R. lamina

Rey Auditory Verbal Learning Test
Reye-like syndrome
Reye syndrome
Reynolds
R. number
R. skull traction tongs

Rey-Osterrieth complex
RF
radiofrequency
RF coil
RF electrocoagulation
RF pulse

RFG-3C radiofrequency lesion generator system
RFLP
restriction fragment length polymorphism

RGC
retinal ganglion cell

rhabdoid tumor
rhabdomancy
rhabdomyolysis
rhabdomyoma
rhabdomyosarcoma
intrasellar r.

rhabdovirus infection
rhenium-186
rheoencephalogram
rheoencephalography
rheologic therapy
rheolytic catheter
rheonome
rheostasis
rheumatic
r. carditis
r. chorea
r. fever cerebral embolism
r. tetany
r. torticollis

rheumatica
polymyalgia r. (PMR)
tetania r.

rheumatism
lumbar r.

rheumatoid
r. arteritis
r. arthritis
r. factor
r. neuropathy
r. spondylitis

Rheumatrex
rhigosis
rhigotic
rhinal
r. fissure
r. sulcus

rhinalis
sulcus r.

NOTES

rhinencephalic mamillary body
rhinencephalon
rhinitis
vasomotor r.
viral r.
rhinocele
rhinocerebral zygomycosis
rhinolalia aperta
rhinoplasty
external r.
rhinorrhea
cerebrospinal fluid r.
rhinoseptal approach
rhinosinusitis
rhinotomy
lateral r.
rhizolysis
percutaneous glycerol r.
percutaneous radiofrequency r.
percutaneous retrogasserian glycerol r. (PRGR)
rhizomelic chondrodysplasia punctata
rhizomeningomyelitis
rhizopathy
***Rhizopus* infection**
rhizotomy
anterior r.
bilateral ventral r.
chemical r.
Dana posterior r.
dorsal r.
facet r.
Frazier-Spiller r.
glycerol r.
intracranial r.
percutaneous radiofrequency retrogasserian r. (PRFR)
percutaneous retrogasserian glycerol r.
posterior r.
radiofrequency r.
retrogasserian r.
selective dorsal r. (SDR)
thermal r.
trigeminal r.
rho
Spearman r.
r. wave
rho-aminosalicylic acid
Rhodesian trypanosomiasis
Rhodococcus rodochrous
rhombencephali
isthmus r.
tegmentum r.
rhombencephalic
r. gustatory nucleus
r. isthmus
r. tegmentum
rhombencephalitis
rhombencephalon
tegmentum of r.
ventricle of r.
rhombencephalosynapsis
rhombic
rhombocele
rhomboid
r. fossa
medial eminence of r.
r. nucleus
rhomboidalis
nucleus commissuralis r.
sinus r.
rhomboidal sinus
rhomboidea
fossa r.
rhomboideae
eminentia medialis fossae r.
striae medullares fossae r.
sulcus limitans fossae r.
Rhoton
R. ball dissector
R. blunt-ring curette
R. dissecting forceps
R. loop curette
R. microcurette
R. microdissector
R. microhook
R. spatula
R. spoon curette
R. suction tip
Rhoton-Cushing forceps
Rhoton-Merz suction tube
Rhoton-Tew bipolar forceps
rhythm
alpha r.
background r.
Berger r.
beta r.
breach r.
cardiac r.
circadian r.
circannual r.
delta r.
EEG alpha r.
electroencephalogram r.
endogenous circadian r.
fast field-potential r.
focal slowing of background r.
gamma r.
heart r.
idiojunctional r.
infradian r.

r.'s of lags and spurts in development
mu r.
phi r.
pi r.
posterior r.
rolandic mu r.
sleep-wake r.
Society for Light Therapy and Biological R.'s
theta r.
time-locked occipital r.
ultradian r.
well-formed electroencephalogram r.
wicket r.

rhythmic
r. artifact
r. chorea
r. delta activity
r. discharge
r. midtemporal theta of drowsiness (RMTD)
r. movement
r. movement disorder
r. repetitive muscle potential
r. spindle-shaped activity

rhythmical midtemporal discharge

rhythmicity
circadian r.
sleep-wake r.
vegetative circadian r.

rib
r. cranioplasty
r. fracture
r. graft
r. removal

ribavirin

ribbed hook

ribbon
r. blade
r. encephaloduromyosynangiosis
Reil r.

Ribes ganglion

riboflavin deficiency

ribonucleic acid (RNA)

ribosuria

Ribot
R. gradient
R. law
R. law of memory

Richards
R. curette
R. tamp

Richardson-Steele-Oslzewski syndrome

Richards-Rundle syndrome

Riche-Cannieu anastomosis

Richmond
R. bolt
R. subarachnoid screw instrument

Richter laminectomy punch forceps

rickets
tumor-associated r.

rickettsial infection

rickettsii
Rochalimaea r.

Rickham reservoir

Riddoch
R. mass reflex
R. phenomenon

Ridenol

ridge
apical ectodermal r.
mamilloaccessory r.
supraorbital r.
transverse r.
triangular r.

ridging
spondylitic r.

Ridley
R. circle
R. sinus

ridleyi
circulus venosus r.

Riedel thyroiditis

Rieger syndrome

Rienhoff-Finochietto rib spreader

Rienhoff rib spreader

Rift Valley fever

right
r. anterior-temporal negativity
r. basilar mesial temporoparietal cortex
r. brain stroke (RBS)
r. ear advantage
r. frontal craniotomy for gross total resection of tumor
r. frontal lobe
r. frontoparietal infarction
r. hemiplegia
r. hemisphere dominance
r. hepatic vein

NOTES

right *(continued)*
r. parietal lobe syndrome
r. parietal occipital vertex craniotomy
r. sixth nerve palsy
r. temporoparietal craniotomy
r. thalamus
r. thoracic curve
r. thoracic curve scoliosis
r. thoracic curve with hypokyphosis
r. thoracic curve with junctional kyphosis
r. thoracic left lumbar curve pattern
r. thoracic left lumbar scoliosis
r. thoracic left thoracolumbar scoliosis
r. thoracic minor curve pattern
r. ventricle
r. ventricular activation (RVA)
r. and wrong test

right-angle
r.-a. bipolar cautery
r.-a. blunt probe
r.-a. booster clip
r.-a. drill
r.-a. screwdriver

right-ankle bur
right-bearing nystagmus
righting reflex
right-left confusion
right-sided
r.-s. submandibular transverse incision
r.-s. thoracotomy

right-to-left shunt (RLS)
rightward saccade
rigid
r. body transformation matrix
r. curve
r. curve scoliosis
r. dysarthria
r. internal fixation
r. pedicle
r. pedicle screw
r. pupil
r. rod-lens endoscope
r. spine disease
r. spine syndrome
r. ventriculoscope

rigidity
catatonic r.
C-D instrumentation r.
cerebellar r.
clasp-knife r.
cogwheel r.
Cotrel pedicle screw r.
decerebrate r.
decorticate r.
extrapyramidal r.
gamma r.
hemiplegic r.
lead-pipe r.
muscle r.
mydriatic r.
nuchal r.
paratonic r.
spastic r.
spinal fixation r.

Riley-Day syndrome
Riley-Smith syndrome
riluzole
rim
r. degeneration
supraorbital r.

rimula
RIND
resolving ischemic neurologic deficit
reversible ischemic neurologic deficit
reversible ischemic neurologic disability

ring
atrial r.
r. block anesthesia
Brown-Roberts-Wells base r.
Budde halo r.
carotid r.
r. chromosome
Cosman-Roberts-Wells stereotactic r.
cricoid r.
r. curette
dural r.
enhancing r.
Gibbs r.
halo r.
head r.
hemosiderin r.
Kayser-Fleischer corneal r.
Luque r.
platinum r.
proximal carotid r.
tentorial r.
vascular r.
V1 halo r.

ringed formed forceps
Ringer lactate
ring-wall lesion
Rinne test
Rio Bravo virus
RIP
radioimmunoprecipitation

rippling muscle disease
risedronate
rise time
rising phase

risk
r. factors for violence
r. paradigm
r. ratio
risk-benefit
r.-b. assessment
r.-b. profile
r.-b. ratio
Risperdal Consta
Risser-Cotrel body cast
Risser localizer
risus
r. caninus
r. sardonicus
Ritadex
Ritalin LA extended-release capsule
Ritchie index
ritonavir
Ritscher-Schnitzel syndrome
Ritter
R. law
R. opening tetanus
Ritter-Rollet phenomenon
ritual reduction
rivastigmine tartrate
Rivermead
R. ADL index
R. Behavioural Memory Test
R. Mobility Index
R. Motor Assessment
R. Perceptual Assessment Battery
rizatriptan benzoate
R-K needle
RLN
recurrent laryngeal nerve
RLS
restless legs syndrome
right-to-left shunt
rm
repeated measure
RMI
repetitive motion injury
RMS
repetitive motion syndrome
RMT
Recognition Memory Test
RMTD
rhythmic midtemporal theta of drowsiness
RMTD on electroencephalogram
RN
radionucleotide
RN scanning
RNA
ribonucleic acid
R. expression
R. virus
RNL
Reintegration to Normal Living
RNL index
Robaxin
robertsonian chromosome translocation
Robertson pupil
Robert syndrome
Robinow syndrome
Robin sequence micrognathia
Robinson
R. anterior cervical discectomy
R. anterior cervical fusion
robot
Evolution 1 precision r.
Grenoble stereotactic r.
Lausanne stereotactic r.
Long Beach stereotactic r.
Mayo Clinic stereotactic r.
neurosurgical stereotactic r.
stereotactic r.
robotic
r. microscope
r. system
robustus archistriatalis (RA)
ROC
receiver operating characteristic
Rocaltrol
Rochalimaea
R. akari
R. henselae
R. mooseri
R. prowazekii
R. quintana
R. rickettsii
R. tsutsugamushi
Rochester lamina dissector
Rockland-Simpson Dyskinesia Rating Scale
Rocky
R. Mountain spotted fever
R. Mountain spotted fever meningoencephalitis
ROD
relative optical density

NOTES

rod
aluminum master r.
r. bending
r. cell of retina
cerebellomesoencephalic fissure Perspex r.
compression r.
compressive r.
r. contour preparation
Corti r.
Cotrel-Dubousset r.
Delrin r.
distraction r.
double-L spinal r.
Edwards-Levine r.
Edwards modular system universal r.
r. fiber
r. fracture repair
Harrington r.
Hartshill rectangle r.
Isola spinal implant system eye r.
Jacobs locking hook spinal r.
Knodt r.
Kostuik r.
r. linkage
Luque r.
r. migration
modified Harrington r.
Moe r.
olfactory r.
pediatric Cotrel-Dubousset r.
r. placement
precontoured unit r.
r. rotation prevention
screw alignment r.
spinal r.
unit spinal r.
Wiltse system aluminum master r.
Wiltse system spinal r.
rod-hook construct
rodochrous
Rhodococcus r.
rodonalgia
rod-sleeve
Edwards modular system spinal r.-s.
r.-s. instrumentation
Roeder manipulative aptitude test device
roentgen knife stereotactic radiosurgical device
roentgenogram
biplane r.
lateral r.
roentgenographic opaque marker
rofecoxib
Roger
R. reflex
R. symptom
rogerian
Rogozinski spinal rod system
Rohon-Beard cella
ROI
region of interest
Rolandi
substantia gelatinosa R.
rolandic
r. area
r. benign epilepsy of childhood with centrotemporal spike
r. cortex
r. epilepsy
r. epileptiform discharge
r. line
r. mu rhythm
r. paroxysmal focus
r. region
r. seizure
r. vein syndrome
rolandica
zona r.
Roland-Morris disability questionnaire
Rolando
R. angle
R. area
R. cell
R. column
fissure of R.
R. gelatinous substance
R. tubercle
rolandoparietal glioma
role
adultomorphic behavior r.
central r.
etiologic r.
integral r.
intrinsic transverse connector r.
pathophysiological r.
pivotal r.
regulatory r.
r. strain
roll
FLUFTEX gauze r.
laminectomy r.
Roller nucleus
rolling
roll-off filter
Romano-Ward syndrome
Romberg
R. disease
facial hemiatrophy of R.
R. sign
R. spasm

R. symptom
R. syndrome
R. test
R. trophoneurosis

Romberg-Howship symptom

rombergism

rongeur

Adson cranial r.
Bacon cranial r.
Beyer laminectomy r.
bone-biting r.
Bucy laminectomy r.
Cherry-Kerrison laminectomy r.
Cloward disk r.
Cloward-English laminectomy r.
Codman-Harper laminectomy r.
Codman-Kerrison laminectomy r.
Codman-Leksell laminectomy r.
Codman-Schlesinger cervical laminectomy r.
Codman-Schlesinger laminectomy r.
cranial r.
Cushing cranial r.
Cushing intervertebral disk r.
Dahlgren cranial r.
DeVilbiss cranial r.
disk r.
double-action r.
Echlin laminectomy r.
Echlin-Luer r.
Elekta Leksell r.
Ferris Smith-Kerrison laminectomy r.
Fulton laminectomy r.
gooseneck r.
Gruenwald neurosurgical r.
Hajek-Koffler laminectomy r.
Hoen intervertebral disk r.
Hoen pituitary r.
Horsley r.
Hudson cranial r.
Husk bone r.
Jansen r.
Jansen-Middleton r.
Jarit-Kerrison laminectomy r.
Jarit-Liston bone r.
Jarit-Ruskin bone r.
Kerrison r.
Leksell r.
Love-Gruenwald cranial r.
Love-Gruenwald disk r.
Love-Gruenwald pituitary r.
Love-Kerrison laminectomy r.
Love pituitary r.
Mayfield r.
micropituitary r.
Mount laminectomy r.
narrow-bite bone r.
needle-nose r.
Nicola pituitary r.
Oldberg intervertebral disk r.
Oldberg pituitary r.
Olivecrona r.
Peiper-Beyer laminectomy r.
Poppen intervertebral disk laminectomy r.
punch r.
Raney laminectomy r.
Schlesinger intervertebral disk r.
Schlesinger laminectomy r.
Selverstone intervertebral disk r.
Smith-Petersen laminectomy r.
Spence intervertebral disk r.
Spurling-Kerrison laminectomy r.
Stille-Luer r.
Stookey cranial r.
upbiting/downbiting pituitary r.
Watson-Williams intervertebral disk r.
Weil-Blakesley intervertebral disk r.
Yasargil pituitary r.

roof

r. of fourth ventricle
r. nucleus
r. plate

roof-patch graft

room temperature

Roos brachial plexus root retractor

Roosen clamp

root

r. of ansa cervicalis
anterior r.
r. avulsion
conjoined nerve r.
cranial r.
developmental r.
dorsal spinal r.
entering r.
r. entry zone
r. entry-zone lesion
facial r.
r. of facial nerve

NOTES

root *(continued)*
r. filament
ganglion cell of dorsal spinal r.
r. level motor impairment
r. mean square error
nasociliary r.
nerve r.
olfactory r.
r. of olfactory tract, lateral and medial
r. of otic ganglion
r. pain
posterior r.
selective nerve r. (SNR)
r. sleeve fibrosis
spinal nerve r.
symptomatic r.
r. syndrome
trigeminal r.
r. of trigeminal nerve
ventral spinal r.
vestibular r.

rooting reflex

ropinirole
r. hydrochloride
r. monotherapy
r. study

ROS
reactive oxygen species

Rosai-Dorfman disease (RDD)

rose
r. bengal test
R. cephalic tetanus

Rosenbach
R. law
R. sign

Rosenberg-Chutorian syndrome

Rosen bur

Rosenmüller
fossa of R.

Rosenthal
basal vein of R. (BVR)
R. degeneration
R. fiber
R. fiber formation
R. vein

Rosenthal-Rosenthal syndrome

roseola infection

rosette
Homer Wright r.

Rosser crypt hook

Rossolimo
R. contraction
R. reflex
R. sign

rostra (*pl. of* rostrum)

rostrad

rostral
r. basilar artery syndrome
r. brainstem
r. brainstem ischemia
caudal to r.
r. cerebellar peduncle
r. cingulotomy
r. colliculus
r. colliculus commissure
r. interstitial nucleus
r. lamina
r. layer
r. lobe of cerebellum
r. medial prefrontal cortex
r. medullary vellum frenulum
r. midbrain
r. neuropore
r. olivary nucleus
r. posterior fossa
r. spinal axon
r. subcortical target
r. supplementary motor area
r. tegmentum
r. transtentorial herniation
r. ventrolateral medulla

rostral-central tegmentum

rostralis
area hypothalamica r.
brachium colliculi r.
colliculus r.
commissura colliculi r.
frenulum veli medullaris r.
lamina r.
lobulus semilunaris r.
nucleus cuneatus pars r.
nucleus olivaris r.
nucleus reticularis pontis r.
nucleus vestibularis r.
pars anterior commissurae r.
pars posterior commissurae r.
strata colliculi r.
strata grisea et alba colliculi r.
substantia perforata r.

rostrocaudal
r. contact array
r. epidural array

rostrum, pl. **rostra**
r. corporis callosi
r. of corpus callosum
sphenoid r.

Rotablator rotating bur

rotary
r. nystagmus
r. vertigo

rotating
r. hemostatic valve
r. mechanism

rotation
gantry r.
lateral r.
varimax r.
rotational
r. correction
r. injury
rotationally
r. induced shear-strain injury
r. induced shear-strain lesion
rotator
Jarit r.
rotatoria
chorea r.
rotatory
r. epilepsy
r. luxation
r. nystagmus
r. spasm
r. tic
rotavirus encephalitis
Roth
R. disease
R. spot
R. syndrome
Roth-Bernhardt syndrome
rotigotine
Roton sellar punch
rotoscoliosis
rotundum
foramen r.
rotundus
fasciculus r.
Rouget muscle
rouleaux formation
round
r. bur
r. eminence
r. fasciculus
r. hole plate
round-handled forceps
round-tipped periosteal elevator
Roussy-Dejerine syndrome
Roussy-Lévy
R.-L. disease
R.-L. hereditary areflexic dystasia
R.-L. syndrome
router
power r.
routine
complex finger r.
complex hand r.
rovelizumab
Rowland
criteria of R.
Roy-Camille
R.-C. plate
R.-C. posterior screw plate fixation
R.-C. posterior screw plate fixation biomechanics
R.-C. technique
RPLS
reversible posterior leukoencephalopathy syndrome
RPR
rapid plasma reagin
RPR test
RPTP zeta/beta
RR
relapsing-remitting
RRF
ragged red fiber
RRMS
relapsing-remitting multiple sclerosis
RSD
reflex sympathetic dystrophy
RSDS
reflex sympathetic dystrophy syndrome
RSE
rapid spin echo
rSO_2
regional oxygen saturation
rTMS
repetitive transcranial magnetic stimulation
RTPA
recombinant tissue plasminogen activator
RT-PCR
reverse transcriptase polymerase chain reaction
rubber button
rubella
congenital r.
r. panencephalitis
r. vaccination complication
r. virus
rubeosis iridis
ruber
nucleus r.
Rubin vase

NOTES

rubral tremor
rubri
pars parvocellularis nuclei r.
rubrobulbaris
tractus r.
rubrobulbar tract
rubroolivares
fibrae r.
rubroolivary fiber
rubropontine tract
rubropontinus
tractus r.
rubroreticular
r. fasciculus
r. tract
rubroreticulares
fasciculi r.
rubrospinal
r. decussation
r. syndrome
r. tract
rubrospinalis
tractus r.
rubrothalamic
rucksack paralysis
rudimentary sympathetic innervation
rudimentum, pl. **rudimenta**
r. hippocampus
Ruffini
R. corpuscle
R. cylinder
R. ending
flower-spray organ of R.
R. mechanoreceptor
R. organ
rufinamide
Ruggeri
R. reflex
R. sign
Ruggles Surgical Instrument
Rukavina syndrome
Rukavina-type familial amyloid polyneuropathy
rule
Allen r.
Bergman r.
inverse square r.
Jackson r.
r. of Spence
r. of two
ruling in tics
rumination
manie de r.
persistent r.
repetitive r.
ruminative depression
Rum-K
runner
intrinsic-negative r.
intrinsic-positive r.
running commentary hallucination
runs of activity
rupture
aneurysmal r.
annular radial r.
disk r.
intervertebral disk r.
intraoperative r.
longitudinal ligament r.
lumbar disk r.
vein patch r.
ruptured
r. aneurysm
r. disk
Rush Alzheimer Registry
Russell
hooked bundle of R.
R. syndrome
uncinate bundle of R.
uncinate fasciculus of R.
R. viper venom time
Russell-Rubinstein cerebrovascular malformation classification
Russian
R. autumnal encephalitis
R. autumn encephalitis
R. endemic encephalitis
R. forest-spring encephalitis
R. spring-summer encephalitis
R. spring-summer encephalitis (Eastern subtype)
R. spring-summer encephalitis (Western subtype)
R. tick-borne encephalitis
R. vernal encephalitis
Rust
R. disease
R. phenomenon
Ruvalcaba-Myhre syndrome
RVA
right ventricular activation
R_1 wave
R_2 wave

S
  S incision
  S phase cell
  S sleep
S5
  Philips Gyroscan S5, S15
S-100
  S. protein
  S. tumor marker
S15
S-44
  Grass stimulator S.
S-100beta protein
SAB
 subarachnoid block
  SAB anesthesia
sabeluzole
Saber CBF-ICP trauma sensor
Sabin-Feldman dye test
Sabril
sac
  dural s.
  endolymphatic s.
  nasal mucosal s.
  thecal s.
saccade
  contrapulsion of s.
  s. impairment
  leftward s.
  memory-guided s.
  s. paralysis
  rightward s.
  s. velocity
  visually-guided s.
saccadic
  s. abnormality
  s. contraversive head turning
  s. overshooting
  s. palsy
  s. pursuit
  s. pursuit eye movement
  s. slowing
saccharopinuria
saccular
  s. aneurysm
  s. nerve
  s. spot
saccularis
  nervus s.
sacculi
  macula s.
sacculus communis
sacerdotalism
Sachs
  S. brain suction tip
  S. brain suction tube
  S. dural hook
  S. dural separator
  S. nerve separator-spatula
  S. nerve spatula
sacral
  s. agenesis
  s. alar screw
  s. brim target point
  s. dimple
  s. dorsal commissural neuron
  s. dorsal commissural nucleus (SDCN)
  s. foraminal approach
  s. ganglion
  s. hemangioma
  s. meningocele
  s. nerve
  s. nerve root cyst
  s. nerve stimulation
  s. nerve stimulation therapy
  s. parasympathetic nucleus
  s. pedicle screw
  s. pedicle screw fixation
  s. plexopathy
  s. plexus
  s. plexus avulsion
  s. plexus neuropathy
  s. screw placement
  s. segmental nerve stimulation implantable neural prosthesis
  s. spine
  s. spine decompression
  s. spine fixation
  s. spine fusion
  s. spine modular instrumentation
  s. spine stabilization
  s. spine Universal instrumentation
sacrales
  nervi splanchnici s.
  nuclei parasympathici s.
sacralia
  ganglia s.
sacralis
  ansa s.
  plexus s.
  ramus lateralis rami posterioris nervi s.
  ramus medialis rami posterioris nervi s.
  segmentum medullae spinalis s.

sacralium
rami anteriores nervorum s.
rami dorsales nervorum s.
rami posteriores nervorum s.
rami ventrales nervorum s.
sacrifice
carotid artery s.
endovascular carotid s.
sacrococcygeal
s. agenesis
s. myxopapillary ependymoma
s. spine
s. teratoma
sacroiliac joint
sacroiliitis
sacrolisthesis
sacrolumbar
sacroposterior (SP)
sacrosanct
sacrospinalis muscle
sacrum fusion screw fixation
SAD
sleep apnea syndrome
saddle
Cloward surgical s.
s. coil
s. nose deformity
tubercle of s.
saddle-area sensory loss
saddleback fever
saddle-shaped anesthesia
S-adenosylmethionine (SAM, SAMe)
S-adenosylmethionine (SAM, SAMe)
S-adenosyl-*l*-methionine
Saenger
S. reflex
S. sign
Saethre-Chotzen syndrome
Safe-T-Wheel pinwheel
safrazine
sagittal
s. anatomic alignment
s. craniosynostosis
s. deformity
s. groove
s. orientation
s. pedicle angle
s. pedicle diameter
s. plane
s. plane instability
s. plexus
s. projection
s. sinus
s. sinus thrombosis
s. slice fracture
s. spin-echo image
s. synostosis
s. T1-weighted SE image
s. T1-weighted spin echo image
saguli
nucleus s.
sagulum nucleus
SAH
subarachnoid hemorrhage
angiogram-negative SAH
sailatoria
chorea s.
Saint
S. Anthony dance
S. Guy dance
S. Louis encephalitis
S. Louis encephalitis virus
S. Vitus dance
Sakoda complex
salaam
s. attack
s. convulsion
s. spasm
Sala cell
salax
paroniria s.
salbutamol
Salibi carotid artery clamp
salicylate
magnesium s.
potassium s.
serum s.
sodium s.
s. toxic effect
triethanolamine s.
salience
emotional s.
salient loading
saline
s. injection
phosphate-buffered s. (PBS)
preservative-free normal s.
s. torch
saline-soaked sponge
salivary
s. gland
s. gland dysfunction
s. nucleus
saliva screen for alcohol
salivatory nucleus
Salla disease
Salmonella
salmonellosis
nontyphoidal s.
Salmonine Injection
Salmon Rickham ventriculostomy reservoir
Salpix

salt
Earle s.'s
s. wasting
saltation
saltatorial
saltatoric
saltatory
chorea s.
s. conduction
s. spasm
SAM
S-adenosylmethionine
synthetic aperture magnetometry
samarium-EDTMP
SAMe
S-adenosylmethionine
SAM-e
sampling
chorionic villus s. (CVS)
petrosal sinus s.
Samuels-Weck hemoclip
sanatorium disease
sand
s. body
brain s.
s. tumor
Sandhoff disease
Sandifer syndrome
Sandostatin
sandwich
fascia-muscle-fascia s.
Sanfilippo
S. disease
S. syndrome
Sanger Brown ataxia
sanguinis
ictus s.
Sano clip applier
Sansert
Santavuori disease
Santavuori-Haltia disease
Santavuori-Haltia-Hagberg disease
Santorini plexus
SaO2
saturation of oxygen
sapheni
falciformis hiatus s.
rami cutanei cruris medialis nervi s.
ramus infrapatellaris nervi s.
saphenous
s. nerve
s. vein
s. vein bypass graft
s. vein patch graft
saphenus
cornu inferius hiatus s.
nervus s.
sapophore group
saposin B
Sapporo shunt tube
saquinavir
SARA
SQUID array for reproductive assessment
sarcoglia
sarcoglycan deficiency
sarcoid
s. neuropathy
s. polyneuropathy
sarcoidosis
intracranial s.
s. neuromuscular involvement
s. peripheral neuropathy
sarcolemma membrane
sarcoma
angiolithic s.
Ewing s.
fibrous s.
granulocytic s.
juxtacortical s.
Kaposi s.
orbital granulocytic s.
osteogenic s.
perithelial small cell s.
reticulum cell s.
sarcomatous
s. leptomeningitis
s. tumor
sarcomere
sarcoplasmic reticulum
sarcosinemia
sarcotubular myopathy
Sardinian multiple sclerosis
sardonic
sardonicus
risus s.
trismus s.
sartorius nerve
Sassouni analysis

NOTES

satellite
s. cell
s. potential
satellitosis
satiety center
satumomab pendetide
saturation
arterial oxygen s.
jugular bulb venous oxygen s.
nocturnal oxygen s.
s. of oxygen (SaO2)
partial s.
receiver s.
s. recovery
regional oxygen s. (rSO_2)
s. transfer
venous oxygen s.
Saturday night palsy
saturnine
s. encephalopathy
s. tremor
Saunders cervical HomeTrac
saver
Cell S.
intraoperative cell s.
saw
Adson wire s.
Bier s.
Cushing s.
DeMartel wire s.
Gigli s.
Midas Rex craniotomy s.
Olivecrona-Gigli s.
Olivecrona wire s.
spinal s.
threadwire s.
Triton reciprocating s.
undercutting s.
sawtooth wave
Sayk preparation of cerebrospinal fluid
Sayre head sling (SHS)
SCA
SCA gene (SCA 1-7)
SC-AcuFix Anterior Cervical Plate System
scala, pl. **scalae**
Löwenberg s.
s. media
s. vestibuli
scale
Abnormal Involuntary Movement S.
absolute s.
Alzheimer Disease Assessment S. (ADAS)
Alzheimer Disease Rating S. (ADRS)
American Musculoskeletal Tumor Society rating s.
American Spinal Injury Association/International Medical Society of Paraplegia Impairment S.
AO s.
Aphasia Language Performance S.
Ashworth s.
Barratt s.
Barthel Activities of Daily Living S.
Basic Living Skills S.
Behavior Pathology in Alzheimer's Disease Rating S.
Berg Balance S. (BBS)
Blessed-Roth Dementia S.
Bricklin Perceptual S.
Brief Cognitive Rating S.
British Ability S.
Brown-Goodwin s.
Buss-Durkee s.
CDR S.
Chapman S.
Clinical Adaptive Test/Clinical Linguistic and Auditory Milestone S. (CAT/CLAMS)
Clinical Dementia Rating S.
Clinical Global Improvement S.
Clinical Linguistic Auditory Milestone S.
Clinician Global Rating S.
clinician-rated s.
clinician rating s.
Cognitive Abilities S.
coma s.
Community-Oriented Programs Environment S.
Comprehensive Level of Consciousness S.
Conversational Skills Rating S.
Daily Rating S.
DBD S.
Delirium Rating S. (DRS)
Dementia Mood Assessment S.
Derogatis Affects Balance S.
Differential Ability S.
digital vernier s.
Edinburgh 2 Coma S.
efficacy s.
Engel Seizure Outcome S.
Epworth Sleepiness S. (ESS)
EuroQol visual analog s.
Expanded Disability Status S. (EDSS)
Fahn-Tolosa-Marin Tremor Rating S.

FIRO Awareness S.
Frankel s.
Functional Ergonomic Prolo S.
Gait Abnormality Rating S.
Geriatric Depression S.
Gesell Developmental S.
Glasgow Outcome S.
global clinician-rated s.
global dementia rating s.
Global Deterioration S. (GDS)
Gracely Pain S.
Hachinski Ischemic S.
Hague Seizure Severity S.
Hasegawa Dementia S.
Hoehn and Yahr s.
Hollingshead-Redlich s.
House-Brackmann Facial Nerve Function Grading S.
House-Brackmann Grading S.
Hunt-Hess subarachnoid hemorrhage s.
Injury Severity S.
Internal State S.
Iowa Conners s.
Karnofsky Performance S.
Karnofsky rating s.
Kurtzke Expanded Disability Status S.
Kurtzke multiple sclerosis disability s.
Leeds Anxiety S.
Level of Functioning S.
Liebowitz Social Anxiety S.
linear s.
manual vernier s.
Maryland coma s.
Memorial Delirium Assessment S. (MDAS)
Memorial Symptom Assessment S.
Modified Rankin S.
modified Simpson-Angus Rating S.
Morgan-Russell s.
National Institutes of Health Stroke S. (NIHSS)
Neurosurgical Cervical Spine S.
New York University Parkinson's Disease S.
Orpington Prognosis S.
Parkinson Disease Quality of Life S. (PDQUALIF)
PD Quality of Life S. (PDQUALIF)
Physicians' Global Rating S.
7-point s.
Positive and Negative Stroke S.
Positive and Negative Syndrome S. (PANSS)
Positive and Negative Syndrome S.-Component Excited (PANSS-EC)
Prognostic S.
Progressive Deterioration S.
Prolo function-economic rating s.
psychopathology rating s.
Pyramid S.
Quality of Crisis Support s.
Quality of Life S.
Reaction Level S.
Revised Physical Anhedonia S.
Rockland-Simpson Dyskinesia Rating S.
Scandinavian Stroke S. (SSS)
Sheehan's Disability S.
Shipley-Hartford S.
Smith Extrapyramidal S.
Spetzler-Martin grading s.
Stanford Sleepiness S.
state-dependent psychopathology rating s.
St. Paul-Ramsey S.
Strauss-Carpenter s.
Stroke Impact S. (SIS)
Teasdale and Jennett s.
Three-Item Delirium S.
Thurston s.
total s.
Tourette Syndrome Association Unified Tic Rating S.
Tremor Clinical Rating S.
Unified Huntington Disease Rating S. (UHDRS)
Unified Parkinson Disease Rating S. (UPDRS)
UPDRS s.
verbal analog pain s.
Vineland percentile s.
visual analog s. (VAS)
Wechsler Adult Intelligence S. (WAIS)
Wechsler Intelligence S. for Children-Revised (WISC-R)

S

NOTES

scale *(continued)*
Wechsler Intelligence S. for Children-Revised, Version III (WISC-III)
Wechsler Memory S. for Children, Russell version (WMS-R)
WFNS s.
World Federation of Neurological Surgeons scale
World Federation of Neurological Surgeons s. (WFNS scale)
Yale Global Tic Severity S. (YGTSS)
Yale Tic Severity S.
Young Mania Rating S. (YMRS)
Zung Anxiety S.

scaled stereotactic atlas section

scalenectomy

scalenotomy

scalenus
s. anterior syndrome
s. anticus
s. anticus muscle

scalp
s. clip
s. clip applicator
s. clip forceps
s. closure
s. contusion
s. EEG monitoring
s. electrical potential
s. electrode
s. flap
s. flap forceps
s. hematoma
s. ictal electroencephalography
s. incision
s. infection
s. laceration

scalp-derived EEG activity

scalp-EEG

scalp-sphenoidal electroencephalography

scan
attenuation coefficient on MRI s.
attenuation value on MRI s.
baseline s.
bone density s.
bone-window CT s.
brain SPECT s.
CAT s.
computerized tomography s.
contrast-enhanced CT s.
CT s.
echo planar diffusion- and perfusion-weighted imaging s.
fast spin echo s.
fluorodopa positron emission tomographic s.
gallium s.
instant s.
longitudinal s.
MRI s.
nuclear MR s.
PET s.
radioisotope s.
radionuclide bone s.
sequential computed tomographic s.
single photon emission CT s.
SPECT s.
standardized A s.
1.5-Tesla General Electric signa s.
s. time
triple phase bone s.
T1-weighted inversion recovery s.
T2-weighted magnetic resonance s.

scandale
succes de s.

Scandinavian Stroke Scale (SSS)

scanner
s. assisted target localization
ATL real-time Neurosector s.
General Electric CT 9800 s.
General Electric Hi-Speed Advantage helical s.
General Electric Hi-Speed Spiral CT S.
General Electric Signa 1.5-Tesla magnetic resonance s.
Magnetom Open s.
Magnetom Vision s.
OctreoScan s.
Picker s.
Siemens Magnetom Harmony s.
Siemens Vision s.
Sigma .15T s.
SilkTouch CO_2 laser s.
SwiftLase s.
Vista American Health 0.5 Tesla MRI s.

scanning
CAT s.
computerized axial tomography s.
confocal laser s.
diffusion-weighted s.
duplex s.
s. electron microscopy
functional activation PET s.
GE Signa s.
GE Vector s.
line s.
point s.
radionucleotide s.
RN s.

s. speech
XeCT s.
xenon CT s.
xenon-enhanced CT s.
scaphocephaly
scaphohydrocephalus
scaphohydrocephaly
scapulae
levator s.
nervus dorsalis s.
scapular
s. nerve
s. reflex
scapulohumeral
s. atrophy
s. muscular dystrophy
s. reflex
scapuloperiosteal reflex
scapuloperoneal
s. muscular atrophy
s. muscular dystrophy
s. syndrome
scar
glia s.
hemosiderin s.
Scaramella procedure
scarf sign
scarlatiniform rash
Scarpa
S. ganglion
S. method
S. nerve
scarring
glial s.
scatter
intratest s.
scatteration
scattered
s. dysrhythmic slow activity
s. dysrhythmic slow activity on EEG
scattergram
scattering
Compton s.
scavenger
free radical s.
SCD
spinocerebellar degeneration
Scedosporium apiospermum
scelalgia
scelotyrbe
Sceratti arc
SCG
superior cervical ganglion
Schacher ganglion
Schaffer
S. collateral
S. collateral cell
Schäffer reflex
Schaltenbrand-Wahren stereotactic atlas
Scharff microbipolar and suction forceps
Schaumberg disease
schedule
altered sleep s.
S.'s for Clinical Assessment in Neuropsychiatry
Glasgow Assessment S.
s. II substance
medical taper s.
medication taper s.
regular eating s.
regular sleeping s.
regular waking s.
sleep-wake s.
work s.
Scheie
S. disease
S. syndrome
schema, pl. **schemata**
body s.
Kraepelin s.
schematic mental model
schenckii
Sporothrix s.
Scheuermann
S. disease
S. kyphosis
Schiefferdecker disk
Schiff-Sherrington phenomenon
Schilder
S. aminoaciduria
S. disease
S. encephalitis
Schilling test
Schindler disease
Schinzel-Giedion syndrome
Schirmer
S. syndrome
S. test
schismatize
schistorrhachis

NOTES

Schistosoma mansoni
schistosomiasis
schizaxon
schizencephalic
s. microcephaly
s. porencephaly
schizencephaly
schizogyria
Schizophyllum commune
Schlesinger
S. intervertebral disk rongeur
S. laminectomy rongeur
S. phenomenon
S. sign
Schlichter test
Schloffer operation
Schlösser treatment
Schmidt-Fischer angle
Schmidt-Lanterman
S.-L. cleft
S.-L. incisure
S.-L. segment
Schmidt vagoaccessory syndrome
Schmiedel ganglion
Schmieden-Taylor dissector
Schmitt disease
Schmorl
S. node
S. nodule
Schneider first rank symptom
Schnidt clamp
Schober measurement
Scholz disease
Schramm phenomenon
Schreiber maneuver
Schrötter chorea
Schüller-Christian syndrome
Schüller phenomenon
Schultze
S. bundle
S. cell
comma bundle of S.
comma tract of S.
S. comma tract
S. scissors
S. sign
Schultze-Chvostek sign
Schütz
S. bundle
S. fasciculus
S. Measures
tract of S.
S. tract
Schwabach test
Schwalbe
S. corpuscle
S. fissure
S. foramen
S. nucleus
S. space
Schwann
S. cell
S. cell body
S. cell differentiation
S. cell marker
S. cell origin
S. cell tumor
S. cell unit
S. membrane
S. nucleus
sheath of S.
S. white substance
Schwann-cell implant
schwannoglioma
schwannoma
acoustic s.
cerebellopontine angle s.
intracranial s.
intralabyrinthine s.
intraosseous s.
jugular foramen s.
nonacoustic s.
spinal intradural s.
synchronous facial s.
trigeminal s.
vestibular s.
schwannomin
schwannosis
Schwartz
S. aneurysm clip
S. laminectomy retractor
S. temporary intracranial artery clamp
S. tractotomy
Schwartz-Jampel syndrome
SCI
spinal cord injury
sciatic
s. nerve
s. nerve lesion
s. nerve trauma
s. neuralgia
s. neuritis
s. notch syndrome
s. pain
s. plexus
s. scoliosis
sciatica
sciaticus
nervus s.
scientific empiricism
scieropia
scintiangiography

scintigram
^{99m}Tc-HMPAO leukocyte s.
scintigraphy
Ga s.
indium-111 octreotide s.
leukocyte s.
regional cerebral blood flow s.
^{99m}Tc-HMPAO leukocyte s.
^{201}Tl s.
scintillating visual scotoma
scintillation camera
scintiphoto
scissoring walk
scissors
Adson ganglion s.
alligator MacCarty s.
Aslan endoscopic s.
bipolar cautery s.
Codman s.
Dandy neurological s.
Dandy neurosurgical s.
Dandy trigeminal nerve s.
DeBakey endarterectomy s.
Decker alligator s.
Decker microsurgical s.
dural s.
Frazier dural s.
s. gait
Harrington s.
Jacobson microneurosurgical s.
Jannetta-Kurze dissecting s.
Jansen-Middleton s.
Kurze dissection s.
Malis bipolar cautery s.
Malis neurological s.
Mayo s.
Metzenbaum s.
Micro-Two s.
Nicola s.
Olivecrona dura s.
Olivecrona trigeminal s.
Schultze s.
Smellie s.
Strully dural s.
Strully neurological s.
Sweet pituitary s.
Taylor brain s.
Taylor dural s.
Toennis dissecting s.
Yasargil bayonet s.

SCIWORA
spinal cord injury without radiographic abnormality
scleractinian coral
sclerencephalia
sclerencephaly
scleritis
sclerodactylia
sclerodactyly, telangiectasia
scleroderma
sclerodermatomyositis
sclérose en plaque
sclerosing
s. leukoencephalitis
s. panencephalitis
sclerosis, pl. **scleroses**
acute lateral s. (ALS)
Alzheimer s.
Ammon horn s.
amyotrophic lateral s. (ALS, AML)
ash-leaf spot in tuberous s.
Baló concentric s.
Bourneville tuberous s.
Canavan s.
cerebral s.
combined s.
concentric s.
congenital hippocampal s.
diffuse cerebral s.
diffuse infantile familial s.
discogenic s.
disseminated s.
epidemic multiple s.
Erb s.
Evers diet for multiple s.
familial amyotrophic lateral s. (FALS)
familial centrolobar s.
familial form of amyotrophic lateral s.
focal s.
hippocampal s.
hippocampus s.
human herpesvirus 6/multiple s. (HHV6-MS)
insular s.
ipsilateral mesial temporal s.
Krabbe diffuse s.
laminar cortical s.
lateral spinal s.
lobar s.

NOTES

sclerosis *(continued)*
MacDougall diet for multiple s.
mantle s.
mesial temporal s.
multiple s. (MS)
myelinoclastic diffuse cerebral s.
Pelizaeus-Merzbacher s.
posterior spinal s.
posterolateral s.
primary lateral s.
progressive systemic s.
relapsing-remitting multiple s. (RRMS)
Sardinian multiple s.
secondary progressive multiple s. (SPMS)
subchondral s.
sudanophilic cerebral s.
systemic s.
tuberous s.
ventrolateral s.
s. of white matter
sclerotic
s. area
s. plaque
sclerotome area
SCM
sternocleidomastoid
SCN1B gene
scoliosis
adult s.
compensatory s.
congenital s.
degenerative lumbar s.
double major curve s.
double thoracic curve s.
fracture with s.
idiopathic thoracic s.
King type II, V s.
Lenke classification of adolescent idiopathic s.
lumbar s.
neuromuscular s.
osteopathic s.
paralytic s.
right thoracic curve s.
right thoracic left lumbar s.
right thoracic left thoracolumbar s.
rigid curve s.
sciatic s.
thoracic curve s.
thoracolumbar idiopathic s.
thoracolumbar spine s.
scoliotic
s. curve fixation
scombroid
scoop
Cushing pituitary s.
Scoville intervertebral disk s.
Yasargil s.
scopolamine
score
Abbreviated Injury S.
Abnormal Involuntary Movement S.
Acute Physiology S.
Barnes global s.
Champion Trauma S.
Children's Coma S.
cognitive s.
conservative cutoff s.
cutoff s.
elevated s.
emotional memory s.
end-point CGI s.
event recall s.
factor s.
general knowledge s.
Glasgow Coma S. (GCS)
Glasgow Outcome S. (GOS)
global AIMS s.
global clinical impression s.
Global Tic Rating s.
Hachinski ischemic s.
Hopkins Symptom Checklist–90 Total S.
House-Brackmann S.
Impairment Rating s.
ipsative s.
Karnofsky performance s. (KPS)
Kurtzke s.
Lahey s.
logarithm of the odds s.
logical memory subtest s.
mean total weighted sum s.
mean weighted s.
neurofibrillary tangle s.
objective motor s.
Oswestry s.
peak s.
Performance Scale S.'s
positive s.
Q s.
RAATE s.
raw Q s.
Revised Trauma S.
Simpson-Angus total s.
standard s.
stroke s.
subtest scale s.
T s.
total AIMS s.
total emotional memory s.
total symptom s.

total weighted sum s.
UPDRS OFF s.
verbal recall s.
verbal weighted sum s.
Wada memory s.
weighted sum s.
scoring coefficient
scotodinia
scotoma, pl. **scotomata**
scotomata of action
bilateral centrocecal s.
cecocentral s.
flittering s.
hemianopic s.
homonymous scintillating s.
paracentral s.
scintillating visual s.
Scott
S. cannula
S. silicone ventricular catheter
scotty dog sign
Scoville
S. blade
S. brain clip-applying forceps
S. brain spatula
S. brain spatula forceps
S. cervical disk retractor
S. clip
S. clip-applying forceps
S. dissector
S. hemilaminectomy retractor
S. intervertebral disk scoop
S. nerve root hook
S. nerve root retractor
S. ruptured disk curette
S. skull trephine
S. ventricular needle
Scoville-Haverfield hemilaminectomy retractor
Scoville-Richter laminectomy retractor
scrapie form
scratching automatism
scratch reflex
screener
Closed Head Injury S.
screening
anencephaly s.
bone density s.
developmental disorder s.
Down syndrome s.
genetic s.
metabolic disorder s.
Tay-Sachs disease s.
S. Test for the Assignment of Remedial Treatments
urine s.
Wyatt s.
screw
alar s.
s. alignment bar
s. alignment rod
s. angulation
s. backout
bone s.
s. breakage
Camino subdural s.
cancellous s.
Caspar cervical s.
cortical s.
Cotrel pedicle s.
Edwards sacral s.
s. fixation
iliac s.
iliosacral s.
s. implantation
s. insertion
s. insertion technique
Isola spinal implant system iliac s.
KLS-Martin center-drive s.
Kostuik s.
Leibinger Micro Plus s.
Lorenz cranial s.
lumbar pedicle s.
Micro Plus s.
Mille Pattes s.
Mini Würzburg s.
Moss-Miami polyaxial s.
pedicle s.
s. plate approach
polyaxial s.
s. position perioperative monitoring
s. pullout
rigid pedicle s.
sacral alar s.
sacral pedicle s.
set s.
s. stabilization
stainless steel s.
Steinhauser cranial s.
s. stripout
subarachnoid s.
subdural pressure s.

NOTES

screw *(continued)*
superior thoracic pedicle s.
Synthes s.
Texas Scottish Rite Hospital pedicle s.
thoracolumbar pedicle s.
TiMesh s.
transarticular s.
transpedicular s.
triangulated pedicle s.
tulip pedicle s.
Vari-Angle s.
screwdriver
right-angle s.
Stab-and-Grab s.
screw-to-screw compression construct
scriptorius
calamus s.
tric s.
Script Stat, Inc. dispensing system
scrivener's palsy
scrotal nerve
scrub typhus
scurrile
scurrility
Scutellaria lateriflora
SD
semantic dementia
sleep deprivation
stimulus drive
SDAT
senile dementia of the Alzheimer's type
SDAVF
spinal dural arteriovenous fistula
SDCN
sacral dorsal commissural nucleus
SDEEG
stereotactic depth electroencephalogram
stereotactic depth electroencephalography
SDR
selective dorsal rhizotomy
SDS
Shy-Drager syndrome
sodium dodecyl sulfate
SDS-PAGE
sodium dodecyl sulfate polyacrylamide
SE
Myoclonic SE
sealant
FloSeal Matrix hemostatic s.
FocalSeal-S-surgical s.
tissue fibrin s.
seamstress's cramp
Seashore test
seasonal
s. migraine
s. migraine headache
seat
Wayne laminectomy s.
seatbelt fracture
Seattle Longitudinal Study
sebaceous adenoma
sebaceum
adenoma s.
sebaceus
seborrheic keratosis
Sechrist monoplace hyperbaric chamber
Seconal
second
s. cervical nerve
s. cranial nerve [CN II]
s. harmonic imaging (SHI)
s. impact syndrome
s. somatosensory area
s. temporal convolution
s. visual area
secondarily generalized tonic-clonic seizure
secondary
s. axotomy
s. bilateral synchrony
s. degeneration
s. delirium
s. disorder
s. drive
s. dual pathology
s. dystonia
s. effect
s. encephalitis
s. ending
s. epileptogenesis
s. epileptogenic focus
s. fissure of cerebellum
s. generalized epilepsy
s. headache
s. hydrocephalus
s. posttraumatic syringomyelia
s. process
s. progressive multiple sclerosis (SPMS)
s. seizure
s. sensory cortex
s. sensory neuron
s. sensory nucleus
s. somatosensory area
s. somatosensory cortex
s. symptom
s. synaptic cleft
s. verbal memory
s. visual area
s. visual cortex
second-degree nystagmus

second-line
s.-l. agent
s.-l. therapy
second-messenger molecule
second-order neuron
Secor system
secretase
alpha s.
beta s.
gamma s.
secret curette
secreted
s. protein acidic and rich in cysteine
regulated on activation, normal T-cell expressed, and s. (RANTES)
secretin
secreting glial pseudocyst
secretion
androgen s.
gastrointestinal s.
leptin s.
ovarian androgen s.
progesterone s.
secretomotor nerve
secretomotory
secretory
s. function
s. meningioma
s. nerve
section
attached cranial s.
axial s.
callosal s.
coronal s.
detached cranial s.
histologic s.
midsagittal s.
parasagittal s.
permanent s.
pituitary stalk s.
scaled stereotactic atlas s.
trigeminal root s.
vestibular nerve s.
sectioning
cryomicrotome s.
sectoranopia
quadruple s.
SecureStrand
S. cable
S. cervical fusion system
Sedan cannula
Sedan-Nashold needle
sedation
preoperative s.
prolonged s.
sedation/apathy
sedative
s. activity
s. antihistamine
s. hallucinogen
hypnotic s.
s. property
seed
^{125}I s.
radioactive yttrium s.
seeding
subarachnoid s.
surgical s.
SEEG
stereoelectroencephalography
Seeligmüller sign
seesaw nystagmus (SSN)
SEF
spectral edge frequency
supplementary eye field
Seglas-type paranoia
segment
adrenal s.
clinoidal s.
exiting s.
globus pallidus external s.
globus pallidus internal s.
initial s.
interannular s.
internodal s.
intradural s.
Lanterman s.
M s.
M2 artery s.
medullary s.
motion s.
neural s.
ophthalmic s.
P s.
Ranvier s.
Schmidt-Lanterman s.
s. of spinal cord
sympathetic s.
traversing s.
segmenta
s. cervicalia 1–8

S

NOTES

segmenta *(continued)*
s. cervicalia medullae spinalis
s. coccygea medullae spinalis
s. lumbalia medullae spinalis
s. medullae spinalis
s. sacralia medullae spinalis
s. thoracica medullae spinalis
segmental
s. anesthesia
s. arterial disorganization
s. compression construct
s. demyelinating polyneuropathy
s. demyelination
s. dystonia
s. ectasia
s. fixation
s. medullary reflex
s. neuritis
s. neurofibromatosis
s. neuropathy
s. registration
s. sensory disassociation with brachial muscular atrophy
s. spinal instrumentation
s. vulnerability
segmentary
s. response
s. syndrome
segmentation
volume s.
segmentum
s. coccygea 1–3
s. internodale
s. lumbalia 1–5
s. lumbaria
s. medullae spinalis
s. medullae spinalis cervicalia
s. medullae spinalis coccygea
s. medullae spinalis lumbalis
s. medullae spinalis sacralis
s. medullae spinalis thoracica
s. sacralia 1–5
s. thoracica 1–12
segregation
mitotic s.
Séguin
S. sign
S. signal symptom
SEH
spinal epidural hematoma
seine kinase
seipin gene
Seitelberger disease
seizure
absence s.
s. activity
afebrile s.
affective symptom of s.
alcohol-related s.
alcohol withdrawal s.
alimentary s.
amygdala s.
anosognosic s.
astatic s.
atonic s.
atypical absence s.
atypical petit mal s.
audiogenic s.
auditory s.
automotor s.
autonomic s.
catamenial s.
cerebellar fit s.
chemically-induced s.
childhood absence epilepsy with generalized tonic-clonic s.
clinical s.
clonic s.
clonicotonic s.
complex febrile s.
complex motor s.
complex partial nocturnal s.
convulsive s.
dileptic s.
drop s.
drug-resistant localization-related s.
early s.
eclamptic s.
electroconvulsive s.
electrodecremental s.
electrographic s.
encephalotrigeminal angiomatosis s.
epileptic s.
s. evaluation
evoked s.
s. exacerbation
extratemporal s.
febrile s.
fictitious s.
first-trimester maternal s.
focal motor s.
s. foci resection
frontal lobe s.
gelastic s.
generalized atypical absence s.
generalized epilepsy plus febrile s.
generalized tonic-clonic s. (GTCS)
grand mal s.
habitual s.
hippocampal slice model of s.
HIV-related s.
hypermotor s.
hyperventilation s.
hypoglycemic s.

hypomotor s.
hysterical s.
ictal confusional s.
idiopathic s.
International Classification of S.'s
intractable partial s.
jacksonian s.
Janz juvenile myoclonic s.
juvenile absence s.
kindled s.
late s.
laughing s.
localization-related s.
major motor s.
s. management
maximal electroshock s. (MES)
maximal electroshock-induced s.
medically refractory partial s.
midtemporal s.
minor motor s.
s. monitoring
motor s.
myoclonic-astatic petit mal s.
negative myoclonic s.
neonatal drug addiction s.
neonatal hypoglycemic s.
new-onset s.
nicotine-induced s.
nocturnal s.
nonconvulsive s.
nonepileptic s.
occipital lobe s.
opioid peptide in s.
partial complex s.
partial-onset s.
s. pattern
petit mal s.
phantom absence s.
postischemic s.
postmenopausal s.
postpump s.
premature infant s.
primary generalized s.
primary idiopathic s.
pseudoepileptic s.
psychic s.
psychogenic nonepileptic s.
psychomotor s.
pyridoxine-deficiency s.
reactive s.
s. recurrence
refractory localization-related s.
remote symptomatic s.
rolandic s.
secondarily generalized tonic-clonic s.
secondary s.
serial motor s.
simple febrile s.
simple partial s.
single s.
sound-sensitive s.
subclinical s.
subtle s.
supplementary motor s.
sylvian s.
symptomatic s.
temporal lobe s.
tonic s.
tonic-clonic s.
Torric-Clount s.
s. trigger
typical absence s.
unclassified epileptic s.
unprovoked s.
versive s.
vestibulogenic s.
video monitoring of s.

seizure-free
s.-f. outcome
s.-f. state

seizurelike
s. activity
s. phenomenon

sejunction

selachian

Seldinger
S. angiogram
S. method
S. retrograde wire/intubation technique

selection
bone plate s.
Edwards modular system construct s.
internal s.
ligand s.
slice s.

selective
s. amnesia
s. auditory agnosia
s. dorsal rhizotomy (SDR)

NOTES

selective *(continued)*
s. embolization
s. estrogen receptor modulator (SERM)
s. excitation
s. focusing on environmental stimulus
s. imaging and graphics for stereotactic surgery (SIGSS)
s. irradiation
s. memory
s. microadenomectomy
s. nerve root (SNR)
s. norepinephrine reuptake inhibitor
s. phosphodiesterase inhibitor
s. relaxation enhancement
S. Reminding Test
s. serotonin reuptake inhibitor (SSRI)
s. speech perception alteration
s. thoracic spine fusion
s. T2 shortening
s. vagotomy
selectivity
mesolimbic s.
selector
Leksell s.
S. ultrasonic aspirator
selegiline patch
self-adhering electrode
self-attaching electrode
Self-Description Inventory
self-induced
s.-i. artefactual skin disease
s.-i. dermatitis artefacta
s.-i. epilepsy
self-object transference
self-perceived cognitive disorder
self-perpetuated disease
self-retaining brain retractor
self-stopping drill point
self-sustaining hyperexcitability
sella
ballooning of the s.
diaphragm of s.
empty s.
s. punch forceps
tuberculum s.
s. turcica
s. turcica diaphragm
sellae
diaphragma s.
sellar
s. aneurysm
s. cyst
s. entrance
s. gangliocytoma
s. punch
s. region
s. tumor
sellaris
pars s.
Selter disease
Selverstone
S. clamp
S. cordotomy hook
S. intervertebral disk rongeur
S. Semmes curette sensor
SEM
standard error of the mean
semantic
s. aphasia
s. cue
s. cueing
s. dementia (SD)
s. memory
s. memory function
s. memory impairment
s. process
Semap
semialdehyde
succinic s.
semicircular
s. canal
s. duct
semicirculares
crura ossea canales s.
ductus s.
semicircularis
crus membranaceum commune ductus s.
crus membranaceum simplex ductus s.
ductus s.
tenia s.
semicircularium
canalium s.
ductuum s.
semicoma
semicomatose
semiconscious
semi-Fowler position
semiinvasive electrode
semilunar
s. fasciculus
s. ganglion
s. lobe
s. lobule
s. notch
s. nucleus of Flechsig
s. tract
semilunare
velum s.

semilunares
lobuli s.
semilunaris
fasciculus s.
hiatus s.
nucleus s.
semimembranosus reflex
seminoma
intracranial s.
semiology
ictal s.
semioval center
semiovale
centrum s.
Vicq d'Azyr centrum s.
semiplegia
semipurposeful
s. activity
s. behavior
semisleep
state of s.
semispinalis capitis
semisynthetic sphingolipid
semitendinosus reflex
Semliki Forest encephalitis
Semmes curette
Semmes-Weinstein esthesiometer
Semon-Hering theory
Semon law
semustine
senectitude
senescence
motor neuron s.
senescent
s. fibroblast
s. forgetfulness
senile
s. chorea
s. delirium
s. dementia
s. dementia of the Alzheimer's type (SDAT)
s. gait disorder
s. leukoencephalopathic lesion
s. memory
s. neuropathy
s. paranoid state
s. paraplegia
s. plaque
s. tremor
Senn retractor
sensate focus approach
sensation
abnormal tactile s.
cincture s.
cutaneous s.
delayed s.
dysesthesic s.
epicritic s.
general s.
girdle s.
objective s.
pin s.
pins-and-needles s.
primary s.
referred s.
reflex s.
special s.
subjective s.
transferred s.
vascular s.
sense
s. of alienation
body s.
contact s.
s. of control
distance s.
s. epithelium
s. of equilibrium
s. of fatigue
internal s.
joint s.
kinesthetic s.
motion s.
movement s.
muscle s.
muscular s.
obstacle s.
s. organ
organ of special s.
pain s.
position s.
posture s.
pressure s.
proprioceptive s.
seventh s.
sixth s.
somatic s.
space s.
special s.
static s.
tactile s.

NOTES

sense *(continued)*
taste s.
temperature s.
thermal s.
thermic s.
time s.
vestibular s.
vibration s.
visceral s.
weight s.
s. of wellness
s. of wholeness
sensibility
articular s.
bone s.
common s.
cortical s.
deep s.
dissociation s.
electromuscular s.
epicritic s.
mesoblastic s.
pallesthetic s.
proprioceptive s.
protopathic s.
splanchnesthetic s.
vibratory s.
sensible hemideficit
sensiferous
sensigenous
sensimeter
sensitiva
trichosis s.
sensitive
s. measure
s. plane
s. point
s. volume
sensitivity
age-associated s.
cold s.
enhanced s.
feedback s.
high s.
loss of s.
neuroleptic s.
pharmacologic s.
proportional s.
s. threshold
warm s.
sensitization
central s.
peripheral nociceptor s.
sensomobile
sensomobility
sensomotor
sensor
CardioSearch s.
DC SQUID s.
DermaTemp infrared thermographic s.
disposable Doppler-constant thermocouple s.
MEG s.
Neurotrend s.
Paratrend 7 s.
s. position indicator
Saber CBF-ICP trauma s.
Selverstone Semmes curette s.
telemetric intracranial pressure s.
Watson angular rate s.
zero drift of the s.
sensoria
decussatio s.
ganglia craniospinalia s.
organa s.
sensorial area
sensoriale
ganglion s.
sensoriglandular
sensorimotor
s. area
s. axonal polyneuropathy
s. grating
s. period
s. peripheral neuropathy
sensorimuscular
sensorineural
s. acuity level masking technique
s. deafness
sensorium commune
sensorius
nervus s.
sensorivascular
sensorivasomotor
sensory
s. alexia
s. amusia
s. aphasia
s. apraxia
s. association area
s. ataxia
s. aura
s. axon
s. cell
s. compound action potential
s. compound action potential amplitude
s. cortex
s. crossway
s. decussation of medulla oblongata
s. deficit
s. deprivation

s. dimension
s. distribution
s. dysprosody
s. dystaxia
s. epithelium
s. evoked potential (SEP)
s. function
s. ganglion of cranial nerve
s. ganglion of encephalic nerve
s. gating
s. hair
s. image
s. impairment
s. inattention
s. information
s. integration dysfunction
s. interface
s. jacksonian attack
s. latency
s. load
s. loss
s. myelinated fiber
s. nerve action potential (SNAP)
s. nerve action potential amplitude
s. neurogenic arthropathy
s. neuron
s. neuronopathy
s. neuron-specific G protein-coupled receptor (SNSRs)
s. neuropathy
s. nucleus
s. organ
s. overload
s. paralysis
s. pathway
S. Perceptual Examination
s. phantom
s. precipitated epilepsy
s. process
s. processing area
s. region
s. root of ciliary ganglion
s. root of mandibular nerve
s. root of otic ganglion
s. root of spinal nerve
s. root of submandibular ganglion
s. root of trigeminal nerve
s. speech center
s. tract
s. transduction

sensory-deprivation nystagmus

sensory-motor
s.-m. behavior
s.-m. strip
s.-m. stroke

sensory-motor-autonomic neuropathy

sensual dysarthria

sensuosity

sensuum
organa s.

senticosus
Eleutherococcus s.

SentiLite
S. EEG monitor
S. neurological monitor

sentinel
s. leak
s. spinous process fracture

Sentinel-4 neurological monitor

Sentinel system

Seoul virus

SEP
sensory evoked potential
pudendal SEP

separans
funiculus s.

separation
articular mass s.
atlantoaxial s.
atlantooccipital s.
pontomedullary s.

separator
Davis dural s.
Davis nerve s.
Dorsey dural s.
dural s.
Frazier dural s.
Hoen dural s.
Horsley dural s.
Hunter dural s.
Sachs dural s.
synovial s.
Woodson dural s.

separator-spatula
Davis nerve s.-s.
Sachs nerve s.-s.
Woodson dural s.-s.

SEPNR
spinally elicited peripheral nerve response

septa (*pl. of* septum)

NOTES

S

septal
s. area
s. nucleus
s. region
septation
intraventricular s.
septi
nuclei triangularis s.
nucleus accumbens s.
septic
s. embolus
s. encephalitis
s. meningitis
s. shock
s. thrombosis
s. venous vasculitis
septicemia
septineuritis
Nicolau s.
septofimbrial nucleus
septomarginal
s. fasciculus
s. tract
septomarginalis
fasciculus s.
septooptic dysplasia
septooptic-pituitary dysplasia
septum, pl. **septa**
s. cervicale intermedium
intermediate cervical s.
s. lingua
lingual s.
s. lucidum
s. medianum dorsale medullae spinalis
s. medianum posterius medullae spinalis
s. pellucidum
s. pellucidum cave
precommissural s.
subarachnoidal s.
s. of tongue
transparent s.
transverse s.
triangular nucleus of s.
s. verum
sequela, pl. **sequelae**
caffeine s.
caffeine-related s.
clinical s.
clinically adverse s.
neurobehavioral s.
postpolio s.
sequence
Carr-Purcell s.
Carr-Purcell-Meiboom-Gill s.
fast low-angle shot s.
fast spin-echo inversion recovery s.
gradient-refocused s.
hemisphere s.
magnetization-prepared rapid acquisition gradient echo s. (MPRAGE)
s. polymorphism
pulse s.
pulse-gated cine phase contrast s.
short-tau inversion recovery MRI s.
SPGR s.
spin-density s.
spin-warp pulse s.
spoiled gradient echo s.
stimulated spin-echo s.
STIR s.
three-dimensional spoiled GRASS s.
s. time
T2-weighted spin echo s.
sequencing
s. deletion breakpoint
s. task
sequential
s. compression device
s. computed tomographic scan
s. diagrammatic reformulation
s. dose
s. gradient-recalled acquisition in the steady state
s. GRASS
s. opposition finger movement
s. plane imaging
s. point imaging
s. ultrasonography
sequestrate
sequestrated disk
sequestrectomy
Williams s.
SER
somatosensory evoked response
sera (*pl. of* serum)
Serax
serial
s. CT
s. imaging
s. motor seizure
s. percutaneous needle drainage
s. position effect
s. reaction time (SRT)
series
Leksell gamma knife target s.
serine
s. protease
s. proteinase
Serlect
SERM
selective estrogen receptor modulator

seroepidemiological study
seronegative
s. myasthenia gravis
s. spondyloarthropathy
Seroquel
serosa
s. meningitis
meninx s.
serositis
serotonergic
s. activity
s. agent
s. dorsal raphe
s. pathway
s. side effect
s. system
serotonin
s. antagonist
s. excess disorder
s. 5-HT1
s. 5-HT_2 receptor
s. 5-HT receptor agonist
s. norepinephrine reuptake inhibitor
s. receptor assay
s. stimulation
s. syndrome
s. system
serotonin/dopamine antagonist
serotoninergic
s. cell body
s. syndrome
serous
s. apoplexy
s. meningitis
serpentine aneurysm
serpiginous mass
Serralnyl suture
Serralsilk suture
serrated action potential
serration
dentated s.
sertindole
Sertoli cell
sertraline hydrochloride
serum, pl. **sera**
s. albumin
s. ammonia level
s. androgen level
s. bicarbonate
s. bromide
s. caffeine level
s. calcium
s. ceruloplasmin
s. chloride
s. copper
s. cotinine
s. creatinine kinase
s. enzyme determination
s. ferritin
s. folate
s. folic acid
s. folic acid level
s. glutamic oxaloacetic transaminase
s. glutamic-pyruvic transaminase
s. glutamyl transaminase
s. heavy metal intoxication
s. lipid
s. lipid concentration
s. marker
s. neopterin
s. neuritis
s. neuron-specific enolase
s. phosphorus
s. potassium
s. prolactin
s. protein
s. protein binding
s. salicylate
s. sickness peripheral neuropathy
s. sodium
s. vitamin B12
s. von Willebrand factor
service
sleep disorder s.
servomechanism
Serzone
sestamibi
technetium 99m s.
set
abract s.
aluminum contouring template s.
Bremer halo crown traction s.
empty s.
Greenberg retractor s.
Hudson cranial drill s.
Mira Mark III cranial drill s.
Mira Mark V craniotome s.
Mullan percutaneous trigeminal ganglion microcompression s.
s. screw
SWAP item s.
SWAP-200 item s.

NOTES

SET therapy
setting-sun sign
settling
cranial s.
seventh
s. cranial nerve [CN VII]
s. cranial nerve transposition
s. nerve palsy
s. sense
severe
s. childhood autosomal recessive muscular dystrophy
s. degenerative disk disease
s. head injury
s. impairment
s. kyphoscoliosis
s. postanoxic encephalopathy
s. rigid right thoracic curve
severity
APACHE II measure of disease s.
baseline s.
dementia s.
depression s.
hyperintensity s.
objective s.
s. of worry
sevoflurane anesthesia
sewing spasm
sex
s. headache
s. hormone
s. hormone-binding globulin (SHBG)
sex-behavior center
sexual
s. differentiation
s. motive state
s. neurasthenia
s. reflex
s. side effect
sexuality conversion therapy
SF
Kaochlor SF
SFEMG
single fiber electroencephalography
single fiber EMG
SF-MPQ
Short-Form McGill Pain Questionnaire
SFN
small-fiber neuropathy
SFr-TMS
slow frequency repetitive transcranial magnetic stimulation
slow frequency repetitive transcranial magnetic stimulation (SFr-TMS)
slow frequency repetitive transcranial magnetic stimulation (SFr-TMS)
SGPG
sulfated glucuronyl paragloboside
shadow
plaque s.
shadowing
acoustical s.
shaft
dendritic s.
shagreen
s. patch
s. spot
shaken baby syndrome
shaken-impact syndrome
shaking palsy
shallow
sham block
shame attenuation
sham-movement vertigo
shampoo
chlorhexidine s.
shank clipping
Shannon bur
shape
s. analysis
dendritic s.
s. property
Shapiro-Wilk test
sharing
Edwards modular system load s.
sharpen
Sharplan
S. laser
S. Ultra ultrasonic aspirator
sharp wave
sharp-wave complex
shaver
FESS s.
shaving cramp
Shaw
S. aneurysm needle
S. catheter
SHBG
sex hormone-binding globulin
Shealy theory
shearing
s. force
s. injury
shear-strain deformation
shear stress
sheath
arachnoid s.
Avanti s.
axillary s.
carotid s.

dural s.
femoral introducer s.
ganglionic cyst in synovial tendon s.
Henle s.
s. of Key and Retzius
lamellar s.
Mauthner s.
medullary s.
myelin s.
nerve s.
outer mesaxon of the myelin s.
perivascular s.
s. of Schwann
s. tumor
Shedler-Western Assessment Procedure-200
Sheehan's Disability Scale
Sheehan syndrome
sheet
beta-B-structure s.
beta-pleated s.
MacroPore s.
Sheffield
S. collimator helmet
S. gamma unit
Sheldon hemilaminectomy retractor
Sheldon-Spatz vertebral arteriogram needle
Sherrington
S. law
S. phenomenon
***shh* gene**
SHI
second harmonic imaging
shield
designs for vision side s.
Faraday s.
shielding
magnet s.
shift
brain s.
chemical s.
fat/water chemical s.
field s.
frequency s.
gaze refixational s.
midline s.
s. of midline structure
phase s.
transmembrane ionic s.
s. work-related sleep disorder
s. work sleep disorder
shiga toxin
***Shigella dysenteriae* infection**
Shiley
S. catheter
S. catheter distention system
S. distention kit
Shiley-Infusaid pump
shim coil
shimmering light with aura
shingle
optical s.
shingles-related stroke
Shipley-Hartford Scale
Shirley drain
shivering thermogenesis
shock
anaphylactic s.
break s.
cardiogenic s.
deferred s.
delayed s.
delirious s.
hemorrhagic s.
hypovolemic s.
primary s.
reversible s.
septic s.
spinal s.
vasogenic s.
short
s. association fiber
s. EEG epoch FFT analysis
s. gyrus of the insula
s. insular gyrus
s. inversion recovery imaging
s. pulse repetition time/echo time
s. pulse repetition time/echo time image
s. pulse repetition time/short echo time
s. root of ciliary ganglion
s. segment spinal fusion
s. sleep (SS)
s. sleeper
s. TI inversion recovery (STIR)
s. time inversion recovery
short-acting
s.-a. benzodiazepine
s.-a. block

NOTES

short-acting *(continued)*
s.-a. hypnotic agent
s.-a. local anesthetic
shortening
selective T2 s.
T2 s.
Short-Form McGill Pain Questionnaire (SF-MPQ)
short-lasting
s.-l. unilateral neuralgiform headache with conjunctival injection and tearing
s.-l. unilateral neuralgiform pain
s.-l. unilateral neuralgiform pain with conjunctival injecting and tearing (SUNCT)
short-latency SSEP
short-tau
s.-t. inversion recovery
s.-t. inversion recovery MRI sequence
short-term
s.-t. declarative memory
s.-t. hypoxia
s.-t. insomnia
s.-t. potentiation (STP)
s.-t. therapy
s.-t. treatment
s.-t. vasomotor tone
s.-t. visual memory
shot
fast low-angle s. (FLASH)
shoulder-girdle
s.-g. neuritis
s.-g. syndrome
shoulder-hand syndrome
shrinkage
neuronal s.
shrinking retrograde amnesia
SHS
Sayre head sling
sleep hypopnea syndrome
SH-SY5Y cell line
shunt
Accura s.
artery-to-vein s.
AV s.
s. blockage
cerebrospinal fluid s.
cisterna-atrial s.
cisternal-peritoneal s.
cisternal-pleural s.
CSF s.
cystoatrial s.
Delta valve in ventriculoperitoneal s.
Denver hydrocephalus s.
Diamond valve flow-regulating s.
Edwards/Barbaro syringo-peritoneal s.
s. filter
Hakin-Cortis ventriculoperitoneal s.
Heyer-Schulte neurosurgical s.
intratumoral arteriovenous s.
Javid s.
left-to-right s.
lumbar arachnoid peritoneal s.
lumbar-peritoneal s.
lumbo-atrial s.
lumboperitoneal s.
s. nephritis
Ommaya ventriculoperitoneal s.
percutaneous thecoperitoneal s.
portosystemic s.
posterior fossa-atrial s.
Pruitt-Inahara s.
Pudenz s.
pulmonary arteriovenous s.
Raimondi low pressure s.
right-to-left s. (RLS)
Spetzler lumboperitoneal s.
spinal cord arteriovenous s.
subdural-pleural s.
subduroperitoneal s.
Sundt carotid s.
Sundt loop s.
syringoperitoneal s.
syringosubarachnoid s.
syrinx s.
s. tap
thecoperitoneal Pudenz-Schulte s.
Torkildsen s.
T-shaped Edwards-Barbaro syringeal s.
T-tube s.
valve-regulated s.
ventriculoatrial s.
ventriculocisternal s.
ventriculoperitoneal s.
ventriculopleural s.
ventriculosubgaleal s.
ventriculovenous s.
VJ s.
VP s.
zero ICP ventricle s.
shunted hydrocephalus
shunting
lumbar-peritoneal s.
syringosubarachnoid s.
ventriculoamniotic s.
ventriculoperitoneal s.
Shy-Drager
S.-D. disease

S.-D. neuropathy
S.-D. syndrome (SDS)

SIADH
syndrome of inappropriate secretion of antidiuretic hormone

sialic acid

sialidase gene

sialidosis

sialocele

sialodochitis

sialorrhea

sialosis

sialuria

siboroxime
technetium 99m s.

Sicard syndrome

sicca
hypophysis s.
keratoconjunctivitis s.

sick
s. headache
s. sinus syndrome

sickle
s. cell trait
s. flap

sickness
acute African sleeping s.
acute mountain s. (AMS)
African sleeping s.
chronic African sleeping s.
decompression s.
decompressive s.
East African sleeping s.
S. Impact Profile (SIP)
Jamaican vomiting s.
laughing s.
motion s.
sleeping s.
West African sleeping s.

sidebent
extended, rotated, s. (ERS)
extended, rotated, s. left (ERSL)
extended, rotated, s. right (ERSR)

side-cutting cannula

side-glance

side-opening laminar hook

side-port flat-bottomed Ommaya reservoir

siderosis
superficial s.

Siegert sign

Siemens
S. couch
S. Magnetom Harmony scanner
S. Neurostar digital subtraction angiographic system
S. somatoma plus DCT system
S. Somatom Plus
S. Vision scanner
S. Vision system

Siemerling-Creutzfeldt disease

Siemerling nucleus

sighing dyspnea

sight blindness

sigma
s. activity
S. .15T scanner

sigmoid
s. sinus (SS)
s. sinus retraction

sigmoideus
sinus s.

sign
Abadie s.
alien hand s.
alien limb s.
André Thomas s.
anterior tibialis s.
anticus s.
Babinski s.
Baillarger s.
Bamberger s.
Bamberger-Pins-Ewart s.
Barré pyramidal s.
Bastian-Bruns s.
Battle s.
Bechterew s.
Beevor s.
Bell s.
Berger s.
Biernacki s.
Biot breathing s.
s. blindness
Bonhoeffer s.
Bonnet s.
Bordier-Frequentänkel s.
Bouchet-Gsell s.
Bragard s.
brim s.
Brown-Séquard s.
Brudzinski s.
Bruns s.

NOTES

sign *(continued)*
buckling s.
Cantelli s.
cap s.
Castellani-Low s.
Chaddock s.
Charcot s.
Chvostek s.
Chvostek-Weiss s.
clinical s.
cogwheel s.
Collier s.
contralateral s.
cotton wool s.
coughing s.
cracked pot s.
cranial cracked pot s.
Crichton-Browne s.
crossed adductor s.
Crowe s.
Cupid's bow s.
Czarnecki s.
Dejerine s.
Demianoff s.
doll's eye s.
double fragment s.
Duchenne s.
Duckworth s.
early warning s.
empty delta s.
empty sella s.
empty triangle s.
Erb s.
Erben s.
Erb-Westphal s.
Escherich s.
external malleolar s.
extrapyramidal s. (EPS)
eyelash s.
facial s.
Fajersztajn crossed sciatic s.
false localizing s.
Falx s.
fan s.
flat tire s.
forearm s.
formication s.
Fränkel s.
Froment paper s.
Froment prehensile thumb s.
Goldstein toe s.
Goldthwait s.
Gordon s.
Gorlin s.
Gottron s.
Gowers s.
Graefe s.
Grasset s.
Grasset-Bychowski s.
Grasset-Gaussel-Hoover s.
Griesinger s.
Guilland s.
Gunn s.
Hahn s.
Heilbronner s.
Hirschberg s.
Hitzelberger s.
Hochsinger s.
Hoffmann s.
Holmes s.
Homans s.
Hoover s.
Horsley s.
Hoyt-Spencer s.
Huntington s.
Hutchinson s.
hyperkinesis s.
interossei s.
ipsilateral cerebellar s.
ipsilateral corticospinal tract s.
Jackson s.
Joffroy s.
jugular s.
Kernig s.
Kernohan s.
Kerr s.
Kleist s.
Klippel-Weil s.
Lasègue s.
leg s.
Legendre s.
Leichtenstern s.
Leri s.
Leser-Trélat s.
Lhermitte s.
Lichtheim s.
Linder s.
Livierato s.
local s.
Lust s.
Macewen s.
Magendie-Hertwig s.
Magnan s.
Mannkopf s.
Marie-Foix s.
Marie quadrilateral s.
Marinesco s.
Masini s.
matchbox s.
Mayerson s.
medullary s.
Mendel-Bekhterev s.
meningeal s.
mesencephalic s.

Minor s.
motor s.
Myerson s.
neck s.
Negro s.
Néri s.
neurologic s.
Oppenheim s.
orbicularis s.
s. of the orbicularis
Parinaud s.
Parkinson s.
Parrot s.
pathognomonic s.
Patrick s.
pearl-and-string s.
Pende s.
peroneal s.
Pfuhl s.
Phalen s.
Piltz s.
Piotrowski s.
pontine s.
Pool-Schlesinger s.
Prévost s.
procerus s.
pronation s.
pseudo-Graefe s.
pyramid s.
pyramidal tract s.
Queckenstedt s.
radialis s.
Radovici s.
Remak s.
reservoir s.
Revilliod s.
Romberg s.
Rosenbach s.
Rossolimo s.
Ruggeri s.
Saenger s.
scarf s.
Schlesinger s.
Schultze s.
Schultze-Chvostek s.
scotty dog s.
Seeligmüller s.
Séguin s.
setting-sun s.
Siegert s.
Signorelli s.
Simon s.
soft s.
Souques s.
spine s.
Spurling s.
stairs s.
Stellwag s.
Stewart-Holmes s.
Straus s.
string s.
Strümpell s.
Summerskill s.
sunset s.
swinging-flashlight s.
telltale s.
Theimich lip s.
Thomas s.
Throckmorton s.
tibialis s.
Tinel s.
toe s.
tram track s.
Trendelenburg s.
Trousseau s.
Turyn s.
Uhthoff s.
upper extremity pronator s.
upper extremity scarf s.
Vanzetti s.
von Graefe s.
Waddell s.
Wartenberg s.
Weber s.
Weiss s.
Wernicke s.
Westphal s.
Westphal-Erb s.

signal
s. analysis
anchorage-dependent s.
astrocytic s.
contralateral routing of s.
costimulatory s.
s. detection
feedback s. (FBS)
s. filtering
free induction s.
high-density transient s.
high-intensity s.
s. hyperintensity
increased s.

NOTES

signal *(continued)*
s. intensity curve
intracellular s.
leptin s.
s. loss
magnetic resonance s.
microembolic s.
neuronal s.
N-terminal s.
nuclear s.
s. processing
s. recognition particle (SRP)
repulsive axon guidance s.
s. strength
s. symptom
s. transducing receptor
s. transducing receptor component
s. transduction
s. transduction inhibitor
s. transduction pathway
vestibulospinal s.
s. void
s. voltage waveform
signaling
chemical s.
downstream s.
inside-out s.
outside-in s.
oxidative stress s.
signal-noise characteristic
signal-to-noise
s.-t.-n. ratio (SNR)
s.-t.-n. threshold
Signa 1.5 Tesla unit
significant
s. displacement
s. range
s. subjective distortion
Signorelli sign
SIGSS
selective imaging and graphics for stereotactic surgery
Silapap
Children's S.
Infant's S.
Silastic
S. catheter
S. device
S. sponge
S. stent
S. tube
S. wick
sildenafil
silence
electrical s.
electrocerebral s. (ECS)
silent
s. area
s. infarction
s. microembolism
s. period
s. stroke
silicone
s. balloon
Codman ventricular s.
s. implant
s. sponge
siliqua olivae
SilkTouch CO_2 laser scanner
silly
Silverman placement of electrode
silver-silver chloride electrode
silver-staining nucleolar organizer region (AgNOR)
simethicone
aluminum hydroxide with magnesium hydroxide and s.
simiae
Herpesvirus s.
simian
s. crease
s. fissure
s. hand
s. line
s. virus 40 (SV40)
similarity
vocabulary, information, block (design), and s.'s (*pl. of* vibs)
Simmerlin dystrophy
Simmer paralysis
Simmons
S. catheter
S. cervical spine fusion
S. method
S. plating system
Simon
S. sign
S. task
simple
s. absence
s. chorea
s. decompression
s. febrile seizure
s. hallucination
s. lobule
s. membranous limb of semicircular duct
s. partial seizure
s. partial status
s. primitive aura
s. reflex
s. skull fracture

simplex
crus membranaceum s.
herpes s.
lobulus s.
toxoplasmosis, other infections, rubella, cytomegalovirus, and herpes s. (TORCH)
Simpson
S. catheter
S. Grade
S. grading
Simpson-Angus total score
simulation
conscious s.
simulator
BTE Work S.
Tepper proprioceptor s.
simulee
folie s.
simulis
simultanagnosia, simultagnosia
simultanee
folie s.
simultaneous volume imaging
Simvastatin Survival Study
sinal dura mater filament
sincalide
sinciput
sine delirium
Sinemet CR
Sinequan
singe
main en s.
single
s. bur hole procedure
s. enhancing CT lesion
s. fiber electroencephalography (SFEMG)
s. fiber EMG (SFEMG)
s. hook retractor
s. photon emission computed tomography (SPECT)
s. photon emission CT scan
s. point mutation
s. seizure
s. synostosis
single-agent oral strategy
single-fiber
s.-f. electromyography
s.-f. EMG
single-fraction radiation
single-level
s.-l. decompressive laminectomy
s.-l. spinal fusion
single-rod construct
single-voxel
s.-v. magnetic resonance spectroscopy (SV-MRS)
s.-v. technique
sinica
Ephedra s.
sinistral
sinistrality
sinistrocerebral
sinistromanual
sinistropedal
sinodural angle
sinogenic meningitis
Sinografin
sinography
sinonasal
s. cavity
s. psammomatoid ossifying fibroma
sinovenous
s. occlusion
s. stroke
s. thrombosis
sinus
anterior intercavernous s.
Breschet s.
s. cavernosus
cavernous s.
cerebral s.
circular s.
s. circularis
confluence of s.
cranial dermal s.
dermal s.
dilated intercavernous s.
dural venous s.
s. of dura mater
endodermal s.
ethmoid s.
s. headache
Henle rhomboid s.
s. histiocytosis
inferior longitudinal s.
inferior petrosal s.
inferior sagittal s.
s. intercavernosus anterior
s. intercavernosus posterior
intercavernous s.

S

NOTES

sinus *(continued)*
intracranial venous s.
lateral s.
marginal s.
s. marginalis
maxillary s.
nasal s.
s. nerve of Hering
neurodermal s.
occipital s.
s. occipitalis
occluded s.
s. occlusion
paranasal s.
parasinoidal s.
s. pericranii
petrosal s.
petrosquamosal s.
petrosquamous s.
s. petrosus inferior
s. petrosus superior
s. phlebitis
pilonidal s.
posterior intercavernous s.
s. rectus
s. reflex
rhomboidal s.
s. rhomboidalis
Ridley s.
sagittal s.
s. sagittalis inferior
s. sagittalis superior
sigmoid s. (SS)
s. sigmoideus
space of the cavernous s.
sphenoid s.
sphenoidal s.
sphenoparietal s.
s. sphenoparietalis
sphenotemporal s.
spinal dermal s.
s. squeeze
straight s.
subarachnoidal s.
superior longitudinal s.
superior petrosal s. (SPS)
superior sagittal s.
tentorial s.
thrombosis of venous s.
transverse s. (TS)
s. transversus durae matris
s. venosi duralis
venous dural s.

sinusitis

sinusoidal

sinus-vein thrombosis

sinuum
confluens s.

sinuvertebral nerve

SIP
Sickness Impact Profile

SIS
Stroke Impact Scale

SI, SII area

site
binding s.
dopamine uptake s.
enzymatic binding s.
graft s.
high-affinity binding s.
hook s.
uptake s.

sitieirgia

sitting
s. balance
s. position

situ
carcinoma in s.

situation
s. neurosis

situational
s. neurosis
s. stress reaction
s. tic variation
s. variable

sixth
s. cranial nerve [CN VI]
s. cranial nerve palsy
s. sense
s. ventricle

size
effect s.
fiber s.
internal architecture neuronal s.
neuronal s.
optimal group s.

sizer-dissector
Mizuho aneurysm s.-d.

SjO_2
jugular bulb oxyhemoglobin saturation monitoring

Sjogren-Larsson syndrome

Sjögren syndrome

Sjöqvist tractotomy

skein
choroid s.

skeletal
s. amyloidosis
s. deformity
s. muscle
s. muscle injury

Skelid

skill
abstraction s.
ambulation s.
basic s.
Brigance Diagnostic Comprehensive Inventory of Basic S.'s
Brigance Diagnostic Inventory of Basic S.'s
Brigance Diagnostic Inventory of Essential S.'s
Canadian Test of Basic S.'s, Forms 7 and 8
Canadian Test of Cognitive S.'s
Clinical Observations of Motor and Postural S.'s
communication s.
graphomotor s.
improved communication s.
perceptual motor s.
perspective-taking s.
physical s.
spatial conceptualization s.
visuoconstruction s.
visuomotor problem-solving s.
visuospatial s.
vocabulary s.
skilled finger movement
skin
s. conductance response
s. depth
s. flap
glabrous s.
glossy s.
s. graft harvesting pain
s. incision
s. reflex
skin-muscle reflex
skin-pupillary reflex
Skiodan
skip lesion
SK-N-SH cell
Skoog release of Dupuytren contracture
Skoptsy
skull
s. base
s. bone graft
cloverleaf s.
s. fracture
hemihypertrophied s.
maplike s.
s. plate
s. punch
steeple s.
tower s.
s. transillumination
skull-base
endoscopic s.-b.
s.-b. malignancy
s.-b. surgery
skullcap
skull-stripped
Skytron bed
slant
antimongoloid s.
slap
foot s.
slattern
slatternly
SLE
systemic lupus erythematosus
sleep
s. activity
American Association for the Psychophysiological Study of S.
s. apnea syndrome (SAD)
s. architecture
s. attack
benign epileptiform transient of s.
s. bruxism
crescendo s.
curtailed s.
s. cycle
decreased need for s.
s. deficit
delta s.
s. deprivation (SD)
desynchronized s.
s. diary
disorder of initiation and maintenance of s.
s. disorder service
s. disruption
s. dissociation
s. disturbance
disturbed s.
dreaming s.
s. drive
s. efficiency
electrical status epilepticus of s.
electrical status epilepticus during slow s.
electrotherapeutic s.

S

NOTES

sleep *(continued)*
s. epilepsy
epilepsy with continuous spikes and waves during s.
erratic s.
s. feature
s. fragmentation
fragmentation of nocturnal s.
function of s.
s. hallucination
S. Heart Health Study
s. hygiene abnormality
s. hyperhidrosis
s. hypopnea syndrome (SHS)
s. hypoventilation syndrome
s. inertia
s. initiation insomnia
s. latency
light s.
s. log
long s. (LS)
s. maintenance insomnia
s. myoclonus
nocturnal s.
nonrapid eye movement s.
non-REM s.
s. onset period (SOP)
orthodox s.
overconcern with s.
paradoxical s.
s. paralysis
paroxysmal s.
periodic limb movement of s. (PLMS)
periodic limb movement during s. (PLMS)
s. phase delay syndrome
s. position indicator (SPI)
positive occipital sharp transients of s. (POSTS)
s. problem
prolonged nocturnal s.
s. psychogenic disorder
s. quality
rapid eye movement s.
S. Research Society
s. restriction therapy
S s.
short s. (SS)
slow-wave s. (SWS)
s. spindle
s. stage 1–4
stage 1–4 s.
s. state
supine s.
synchronized s.
s. technique
s. terror disorder

sleep-awake
s.-a. activity inventory
s.-a. cycle

sleep-deprived EEG

sleeper
long s.
short s.

sleep-generating center

sleepiness
daytime s.
disorder of excessive s.
diurnal s.
excessive daytime s. (EDS)
pathological s.

sleeping sickness

sleepless

sleeplessness
s. associated with acute emotional conflicts or reaction
s. associated with conditional arousal
s. associated with intermittent emotional conflicts or reaction

sleep-onset
s.-o. association disorder
s.-o. rapid eye movement

sleep-related
s.-r. asthma
s.-r. breathing disorder (SRBD)
s.-r. epilepsy
s.-r. headache
s.-r. respiratory disturbance
s.-r. respiratory dysregulation

sleep-starts disorder

sleep-state misconception

sleeptalking disorder

sleep-wake
s.-w. cycle
s.-w. cyclicity
s.-w. rhythm
s.-w. rhythmicity
s.-w. schedule
s.-w. schedule disturbance
s.-w. transition disorder

sleepwalker

sleepwalking

sleeve
arachnoid s.
arachnoidal root s.
s. graft
polyethylene s.

slender
s. fasciculus
s. lobule

SLEV
St. Louis encephalitis virus
slice
corticostriatal s.
digital subtraction venous angiography s.
s. fracture
hippocampal s.
s. selection
three-dimensional s.
slice-select encoding gradient
slide
Superfrost microscope s.
Slimline clip
Slim-Loc anterior cervical plate system
sling
clip-reinforced cotton s.
fascia lata s.
Sayre head s. (SHS)
slipped disk
slit
s. hemorrhage
s. valve
s. ventricle
s. ventricle syndrome
slit-lamp examination
SLN
superior laryngeal nerve
slope
gradient s.
Slosson
slot fracture
slotted
s. hammer
s. suction tip
slow
s. axonal transport
s. channel syndrome
s. component neuropathy
s. double taper
s. frequency repetitive transcranial magnetic stimulation (SFr-TMS)
s. frequency wave
s. lateral eye movement
s. metabolizer patient
s. rolling eye movement
s. wave activity (SWA)
s. wave complex
slowed mentation
slowing
age-dependent s.
cognitive s.
diffuse bilateral s.
focal s.
frontotemporal s.
generalized s.
intermittent focal s.
motor s.
motoric s.
physiologic s.
postictal s.
psychomotor s.
saccadic s.
temporal s.
slowly adaptic receptor
slow-virus infection
slow-wave
s.-w. abnormality
s.-w. generation
s.-w. sleep (SWS)
s.-w. stupor
Sluder
S. neuralgia
S. syndrome
***slug* gene**
Sluijter-Mehta SMK-C10 cannula
Sluyter-Mehta thermocouple electrode
Sly disease
SMA
spinal muscular atrophy type 1–4
supplementary motor area
small
s. angle double incidence angiogram
s. cell carcinoma
s. centrum ovale infarction
s. deep recent infarction
s. intensely fluorescent cell
s. lacunar infarction
s. motor unit potential
s. sciatic nerve
s. sharp spike
s. volume correction (SVC)
small-bowel carcinoid tumor
small-fiber
s.-f. dysfunction
s.-f. neuropathy (SFN)
small-penetrator infarction (SPI)
smallpox vaccination complication
small-step gait

NOTES

small-vessel
s.-v. disease
s.-v. infarction
S.M.A.R.T. stent
SmartStent delivery device
smear
acid-fast bacilli s.
fungal s.
Tzanck s.
smell
s. blindness
s. brain
s. disorder
S. Identification Test
nerve of s.
organ of s.
smell-brain
Smellie scissors
SMI 5000 bed
Smiley-Williams arteriogram needle
Smith
S. air craniotome
S. Extrapyramidal Scale
S. nerve root suction retractor
Smith-Lemli-Opitz syndrome
Smith-Magenis syndrome
Smith-Petersen laminectomy rongeur
Smith-Robinson
S.-R. operation
S.-R. procedure
S.-R. technique
Smithwick
S. button hook
S. dissector
S. ganglion hook
S. sympathectomy
S. sympathectomy hook
SMK
S. C5 with a 2-mm exposed tip cannula
S. electrode
***SMN* gene**
SMN system
smoker's stroke
smoking-related reduction
SMON
subacute myelooptic neuropathy
subacute myelopticoneuropathy
smooth
s. endoplasmic reticulum
s. muscle
s. muscle proliferation
s. muscle tumor
s. pursuit
s. pursuit defect
s. pursuit eye movement
SN
substantia nigra
SNAP
sensory nerve action potential
SNAP amplitude
SNAP on electromyogram
snap finger
snapping reflex
snapshot
cross-sectional s.
snarl
myasthenia s.
SNc
substantia nigra pars compacta
SNE
subacute necrotizing encephalomyelopathy
Sneddon syndrome
Snellen reflex
sniff test
snore
s. guard
S. Guard mandibular repositioning device
SnoreSat Sleep Recorder
snoring
Sno-Traks wheelchair chain
snout reflex
snowshoe hare virus
SNP
sodium nitroprusside
SNR
selective nerve root
signal-to-noise ratio
sNr
substantia nigra pars reticulata
SNSRs
sensory neuron-specific G protein-coupled receptor
snuff
snuffbox
anatomical s.
soaked
s. fat plug
s. muscle plug
Soaker catheter
soapsuds cyst
social
s. cognition
s. deprivation syndrome
s. impairment
s. learning theory
s. relations deficit
s. status
s. stress and functionality inventory
s. therapy
s. toxicity

s. undesirable
s. viscosity
s. welfare
s. Zeitgebers
social-breakdown syndrome
social-isolation syndrome
socially dysfunctional
societal force
Society
American Pain S.
American Thoracic S.
Behavior Therapy and Research S.
European Sleep Research S.
International Headache S. (IHS)
Latin American Sleep S.
S. for Light Therapy and Biological Rhythms
S. for Quantitative Analyses of Behavior
Sleep Research S.
World Federation of Neurosurgical S.'s (WFNS)
Socon spinal system
SOD
superoxide dismutase
sodium
s. acetate
s. aminobenzoate
s. amytal
s. ascorbate
s. bicarbonate
s. bromide
cefalothin s.
s. channel beta subunit
s. channel disorder
s. chloride
danaparoid s.
dantrolene s.
divalproex s.
s. dodecyl sulfate (SDS)
s. dodecyl sulfate polyacrylamide (SDS-PAGE)
s. dodecyl sulfate-polyacrylamide gel electrophoresis
extended phenytoin s.
high s.
s. imbalance
indigotin disulfonate s.
ioxaglate s.
s. lactate
liothyronine s.
methotrexate s.
Nembutal S.
s. nitroprusside (SNP)
s. oxylate
s. phosphate
photofrin porfimer s.
s. salicylate
serum s.
technetium 99m pertechnetate s.
thiopental s.
s. thiosalicylate
s. thiosulfate
sodium-potassium ATPase
sodium-responsive periodic paralysis
sodium-water retention
Soemmerring
S. ganglion
S. spot
SOF
superior orbital fissure
Sofamor-Danek Stealth System
Sofamor spinal instrument device
Sof-Rol dressing
soft
s. disk herniation
s. line
s. palate retraction
s. psychotic-like phenomenon
s. sign
s. sign in neurologic examination
s. tissue abnormality
s. tissue dissection
s. tissue injury
s. tissue stretching
softening
s. of brain
hemorrhagic s.
pyriform s.
red s.
white s.
yellow s.
Softplate
soft-tissue contrast
software
BrainVoyager s.
StatView 4.51 s.
three-dimensional postprocessing s.
Sof-Wick dressing
Sofwire spinal fixation
Sokoda complex

NOTES

solar
s. ganglion
s. plexus
sole
s. nucleus
s. plate
s. tap reflex
solenoid coil
sole-plate ending
solid-phase extraction (SPE)
solid-state
s.-s. coagulator
s.-s. instrument
solitarii
nuclei s.
nuclei tractus s.
nucleus tractus s.
solitariospinalis
tractus s.
solitariospinal tract
solitarius
fasciculus s.
funiculus s.
nucleus s.
tractus s.
solitary
s. aggressive type conduct disorder
s. bundle
s. extranodal lymphoma
s. fasciculus
s. fibrous tumor
s. hydatid cyst
s. neurofibroma
s. tract
solium
Taenia s.
Solomon-Bloembergen equation
Solstice balloon
SolTab
Remeron S.
Solu-Biloptin
soluble specific substance (SSS)
solute transport
solution
10% acetylcysteine 0.05% isoproterenol hydrochloride s.
ferumoxide injectable s.
[^{18}F] fluoride s.
Formula EM oral s.
Hanks buffered saline s.
hydroxyethyl methacrylate polymerizing s.
image guided s.
major s.
volumetric s. (VS)
Zenker s.
solution-focused therapy
Solutrast
solvent
organic s.
solving
frontal-lobe abstraction/problem s.
rational problem s.
Somanetics
S. INVOS 3100 cerebral oximeter
S. INVOS cerebral oximeter device
SomaSensor device
somata
neuronal s.
somatagnosia agnosia
somatalgia
somatesthesia
somatesthetic area
somatic
s. afferent fiber
s. block
s. category
s. depression
s. efferent fiber
s. motor component
s. motor neuron
s. motor nucleus
s. muscle
s. nerve
s. nerve fiber
s. nervous system
s. neurofiber
s. neurologic manifestation
s. pain
s. problem
s. sense
s. sensory component
s. sensory cortex
somaticae
neurofibrae s.
Somatics monitoring electrode
somatization disorder
somatizing
somatochrome
somatodendritic excitability
somatoform
s. disorder
s. pain
somatognosis
somatointestinal reflex
Somatom DR1
somatoparaphrenia
somatosensory
s. area
s. aura
s. cortex
s. cortices of the right hemisphere of the brain
s. cued task

s. dysfunction
s. evoked magnetic
s. evoked potential (SSEP)
s. evoked potential monitoring
s. evoked response (SER)
s. homunculus
s. map
s. mapping
s. plasticity
somatosexuality
somatostatin
somatotopagnosis
somatotopic
somatotopographic reorganization
somatotopy
somatotroph
s. cell
s. hyperplasia
somatotropin
somatotypology
somesthesia
somesthetic
s. area
s. cortex
s. dysarthria
s. neuron
s. relay nucleus
s. system
SOMI
sternooccipital-mandibular immobilization
SOMI Jr. brace
somite
embryonic cervical s.
sommeil
tic de s.
somnambulance
somnambulant
somnambulate
somnambulic epilepsy
somnambulism
somnambulist
somnocinematograph
somnofluoroscopy
somnolence
daytime s.
disorder of excessive s.
excessive daytime s.
s. syndrome
treatment-emergent s.
somnolency
somnolent
somnolentia
somnoplasty
Sonata
Songer
S. cable
S. cable system
sonic
s. hedgehog gene
s. stereometry
Sonneberg neurectomy
Sonocut ultrasonic aspirator
sonography
color-flow Doppler s.
Doppler s.
TCD s.
transcranial color-coded duplex s.
transcranial color-coded real-time s.
sonomotor response
sonophobia
Sonopuls 190
sonorous
Sono-Stat Plus sound device
SonoWand
S. intraoperative imaging system
S. ultrasound-based neuronavigation system
SOP
sleep onset period
Sophy mini programmable pressure valve
sopor
soporific
soporose, soporous
soretolide
sorrow-provoking stimulus
sosies
illusion des s.
sotalol
soteira
Sotos syndrome
sound
coconut s.
contralateral routing of s.
pulse synchronous s.
sound-sensitive seizure
Souques
S. phenomenon
S. sign
source
Arclite 20,000 light s.

NOTES

source *(continued)*
embolic s.
external s.
s. image
interstitial radiation s.
Maxenon 300 watt xenon light s.
Maxillume 250 watt quartz halogen light s.
Minimax 200 watt light s.
spike s.
Zeiss Super Lux 40 light s.
201-source
201-s. cobalt-60 gamma knife
201-s. cobalt-60 gamma unit
South African tick-bite fever
Southern blot
Southwestern immunohistochemistry
SP
sacroposterior
space
anterior cavernous sinus s.
arachnoid s.
brain s.
s. of the cavernous sinus
s. context
craniospinal s.
dead s.
detail response to small white s.
disk s.
dorsal subcutaneous s.
enclosed s.
epicerebral s.
epidural s.
epispinal s.
extracellular s.
extradural s.
frontal interhemispheric s.
His perivascular s.
incisural s.
intercrural s.
interpeduncular s.
Magendie s.
Malacarne s.
Marie quadrilateral s.
Meckel s.
oropharyngeal airway s.
parasinoidal s.
perforated s.
perineuronal s.
perioptic subarachnoid s.
perivascular s.
retropharyngeal s.
Schwalbe s.
s. sense
subarachnoid s.
subdural s.
subepicranial s.
subgaleal s.
synaptic s.
Talairach s.
Tarin s.
Virchow-Robin s.
***k*-space**
space-occupying brain lesion
3-SPACE Polhemus digitizing system
spacer
Allograft s.
ceramic vertebral s.
methylmethacrylate s.
telescopic plate s.
SPAMM
spatial modulation of magnetization
span
auditory s.
life s.
liver s.
spanning
transmembrane s.
SPAR
Spastic Paraplegia, Ataxia, Mental Retardation
sparing
macular s.
spark-gap instrument
spasm
affect s.
athetoid s.
Bell s.
canine s.
carpopedal s.
cervical muscle s.
clonic s.
convergence s.
cryptogenic hemifacial s.
cynic s.
dancing s.
dystonic s.
epileptic s.
facial habit s.
fixed s.
functional s.
habit s.
hemifacial s. (HFS)
infantile s.
intention s.
jackknife s.
lightning attacks in infantile s.
lock s.
malleatory s.
massive s.
masticatory s.
mimic s.
mixed s.
mobile s.

muscle s.
myopathic s.
near reflex s.
nictitating s.
nodding s.
occupational s.
paraplegic s.
phonatory s.
phonic s.
progressive torsion s.
reflex s.
retrocollic s.
Romberg s.
rotatory s.
salaam s.
saltatory s.
sewing s.
spasmogenic s.
spasmophile s.
synclonic s.
tailor's s.
tetanic s.
s.'s and tics
tonic s.
tonoclonic s.
torsion s.
toxic s.
vascular s.
vasomotor s.
winking s.

spasmodic
s. apoplexy
s. diathesis
s. mydriasis
s. tic
s. torticollis

spasmodica
dysarthria syllabaris s.
tabes s.

spasmogen

spasmogenic spasm

spasmology

spasmolygmus

spasmolysis

spasmolytic

spasmophile spasm

spasmophilia

spasmophilic diathesis

spasmus
s. agitans
s. caninus
s. coordinatus
s. mutans nystagmus
s. nictitans
s. nutans

spastic
s. abasia
s. aphonia
s. ataxia
s. bulbar palsy
s. cerebral palsy
s. diplegia
s. dysarthria
s. dystonia
s. equinus foot
s. gait
s. hemiparesis
s. hemiplegia
s. hyperreflexia
s. miosis
s. monoplegia
s. mydriasis
s. paraparesis
s. paraplegia
S. Paraplegia, Ataxia, Mental Retardation (SPAR)
s. paresis
s. quadriparesis
s. quadriplegia
s. rigidity
s. spinal paralysis

spastica
dysphonia s.
torticollis s.

spasticity
Ashworth score of muscle s.
clasp-knife s.
sphincter s.
s. vertical suspension test

spatia (*pl. of* spatium)

spatial
s. agraphia
s. conceptualization
s. conceptualization skill
s. frequency
s. frequency grating
s. homogeneity
s. localization
s. memory
s. modulation of magnetization (SPAMM)
s. perception

NOTES

spatial *(continued)*
s. planning
s. response
s. span backward (SSB)
s. span forward (SSF)
S. Span Test
spatial-temporal context
spatiotemporal
s. brain mapping
s. source analysis
spatium, pl. **spatia**
s. epidurale
s. extradurale
s. leptomeningeum
s. peridurale
s. subarachnoideum
s. subdurale
spatula
brain s.
Children's Hospital brain s.
curved-tipped s.
Cushing brain s.
Davis brain s.
Davis nerve s.
D'Errico brain s.
s. dissector
double-vector brain s.
duck-billed anodized s.
House-Fisch dural s.
Jacobson endarterectomy s.
Mayfield brain s.
Olivecrona brain s.
Peyton brain s.
Rainin clip-bending s.
Ray brain s.
rectangular brain s.
Rhoton s.
Sachs nerve s.
Scoville brain s.
S-shaped brain s.
tapered brain s.
Weary brain s.
SPE
solid-phase extraction
Speare dural hook
Spearman
S. correlation coefficient
S. rho
S. two-factor theory
spear tackler's spine
special
s. sensation
s. sense
s. somatic afferent (SSA)
s. somatic afferent column
s. visceral efferent column
s. visceral efferent nucleus
s. visceral motor nucleus
species
allopatric s.
reactive oxygen s. (ROS)
specific
s. absorption rate
s. curve
s. effect
s. irritability
s. sensory cue
s. symptom
s. system
specificity
criterion of s.
neuronal s.
specimen
flash-frozen tumor s.
s. staining
speckle
laser s.
SPECT
single photon emission computed tomography
SPECT analysis
dual-isotope SPECT
high-resolution brain SPECT
SPECT image
SPECT scan
^{99m}Tc HMPAO SPECT
^{201}Tl SPECT
spectra (*pl. of* spectrum)
spectral
s. analysis
s. density
s. density function
s. edge frequency (SEF)
s. peak frequency of activity
s. velocity
spectrometer
mass s.
spectrometry
gas chromatography mass s.
spectrophotometer
Hitachi s.
spectrophotometric assay
spectrophotometry
reflectance s.
spectropolarimeter
Jasco S.
spectroscopy
Fourier s.
laser Doppler s.
magnetic resonance s. (MRS)
MR s.
near-infrared s. (NIRS)

phosphorus nuclear magnetic resonance s.
point-resolved s. (PRESS)
proton magnetic resonance s.
proton nuclear magnetic resonance s.
single-voxel magnetic resonance s. (SV-MRS)
in vivo ′H magnetic resonance s.
in vivo optical s. (INVOS)
s. voxel

spectrum, pl. **spectra**
s. disorder
Doppler frequency s.
fortification s.
impulsive s.
proton s.
in vitro spectra

speculum
bivalved s.
Cushing-Landolt s.
Halle nasal s.
Hardy bivalve s.
Killian septum s.
Landolt pituitary s.
transsphenoidal s.

speech
absent s.
s. apraxia
s. aprosody
aprosody of s.
s. arrest
s. center
cerebellar s.
cluttering in s.
s. developmental disorder
digressed s.
s. discrimination test
disorganized s.
s. disturbance
s. dyspraxia
echo s.
excessive s.
explosive s.
external s.
fluent s.
s. hallucination
ictal s.
increased s.
s. and language cluttering
s. and motor mapping
narrative s.
overabstract s.
s. pattern
s. perception
s. perception region
s. perception system
poverty of s.
pressure of s.
s. processing
s. processing alteration
s. processing impairment
pseudobulbar s.
rate of s.
s. reception threshold
s. recognition threshold
scanning s.
spoken s.
staccato s.
s. structure
subvocal s.
syllabic s.
telegraphic s.
s. tracking
s. tracking alteration
s. tracking task
unstoppable flow of s.

Speech-Sounds Perception Test

speed
s. of conduction
mental s.
s. of processing
psychomotor s.

speed-dependent treadmill training (STT)

SpeedReducer instrument

spelencephaly

spell
akinetic drop s.
apnea-like s.
breath-holding s.
neonatal breath-holding s.
nocturnal s.
staring s.

Spemann organizer

Spence
S. intervertebral disk rongeur
rule of S.

Spencer
S. biopsy forceps
S. probe depth electrode

Spens syndrome

NOTES

spermatic
s. nerve
s. plexus
spes phthisica
Spetzler
S. lumboperitoneal shunt
S. Microvac suction tube
S. system
S. titanium aneurysm clip
Spetzler-Martin
S.-M. classification
S.-M. classification of arteriovenous malformation
S.-M. grade
S.-M. grade III medium-size lesion with deep venous drainage
S.-M. grade II small lesion with deep venous drainage
S.-M. grading scale
S.-M. grading system
SpF spinal fusion stimulator
SpF-XL stimulator
SPGR sequence
S-phase fraction
sphenocavernous syndrome
sphenoethmoidal
s. encephalocele
s. meningoencephalocele
s. recess
sphenoethmoidectomy
sphenoid
s. encephalocele
s. mucocele
s. ridge meningioma
s. rostrum
s. sinus
s. wing
s. wing dysplasia
s. wing meningioma
sphenoidal
s. electrode
s. electrode insertion
s. encephalocele
s. fossa
s. herniation
s. sinus
sphenoidale
planum s.
sphenoidectomy
sphenoiditis
sphenoidostomy
sphenoidotomy
sphenomaxillary
s. encephalocele
s. ganglion
sphenooccipitalis
fissura s.
sphenoorbital
s. encephalocele
s. meningioma
s. meningoencephalocele
sphenopalatine
s. ganglion
s. ganglionectomy
s. nerve
s. neuralgia
s. test
sphenoparietalis
sinus s.
sphenoparietal sinus
sphenopharyngeal meningoencephalocele
sphenotemporal sinus
sphere
infrared light-reflecting s.
oriented in all s.'s
spheresthesia
spherical
s. bur
s. coordinate representation
s. nucleus
spherule
Fulci s.
sphincter
anal s.
s. ani nerve
s. spasticity
urinary s.
sphingolipid
s. metabolism disorder
semisynthetic s.
sphingolipidosis
cerebral s.
sphingomyelinase
sphingomyelin lipidosis
sphingosine
Sphrintzen syndrome
SPI
sleep position indicator
small-penetrator infarction
spicule
spider cell
Spiegelberg
S. epidural balloon
S. intracranial pressure monitoring system
Spiegel-Wycis human apparatus
Spielmeyer acute swelling
Spielmeyer-Sjögren disease
Spielmeyer-Vogt disease
Spielmeyer-Vogt-Sjögren disease
Spigelius lobe
spike
anterior temporal focal s.

benign childhood epilepsy with centrotemporal s.
benign partial epilepsy with centrotemporal s. (BPECTS)
chasing s.
s. detection
s. discharge
s. frequency
high-voltage centrotemporal s.
injury s.
interictal epileptiform s.
middle temporal focal s.
peak absorption s.
s. potential
preexcision s.
rolandic benign epilepsy of childhood with centrotemporal s.
small sharp s.
s. source
train of s.
wicket s.

spike-and-wave
s.-a.-w. complex
s.-a.-w. electroencephalographic discharge
s.-a.-w. pattern
s.-a.-w. trait

spike-initiation zone

spikelike artifact

spike-wave
s.-w. complex
s.-w. discharge

spiking activity

Spiller-Frazier
S.-F. neurotomy
S.-F. technique

spin
s. density
s. echo
s. magnetization
nuclear s.
s. velocity

spina, pl. **spinae**
s. bifida
s. bifida anterior
s. bifida aperta
s. bifida cystica
s. bifida manifesta
s. bifida myelomeningocele
s. bifida occulta
s. bifida posterior
canalis centralis medullae spinae
s. dorsalis

spinal
s. accessory nerve-facial nerve anastomosis
s. accessory palsy
s. anesthesia
s. angiography
s. apoplexy
s. arachnoid
s. arachnoid mater
s. arteriography
s. arteritis
s. ataxia
s. automatism
s. blastomycosis
s. canal
s. canal hydatid cyst
s. catheter
s. column
s. cord
s. cord abscess
s. cord angioma
s. cord arachnoid cyst
s. cord arachnoiditis
s. cord arteriovenous malformation
s. cord arteriovenous shunt
s. cord arteritis
s. cord artery
s. cord blood supply
s. cord compression
s. cord concussion
s. cord contusion
s. cord disease
s. cord disorder
s. cord function intraoperative monitoring
s. cord hemisection
s. cord hemorrhage
s. cord infarction
s. cord infection
s. cord inflammation
s. cord injury (SCI)
s. cord injury trauma
s. cord injury without radiographic abnormality (SCIWORA)
s. cord lateral horn
S. Cord Motor Index and Sensory Indices
s. cord neoplasm
s. cord pain

NOTES

spinal *(continued)*
s. cord reticular formation
s. cord segmentation in embryonic development
s. cord stimulation
s. cord terminal cone
s. cord terminal ventricle
s. cord tumor
s. cord ventral horn
s. cord ventricular funiculus
s. cord white matter blood flow
s. coronal plane deformity
s. decompression
s. deformity/instability
s. deformity treatment
s. dermal sinus
s. dermal sinus tract
s. disk degeneration
s. disk prosthesis
s. disk replacement
s. drainage
s. dural arteriovenous fistula (SDAVF)
s. dysraphism
s. embolism
s. endodermal cyst
s. ependymoma
s. epidural abscess
s. epidural angiolipoma
s. epidural hematoma (SEH)
s. epidural hemorrhage
s. evaluation myelography
s. extradural arachnoid pouch
s. fixation
s. fixation rigidity
s. fluid
s. fluid analysis
s. fusion
s. fusion gouge
s. fusion pathomechanics
s. fusion technique
s. hemangioblastoma
s. hemianesthesia
s. hemiplegia
s. herniation
s. implant design
s. implant load to failure
s. injury operative stabilization
s. instability
s. instrumentation
interspinous segmental s.
s. intradural schwannoma
s. lamina
s. lamina II
s. lemniscus
s. lesion
s. level
s. lipoma
s. mechanics
s. meningitis
s. meningocele
s. metastasis
s. metastatic disease
s. monosynaptic reflex
s. muscular atrophy type 1–4 (SMA)
s. needle
s. nerve level motor impairment
s. nerve plexus
s. nerve root
s. nerve root filament
s. neurenteric cyst
s. neurofibroma
s. nucleus of accessory nerve
s. nucleus of trigeminal nerve
s. nucleus of the trigeminus
s. osteomyelitis
s. osteotomy stabilization
s. pachymeningitis
s. paralysis
s. paralytic poliomyelitis
s. perforating forceps
s. pia mater
s. puncture
s. puncture headache
s. pyramidotomy
s. range of motion (SROM)
s. reflex arc
s. reticular formation
s. rod
s. rod cross-bracing
s. saw
s. segmental myoclonus
s. sensory evoked potential
s. shock
s. stenosis
s. stroke
s. subarachnoid block
s. subarachnoid hemorrhage
s. subdural hemorrhage
s. synovial cyst
s. syphilis
s. tap
s. teratoma
s. tractotomy
s. tract of trigeminal nerve
s. trigeminal nucleus
s. tuberculosis
ventral derotating s.
s. wind-up

SpinaLase neodymium:yytrium-aluminum-garnet (Nd:YAG) surgical laser system

spinale
filum s.
nucleus retrodorsolateralis medullae s.
tache s.

spinales
nervi s.
nucleus posteromedialis medullae s.
radices s.

spinalis
apex cornus dorsalis medullae s.
apex cornus posterioris medullae s.
arachnoidea mater s.
basis cornus dorsalis medullae s.
basis cornus posterioris medullae s.
canalis centralis medullae s.
cervix cornus dorsalis medullae s.
cervix cornus posterioris medullae s.
chorda s.
columna anterior medullae s.
columna dorsalis medullae s.
columnae griseae medullae s.
columna intermedia medullae s.
columna intermediolateralis medullae s.
columna posterior medullae s.
columna ventralis medullae s.
commissura alba anterior medullae s.
commissura alba posterior medullae s.
commissura grisea anterior medullae s.
commissura grisea anterior/posterior medullae s.
commissura grisea posterior medullae s.
commotio s.
cornu anterius medullae s.
cornu dorsalis medullae s.
cornu laterale medullae s.
cornu posterius medullae s.
cornu ventrale medullae s.
dura mater s.
fasciculus gracilis medullae s.
fasciculus proprius anterior medullae s.
fasciculus proprius dorsalis medullae s.
fasciculus proprius lateralis medullae s.
fasciculus proprius posterior medullae s.
fila radicularia nervi s.
filum durae matris s.
fissura mediana anterior medullae s.
fissura mediana ventralis medullae s.
formatio reticularis medullae s.
funiculi medullae s.
funiculus ventralis medullae s.
ganglion sensorium nervi s.
hydrocele s.
laminae s.
lamina s. II
lemniscus s.
medulla s.
meningitis serous s.
nucleus accessorius columnae anterioris medullae s.
nucleus anterolateralis medullae s.
nucleus centralis medullae s.
nucleus dorsolateralis medullae s.
nucleus dorsomedialis medullae s.
nucleus intermediomedialis medullae s.
nucleus phrenicus columnae anterioris medullae s.
nucleus posterolateralis medullae s.
nucleus retroposterolateralis medulla s.
nucleus ventrolateralis medullae s.
nucleus ventromedialis medullae s.
pars cervicalis medullae s.
pars coccygea medullae s.
pars lumbalis medullae s.
pars sacralis medullae s.
pars thoracica medullae s.
pia mater s.
radix anterior nervi s.
radix dorsalis nervi s.
radix motoria nervi s.
radix posterior nervi s.
radix sensoria nervi s.
radix ventralis nervi s.
ramus albus nevi s.
ramus anterior nervi s.
ramus communicans albus nervi s.

NOTES

spinalis *(continued)*
ramus communicans griseus nervi s.
ramus dorsalis nervi s.
ramus griseus nervi s.
ramus meningeus nervi s.
ramus posterior nervi s.
ramus recurrens nervi s.
ramus ventralis nervi s.
segmenta cervicalia medullae s.
segmenta coccygea medullae s.
segmenta lumbalia medullae s.
segmenta medullae s.
segmenta sacralia medullae s.
segmenta thoracica medullae s.
segmentum medullae s.
septum medianum dorsale medullae s.
septum medianum posterius medullae s.
substantia alba medullae s.
substantia gelatinosa centralis medullae s.
substantia gelatinosa cornu posterioris medullae s.
substantia grisea medullae s.
substantia intermedia centralis medullae s.
substantial visceralis secundaria medullae s.
sulcus dorsolateralis medullae s.
sulcus intermedius dorsalis medullae s.
sulcus intermedius posterior medullae s.
sulcus medianus dorsalis medullae s.
sulcus medianus posterior medullae s.
sulcus posterolateralis medullae s.
sulcus ventrolateralis medullae s.
tabes s.
theca medullare s.
truncus nervi s.
ventriculus terminalis medullae s.

spinalium
ansae nervorum s.
plexus nervorum s.
rami communicantes nervorum s.

spinally elicited peripheral nerve response (SEPNR)

SpinaLogic bone growth stimulator

spin-density sequence

spindle
alpha s.
s. cell
s. coma
EEG alpha s.
Kühne s.
muscle s.
neuromuscular s. (NMS)
neurotendinous s.
sleep s.
tendon s.

spindle-celled layer

spindle-cell tumor

spindle-shaped cyst

SPINE
CID Picture SPINE

spine
bamboo s.
caroticojugular s.
cervical s.
cleft s.
dendritic s.
dorsal s.
Henle s.
internal fixation of s.
kinetic cervical s.
laminectomized s.
lower cervical s.
lower lumbar s.
lower thoracic s.
osteoporotic s.
poker s.
sacral s.
sacrococcygeal s.
s. sign
spear tackler's s.
suprameatal s.
thoracic s.
thoracolumbar s.
s. tuberculosis
tumor metastatic to s.
upper thoracic s.
variable screw placement system-instrumented lumbar s.

SpineCATH

spin-echo
s.-e. imaging
long pulse repetition time/long echo time s.-e.
s.-e. T1-weighted plan image

spineless

SpineLink system

spinescope
Clarus s.

SpineStat probe

spinifugal

spinipetal

spin-lattice
s.-l. relaxation
s.-l. relaxation time

spinoadductor reflex

spinobulbar
spinocerebellar
s. ataxia
s. ataxia type 1
s. degeneration (SCD)
s. tract
spinocerebellum
spinocervicalis
tractus s.
spinocervical tract
spinocervicothalamic tract
spinocollicular
spinocortical
spinocranial meningioma
spinocuneatae
fibrae s.
spinocuneate fiber
spinogalvanization
spinogracile fiber
spinograciles
fibrae s.
spinography
digitized s.
spinohypothalamicae
fibrae s.
spinohypothalamic fiber
spinolamellar line
spinomesencephalicae
fibrae s.
spinomesencephalic fiber
spinomuscular paralysis
spinoolivares
fibrae s.
spinoolivaris
tractus s.
spinoolivary
s. fiber
s. tract
spinoolivocerebellar tract
spinopelvic
s. transiliac fixation (STIF)
s. transiliac fixation technique
spinoperiaqueductales
fibrae s.
spinoperiaqueductal fiber
spinopetal
spinopontine degeneration
spinoreticular
s. fiber
s. tract
spinoreticulares
fibrae s.
spinoreticularis
tractus s.
spinospinalis tract
spinosum
foramen s. (FS)
spinosus
nervus s.
spinotectal
s. fiber
s. tract
spinotectales
fibrae s.
spinotectalis
tractus s.
spinothalamic
s. cordotomy
s. fiber
s. relay
s. tract
s. tractotomy
spinothalamicus
tractus s.
spinous
s. interlaminar line
s. process
s. process fracture
s. process plate
s. process-splitting laminoplasty
s. process wire
s. process wiring
spinovestibularis
tractus s.
spinovestibular tract
spin-spin
s.-s. coupling
s.-s. relaxation
s.-s. relaxation time
spin-warp
s.-w. imaging
s.-w. pulse sequence
spiny neuron
spiral
Archimedes s.
s. cochlear ganglion
S. Flute cranioblade
s. foraminous tract
s. ganglion of cochlea
s. membrane

NOTES

spiral *(continued)*
s. organ
Perroncito s.
spirale
organum s.
spiramycin
spirochetal
s. aneurysm
s. infection
spirochete
spirohydantoin
spirolactone
spirometry
spiromustine
spironolactone
hydrochlorothiazide and s.
Spitz-Holter shunt system
Spitzka
S. marginal tract
S. marginal zone
S. nucleus
Spitzka-Lissauer
S.-L. column
S.-L. tract
SPL
superior parietal lobule
splanchnesthesia
splanchnesthetic sensibility
splanchnic
s. anesthesia
s. ganglion
s. motor component
s. nerve
s. sensory component
splanchnicectomy
splanchnici
ganglion nevi s.
splanchnicotomy
splanchnicum
ganglion thoracicum s.
splendens
splenectomy
splenia
splenial
s. artery
s. gyrus
splenicus
plexus s.
splenium
callosal s.
s. corporis callosi
s. of corpus callosum
s. tissue
splenius
s. capitus
s. cervicis
splenomegaly
splicing
exon s.
splinter hemorrhage
split
s. bone graft reconstruction
s. brain
s. calvarial graft
s. notochord syndrome
palatal s.
vermian s.
split-brain syndrome
split-cord malformation
split-half reliability
split-thickness calvarial graft
SPM
statistical parametric map
SPMS
secondary progressive multiple sclerosis
spoiled
s. gradient echo
s. gradient echo sequence
spoiling
radiofrequency s.
spoken
s. language disorder
s. language impairment
s. speech
spondylalgia
spondylarthritis
spondylectomy
spondylitica
psoriasis s.
spondylitic ridging
spondylitis
ankylosing s.
cryptococcal s.
s. deformans
Kümmell s.
rheumatoid s.
tuberculous s.
spondyloarthropathy
seronegative s.
s. syndrome
spondylocace
spondylo construct
spondylodesis
ventral derotation s. (VDS)
spondylodiskitis
spondylolisthesis
degenerative s.
dysplastic s.
grade IV s.
high-grade s.
isthmic s.
pathologic s.
postlaminectomy two-level s.
s. reduction

s. reduction fixation
symptomatic s.
traumatic s.
s. with significant displacement
spondylolisthetic crisis
spondylolysis
spondylomalacia
spondylopathy
spondyloptosis
spondylopyosis
spondyloschisis
spondylosis
cervical s.
s. deformans
degenerative s.
hyperostotic s.
lumbar s.
thoracolumbar s.
spondylosyndesis
spondylotic
s. caudal radiculopathy
s. headache
s. myelopathy
spondylotomy
sponge
absorbable gelatin s.
gelatin s.
Ivalon embolic s.
Ray-Tec s.
saline-soaked s.
Silastic s.
silicone s.
sponge-holding forceps
spongiform
s. leukodystrophy
s. virus encephalopathy
spongioblast
spongioblastoma
polar s.
s. polare
unipolar s.
s. unipolare
spongiocyte
spongiosa
substantia s.
spongiosis
spongiosus
status s.
spongy
s. bone
s. degeneration
s. degeneration of infancy
s. degeneration leukodystrophy
s. substance
spontaneous
s. activity
s. echo contrast
s. exacerbation
s. flexion
s. improvement
s. intracranial hypotension
s. nystagmus
s. occlusion of the circle of Willis
s. panic attack
s. spinal epidural hematoma (SSEH)
spoon
brain s.
Cushing brain spatula s.
Cushing pituitary s.
Hardy pituitary s.
pituitary s.
Ray brain spatula s.
sporadic
s. ataxia
s. depression
s. fatal insomnia prion protein gene
Sporothrix schenckii
sports-related spinal injury
spot
acoustic s.
ash-leaf s.
blind s.
Brushfield s.
café au lait s.
central direct current bright s.
cherry-red s.
cotton-wool s.
Graefe s.
hot s.
hypnogenic s.
pain s.
Roth s.
saccular s.
shagreen s.
Soemmerring s.
temperature s.
Trousseau s.
utricular s.
warm s.
yellow s.

NOTES

spotted fever
spray
air plasma s.
butorphanol tartrate nasal s.
dihydroergotamine mesylate nasal s.
Miacalcin Nasal S.
oxymetazoline nasal s.
spread
centripetal s.
spreader
Bailey rib s.
Blount laminar s.
Bobechko s.
Burford-Finochietto rib s.
Caspar disk space s.
Cloward cervical vertebra s.
Cloward lamina s.
Davis rib s.
DeBakey rib s.
Doyen rib s.
Favaloro-Morse sternal s.
Finochietto rib s.
Gerbode-Burford rib s.
Haight-Finochietto rib s.
Haight rib s.
Harken rib s.
Harrington s.
Inge cervical lamina s.
Inge laminectomy s.
lamina s.
Landolt s.
Lemmon sternal s.
Lilienthal rib s.
Miltex rib s.
Morse sternal s.
Nelson rib s.
Rehbein rib s.
Rienhoff-Finochietto rib s.
Rienhoff rib s.
Texas Scottish Rite Hospital eyebolt s.
Tuffier rib s.
vertebra s.
Weinberg rib s.
Wilson rib s.
Wiltberger spinous process s.
spreading
s. cortical depression theory
s. depression
spring
coiled s.
compression s.
s. finger
Gruca-Weiss s.
internal fixation s.
s. mechanism
springing mydriasis
springlike phenomenon
spring-loaded electrode
Sprotte
S. epidural needle
S. spinal needle
sprouting
collateral nerve s.
hippocampal s.
mossy fiber s.
neuronal s.
regenerate nerve s.
sympathetic s.
synaptic s.
sprue peripheral neuropathy
SPS
superior petrosal sinus
spur
calcarine s.
Morand s.
traction s.
spurious
s. finding
s. meningocele
s. torticollis
Spurling
S. maneuver
S. nerve root retractor
S. sign
S. test
Spurling-Kerrison laminectomy rongeur
Spurr epoxy resin
squamous cell carcinoma
square
nonlinear least s. (NLS)
s. wave
square-ended hook
square-wave jerk
squeeze
sinus s.
s. technique
SQUID
superconducting quantum interference device
SQUID array for reproductive assessment (SARA)
SR
sustained release
SRBD
sleep-related breathing disorder
Src inhibitor
SREDA
subclinical rhythmic EEG discharge of adults
SREDA on electroencephalogram
SRF
sustained high-frequency repetitive firing

SROM
spinal range of motion
SRP
signal recognition particle
SRS
stereotactic radiosurgery
SRT
serial reaction time
SS
short sleep
sigmoid sinus
SSA
special somatic afferent
SSB
spatial span backward
SSC
superior semicircular canal
SSEH
spontaneous spinal epidural hematoma
SSEP
direct cortical stimulation and somatosensory evoked potential
somatosensory evoked potential
short-latency S.
SSF
spatial span forward
SSH
suppression subtractive hybridization
S-shaped brain spatula
SSI
anterior-posterior fusion with S.
SSN
seesaw nystagmus
SSPE
subacute sclerosing panencephalitis
SSPT
steady-state probe topography
SSR
steady-state response
SSR on electromyogram
SSRI
selective serotonin reuptake inhibitor
SSRI-induced bruxism
SSS
Scandinavian Stroke Scale
soluble specific substance
SSS on electroencephalogram
SST
stereotactic subcaudate tractotomy
St.
St. George Anxiety Questionnaire
St. John's Wort
St. Louis encephalitis
St. Louis encephalitis virus (SLEV)
St. Martin disease
St. Paul-Ramsey Scale
STA
superficial temporal artery
Stab-and-Grab screwdriver
stability
clinical s.
lumbar spine rotational s.
orthostatic s.
temporal s.
stabilization
anterior internal s.
anterior short-segment s.
s. approach
atlantoaxial s.
atlantooccipital s.
cervical spine s.
cervicothoracic junction s.
flexion-compression spine injury s.
fracture s.
iliac crest bone graft s.
lower cervical spine posterior s.
lumbar spine s.
mood s.
occipitocervical s.
odontoid fracture s.
posterior lower cervical spine s.
reduction s.
sacral spine s.
screw s.
spinal injury operative s.
spinal osteotomy s.
subluxation s.
thoracolumbar spine s.
TSRH crosslink s.
wire s.
stable
s. cervical spine injury
s. xenon CT
staccato speech
Stackable Cage corpectomy
Staderini nucleus
stage
Braak s.
concrete operational s.
confrontation s.
delta activity of s.
ideoplastic s.

NOTES

stage *(continued)*
initial s.
manipulation s.
postambivalent phase s.
preclinical s.
premonitory s.
s. 1–4 sleep
sleep s. 1–4
staged
s. bilateral stereotactic thalamotomy
s. embolization
staging
Hoehn and Yahr Parkinson s.
neuraxis s.
stagnant hypoxia
Stagnara wake-up test
stain
acid-fast s.
CSF Gram s.
Elastica-Masson s.
Elastica van Gieson s.
eosin s.
Fite s.
Gomori trichome s.
Gordon and Sweet silver reticulin s.
Gram s.
Grocott s.
hematoxylin-eosin s.
Hortega neuroglia s.
Klüver-Barrera Luxol fast blue s.
Masson-Fontana s.
Masson trichrome s.
myelin tissue s.
periodic acid-Schiff-hematoxylin s.
Perls s.
port wine s.
reticulum s.
trichrome s.
staining
CD34 s.
Golgi s.
immunoperoxidase s.
specimen s.
Sudan black s.
terminal deoxynucleotidyl transferase-mediated dUTP nick end-labeling s.
Weigert s.
stainless
s. steel equipment
s. steel preformed skull plate
s. steel screw
staircase phenomenon
stairs sign
stalk
cerebral s.
hypophysial s.
hypophysial s.
infundibular s.
neural s.
pineal s.
pituitary s.
s. of thalamus
STA-MCA
superficial temporal artery to middle cerebral artery
superficial temporal artery-middle cerebral artery
superior temporal artery-middle cerebral artery
STA-MCA anastomosis
STA-MCA bypass
stammer
stammering of the bladder
stance
adultomorphic s.
walking s.
stand
Brown-Roberts-Wells floor s.
Contraves s.
Yasargil OptiMat floor s.
standard
s. antipsychotic therapy
s. bone algorithm program
s. care
s. of care
s. dose
s. dose administration
s. error of the mean (SEM)
s. kinetic model
s. laboratory test
s. rating procedure
s. retroperitoneal flank approach
s. retroperitoneal flank incision
s. score
s. thoracotomy
s. Würzburg titanium mini-plating system
standardized
s. A scan
s. assessment
S. Assessment of Concussion
standing balance
Stanford
S. Acute Stress Reaction Questionnaire
S. Sleepiness Scale
stanozolol
STA-PCA
superficial temporal artery-posterior cerebral artery
STA-PCA bypass

stapedial
- s. artery
- s. nerve

stapedius
- s. muscle fatigue
- s. nerve
- nervus s.

stapes
- footplate of the s.
- s. reflex

Staphcillin

staphylococcal meningitis

staphylococci
- coagulase-negative s.
- methicillin-resistant s.

Staphylococcus
- *S. aureus*
- *S. epidermidis*
- *S. pneumoniae*

staphyloma

staphyloplegia

star
- s. array
- optic disk edema with a macular s.

stare
- manic s.
- postbasic s.

staring spell

Starling reflex

START kit

startle
- s. disease
- s. epilepsy
- s. reaction
- s. reaction/response
- s. reflex
- s. syndrome

STA-SCA

superficial temporal artery-superior cerebellar artery
- STA-SCA bypass

stasis
- s. retinopathy
- venous s.

state
- absent s.
- active s.
- acute confusional s.
- affective s.
- s. of alertness
- alpha s.
- amnestic s.
- anelectrotonic s.
- apallic s.
- appetitive s.
- calm wakefulness s.
- catelectrotonic s.
- central excitatory s.
- cognitive s.
- confabulatory amnestic s.
- confusional s.
- convulsive s.
- crepuscular s.
- decerebrate s.
- decorticate s.
- deefferented s.
- depressive mixed s.
- dreamlike s.
- dreamy s.
- drug-induced hallucinatory s.
- drug-induced paranoid s.
- drug-induced semihypnotic s.
- drug-like desire s.
- dysphoric manic s.
- elusive illness s.
- epileptic clouded s.
- epileptic twilight s.
- explosive psychotic s.
- s. factor
- general mood s.
- gradient-recalled acquisition in the steady s. (GRASS)
- homozygous s.
- hyperadrenergic s.
- hypercoagulable s.
- hyperdopaminergic s.
- hypnagogic s.
- hypnoidal s.
- hysterical fugue s.
- hysteric coma-like s.
- lacunar s.
- local excitatory s.
- s. of mindful relaxation
- minimally conscious s.
- mixed bipolar s.
- mood s.
- negative myoclonus s.
- neuroexcitatory s.
- neurotic anxiety s.
- neurotic depressive s.
- oxidation s.

NOTES

state *(continued)*
paranoid s.
pathological mood s.
permanent vegetative s.
persistent vegetative s. (PVS)
psychological s.
refractory s.
resting s.
seizure-free s.
s. of semisleep
senile paranoid s.
sequential gradient-recalled acquisition in the steady s.
sexual motive s.
sleep s.
subacute delirious s.
subacute irritable depressive s.
subcortical dysexecutive s.
trancelike s.
twilight s.
vegetative s.
visceral emotional s.
state-dependent
s.-d. measure
s.-d. psychopathology rating scale
statement
SWAP-200 s.
state-of-the-art
s.-o.-t.-a. analysis
s.-o.-t.-a. analysis technique
state-trait interaction
static
s. acoustic impedance
s. allodynia
s. ataxia
s. convulsion
s. and dynamic sitting balance
s. and dynamic standing balance
s. hyperplasia
s. intervention
s. magnetic field
s. reflex
s. sense
s. spastic quadriplegia
s. standing balance
s. tremor
stationary visual stimulus
station test
statistical
s. artifact
s. parametric map (SPM)
statoacoustic
s. nerve
s. organ
statoacusticus
nervus s. [CN VIII]
statokinetic reflex
statotonic reflex
status
acute change in mental s.
altered mental s.
s. aura
s. cataplecticus
s. choreicus
cognitive s.
complex partial s.
s. convulsivus
s. cribalis
s. cribrosus
s. criticus
s. dysmyelinatus
s. dysmyelinisatus
s. dysraphicus
s. epilepticus
functional s.
general cognitive s.
s. hemicranicus
s. hypnoticus
s. lacunaris
s. lacunosus
s. marmoratus
s. migrainosus
s. nervosus
nutritional s.
pressure autoregulatory s.
proband s.
prognostic s.
psychomotor s.
s. raptus
simple partial s.
social s.
s. spongiosus
suicide s.
s. typhosus
s. vertiginosus
visuomotor s.
widowed s.
StatView 4.51 software
stauroplegia
staurosporine
stavudine
steady-state
s.-s. dose
s.-s. free precession
s.-s. method
s.-s. probe topography (SSPT)
s.-s. regimen
s.-s. response (SSR)
s.-s. visual evoked potential
steal
cerebral ischemia s.
s. effect
s. index
intracerebral s.

s. phenomenon
subclavian s.
vascular s.
Stealth Image Guided System
StealthStation
S. image-interactive system
S. system real-time guidance
S. treatment guidance platform
steam-shaping mandrel
steamy
steatosis
microvesicular s.
Stecher arachnoid knife
Steele-Richardson-Olszewski
S.-R.-O. disease
S.-R.-O. syndrome
steep-dose gradient
steeple skull
Steffee
S. instrumentation
S. pedicle screw-plate system
S. plate
S. plating
Steinert
S. disease
S. myotonic dystrophy
Steinhauser cranial screw
Stein-Leventhal syndrome
Steinmann pin
stellate
s. astrocyte
s. cell of cerebral cortex
s. ganglion
s. ganglion block
s. neuron
s. skull fracture
stellatum
ganglion s.
stellectomy
Stellwag sign
stem
brain s.
s. cell transplantation
gaze mechanism in brain s.
infundibular s.
s. serotonergic cell
stem-completion test
stenogyria
Stenosimeter
stenosis, pl. **stenoses**
acquired spinal s.
aqueductal s.
asymptomatic carotid artery s.
canal s.
carotid artery s.
cervical spinal s.
foraminal s.
high-grade s.
lateral recess s.
lumbar spinal s.
spinal s.
stomal s.
thoracolumbar spinal canal s.
stenostenosis
Stensen duct
stent
Acculink s.
AVE GFX s.
Gianturco-Roubin II s.
Jostent graft s.
Memotherm s.
NIR Royal Advanced s.
Palmaz s.
Palmaz-Schatz s.
Silastic s.
S.M.A.R.T. s.
Symbiot covered s.
Wallstent s.
stenting
vertebral origin angioplasty and s.
stent-supported coil embolization
stepdown connector
Stephenson-Gibbs reference electrode
Stephen syndrome
steppage gait
stepping response
stercoralis
Strongyloides s.
stereoadapter
Laitinen s.
stereoagnosis
stereoanesthesia
stereocognosy
stereoelectroencephalography (SEEG)
stereoencephalometry
stereoencephalotomy
stereognosis
stereognostic
stereoguide collimator
stereo-isomer
stereomagnification angiography

S

NOTES

stereometry
sonic s.
stereoselective glomerulus
stereotactic, stereotaxic
s. anatomic target localization
s. angiography
s. anteroposterior and lateral metrizamide ventriculography
s. arc
s. atlas
s. biopsy
s. biopsy exploration
s. brachytherapy
s. catheter drainage
s. cingulotomy
s. coordinate system
s. cordotomy
s. depth electroencephalogram (SDEEG)
s. depth electroencephalography (SDEEG)
s. frame
s. gamma radiation
s. gamma unit
s. guidance
s. guide
s. injection DTI-015
s. instrument
s. instrumentation
s. intracystic injection
s. intratumoral photodynamic therapy
s. irradiation
s. lesionectomy
s. linear accelerator
s. linear accelerator radiotherapy
s. localization
s. microsurgical approach
s. microsurgical craniotomy
s. needle aspiration
s. neurosurgery
s. operation
s. pallidotomy
s. PET image
s. puncture
s. radiation therapy treatment
s. radiosurgery (SRS)
s. retractor
s. robot
s. subcaudate tractotomy (SST)
s. surgery
s. surgical ablation
s. surgical guidance system
s. technique
s. thalamotomy
s. thermocoagulation
s. tractotomy
s. VL thalamotomy
stereotactic-assisted
s.-a. radiation therapy
s.-a. radiation therapy kit
stereotactic-focused radiation therapy
stereotactic-guided craniotomy
stereotaxic (*var. of* stereotactic)
stereotaxis
stereotaxy
frame s.
frameless s.
functional s.
volumetric s.
stereotyped
s. movement
s. movement disorder
stereotypic movement
Steri-Dent dry heat sterilizer
sterile
s. abscess
s. meningitis
s. meningoencephalitis
sterilizer
Steri-Dent dry heat s.
Steripaque
Steripaque-BR
Steripaque-V
Steritek ICP mini monitor
sternal
s. occipital mandibular immobilization
s. puncture
sternobrachial reflex
sternocleidomastoid (SCM)
branch to s.
s. muscle
s. muscle testing in spinal accessory nerve examination
s. muscle weakness
sternohyoid muscle
sternomastoid muscle
sternooccipital-mandibular immobilization (SOMI)
sternooccipitomanubrial immobilizer
sternothyroid muscle
sternotomy
sternum-splitting approach
sternutatory
s. absence
s. reflex
steroid
s. dosage
s. hormone
lumbar epidural s.
s. therapy
steroid-induced osteoporosis

steroid-sensitive neuropathy
stethoparalysis
stethospasm
Stevens-Johnson syndrome
Stewart-Holmes sign
Stewart-Morel syndrome
STGC
syncytiotrophoblastic giant cell
Stickler syndrome
sticky platelet syndrome
STIF
spinopelvic transiliac fixation
STIF technique
stiff-baby syndrome
stiffening
bilateral tonic s.
stiff-man syndrome
stiffness
axial s.
fusion s.
hemiparkinsonian s.
neck s.
torsional s.
stiff-person syndrome
stigma, pl. **stigmata**
medication s.
Stille bur
Stille-Luer rongeur
Stilling
S. column
S. fiber
S. fleece
S. gelatinous substance
S. nucleus
S. raphe
STIM neuromuscular stimulation system
Stimson dressing
stimulant
chimeric s.
dopaminergic s.
s. therapy
s. treatment
stimulant-dependent sleep disorder
stimulated spin-echo sequence
stimulating electrode
stimulation
s. adjustment
antidromic s.
areal s.
audiovisual s.
audio-visual-tactile s.
brain s.
carotid baroceptor s.
click s.
condensation s.
s. condition
conditioned s.
cutaneous electrical s.
deep brain s. (DBS)
direct brain s.
dopamine s.
dorsal column s.
dorsal cord s.
electrical cortical s.
electromyogram-triggered neuromuscular s. (EMG-triggered neuromuscular stimulation)
electrophysiological s.
EMG-triggered neuromuscular s.
electromyogram-triggered neuromuscular stimulation
emotional s.
epileptogenic s.
extraspinal nerve s.
fast-frequency repetitive transcranial magnetic s.
s. fatigability
fixed dose s.
functional electrical s.
functional neuromuscular s.
galvanic vestibular s.
high-intensity click s.
intermittent photic s.
intraoperative cortical s.
intraoperative electrical cortical s. (IOECS)
macro s.
macroelectrical s.
magnetoelectric s.
s. mapping
minimizing s.
neck s.
neuromuscular electrical s.
nociceptive s.
noninvasive carotid baroceptor s.
nonspecific s.
optokinetic s. (OKS)
paradoxical s.
s. parameter
paraspecific s.
percutaneous s.
perivascular nerve-ending s.

NOTES

stimulation *(continued)*
s. PET study
photic s.
post hoc s.
postsynaptic s.
presynaptic s.
s. program in cerebral palsy
punctual s.
ramp s.
rarefaction s.
repetitive nerve s.
repetitive transcranial magnetic s. (rTMS)
sacral nerve s.
serotonin s.
spinal cord s.
STN s.
subthalamic nucleus deep brain s. (STN-DBS)
supramaximal rapid s.
supranormal s.
sympathetic s.
tactile s.
tetanic s.
thalamic s.
therapeutic electric s.
therapeutic electrical s.
thorax s.
threshold electrical s. (TES)
thyrotropin-releasing hormone s.
s. time
transcranial high-frequency repetitive electrical s.
transcranial magnet s. (TMS)
transcranial magnetic s.
transcutaneous electrical nerve s.
transcutaneous nerve s.
transfer direct current s.
trigeminal s.
vagal nerve s. (VNS)
vagus nerve s. (VNS)

stimulation-related adverse effect

stimulator
Axostim nerve s.
Caldwell High Speed Magnetic s.
constant current s.
dorsal column s.
eight-channel muscle s.
electronic s.
EMG s.
Hilger facial nerve s.
Intrel II spinal cord s.
magnetic s.
Magstim 200 s.
Micro-Z neuromuscular s.
monopolar cathodal s.
nerve s.
Neurosign 100 constant current s.
Ojemann cortical s.
Orthofix Cervical-Stim s.
SpF spinal fusion s.
SpF-XL s.
SpinaLogic bone growth s.
Toennis ES standalone constant-current electrical s.
vagus nerve s.

stimulatory effect

stimulus, pl. **stimuli**
adequate s.
ambiguous external s.
anxiogenic s.
anxiolytic s.
s. artifact
binocular flash s.
chemosensory s.
condition s. (CS)
conditioned s.
costimulatory s.
discriminant s.
s. drive (SD)
s. duration
emotive s.
excitatory s.
external speech s.
heterologous s.
homologous s.
inadequate s.
ionic s.
liminal s.
maximal s.
Michotte visual s.
novel s.
stimuli paradigm
patterned s.
pattern-reversal s.
perceptual emotive s.
pharmacological s.
photic s.
precipitating s.
rarefaction s.
real-life s.
reinforcing s.
selective focusing on environmental s.
s. sensitive myoclonus
sorrow-provoking s.
stationary visual s.
subliminal s.
subthreshold s.
summation of s.
supraliminal s.
supramaximal s.
suprathreshold s.
tactile s.

test s.
s. threshold
train-of-four s.
unconditioned s.
s. word
stimulus-control therapy
stimulus-response time
stinger injury
STIR
short TI inversion recovery
S. sequence
stiripentol
STM
supratentorial meningioma
STN
subthalamic nucleolus
subthalamic nucleus
STN stimulation
STN-DBS
subthalamic nucleus deep brain stimulation
stochastic resonance
stock
bone s.
stocking
s. anesthesia
Orthawear antiembolism s.'s
Vairox high compression vascular s.'s
stocking-and-glove
s.-a.-g. anesthesia
s.-a.-g. distribution
stocking-glove sensory loss
Stoffel operation
stoichiometric change
stoker's cramp
Stokes-Adams
S.-A. attack
S.-A. disease
S.-A. syndrome
Stokes law
stoma blast
stomachal vertigo
stomal stenosis
stomatitis
stomodeum
Stookey
S. cranial rongeur
S. reflex
Stookey-Scarff operation
stopcock
Luer-Lok s.
stopping
stop-start technique
storage disease
store
cellular s.
high-energy cellular s.
storiform
s. pattern
s. whorl
Storz
S. Microsystem microplate
S. Microsystems cranial fixation plate
S. Microsystems drill bit
STP
short-term potentiation
strabismus
convergent s.
kinetic s.
Strachan syndrome
straight
s. aneurysm clip
s. cannula with locking dilator
s. connector
s. filament
s. gyrus
s. incision
s. knot-tying forceps
s. leg raising test
s. line bayonet forceps
s. microscissors
s. needle
s. needle electrode
s. nerve hook
s. ring curette
s. sinus
straightening cannula
straight-in ventriculostomy
strain
alpha wave s.
s. birefringence
s. gauge
role s.
strangalesthesia
strap
Flushmesh s.
s. muscle
strata (*pl. of* stratum)

NOTES

strategy
acceptance s.
adjunctive s.
age-appropriate s.
antisense s.
candidate-gene s.
coactive s.
combination s.
dose reduction s.
genetic s.
loading s.
low-dose s.
memory retrieval s.
minimalist surgical s.
optimal treatment s.
single-agent oral s.
therapeutic s.
treatment s.
visual representation s.
strati
stratification
Davidoff age s.
population s.
post hoc s.
stratum, pl. **strata**
Strata adjustable Delta valve
s. album profundum
s. cerebrale retinae
s. cinereum colliculi superioris
s. colliculi rostralis
s. colliculi superioris
s. ganglionare nervi optici
s. ganglionare retinae
s. ganglionicum
s. gangliosum cerebelli
s. granulare
s. granulosum corticis cerebelli
s. grisea et alba colliculi rostralis
s. grisea et alba colliculi superioris
s. griseum colliculi superioris
s. griseum intermedium
s. griseum intermedium colliculus superioris
s. griseum medium
s. griseum profundum
s. griseum profundum colliculis superioris
s. griseum profundum colliculi superioris
s. griseum superficiale
s. griseum superficiale colliculi superioris
s. gyri dentati
s. hippocampus
s. interolivare lemniscus
s. limitans externum
s. limitans internum
s. lucidum hippocampus
s. magnocellularia
s. medullare intermedium
s. medullare intermedium colliculi superioris
s. medullare profundum
s. medullare profundum colliculi superioris
s. moleculare
s. moleculare corticis cerebelli
s. moleculare et substratum lacunosum
s. moleculare hippocampus
s. moleculare retinae
s. multiforme
s. neuroepitheliale retinae
s. neurofibrarum
s. neuronorum piriformium
s. nucleare externum
s. nucleare externum et internum retinae
s. nucleare internum
s. nucleare internum retinae
s. nuclearia externa et interna retinae
s. opticum
s. opticum colliculi superioris
s. oriens
s. oriens hippocampus
s. parvocellularia
s. pigmenti bulbus
s. pigmenti retinae
s. plexiforme cerebelli
s. plexiforme externum
s. plexiforme externum et internum retinae
s. plexiforme internum
s. purkinjense corticis cerebelli
s. pyramidale
s. pyramidale hippocampus
s. radiatum
s. radiatum hippocampus
s. segmentorum externorum et internorum
s. zonale
s. zonale colliculi superioris
s. zonale thalami
Strauss-Carpenter scale
Straus sign
streak
angioid s.
fatty s.
meningitic s.
primitive s.
stream
dorsal s.

primate dorsal s.
ventral s.
streaming
s. birefringence
intravascular s.
strength
axial gripping s.
bending s.
bone-screw interface s.
C-D instrumentation fixation s.
Cotrel pedicle screw fixation s.
field s.
human s.
masseter s.
motor s.
muscle s.
pedicle screw pullout s.
psychological s.
pullout s.
signal s.
torsional gripping s.
strength-duration curve
streptococcal
s. infection
s. meningitis
streptococci
microaerophilic s.
pediatric autoimmune neuropsychiatric disorder associated with s. (PANDAS)
viridans s.
Streptococcus
S. agalactiae
S. pneumoniae
S. pyogenes
S. viridans
streptococcus
group A beta-hemolytic s.
group B s.
streptodornase
streptokinase
streptomycin
stress
acute foot-shock s.
heat s.
ischemic s.
major life s.
measured s.
oxidative s.
s. reaction
s. relaxation
shear s.
tensile s.
transient emotional s.
s. ulcer
stressed-induced iNOS
stressful
stress-illness process
stressor
childhood s.
cumulative s.
disaster s.
educational s.
life s.
stretch
s. receptor
s. reflex
s. reflex pathway
stretching
polyglutamine s.
soft tissue s.
s. syncope
stria, pl. **striae**
acoustic s.
anterior acoustic s.
auditory s.
s. cochlearis anterior
s. cochlearis intermedia
s. cochlearis posterior
s. diagonalis
diagonalis s.
striae distensae
s. fornicis
Gennari s.
intermediate acoustic s.
s. of internal granular layer
s. internal pyramidal layer
s. of internal pyramidal layer
Kaes s.
Kaes-Bechterew s.
s. laminae granularis externae
s. laminae granularis internae
s. laminae molecularis
s. laminae plexiformis
s. laminae pyramidalis internae
Lanci s.
striae lancisi
lateral longitudinal s.
lateral olfactory s.
s. longitudinalis lateralis
s. longitudinalis lateralis corporis callosi

NOTES

stria *(continued)*
s. longitudinalis medialis
s. longitudinalis medialis corporis callosi
medial longitudinal s.
medial olfactory s.
striae medullares
striae medullares acusticae
striae medullares fossae rhomboideae
striae medullares ventriculi quarti
s. medullaris
s. medullaris thalami
s. of molecular layer
molecular layer s.
nucleus of lateral olfactory s.
s. occipitalis
striae olfactoriae
s. olfactoria lateralis
s. olfactoria medialis
olfactory s.
posterior acoustic s.
tectal s.
s. tectum
terminal s.
s. terminalis
s. terminalis fiber
ventral acoustic s.
s. ventriculi tertii

striatae
venae s.

striatal
s. dopamine
s. dopaminergic abnormality
s. dopamine transporter density
s. hand
s. lesion
s. metabolism
s. neuron
s. receptor
s. target
s. toe

striate
s. area
s. body
s. cortex
s. hemorrhage
s. nucleus
s. vein

striated muscle

striati
cauda s.
lamina medullaris lateralis corporis s.
lamina medullaris medialis corporis s.

striation

striational autoantibody

striatocapsular infarction

striatocerebellar tremor

striatofrontal
s. circuitry
s. dysfunction

striatonigral
s. degeneration
s. degeneration type
s. fiber

striatum
corpus s.
dorsal s.
s. dorsale
lateral medullary lamina of corpus s.
medial medullary lamina of corpus s.
vein of corpus s.
ventral s.
s. ventrale

striatus-orbitofrontal metabolism

stricture
clip-induced s.

stridor
nocturnal s.

string sign

striocerebellar tremor

striomotor column

strionigral tract

striosome patch

strip
AdTech electrode s.
motor s.
sensory-motor s.

stripe
s. area
s. of Gennari
occipital s.
Vicq d'Azyr s.

stripout
screw s.

stroboscope

stroboscopic light activating technique

stroke
acute s.
S. and the Alzheimer Disease and Related Disorders Association
anterior circulation s.
cardioembolic s.
caudal s.
completed s.
S. Data Bank Neurologic Rush Alzheimer Registry Examination
developing s.
embolic s.
hemisphere s.

hemorrhagic s.
S. Impact Scale (SIS)
ipsilateral s.
ischemic s.
lacunar s.
migraine-induced s.
National Institute of Neurological and Communicative Disorders and S. (NINCDS-ADRDA)
National Institute of Neurological Disorders and S. (NINDS)
paralytic s.
progressing s.
s. prophylaxis
pure hemisensory s.
pure sensory s.
Randomized Trial of Tirilazad Mesylate in Patients With Acute S. (RANTTAS)
retinal s.
right brain s. (RBS)
s. score
sensory-motor s.
shingles-related s.
silent s.
sinovenous s.
smoker's s.
spinal s.
s. syndrome
thalamic s.
thromboembolic s.
thrombotic s.

strokectomy
stroke-in-evolution
strokelike episode
stroma, pl. **stromata**
s. ganglii
s. ganglionicum
nerve s.
tumor s.

Stromeyer cephalhematocele
Strong Vocational Interest Blank (SVIB)
Strongyloides stercoralis
strongyloidiasis
strontium-89
Stroop task
structural
s. abnormality
s. brain lesion
s. change
s. family therapy
s. gene
s. intracranial disease
s. magnetic resonance imaging
s. malformation
s. MRI
s. neuroimaging

structure
alteration of memory s.
brain s.
cortical s.
dorsal stream s.
dysphoric character s.
hypoactive limbic s.
intraarachnoid neurovascular s.
ipsilateral mesial temporal s.
limbic system s.
medial temporal s.
mesencephalic premotor s.
mesial cerebral s.
narcissistic character s.
nervous system s.
neural s.
neuronal s.
shift of midline s.
speech s.
subcortical s.
white matter s.

Strully
S. dural hook
S. dural scissors
S. neurological scissors

Strümpell
S. disease
S. phenomenon
S. reflex
S. sign

Strümpell-Leichtenstern
S.-L. disease
S.-L. encephalitis

Strümpell-Lorrain disease
Strümpell-Marie disease
Strümpell-Westphal disease
strut
allograft s.
corticocancellous s.
s. fusion technique
s. graft
s. grafting
miniplate s.

Struthers ligament

NOTES

strychnine
lysergic acid diethylamide and s.
Stryker
S. bed
S. drill
S. frame
STS
superior temporal sulcus
STT
speed-dependent treadmill training
Stuart-Power factor
Stuck laminectomy retractor
Student-Newman-Keuls test
Student *t* test
study
AANS/CNS Joint Section Lumbar Disc Herniation S.
Affect Grid s.
air contrast s.
antiphospholipid antibodies in stroke s.
asymptomatic carotid atherosclerosis s.
autopsy-based neurochemical s.
autoradiographic s.
biochemical s.
biophysical s.
Brain Matters Stroke Initiative Edinburgh Artery S.
brain perfusion s.
brain potential s.
brain structure s.
Bronx Aging S.
cabergoline s.
Carotid Artery Stenosis with Asymptomatic Narrowing: Operation Versus Aspirin S. (CASANOVA)
case s.
CBF s.
cerebral blood flow s.
chromosome s.
clinical comparison s.
clinicopathologic s.
cross-over s.
cross-sectional s.
double-blind drug s.
early treatment diabetic retinopathy s.
ECA s.
efficacy s.
electrodiagnostic s.
electroencephalogram s.
electrophysiologic s.
empirical s.
epidemiological s.
Epidemiological Catchment Area S.
event-related brain potential s.
experimental s.
first seizure s. (FIR.S.T.)
fluorodeoxyglucose PET s.
Framingham Eye S.
Framingham Heart S.
functional brain imaging s.
functional MRI s.
GenePD s.
Global Burden of Disease S.
histochemical s.
ICA-occluded stable Xe/CT CBF s.
imaging s.
immunohistochemical s.
indium-diethylene triamine pentaacetic acid s.
Isle of Wight S.
laboratory s.
Life Span S.
light microscopy s.
long-term naturalistic s.
Marcé s.
Mayo Asymptomatic Carotid Endarterectomy S.
metrizamide contrast s.
MIRAGE s.
morphologic s.
motor nerve conduction s. (MNSC)
National Acute Spinal Cord Injury S.'s (NASCIS)
National Comorbidity S.
National Treatment Improvement Evaluation S.
naturalistic followup s.
nerve conduction s. (NCS)
nerve conduction velocity s.
neural crest tumor localization s.
neural imaging s.
neuroendocrine tumor localization s.
neuroimaging s.
New York Longitudinal S.
noninvasive brain imaging s.
nonphantom s.
Northern Manhattan Stroke S.
Olmsted County S.
Operation Versus Aspirin s.
Oregon Brain Aging S. (OBAS)
outcome s.
Parkinson Research The Organized Genetic Initiative s.
pathological s.
phenotypic s.
pheochromocytoma and neuroblastoma localization s.
placebo-controlled drug s.
polysomnographic s.
postmortem s.

pramipexole s.
PROGENI s.
radionuclide s.
RANTTAS s.
resting PET s.
ropinirole s.
Seattle Longitudinal S.
seroepidemiological s.
Simvastatin Survival S.
Sleep Heart Health S.
stimulation PET s.
TEVA s.
time-motion s.
Tirilazad Efficacy Stroke S. (TESS)
ultrastructural s.
in vitro molecular s.
Wisconsin Sleep Cohort S.
XeCT CBF s.

stump
distal sympathetic s.
s. embolization syndrome
s. hallucination
jumpy s.
nerve s.
s. neuralgia
s. neuroma

stupor
benign s.
catatonic s.
daytime s.
depressive s.
frank catatonic s.
idiopathic recurring s.
malignant s.
psychomotor s.
slow-wave s.

Sturge
S. disease
S. syndrome

Sturge-Kalischer-Weber syndrome

Sturge-Weber
S.-W. disease
S.-W. syndrome (SWS)

Sturge-Weber-Dimitri syndrome

stutter

stylet, stylette
Frazier s.

styloglossus muscle

stylohyoid
s. muscle
s. nerve

stylomastoid foramen

stylopharyngeal nerve

stylopharyngeus muscle

styloradial reflex

stylus-type sensor wand

subacute
s. angle closure glaucoma
s. cerebellar degeneration
s. combined degeneration
s. combined degeneration of the spinal cord
s. delirious state
s. demyelinating neuropathy
s. hemorrhage
s. inclusion body encephalitis
s. irritable depressive state
s. measles encephalitis
s. meningitis
s. meningitis syndrome
s. myelooptic neuropathy (SMON)
s. necrotic myelopathy
s. necrotizing encephalomyelitis
s. necrotizing encephalomyelopathy (SNE)
s. necrotizing encephalopathy
s. necrotizing myelitis
s. necrotizing myelopathy
s. polyneuropathy
s. psychoorganic syndrome
s. sclerosing leukoencephalitis
s. sclerosing leukoencephalopathy
s. sclerosing panencephalitis (SSPE)
s. spongiform encephalopathy

subacute myelooopticoneuropathy (SMON)

subarachnoid
s. block (SAB)
s. bolt
s. cavity
s. cistern
s. cysticerci
s. hemorrhage (SAH)
s. lipoma
s. screw
s. seeding
s. space
s. space metastasis

subarachnoidal
s. cistern

NOTES

subarachnoidal *(continued)*
s. septum
s. sinus
subarachnoidea
cavitas s.
subarachnoideae
cisternae s.
subarachnoideales
cisternae s.
subarachnoid-ependymal cyst
subarachnoideum
cavum s.
spatium s.
subarachoidealis
cavitas s.
subcaeruleus nucleus
subcalcarine
subcallosa area s.
subcallosa
area s.
s. area subcalcarine
subcallosal
s. area
s. fasciculus
s. gyrus
s. layer
subcallosus
fasciculus s.
gyrus s.
subcapsular epithelium
subcaudate tractotomy
subcellular localization
subceruleus
nucleus s.
subchondral sclerosis
subchoroidal approach
subclassification
subclavia ansa s.
subclavia
ansa s.
s. ansa subclassification
subclavian
s. artery
s. loop
s. nerve
s. steal
s. steal syndrome
subclavius
s. nerve
nervus s.
plexus s.
subclinical
s. absence
s. depressive symptom
s. neuropathy
s. range
s. rhythmic EEG discharge
s. rhythmic EEG discharge of adults (SREDA)
s. rhythmic epileptiform discharge of adult
s. seizure
s. status epilepticus induced by sleep in children
s. syndrome
subcollateral gyrus
subcommissurale
organum s.
subcommissural organ
subconjunctival hemorrhage
subcoracoid-pectoralis minor tendon syndrome
subcortex
subcortical
s. arteriosclerotic
s. arteriosclerotic encephalopathy
s. atrophy
s. band heterotopia/double cortex
s. cerebrovascular disease
s. condition
s. deficit
s. dysequilibrium
s. dysexecutive state
s. dysfunction model
s. ectopic cortex
s. encephalomalacia
s. gray matter
s. gray matter area
s. gray matter hyperintensity
s. gray region
s. hemorrhage
s. hyperintensity
s. infarction
s. ischemic vascular dementia
s. laminar heterotopia
s. lesion
s. leukoencephalopathy
s. limbic nucleus
s. motor aphasia
s. nature
s. pathology
s. protoplasmic astrocytoma
s. sensory aphasia
s. small vessel disease
s. structure
s. syndrome
s. vascular encephalopathy
subcortical-frontal lobe abnormality
subcorticalis chronica encephalitis
subcostal nerve
subcranial
subcuneiformis
nucleus s.
subcuneiform nucleus

subcutaneous
s. lipoma
s. pentylenetetrazol seizure test
s. sacrococcygeal myxopapillary ependymoma
subdelirium
subdermal plexus
subdivision
hippocampal formation s.
subdural
s. abscess
s. button
s. cavity
s. effusion
s. effusion with hydrocephalus
s. electrode array
s. electrode placement
s. electroencephalography
s. empyema
s. grid
s. grid electrode
s. grid implantation
s. hematoma
s. hematorrhachis
s. hemorrhage
s. hygroma
s. ICP monitoring
s. meningioma
s. peritoneal
s. pressure screw
s. space
s. strip electrode
s. tap
s. tumor
subdurale
cavum s.
spatium s.
subdural-pleural shunt
subduroperitoneal shunt
subendocardial myocardial infarction
subendymal
subependymal
s. diffuse heterotopia
s. extension
s. giant cell astrocytoma
s. glomerate astrocytoma
s. hamartoma
s. hemorrhage
s. mixed glioma
s. tuber
s. tumor
subependymoma
subepicranial space
subepicranium
subfalcial herniation
subfalcine herniation
subfolium
subformicale
subfornicale
organum s.
subfornical organ
subfrontal
s. craniotomy
s. fissure
s. meningioma
s. transbasal approach
s. translamina terminalis approach
subgaleal
s. abscess
s. drain
s. emphysema
s. hematoma
s. hemorrhage
s. space
subgenual cingulate region
subglial cerebrospinal fluid
subgrundation
subhyaloid hemorrhage
subhypoglossalis
nucleus s.
subhypoglossal nucleus
subicular region
subiculum, pl. **subicula**
s. cornu ammonis
s. hippocampus
s. promontorii
subintimal hemorrhage
subitum
exanthem s.
subjective
s. depression
s. distortion
s. effect
s. insomnia
s. mood change
s. sensation
s. vertigo
s. vision
s. well-being
sublabial
s. midline rhinoseptal approach

NOTES

sublabial *(continued)*
s. transseptal transsphenoidal approach
sublaminar
s. fixation
s. wire
s. wiring
sublenticular
s. limb of internal capsule
s. part of internal capsule
sublentiform limb of internal capsule
sublexical process
subligamentous disk herniation
subliminal stimulus
sublingual
s. ganglion
s. nerve
s. nucleus
sublinguale
ganglion s.
sublingualis
nervus s.
radix parasympathica ganglii s.
subluxation
atlantoaxial s.
cervical s.
degenerative s.
s. stabilization
unilateral interfacetal dislocation or s.
vertebral s.
submandibulare
ganglion s.
rami ganglionares nervi lingualis ad ganglion s.
ramus sympathicus ad ganglion s.
submandibular ganglion
submandibularis
radix parasympathica ganglii s.
radix sensoria ganglii s.
rami glandulares ganglii s.
submaxillary
s. ganglion
s. nerve
submucosus
plexus (nervosus) s.
submucous intestinal plexus
subneural
s. apparatus
s. cleft
subnucleus
amygdala s.
s. caudalis
suboccipital
s. craniectomy
s. craniotomy
s. decompression
s. encephalocele
s. headache
s. nerve
s. neuralgia
s. neuritis
s. Ommaya reservoir
s. posterior fossa approach
s. transmeatal approach
suboccipitale
malum vertebrale s.
suboccipitalis
nervus s.
suboptimal treatment
subparabrachialis
nucleus s.
subparabrachial nucleus
subparalytic
subparietalis
sulcus s.
subparietal sulcus
subperiosteal
s. corticotomy
s. cyst
s. dissection
s. hematoma
subpial transection
subplatysmal plane
subpopulation
neuronal s.
subretinal neovascularization
subsartorial plexus
subscale
ADAS noncognitive s.
Alzheimer disease noncognitive s.
nonturbulence s.
subscapulares
nervi s.
subscapular nerve
subsensitization of presynaptic
subserosus
plexus s.
substance
anterior perforated s.
basophil s.
basophilic s.
black s.
central gray s.
central and lateral intermediate s.
chromophil s.
exophthalmos-producing s. (EPS)
gelatinous s.
gray s.
I s.
s. induced delirium
innominate s.
s. intoxication
lateral intermediate s.

medullary s.
neurosecretory s.
Nissl s.
s. P
periaqueductal gray s.
periventricular gray s.
posterior perforated s.
prelipid s.
Reichert s.
reticular s.
Rolando gelatinous s.
schedule II s.
Schwann white s.
soluble specific s. (SSS)
spongy s.
Stilling gelatinous s.
tigroid s.
transmitter s.
vasoactive s.
white s.
s. withdrawal

substance-induced organic mental disorder

substance-related syndrome

substantia, pl. **substantiae**
s. alba
s. alba medullae spinalis
basal s.
s. basalis
s. basophilia
s. cinerea
s. ferruginea
s. gelatinosa
s. gelatinosa centralis
s. gelatinosa centralis medullae spinalis
s. gelatinosa cornu posterioris medullae spinalis
s. gelatinosa Rolandi
s. grisea
s. grisea centralis
s. grisea medullae spinalis
s. grisea periaqueductalis
s. innominata
s. innominata of Reichert
s. innominata of Reil
s. intermedia centralis
s. intermedia centralis et lateralis
s. intermedia centralis medullae spinalis
s. medullaris
s. nigra (SN)
s. nigra disorder
s. nigra pars compacta (SNc)
s. nigra pars reticulata (sNr)
s. perforata anterior
s. perforata interpeduncularis
s. perforata posterior
s. perforata rostralis
s. reticularis
s. spongiosa
s. trabecularis

substantial visceralis secundaria medullae spinalis

substitute
Allomatrix bone s.
human dural s.

substituted benzamide

substitutive agent therapy

substrate
artificial blood s.
biologic s.
brain s.
neural s.
permissive s.
s. transport

subsultus
s. clonus
s. tendinum

subsynaptic web

subsyndromal
s. depression
s. mood symptom

subsystem
cognitive s.
parallel s.
visual s.

subtalar arthralgia

subtemporal
s. basal approach
s. decompression
s. dissection
s. fissure
s. infratemporal approach
s. keyhole approach

subtentorial lesion

subtest scale score

subtetanic

subthalamic
s. fasciculus
s. nucleolus (STN)
s. nucleus (STN)

NOTES

subthalamic *(continued)*
s. nucleus deep brain stimulation (STN-DBS)
s. tegmentum
subthalamicum
corpus s.
subthalamicus
fasciculus s.
nucleus s.
subthalamus
subtherapeutic dose
subthreshold stimulus
subtle
s. memory problem
s. seizure
subtraction
s. ictal ethyl cysteinate dimer single photon emission computed
s. imaging
s. technique
subtrapezius plexus
subtype
clinical s.
glutamate receptor s.
motor s.
subungual fibroma
subunit
glutamide receptor s.
receptor s.
sodium channel beta s.
subventricular zone
subvocal speech
subvoxel registration
subwakefulness syndrome
succedaneum
caput s.
succes de scandale
succimer
technetium 99m s.
succinate
chloramphenicol sodium s.
cortisol and sodium s.
frovatriptan s.
methylprednisolone and sodium s.
succinic semialdehyde
succinimides
succinylcholine
succulente
main s.
succumb
sucker
s. apparatus
s. foot
s. process
suck reflex
suction
s. cautery
s. dissection
Ferguson s.
Frazier s.
s. injury
s. ophthalmodynamometry
s. Regugauge regulator
s. tube
suction-irrigator
Brackmann s.-i.
Kurze s.-i.
Sudan black staining
sudanophilic
s. cerebral sclerosis
s. leukodystrophy
sudden
s. infant death syndrome
s. unexplained death in epilepsy (SUDEP)
s. and unexplained death in epilepsy patient (SUDEP)
sudden-onset headache
Sudeck
S. atrophy
S. syndrome
SUDEP
sudden unexplained death in epilepsy
sudden and unexplained death in epilepsy patient
sudomotor
s. component
s. fiber
s. nerve
sudorific center
Suetens-Gybels-Vandermeulen angiographic localizer
sufentanil citrate
suffocation hysterica
sugar block
Sugita
S. aneurysm clip
S. cross-legged clip
S. fork
S. head clamp
S. headframe
S. head holder
S. headholder
S. multipurpose head frame
S. retractor
S. side-curved bayonet clip
S. temporary straight clip
S. Titanium
Sugita-Ikakogyo clip
suicidal depressed patient
suicide
s. headache
s. potential
s. status

s. survivor syndrome
s. victim
s. vulnerability
sulbactam
sulcal
s. atrophy
s. enlargement
s. prefrontal cortex
sulci (*pl. of* sulcus)
sulcocommissural artery
sulcomarginalis
fasciculus s.
sulcomarginal tract
sulculus
pontopeduncular s.
sulcus, pl. **sulci**
anterior intermediate s.
anterior parolfactory s.
anterolateral s.
s. anterolateralis
s. anterolateralis medullae oblongatae
artery of central s.
artery of postcentral s.
artery of precentral s.
s. basilaris
s. basilaris pontis
basilar pontine s.
bulbopontine s.
s. bulbopontis
calcarine s.
s. calcarinus
callosal s.
callosomarginal s.
s. callosomarginalis
central cerebral s.
s. centralis
s. centralis cerebri
s. centralis insula
cerebellar s.
cerebral s.
s. cerebrales
s. cerebrales
chiasmatic s.
s. chiasmatis
cingulate s.
s. cinguli
s. of cingulum
s. circularis insula
collateral s.
s. collateralis
s. corporis callosi
s. of corpus callosum
cortical s.
dorsal intermediate s.
dorsal median s.
dorsolateral s.
s. dorsolateralis medullae oblongatae
s. dorsolateralis medullae spinalis
s. effacement
fimbriodentate s.
s. fimbriodentatus
s. frontalis inferior
s. frontalis medius
s. frontalis superior
s. frontomarginalis
s. habenula
habenular s.
s. habenularis
hippocampal s.
s. hippocampalis
s. hippocampus
hypothalamic s.
s. hypothalamicus
inferior frontal s.
inferior temporal s.
s. interlobares cerebri
s. intermedius anterior
s. intermedius dorsalis medullae spinalis
s. intermedius posterior
s. intermedius posterior medullae spinalis
interparietal s.
intragracile s.
s. intragracilis
intraparietal s.
s. intraparietalis
lateral cerebral s.
s. lateralis anterior
s. lateralis mesencephali
s. lateralis pedunculi cerebri
s. lateralis posterior
lateral occipital s.
s. limitans
s. limitans fossae rhomboideae
s. limitans of insula
s. limitans ventriculi quarti
limiting s.
lunate s.
s. lunatus

NOTES

sulcus *(continued)*
s. lunatus cerebri
marginal branch of cingulate s.
s. marginalis
s. medialis cruris cerebri
median frontal s.
s. medianus dorsalis medullae oblongatae
s. medianus dorsalis medullae spinalis
s. medianus posterior medullae oblongatae
s. medianus posterior medullae spinalis
s. medianus ventriculi quarti
medullopontine s.
middle frontal s.
middle temporal s.
Monro s.
s. nervi oculomotorii
s. nervi petrosi majoris
s. nervi petrosi minoris
s. occipitalis lateralis
s. occipitalis superior
s. occipitalis transversus
occipitotemporal s.
s. occipitotemporalis
oculomotor s.
s. oculomotorius
s. of the oculomotor nerve
s. olfactorius
s. olfactorius lobi frontalis
olfactory s.
orbital s.
s. orbitales
s. orbitales lobi frontalis
paracentral s.
s. paracentralis
s. paraolfactorii
parietooccipital s.
s. parietooccipitalis
s. parolfactorius anterior
s. parolfactorius posterior
parolfactory s.
polar s.
pontobulbar s.
pontomedullary s.
postcentral s.
s. postcentralis
postclival s.
posterior intermediate s.
posterior parolfactory s.
posterolateral s.
s. posterolateralis
s. posterolateralis medullae oblongatae
s. posterolateralis medullae spinalis
postnodular s.
postpyramidal s.
precentral s.
s. precentralis
prechiasmatic s.
s. prechiasmaticus
s. prechiasmatis
preclival s.
prepyramidal s.
prerolandic s.
Reil s.
s. retroolivaris
rhinal s.
s. rhinalis
subparietal s.
s. subparietalis
superior frontal s.
superior occipital s.
superior temporal s. (STS)
suprasplenial s.
s. sylvii
s. temporales transversi
s. temporalis inferior
s. temporalis medius
s. temporalis superior
s. temporalis transversus
transverse occipital s.
transverse temporal s.
Turner s.
s. valleculae
s. ventralis
ventrolateral s.
s. ventrolateralis medullae oblongatae
s. ventrolateralis medullae spinalis
vermicular s.
s. verticalis

sulfadoxine
pyrimethamine s.

sulfamethoxazole

sulfatase
s. A
N-acetylgalactosamine-4-sulfate s.
N-acetylglucosamine-6-sulfate s.
s. A deficiency
cerebroside s.
galactose-6-sulfate s.
iduronate s.

sulfate
amphetamine s.
barium s.
bleomycin s.
dehydroepiandrosterone s. (DHEA-S, DHGA)
dermatan s.
dimethylamine s. (DMAS)
ephedrine s.

guanethidine s.
heparin s.
iron ferrous s.
keratan s.
magnesium s.
sodium dodecyl s. (SDS)
tranylcypromine s.
vinblastine s.
vincristine s.
sulfate-3-glucuronyllactosaminyl paragloboside
sulfate-3-glucuronyl paragloboside
sulfated glucuronyl paragloboside (SGPG)
sulfatide
s. accumulation
s. lipidosis
sulfatidosis
sulfinpyrazone
sulfite oxidase deficiency aminoaciduria
sulfoglucuronyl lactosaminyl paragloboside
sulfonamide peripheral neuropathy
sulfonylurea (SUR)
sulfosuccinate
dioctyl sodium s.
sulfoxide
dimethyl s. (DMSO)
sulodexide
sumatriptan succinate injection
summation of stimulus
summer encephalitis
Summerskill sign
Summit occipito-cervico-thoracic spinal fixation system
sunburst mechanism
SUNCT
short-lasting unilateral neuralgiform pain with conjunctival injecting and tearing
Sunderland classification
sundowner effect
sundowning
s. behavior
s. syndrome
Sundt
S. AVM microclip system
S. booster clip
S. carotid shunt
S. carotid ulceration classification
S. cross-legged clip
S. loop shunt
S. straddling clip
Sundt-Kees
S.-K. encircling patch clip
S.-K. graft clip
S.-K. Slimline clip
sunset sign
Sun Sparc Station 10
SUN workstation
superactivity
phosphoribosyl pyrophosphate synthetase s.
superantigen
superconducting
s. magnet
s. quantum interference device (SQUID)
superconductor
Type 2 s.
superficial
s. cerebral vein
s. gray layer of superior colliculus
s. middle cerebral vein
s. origin
s. petrosal nerve
s. reflex
s. siderosis
s. siderosis of the central nervous system
s. temporal artery (STA)
s. temporal artery to middle cerebral artery (STA-MCA)
s. temporal artery-middle cerebral artery (STA-MCA)
s. temporal artery to middle cerebral artery bypass
s. temporal artery-posterior cerebral artery (STA-PCA)
s. temporal artery to posterior cerebral artery bypass
s. temporal artery-superior cerebellar artery (STA-SCA)
s. temporal artery to superior cerebral artery bypass
s. temporal plexus
s. temporal vein
superficiale
stratum griseum s.
superficiales
venae cerebri s.

NOTES

superficialis
fibrae pontis s.
nervus fibularis s.
nervus peroneus s.
rami musculares nervi peronei s.
vena cerebri media s.
superfine fiberscope
superfrontal fissure
Superfrost microscope slide
superior
s. alternating hemiplegia
s. anastomotic vein
s. aperture of axillary fossa
area vestibularis s.
arteria cerebelli s.
s. basal vein
s. central raphe nucleus
s. central tegmental nucleus
s. cerebellar artery
s. cerebellar artery syndrome
s. cerebellar peduncle
s. cerebral vein
s. cervical ganglion (SCG)
s. cervical ganglionectomy
s. choroid vein
s. cistern
s. colliculus
s. colliculus layer
fasciculus longitudinalis s.
fasciculus occipitofrontalis s.
fissura posterior s.
s. fovea
s. frontal convolution
s. frontal gyrus
s. frontal sulcus
s. ganglion of glossopharyngeal nerve
s. ganglion of vagus nerve
gyrus frontalis s.
gyrus temporalis s.
s. hemorrhagic polioencephalitis
s. hemorrhoidal plexus
s. hypophysial artery
s. intradural approach
s. laryngeal artery
s. laryngeal nerve (SLN)
s. laryngeal nerve external branch
s. limb of ansa cervicalis
lobulus parietalis s.
lobulus semilunaris s.
s. longitudinal fasciculus
s. longitudinal sinus
s. long-term memory
macula cribrosa s.
s. medullary velum
s. mesenteric artery syndrome
s. mesenteric ganglion
nervus cardiacus cervicalis s.
nervus cutaneous brachii lateralis s.
nervus gluteus s.
nervus laryngealis s.
nervus laryngeus s.
nucleus centralis tegmenti s.
nucleus linearis s.
nucleus olivaris s.
nucleus salivarius s.
nucleus salivatorius s.
nucleus vestibularis s.
s. oblique tendon sheath syndrome
s. occipital gyrus
s. occipital sulcus
s. occipitofrontal fasciculus
oliva s.
s. olivary complex
s. olivary nucleus
s. olive
s. ophthalmic vein
s. ophthalmic vein approach
s. orbital fissure (SOF)
s. paraplegia
s. parietal gyrus
s. parietal lobule (SPL)
s. part of vestibulocochlear nerve
s. peduncle of thalamus
pedunculus cerebellaris s.
s. periventricular white matter
s. petrosal sinus (SPS)
plexus dentalis s.
plexus hypogastricus s.
plexus mesentericus s.
plexus rectalis s.
s. pontine syndrome
s. pulmonary sulcus tumor
s. quadrigeminal brachium
s. rectus muscle
s. root of ansa cervicalis
s. root of cervical loop
s. root of vestibulocochlear nerve
s. sagittal sinus
s. sagittal sinus occlusion
s. salivary nucleus
s. salivatory nucleus
s. semicircular canal (SSC)
s. semilunar lobule
sinus petrosus s.
sinus sagittalis s.
sulcus frontalis s.
sulcus occipitalis s.
sulcus temporalis s.
s. surface of cerebellar hemisphere
tela choroidea s.
s. temporal artery-middle cerebral artery (STA-MCA)

s. temporal artery-middle cerebral artery anastomosis
s. temporal auditory cortical area
s. temporal convolution
s. temporal fissure
s. temporal lobe gyrus
s. temporal plane
s. temporal sulcus (STS)
s. thalamostriate vein
s. thoracic pedicle screw
s. thyroid artery
s. thyroid plexus
s. thyroid vein
s. vein of cerebellar hemisphere
s. vein of vermis
vena anastomotica s.
s. vena cava syndrome
vena choroidea s.
vena thalamostriata s.
vena vermis s.
s. vestibular area
s. vestibular nucleus

superiores
nervi alveolares s.
nervi clunium s.
rami clunium s.
rami dentales superiores plexus dentalis s.
rami gluteales s.
venae cerebelli s.
venae cerebri s.
venae hemispherii cerebelli s.

superior-inferior submucous tunnel

superioris
brachium colliculi s.
cisterna s.
commissura colliculi s.
frenulum veli medullaris s.
nucleus reticularis intermedius pontis s.
rami gingivales superiores plexus dentalis s.
rami laryngopharyngei ganglii cervicalis s.
ramus externus nervi laryngei s.
ramus internus nervi laryngei s.
strata colliculi s.
strata grisea et alba colliculi s.
stratum cinereum colliculi s.
stratum griseum colliculi s.
stratum griseum intermedium colliculus s.
stratum griseum profundum colliculi s.
stratum griseum profundum colliculis s.
stratum griseum superficiale colliculi s.
stratum medullare intermedium colliculi s.
stratum medullare profundum colliculi s.
stratum opticum colliculi s.
stratum zonale colliculi s.

superiorum
decussatio pedunculorum cerebellarium s.

superius
brachium quadrigeminum s.
frenulum veli medullaris s.
ganglion cervicale s.
ganglion mesentericum s.
velum medullare s.

supermotility

superolateral
s. cerebral surface
s. face of cerebral hemisphere
s. surface of cerebrum

superomedialis
margo s.

superoxide
s. anion
s. anion radical
s. dismutase (SOD)

superparamagnetic iron oxide

superparamagnetism

superselective
s. angiography
s. catheterization
s. embolization

supersensitivity
disuse s.

SupHypArt

supination reflex

supinator
s. jerk
s. longus reflex

supine
s. position
s. sleep

supplemental steroid hormone

S

NOTES

supplementary
s. eye field (SEF)
s. motor area (SMA)
s. motor area epilepsy
s. motor cortex
s. motor seizure
supplementation
glycine s.
oral s.
supply
cochlear vascular s.
collateral blood s.
spinal cord blood s.
support
youth self s.
supporter
Malis vessel s.
suppressant
vestibular s.
suppression
apoptosis s.
bone marrow s.
burst s.
medication-induced REM sleep s.
postictal s.
rebound s.
s. subtractive hybridization (SSH)
vestibuloocular reflex s.
suppressor area
suppurative
s. cerebritis
s. encephalitis
suprabrow
s. approach
s. transorbital roof craniotomy
supracallosal gyrus
supracerebellar
s. approach
infratentorial s.
supracerebral
suprachiasmatic nucleus
suprachiasmaticus
nucleus s.
supraclavicular
s. approach
s. nerve
s. point
supraclaviculares
nervi s.
supraclinoid
s. aneurysm
s. internal carotid artery
supraglottic pressure
supraglottis
supralemniscalis
nucleus s.
supralemniscal nucleus
supraliminal stimulus
supramammillaris
nucleus s.
supramammillary nucleus
supramarginal
s. convolution
s. gyrus
supramarginalis
gyrus s.
supramastoid crest
supramaximal
s. rapid stimulation
s. response
s. stimulus
suprameatal spine
supraneuroporica
lamina s.
supranormal stimulation
supranuclear
s. gaze palsy
s. lesion
s. ophthalmoplegia
s. paralysis
s. vertical gaze impairment
supraoptic
s. commissure
s. fiber
s. nucleus
s. nucleus of hypothalamus
s. recess
s. region
supraopticae
commissurae s.
fibrae s.
supraopticohypophyseal tract
supraopticohypophysiales
fibrae s.
supraopticohypophysialis
tractus s.
supraopticohypophysial tract
supraopticus
nucleus s.
recessus s.
supraorbital
s. nerve
s. neuralgia
s. pericranial flap
s. point
s. pterional approach
s. reflex
s. ridge
s. rim
supraorbitalis
nervus s.
ramus lateralis nervi s.
ramus medialis nervi s.
suprapatellar reflex

suprapinealis
recessus s.
suprapineal recess
suprapubic reflex
supraradial plexus
suprarenal ganglion
suprarenalis
plexus s.
suprascapular
s. nerve
s. nerve entrapment
s. neuropathy
suprascapularis
nervus s.
suprasegmental parameter
suprasellar
s. adenoma
s. aneurysm
s. area
s. capsule
s. cistern
s. cyst
s. extension
s. lesion
s. mass
s. meningioma
s. region
suprasplenial sulcus
suprastriate layer
suprasylvian
supratentorial
s. approach
s. arteriovenous malformation
s. astrocytoma
s. brain
s. cavernous angioma
s. craniotomy
s. dura
s. glioma
s. lobar ependymoma
s. mass
s. meningioma (STM)
s. oligodendroglioma
s. primary malignant brain tumor
s. primitive neuroectodermal tumor
s. structural lesion
s. subdural hemorrhage
s. system
supratherapeutic concentration
suprathreshold stimulus
supratrochlearis
nervus s.
supratrochlear nerve
supraumbilical reflex
supreme intercostal artery
Suprol
SUR
sulfonylurea
sural
s. cutaneous nerve
s. nerve biopsy
s. nerve bridge graft
s. nerve cable graft
s. sensory nerve
s. sensory potential
suralis
nervus s.
rami calcanei laterales nervi s.
Suramin
surface
s. affability
s. coil
s. coil array
s. coil MR
s. coil spectroscopic imaging
s. electrode
s. epitope
s. fiducial marker
inferior cerebral s.
s. landmark
medial cerebral s.
mesial s.
s. reconstruction
s. scalp electroencephalogram
superolateral cerebral s.
tentorial s.
s. thalamic vein
s. vessel registration
Surgairtome II drill halo
surgeon
American Association of Neurological Surgeons/Congress of Neurological S.'s (AANS/CNS)
surgery
acoustic neuroma s.
adult scoliosis s.
aneurysm s.
anterior cervical spine s.
anterior cervicothoracic junction s.
anterior cranial fossa s.
anterior lower cervical spine s.

NOTES

surgery *(continued)*
cerebellopontine angle s.
cervical decompression s.
cervicothoracic junction s.
computer-assisted stereotactic s. (CASS)
craniofacial s.
cytoreductive s.
decompressive s.
direct vision s.
DREZ s.
ECA-PCA bypass s.
endoscopic sinus s.
endoscopic skull-base s.
epilepsy s.
extracranial-intracranial bypass s.
Foundation for International Education in Neurological S. (FIENS)
gastric bypass s.
hypotensive s.
International Cooperative Study on the Timing of Aneurysm S.
intradural tumor s.
intraorbital s.
keyhole s.
laser s.
lower posterior lumbar spine and sacrum s.
microscopic endoscopy s.
minimum incision s.
naked-eye direct vision s.
nasal s.
neuronavigator-guided brain s.
Novalis shaped beam s.
palatal s.
Pitanguy plastic s.
posterior cervical spine s.
posterior lower cervical spine s.
posterior lumbar interbody fusion s.
posterior lumbar spine and sacrum s.
posterior upper cervical spine s.
resective epilepsy s.
selective imaging and graphics for stereotactic s. (SIGSS)
skull-base s.
stereotactic s.
telepresence s.
thoracic and thoracolumbar spine s.
tongue reduction s.
transsphenoidal s.
vascular s.

Surgica K6 laser

surgical
s. anatomy
s. correction
s. decompression
s. dressing
s. epilepsy
s. exposure
s. hearing loss
S. Interbody Research Group
s. microscope
s. microscope navigator system (SMN system)
s. procedure
s. resection
s. seeding
s. technique

Surgicel
S. fibrillator absorbable hemostat
S. Nu-Knit dressing

Surg-I-Loop

SurgiScope
S. image-guided system
S. robotic microscope
S. stereotactic system

Surgi-Spec telescope

Surgivac drain

Surmontil

Surrogate Outcome Measure

surveillance
s. imaging
s. protocol

survival
cell s.
s. motor neuron gene
overall s.
progression-free s.
s. time

survivor
Alzheimer s.
trauma s.

Susac syndrome

susceptibility
s. agent
s. artifact
s. effect
environmental s.
s. factor
genetic s.
magnetic s.

suspended embryonic astrocyte

suspenopsia

suspension
Alksne iron s.
hyoid s.
magnesium hydroxide s.

sustained
s. ankle clonus
s. compliance
s. fatigability

s. high-frequency repetitive firing (SRF)
s. release (SR)
sustentacular fiber of retina
sustention/intention tremor
Sustiva
suture
American silk s.
Bondek s.
s. clamp
coronal s.
cranial s.
Czerny s.
s. diastasis
dural tack-up s.
lambdoidal s.
Mersilk black silk s.
metopic s.
Micrins microsurgical s.
Millipore s.
nerve s.
Nurolon s.
occipitomastoid s.
parietosquamous s.
petrosquamous s.
polypropylene s.
PremiCron nonabsorbable s.
pterygomaxillary s.
retracting s.
Serralnyl s.
Serralsilk s.
tacking s.
tension s.
tentalum wire tension s.
tympanosquamous s.
Vicryl Rapide s.
suturectomy
Suzuki classification
SV40
simian virus 40
SV40 tumor antigen immortalized cell
SVC
small volume correction
SVIB
Strong Vocational Interest Blank
SV-MRS
single-voxel magnetic resonance spectroscopy
SWA
slow wave activity
swallowing
s. automatism
s. center
s. disorder
s. reflex
s. threshold
swallow syncope
Swan-Ganz catheter
swan-neck
s.-n. deformity
s.-n. deformity reduction
Swanson scaphoid awl
SWAP
S. item set
S. procedure
SWAP-200
S. assessment procedure
S. item set
S. statement
Swash-Schwartz disease
sway velocity
sweat center
sweating test
Swedish gamma knife group
Sweet
S. disease
S. pituitary scissors
S. two-point discrimination
swelling
blennorrhagic s.
brain s.
optic disk s.
psychomotor s.
Spielmeyer acute s.
tympanic s.
SwiftLase scanner
swim-goggle headache
swimmer's view
swineherd disease
swinging-flashlight
s.-f. sign
s.-f. test
switch
postictal blood flow s.
swollen axon
SWS
slow-wave sleep
Sturge-Weber syndrome
Sydenham
S. chorea
S. disease

NOTES

sylaminoimidazole carboxylase
syllabic
s. blindness
s. speech
sylleptic argument
sylvian
s. angle
s. approach
s. aqueduct
s. aqueduct syndrome
s. cistern
s. dissection
s. fissure
s. fossa
s. hematoma
s. line
s. operculum
s. point
s. seizure
s. ventricle
sylvian/rolandic junction
sylvii
aqueductus s.
cistern s.
cisterna fossae s.
sulcus s.
vallecula s.
Sylvius
S. angle
aqueduct of S.
fissure of S.
fossa of S.
iter of S.
ventricle of S.
S. ventricle
Symadine
Symax-SR caplet
Symbiot covered stent
symbolism
Symmetrel
symmetric
s. distal neuropathy
s. polyneuropathy
symmetrical
s. diffuse neuropathy
s. sacral plate
s. sensory polyneuropathy
s. thoracic vertebral plate
symmetry
S. angioplasty balloon
Hermetian s.
Symonds headache
sympathectomy
cervical perivascular s.
chemical s.
s. effect
Leriche s.
lumbar s.
percutaneous radiofrequency s.
periarterial s.
permanent s.
presacral s.
radiofrequency thoracic s.
Smithwick s.
thoracic endoscopic s.
three-portal video-assisted thoracoscopic s.
video-assisted endoscopic s.
visceral s.
sympathetectomy
sympathetic
s. blockade
s. chain
s. discharge
s. dystrophy syndrome
s. ganglion
s. hypertonia
s. imbalance
s. iridoplegia
s. meningitis
s. nerve
s. nerve ending
s. nervous system
s. neuroblast
s. output
s. part
s. plexus
s. reflex dystrophy
s. segment
s. skin response
s. sprouting
s. stimulation
s. trunk
sympathetica
ptosis s.
sympathetically
s. independent pain syndrome
s. mediated pain syndrome
sympathetic-nervous-system-medicated vasoconstriction
sympatheticotonic type
sympatheticum
ganglion s.
sympatheticus
truncus s.
sympathetoblastoma
sympathica
meningitis s.
pars s.
sympathicectomy
sympathici
ganglia trunci s.
rami interganglionares trunci s.
sympathicoblast

sympathicoblastoma
sympathicogonioma
sympathicolysis
sympathicolytic
sympathicomimetic
sympathiconeuritis
sympathicopathy
sympathicotonia
sympathicotonic
sympathicotripsy
sympathicotrope
sympathicotropic
sympathicum
  ganglion s.
sympathicus
  truncus s.
sympathoadrenomedullary response
sympathoblastoma
sympathogonioma
sympatholytic
sympathomimetic
  s. agent
  s. drug
  s. toxicity
sympathomimetic-induced thermogenesis
sympathotonic orthostatic hypotension
Symphony platelet concentrate system
symptom
  affective s.
  s. amplification
  Anton s.
  arousal s.
  array of s.
  s. assessment
  behavioral s.
  bodily s.
  body-related obsessive-like s.
  Bonhoeffer s.
  Brauch-Romberg s.
  s. categorization
  S. Checklist-90
  S. Checklist 90-Revised Global Severity Index
  clinical s.
  clinician-rated cognitive s.
  cluster of s.
  cluster C, D s.
  cognitive s.
  cranial autonomic s.
  s. crystallization
  debilitating dysphoric s.
  s. dimension
  disaster-related avoidant s.
  disaster-related intrusive s.
  discrete s.
  disorganization s.
  dissociation s.
  drug-induced negative s.
  eclamptic s.
  Epstein s.
  s. exacerbation
  extrapyramidal s. (EPS)
  extrapyramidal syndrome s.
  first-rank s.
  Frenkel s.
  generic negative s.
  Gordon s.
  Haenel s.
  hyperarousal s.
  induced factitious s.
  intrusive s.
  Kerandel s.
  s. level
  longstanding s.
  Macewen s.
  manifest s.
  s. measure
  migrainous s.
  mild subsyndromal s.
  multiple medically unexplained s.
  neurobehavioral s.
  neurologic s.
  numbing s.
  parkinsonian s.
  positive s.
  postspell s.
  posttraumatic stress s.
  precursory s.
  premonitory s.
  primary enduring negative s.
  primary nonenduring negative s.
  prodromal psychotic s.
  s. profile
  s. progression
  psychological s.
  recurring s.
  s. reduction
  Remak s.
  residual negative s.
  residual positive s.
  Roger s.
  Romberg s.

NOTES

symptom *(continued)*
Romberg-Howship s.
Schneider first rank s.
secondary s.
Séguin signal s.
signal s.
specific s.
subclinical depressive s.
subsyndromal mood s.
tic s.
total s.
Trendelenburg s.
Ulthoff s.
vegetative s.
visual s.
Wartenberg s.
worrying s.
s. worsening
symptomatic
s. depression
s. dystonia
s. extrapulmonary disease
s. headache
s. hydrocephalus
s. neuralgia
s. palatal tremor
s. paramyotonia
s. partial epilepsy
s. patient
s. perspective
s. root
s. seizure
s. spondylolisthesis
s. tetany
s. torticollis
symptom-related predictor
synalgia
synalgic
synangiosis
synaphoceptor
synapse
axoaxonic s.
axodendritic s.
axodendrosomatic s.
axosomatic s.
dendrodendritic s.
electrotonic s.
Gray type I, II s.
hebbian potentiation of s.
inhibitory s.
loop s.
s. loss
pericorpuscular s.
s. plasticity
s. redundancy
viable s.
synapsis
synaptic
s. activity
s. bouton
s. cleft
s. conduction
s. connection
s. degeneration
s. density
s. ending
s. glomerulus
s. knob
s. membrane
s. pathway
s. plasticity
s. space
s. sprouting
s. terminal
s. terminal
s. trough
s. vesicle
synaptogenesis
dendrite s.
synaptology
synaptophysin
synaptosome
s. associated protein
brain s.
syncheiria
synchiria
synchondrosis
synchrocyclotron operation
SynchroMed
S. drug administration device
S. model 8611H prototype implantable pump
synchronization
thalamocortical s.
synchronized
s. neuronal discharge
s. sleep
synchronous
s. bilateral PLED
s. corticofugal epileptic discharge
s. epileptiform activity
s. facial schwannoma
s. lesion
s. reflex
s. spike-and-wave discharge
synchrony
bilateral s.
interhemispheric s.
secondary bilateral s.
syncinesis
synclonic spasm
synclonus

syncopal
s. migraine
s. migraine headache
syncope
Adams-Stokes s.
cardiac s.
carotid sinus s.
carotid-sinus hypersensitivity-induced s.
convulsive s.
cough s.
digital s.
hysterical s.
laryngeal s.
local s.
micturition s.
near s.
neurally mediated s.
neurocardiogenic s.
orthostatic s.
postural s.
reflex s.
reflexogenic s.
stretching s.
swallow s.
tussive s.
vasodepressor s.
vasomotor s.
vasovagal s.
syncopic
syncytial
s. island
s. meningioma
syncytiotrophoblastic giant cell (STGC)
syncytium
syndactyly
syndesmosis
syndromal
s. depression
s. pattern
syndrome
Aarskog-Scott s. (AAS)
ABC s.
angry backfiring C nociceptor
abolic s.
acarinatum s.
acquired epileptiform opercular s.
acquired hepatocerebral s.
acquired immunodeficiency s. (AIDS)
acrocallosal s.
acromegaloid-hypertelorism-pectus carinatum s.
acroparesthesia s.
acute brain s.
acute disconnection s.
acute organic brain s.
acute psychoorganic s.
Adams-Stokes s.
Adie tonic pupil s.
adiposogenital s.
adult respiratory distress s.
adult Reye s. (ARS)
advanced sleep-phase s. (ASPS)
age-dependent epilepsy s.
agitated delirium s.
Aicardi s.
Aicardi-Goutieres s.
akinetic-rigid s.
Alagille s.
Alajouanine s.
Albright s.
Aldrich s.
Alice in Wonderland s.
alien hand s.
Allgrave s.
Alport s.
ALS-like s.
Alstrom-Hallgren s.
alveolar hypoventilation s.
amnesic s.
amnestic s.
anatomicoclinical s.
Andermann s.
Andersen s.
Anderson s.
Andrade s.
aneusomy s.
Angelman s. (AS)
Angelucci s.
angular gyrus s.
anterior bulb s.
anterior cervical cord s.
anterior cingulate prefrontal s.
anterior cord s.
anterior cornual s.
anterior interosseus s.
anterior spinal artery s.
anterior spinal cord s.
anterior vermis s.
antiepileptic drug hypersensitivity s.
antiphospholipid s.

NOTES

syndrome *(continued)*
Antley-Bixler s.
Anton s.
Anton-Babinski s.
aortic arch s.
apallic s.
Apert s.
Arnold-Chiari s.
Arnold nerve reflex cough s.
arterial thoracic outlet s.
Asperger s.
ataxia telangiectasia s.
auriculotemporal nerve s.
Autley-Bixler s.
Avellis s.
axonopathic neurogenic thoracic outlet s.
Babinski s.
Babinski-Nageotte s.
Balint s.
Baller-Gerold s.
Baltic s.
Bannayan s.
Bannwarth s.
barber chair s.
Bardet-Biedl s.
Barlow s.
Barré-Lieou s.
Barth s.
Bartter s.
basal cell nevus s.
basal ganglia s.
basilar artery thrombosis s.
Bassen-Kornzweig s.
Basser s.
Behçet s.
Benedikt s.
benzodiazepine discontinuation s.
Beradinelli s.
Bernard s.
Bernard-Horner s.
Bernhardt-Roth s.
Bessman-Baldwin s.
Beuren s.
Biedl-Moon-Laurence s.
Biemond s.
bilateral acoustic neuroma s.
Bing-Horton s.
Bing-Neel s.
biopercular s.
Björeson s.
Bloch-Sulzberger s.
Bloom s.
blue diaper s.
bobble-head doll s.
body of Luys s.
Bonhoeffer s.
Bonnet-Dechaume-Blanc s.
Bonnevie-Ullrich s.
Bonnier s.
Börjeson-Forssman-Lehmann s.
brachial-basilar insufficiency s.
brachialgia and cord s.
Brachmann-de Lange s.
Bradbury-Eggleston s.
brainstem s.
Brauch-Romberg s.
bright thalamus s.
Briquet s.
Brissaud s.
Brissaud-Marie s.
Brissaud-Sicard s.
Broca s.
Brown s.
Brown-Séquard s.
Brown-Vialetto-van Laere s.
Brueghel s.
Bruns s.
Brushfield-Wyatt s.
bulbar s.
burner s.
burning feet s.
burning hands s.
C2 s.
Call-Fleming s.
Camurati-Engelmann s.
Canto-Rapin s.
cardiofacial s.
carotid sinus s.
carpal tunnel s. (CTS)
Carpenter s.
Carpenter-Philappart s.
cataract-oligophrenia s.
cauda equina s.
caudal regression s.
cavernous sinus s.
Cayler s.
central alveolar hypoventilation s.
central anticholinergic s.
central cord injury s.
central hypoventilation s.
central sleep apnea s.
cerebellar cognitive affective s.
cerebellar hemisphere s.
cerebellar hemorrhage s.
cerebellomedullary malformation s.
cerebellopontine angle s.
cerebral salt wasting s.
cerebral steal s.
cerebrofaciothoracic dysplasia s.
cerebrohepatorenal s.
cerebrovascular s.
cervical compression s.
cervical disk s.

cervical fusion s.
cervical rib and band s.
cervical tension s.
cervicobrachial s.
Cestan s.
Cestan-Chenais s.
Cestan-Raymond s.
Charcot-Marie s.
Charcot-Weiss-Baker s.
CHARGE s.
Charles Bonnet s.
Charlevoix-Saguenay s.
Charlin s.
Chediak-Higashi s.
cherry-red spot myoclonus s.
Chiari II s.
chiasma s.
Chiasmal s.
chiasmatic s.
childhood-onset Tourette s.
Chinese paralytic s.
choreic s.
chronic fatigue and immune dysfunction s.
chronic hyperventilation s.
chronic paroxysmal hemicrania-tic s. (CPH-tic syndrome)
Churg-Strauss s.
classic cervical rib s.
Claude s.
Claude-Bernard s.
Clerambault s.
clinical s.
clinically isolated s.
closed head s.
cloverleaf skull s.
clumsy child s.
clumsy hand s.
cluster-tic s.
Cobb s.
cochleovestibular compression s.
Cockayne s.
Coffin-Lowry s. (CLS)
Coffin-Siris s.
Cogan s.
Cohen s.
Collet s.
Collet-Sicard s.
compartment s.
complex regional pain s.
compression s.
congenital bilateral perisylvian s.
congenital central hypoventilation s.
congenital Horner s.
congenital myasthenic s. (CMS)
Conradi s.
Conradi-Hünermann s.
Constantinidis-Wisniewski s.
continuous muscle activity s.
continuous muscle fiber activity s.
conus medullaris s.
cord s.
corpus striatum s.
cortical s.
cortical disconnection s.
Costen s.
costoclavicular s.
coxsackievirus infection paralytic s.
CPH-tic s.
  chronic paroxysmal hemicrania-tic syndrome
craniocerebellocardiac s.
creatinine deficiency s.
CREST s.
cri du chat s.
Crigler-Najjar s.
crocodile tears s.
Crouzon s.
Crow-Fukase s.
crying-cat s.
CSF-pressure s.
cubital tunnel s.
Curschmann-Steinert s.
Cushing s.
DaCosta s.
DAF s.
  down-gaze paralysis, ataxia/athetosis and foam cell
Dandy-Walker s.
Davidenkow s.
Davidoff-Dyke-Masson s.
deafferentation pain s.
Debre-Sémélaigne s.
deficit s.
Dejerine anterior bulb s.
Dejerine-Klumpke s.
Dejerine-Roussy s.
Dejerine-Sottas s.
Dejerine-Thomas s.
delayed sleep-phase s.
delusional and hallucinatory s.
delusional misidentification s.

NOTES

syndrome *(continued)*
dementia s.
de Morsier s.
denervation pain s.
Denis Browne s.
Denny-Brown s.
depressive s.
De Sanctis-Cacchione s.
De Toni-Fanconi s.
developmental quotient in Down s.
dialysis dysequilibrium s.
dialysis encephalopathy s.
DiGeorge s.
DiMauro s.
disconnection s.
disk s.
disputed neurogenic thoracic outlet s.
Divry-van Bogaert s.
DNA repletion s.
Doose s.
dorsal column s.
dorsal mesencephalic s.
dorsal midbrain s.
dorsolateral prefrontal s.
dorsomedial mesencephalic s.
Down s.
Dravet s.
droopy shoulder s.
drug-induced organic personality s.
dry eye s.
Duane retraction s.
Duchenne s.
Duchenne-Davidoff-Masson s.
Duchenne-Erb s.
Duncan s.
Dyke-Davidoff s.
Dyke-Davidoff-Mason s.
Dyken s.
Dyken-Edathodu s.
Dyken-Wisniewski s.
dysexecutive s.
dysgenetic s.
dysmnesic s.
Eagle s.
Eaton-Lambert s.
ectopic ACTH s.
effort s.
Ehlers-Danlos s. (EDS)
eight-and-a-half s.
Eisenlohr s.
Ekbom s.
elfin facies s.
E-M s.
empty sella s.
encephalotrigeminal vascular s.
eosinophilia-myalgia s.
epiconus s.
epidermal nevus s.
epilepsy s.
episodic dyscontrol s.
Erb-Duchenne s.
Escobar s.
exploding head s.
extrapyramidal s.
facet s.
facet joint s.
Fahr s.
failed back s. (FBS)
failed back surgery s.
familial dysautonomia s.
familial restless leg s.
Fanconi s.
fatty degeneration in Reye s.
FAV s.
Fazio-Londe s.
Felty s.
fetal alcohol s. (FAS)
fetal valproic acid s.
FG s.
Figueira s.
filum terminale s.
Fischer s.
Fisher s.
flashing pain s.
flat back s.
floppy head s.
floppy infant s.
flu-like s.
Flynn-Aird s.
focal brain s.
Foix s.
Foix-Alajouanine s.
Foix-Cavany-Marie s.
Förster s.
Foster Kennedy s.
Foville s.
fragmented s.
Frey s.
Friderichsen-Waterhouse s.
Friedmann vasomotor s.
Frohlich s.
Froin s.
frontal lobe s.
Fryns s.
Fukuhara s.
Fukuyama s.
full s.
full-blown s.
fulminant neuroleptic malignant s.
functional psychiatric s.
Garcin s.
Gardner s.
Gass s.

Gélineau s.
Gerstmann s.
Gerstmann-Sträussler s.
Gerstmann-Sträussler-Scheinker s.
Giessing s.
Gilles de la Tourette s.
glioma-polyposis s.
Godtfredsen s.
Goebel s.
Goldberg-Shprintzen s.
Goldenhar s.
Goldenhar-Gorlin s.
gold-myokymia s.
Goliath s.
Gorlin s.
Gowers s.
Gradenigo s.
gray baby s.
Greig cephalopolysyndactyly s.
Gubler s.
Guillain-Barré s.
Guillain-Barré-Strohl s.
Guillain-Garcin s.
Gunn s.
gustatory sweating s.
Haddad s.
Hajdu-Cheney s.
Hakim s.
half base s.
Hallermann-Streiff s.
Hallervorden s.
Hallervorden-Spatz s.
hallucinatory transient organic s.
hand-shoulder s.
Harris s.
headache s.
head-bobbing doll s.
Heidenhain s.
hemibasal s.
hemichorea-hemiballism s.
hemineglect s.
hemipontine s.
hemisensory s.
hemispheric disconnection s.
hemolytic uremia s.
hemolytic-uremic s.
hereditary ataxic s.
hereditary spinocerebellar ataxia s.
herniation s.
Herrmann s.
HHE s.
Hick s.
HID s.
Hoffmann-Werdnig s.
Holmes-Adie s.
Homén s.
Hopkins s.
Horner s.
Horner-Bernard s.
Horton s.
Hunt s.
Hunter s.
Hunter-McAlpine s.
Hurler s.
Hurler-Scheie s.
Hutchison s.
hyperabduction s.
hypereosinophilic s.
hyperkinetic s.
hyperosmolar hyperglycemic nonketotic s.
hyperperfusion s.
hypertrophied frenula s.
hyperviscosity s.
hypokinetic s.
hypoperfusion s.
hypophysial s.
hypophysiosphenoidal s.
hypothalamic savage s.
idiopathic generalized epilepsy s.
idiopathic Parsonage-Turner s.
iliac crest s.
s. of inappropriate secretion of antidiuretic hormone (SIADH)
indifference to pain s.
indomethacin-responsive headache s.
infectious polyneuritis s.
inferior pontine s.
infratentorial neoplastic s.
infratentorial structural s.
insufficient sleep s.
insular-opercular s.
interictal behavior s.
intermediolateral mesencephalic s.
internal capsule s.
International Classification of Epilepsies and Epileptic S.'s
intracranial steal s.
inverse Anton s.
inversed jaw-winking s.
irritable s.
Isaacs s.

NOTES

syndrome *(continued)*
Isaacs-Mertens s.
jabs and jolts s.
Jackson-Weiss s.
Jacod s.
Jahnke s.
Janz s.
s. of Janz
Jarcho-Levin s.
jaw-winking s.
Jefferson s.
jerking stiff-person s.
Jervell-Lange-Nielsen s.
Johanson-Blizzard s.
Joubert s.
jugular foramen s.
Kahn s.
Kallmann s.
Kartagener s.
Kasabach-Merritt s.
Kearns-Sayre s.
Kennedy s.
Kernohan notch s.
Kerns-Sayre s.
Kiloh-Nevin s.
Kinsbourne s.
Kleine-Levin s.
Klippel-Feil s.
Klippel-Trenaunay s.
Klippel-Trenaunay-Weber s.
Klumpke-Dejerine s.
Klüver-Bucy s.
Kocher-Debré-Semelaigne s.
Koerber-Salus-Elschnig s.
Kohlmeier-Degos s.
Korsakoff s.
Krabbe s.
K's s.
Kugelberg-Welander s.
Labbé neurocirculatory s.
labyrinthine concussion s.
lacunar s.
Lambert s.
Lambert-Eaton s. (LES)
Lambert-Eaton myasthenic s. (LEMS)
Lance-Adams s.
Landau s.
Landau-Kleffner s.
Landry s.
Landry-Guillain-Barré s.
Landry-Guillain-Barré-Strohl s.
Langer-Giedion s.
Lasègue s.
Lasègue s. I, II
lateral inferior pontine s.
lateral medullary s.
lateral midpontine s.
lateral superior pontine s.
late whiplash s.
Laurence-Biedl s.
Laurence-Moon s.
Laurence-Moon-Bardet-Biedl s.
Laurence-Moon-Biedl s.
Lawford s.
Leigh s.
Lemieux-Neemeh s.
Lennox s.
Lennox-Gastaut s.
Leopard s.
Leriche s.
Lesch-Nyhan s.
Levine-Critchley s.
Lévy-Roussy s.
Leyden-Möbius s.
Lichtheim s.
Li-Fraumeni s.
lissencephalic s.
lissencephaly s.
locked-in s.
loculation s.
Louis-Bar s.
low back s.
Lowe s.
lower motor neuron s.
lower radicular s.
Lowry-MacLean s.
lumbar flat back s.
lumbar theco-peritoneal shunt s.
luxury perfusion s.
Lyell s.
Mackenzie s.
Mad Hatter s.
Maffucci s.
Magendie-Hertwig s.
MAGIC s.
magnesium deficiency infantile tremor s.
major psychiatric s.
malignant neuroleptic s.
malnutrition infantile tremor s.
manic s.
man-in-a-barrel s.
mapped epilepsy s.
Marchiafava-Bignami s.
Marcus Gunn s.
Marfan s.
marfanoid craniosynostosis s.
Marin Amat s.
Marinesco-Garland s.
Marinesco-Sjögren s.
marker X s.
Maroteaux-Lamy s.
Martin-Bell s.

maternal deprivation s.
May-White s.
McLeod s.
Meckel-Gruber s.
medial frontal lobe s.
medial inferior pontine s.
medial medullary s.
median cleft face s.
median face s.
medication-induced depressive s.
medullary s.
Meige s.
MELAS s.
Melkersson s.
Melkersson-Rosenthal s.
Melnick-Fraser s.
Ménière s.
Menkes kinky hair s.
Meretoja s.
MERRF s.
MERRLA s.
metameric s.
microvascular compression s.
middle radicular s.
midface hypoplasia s.
midline s.
midpontine s.
Millard-Gubler s.
Miller-Dieker s.
Miller-Fisher s. (MFS)
Miller-Fisher variant of Guillain-Barré s.
Milles s.
Möbius s.
Moersch-Woltmann s.
Monakow s.
Mondini s.
Morgagni s.
Morgagni-Adams-Stokes s.
morning glory s.
Morquio s.
Morquio s. type A, B
Morvan s.
motor system s.
Mount s.
Mount-Reback s.
moyamoya s.
mtDNA depletion s.
mucocutaneous lymph node s.
multiple mucosal neuroma s.
multiple operations s.
MURCS s.
myasthenic s.
myelopathy s.
myoclonic encephalopathy s.
myoclonic epilepsy with ragged red fiber s.
myofascial s.
myokymia-cramp s.
Naffziger s.
Nager Miller s.
neck-tongue s.
needle-in-the-eye s.
Negri-Jacod s.
Nélaton s.
Nelson s.
neonatal abstinence s.
neonatal withdrawal s.
nerve compression s.
Neuhauser s.
neural crest s.
neuralgic pain s.
neurocutaneous s.
neuroleptic malignant s. (NMS)
neurologic s.
neuromusculoskeletal s.
nevoid basal cell carcinoma s.
Nijmegen breakage s.
nocturnal eating s.
nonlacunar s.
nonpsychotic posttraumatic brain s.
nonpsychotic severity psychoorganic s.
Noonan s.
Norman-Roberts s.
Norman-Wood s.
Nothnagel s.
numb cheek s.
numb chin s.
Nyssen-van Bogaert s.
obesity hypoventilation s.
obstructive sleep apnea s. (OSAS)
obstructive sleep apnea-hypopnea s. (OSAHS)
ocular ischemic s.
ocular motor s.
oculocerebrorenal s.
oculopharyngeal s.
Oden s.
old-sergeant s.
Omersch-Woltman s.
one-and-a-half s.

NOTES

syndrome *(continued)*
Oppenheim s.
opsoclonus-myoclonus s. (OMS)
optic chiasmal s.
opticocerebral s.
opticopyramidal s.
optic tract s.
oral-facial-digital s.
orbital apex s.
orbital floor s.
orbitofrontal s.
organic affective s.
organic amnestic s.
organic brain s. (OBS)
organic delusional s.
organic hallucinosis s.
organic mental s.
organic mood s.
Osler-Rendu-Weber s.
osmotic demyelination s.
outlet s.
overdrainage s.
painful leg and moving fingers s.
painful leg and moving toes s.
palatal s.
paleostriatal s.
pallidal s.
Pallister-Hall s.
Pallister-Killian s.
Pancoast s.
paramedian mesencephalic s.
paraneoplastic s.
paraneoplastic neurologic s.
paraneoplastic pain s.
paranoid-type psycho-organic s.
paratrigeminal s.
parietal lobe s.
Parinaud s.
Parkes Weber s.
parkinsonian s.
Parkinson-plus s.
Parry-Romberg s.
Parsonage-Aldren-Turner s.
Parsonage-Turner s.
Patau s.
Payne s.
Pearson s.
Pena-Shokeir s.
Pendred s.
Pepper s.
peripheral nerve entrapment s.
peripheral neuropathic pain s.
Petit s.
petrosphenoid s.
Pfeiffer s.
phantom shock s.
Phineas Gage s.
phonologic syntactic s.
phosphate-wasting s.
Pick s.
piriformis s.
Pitt-Rogers-Dank s.
POEMS s.
Poland s.
polycystic ovary s.
pontine s.
postadrenalectomy s.
postconcussion s.
postcontusional brain s.
postencephalitic behavior s.
posterior column s.
posterior cord s.
posterior fossa s.
posterior inferior cerebellar artery s.
posterior joint s.
posterior leukoencephalopathy s.
posterior spinal cord s.
posterior vermis s.
posthypophysectomy traction s.
postlaminectomy s.
postleucotomy s.
postlobotomy s.
postlumbar puncture s.
postmalaria neurologic s.
postpartum s.
postpartum pituitary necrosis s.
postpolio s.
postpoliomyelitis s.
postrape s.
posttorture s.
posttraumatic amnestic s.
posttraumatic brain s.
posttraumatic neck s.
posttraumatic pain s.
postural orthostatic tachycardia s.
Potter s.
Potzl s.
Pourfour du Petit s.
Prader-Willi s.
premotor s.
presynaptic congenital myasthenic s.
pretectal s.
primary antiphospholipid antibody s.
primary fibromyalgia s.
primary Sjögren s.
primary trunk s.
pronator teres s.
Proteus s.
pseudo-battered child s.
pseudo-Hurler s.
pseudotrisomy 13 s.
pseudo-Wernicke s.
pseudo-Zellweger s.

psychiatric s.
psychogenic effort s.
psychoorganic s.
psychotic brain s.
punch-drunk s.
putatively poor-prognosis deficit s.
Putnam-Dana s.
s. of the pyramid
radicular s.
radiculomedullary s.
Raeder paratrigeminal s.
Rambaud s.
Ramsay Hunt s., type I, II
rapid time-zone change s.
Rasmussen s.
Raymond s.
Raymond-Cestan s.
Raynaud s.
red man s.
red neck s.
reflex sympathetic dystrophy s. (RSDS)
Refsum s.
Reichert-Mundinger s.
Reiter s.
repetitive motion s. (RMS)
residual autoparalytic s.
restless leg s.
restless legs s. (RLS)
retroparotid space s.
Rett s.
reversible posterior leukoencephalopathy s. (RPLS)
revolving door s.
Reye s.
Reye-like s.
Richardson-Steele-Oslzewski s.
Richards-Rundle s.
Rieger s.
right parietal lobe s.
rigid spine s.
Riley-Day s.
Riley-Smith s.
Ritscher-Schnitzel s.
Robert s.
Robinow s.
rolandic vein s.
Romano-Ward s.
Romberg s.
root s.
Rosenberg-Chutorian s.
Rosenthal-Rosenthal s.
rostral basilar artery s.
Roth s.
Roth-Bernhardt s.
Roussy-Dejerine s.
Roussy-Lévy s.
rubrospinal s.
Rukavina s.
Russell s.
Ruvalcaba-Myhre s.
Saethre-Chotzen s.
Sandifer s.
Sanfilippo s.
scalenus anterior s.
scapuloperoneal s.
Scheie s.
Schinzel-Giedion s.
Schirmer s.
Schmidt vagoaccessory s.
Schüller-Christian s.
Schwartz-Jampel s.
sciatic notch s.
second impact s.
segmentary s.
serotonin s.
serotoninergic s.
shaken baby s.
shaken-impact s.
Sheehan s.
shoulder-girdle s.
shoulder-hand s.
Shy-Drager s. (SDS)
Sicard s.
sick sinus s.
Sjögren s.
Sjogren-Larsson s.
sleep apnea s. (SAD)
sleep hypopnea s. (SHS)
sleep hypoventilation s.
sleep phase delay s.
slit ventricle s.
slow channel s.
Sluder s.
Smith-Lemli-Opitz s.
Smith-Magenis s.
Sneddon s.
social-breakdown s.
social deprivation s.
social-isolation s.
somnolence s.
Sotos s.

S

NOTES

syndrome *(continued)*
Spens s.
sphenocavernous s.
Sphrintzen s.
split-brain s.
split notochord s.
spondyloarthropathy s.
startle s.
Steele-Richardson-Olszewski s.
Stein-Leventhal s.
Stephen s.
Stevens-Johnson s.
Stewart-Morel s.
Stickler s.
sticky platelet s.
stiff-baby s.
stiff-man s.
stiff-person s.
Stokes-Adams s.
Strachan s.
stroke s.
stump embolization s.
Sturge s.
Sturge-Kalischer-Weber s.
Sturge-Weber s. (SWS)
Sturge-Weber-Dimitri s.
subacute meningitis s.
subacute psychoorganic s.
subclavian steal s.
subclinical s.
subcoracoid-pectoralis minor tendon s.
subcortical s.
substance-related s.
subwakefulness s.
sudden infant death s.
Sudeck s.
suicide survivor s.
sundowning s.
superior cerebellar artery s.
superior mesenteric artery s.
superior oblique tendon sheath s.
superior pontine s.
superior vena cava s.
Susac s.
sylvian aqueduct s.
sympathetically independent pain s.
sympathetically mediated pain s.
sympathetic dystrophy s.
syringomyelic cord s.
Tapia s.
tarsal tunnel s.
tegmental s.
Terson s.
tethered spinal cord s.
thalamic pain s.
Thévenard s.
thoracic outlet s. (TOS)
thyrohypophysial s.
tight filum terminale s.
tin ear s.
Tolosa-Hunt s.
top of the basilar s.
TORCH s.
Torré s.
Torsten Sjögren s.
Tourette s.
toxic shock s.
trapped ventricle s.
Treacher Collins s.
s. of the trephined
triangular s.
trisomy 8, 13, 20, 21 s.
trisomy C, D s.
trisomy 9 mosaic s.
Trousseau s.
true neurogenic thoracic outlet s.
tuberous sclerosis s.
Turcot s.
Ulrich-Turner s.
unilateral facial pain s.
Unverricht-Lundborg s.
upper airway resistance s. (UARS)
upper radicular s.
Usher s.
uveomeningoencephalic s.
vaccine-associated Guillain-Barré s.
vagoaccessory s.
vagoaccessory-hypoglossal s.
Vail s.
Van Allen s.
van der Knaap s.
van-Dyke-Hansen s.
vasovagal s.
ventral medial mesencephalic s.
Vernet s.
vertebrobasilar s.
vertebrogenic pain s.
very low density s.
VHL s.
vibration s.
Villaret s.
Villaret-Mackenzie s.
visual paraneoplastic s.
Vogt s.
Vogt-Koyanagi-Harada s.
von Hippel-Lindau s.
Walker-Warburg s.
Wallenberg s.
Warburg s.
warfarin s.
Waring blender s.
wasting s.
Waterhouse-Friderichsen s.

Watson s.
Weber s.
Weber-Leyden s.
Welander s.
Wermer s.
Wernicke s.
Wernicke-Korsakoff s.
West s. (WS)
whiplash shaken infant s.
white-out s.
Wildervanck s.
Williams s.
Wilson s.
Wisniewski s.
withdrawal emergent s.
Wohlfart-Kugelberg-Welander s.
Wolf-Hirschhorn s.
Wolfram s.
Wright s.
Wyburn-Mason s.
X-linked lymphoproliferative s.
XXX s.
yo-yo s.
Zellweger s.
Zinsser-Cole-Engman s.
Zollinger-Ellison s.

syndromic
s. depression
s. pattern

synecdoche

synencephalocele

synergia

synergic control

synergistic divergence

synergy
gene s.
S. neurostimulation system
S. Versitrel neurostimulator

synesthesia
s. algica
auditory s.

synesthesialgia

synkinesia

synkinesis

synostosis
coronal s.
cranial s.
lambdoid s.
metopic s.
multiple s.
sagittal s.
single s.
tribasilar s.
unicoronal s.

synovial
s. cyst
s. separator

synovitis
pigmented villonodular s. (PVS)

synphilin-1

synreflexia

syntactical aphasia

syntactic manipulation

syntagmatic response

syntaxic mode

synthase
endothelial nitric oxide s.
immunologic nitric oxide s.
isoform of NO s. (iNOS)
neuronal nitric oxide s. (nNOS)
nitric oxide s. (NOS)

Synthes
S. cervical plate
S. guide pin
S. Microsystem cranial fixation plate
S. Microsystem drill bit
S. Microsystem microplate
S. screw
S. universal spinal system
S. USS

synthesis
adenosine triphosphate s.
de novo s.
dopamine s.
fibronectin s.
Fourier s.
heme s.
illegal drug s.
intrathecal immunoglobulin s.
protein s.

synthetase
alanyl-tRNA s.
glutathione s.
holocarboxylase s.

synthetic
s. aperture magnetometry (SAM)
s. corticotropin-releasing factor
s. progesterone

synuclein pathology

syphilis
cerebrospinal s.

NOTES

syphilis *(continued)*
Hutchison triad in s.
meningeal s.
meningovascular s.
parenchymatous s.
spinal s.
syphilitic
s. amyotrophy
s. cerebral hypertrophic pachymeningitis
s. meningoencephalitis
s. meningomyelitis
s. meningovasculitis
s. myelitis
s. neuritis
s. osteonecrosis
s. paraplegia
Syracuse
S. anterior I-plate
S. anterior I-plate insertion
syringeal
syringe grip
syringes (*pl. of* syrinx)
syringobulbia
syringocele
syringocephalus
syringocisternostomy
syringocoele
syringocystadenoma
syringoencephalia
syringoencephalomyelia
syringohydromyelia
syringoid
syringomeningocele
syringomyelia
ape hand of s.
cervical s.
secondary posttraumatic s.
traumatic s.
syringomyelia-Chiari complex
syringomyelic
s. cavity
s. cord syndrome
s. dissociation
s. hemorrhage
syringomyelobulbia
syringomyelocele
syringomyelomeningocele
syringomyelus
syringoperitoneal shunt
syringopontia
syringosubarachnoid
s. shunt
s. shunting
syrinx, pl. **syringes**
s. cavity
s. drainage
s. formation
s. shunt
Syrup
Mestinon S.
system
ABC anterior cervical plating s.
Accusway balance measurement s.
Acraclip scalp clip s.
Acragun system
ACT s.
Activa Tremor Control S.
adaptive control of thought s.
adrenergic s.
angiographic reference s.
AngioJet rapid thrombectomy s.
Anspach 65K instrument s.
Anspach 65K neuro s.
anterior Kostuik-Harrington distraction s.
anterolateral s.
antioxidant s.
arc-centered guidance s.
arc guidance s.
arc-quadrant stereotactic s.
arc radius s.
Ariel computerized exercise s.
ascending neurotransmitter s.
ascending reticular activating s. (ARAS)
ascending reticular arousal s.
Aspen ultrasound s.
association s.
Atavi atraumatic spine fusion s.
Atlantis anterior cervical plate s.
auditory s.
automatic positioning s.
autonomic division of nervous s.
autonomic nervous s. (ANS)
autonomic part of peripheral nervous s.
axial spinal s.
Bactiseal antimicrobial impregnated catheter s.
BAK/Cervical Interbody Fusion S.
BAK/C Interbody Fusion S.
Balance Master-training and assessment s.
behavior s.
Betaseron needle-free delivery s.
bilateral variable screw placement s.
Biojector 2000 needle-free injection management s.
BIOWARE software for Biodex isokinetic exercise s.
Boston Classification S.
brain cooling s.

brain dopaminergic s.
BrainLAB VectorVision neuronavigational s.
brain neurochemical s.
BrainSCAN computer planning s.
BrainSCAN Linac radiosurgery s.
Bremer halo crown s.
Brown-Roberts-Wells arc s.
Brown-Roberts-Wells stereotactic s.
Bruker Biospec s.
Bruker S 200 MR s.
Bryan Cervical Disc S.
Budde halo retractor s.
Budde surgical s.
bulbosacral s.
Camino intracranial pressure monitoring s.
CASS whole-brain mapping s.
CD Horizon Sextant percutaneous screw-rod s.
cellular s.
central cholinergic s.
central nervous s. (CNS)
central vestibular s.
centrencephalic integrating s.
cerebrospinal s.
cholinergic s.
classification s.
CMS AccuProbe 450 s.
Coblation-based spinal surgery s.
Codman anterior cervical plate s.
Codman Bactiseal antimicrobial impregnated catheter s.
Codman neurological headrest s.
Compass arc-quadrant stereotactic s.
Compass frame-based stereotactic s.
computer-assisted image-guided s.
computer-controlled neurological stimulation s.
conceptual s.
Cordis-Hakim shunt s.
Cosman-Roberts-Wells stereotactic s.
Cotrel-Dubousset distraction s.
Cotrel-Dubousset screw-rod s.
cranial osteosynthesis s.
cranial plating s.
craniomaxillofacial plating s.
craniosacral nervous s.
CRW arc s.
CRW stereotactic s.
C-Tek anterior cervical plate s.
CUSA CEM s.
CyberKnife robotic radiosurgery s.
CyberKnife stereotactic radiosurgery/radiotherapy s.
Cygnus PFS Image-Guided s.
Das-Naglieri Cognitive Assessment S.
data acquisition s.
Daumas-Duport s.
DePuy AcroMed DOC ventral cervical stabilization s.
Developmental Observation Checklist S.
Diaspan instrumentation s.
Diaspan screw-rod s.
Dingman oral retraction s.
DOC ventral cervical stabilization s.
Dogbone anterior cervical plate fixation s.
dopamine s.
dopamine-modulating transmitter s.
dopaminergic s.
"double donut" s.
double-pore vent s.
drug risk analysis message s.
Dual Quattrode spinal cord stimulation s.
DYNA-LOC anterior fixation s.
dysfunctional dopamine s.
EasyGuide Neuro image-guided surgery s.
ECL chemiluminescence s.
Edwards modular s.
Elan-E electronic motor s.
Electri-Cool cold therapy s.
Embolyx liquid embolic s.
Endeavor Instructional Rating S.
endocrine s.
entorhinal-hippocampal s.
Envision anterior cervical plate s.
E9000 Power S.
Epstein staging s.
Equinox EEG neuromonitoring s.
ertotropid s.
esthesiodic s.
Exner's Comprehensive S.
external support s.
exteroceptive nervous s.
exterofective s.
extracorticospinal s.

NOTES

system *(continued)*
extralemniscal s.
extrapyramidal motor s.
E-Z flap cranial flap fixation s.
feedback s.
fetal cerebrovascular s.
Fischer stereotaxy s.
flavin-containing mono-oxygenase metabolic s.
F.L. Fischer modular stereotaxy s.
FluoroNav virtual fluoroscopic s.
FluoroNav virtual fluoroscopy s.
fluoroptic thermometry s.
frameless stereotaxy s.
Freehand neuroprosthetic s.
Galassi classification s.
gamma efferent s.
gamma motor s.
Gardner and Robertson classification s.
GE 9800 CT s.
GFX II balloon and stent s.
GliaSite radiation therapy s.
glucose-6-phosphate transport s.
gNomos stereotactic s.
Golgi s.
Gordon Diagnostic S.
granulomatous angiitis of the central nervous s.
Greenberg retracting s.
Haid universal bone plate s.
Hakim programmable valve s.
Halifax interlaminar clamp s.
halo retractor s.
Hannover s.
Harrington rod and hook s.
heads-up imaging s.
Hematome s.
hemodynamic s.
hemoglobin glutamer-250[bovine] oxygen-based therapeutic s.
Hemopure oxygen-based therapeutic s.
Hermetic external ventricular drainage s.
Hermetic II drainage management s.
Hermetic lumbar drainage s.
high-force Sundt clip s.
high-resolution brain SPECT s.
s. high-speed microdrill
humoral immune s.
Hunt-Hess aneurysm grading s.
hypophyseoportal s.
hypophysial portal s.
hypothalamic-pituitary s.
hypothalamic-pituitary-adrenocortical s.
hypothalamohypophysial portal s.
immune s.
incentive s.
Indiana tome carpal tunnel release s.
InFix interbody fusion s.
Innovative Magnetic Resonance Imaging S.
Instatrak guidance s.
integrated ECT s.
interactive voice response s.
internal fixation plate-screw s.
interoceptive nervous s.
interofective s.
intraspinal drug infusion s.
Intrel II spinal cord stimulation s.
involuntary nervous s.
INVOS 3100 cerebral oximeter monitoring s.
irrigation bipolar s.
ISG Wand navigation s.
Isola spinal implant s.
isolated angiitis of the central nervous s.
Itrel 3 Spinal Cord Stimulation S.
juvenile justice s.
Kaneda anterior spinal s.
Kaneda anterior spinal/scoliosis s.
Kaneda SR spinal s.
K-Centrum anterior spinal fixation s.
Kelly-Goerss COMPASS stereotactic s.
Kelly stereotactic s.
Kernohan s.
Komet K-wire/Steinman pin and delivery tray s.
Komet Medical/Brasseler USA XK-95 high-speed drill s.
Komet XK-95 high-speed surgical drill s.
Kostuik-Harrington distraction s.
Ladd fiberoptic s.
Laitinen stereotactic s.
lateralized brain language s.
LDD delivery s.
Legend high speed pneumatic s.
Leibinger titanium mini-Würzburg implant s.
Leksell Micro-Stereotactic s.
lemniscal s.
Lenke scoring s.
limbic s.
LINAC-based radiosurgical s.
LINAC radiosurgery s.

linear accelerator s.
Liquid Embolic S.
Lorenz Neuro/skull base titanium osteosynthesis s.
3M Agee carpal tunnel release s.
Magellan electromagnetic navigation s.
Magerl hook-plate s.
Magerl plate-screw s.
MAGNES MEG s.
Magnetom SP 4000 1.5-Tesla s.
magnocellular visual s.
malevolent thought s.
Malis CMC-III electrosurgical s.
mammalian olfactory s.
mammalian vomeronasal s.
M-2 anterior plate s.
maxillofacial plating s.
Mayfield headrest s.
Mayfield surgical s.
McGuire screw s.
MED s.
MED^{next} bone dissecting s.
medial temporal memory s.
medical value s.
Medisorb drug delivery s.
Medtronic Midas Rex Legend s.
MEG head-based coordinate s.
memory s.
mesocortical dopaminergic s.
mesolimbic dopamine s.
metameric nervous s.
METRx s.
microcatheter s.
MicroChoice electric powered surgical s.
microelectromechanical s. (MEMS)
microendoscopic discectomy s.
MicroGuide microelectrode recording s.
microMax drill s.
Micro-Plus titanium plating s.
Midas Rex instrumentation s.
Midas Rex power s.
Mini Würzburg implant s.
MKM stereotactic image-guided s.
Moe s.
Monarch spinal s.
monoaminergic s.
monocular heads-up display imaging s.
Moss-Miami spinal s.
motor s.
MPM I multi-parameter monitoring s.
MultiDop XS s.
muscle tone inhibitor s.
NCP S.
needle trephination s.
nervous s.
neural s.
NeuroCybernetic Prosthesis S. (NPS)
NeuroLink II EEG data acquisition s.
Neuropak 8 s.
NEURO-SAT frameless isocentric stereotactic s.
NeuroTrek microelectrode recording s.
Neurotrend continuous multiparameter s.
Neuroview integrated visualization s.
Nicolet Viking II electrophysiologic s.
nigrostriatal dopamine s.
nigrostriatal dopaminergic s.
Nishioka s.
nonspecific s.
NS2000 bipolar generator s.
oculomotor s.
olfactory s.
ophthalmic s.
OPMI Vario/NC 33 s.
OPTAx s.
optical s.
Optotrak motion and position measurement s.
OSI modular table s.
OSV II Smart Valve s.
Parastep I S.
parasympathetic nervous s.
Patil stereotactic s. II
PEAK polyaxial anterior cervical fixation s.
pedal s.
Pelorus surgical s.
perimedullary venous s.
peripheral nervous s. (PNS)
peripheral part of nervous s.
peripheral vestibular s.

S

NOTES

system *(continued)*
phased-array color-flow ultrasound s.
Phoenix fifth ventricle s.
photonic radiosurgical s.
Photon Radiosurgery S.
pituitary portal s.
plasma fibrinolytic enzyme s.
polar coordinate s.
Polaris camera s.
posterior rod s.
Premier anterior cervical plate s.
pressoreceptor s.
primary angiitis of the central nervous s.
Profile anterior plate s.
projection s.
proprioceptive nervous s.
propriospinal s.
protease-linked activation cloning s. (PLACS)
Providence scoliosis s.
Pudenz-Heyer shunt s.
Puno-Winter-Byrd s.
pursuit s.
pyramidal s.
Quantitative Scoring S.
radiofrequency needle electrode s.
Radiofrequency Triage S. (RAFTS)
Regulus frameless stereotactic s.
Reichert stereotaxy s.
respiratory s.
reticular activating s. (RAS)
reward s.
RFG-3C radiofrequency lesion generator s.
robotic s.
Rogozinski spinal rod s.
SC-AcuFix Anterior Cervical Plate S.
Script Stat, Inc. dispensing s.
Secor s.
SecureStrand cervical fusion s.
Sentinel s.
serotonergic s.
serotonin s.
Shiley catheter distention s.
Siemens Neurostar digital subtraction angiographic s.
Siemens somatoma plus DCT s.
Siemens Vision s.
Simmons plating s.
Slim-Loc anterior cervical plate s.
SMN s.
surgical microscope navigator system
Socon spinal s.
Sofamor-Danek Stealth S.
somatic nervous s.
somesthetic s.
Songer cable s.
SonoWand intraoperative imaging s.
SonoWand ultrasound-based neuronavigation s.
3-SPACE Polhemus digitizing s.
specific s.
speech perception s.
Spetzler s.
Spetzler-Martin grading s.
Spiegelberg intracranial pressure monitoring s.
SpinaLase neodymium:yytrium-aluminum-garnet (Nd:YAG) surgical laser s.
SpineLink s.
Spitz-Holter shunt s.
standard Würzburg titanium mini-plating s.
Stealth Image Guided S.
StealthStation image-interactive s.
Steffee pedicle screw-plate s.
stereotactic coordinate s.
stereotactic surgical guidance s.
STIM neuromuscular stimulation s.
Summit occipito-cervico-thoracic spinal fixation s.
Sundt AVM microclip s.
superficial siderosis of the central nervous s.
supratentorial s.
surgical microscope navigator s. (SMN system)
SurgiScope image-guided s.
SurgiScope stereotactic s.
sympathetic nervous s.
Symphony platelet concentrate s.
Synergy neurostimulation s.
Synthes universal spinal s.
table-fixed retractor s.
Talairach bicommissural reference s.
Talairach stereotactic s.
Talairach-Tournoux s.
Taylor and Abrams diagnostic s.
TCD100M digital transcranial Doppler s.
Tech-Attach connection s.
Telefactor beehive s.
Telescopic Plate Spacer spinal s.
temporolimbic s.
Tesla MRI s.
Texas Scottish Rite Hospital crosslink s.
Texas Scottish Rite Hospital screw-rod s.

thermoregulatory s.
Thompson-Farley spinal retractor s.
thoracolumbar s.
thoracolumbosacroiliac implant s.
Thoracoport trocar s.
TiMesh titanium bone plating s.
TiMX low back s.
titanium hollow screw plate s.
titanium micro s.
transdermal methylphenidate s.
transmitter s.
TS s.
1.5-T Signa imaging s.
TSRH universal spinal instrumentation s.
ubiquitin-proteosome s. (UPS)
UltraPower basic drill s.
UltraPower bur guard drill s.
UltraPower revision drill s.
UltraPower surgical drill s.
unilateral variable screw placement s.
Universal bone screw insertion/extraction s.
Universal cannulated screw s.
Valleylab CUSA CEM s.
value s.
valve s.
variable screw placement s.
Varigrip spine fixation s.
VectorVision image guided surgery s.
vegetative nervous s.
VenaFlow Compression s.
venous s.
Ventrix fiberoptic ventricular drainage s.
Ventrix fiberoptic ventricular monitoring s.
Ventrix tunnelable ventricular ICP monitoring and drainage s.
Ventrix tunnelable ventricular intracranial pressure monitoring s.
vergence s.
VertAlign spinal support s.
vertebrobasilar s.
Vertex reconstruction s.
vestibular s.
Viewing Wand image guided s.
viral vector s.
visceral nervous s.
visual s.
V-tunnel drill s.
welfare s.
wet bipolar s.
whole-cortex MEG/EEG s.
Wiltse s.
Winquest tibial/femoral extraction s.
Winquist tibial/femoral extraction s.
Würzburg implant s.
Würzburg titanium plating s.
Xia hook s.
Xia spinal s.
X-Trel spinal cord stimulation s.
ZD stereotactic s.
Zeiss Image Guided S.
Zeiss OpMi CS-NC2 surgical microscope s.
Zeiss stereotactic tool navigator s.
ZEPHIR s.
Zephyr anterior cervical plate s.
Zeppelin micro-motor s.
Z-plate fixation s.

systema, pl. **systemata**
s. nervosum
s. nervosum autonomicum
s. nervosum centrale
s. nervosum periphericum

systematic
s. drug administration
s. family therapy
s. followup
s. vertigo

systematique
delire chronique a evolution s.

systematis
pars abdominalis s.

systemic
s. giant cell disorder
s. impact
s. inflammatory disease
s. lupus erythematosus (SLE)
s. mastocytosis
s. multifocal fibrosclerosis
s. myelitis
s. myelopathy
s. sclerosis
s. vasculature
s. vasculitis

NOTES

S

T
T cell
T fiber
T myelotomy
T ratio
T score
T score elevation
T1
T1 relaxation
T1 weighting
1.5-T
1.5-T imager
1.5-T Signa imaging system
T2
T2 relaxation
T2 relaxation rate
T2 shortening
T2 weighting
T_3
3,5,3′-triiodothyronine
T_4
thyroxine
T_1 relaxation constant
T_2 relaxation constant
tabes
t. diabetica
t. dorsalis
t. ergotica
Friedreich t.
peripheral t.
t. spasmodica
t. spinalis
tabetic
t. arthropathy
t. crisis
t. cuirass
t. dissociation
t. gait
t. mask
t. neurosyphilis
t. otalgia
t. pain
tabetiform
table
activator t.
American Sterilizer operating t.
Jackson spine t.
T-shaped Edwards-Barbaro syringeal shunt t.
table-fixed retractor system
tablet
20-20 t.
357 HR Magnum t.
Koala Pad graphics t.
Overtime t.
taboparalysis
taboparesis
tabula interna
tabulation
allophone t.
Tac
T. gel for EMS unit
T. gel for TENS unit
tache
t. cerebrale
t. méningéale
t. motrice
t. spinale
Tachistoscopic constant reading test
tachistoscopy viewing
tachykinin
tachyphemia
tacking suture
tacrine HCl
tacrolimus
TACTICON peripheral neuropathy screening device
tactile
t. agnosia
t. alexia
t. amnesia
t. anesthesia
t. anomia
t. aphasia
t. bisection task
t. cell
t. corpuscle
t. disk
t. hallucination
t. hyperesthesia
t. image
t. meniscus
T. Naming Test
t. organ
t. pain
T. Perception Test
T. Performance Test
t. pricklings with aura
t. receptor
t. sense
t. stimulation
t. stimulus
t. transfer deficit
tactile-kinesthetic training
tactometer
tact operant
Tactual Performance Test

tactus
corpuscula t.
corpusculum t.
meniscus t.
organum t.
taenia
t. choroidea
t. fornicis
t. of fornix
t. pontis
t. tela
t. thalami
t. ventriculi quarti
taeniae acusticae
Taenia solium
taeniola
t. corporis callosi
t. corporis callosi of Reil
taftian
t. theory
t. therapy
Tag complex
tail
t. of caudate nucleus
t. of dentate gyrus
dural t.
embryonic t.
tailor's
t. cramp
t. spasm
Takayasu
T. arteritis
T. disease
Talairach
T. bicommissural reference system
T. space
T. stereotactic frame
T. stereotactic system
T. whole-brain mapping
Talairach-Tournoux system
talampanel
Talbieh Brief Distress Inventory
talipes
talipexole
Talma disease
talocalcaneal
anteroposterior t.
Tamaki endoscope
tamoxifen therapy
tamp
KyphX inflatable bone t.
Richards t.
tampon
Merocel t.
TAN
tropical ataxic neuropathy
Tanacetum parthenium
tandem
t. clipping technique
t. connector
t. double mutation
tangential
t. incision
t. nerve fiber
t. neurofiber
tangentiales
neurofibrae t.
TANGENT posterior impacted instrument kit
tangent screen examination
tangere
noli me t.
Tangier
T. disease
T. peripheral neuropathy
tangle
t. fragment
intraneural neurofibrillary t.
intraneuronal fibrillary t.
neurofibrillary t.
tannate
vasopressin t.
tantalum
t. cranioplasty
t. mesh
t. powder contrast agent
t. preformed skull plate
tanycyte
tap
bloody t.
front t.
glabellar t.
heel t.
shunt t.
spinal t.
subdural t.
tape
Mersiline t.
taper
double t.
slow double t.
tapered
t. blade
t. brain spatula
tapering
drug t.
medication t.
tapetum
t. corporis callosi
t. nigrum
t. oculi
Tapia
T. syndrome
T. vagohypoglossal palsy

tapir
bouche de t.
t. mouth
tapping memory
TaqIA
allele A2 of T.
Tarasoff principle
tarbagan
tarda
epilepsia t.
neurosis t.
tardive
t. dystonia
t. movement
myoclonus t.
t. myoclonus
t. oral dyskinesia
t. orobuccal dyskinesia
t. tic
t. tremor
tardy
t. epilepsy
t. median palsy
t. ulnar nerve palsy
target
t. acquisition
brain t.
bullying t.
intramodal t.
t. localization
t. localization error
t. population
t. rash
t. registration error (TRE)
retinofugal t.
rostral subcortical t.
striatal t.
therapeutic t.
t. velocity
t. weight
targeted
t. approach
t. brain biopsy
t. intervention
targeting
angiographic t.
multiple t.
targetry
angiographic t.
Tarin
T. fascia
T. recess
T. space
T. tenia
T. valve
tarini
valvula semilunaris t.
velum t.
Tarinus valve
Tarlov cyst
tarsal
t. tunnel
t. tunnel syndrome
tarsophalangeal reflex
tarsorrhaphy
bilateral temporary t.
lateral t.
tartrate
butorphanol t.
ergotamine t.
levallorphan t.
metoprolol t.
rivastigmine t.
thorium t.
zolpidem t.
task
auditory continuous performance t.
auditory three-stimuli oddball t.
chronometric and force generation t.
cognitive t.
complex t.
developmental t.
dot-probe t.
Eriksen t.
handgrip t.
t.'s of independent living
light-prompted button t.
memory t.
motor t.
negative priming t.
neuropsychologically relevant t.
nonverbal tactile attention t.
novel memory t.
novel recall t.
t. paradigm
t. performance
practiced t.
sequencing t.
Simon t.
somatosensory cued t.
speech tracking t.

NOTES

task *(continued)*
Stroop t.
tactile bisection t.
theory of mind t.
transitive inference t.
two-stimuli t.
visually guided pointing t. (VGPT)
work-related t.
task-accuracy
continuous performance t.-a.
task-efficiency
continuous performance t.-e.
task-specific tremor
taste
t. blindness
t. bud
t. cell
color t.
t. corpuscle
t. disorder
franklinic t.
t. hair
organ of t.
t. pore
t. receiving area
t. sense
TAT
thematic apperception test
tau
fetal t.
t. gene
hyperphosphorylated t.
t. phosphorylation
t. processing
t. protein
tau-negative nerve cell
tauopathy
tautological
tautology
tautomeral cell
tautomeric fiber
taxometric analysis
taxonomic research
taxonomy of anger disorder
Taylor
T. and Abrams diagnostic system
T. brain scissors
T. Complex Figure task performance
T. dural scissors
T. halter device
occipital cortical dysplasia of T.
T. percussion hammer
T. retractor
T. series linearization method
Tay-Sachs
T.-S. disease
T.-S. disease screening
TBI
traumatic brain injury
^{99m}Tc
technetium-99m
^{99m}Tc HMPAO SPECT
^{99m}Tc HMPAO T/C ratio
Tc-99m HMPAO cerebral perfusion SPECT imaging
TCA
tricarboxylic acid
TCB
transcallosal band
TCC
traditional circulatory criteria
TCD
transcranial Doppler
TCD probe
TCD pulsatility index
TCD recanalization
TCD sonography
TCD ultrasound
TCD100M digital transcranial Doppler system
TCDB
trauma coma databank
T-cell
T.-c. alpha chemoattractant (ITAC)
T.-c. function
^{99m}Tc-hexamethylpropyleneamine oxime
TcHIDA
^{99m}Tc-HMPAO
-H. leukocyte scintigram
-H. leukocyte scintigraphy
-H. SPECT imaging
TCI
transient cognitive impairment
TCOF1 gene
TCT
transcallosal conduction time
TE
echo time
toxoplasmic encephalitis
Te
effective half time
tellurium
tear
annular t.
intraoperative dural t.
teardrop
t. dissector
t. fracture

tearing
  short-lasting unilateral neuralgiform headache with conjunctival injection and t.
  short-lasting unilateral neuralgiform pain with conjunctival injecting and t. (SUNCT)
Teasdale and Jennett scale
teboroxime
  technetium 99m t.
TECA-TD20 EMG machine
Tech-Attach connection system
Techneplex
Technescan MAG3
technetium
  t. albumin colloid
  t. etidronate
  t. 99m albumin aggregated
  t. 99m bicisate
  t. 99m disofenin
  t. 99m ferpentetate
  t. 99m furifosmin
  t. 99m glucepate
  t. 99m HIDA
  t. 99m iron-ascorbate-DTPA
  t. 99m lidofenin
  t. 99m macroaggregated albumin
  t. 99m medronate
  t. 99m mertiatide
  t. 99m, or 99mTc
  t. 99m oxidronate
  t. 99m pertechnetate sodium
  t. 99m PIPIDA
  t. 99m pyrophosphate
  t. 99m sestamibi
  t. 99m siboroxime
  t. 99m succimer
  t. 99m sulfur colloid
  t. 99m teboroxime
  t. 99m tetrofosmin
  t. stannous pyrophosphate
^{99m}technetium
technetium-gagged Cardiolite
technetium-99m (^{99m}Tc)
technique
  Abbott fluorescence polarization immunoassay t.
  active t.
  Agee t.
  angiographic road-mapping t.
  Arana-Iniquez intracranial cyst removal t.
  Asher physical build assessment t.
  avidin-biotin stain t.
  Barbour t.
  Bayesian t.
  biportal t.
  blood oxygenation level-dependent contrast t.
  Bohlman cervical fusion t.
  boost irradiation t.
  Brooks t.
  Brown-Roberts-Wells t.
  carotid preservation t.
  cervical screw insertion t.
  cervical spondylotic myelopathy fusion t.
  chromosomal banding t.
  clinical monitoring t.
  Cloward t.
  Cobb t.
  cognitive t.
  composite addition t.
  Cone-Grant t.
  continuous-wave t.
  contoured anterior spinal plate t.
  Cushing t.
  decortication t.
  destructive interference t.
  direct screw fixation t.
  Dolenc t.
  double-rod t.
  Dowling intracranial cyst removal t.
  Drake tandem clipping t.
  drilling t.
  Drummond spinous wiring t.
  effective t.
  electroencephalogram BEAM t.
  electroencephalogram brain electrical activity method t.
  endovascular t.
  entubulation t.
  facet excision t.
  fast gradient recalled spectroscopic imaging t.
  fat-suppression t.
  fiber dissection t.
  finger fracture t.
  fixation t.
  Flamm t.

NOTES

technique *(continued)*
flow detection t.
Fourier transform t.
frameless stereotactic t.
functional imaging t.
fusion t.
Gallie-Rodgers t.
Gallie wiring t.
gradient recalled echo t.
Håkanson t.
Halstead modified t.
Harms t.
Harriluque t.
Hartel t.
Hirsch endonasal t.
homogenate t.
Hood masking t.
Hunt-Early t.
hyperventilation activating t.
immunoelectrotransfer blot t.
immunohistochemical t.
implantation t.
interspinous segmental spinal instrumentation t.
intravenous oxygen-15 water bolus t.
ipsilateral transcallosal t.
Jacobs locking hook spinal rod t.
Kennerdell-Maroon t.
Lamaze t.
Leksell t.
loss-of-resistance t.
Luque instrumentation concave t.
Luque instrumentation convex t.
Luque sublaminar wiring t.
macroelectrode t.
mandibular swing t.
Margrel transfacetal screw t.
Meyer sublaminar wiring t.
midface degloving t.
Mille Pattes t.
mini-open t.
t. of Miyazaki and Kato
modified Gilsbach t.
molecular diagnostic t.
monitoring t.
morphometric t.
multivariate t.
multivoxel t.
O-PET t.
Ouchterlony double diffusion t.
oxalate pryoantimonate t.
PET t.
phase-contrast t.
photic stimulation activating t.
picture in picture t.
polymerase chain reaction t.
positron emission tomography t.
posterolateral costotransversectomy t.
postmortem t.
preservation t.
pressure distension t.
Q-sort t.
quantitative morphometric t.
recombinant DNA t.
reduction t.
Reichert-Mundinger t.
Roy-Camille t.
screw insertion t.
Seldinger retrograde wire/intubation t.
sensorineural acuity level masking t.
single-voxel t.
sleep t.
Smith-Robinson t.
Spiller-Frazier t.
spinal fusion t.
spinopelvic transiliac fixation t.
squeeze t.
state-of-the-art analysis t.
stereotactic t.
STIF t.
stop-start t.
stroboscopic light activating t.
strut fusion t.
subtraction t.
surgical t.
tandem clipping t.
terminal deoxynucleotide transferase-mediated nick end labeling t.
thin-slab acquisition t.
thoracolumbar spondylosis surgical t.
tilted optimized nonsaturating excitation t.
time-of-flight t.
Todd-Wells t.
transcortical t.
transfemoral artery t.
transsylvian transsulcal t.
triple-wire t.
vagus nerve stimulation t.
Whitesides-Kell cervical t.
whole-cell patch clamp t.
wire removal t.
^{133}Xe intravenous injection t.

technology
Cogent microillumination t.
information t.
minimal access spinal t. (MAST)
NeuroMate robotic t.
wafer t.

work evaluation systems t.
Zydis drug delivery t.
tecta (*pl. of* tectum)
tectal
t. glioma
t. lesion
t. lipoma
t. nucleus
t. plate
t. plate tumor
t. stria
tecti
lamina t.
nucleus t.
tectobulbaris
tractus t.
tectobulbar tract
tectocerebellar
t. dysraphism
t. tract
tectoolivares
fibrae t.
tectoolivary fiber
tectopontinae
fibrae t.
tectopontine
t. fiber
t. tract
tectopontinus
tractus t.
tectoreticulares
fibrae t.
tectoreticular fiber
tectospinal
t. decussation
t. tract
tectospinalis
tractus t.
tectum, pl. **tecta**
lamina of mesencephalic t.
t. mesencephali
t. mesencephalicum
t. of midbrain
optic t.
stria t.
tenia t.
teddy bear gait
Teflon
T. mesh
T. mesh reinforcement
T. tube graft
Teflon-coated brain retractor
tegmen
t. cruris
t. ventriculi quarti
tegmenta (*pl. of* tegmentum)
tegmental
t. decussation
t. field of Forel
t. glioma
t. mesencephalic paralysis
t. pedunculopontine reticular nucleus
t. radiation
t. syndrome
t. tract
tegmentales
decussationes t.
tegmenti
decussationes t.
nuclei t.
tractus centralis t.
tegmentoreticular tract
tegmentorum
decussationes t.
tegmentospinal tract
tegmentotomy
tegmentum, pl. **tegmenta**
lateral dorsal t.
t. mesencephali
mesencephalic t.
t. mesencephalicum
t. of midbrain
midbrain t.
pedunculopontine t.
t. of pons
pontine t.
t. pontis
t. rhombencephali
rhombencephalic t.
t. of rhombencephalon
rostral t.
rostral-central t.
subthalamic t.
ventral t.
Tegopen
Tegretol
teichopsia
Tektronix 2214 oscilloscope
tela, pl. **telae**
t. choroidea
t. choroidea of fourth ventricle

NOTES

tela *(continued)*
t. choroidea inferior
t. choroidea of lateral ventricle
t. choroidea superior
t. choroidea of third ventricle
t. choroidea ventriculi lateralis
t. choroidea ventriculi quarti
t. choroidea ventriculi tertii
taenia t.
tenia t.
t. vasculosa
telalgia
telangiectasia
ataxia t.
calcinosis, Raynaud phenomenon, esophageal motility disorders, sclerodactyly, and t. (CREST)
capillary t.
cephalooculocutaneous t.
hereditary hemorrhagic t.
sclerodactyly, t.
telangiectasis, pl. **telangiectases**
telangiectatic
t. angiomatosis
t. change
t. discectomy vessel
t. glioma
telangiectodes
glioma t.
neuroma t.
Telebrix
teleceptive
teledendrite
teledendron
Telefactor beehive system
telegraphic speech
telemetric intracranial pressure sensor
telemetry
closed-circuit-television electroencephalographic t.
telencephali
fasciculus medialis t.
fibrae associationis t.
fibrae commissurales t.
telencephalic
t. flexure
t. vein
t. ventriculofugal artery
t. vesicle
telencephalization
telencephalon
teleneurite
teleneuron
teleophobia
teleopsia
Telepaque
telepresence surgery
teleradiotherapy unit
telereceptor
telergy
telescope
High-Vision surgical t.
Luxtec illuminated surgical t.
Surgi-Spec t.
telescopic
t. plate spacer
T. Plate Spacer spinal system
telesensor
in-line t.
Osaka t.
Telestill photo adapter
teletactor
televised
t. radiofluoroscopic control
t. radiofluoroscopy
television-induced epilepsy
telltale sign
tellurium (Te)
telodendria
telodendron
teloglia
teloreceptor
telovelotonsillar
temazepam
TeMEP
transcranial motor evoked potential
temerity
Temodar
temozolomide
temperature
core t.
t. fluctuation
intracranial pressure-t. (ICP-T)
t. irritation
repetitive temporalis muscle t.
room t.
t. sense
t. spot
temporalis muscle t.
temperature-sensitive neural progenitor
Tempium
template
Damasio and Damasio t.
diagnostic t.
Marchac forehead t.
Temple-Fay laminectomy retractor
temporal
t. arachnoid cyst
t. arteritis
t. artery
t. artery biopsy
t. bone
t. bone jugular incisure
t. characteristic

t. cortex
t. cortex damage
t. course
t. dispersion
t. dynamic
t. fossa
t. fossa floor
t. gyrus
t. headache
t. horn
t. horn atrophy
t. horn neoplasm
left planum t.
t. lobe
t. lobe abscess
t. lobe atrophy
t. lobectomy
t. lobe dysfunction
t. lobe epilepsy
t. lobe herniation
t. lobe impairment
t. lobe infarction
t. lobe metabolism
t. lobe radiation
t. lobe retraction
t. lobe seizure
t. lobe tumor
medial superior t.
t. neocortical association area
t. nerve
t. operculum
t. pattern
t. pole
t. pole of cerebrum
t. processing
t. processing acuity (TPA)
t. resection
t. slowing
t. speech region
t. stability
t. tissue

temporal-cerebral arterial anastomosis

temporale
operculum t.
planum t.

temporalis
impressio trigeminalis ossis t.
impressio trigemini ossis t.
incisura jugularis ossis t.
lobus t.
t. muscle
t. muscle temperature
polus t.
processus intrajugularis ossis t.
Tutoplast fascia t.

temporary
t. clip
t. percutaneous SCS electrode
t. personality disorder

temporofrontal tract

temporolimbic
t. epilepsy
t. system

temporomandibular
t. joint
t. joint arthralgia
t. joint dislocation

temporomesial region

temporooccipital craniotomy

temporoparietal
t. aphasia
t. association area
t. defect
t. hypoperfusion
t. junction (TPJ)

temporopolar artery (TPA)

temporopontinae
fibrae t.

temporopontine
t. fiber
t. tract

temporopontinus
tractus t.

temporospatial orientation disturbance

temporosuboccipital bone graft

TEN
toxic epidermal necrolysis

tendency
cognitive t.
dissociative t.

tender
t. line
t. point
t. zone

tendineus
annulus t.

tendinum
subsultus t.
tremor t.

tendo Achillis reflex

tendon
t. jerk

T

NOTES

tendon *(continued)*
t. reaction
t. reflex
t. spindle
Tutoplast anterior tibialis t.
tendril fiber
tenebric vertigo
tenia, pl. **teniae**
teniae acusticae
t. choroidea
t. fimbria
t. of fourth ventricle
t. hippocampus
medullary t.
t. semicircularis
Tarin t.
t. tectum
t. tela
t. terminalis
t. thalami
thalamic t.
t. ventriculi quarti
t. ventriculi tertii
teniola corporis callosi
Ten-K
tenoreceptor
Tenoretic
tenosynovectomy
tenoxicam
tensa
pars t.
tensile stress
Tensilon
T. Injection
T. test
tensiometer
tension
conjugal t.
t. hydrocephalus
oxygen t.
t. pneumocephalus
t. suture
tension-type headache
tension-vascular headache
tensor
t. tympani
t. tympani nerve
t. veli palatini
t. veli palatini nerve
tentalum wire tension suture
tenth
tenth cranial nerve [CN X]
tentorial
t. angle
t. apex meningioma
t. draining group
t. herniation
t. hiatus
t. incisura
t. incisure
t. leaf meningioma
t. nerve
t. plexus
t. pressure
t. ring
t. sinus
t. surface
t. traversal
tentorii
incisura t.
tentorium
cerebellar t.
t. cerebelli
t. of hypophysis
notch of t.
Tenuate Dospan
tenuis
meninx t.
TEP
trigeminal evoked potential
Tepanil
tephromalacia
tephrylometer
Tepper proprioceptor simulator
teratoid-rhabdoid tumor
teratoid tumor
teratoma
atypical t.
HCG-secreting suprasellar immature t.
malignant t.
pineal region t.
sacrococcygeal t.
spinal t.
Terazoff Act
terbutaline
terebrating pain
teres
eminentia t.
funiculus t.
t. major muscle
terete eminence
terfenadine
tergiversate
terminal
t. anoxia
axon t.
t. bouton
cerebrocortical nerve t.
t. cylinder
delire t.
t. deoxynucleotide transferase-mediated nick end labeling (TUNEL)

t. deoxynucleotide transferase-mediated nick end labeling technique
t. deoxynucleotidyl transferase-mediated dUTP nick end-labeling (TUNEL)
t. deoxynucleotidyl transferase-mediated dUTP nick end-labeling staining
t. filament
t. filum
t. ganglion
t. hydrolase
t. latency
motor nerve t.
t. myelocystocele
t. nerve
t. nerve corpuscle
t. nucleus
t. organ
t. plate
presynaptic t.
t. QST
t. region
t. stria
synaptic t.
synaptic t.
t. thread
t. vein
t. ventricle
t. ventriculostomy

terminale
corpusculum nervosum t.
dural part of filum t.
filum t.
ganglion t.
pial part of filum t.
velum t.

terminales
nuclei t.

terminalia
corpuscula nervosa t.

terminalis
bed nucleus of stria t.
cisterna laminae t.
cistern of lamina t.
conus t.
fibrae striae t.
lamina t. (LT)
nervus t.
nucleus striae t.
organum vasculosum of lamina t.
organum vasculosum laminae t.
pars duralis fili t.
pars pialis fili t.
primitive lamina t.
stria t.
tenia t.
vascular organ of lamina t.
vena t.
ventriculus t.

terminate

terminatio

termination

terminationes nervorum liberae

terminationis
nuclei t.
nucleus t.

terminaux
bouton t.
pieds t.

terra firma

terrestial

terreus
Aspergillus t.

Terson syndrome

tertii
plexus choroideus ventriculi t.
ramus choroidei ventriculi t.
stria ventriculi t.
tela choroidea ventriculi t.
tenia ventriculi t.

tertius
nervus occipitalis t.
ventriculus t.

TES
threshold electrical stimulation

1.5-Tesla General Electric signa scan

Tesla MRI system

TESS
Tirilazad Efficacy Stroke Study

Tessier osteotomy

test
ability t.
ABLA t.
Ad7C cerebrospinal fluid t.
ADL t.
adrenaline-Mecholyl t.
Adson t.
air conduction t.
Alcock t.
Allen t.

NOTES

test *(continued)*
alpha t.
alternate binaural loudness balance t.
amobarbital t.
ancillary t.
Anstie t.
anti-GM_1 antibody t.
antimicrobial susceptibility t.
antinuclear antibody t.
axial manual traction t.
axon reflex t.
Ayer t.
Ayer-Tobey t.
Babinski t.
Balance subscale of the Fugl-Meyer t. (FM-B)
t. balloon occlusion
balloon occlusion t.
Bankson Language T. 2
Bárány pointing t.
baseline t.
Bekhterev t.
Bender Gestalt Visual Motor t.
Benton Visual Form Discrimination t.
Benton Visual Retention T. (BVRT)
Bero t.
Bielschowsky head tilt t.
binaural distorted speech t.
blind t.
Bloomer Learning t.
Box and Block timed manipulation t.
Bragard sign t.
bromocriptine t.
Buschke Free and Cued Selective Reminding t.
Buschke-Fuld Selective Memory t.
caloric t.
Canadian Cognitive Abilities T., Form 7
cardiac function t.
Carrow Auditory-Visual Abilities t.
category fluency t.
7C Gold t.
chi-square t.
Cognitive Abilities T., Form 5
complement fixation antibody t.
Contextual Memory t.
contralateral straight leg raising t.
Controlled Oral Word Association t.
Coombs t.
countercurrent immunoelectrophoresis t.
cover t.
CO_2-withdrawal seizure t.
C-reactive protein t.
Creative Reasoning t.
Crithidia IFA t.
cryptococcal polysaccharide antigen t.
DAP t.
Deductive Reasoning t.
Delayed List Recall t.
Denver-II Developmental screening t.
dexamethasone suppression t.
Deyerle sciatic tension t.
Discourse Comprehension t.
Dix-Hallpike t.
Dunnett t.
Ebbinghaus t.
edrophonium chloride t.
electrophysiologic t.
electrophysiology t.
Elihorn Maze t.
ELISA t.
Elsberg t.
Ennis-Weir Critical Thinking Essay t.
excitability t.
eye blink conditioning t.
femoral nerve stretch t.
ferritin t.
finger-nose t.
Finger Tapping t.
finger-to-finger t.
finger-to-nose t.
Fisher exact t.
fluorescent treponemal antibody absorption t.
forced choice of recognition t.
Frenchay Aphasia Screening t.
F-wave t.
Gaenslen t.
Galveston Orientation and Awareness t.
glycerol t.
Goldscheider t.
grip-strength t.
Guthrie t.
Hallpike t.
Halstead-Wepman Aphasia Screening t.
Hammill Multiability Achievement t.
Hand Dynamometer t.
Hand T., Revised 1983
Harding W87 t.
Hausa Speaking t.
head-dropping t.

heel-knee t.
heel-knee-shin t.
heel-tap t.
heel-to-knee-to-toe t.
heel-to-shin t.
Hendler t.
Hess screen t.
Hirschberg t.
Hollander t.
Holter monitor t.
homovanillic acid t.
H-wave t.
hyperventilation t.
incomplete-sentence t.
insulin hypoglycemia t.
internal carotid balloon t.
ischemic forearm exercise t. (IFET)
isoproterenol tilt table t.
Janet t.
Jolly t.
Katzman t.
Kennedy disease t.
Kernig t.
Krimsky t.
Kruskal-Wallis t.
Kruskal-Wallis H t.
Kveim t.
labyrinthine fistula t.
Lasègue t.
latex particle agglutination t.
L-dopa stimulation t.
leg-raising t.
letter fluency t.
Liddle dexamethasone suppression t.
lidocaine t.
Linder t.
liver function t.
Lombard voice-reflex t.
maintenance of wakefulness t. (MWT)
Mann-Whitney t.
Mantoux interdermal tuberculin skin t.
Matas t.
melatonin t.
Mental Alternation t.
MES t.
metyrapone t.
MFD t.
MicroFET2 muscle t.
microhemagglutination-*T. pallidum* t.
Miller-Fisher t.
M'Naghten t.
morphine-naloxone t.
multiple sleep latency t. (MSLT)
Naffziger t.
neostigmine t.
neuroendocrine t.
neuropsychologic t.
Newman-Keuls t.
nose spray t.
Nymox urinary t.
oculocephalic t.
Paced Auditory Serial Addition t.
Pachon t.
palmomental t.
Patrick t.
perceptual-identification t.
Phalen t.
Photoarticulation t.
pointing t.
post hoc t.
Proetz t.
projective t.
prone straight leg raising t.
Prostigmin t.
psychologic t.
pull t.
Q t.
quantitative sensory t. (QST)
Quantitative Sudomotor Axon Reflex t. (Q-SART)
Queckenstedt t.
Queckenstedt-Stookey t.
Quick Neurological Screening t.
recognition t.
Recognition Memory T. (RMT)
Rey Auditory Verbal Learning t.
right and wrong t.
Rinne t.
Rivermead Behavioural Memory t.
Romberg t.
rose bengal t.
RPR t.
Sabin-Feldman dye t.
Schilling t.
Schirmer t.
Schlichter t.
Schwabach t.
Seashore t.
Selective Reminding t.
Shapiro-Wilk t.

NOTES

test *(continued)*
Smell Identification t.
sniff t.
spasticity vertical suspension t.
Spatial Span t.
speech discrimination t.
Speech-Sounds Perception t.
sphenopalatine t.
Spurling t.
Stagnara wake-up t.
standard laboratory t.
station t.
stem-completion t.
t. stimulus
straight leg raising t.
Student-Newman-Keuls t.
Student *t* t.
subcutaneous pentylenetetrazol seizure t.
sweating t.
swinging-flashlight t.
t t.
Tachistoscopic constant reading t.
Tactile Naming t.
Tactile Perception t.
Tactile Performance t.
Tactual Performance t.
Tensilon t.
thematic apperception t. (TAT)
thenar weakness t.
thermoregulatory sweat t.
three-tube t.
three-word recall t.
thyroid function t.
TIB t.
tilt-table t.
Tobey-Ayer t.
TPI t.
transmission dysequilibrium t.
Treponema pallidum immobilization t.
Tukey t.
tuning fork t.
tyramine challenge t.
VASC t.
VDRL t.
Venereal Disease Research Laboratory t.
vertical suspension t.
very short Minnesota Differential Aphasia t.
von Frey t.
Wada memory t.
Waddell t.
Warrington Recognition Memory t.
Watson-Schwartz t.
Weber t.
Wechsler Individual Achievement T. (WIAT)
Weinstein Enhanced Sensory t.
Wide Range Achievement T., Revised (*pl. of* WRAT-R)
Wilcoxon rank sum t.
X-O t.

tester
Komet medical battery t.
West hand and foot nerve t.

testicular
t. atrophy
t. compression reflex
t. insufficiency

testing
adult Wada t.
Amsler grid t.
autoantibody assay t.
biomechanical t.
caloric t.
cerebellar aggregation culture for teratogenicity t.
cognitive t.
conduction t.
confrontation t.
continuous cognitive t.
coordination t.
corneal reflex t.
Diamox challenge t.
electrodiagnostic t.
flexion reflex t.
head-up tilt t.
hypoglossal nerve t.
intraarterial Amytal t.
intracarotid amobarbital t.
intracarotid sodium Amytal memory t.
Medical Research Council scale for strength t.
MRC scale for strength t.
multiple-choice t.
neuropsychologic t.
pediatric Wada t.
post hoc t.
provocative t.
random urine t.
reflex t.
urine t.
visual field t.
Wada language lateralization t.
Wada language and memory t.

testobulbar tract

testosterone enanthate

testosterone-estradiol-binding globulin

Tesuloid

tetani
Clostridium t.

tetania
t. epidemica
t. gastrica
t. gravidarum
t. neonatorum
t. parathyreopriva
t. rheumatica
tetanic
t. contraction
t. convulsion
t. spasm
t. stimulation
tetaniform
tetanigenous
tetanilla
tetanism
tetanization
tetanize
tetanode
tetanoid
t. chorea
t. paraplegia
tetanometer
tetanomotor
tetanospasmin
tetanus
t. anticus
t. antitoxin
apyretic t.
benign t.
cephalic t.
cerebral t.
complete t.
t. completus
t. dorsalis
drug t.
extensor t.
flexor t.
generalized t.
head t.
hydrophobic t.
imitative t.
intermittent t.
local t.
neonatal t.
t. neonatorum
physiologic t.
t. posticus
Ritter opening t.
Rose cephalic t.
toxic t.
t. toxoid
traumatic t.
tetany
t. of alkalosis
duration t.
epidemic t.
gastric t.
hyperventilation t.
hypoparathyroid t.
infantile t.
latent t.
manifest t.
neonatal t.
parathyroid t.
parathyroprival t.
postoperative t.
rheumatic t.
symptomatic t.
tethered
t. conus medullaris
t. spinal cord
t. spinal cord syndrome
tetrabenazine
tetrabromophenolphthalein
tetrad
narcoleptic t.
tetrahydroaminoacridine
tetrahydrobiopterin
tetrahydrocannabinol
tetrahydronaphthalene
tetrahydropyridine
tetraiodophenolphthalein
tetraparalysis
tetraparesis
tetrapeptide
cholecystokinin t. (CCK-4)
tetraplegia
tetraplegic
tetrathiomolybdate
ammonium t.
tetrodotoxin (TTX)
tetrofosmin
technetium 99m t.
TEVA study
Tew cranial spinal retractor
Texas
T. Scottish Rite Hospital (TSRH)
T. Scottish Rite Hospital buttressed laminar hook
T. Scottish Rite Hospital circular laminar hook

NOTES

Texas *(continued)*
T. Scottish Rite Hospital corkscrew device
T. Scottish Rite Hospital crosslink
T. Scottish Rite Hospital crosslink system
T. Scottish Rite Hospital double-rod construct
T. Scottish Rite Hospital eyebolt spreader
T. Scottish Rite Hospital hook holder
T. Scottish Rite Hospital hook inserter
T. Scottish Rite Hospital I-bolt
T. Scottish Rite Hospital instrumentation
T. Scottish Rite Hospital mini-corkscrew device
T. Scottish Rite Hospital pedicle hook
T. Scottish Rite Hospital pedicle screw
T. Scottish Rite Hospital rod fixation
T. Scottish Rite Hospital screw-rod system
T. Scottish Rite Hospital trial hook
T. Scottish Rite Hospital wrench

text blindness

TFC
threaded fusion cage
Ray TFC

TFNE
transient focal neurologic event

6TG
6-thioguanine

TGA
transient global amnesia

TGF
transforming growth factor

T-group

thalamectomy

thalamencephalic

thalamencephalon

thalami
laminae medullares t.
nuclei anteriores t.
nuclei dorsales t.
nuclei intralaminares t.
nuclei mediales t.
nuclei paraventriculares t.
nuclei posteriores t.
nuclei pulvinares t.
nuclei ventrales t.
nuclei ventrales laterales t.
nuclei ventrales mediales t.
nucleus anterodorsalis t.
nucleus anteroinferior t.
nucleus anteromedialis t.
nucleus anterosuperior t.
nucleus anteroventralis t.
nucleus arcuatus t.
nucleus centralis lateralis t.
nucleus centralis medialis t.
nucleus centromedianus t.
nucleus dorsalis lateralis t.
nucleus lateralis dorsalis t.
nucleus medialis centralis t.
nucleus paracentralis t.
nucleus parafascicularis t.
nucleus parataenialis t.
nucleus paraventricularis posterior t.
nucleus reticularis t.
nucleus reticulatus t.
nucleus ventralis anterior t.
nucleus ventralis intermedius t.
nucleus ventralis posterior t.
nucleus ventralis posterior intermedius t.
nucleus ventralis posterolateralis t.
nucleus ventralis posteromedialis t.
pulvinar t.
radiatio inferior t.
stratum zonale t.
stria medullaris t.
taenia t.
tenia t.
tuberculum anterius t.

thalamic
t. aphasia
t. astrocytoma
t. circulation
t. fasciculitis
t. fasciculus
t. glioma
t. gustatory nucleus
t. hemorrhage
t. hyperesthetic anesthesia
t. infarction
t. lesion
t. neglect
t. pain
t. pain syndrome
t. peduncle
t. radiation
t. region
t. relay
t. response
t. reticular neuron
t. stimulation
t. stroke

t. tenia
t. tumor
thalamici
rami t.
thalamic-subthalamic hemorrhage
thalamicus
fasciculus t.
ramus t.
thalamocaudate
t. arteriovenous malformation
t. artery
thalamocortical
t. axon
t. connection
t. excitability
t. fiber
t. network
t. pathway
t. projection
t. relay
t. synchronization
thalamogeniculate artery
thalamolenticular
thalamomamillaris
fasciculus t.
thalamomamillary bundle
thalamomammillaris
fasciculus t.
thalamoolivary tract
thalamoparietales
fibrae t.
thalamopeduncular infarction
thalamoperforating artery
thalamoperforator
thalamostriate
t. radiation
t. vein
thalamotegmental
thalamotemporal radiation
thalamotomy
anterior t.
dorsomedial t.
gamma t.
staged bilateral stereotactic t.
stereotactic t.
stereotactic VL t.
ventrolateralis t.
Vim t.
VL t.
thalamus
anterior nuclei of t.
anterior nucleus of t.
anterior peduncle of t.
anterior tubercle of t.
anterodorsal nucleus of t.
anteromedial nucleus of t.
arcuate nucleus of t.
caudal peduncle of t.
central lateral nucleus of t.
central peduncle of t.
dorsal t.
t. dorsalis
dorsal nucleus of t.
lateral nucleus of t.
medial central nucleus of t.
medial dorsal nucleus of t.
medial nucleus of t.
medullary lamina of t.
medullary layer of t.
medullary stria of t.
medullary taenia of t.
motor t.
optic t.
paracentral nucleus of t.
paramedian t.
posterior medial nucleus of t.
posterior nuclear complex of the t.
posterior peduncle of t.
pulvinar nucleus of t.
reticular nucleus of t.
right t.
stalk of t.
superior peduncle of t.
t. tissue
ventral t.
ventral anterior nucleus of t.
ventral anterior nucleus of t.
ventral intermediate nucleus of t.
t. ventralis
ventral lateral t.
ventral lateral complex of the t.
ventral lateral nucleus of t.
ventral medial complex of the t.
ventral nuclei of t.
ventral nucleus of t.
ventral posterior intermediate nucleus of t.
ventral posterior lateral nucleus of t.
ventral posterior nucleus of t.
ventral posterolateral nucleus of t.
ventral posterolateral nucleus of t.

T

NOTES

thalamus *(continued)*
ventral posteromedial nucleus of t.
ventral posteromedial nucleus of t.
ventrobasal complex of the t.
ventrointermediate t.
Vim t.
zonal layer of t.
thalassemia
thalidomide
thallium
t. intoxication
t. peripheral neuropathy
t. poisoning
t. polyneuropathy
thallium-201 (^{201}Tl)
thalposis
thalpotic
THAM-E Injection
THAM Injection
thanatobiologic
thanatognomonic
thanatopsis
thanatotic
T-handle
T.-h. bone awl
T.-h. Jacob chuck
T.-h. nut wrench
T.-h. screw wrench
T-handled
T.-h. nut wrench
T.-h. screw wrench
Thane method
theca, pl. **thecae**
t. medullare spinalis
t. vertebralis
thecal
t. abscess
t. puncture
t. sac
t. sac compression
thecoperitoneal Pudenz-Schulte shunt
Theimich lip sign
thematic
t. apperception test (TAT)
t. paraphasia
thenar
t. eminence
t. weakness test
theophany
theophylamine
theophylline
theoretical
t. orientation
t. understanding
theory
advanced wakefulness t.
affective arousal t.
avalanche t.
Burn and Rand t.
Cannon t.
Cannon-Bard t.
causal-attributional t.
clinical t.
convergence-projection t.
deontologic t.
emotive t.
ERG t.
etiology t.
existential-humanistic t.
flow t.
gate t.
gate-control t.
Golgi t.
injury-healing t.
local circuit t.
mass action t.
McLone and Knepper etiological t.
Melzack and Wall gate t.
t. of mind task
mnemic t.
t. of mnemism
mnemism t.
neuron t.
personality t.
relaxation t.
Semon-Hering t.
Shealy t.
social learning t.
Spearman two-factor t.
spreading cortical depression t.
taftian t.
thermostat t.
vasogenic t.
Wolff vasogenic t.
Wollaston t.
Young-Helmholtz trichromacy t.
Thera
T. Cane
T. Pulse bed
therapeutic
t. advantage
t. agent
t. agent-related neuropathy
t. approach
t. connection
t. contribution
t. efficacy
t. electrical stimulation
t. electric stimulation
t. embolism
t. embolization
t. exploration
t. malaria
t. measure

t. outcome
t. profile
t. range
t. response
t. school placement
t. strategy
t. target
t. vocational placement

therapy
abortive t.
Activa Tremor Control T.
adjuvant t.
adjuvant whole-brain radiation t.
albendazole t.
analytic t.
analytical t.
anticoagulation t.
anticonvulsant t.
antifibrinolytic t.
antimicrobial t.
antimigraine t.
antioxidant t.
antiplatelet t.
antiretroviral t.
antiviral t.
attractor field t. (AFT)
behavior modification t.
boron neutron capture t. (BNCT)
Bragg peak proton beam t.
brain gene t.
bright light t.
cellular t.
cerebral protective t.
chelation t.
cholinergic t.
cholinomimetic t.
chronic corticosteroid t.
cloaca t.
clozapine t.
cognitive t.
cognitive analytic t.
cognitive behavioral group t.
cognitive enhancement t.
computer-aided t.
computer-guided t.
constrained induced t.
constraint-induced t.
convulsive t.
corticosteroid t.
cytosine arabinoside t.
disease-modifying t.
disease-modifying agent t. (DMA therapy)
DMA t.
disease-modifying agent therapy
dopaminergic t.
electric differential t.
electroconvulsive t.
electrotherapeutic sleep t.
emotional control t.
emotional release t.
empirical t.
endovascular t.
estrogen replacement t. (ERT)
FearFighter computer program tailored for specific fear t.
first-line t.
fluorouracil t.
focused radiation t.
functional occupational t. (FOT)
gene t.
Gerson t.
global gene replacement t.
granulocyte-macrophage colony-stimulating factor immunogene t. (GM-CSF)
HBO t.
hyperbaric oxygen therapy
highly active antiretroviral t. (HAART)
hormonal t.
hormone replacement t. (HRT)
hyperbaric oxygen t. (HBO therapy)
hypertensive, hypervolemic, hemodilutional t.
image-guided minimally invasive t. (IGMIT)
immunosuppressive t.
implosion t.
inadequate t.
intensity modulated radiation t.
interstitial radiation t.
intradiscal electrothermal t. (IDET)
intrathecal drug t.
intravenous immune globulin humoral t.
iron replacement t.
isoniazid t.
IT-MS infusion t.
language t.
localized restorative central nervous system gene t.

T

NOTES

therapy *(continued)*
magnetic seizure t.
melatonin-replacement t.
molecular-based conceptual t.
motivational enhancement t.
multidimensional family t.
multimodal t.
multisystem t.
multisystemic t.
occupational t.
oral appliance t.
oxygen t.
photodynamic t.
photoradiation t.
physical t.
pituitary replacement t.
positional t.
prophylactic anticonvulsant t.
psychotherapeutic t.
psychovisual t.
radiation t.
reality t.
reflex t.
regressive electric shock t. (REST)
retrogasserian anhydrous glycerol injection t.
rheologic t.
sacral nerve stimulation t.
second-line t.
SET t.
sexuality conversion t.
short-term t.
sleep restriction t.
social t.
solution-focused t.
standard antipsychotic t.
stereotactic-assisted radiation t.
stereotactic-focused radiation t.
stereotactic intratumoral photodynamic t.
steroid t.
stimulant t.
stimulus-control t.
structural family t.
substitutive agent t.
systematic family t.
taftian t.
tamoxifen t.
third-line t.
thrombolytic t.
transvenous t.
Triple-H t.
ultrasonic t.
video t.
viral vector-mediated t.
virtual reality t.
VNS t.
whole-brain radiation t. (WBRT)
x-ray t. (XRT)

thermal
t. ablation
t. anesthesia
t. drive
t. lesioning
t. receptor
t. rhizotomy
t. sense

thermalgesia

thermalgia

thermanalgesia

thermanesthesia

thermesthesia

thermesthesiometer

thermhyperesthesia

thermhypesthesia

thermic
t. anesthesia
t. sense

thermistor
t. electrode
T. needle

thermistry

thermoalgesia

thermoanalgesia

thermoanesthesia

thermoceptor

thermocoagulation
percutaneous t.
radiofrequency t.
stereotactic t.

thermocouple
copper-constantan t.

thermoeffector
t. activity
antagonistic t.
t. function
t. response

thermoesthesia

thermoesthesiometer

thermoexcitory

thermogenesis
catecholamine-induced t.
nonshivering t.
normal t.
shivering t.
sympathomimetic-induced t.

thermogenic
t. component
t. effect
t. mechanism
t. tissue mass

thermography
infrared t. (IRT)

thermohyperalgesia

thermohyperesthesia
thermohypesthesia
thermohypoesthesia
thermoluminescent dosimeter
thermoneutrality
thermoregulatory
t. center
t. function
t. property
t. response
t. sweat test
t. system
thermorhizotomy
thermosensory
t. information
t. property
thermostat
hypothalamic t.
t. theory
theta
t. activity
t. peak frequency
t. response
t. rhythm
t. wave
Thévenard syndrome
thiabendazole
thiamine
t. deficiency
t. deficiency encephalopathy
thiamylal
thiazide-induced hypokalemia
thickening
hyaline t.
myxomatous t.
thickness
lumbosacral junction cortical t.
preinduction t.
thick-skinned
thick-witted
thienobenzodiazepine
thigh
driver's t.
Heilbronner t.
thigh-high alternating compression air boot
thigmesthesia
thinking
abnormal t.
clinical t.
disorganized t.
magic t.
obsessional t.
paleologic t.
paralogical t.
paranoid t.
trouble t.
thin-layer agarose gel electrophoresis
thin-section image
thin-slab acquisition technique
thin-wall introducer catheter
thioflavin-positive fibril
6-thioguanine (6TG)
thiopental sodium
thiophene
analog of phencyclidine t.
phencyclidine t.
thioridazine
thiosalicylate
sodium t.
thiosulfate
sodium t.
thiotepa
thiothixene
thioxanthene
third
t. cranial nerve [CN III]
law of t.'s
t. nerve avulsion
t. nerve palsy
t. temporal convolution
t. ventricle
t. ventricle floor
t. ventricular hemangioblastoma
t. ventriculostomy
t. visual area
third-degree continuous spontaneous nystagmus
third-generation
t.-g. cephalosporin
t.-g. Neutraceuticals
third-line therapy
third-person auditory hallucination
third-rate
thirst center
thirteen
Thixokon
thixophobia
Thomas sign
Thompson carotid clamp
Thompson-Farley spinal retractor system

NOTES

Thomsen
T. disease
T. dystrophy
thoracalis
plexus aorticus t.
thoracic
t. aortic plexus
t. column
t. curve scoliosis
t. dermatome
t. discectomy
t. disk herniation
t. duct injury
t. endoscopic sympathectomy
t. hypokyphosis
t. interspace
t. kyphosis
t. meningioma
t. nucleus
t. outlet
t. outlet syndrome (TOS)
t. part of aorta
t. part of esophagus
t. part of spinal cord
t. part of thoracic duct
t. pedicle
t. pedicle marker
t. spinal fusion
t. spine
t. spine biopsy
t. spine decompression
t. spine fracture
t. spine injury
t. spine lordosis
t. spine pedicle diameter
t. spine scoliotic deformity
t. spine vertebral osteosynthesis
t. splanchnic ganglion
t. splanchnic nerve
t. and thoracolumbar spine surgery
t. tumor
t. vertebra
thoracica
columna t.
ganglia t.
segmentum t. 1–12
segmentum medullae spinalis t.
thoracici
nervi cardiaci t.
pars cervicalis ductus t.
pars thoracica ductus t.
rami cardiaci t.
ramus lateralis rami posterioris nervi t.
ramus medialis rami posterioris nervi t.
thoracicorum
rami anteriores nervorum t.
rami dorsales nervorum t.
rami oesophageales gangliorum t.
rami posteriores nervorum t.
rami pulmonales thoracici gangliorum t.
rami ventrales nervorum t.
thoracicus
nucleus t.
plexus aorticus t.
thoracoabdominal approach
thoracodorsalis
nervus t.
thoracodorsal nerve
thoracolumbar
t. burst fracture
t. curve
t. degenerative disease
t. gibbus deformity
t. idiopathic scoliosis
t. junction
t. junction surgical exposure
t. kyphoscoliosis
t. kyphosis
t. pedicle screw
t. retroperitoneal approach
t. spinal canal stenosis
t. spine
t. spine anterior exposure
t. spine decompression
t. spine flexion-distraction injury
t. spine fracture-dislocation
t. spine scoliosis
t. spine stabilization
t. spine vertebral osteosynthesis
t. spondylosis
t. spondylosis surgical technique
t. standing orthosis
t. system
t. trauma
t. vertebra
thoracolumbosacral
t. orthosis
t. plate
thoracolumbosacroiliac
t. implant system
t. implant system thread
Thoracoport trocar system
thoracostomy
thoracotomy
left-sided t.
right-sided t.
standard t.
thorax stimulation
Thorazine

thorium
t. dioxide
t. tartrate
thorn
dendritic t.
Thornton-Griggs-Moxley disease
thorny
Thorotrast
thoroughness, reliability, efficiency, analytic
Thor-Prom
thousand-hands Kannon universal headframe
thread
neuropil t.
polyene t.
terminal t.
thoracolumbosacroiliac implant system t.
threaded fusion cage (TFC)
threadwire saw
three
t. axis gradient coil
t. strikes law
three-color FACScan-analysis
three-column
t.-c. cervical spine injury
t.-c. concept
three-dimensional (3D)
t.-d. acquisition
t.-d. analysis
t.-d. computed tomographic angiography (3D-CTA)
t.-d. digitizer neuronavigator
t.-d. fast low-angle shot imaging
t.-d. Fourier transform (3DFT)
t.-d. Fourier transform gradient-echo imaging
t.-d. neuroimaging
t.-d. postprocessing software
t.-d. reconstruction
t.-d. slice
t.-d. sonic digitizer
t.-d. SPECT phantom
t.-d. spoiled GRASS sequence
t.-d. target definition
Three-Item Delirium Scale
three-point
t.-p. bending moment
t.-p. headholder
t.-p. skull clamp
three-portal video-assisted thoracoscopic sympathectomy
three-repeat isoform
three-stimulus paradigm
three-tube test
three-word recall test
threonine kinase
threonyl
threshold
absolute t.
afterdischarge t.
arousal t.
auditory t.
t. of consciousness
convulsant t.
current perception t. (CPT)
differential t.
double-point t.
t. electrical stimulation (TES)
electroshock seizure t.
insular t.
t. of island of Reil
low anger t.
motor t.
neuron t.
null-condition detection t.
pain intensity t.
relational t.
resolution t.
sensitivity t.
signal-to-noise t.
speech reception t.
speech recognition t.
stimulus t.
swallowing t.
touch perception t. (TPT)
throbbing
t. headache
Throckmorton
T. reflex
T. sign
thrombin
topical t.
Thrombinar
thrombin-soaked Gelfoam
thromboangiitis obliterans
thrombocythemia
thrombocytopenia
neonatal alloimmune t.
t. venous-sinus

NOTES

thrombocytosis
essential t.
thromboelastography
thromboembolectomy
thromboembolic stroke
thromboembolism
Thrombogen
thrombogenic
t. coil
t. ferrous mixture
thrombolysis
intraluminal t.
thrombolytic therapy
thrombomodulin-protein
thrombophlebitis
cavernous sinus t.
thromboplastin
plasma t.
thrombosed
t. giant aneurysm
t. thick-walled vein
thrombosinusitis
thrombosis, pl. **thromboses**
acute t.
arterial t.
catheter-induced subclavian vein t.
cavernous sinus t.
cerebral artery t.
cerebral vein t.
cerebral venous t.
cerebrovascular arterial t.
cerebrovascular venous t.
cortical venous t.
deep vein t.
deep venous t.
dural venous sinus t.
fistula-induced sinus t.
iliofemoral t.
intracranial sinus t.
lateral sinus t.
marantic t.
marasmic t.
middle cerebral artery t. (MCAT)
sagittal sinus t.
septic t.
sinovenous t.
sinus-vein t.
venous t.
venous sinus t.
t. of venous sinus
wire t.
thrombospondin
Thrombostat
thrombotic
t. apoplexy
t. hydrocephalus
t. occlusion
t. stroke
t. thrombocytopenic purpura
thromboxane
t. synthase inhibitor
thrombus, pl. **thrombi**
chronic t.
longitudinal sinus t.
marantic t.
marasmic t.
mural t.
thrusting
tongue t.
thumbprinting appearance
thumb reflex
Thumb-Saver introducer clamp
thunderclap headache
Thurstone
Thurston scale
Thymapad stimulus electrode
Thymatron DGx
thymectomy
thymergasia
thymic
t. involution
t. myoid cell
thymine
thymineruaciluria
thymocyte apoptosis
thymogenic drinking
thymoleptic
thymoma
thymopathy
Thypinone
thyrocervical trunk of subclavian artery
thyroglobulin
thyroglossal duct cyst
thyrohypophysial syndrome
thyroid
t. cartilage
t. deficiency
t. function test
t. gland
t. orbitopathy
thyroideae
cartilaginis t.
cornu inferius cartilaginis t.
thyroiditis
autoimmune t.
Riedel t.
thyroid-stimulating
t.-s. hormone (TSH)
t.-s. hormone level
thyrotoxic
t. coma
t. encephalopathy
t. myopathy
t. periodic paralysis (TPP)

thyrotoxicosis
apathetic t.
endogenous t.
thyrotoxicosis-induced
t.-i. chorea
t.-i. choreoathetosis
thyrotroph cell
thyrotrophic axis
thyrotropin
thyrotropin-producing adenoma
thyrotropin-releasing
t.-r. hormone (TRH)
t.-r. hormone stimulation
thyroxine (T_4)
Thytropar
TIA
transient ischemic attack
tiagabine
t. HCl
t. hydrochloride
tiapride
Tibex
tibial
t. nerve
t. phenomenon
tibialis
nervus t.
rami calcanei mediales nervi t.
rami musculares nervi t.
t. sign
tibiarum
anxietas t.
tibioadductor reflex
TIB Test
tic
chronic t.
compulsive spasms and t.
convulsive t.
t. convulsive with coprolalia
t. de sommeil
diaphragmatic t.
t. douloureux
facial t.
glossopharyngeal t.
habit t.
local t.
maladie des t.
mimic t.
psychic t.
rotatory t.
ruling in t.
spasmodic t.
spasms and t.
t. symptom
tardive t.
TICA
traumatic intracranial aneurysm
tick-borne
t.-b. encephalitis (Central European subtype)
t.-b. encephalitis (Eastern subtype)
t.-b. meningopolyneuritis
tick paralysis
tic-like
tic-related obsessive-compulsive disorder
tidal volume (VT)
tidembersat
Tiedemann nerve
tier
Adson knot t.
Tigan
tight
t. brain
t. filum terminale syndrome
t. junctioned endothelium
tightener
Love-Adson wire t.
tigretier
tigroid
t. body
t. mass
t. substance
tigrolysis
TIL
tumor-infiltrating leukocyte
tumor-infiltrating lymphocyte
Tilcotil
tile plate facet replacement
tilt
head t.
head-down t. (HDT)
T. and Turn Paragon bed
tilted optimized nonsaturating excitation technique
tilting of visual image
tilt-table test
tiludronate
time
Achilles tendon reflex t.
acquisition t.
association t.
t. axis

NOTES

time *(continued)*
biologic t.
bleeding t.
central somatosensory conduction t.
cochlear response t.
conduction t.
t. constant
t. context
correlation t.
dilute Russell Viper Venom t. (DRVVT)
echo t. (TE)
effective half t. (Te)
image acquisition t.
inertia t.
interhemispheric propagation t.
interpulse t.
t. interval
inversion t.
kaolin clotting t.
long pulse repetition time/long echo t.
mass doubling t.
non-paretic eye valid reaction t.
partial thromboplastin t. (PTT)
phrenic nerve conduction t.
t. point
processing t.
prothrombin t. (PT)
proton relaxation t.
pulse repetition t.
pulse transit t.
reaction t.
recognition t.
relaxation t.
repetition t.
response processing t.
rise t.
Russell viper venom t.
scan t.
t. sense
sequence t.
serial reaction t. (SRT)
short pulse repetition time/echo t.
short pulse repetition time/short echo t.
spin-lattice relaxation t.
spin-spin relaxation t.
stimulation t.
stimulus-response t.
survival t.
total sleep t.
transcallosal conduction t. (TCT)
vigilance reaction t.
time-density curve
time-locked occipital rhythm
time-motion study
time-of-flight
t.-o.-f. angiography
t.-o.-f. effect
t.-o.-f. positron emission tomographic camera
t.-o.-f. technique
time-on-task effect
time-out
involuntary t.-o.
voluntary t.-o.
TiMesh
TiMesh hardware
TiMesh screw
TiMesh titanium bone plating system
Timespan
Mestinon T.
time-variance imaging (TVI)
timing
circadian t.
t. of decompression
Timofeew corpuscle
timolol maleate
TIMP
tissue inhibitor of metalloproteinase
TiMX low back system
Tindal
tin ear syndrome
Tinel sign
tingling with aura
tinnitus
objective pulsatile t.
pulsatile t.
tip
Adson brain suction t.
bipolar diathermy forceps t.
CUSA t.
Ferguson brain suction t.
forceps t.
Frazier suction t.
French t.
Japanese suction t.
multipore suction t.
t. of posterior horn
Rhoton suction t.
Sachs brain suction t.
slotted suction t.
volar t.
Tipramine
Tirilazad Efficacy Stroke Study (TESS)
Tisokinase native t-PA
Tisseel artificial dura
Tissucol
tissue
adipose t.
Antoni A, B t.
areolar t.

autologous adrenal medullary t.
brain t.
caudate t.
cingulate t.
connective t.
cortical t.
cryopreserved t.
t. culture
distensible t.
epivaginal connective t.
t. factor pathway inhibitor
fetal mesencephalic t.
t. fibrin sealant
t. forceps
gray matter t.
t. hyperperfusion
t. implant
t. inhibitor of metalloproteinase (TIMP)
insular cortex t.
Kuhnt intermediary t.
t. magnetic susceptibility artifact
mesencephalic t.
nervous t.
occipital cortex t.
parietal t.
partial oxygen pressure of brain t. ($PbrO_2$)
peripheral t.
pharyngeal t.
pial t.
t. plane dissector
t. plasminogen activator (TPA, t-PA)
postmortem brain t.
t. respiration
splenium t.
temporal t.
thalamus t.
t. transplantation
t. welding
white matter t.

tissue-based monoamine oxidase assay

Tissue-Guard bovine pericardial patch

tissue-type

t.-t. metabolic response
t.-t. PA

Tissuewax paraffin

titanium

t. alloy needle
t. aneurysm clip
t. cable
t. construct
t. hollow screw plate system
t. microconnector
t. micromesh
t. micro system
t. mini bur hole cover
t. mini bur hole covering
t. miniplate
t. plate
Sugita T.
t. wire
t. wound retractor

titer

complement fixation antibody t.

titillate

titillating

titillation

titubation

tizanidine hydrochloride

^{201}Tl

thallium-201
^{201}Tl chloride
^{201}Tl scintigraphy
^{201}Tl SPECT

TMB

transient monocular blindness

TMP

transmembrane potential

TMS

transcranial magnet stimulation

TN

trigeminal neuralgia

TNF

tumor necrosis factor

TNF-alpha

tumor necrosis factor-alpha

TNFR

tumor necrosis factor receptor

TNP-470

***TOAD-64* gene**

tobacco-alcohol amblyopia

tobacism

tobacosis

Tobey-Ayer test

tobramycin

tocopherol

alpha t.

TOCP neuropathy

NOTES

Todd
T. body
T. postepileptic paralysis
Todd-Wells
T.-W. apparatus
T.-W. stereotactic frame
T.-W. technique
toe
t. clonus
t. drop
t. phenomenon
t. reflex
t. sign
striatal t.
Toennis
T. dissecting scissors
T. dura dissector
T. dura knife
T. dural hook
T. ES standalone constant-current electrical stimulator
T. tumor forceps
Toennis-Adson dissector
toe-walking
Tofranil
Toft spinal correction treatment
togavirus infection
tolazamide
tolbutamide
tolcapone
tolfenamic acid
Tolinase
tolmetin
Tolosa-Hunt syndrome
tolterodine
toluidine blue-stained
tomaculous neuropathy
tomentum
Tomkins-Horn
tomogram
open-mouthed anteroposterior t.
tomograph
CTI-Siemens 933 t.
PC-2048B positron emission t.
Tomomatic 64 single photon emission computed t.
tomographic
vasodilator-stimulated rCBF single photon emission computed t.
tomography
automate computed axial t.
cerebrovascular computed t.
computed t. (CT)
computed axial t. (CAT)
computerized axial t.
cranial computed t.
dynamic single photon emission computed t.
emission computed t.
fluorodopa positron emission t.
head computed t.
infusion computed t.
magnetic resonance t. (MRT)
plain t.
positive emission t. (PET)
positron emission t. (PET)
preoperative t.
single photon emission computed t. (SPECT)
volumetric computed t.
xenon computed t.
xenon-enhanced computed t. (XeCT)
Tomomatic 64 single photon emission computed tomograph
Tomoscan
Philips T.
tomoxetine
tonaphasia
tone
airway muscle t.
dopaminergic t.
low EMG t.
muscle t.
resting t.
short-term vasomotor t.
upper airway muscular t.
vascular t.
viscerosomatic t.
tongs
Cherry traction t.
Cone skull traction t.
Crutchfield-Raney skull traction t.
Crutchfield skeletal traction t.
Crutchfield skull traction t.
Edmonton extension t.
Gardner-Wells t.
Mayfield t.
Reynolds skull traction t.
tongue
t. of cerebellum
chameleon t.
galloping t.
t. phenomenon
t. reduction surgery
t. retainer
septum of t.
t. thrusting
trombone tremor of t.
tongue-in-groove operation
tongue-locking device
tongue-retaining device

tonic
t. block
t. contraction
t. control
t. convulsion
t. drop attack
t. epilepsy
t. inhibitor control
t. phase
t. pupil
t. reflex
t. seizure
t. spasm
t. status epilepticus
tonically dilated pupil
tonic-clonic
t.-c. activity
generalized t.-c. (GTC)
t.-c. seizure
t.-c. status epilepticus
tonicoclonic
tonoclonic spasm
tonogenic
tonometry
tonotopic
tonotopocity
tonotopy
tonsil
cerebellar t.
t. of cerebellum
herniation of cerebellar t.'s
tonsilla, pl. **tonsillae**
t. cerebelli
tonsillar
t. herniation
t. nerve
t. plexus
tonus
myogenic t.
neurogenic t.
tool
Auto Segmentation software t.
communication t.
genetic t.
MMS-900 balancing t.
relationship t.
Tool-Proxy
tooth
t. atrophy
T. disease
top
t. of the basilar syndrome
circular laminar hook with offset t.
topagnosia
topagnosis
topalgia
Topamax
top-down
t.-d. organization of memory
t.-d. regulation
topectomy
top-entry
t.-e. (open body) hook
t.-e. (open body) hook torque
topesthesia
tophaceous gout
tophus
topical
t. clonidine
t. thrombin
topiramate monotherapy
topoanesthesia
topognosia
topognosis
topographical agnosia
topographic memory loss
topography
steady-state probe t. (SSPT)
topology
toponarcosis
toposcope
toposcopic catheter
topothermesthesiometer
toppling gait
Toradol
TORCH
toxoplasmosis, other infections, rubella, cytomegalovirus, and herpes simplex
TORCH syndrome
torch
saline t.
torcular
t. epidermoid
t. herophili
t. meningioma
Torg ratio
Toriello-Carey agnesis
Torkildsen
T. operation
T. shunt
T. ventriculocisternostomy

NOTES

torlone fixation pin
tornado epilepsy
Tornwaldt cyst
Torpedo electroplaque
torpidity mental torticollis
torpillage
torpor
torque
top-entry (open body) hook t.
unwanted screw t.
torque-pulse perturbation
Torré syndrome
Torric-Clount seizure
torsades
t. de pointes
t. de pointes arrhythmia
torsion
t. disease of childhood
t. dystonia
t. neurosis
t. spasm
torsional
t. abnormality
t. gripping strength
t. nystagmus
t. stiffness
torsionometer
Torsten Sjögren syndrome
torti
pili t.
torticollar
torticollis
benign paroxysmal t.
dermatogenic t.
dystonic t.
fixed t.
hysterical t.
intermittent t.
labyrinthine t.
neurogenic t.
ocular t.
paroxysmal t.
psychogenic t.
rheumatic t.
spasmodic t.
t. spastica
spurious t.
symptomatic t.
torpidity mental t.
tortipelvis
tortuosity
toruloma
TOS
thoracic outlet syndrome
tosylate
daledalin t.
total
t. agenesis
t. AIMS score
t. aphasia
t. body neutron activation analysis
t. emotional memory score
t. fractional regional brain volume
t. hypophysectomy
t. monocular blindness
t. neuroleptic dosage
t. parenteral nutrition (TPN)
t. pituitary ablation
t. scale
t. sleep time
t. symptom
t. symptom score
t. weighted sum score
totalis
alopecia capitis t.
ophthalmoplegia t.
rachischisis t.
toto
in t.
touch
t. cell
t. corpuscle
organ of t.
t. perception threshold (TPT)
t. receptor
touched
toucher
delire de t.
toucherism
Tourette
T. disease
Gilles de la T.
T. syndrome
T. Syndrome Association Unified Tic Rating Scale
tourniquet
Drake t.
t. ischemia
Tournoux
atlas of Talairach and T.
tower skull
toxemia
cerebropathia psychica t.
toxic
t. amblyopia
t. delirium
t. dementia
t. epidermal necrolysis (TEN)
t. exposure
t. headache
t. hepatitis
t. hydrocephalus
t. hypoxia

t. metabolite
t. neuritis
t. neuropathy
t. nystagmus
t. paraplegia
t. retinoneuropathy
t. shock syndrome
t. side effect
t. spasm
t. tetanus
t. vertigo

toxicity
acute neuronal t.
alcohol t.
aluminum t.
caffeine t.
central anticholinergic t.
dose-limiting t.
drug t.
epinephrine t.
glutamate t.
hexachlorophene t.
hydrazine t.
manganese t.
mercury t.
methyl alcohol t.
norepinephrine t.
propylene glycol t.
social t.
sympathomimetic t.

toxicophobia

toxicus
Gambierdiscus t.

toxin
bacterial t.
botulinum A t.
botulinum t. type A, B
botulism t.
endogenous benzodiazepine-like t.
manganese t.
mercury t.
metallic t.
methyl alcohol t.
shiga t.
uremic t.

toxin-induced sleep disorder

Toxocara canis

toxocariasis

toxoid
tetanus t.

Toxoplasma gondii

toxoplasmic
t. encephalitis (TE)
t. encephalomyelitis
t. meningoencephalitis

toxoplasmosis
acquired t.
AIDS-related t.
cerebral t.
congenital t.
intramedullary t.
t., other infections, rubella, cytomegalovirus, and herpes simplex (TORCH)
t., other infections, rubella, cytomegalovirus infection, herpes

TPA
temporal processing acuity
temporopolar artery
tissue plasminogen activator

t-PA
tissue plasminogen activator
Tisokinase native t.-P.

TPI test

TPJ
temporoparietal junction

T-plate

TPN
total parenteral nutrition

TPP
thyrotoxic periodic paralysis

TPT
touch perception threshold

trabecula, pl. **trabeculae**
arachnoid t.
nondecalcified t.

trabecular bone

trabecularis
substantia t.

trace
t. conditioned reflex
memory t.

tracer
flow t.
radioactive t.

trachea

tracheal injury

trachelagra

trachelism

trachelismus

trachelocyrtosis

trachelodynia

NOTES

trachelokyphosis
trachelology
tracheostomy
tracing
dipole t.
track
CD t.
tracker
T. Excel microcatheter
T. infusion catheter
Polaris position t.
Tracker-10 catheter
Tracker-18 catheter
tracking
eye t.
speech t.
Tracrium
tract
accessory nucleus of optic t.
anterior corticospinal t.
anterior pyramidal t.
anterior raphespinal t.
anterior spinocerebellar t.
anterior spinothalamic t.
anterior trigeminothalamic t.
anterolateral t.
Arnold t.
ascending t.
association t.
auditory t.
Bekhterev t.
Bruce t.
t. of Bruce and Muir
bulbar t.
bulboreticulospinal t.
bulbothalamic t.
Burdach t.
caerulospinal t.
central tegmental t.
cerebellorubral t.
cerebellorubrospinal t.
cerebellospinal t.
cerebellotegmental t.
cerebellothalamic t.
Collier t.
corticobulbar t.
corticohypothalamic t.
corticomesencephalic t.
corticopontine t.
corticorubral t.
corticospinal t.
crossed pyramidal t.
cuneocerebellar t.
deiterospinal t.
dentatothalamic t.
Dieters t.
direct pyramidal t.
dorsal column sensory t.
dorsal spinocerebellar t.
dorsal trigeminothalamic t.
dorsolateral t.
external corticotectal t.
extracorticospinal t.
fastigiobulbar t.
fastigiospinal t.
fiber sensory t.
Flechsig t.
frontopontine t.
frontotemporal t.
geniculocalcarine t.
geniculostriate t.
t. of Goll
Gowers t.
habenulointerpeduncular t.
habenulopeduncular t.
habenulothalamic t.
Helwig t.
Hoche t.
hypothalamohypophysial t.
hypothalamospinal t.
intermediolateral t.
internal corticotectal t.
interpositospinal t.
interstitiospinal t.
lateral corticospinal t.
lateral olfactory t.
lateral pyramidal t.
lateral raphespinal t.
lateral reticulospinal t.
lateral root of optic t.
lateral spinothalamic t.
lateral vestibulospinal t.
Lissauer t.
Loewenthal t.
mamillopeduncular t.
mamillotegmental t.
mamillothalamic t.
Marchi t.
medial reticulospinal t.
medial root of optic t.
medial vestibulospinal t.
medullary reticulospinal t.
medullary solitary t.
Meynert t.
Monakow t.
motor t.
t. of Münzer and Wiener
neospinothalmic t.
nerve t.
nigrostriatal t.
nigrostriate t.
nucleus of the lateral olfactory t.
nucleus of solitary t.
occipitocollicular t.

occipitopontile t.
occipitopontine t.
occipitotectal t.
olfactory t.
olivocerebellar t.
olivocochlear t.
olivospinal t.
optic t.
paraventriculohypophysial t.
parietopontine t.
pontoreticulospinal t.
posterior spinocerebellar t.
posterior trigeminothalamic t.
posterolateral t.
prepyramidal t.
pyramidal t.
reticulocerebellar t.
reticulospinal t.
rubrobulbar t.
rubropontine t.
rubroreticular t.
rubrospinal t.
Schultze comma t.
t. of Schütz
Schütz t.
semilunar t.
sensory t.
septomarginal t.
solitariospinal t.
solitary t.
spinal dermal sinus t.
spinocerebellar t.
spinocervical t.
spinocervicothalamic t.
spinoolivary t.
spinoolivocerebellar t.
spinoreticular t.
spinospinalis t.
spinotectal t.
spinothalamic t.
spinovestibular t.
spiral foraminous t.
Spitzka-Lissauer t.
Spitzka marginal t.
strionigral t.
sulcomarginal t.
supraopticohypophyseal t.
supraopticohypophysial t.
tectobulbar t.
tectocerebellar t.
tectopontine t.
tectospinal t.
tegmental t.
tegmentoreticular t.
tegmentospinal t.
temporofrontal t.
temporopontine t.
testobulbar t.
thalamoolivary t.
transverse peduncular t.
triangular t.
trigeminospinal t.
trigeminothalamic t.
tuberohypophysial t.
tuberoinfundibular t.
Türck t.
urinary t.
ventral raphespinal t.
ventral spinocerebellar t.
ventral spinothalamic t.
ventral trigeminothalamic t.
vestibulocerebellar t.
vestibulospinal t.
Vicq d'Azyr t.
Waldeyer t.

traction
Ace Trippi-Wells tong cervical t.
Ace universal tong cervical t.
t. anchor
axial t.
bipolar vertebral t.
Bremer halo crown t.
Crile head t.
device for transverse t. (DTT)
t. neuritis
t. response of infant
t. spur
transverse t.

tractotomy
anterolateral t.
bulbar cephalic pain t.
intramedullary t.
medullary t.
mesencephalic t.
pontine t.
pyramidal t.
Schwartz t.
Sjöqvist t.
spinal t.
spinothalamic t.
stereotactic t.
stereotactic subcaudate t. (SST)

NOTES

tractotomy *(continued)*
subcaudate t.
trigeminal t.
Walker t.
tractus
t. anterolaterales
t. bulboreticulospinalis
t. caeruleospinalis
t. centralis tegmenti
t. cerebellorubralis
t. cerebellothalamicus
t. corticobulbaris
t. corticopontini
t. corticospinalis
t. corticospinalis anterior
t. corticospinalis lateralis
t. corticospinalis ventralis
t. descendens nervi trigemini
t. dorsolateralis
t. fastigiobulbaris
t. fastigiospinalis
t. frontopontinus
t. habenulointerpeduncularis
t. habenulopeduncularis
t. hypothalamohypophysialis
t. interpositospinalis
t. interstitiospinalis
t. mesencephalicus nervi trigemini
t. occipitopontinus
t. olfactorius
t. olivocerebellaris
t. olivocochlearis
t. opticus
t. paraventriculohypophysialis
t. parietopontinus
t. pontoreticulospinalis
t. posterolateralis
t. pyramidalis
t. pyramidalis anterior
t. pyramidalis lateralis
t. pyramidalis ventralis
t. raphespinalis anterior
t. raphespinalis lateralis
t. reticulospinalis
t. reticulospinalis anterior
t. reticulospinalis ventralis
t. retrobulbaris
t. rubrobulbaris
t. rubropontinus
t. rubrospinalis
t. solitariospinalis
t. solitarius
t. solitarius medullae oblongatae
t. spinalis nervi trigeminalis
t. spinalis nervi trigemini
t. spinocerebellaris anterior
t. spinocerebellaris dorsalis
t. spinocerebellaris posterior
t. spinocerebellaris ventralis
t. spinocervicalis
t. spinoolivaris
t. spinoreticularis
t. spinotectalis
t. spinothalamicus
t. spinothalamicus anterior
t. spinothalamicus lateralis
t. spinothalamicus ventralis
t. spinovestibularis
t. spiralis foraminosus
t. spiralis foraminulosus
t. supraopticohypophysialis
t. tectobulbaris
t. tectopontinus
t. tectospinalis
t. tegmentalis centralis
t. temporopontinus
t. trigeminospinalis
t. trigeminothalamicus
t. trigeminothalamicus anterior
t. trigeminothalamicus posterior
t. tuberoinfundibularis
t. vestibulospinalis
t. vestibulospinalis lateralis
t. vestibulospinalis medialis
traditional
t. circulatory criteria (TCC)
t. limbic circuit
t. neuroleptic
t. neuroleptic agent
tragus
ipsilateral t.
trailing
train
orphan t.
t. of spike
trained reflex
training
American Association of Directors of Psychiatric Residency T. (AADPRT)
anxiety control t.
biologic t.
body weight-supported treadmill t.
habit reversal t.
speed-dependent treadmill t. (STT)
tactile-kinesthetic t.
train-of-four stimulus
trait
abnormal t.
t. characteristic
cluster B t.
dependence t.
egosyntonic t.
ergic t.

identified t.
impulsive-aggressive t.
premorbid personality t.
psychopathic t.
sickle cell t.
spike-and-wave t.
trait-level region abnormalities
traitor
trajectory
behavioral t.
cognitive t.
emotional t.
operative t.
tramadol
tram track sign
trancelike state
tranexamic acid
transaminase
alanine t.
GABA t.
gamma aminobutyric acid t. (GABA-T)
glutamyl t.
serum glutamic oxaloacetic t.
serum glutamic-pyruvic t.
serum glutamyl t.
transantral
t. ethmoidal approach
t. ethmoidal orbital decompression
transarterial platinum coil embolization
transarticular
t. screw
t. screw fixation
transaxonal ephaptic transmission
transbasal
transcallosal
t. band (TCB)
t. conduction delay
t. conduction time (TCT)
t. interforniceal corridor
t. interforniceal-transforaminal microsurgical approach
t. interhemispheric
t. transforaminal approach
transcalvarial
transcapsular gray bridge
transcarbamoylase
ornithine t.
transcarbamylase
ornithine t.
transcardiac perfusion
transcatheter obliteration
transcavernous transpetrous apex approach
Transcend
T. microguidewire
T. 14 wire
transcendentalism
transcerebellar
t. diameter
t. hemispheric approach
transcervical
transchoroidal approach
transcochlear approach
transcortical
t. aphasia
t. apraxia
t. incision
t. technique
t. transventricular approach
transcranial
t. B-mode ultrasound
t. color-coded duplex sonography
t. color-coded real-time sonography
t. Doppler (TCD)
t. Doppler B mode
t. Doppler ultrasonography
t. frontofacial advancement
t. frontotemporoorbital approach
t. high-frequency repetitive electrical stimulation
t. magnetic stimulation
t. magnet stimulation (TMS)
t. motor evoked potential (TeMEP)
t. orbital exploration
t. real-time color Doppler imaging
t. resection
t. skull-base endoscopy
transcription
broad phonemic t.
t. factor
transcubital approach
transcutaneous
t. carbon dioxide monitoring
t. electrical nerve stimulation
t. nerve stimulation
t. oxygen monitoring
transcytosis
blood-brain t.
bulk flow t.
transdermal
Duragesic T.

NOTES

transdermal *(continued)*
t. methylphenidate system
t. patch
transdiaphragmatic pressure
transdominance
transducer
bur hole t.
t. cell
Combitrans t.
Drager MTC t.
force t.
intrasinus t.
neuro convex t.
neuroendocrine t.
piezoresistive t.
Transpac IV pressure t.
transducer-measured intracranial venous pressure
transducer-tipped catheter
transduction
chemical-mechanical t.
pain t.
phospholipid-related signal t.
sensory t.
signal t.
transdural
transection
fiber tract t.
t. hook
multiple subpial t. (MST)
subpial t.
transendothelial migration
transentorhinal region
transethmoidal encephalocele
transethmosphenoidal hypophysectomy
transfacial transclival approach
transfectant
transfected fibroblast
transfemoral
t. artery technique
t. catheter
transfer
t. deficit
t. direct current stimulation
immunostimulatory gene t.
interdigital t.
linear energy t. (LET)
saturation t.
vector-mediated gene t.
virus-mediated gene t.
transferase
chloramphenicol acetyl t. (CAT)
uridine glucuronyl t.
transferase-mediated dUTP-digoxigenin nick end-labeling (TUNEL)
transference
idealizing t.
self-object t.
twinship t.
transferred
t. sensation
transferrin
anti-human t.
carbohydrate-deficient t.
transfix
transfontanel Doppler ultrasound
transforaminal herniation
transform
fast Fournier t. (FFT)
Fourier t.
I-o t.'s
isotropic three-dimensional Fourier t.
multidimensional Fourier t.
three-dimensional Fourier t. (3DFT)
two-dimensional Fourier t. (2DFT)
transformation
hemorrhagic t. (HT)
Z score t.
transformational
transforming
t. growth factor (TGF)
t. growth factor beta
transfrontal
t. approach
transfrontonasoorbital approach
transfusion
albumin t.
autologous blood t.
fetal t.
transgender
transgene
nonselective expression of t.
transgenic
transgress
transient
alpha t.
t. brain stem ischemia
t. cognitive impairment (TCI)
t. disorder
t. dystonia
t. emotional disturbance
t. emotional stress
t. facial paresthesia
t. flaccid paralysis
t. focal neurologic event (TFNE)
t. global amnesia (TGA)
t. hemiparesis
t. hemisphere attack
t. ischemic attack (TIA)
t. leukopenia
t. monocular blindness (TMB)
t. monocular visual loss
t. neonatal myasthenia gravis

t. nystagmus
t. plexus injury
positive occipital sharp t.
t. signal abnormality
t. tic disorder of childhood
t. visual phenomenon
t. voltage
transillumination
t. microscopy
skull t.
transinsular
transisthmian
transitional
t. convolution
t. gyrus
t. meningioma
t. vertebra
transitive
t. inference task
t. limb movement
transitivism
transitivity
transketolase
translabyrinthine
t. and suboccipital approach
t. transotic approach
translation
coronal plane deformity sagittal t.
translational
t. fracture
t. position
translocation
robertsonian chromosome t.
transmandibular glossopharyngeal approach
transmantle pressure gradient
transmaxillosphenoidal approach
transmembrane
t. ionic shift
t. potential (TMP)
t. spanning
transmissible
t. neurodegenerative disease
t. spongiform viral encephalopathy
transmission
autosomal dominant t.
cholinergic t.
depolarization-dependent synaptic t.
diffusion t.
duplex t.
t. dysequilibrium test
ephaptic t.
extrastriatal dopamine t.
familial t.
fetal AIDS t.
GABA-mediated inhibitory synaptic t.
genetic t.
glutamate-mediated excitatory synaptic t.
glutamatergic synaptic t.
impaired neuromuscular t.
indirect genetic t.
neurochemical t.
neurohumoral t.
neuromuscular junction t.
nonsynaptic t.
transaxonal ephaptic t.
volume t.
transmitter
endogenous t.
inhibitory t.
radiofrequency t.
t. substance
t. system
transmitter-gated ion channel
transnasal
t. approach
t. biopsy
t. septal displacement procedure
transnasoorbital approach
transneuronal
t. atrophy
t. degeneration
Transonics flow probe
transopercular hemispherotomy
transoral
t. approach
t. odontoid resection
transorbital
t. leukotomy
t. lobotomy
transosseous venography
Transpac IV pressure transducer
transpalatal approach
transparent
t. septum
transpedicular
t. approach
t. fixation effective pedicle diameter
t. fixation system design

NOTES

transpedicular *(continued)*
t. screw
t. screw-rod fixation
t. spinal instrumentation
transpeptidase
gamma glutamyl t.
transperitoneal approach
transpetrosal approach
transphenoidal cryohypophysectomy
transplant
adrenal body t.
carotid body t.
chromaffin cell t.
fetal neural t.
fetal tissue t.
mesencephalic t.
transplantation
adrenal medulla t.
autologous hematopoietic stem cell t. (AHSCT)
bone marrow t.
brain t.
core assessment program for intracerebral t. (CAPIT)
fetal cell t.
intracranial-extracranial t.
liver t.
neural t.
organ t.
porcine cell t.
stem cell t.
tissue t.
transport
anterograde axonal t.
axonal t.
axoplasmic t.
defective glucose t.
fast axonal t.
glucose t.
retrograde t.
slow axonal t.
solute t.
substrate t.
transporter
amino acid t.
dopamine t. (DAT)
drug t.
glutamate t.
neurotransmitter t.
plasma membrane dopamine t.
transposition
Müller-König t.
seventh cranial nerve t.
vertebral artery t.
transradial cerebral angiography
transsinus approach
transsphenoidal
t. approach
t. bipolar forceps
t. chiasmapexy
t. complication
t. curette
t. encephalocele
t. evacuation
t. hook
t. hypophysectomy
t. meningoencephalocele
t. removal
t. selective adenomectomy
t. speculum
t. surgery
transsternal
transsylvian
t. approach
t. keyhole
t. transsulcal technique
transsynaptic
t. chromatolysis
t. degeneration
transtemporal
t. approach
t. fissure
transtentorial
t. approach
occipital t.
t. uncal herniation
transthalamic
transthoracic
t. approach
t. discectomy
t. vertebral body resection
transthyretin (TTR)
t. protein
transthyretin-associated neuropathic amyloidosis
transtorcular
t. approach
t. embolization
t. occlusion
transuncodiscal approach
transvenous
t. approach
t. therapy
transventricular approach
transversa
crista t.
transversae
fibrae pontis t.
transversalis
crista t.
transverse
t. atlantal ligament
t. bipolar montage

t. cerebral fissure
t. connector
t. cord lesion
t. crest
t. diffusivity
t. fasciculus
t. fiber of pons
t. fissure of cerebellum
t. fissure of cerebrum
t. fixation
t. fixator application
t. fornix
t. gradient coil
t. incision
t. magnetization
t. magnetization phase
t. myelitis
t. myelopathy
t. nerve of the neck
t. occipital sulcus
t. orientation
t. pedicle angle
t. pedicle diameter
t. peduncular tract
t. pontine fiber
t. relaxation
t. relaxation rate
t. rhombencephalic flexure
t. ridge
t. septum
t. sinus (TS)
t. sinus of dura mater
t. sinus occlusion
t. striae of corpus callosum
t. temporal convolution
t. temporal gyri of Heschl
t. temporal gyrus
t. temporal sulcus
t. traction
t. tripolar epidural array
t. velum

transversectomy

transversi
fasciculi t.
gyri temporales t.
sulci temporales t.

transversospinalis muscle group

transversum
velum t.

transversus
sulcus occipitalis t.
sulcus temporalis t.

transvestism

transzygomatic approach

Tranxene

tranylcypromine sulfate

trap-door type flap

trapezius muscle

trapezoid body

trapezoidei
nucleus anterior corporis t.
nucleus dorsalis corporis t.
nucleus lateralis corporis t.
nucleus medialis corporis t.
nucleus ventralis corporis t.

trapezoideum
corpus t.

trapped ventricle syndrome

trapping
aneurysm t.
t. of aneurysm

Traquair
junctional scotoma of T.

Trasylol

Traube-Hering-Mayer
T.-H.-M. wave
T.-H.-M. waves in cerebrospinal fluid

trauma
abdominal t.
acceleration-deceleration forces in craniocerebral t.
amnesia for t.
cervical spine t.
t. characteristic
circumflex nerve t.
t. coma databank (TCDB)
compression-rarefaction strain in craniocerebral t.
cranial nerve t.
t. craniocerebral
craniocerebral drug t.
t. cue
disaster t.
exposure to t.
facial nerve perinatal t.
head t.
intensity of t.
intestinal t.
long-term effects of t.

NOTES

trauma *(continued)*
lumbar spine t.
maxillofacial t.
median nerve t.
nonpenetrating t.
penetrating t.
perinatal craniocerebral t.
peripheral nerve t.
premorbid t.
psychological t.
radial nerve t.
sciatic nerve t.
t. spectrum disorder
spinal cord injury t.
t. survivor
thoracolumbar t.
ulnar nerve t.
vertebral artery t.

TraumaCal

trauma-induced fistula

traumasthenia

traumata

traumatic
t. amnesia
t. anastomosis
t. brachial plexus disorder
t. brain injury (TBI)
t. cervical discopathy
t. cervical disk herniation
T. Coma Data Bank
t. degeneration
t. displacement
t. headache
t. hematoma
t. intracranial aneurysm (TICA)
t. meningeal hemorrhage
t. meningocele
t. myelopathy
t. neurasthenia
t. neuritis
t. neuroma
t. neuropathy
t. neurosis
t. progressive encephalopathy
t. pseudomeningocele
t. spondylolisthesis
t. subarachnoid hemorrhage (TSAH)
t. syringomyelia
t. tetanus

traumatica
cephalhydrocele t.
malacia t.

Traum-Ex

Trautmann triangle

Travasorb

traversal
tentorial t.

traversing segment

traxoprodil mesylate

trazodone

TRE
target registration error

Treacher Collins syndrome

treatment
bacterial meningitis t.
t. completion rate
t. compliance
compression rod t.
t. condition
conventional neuroleptic t.
distraction/compression scoliosis t.
dopaminergic t.
D-penicillamine t.
dual compression scoliosis t.
dystonia t.
t. effectiveness
ethanol t.
fluoxetine t.
gamma-interferon t.
t. gap
Hartel t.
hepatic encephalopathy t.
hypervolemic t.
immunoglobulin t.
insulin coma t.
insulin shock t.
t. intensity-by-time interaction
t. intensity parameter
intravenous immunoglobulin t.
lithium t.
massage t.
Matas t.
microoperative t.
t. model
neuromuscular scoliosis orthotic t.
ongoing neuroleptic t.
t. outcome
t. period
t. phase
phenylketonuria t.
poliomyelitis t.
t. program
t. protocol
t. regimen
t. resistant
t. response rate
Schlösser t.
Screening Test for the Assignment of Remedial T.'s
short-term t.
spinal deformity t.
stereotactic radiation therapy t.
stimulant t.
t. strategy

suboptimal t.
Toft spinal correction t.
tuberculosis meningitis t.
treatment-emergent
t.-e. akathisia
t.-e. asthenia
t.-e. extrapyramidal side effect
t.-e. hypertonia
t.-e. hypomania
t.-e. somnolence
treatment-intolerant patient
tree
dendritic t.
maidenhair t.
neurovascular t.
trefoil tendon deformation
Trélate-Charlin neuralgia
trematode infection
tremblant
delire t.
trembling
hereditary chin t.
t. palsy
tremens
alcoholic delirium t.
delirium t. (DT)
tremogram
tremograph
tremor
action t.
alcoholic withdrawal t.
alternating t.
alternative t.
anticonvulsant medication-induced postural t.
arsenical t.
t. artuum
benign familial essential t.
cerebellar t.
cerebral t.
T. Clinical Rating Scale
coarse t.
continuous t.
drug-induced t.
drug/toxin-induced t.
dystonic t.
enhanced physiologic t.
essential palatal t.
familial cortical t.
fibrillary t.
fine t.
flapping t.
hereditary essential t.
heredofamilial t.
Holmes t.
hysterical t.
intention t.
isometric t.
kinetic t.
t. lingua
mercurial t.
metallic t.
methylxanthine-induced postural t.
t. opiophagorum
orthostatic t.
parkinsonism t.
passive t.
t. pathophysiology
persistent t.
physiologic t.
pill-rolling t.
position-specific t.
postural t.
t. potatorum
primary orthostatic t.
progressive cerebellar t.
psychogenic t.
rest t.
resting t.
rubral t.
saturnine t.
senile t.
static t.
striatocerebellar t.
striocerebellar t.
sustention/intention t.
symptomatic palatal t.
tardive t.
task-specific t.
t. tendinum
volitional t.
wing-beating t.
tremorgram
tremulous
trench lung
Trendar
Trendelenburg
T. gait
T. position
T. sign
T. symptom

NOTES

trending
evoked potential t.
trepan
trepanation
trephination
cranial vault t.
trephine
t. craniotomy
D'Errico skull t.
DeVilbiss skull t.
Galt skull t.
Michele vertebral body t.
Scoville skull t.
trephined
syndrome of the t.
Treponema
T. denticola
T. pallidum
T. pallidum immobilization
T. pallidum immobilization test
Trevor disease
Trexan
TRH
thyrotropin-releasing hormone
triad
Charcot t.
Jacod t.
Luciani t.
narcoleptic t.
trial
clinical t.
controlled medication t.
double-blind placebo t.
European Carotid Surgery T. (ECST)
head-to-head clinical t.
lower hook t.
North American Symptomatic Carotid Endarterectomy T. (NASCET)
open-label t.
placebo-controlled t.
randomized clinical t.
randomized controlled t.
tumor sensitizer t.
upper hook t.
VA Symptomatic T.
t. visit
Trialodine
triamterene
hydrochlorothiazide and t.
triangle
t. of fillet
Glasscock t.
Gombault t.
Gombault-Philippe t.
Guillain-Mollaret t.
hypoglossal t.
interscalene t.
Kawase t.
Mullan t.
opticocarotid t.
paramedian t.
Parkinson t.
Philippe t.
Reil t.
Trautmann t.
Wernicke t.
triangular
t. base transverse bar configuration
t. crest
t. lamella
t. nucleus
t. nucleus of septum
t. part
t. recess
t. ridge
t. septal nucleus
t. syndrome
t. tract
triangulare
velum t.
triangularis
crista t.
nucleus t.
pars t.
recessus t.
triangulated pedicle screw
Triavil
triazolam
triazolobenzodiazepine
tribasilar synostosis
tricarboxylic acid (TCA)
triceps
t. surae jerk
t. surae reflex
trichalgia
trichesthesia
trichilemmoma
trichinellosis
trichinosis
trichlormethiazide
trichloromonofluoromethane
dichlorodifluoromethane and t.
trichodynia
trichoepithelioma
trichoesthesia
trichoesthesiometer
trichofolliculoma
trichorrhexis nodosa
trichosis sensitiva
Trichosporon beigelii

trichrome
Gomori t.
t. stain
tricorn
tricortical iliac crest bone graft
tricresyl phosphate peripheral neuropathy
tric scriptorius
tricyclic
t. dibenzodiazepine derivative
t. drug
t. effect
Tridione
triethanolamine salicylate
triethiodide
gallamine t.
triethylene tetramine dihydrochloride
trifacial
t. nerve
t. neuralgia
trifluoperazine hydrochloride
trifluopromazine
trifluorinated
triflupromazine
trifocal neuralgia
trifurcation of middle cerebral artery
trigeminal
t. branch
t. cave
t. cavity
t. cistern
t. cough
t. cranial nerve
t. crest
t. decompression
t. dermatome
t. electrode
t. eminence
t. evoked potential (TEP)
t. ganglion
t. hypesthesia
t. impression of temporal bone
t. lemniscus
t. mesencephalic nucleus
t. motor dysfunction
t. motor nucleus
t. nerve [CN V]
t. nerve neurinoma
t. neuralgia (TN)
t. neurolysis
t. neuroma
t. neuropathy
t. nucleus caudalis lesioning
t. paralysis
t. rhizotomy
t. root
t. root section
t. schwannoma
t. stimulation
t. tractotomy
t. tubercle
trigeminale
cavum t.
ganglion t.
tuberculum t.
trigeminalis
cavitas t.
lemniscus t.
nervus t.
nuclei nervi t.
nucleus inferior nervi t.
nucleus mesencephalicus t.
nucleus motorius t.
nucleus pontinus nervi t.
nucleus sensorius inferior nervi t.
nucleus tractus mesencephalici nervi t.
tractus spinalis nervi t.
trigemini
nuclei nervi t.
nucleus mesencephalicus nervi t.
nucleus motorius nervi t.
nucleus principalis nervi t.
nucleus sensorius principalis nervi t.
nucleus sensorius superior nervi t.
nucleus spinalis nervi t.
nucleus tractus mesencephali nervi t.
nucleus tractus spinalis nervi t.
radices nervi t.
radix sensoria nervi t.
tractus descendens nervi t.
tractus mesencephalicus nervi t.
tractus spinalis nervi t.
trigeminocerebellar artery
trigeminofacial reflex
trigeminospinalis
tractus t.
trigeminospinal tract

NOTES

T

trigeminothalamic
t. fiber
t. tract
trigeminothalamicus
tractus t.
trigeminovascular pathway
trigeminus
descending nucleus of the t.
main sensory nucleus of the t.
mesencephalic nucleus of the t.
motor nucleus of t.
principal sensory nucleus of the t.
spinal nucleus of the t.
Trigesic
trigger
t. area
t. finger
t. point
t. point neuralgia
seizure t.
t. zone
triggered EMG
TriggerWheel Wand
trigona (*pl. of* trigonum)
trigone
t. of auditory nerve
cerebral t.
collateral t.
t. of fillet
t. of habenula
habenular t.
hypoglossal t.
t. of hypoglossal nerve
interpeduncular t.
t. of lateral lemniscus
lateral lemniscus t.
t. of lateral ventricle
lemniscal t.
Müller t.
oculomotor t.
olfactory t.
pontocerebellar t.
Reil t.
vagal (nerve) t.
t. of vagus nerve
ventricular t.
trigonocephaly
trigonum, pl. **trigona**
t. cerebrale
t. collaterale
t. collaterale ventriculi lateralis
t. habenula
t. hypoglossale
t. lemnisci lateralis
t. lemniscus
t. nervi acustici
t. nervi hypoglossi
t. nervi vagi
t. olfactorium
t. pontocerebellare
t. vagale
t. vagi
t. ventriculi
trihexoside
ceramide t.
trihexosyl ceramide
trihexyphenidyl
t. hydrochloride
triiodobenzoic acid
3,5,3′-triiodothyronine (T_3)
Trilafon
trilaminar myopathy
Trilizad
trill
vocal t.
trimeric form
trimethadione
trimethaphan
trimethobenzamide hydrochloride
trimipramine maleate
Trimstat
trinitrate
glyceryl t.
trinucleotide
t. repeat
t. repeat expansion
triorthocresyl phosphate neuropathy (TOCP neuropathy)
triosephosphate isomerase deficiency
Triosil
tripa ida
tripelennamine
triphasic
t. slow wave activity
t. wave
2,3,5-triphenyltetrazolium chloride (TTC)
triphosphatase
adenosine t. (ATPase)
triphosphate
adenosine t.
deoxynucleside t.
guanosine t. (GTP)
inositol t.
1,4,5-triphosphate
inositol t. (IP_3)
5′-triphosphate
adenosine 5′-t. (ATP)
triple
T. A syndrome gene (AAAS)
t. discharge
t. phase bone scan
t. repeat disorder
triplegia
Triple-H therapy

triple-wire technique
tripoding
tripolar nerve cuff electrode
tripole
guarded t.
narrow t.
triptan rebound headache
Triptil
TripTone Caplets
trismic
trismoid
trismus
t. capistratus
t. dolorificus
t. nascentium
t. neonatorum
t. sardonicus
trisomy
t. C, D syndrome
t. 9 mosaic syndrome
t. 8, 13, 20, 21 syndrome
trisulfapyramidine
triton
T. reciprocating saw
t. tumor
triventricular hydrocephalus
Trivittatus virus
Trk receptor
tRNA
alanine t.
trocar
brain t.
Frazier brain t.
McCain TMJ t.
Paulus t.
pyramidal t.
trochanter reflex
trochlear
t. cranial nerve
t. nerve [CN IV]
t. nerve neoplasm
t. nerve palsy
t. nerve paralysis
t. nerve paresis
t. nucleus
trochlearis
decussatio t.
decussatio nervorum t.
nervus t. [CN IV]
nucleus nervi t.
trochlearium
decussatio fibrarum nervorum t.
Trofan
Trofan-DS
troilism paraphilia
Trolard
vein of T.
T. vein
trombone tremor of tongue
tromethamine
ketorolac t.
Trömner
T. percussion hammer
T. reflex
trophesic
trophesy
trophic
t. change
t. gangrene
trophicity
trophism
trophodermatoneurosis
trophoneurosis
facial t.
lingual t.
muscular t.
Romberg t.
trophoneurotic
t. atrophy
t. leprosy
t. ulcer
trophotropic
t. zone of Hess
tropia
tropical
t. ataxic neuropathy (TAN)
t. myeloneuropathy
t. spastic paraparesis
t. spastic paraparesis/HTLV-I associated myelopathy
t. spastic paraplegia
tropicamide
troponin-tropomyosin complex
trouble thinking
troubling
trough
synaptic t.
trounce
Trousseau
T. phenomenon
T. point

NOTES

Trousseau *(continued)*
T. sign
T. spot
T. syndrome
T. twitching
trovato
truce
truculence
Tru-Cut needle biopsy
true
t. anosmia
t. aphasia
t. component
t. difference
t. dual pathology
t. neurogenic thoracic outlet syndrome
t. neuroma
t. nystagmus
trumpet
truncal
t. apraxia-ataxia
t. ataxia
t. dysmetria
t. vagotomy
truncation artifact
trunci plexus brachialis
truncus
t. arteriosus
t. corporis callosi
t. encephali
t. encephalicus
t. inferior plexus brachialis
t. lumbosacralis
t. medius plexus brachialis
t. nervi accessorii
t. nervi spinalis
t. superior plexus brachialis
t. sympatheticus
t. sympathicus
t. vagalis anterior
t. vagalis posterior
trunk
accessory nerve t.
anterior vagal t.
t. ataxia
communicating branch of sympathetic t.
t. of corpus callosum
encephalic t.
extra point on the back of the t. (Ex-B)
ganglia of sympathetic t.
ganglion of sympathetic t.
lumbosacral t.
meningohypophyseal t.
posterior vagal t.
sympathetic t.
trunnion-guided radiosurgery
Trypanosoma
T. brucei
T. cruzi
trypanosome fever
trypanosomiasis
acute t.
African t.
chronic t.
Cruz t.
East African t.
Gambian t.
Rhodesian t.
West African t.
tryptamine
tryptizol hydrochloride
tryptophan
t. hydroxylase
t. hydroxylase allelic genotype
TS
transverse sinus
TS system
TSAH
traumatic subarachnoid hemorrhage
***TSC1* gene**
***TSC2* gene**
TSH
thyroid-stimulating hormone
T-shaped
T.-s. Edwards-Barbaro syringeal shunt
T.-s. Edwards-Barbaro syringeal shunt table
T.-s. incision
TSRH
Texas Scottish Rite Hospital
T. buttressed laminar hook
T. circular laminar hook
T. crosslink stabilization
T. double-rod construct
Galveston fixation with T.
T. implant
T. instrumentation
T. pedicle hook
T. pedicle screw-laminar claw construct
T. plate
T. rod fixation
T. universal spinal instrumentation system
Tsuji laminaplasty
0.5-T superconducting magnet
tsutsugamushi
Rochalimaea t.

TTC
2,3,5-triphenyltetrazolium chloride
***t* test**
TTR
transthyretin
T-tube shunt
TTX
tetrodotoxin
T-type calcium channel
tube
Adson brain suction t.
air t.
alar lamina of neural t.
alar plate of neural t.
basal lamina of neural t.
basal plate of neural t.
blunt suction t.
Cone suction t.
Dandy suction t.
dorsal plate of neural t.
endoneural t.
endothelin-1 platinum-Dacron microcoil endotracheal t.
endotracheal t.
Ferguson brain suction t.
flow regulated suction t.
Frazier suction t.
Hardy suction t.
malleable multipore suction t.
medullary t.
microbore Tygon t.
nasogastric t.
neural t.
Nishizaki-Wakabayashi suction t.
Rhoton-Merz suction t.
Sachs brain suction t.
Sapporo shunt t.
Silastic t.
Spetzler Microvac suction t.
suction t.
tympanostomy t.
Univent endotracheal t.
ventral plate of neural t.
Yankauer suction t.
Yasargil suction t.
tuber, pl. **tubera**
t. anterius
ashen t.
t. cinereum
t. corporis callosi
cortical t.
t. dorsale
frontal t.
gray t.
subependymal t.
t. valvulae
t. of vermis
t. vermis
tuberales
nuclei t.
tuberalis
pars t.
tuberal nucleus
tubercle
acoustic t.
amygdaloid t.
anterior thalamic t.
ashen t.
auditory t.
Babès t.
t. bacillus
Chassaignac t.
cuneate t.
t. of cuneate nucleus
gracile t.
gray t.
intercolumnar t.
Morgagni t.
nucleus cuneatus t.
nucleus gracilis t.
t. of nucleus gracilis
olfactory t.
pharyngeal t.
posterior thalamic t.
rabic t.
Rolando t.
t. of saddle
trigeminal t.
wedge-shaped t.
tubercula (*pl. of* tuberculum)
tubercular meningitis
tuberculoma
t. en plaque
intracranial t.
tuberculosis
calvarial t.
cerebral t.
t. meningitis
t. meningitis treatment
miliary pulmonary t.
Mycobacterium t.
t. peripheral neuropathy

NOTES

tuberculosis *(continued)*
pulmonary t.
spinal t.
spine t.
tuberculous
t. abscess
t. antigen
t. focus
t. meningitis
t. spondylitis
tuberculum, pl. **tubercula**
t. anterius thalami
t. cinereum
t. cuneatum
t. gracile
t. hypoglossi
t. nuclei cuneati
t. nuclei gracilis
t. olfactorium
t. sella
t. sellae meningioma
t. sellae turcicae
t. sella meningioma
t. trigeminale
tuberin
tuberofundibular
tuberohypophysial tract
tuberoinfundibular
t. pathway
t. tract
tuberoinfundibularis
tractus t.
tuberomammillaris
nucleus t.
tuberomammillary nucleus
tuberosa
urticaria t.
tuberothalamic infarction
tuberous
t. sclerosis
t. sclerosis monster cell
t. sclerosis railroad track appearance
t. sclerosis syndrome
Tubex gauze dressing
tubing
Intramedic PE-50 polyethylene t.
tubular
t. aggregate myopathy
t. necrosis
tubulin assembly
tubulization
tubus medullaris
tuck position
Tuffier
T. laminectomy retractor
T. rib spreader
Tuffier-Raney retractor
tuft
dendritic t.
tufted cell
Tukey test
tulip pedicle screw
tumarcin crisis
tumefaction
tumescent
tumeur perlée
tumor
acidophilic pituitary t.
acoustic nerve sheath t.
ACTH-secreting t.
ACTH-secreting pituitary t.
adrenocorticotrophic hormone-secreting pituitary tumor
adenomatoid odontogenic t.
adhesio interthalamica t.
adrenocorticotrophic hormone-secreting pituitary t. (ACTH-secreting pituitary tumor)
adult granulosa cell t. (AGCT)
aggressive papillary middle ear t.
angioglomoid t.
anterior cingulate gyrus t.
aortic body t.
astrocytic t.
atypical giant cell t.
atypical teratoid/rhabdoid t. (AT/RT)
basiocciput t.
basophilic pituitary t.
t. bed
benign cranial nerve t.
benign lymphoepithelial parotid t.
bone t.
brain t.
brainstem t.
t. bulk
carotid body t.
cartilaginous t.
cavernous sinus t.
central nervous system t.
cerebellar t.
cerebellopontine angle t.
cervical intramedullary t.
cervicomedullary t.
chemoreceptor t.
chiasmatic t.
childhood primitive neuroectodermal t.
chondromatous t.
chromaffin t.
Collins law of survival after brain t.
collision t.

congenital t.
convexity metastatic t.
craniopharyngeal duct t.
Cushing triad in brain t.
dermoid t.
t. differentiating agent
diffuse fibrillary astrocytic t.
diffuse intrinsic brainstem t.
dumbbell t.
dysembryoplastic neuroepithelial t.
eighth nerve t.
endodermal sinus t.
enhancing exophytic t.
t. enucleation
ependymal t.
epidermoid t.
epidural t.
Erdheim t.
t. extension
t. extirpation
extradural t.
extrameatal intracapsular t.
extramedullary spinal cord t.
frontal lobe t.
germ cell t.
giant cell t.
giant glomus t.
giant pituitary t.
glial t.
glomus jugulare t.
glomus vagale t.
granular cell t.
growth-hormone-secreting t.
hour-glass t.
inclusion t.
infiltrating t.
infratemporal fossa t.
infratentorial-Lindau t.
infratentorial neurological t.
interdural t.
intracavernous t.
intracranial t.
intradural t.
intramedullary spinal cord t.
intraorbital granular cell t.
intrasellar growth-hormone-secreting pituitary t.
intraventricular t.
intrinsic brainstem t.
invasive t.
Kernohan classification of brain t.
Koenen t.
leptomeningeal t.
Lindau t.
lumbar t.
lymphoepithelial parotid t.
lymphomatous t.
malignant germ cell t.
margaroid t.
t. marker
McLain-Weinstein classification of spinal t.'s
medullary t.
melanotic neuroectodermal t.
meningeal t.
metastatic brain t.
t. metastatic to spine
midline t.
mixed germ cell t.
mixed pineal t.
t. necrosis
t. necrosis factor (TNF)
t. necrosis factor-alpha (TNF-alpha)
t. necrosis factor receptor (TNFR)
Nelson t.
nerve sheath t.
neuroectodermal t.
neuroepithelial t.
neuronal t.
nongerminoma malignant germ cell t.
occipital lobe t.
optic chiasm t.
optic pathway t.
orbital solitary fibrous t.
Pancoast t.
parachiasmal epidermoid t.
paranasal sinus t.
parasellar t.
parietal lobe t.
parotid t.
pearl t.
pearly t.
pediatric supratentorial hemispheric t.
Pepper t.
peripheral nerve sheath t.
peripheral neuroectodermal t.
petroclival t.
pineal cell t.
pineal parenchymal t.
pineal region t.

NOTES

tumor *(continued)*
pituitary t.
pontine angle t.
posterior fossa t.
Pott puffy t.
primary brain t.
primary neuroectodermal t.
primitive neuroectodermal t. (PNET)
primitive neuroepithelial t.
prolactin-secreting pituitary t.
Rathke pouch t.
recurrent t.
t. resection
rhabdoid t.
right frontal craniotomy for gross total resection of t.
sand t.
sarcomatous t.
Schwann cell t.
sellar t.
t. sensitizer trial
sheath t.
small-bowel carcinoid t.
smooth muscle t.
solitary fibrous t.
spinal cord t.
spindle-cell t.
t. stroma
subdural t.
subependymal t.
superior pulmonary sulcus t.
t. suppressor gene
t. suppressor gene mutation
supratentorial primary malignant brain t.
supratentorial primitive neuroectodermal t.
tectal plate t.
temporal lobe t.
teratoid t.
teratoid-rhabdoid t.
thalamic t.
thoracic t.
triton t.
turban t.
t. vaccine
vascular t.
vasoformative t.
vertebral body t.
visual system t.
t. volume
Wilms t.

tumoral calcinosis
tumor-associated rickets
tumor:cerebellum ratio
tumor:healthy tissue ratio
tumorigenesis
glial t.
tumor-infiltrating
t.-i. leukocyte (TIL)
t.-i. lymphocyte (TIL)
tumor-nerve bundle
tumorous involvement
Tums
tumultuous
TUNEL
terminal deoxynucleotide transferase-mediated nick end labeling
terminal deoxynucleotidyl transferase-mediated dUTP nick end-labeling
transferase-mediated dUTP-digoxigenin nick end-labeling
TUNEL-positive cell
tunicate
tunicin
tuning fork test
Tun-L-Kath epidural catheter
tunnel
t. cell
cubital t.
superior-inferior submucous t.
tarsal t.
t. vision
tunnelable ventricular ICP catheter
tunneled ventriculostomy
Tuohy needle
tupe
tu quoque
turban tumor
turbid
turbidity
turbinectomy
Turbo Tracker catheter
turcica
diaphragm of sella t.
sella t.
turcicae
tuberculum sellae t.
Türck
T. bundle
T. column
T. degeneration
T. fasciculus
T. tract
Turcot syndrome
Turnbull method
turned-on
Turner
intraparietal sulcus of T.
T. marginal gyrus
T. sulcus
turning
saccadic contraversive head t.

turricephaly
Turyn sign
tussive
t. absence
t. syncope
tutamen
tutamina cerebri
Tutoplast
T. anterior tibialis tendon
T. auditory ossicle
T. bone
T. costal cartilage
T. Dura
T. fascia lata
T. fascia temporalis
T. processed allograft
TVI
time-variance imaging
T1-weighted
T.-w. inversion recovery scan
T.-w. magnetic resonance image
T.-w. MR image
T.-w. spin echo
T.-w. spin-echo image
T2-weighted
T.-w. magnetic resonance image
T.-w. magnetic resonance scan
T.-w. MR image
T.-w. spin echo
T.-w. spin-echo image
T.-w. spin echo sequence
T.-w. turbo-gradient image
twice-born
twice-repeated multivariate analysis of variance
twilight state
twin
conjoined t.'s
t. research
twinge
Twin-K
twinship transference
twitch
Cogan lid t.
t. contraction
twitching
phasic t.
Trousseau t.
uremic t.
two
rule of t.
two-column cervical spine injury
two-component microgrip precision control suction unit
two-dimensional (2D)
t.-d. electrophoresis
t.-d. Fourier transform (2DFT)
t.-d. Fourier transform gradient-echo imaging
t.-d. mapping
t.-d. proton echo-planar spectroscopic imaging
twoness
limen to t.
two-stage procedure
two-stimuli task
Tycolet
tying forceps
Tylenol
Tylox
tympana (*pl. of* tympanum)
tympani
anterior canaliculus of chorda t.
chorda t.
communicating branch of otic ganglion to chorda t.
communicating branch of otic ganglion with chorda t.
nervus musculi tensoris t.
pyramis t.
ramus communicans nervi glossopharyngei cum chorda t.
ramus communicans nervi lingualis cum chorda t.
tensor t.
tympanic
t. cavity
t. enlargement
t. ganglion
t. intumescence
t. nerve
t. swelling
tympanica
intumescentia t.
tympanici
ramus tubalis plexus t.
ramus tubarius plexus t.
tympanico
ramus communicans nervi intermedii cum plexu t.

NOTES

T

tympanicum
ganglion t.
glomus t.
tympanicus
nervus t.
plexus t.
tympanometry
tympanophonia
tympanoplasty
tympanosquamous suture
tympanostomy tube
tympanum, pl. **tympana, tympanums**
pyramid of t.
Tyndall effect seen in cerebrospinal fluid
type
amyloidosis-Dutch t.
asthenic t.
Binswanger t.
choleric constitutional t.
dementia Alzheimer t. (DAT)
Dementia of the Alzheimer's T.
dementia frontal t.
function t.
t. 1 G_{M1} gangliosidosis
hereditary cerebral hemorrhage with amyloidosis-Dutch t. (HCHWA-D)
hypercompensatory t.
t. II curve pattern
melancholic t.
paranoid t.
senile dementia of the Alzheimer's t. (SDAT)
striatonigral degeneration t.
T. 2 superconductor
sympatheticotonic t.
typhoid peripheral neuropathy
typhomania
typhosus
status t.
typhus
epidemic t.
t. fever
murine t.
scrub t.
typical
t. absence seizure
t. neuroleptic
typify
typing
genetic t.
HLA DR15 (DR2) t.
tyramine challenge test
tyramine-induced hypertensive crisis
tyropanoate
tyropanoic acid
tyrosine
t. hydroxylase
t. hydroxylase-positive
t. kinase
t. metabolism disorder
t. phosphatase
tyrosine-kinase receptor
tyrosinemia
t. aminoaciduria
premature infant t.
tyrosinosis
Tzanck smear

UARS
upper airway resistance syndrome
UBE3A
UBE3A gene
UBE3A mutation
ubiquitin
u. pathway
u. protein ligase
ubiquitin-activating enzyme E1
ubiquitin-conjugating enzyme E2
ubiquitin-ligase gene
ubiquitin-ligating enzyme E3
ubiquitin-proteosome system (UPS)
UCLA
University of California Los Angeles
UCLA Brain Mapping Center
uEEG ProSystem 5000
U74006F
21-aminosteroid U.
ufologist
ugliness
UHDRS
Unified Huntington Disease Rating Scale
UHMWPE
U. cable
Uhthoff
U. phenomenon
U. sign
UK Parkinson Disease Research Group
UL
unit labyrinthectomy
ulcer
acute decubitus u.
Cushing u.
decubitus u.
neurogenic u.
neurotrophic u.
psychogenic duodenal u.
psychogenic gastric u.
psychogenic peptic u.
stress u.
trophoneurotic u.
ulceration
cerebrovascular u.
genital u.
oral u.
ulegyria
Ullmann line
ulnar
u. nerve
u. nerve entrapment
u. nerve lesion
u. nerve trauma
u. neuropathy
u. reflex
ulnari
ramus communicans nervi mediani com nervo u.
ulnaris
nervi digitales dorsales nervi u.
nervi digitales palmares communes nervi u.
nervi digitales palmares proprii nervi u.
nervus u.
rami musculares nervi u.
ramus dorsalis nervi u.
ramus palmaris nervi u.
ramus profundus nervi u.
ramus superficialis nervi u.
Ulrich disease
Ulrich-Turner syndrome
Ulthoff symptom
Ultracet
ultradian rhythm
Ultradol
ultra high molecular weight polyethylene fiber
ultra-high molecular weight polyethylene fiber cable
ultramicroclip
UltraPower
U. basic drill system
U. bur guard
U. bur guard drill system
U. revision
U. revision drill system
U. surgical drill system
ultrasonic
u. aspirating device
u. dissector
u. localizer
u. probe
u. surgical aspirator
u. therapy
u. wave
ultrasonographic
u. guidance
u. localization
ultrasonography
B-mode u.
cranial u.
Doppler u.
sequential u.
transcranial Doppler u.
ultrasonosurgery

ultrasound
cranial u.
Doppler u.
intraoperative B-mode u.
Intrascan u.
TCD u.
transcranial B-mode u.
transfontanel Doppler u.
ultrasound-guided transfrontal transventricular approach
ultrastructural study
ultraterminal fiber
Umbradil
UMN
upper motor neuron
un-American
unbearable
unbecoming
unbelievable
unbendable
***unc-33* gene**
uncal
u. gyrus
u. transtentorial herniation
uncalis
vena u.
uncharacteristically
unci (*pl. of* uncus)
unciform
u. fasciculus
uncinate
u. attack
u. aura
u. bundle of Russell
u. epilepsy
u. fasciculus of cerebellum
u. fasciculus of Russell
u. fit
u. gyrus
u. process
uncinatus
fasciculus u.
unclassified epileptic seizure
uncompensated hydrocephalus
uncomplaining
uncomplicated
u. arteriosclerotic
u. arteriosclerotic dementia
u. presenile dementia
u. senile dementia
unconditional reflex
unconditioned
u. reflex
u. response
u. stimulus
uncontrollable
uncontrolled
unco-parahippocampectomy
uncotomy
uncovertebral joint hypertrophy
uncus, pl. **unci**
arachnoid of u.
u. band of Giacomini
u. gyri fornicati
u. gyri hippocampus
u. gyri parahippocampalis
u. of temporal lobe
vein of u.
undercutting
cortical u.
u. saw
underlying
u. condition
u. mass lesion
u. sleep-disordered breathing
u. structural lesion
undifferentiated
u. cell adenoma
u. effect
undifferentiated-type
undulant fever
ungues
unguis
u. avis
Haller u.
u. ventriculi lateralis cerebri
unicoronal synostosis
unidirectional nystagmus
Unified
U. Huntington Disease Rating Scale (UHDRS)
U. Parkinson Disease Rating Scale (UPDRS)
Unilab Surgibone bovine bone graft
unilateral
u. anesthesia
u. chorea
u. deficit
u. dystonic posturing
u. electrodecremental event
u. epileptiform activity
u. facial pain syndrome
u. focus of activity
u. gliosis
u. hemilaminectomy
u. hydrocephalus
u. hyperreflexia
u. hypophysectomy
u. interfacetal dislocation or subluxation
u. interictal focal epileptic discharge
u. laminotomy
u. megalencephaly

u. migraine
u. migraine headache
u. optic neuritis
u. pain
u. pedicle cannulation
u. variable screw placement system
u. visual loss
unimodal association cortex
uninhibited neurogenic bladder
uniparental disomy
Unipen
unipolar
u. cell
u. cutting loop
u. neuron
u. patient
u. spongioblastoma
unipolare
spongioblastoma u.
unisensory
unit
adult u.
afferent motor u.
AME microcurrent TENS u.
BICAP u.
Cadwell 5200A somatosensory evoked potential u.
delirium u.
Dial Away Pain 400 electrotherapy u.
Eclipse TENS u.
efferent motor u.
fast motor u.
G5 Fleximatic massage/percussion u.
G5 Vibramatic massage/percussion u.
Hounsfield u. (HU)
internal pulse generating u.
u. labyrinthectomy (UL)
Leksell stereotactic gamma u.
Malis electrocoagulation u.
Maxima II TENS u.
Mayfield radiolucent base u.
motor u. (MU)
polyphasic motor u.
Radionics bipolar coagulation u.
reinnervated motor u.
Schwann cell u.
Sheffield gamma u.
Signa 1.5 Tesla u.
201-source cobalt-60 gamma u.
u. spinal rod
stereotactic gamma u.
Tac gel for EMS u.
Tac gel for TENS u.
teleradiotherapy u.
two-component microgrip precision control suction u.
valve u.
Wright Care TENS u.
ZD-Neurosurgical localizing u.
uniting
u. canal
u. duct
Univent endotracheal tube
universal
U. bone screw insertion/extraction system
U. cannulated screw system
u. instrumentation
u. phobia
U. Spine Classification
University
University of California Los Angeles (UCLA)
University Plate spinal attachment
unmyelinated
u. axon
u. fiber
u. nerve
unnerve
unpatterned flash visual evoked potential
unprovoked seizure
unruptured aneurysm
unshunted hydrocephalus
unspecified
u. aneurysm
u. depression
unsteadiness
postural u.
unstoppable flow of speech
unsuccessful
Unverricht
U. disease
U. myoclonus epilepsy
Unverricht-Lafora disease
Unverricht-Lundborg
U.-L. disease
U.-L. myoclonus epilepsy
U.-L. syndrome

U

NOTES

unwanted screw torque
unyielding
u-PA
urokinase-type plasminogen activator
upbeating nystagmus
UPBEAT program
upbiting/downbiting pituitary rongeur
update
UPDRS
Unified Parkinson Disease Rating Scale
UPDRS OFF score
UPDRS scale
up-front
upkeep
uplift
UPP
uvulopalatoplasty
upper
u. abdominal periosteal reflex
u. airway
u. airway collapse
u. airway muscular tone
u. airway obstruction
u. airway reflex
u. airway resistance
u. airway resistance syndrome (UARS)
u. cervical spine anterior construct
u. cervical spine anterior exposure
u. cervical spine fusion
u. cervical spine posterior construct
u. cervical spine procedure
u. extremity pronator sign
u. extremity scarf sign
u. hand
u. homonymous quadrantanopsia
u. hook trial
u. limb areflexia
u. motoneuron
u. motor neuron (UMN)
u. motor neuron disease
u. motor neuron impairment
u. motor neuron lesion
u. motor neuron paralysis
u. pons
u. radicular syndrome
u. thoracic spine
UPPP
uvulopalatopharyngoplasty
up-regulation
receptor u.-r.
upregulation/downregulation hypothesis
UPS
ubiquitin-proteosome system
upside-down Mooney face
uptake
radioisotope u.
u. site
upward gaze paresis
Uracel
uranoschisis
uratic degeneration
urban
urbanization
ur-defenses
urea
u. blood level
u. cycle
u. cycle disorder
Ureaphil Injection
uremia
u. peripheral neuropathy
uremic
u. amaurosis
u. coma
u. convulsion
u. encephalopathy
u. frost
u. neuropathy
OKT3 u.
u. polyneuropathy
u. toxin
u. twitching
uretericus
plexus u.
ureter injury
ureterolysis
urethral complex
urethrism
urethrismus
urethritis
urethrospasm
uric
u. acid
u. acid level
uridine glucuronyl transferases
urinary
u. creatinine
u. infection in spina bifida cystica
u. porphobilinogen
u. reflex
u. sphincter
u. tract
u. tract function
urine
u. continence
u. coproporphyria
u. screening
u. testing
Uristix
Dextrostix U.
urocrisia

urocrisis
U-rod
compression U.-r.
urogenital atrophy
Urografin
urokinase
u. plasminogen activator receptor
urokinase-type
u.-t. PA
u.-t. plasminogen activator (u-PA)
Uro-KP-Neutral
Uromiro
Uropac
Urovision
urticaria
giant u.
u. gigans
u. gigantea
u. tuberosa
US
Imagent US
USCF II diagnostic catheter
U-shaped scalp flap
Usher syndrome
USS
Synthes USS
ustus
Aspergillus u.
uterovaginalis
plexus u.
Utradol
utricle
utricular
u. nerve
u. reflex
u. spot
utricularis
nervus u.
utriculi
macula u.
utriculoampullaris
nervus u.
utriculoampullarly nerve
utriculofugal
utriculofugally
utriculosaccular duct
utriculosaccularis
ductus u.
utriculus
uveitis
juxtapapillary u.
uveomeningoencephalic syndrome
uveomeningoencephalitis
uvula
bifid u.
u. cerebelli
u. of cerebellum
u. vermis
uvulectomy
uvuli
uvulopalatopharyngoplasty (UPPP)
uvulopalatoplasty (UPP)
laser u. (LUPP)
laser-assisted u. (LAUP)

U

NOTES

μV
microvolt
V1 halo ring
VA
ventriculoatrial
vertebral artery
VA Hospital
VA Symptomatic Trial
vacant
vaccination
v. encephalomyelitis
v. encephalopathy
v. peripheral neuropathy
vaccine
diphtheria, tetanus toxoids, and pertussis v.
tumor v.
vaccine-associated Guillain-Barré syndrome
vaccinia
myelitis v.
vacuo
hydrocephalus ex v.
vacuolar
v. degeneration
v. myelopathy
vacuum
v. disk
v. headache
v. phenomenon
vagal
v. attack
v. lobe
v. nerve implant
v. nerve stimulation (VNS)
v. (nerve) trigone
v. part of accessory nerve
vagale
glomus v.
trigonum v.
vagalis
pars v.
vagectomy
vagi (*pl. of* vagus)
vagina
v. cellulosa
v. externa nervi optici
v. interna nervi optici
vaginae
v. nervi optici
pars anterior fornicis v.
pars anterior fornix v.
pars posterior fornix v.
pars postlaminalis nervi optici v.
vaginal
v. hyperesthesia
v. nerve
v. plexus
vaginales
nervi v.
vaginate
vaginismus
functional v.
vagoaccessorius
vagoaccessory-hypoglossal syndrome
vagoaccessory syndrome
vagoglossopharyngeal
v. neuralgia
vagogram
vagolysis
vagolytic
vagomimetic
vagosplanchnic
vagosympathetic
vagotomy
bilateral v.
highly selective v.
parietal cell v.
posterior truncal v.
selective v.
truncal v.
vagotonia
vagotonic
vagotony
vagotropic
vagovagal
vagus, pl. **vagi**
v. area
v. cranial nerve
v. cranial nerve [CN X]
dorsal motor nucleus of v.
dorsal nucleus of v.
v. eminentia
ganglion inferius nervi v.
ganglion rostralis nervi v.
ganglion superius nervi v.
ganglion of trunk of v.
inferior ganglion of v.
lobus v.
v. nerve examination
v. nerve jugular ganglion
v. nerve rostral ganglion
v. nerve stimulation (VNS)
v. nerve stimulation technique
v. nerve stimulator
v. neuropathy
nuclei nervi v.
nucleus commissuralis nevi v.

V

vagus *(continued)*
nucleus dorsalis nervi v.
nucleus posterior nervi v.
plexus pharyngeus nervi v.
rami bronchiales anteriores nervi v.
rami bronchiales nervi v.
rami bronchiales posteriores nervi v.
rami cardiaci cervicales inferiores nervi v.
rami cardiaci cervicales superiores nervi v.
rami cardiaci thoracici nervi v.
rami celiaci nervi v.
rami gastrici nervi v.
rami renales nervi v.
ramus articularis nervi v.
ramus communicans nervi glossopharyngei ramo auriculari nervi v.
ramus communicans nervi glossopharyngei ramo meningeo nervi v.
ramus communicans nervi intermedii cum nervo v.
ramus meningeus nervi v.
ramus pharyngeus nervi v.
v. reflex
v. stimulator implant
trigonum v.
trigonum nervi v.

Vail
V. neuralgia
V. syndrome

Vairox high compression vascular stockings
valacyclovir
Valentin
V. corpuscle
V. nerve
V. pseudoganglion
V. tympanic ganglion

valepotriate
valerianic acid
valinemia
Valin hemilaminectomy retractor
Valium
vallecula, pl. **valleculae**
v. cerebelli
v. of cerebellum
sulcus valleculae
v. sylvii

Valleix point
Valleylab
V. CUSA CEM system
V. neurosurgical product

vallis
Valmid
valproate
valproate-associated hyperammonemia
valproic
v. acid
v. acid and derivative
v. acid poisoning

valpromide
Valrelease
valrocemide
Valsalva maneuver
valve
ball-in-cone v.
Codman Hakim programmable v.
Codman-Medos programmable v.
Codman slit v.
Cordis-Hakim v.
cruciform slit v.
CRx Diamond v.
Delta v.
Denver v.
differential pressure v.
double spring ball v.
dual-switch v.
Hakim high-pressure v.
Hakim precision v.
Heyer-Pudenz v.
Heyer-Schulte bur hole v.
Holter-Hausner v.
Holter high-pressure v.
Holter medium-pressure v.
Low Profile v.
Medos v.
Medos-Hakim v.
Miethke dual-switch v.
Mishler v.
Novus hydrocephalic v.
Novus mini v.
Orbis-Sigma cerebrospinal fluid shunt v.
v. patency
pedi-gravity assisted v.
Phoenix ancillary v.
Phoenix cruciform v.
programmable v.
prosthetic heart v.
PS Medical Flow Control v.
Pudenz v.
Pudenz-Heyer-Schulte v.
v. replacement
rotating hemostatic v.
slit v.
Sophy mini programmable pressure v.
Strata adjustable Delta v.
v. system
Tarin v.

Tarinus v.
v. unit
Vieussens v.
Willis v.
valve-regulated shunt
valvulae
tuber v.
valvula semilunaris tarini
valvuloplasty
Vamate
van
V. Allen syndrome
V. Allen type familial amyloid polyneuropathy
v. Bogaert-Canavan disease
v. Bogaert disease
v. Bogaert encephalitis
v. Bogaert sclerosing leukoencephalitis
v. der Knaap syndrome
v. der Kolk law
Vancocin
van-Dyke-Hansen syndrome
vanilloid VR1 receptor (VR1)
vaniteuse
folie v.
Vanzetti sign
variable
clinical v.
continuous v.
demographic v.
dynamic v.
v. heavy chain (VH)
v. number tandem repeat (VNTR)
v. screw placement
v. screw placement system
v. screw placement system instrumentation
v. screw placement system-instrumented lumbar spine
v. screw placement system-plated patient
situational v.
v. stereotactic image fusion
v. stiffness microcatheter
variance
analysis of v. (ANOVA)
multiple analysis of v. (MANOVA)
twice-repeated multivariate analysis of v.
Vari-Angle
V.-A. aneurysm clip
V.-A. clip applier
V.-A. clip holder
V.-A. screw
variant
anatomical v.
Becker v.
benign epileptiform v.
bizarre v.
migraine v.
multiple sclerosis v.
neuroectodermal tumor desmoplastic v.
petit mal v.
primitive trigeminal artery v.
v. surface glycoprotein (VSG)
Westphal v.
variation
coefficient of v. (COV)
contingent negative v.
diurnal mood v.
situational tic v.
varicella
congenital v.
v. encephalitis
v. zoster encephalomyelitis
v. zoster virus
v. zoster virus infection
varicella-zoster
v.-z. virus (VZV)
v.-z. virus antigen
v.-z. virus reactivation
varices (*pl. of* varix)
varicose fiber
varicosity
autonomic v.
Varidase
variegate porphyria
Varigrip spine fixation system
varimax rotation
VARIMIC 900 microscope
Vario microscope
varix, pl. **varices**
orbital v.
varolian
varolii
pons v.
VAS
visual analog scale

NOTES

V

vasa
v. recta
v. vasorum
Vasamedics laser Doppler flow probe
VASC test
vascular
v. accident
v. change
v. circle of optic nerve
v. cognitive impairment
v. decompression
v. dementia
v. dissection
v. endothelial growth factor (VEGF)
v. endothelium
v. erosion
v. foot plate
v. fragility
v. groove
v. growth factor
v. hamartoma
v. headache
v. injury
v. intratympanic mass
v. loop
v. malformation
v. meninx
v. myelopathy
v. occlusion
v. organ of lamina terminalis
v. Parkinson disease
v. parkinsonism
v. patch graft
v. perforation
v. plexus
v. ring
v. sensation
v. smooth muscle
v. spasm
v. steal
v. surgery
v. tone
v. tumor
vascularis
pars v.
plexus v.
vascularized split calvarial cranioplasty
vasculature
CNS v.
systemic v.
vasculitic
v. mechanism
v. necrosis
v. neuropathy
vasculitis, pl. **vasculitides**
Churg-Strauss v.
cryoglobulinemic v.
hypersensitivity v.
hypocomplementemic urticarial v.
large vessel v.
leukocytoclastic v.
mesenteric v.
necrotizing v.
pauciimmune necrotizing v.
radiation v.
retinal v.
septic venous v.
systemic v.
vasculomotor
vasculomyelinopathy
vasculopathy
radiation v.
radiation-induced v.
vasculosa
meninx v.
pars v.
tela v.
vasculosum
organum v.
punctum v.
vase
Rubin v.
Vaseline gauze packing
Vaseretic 10-25
Vasiodone
vasoactive
v. effective
v. intestinal peptide
v. intestinal polypeptide (VIP)
v. substance
vasoconstriction
caffeine-induced v.
sympathetic-nervous-system-medicated v.
vasoconstrictive action
vasoconstrictor
v. center
v. nerve
v. pathway
vasodepressor syncope
vasodilatation
hypoxic cerebral v.
mannitol-induced cerebral v.
vasodilating antihypertensive medication
vasodilation
vasodilative
vasodilator
v. center
v. headache
v. nerve
vasodilator-stimulated rCBF single photon emission computed tomographic

vasoformative tumor
vasogenic
v. edema
v. shock
v. theory
vasomotor
v. absence
v. ataxia
v. center
v. change
v. component
v. epilepsy
v. fiber
v. headache
v. imbalance
v. instability
v. ischemia
v. nerve
v. paralysis
v. rhinitis
v. spasm
v. syncope
vasoneuropathy
vasoneurosis
vasopathy
calcifying v.
vasopressin (VP)
arginine v.
desamino-D-arginine v.
v. receptor agonist
v. tannate
vasopressor reflex
vasoreactivity
cerebral v.
vasoreflex
vasoresponsiveness
vasorum
nervi v.
vasa v.
VasoSeal closure device
vasosensory nerve
vasospasm
angiographic v.
arterial v.
cerebral v.
delayed cerebral v.
migraine v.
vasospasm-related hydrocephalus
vasospastic attack
vasostimulant
vasotocin
arginine v.
vasovagal
v. attack
v. epilepsy
v. syncope
v. syndrome
vastus lateralis muscle biopsy
Vater corpuscle
Vater-Pacini
V.-P. body
V.-P. corpuscle
vault
cranial v.
craniosacral v. (CV)
VDRL
Venereal Disease Research Laboratory
VDRL test
VDS
ventral derotation spondylodesis
Vectastain ABC kit
vector
v. diagram
v. field
gene therapy v.
lentiviral v.
M v.
macroscopic magnetization v.
magnetic field v.
nuclear magnetization v.
v. phase
vector-mediated gene transfer
vector-producing cell (VPC)
VectorVision$_2$
VectorVision$_2$ENT
VectorVision$_2$Fluoro
VectorVision image guided surgery system
VectorVision$_2$Spine
vecu
déjà v.
vecuronium bromide
VEE
Venezuelan equine encephalomyelitis
vegetative
v. circadian rhythmicity
v. nervous system
v. state
v. symptom
vegetotherapy

NOTES

VEGF
vascular endothelial growth factor
veil
aqueduct v.
vein
aneurysm of Galen v.
anterior cerebral v.
anterior jugular v.
anterior pontomesencephalic v.
anterior temporobasal v.
arterialized leptomeningeal v.
azygous v.
basal v.
brachiocephalic v.
bridging v.
Browning v.
carotid v.
v. of caudate nucleus
cerebellar v.
v. of cerebellum
cerebral v.
cervical intersegmental v.
choroid v.
cistern of great cerebral v.
common basal v.
v. of corpus striatum
cortical v.
deep cerebral v.
deep middle cerebral v.
diencephalic v.
diploic v.
direct lateral v.
dorsal callosal v.
draining v.
emissary v.
v. of Galen
v. of Galen aneurysm
v. of Galen malformation
great cerebral v.
inferior anastomotic v.
inferior basal v.
inferior cerebral v.
inferior choroid v.
inferior thalamostriate v.
inferior ventricular v.
innominate v.
insular v.
internal cerebral v.
internal jugular v.
intradural draining v.
jugular v.
jugulocephalic v.
v. of Labbé
Labbé v.
lateral atrial v.
lateral direct v.
v. of lateral recess of fourth ventricle
lingual v.
linguofacial v.
maxillary v.
medial atrial v.
v. of medulla oblongata
meningeal v.
meningorachidian v.
mesencephalic v.
middle posterior temporobasal v.
myelencephalic v.
v. of olfactory gyrus
ophthalmic v.
orbital v.
parietal v.
v. patch rupture
peduncular v.
v. of pons
pontine v.
pontomesencephalic v.
posterior callosal v.
v. of posterior horn
posterior marginal v.
posterior pericallosal v.
posterior temporobasal v.
precentral cerebellar v.
prefrontal v.
primitive maxillary v.
radicular v.
right hepatic v.
Rosenthal v.
saphenous v.
v. of septum pellucidum
striate v.
superficial cerebral v.
superficial middle cerebral v.
superficial temporal v.
superior anastomotic v.
superior basal v.
superior cerebral v.
superior choroid v.
superior ophthalmic v.
superior thalamostriate v.
superior thyroid v.
surface thalamic v.
telencephalic v.
terminal v.
thalamostriate v.
thrombosed thick-walled v.
Trolard v.
v. of Trolard
v. of uncus
vertebral v.
vela (*pl. of* velum)
Velban
Veley headrest

vellicate
vellication
vellus olivae inferioris
velocimetry
laser Doppler v.
velocity
absorption v.
average v.
blood v.
blood flow v.
conduction v.
v. encoding
flow v.
glutamate transport v.
maximum saccade peak v.
motor conduction v. (MCV)
nerve conduction v. (NCV)
preserved conduction v.
v. profile
saccade v.
spectral v.
spin v.
sway v.
target v.
velopharyngeal incompetence (VPI)
velum, pl. **vela**
anterior medullary v.
frenulum of superior medullary v.
inferior medullary v.
v. interpositum
v. medullare inferius
v. medullare superius
v. palatinum
posterior medullary v.
v. semilunare
superior medullary v.
v. tarini
v. terminale
transverse v.
v. transversum
v. triangulare
vena, pl. **venae**
v. anastomotica inferior
v. anastomotica superior
venae anteriores cerebri
v. anterior septi pellucidi
v. atrii lateralis
v. atrii medialis
v. basalis
v. cava injury
venae cerebelli inferiores
venae cerebelli superiores
v. cerebri anterior
venae cerebri inferiores
venae cerebri internae
v. cerebri magna
v. cerebri media profunda
v. cerebri media superficialis
venae cerebri profundae
venae cerebri superficiales
venae cerebri superiores
v. choroidea inferior
v. choroidea superior
v. cornus posterioris
venae directae laterales
v. dorsalis corporis callosi
v. gyri olfactorii
venae hemispherii cerebelli inferiores
venae hemispherii cerebelli superiores
venae inferiores cerebelli
venae inferiores cerebri
v. inferior vermis
venae insulares
venae internae cerebri
v. lateralis ventriculi lateralis
v. magna cerebri
v. medialis ventriculi lateralis
v. media profunda cerebri
v. media superficialis cerebri
venae medullae oblongatae
venae mesencephalicae
venae nuclei caudati
venae parietales
venae pedunculares
v. petrosa
venae pontis
v. pontomesencephalica
v. pontomesencephalica anterior
v. posterior corporis callosi
v. posterior septi pellucidi
v. precentralis cerebelli
venae prefrontales
venae profundae cerebri
v. recessus lateralis
v. septi pellucidi anterior
v. septi pellucidi posterior
venae striatae
venae superficiales cerebri
venae superiores cerebelli
venae superiores cerebri

NOTES

vena *(continued)*
v. superior vermis
v. terminalis
venae thalamostriatae inferiores
v. thalamostriata superior
v. uncalis
v. ventricularis inferior
v. vermis inferior
v. vermis superior
VenaFlow Compression system
vendetta
Venereal
V. Disease Research Laboratory (VDRL)
V. Disease Research Laboratory test
Venezuelan
V. equine encephalitis
V. equine encephalomyelitis (VEE)
vengeance
vengeful
venipuncture pain
venlafaxine hydrochloride
venography
digital subtraction v.
epidural v.
magnetic resonance v. (MRV)
transosseous v.
vertebral v.
venorespiratory reflex
venous
v. aneurysm
v. angioma
v. angle
v. dural sinus
v. embolism
v. hypertension
v. lake
v. lake configuration
v. malformation
v. occlusion plethysmography (*pl. of* VOP)
v. occlusive disease
v. outflow obstruction
v. oxygen saturation
v. plexus
v. sinus of dura mater
v. sinus thrombosis
v. stasis
v. stasis retinopathy
v. system
v. thromboembolic disease (VTED)
v. thrombosis
venous-side embolization
venous-sinus
thrombocytopenia v.-s.
ventilation
abnormal v.
assisted v.
controlled mechanical v. (CMV)
high-frequency percussive v. (HFPV)
mechanical v.
negative-pressure v.
noninvasive positive pressure v.
ventilation/perfusion inequality
ventilator
v. alarm
v. weaning
ventilatory
v. support neurologic complication
Ventolin
ventral
v. acoustic stria
v. amygdalofugal pathway
v. anterior nucleus
v. anterior nucleus of thalamus
v. branch of thoracic nerve
v. column of spinal cord
v. derotating spinal
v. derotation spondylodesis (VDS)
v. fasciculus proprius of spinal cord
v. funiculus
v. globus pallidus
v. horn
v. intermediate nucleus (VIM)
v. intermediate nucleus of thalamus
v. intermediate thalamic nucleus
v. lateral complex of the thalamus
v. lateral geniculate nucleus
v. lateral nucleus of thalamus
v. lateral thalamus
v. medial complex of the thalamus
v. medial mesencephalic syndrome
v. medial nuclei of oculomotor nerve
v. median fissure of medulla oblongata
v. median fissure of spinal cord
v. medullary compression
v. mesencephalic dopaminergic cell
v. mesencephalon
v. nuclei of thalamus
v. nucleus of thalamus
v. nucleus of trapezoid body
v. pallidum
v. paraflocculus
v. paralimbic region
v. part of pons
v. plate of neural tube
v. pontine infarction

v. posterior intermediate nucleus of thalamus
v. posterior lateral nucleus of thalamus
v. posterior medial (VPM)
v. posterior nucleus
v. posterior nucleus of thalamus
v. posteroinferior (VPI)
v. posteroinferior nucleus
v. posterolateral (VPL)
v. posterolateral nucleus
v. posterolateral nucleus of thalamus
v. posteromedial nucleus
v. posteromedial nucleus of thalamus
v. premammillary nucleus
v. principal nucleus
v. putamen
v. ramus
v. ramus of thoracic nerve
v. raphespinal tract
v. regimental area
v. respiratory group
v. root of spinal nerve
v. spinal artery occlusion
v. spinal root
v. spinocerebellar tract
v. spinothalamic tract
v. stream
v. striatum
v. tegmental area (VTA)
v. tegmental decussation
v. tegmentum
v. thalamic peduncle
v. tier thalamic nucleus
v. trigeminothalamic tract
v. white column
v. white commissure

ventrale
pallidum v.
striatum v.

ventralis
commissura supraoptica v.
v. intermedius
lamina v.
nucleus v.
nucleus campi v.
nucleus periventricularis v.
nucleus premammillaris v.
v. oralis anterior (Voa)
v. oralis posterior
paraflocculus v.
pedunculus thalami v.
v. posterior lateralis
v. posteromedialis
radix v.
sulcus v.
thalamus v.
tractus corticospinalis v.
tractus pyramidalis v.
tractus reticulospinalis v.
tractus spinocerebellaris v.
tractus spinothalamicus v.

ventricle
Arantius v.
ballooned floor of v.
body of lateral v.
v. of brain
bulb of occipital horn of lateral v.
bulb of posterior horn of lateral v.
central part of lateral v.
cerebral v.
v. of cerebral hemisphere
choroid plexus of fourth v.
choroid plexus of lateral v.
choroid plexus of third v.
choroid tela of fourth v.
choroid tela of third v.
colloid cyst of third v.
cornua of lateral v.
v. of diencephalon
Duncan v.
v. effacement
fifth v.
fourth v.
inferior horn of lateral v.
lateral aperture of fourth v.
lateral aperture of the fourth v.
lateral recess of fourth v.
lateral vein of lateral v.
left v.
limiting sulcus of fourth v.
medial vein of lateral v.
median aperture of fourth v.
median sulcus of fourth v.
medullary striae of fourth v.
pineal v.
v. puncture
v. of rhombencephalon
right v.

NOTES

ventricle *(continued)*
roof of fourth v.
sixth v.
slit v.
spinal cord terminal v.
sylvian v.
v. of Sylvius
Sylvius v.
tela choroidea of fourth v.
tela choroidea of lateral v.
tela choroidea of third v.
tenia of fourth v.
terminal v.
third v.
trigone of lateral v.
vein of lateral recess of fourth v.
Verga v.
Vieussens v.
Wenzel v.
ventricular
v. aqueduct
v. block
v. catheter occlusion
v. catheter reservoir
v. decompression
v. dilatation
v. drainage
v. enlargement
v. ependyma
v. fibrillation
v. fluid
v. ganglion
v. layer
v. needle
v. Ommaya reservoir
v. puncture
v. trigone
v. wall
ventriculitis
ventriculoamniotic shunting
ventriculoatrial (VA)
v. shunt
ventriculoatriostomy
ventriculocisternal shunt
ventriculocisternostomy
Torkildsen v.
ventriculoencephalitis
cytomegalovirus v.
ventriculofugal artery
ventriculogram
iohexol CT v.
ventriculography
air v.
cerebral v.
stereotactic anteroposterior and lateral metrizamide v.
water-soluble contrast v.
ventriculojugular
ventriculomastoidostomy
ventriculomegaly
progressive posthemorrhagic v.
ventriculometry
ventriculoperitoneal
v. shunt
v. shunting
ventriculopleural shunt
ventriculopuncture
ventriculoscope
four-channel Aesculap v.
rigid v.
ventriculoscopy
monoportal v.
ventriculostium
ventriculostomy
v. catheter
endoscopic third v. (ETV)
v. needle
neuroendoscopic third v.
straight-in v.
terminal v.
third v.
tunneled v.
ventriculostomy-related infection
ventriculosubarachnoid
ventriculosubgaleal shunt
ventriculotomy
ventriculovascular shunt procedure
ventriculovenous shunt
ventriculum
iter a tertio ad quartum v.
ventriculus
cornu inferius v.'s
cornu posterius v.'s
v. dexter cerebri
v. lateralis
v. lateralis cerebri
v.'s quarti
v. quartus
v. quartus cerebri
v. quintus
v. sinister cerebri
v. terminalis
v. terminalis medullae spinalis
v. tertius
v. tertius cerebri
trigonum v.'s
Ventrix
V. fiberoptic ventricular drainage system
V. fiberoptic ventricular monitoring system
V. SD fiberoptic subdural ICP catheter

V. tunnelable ventricular ICP monitoring and drainage system
V. tunnelable ventricular intracranial pressure monitoring system
ventrobasal
v. complex of the thalamus
v. nuclei complex
v. nucleus
ventrobasales
nuclei v.
ventrocaudal nucleus
ventrointermediate (Vim)
ventrointermediate thalamus
ventro-intermedius
nucleus v.-i.
ventrolateral
v. nuclear complex
v. nucleus
v. sclerosis
v. sulcus
v. surface of the medulla
ventrolateralis
nucleus hypothalamicus v.
v. thalamotomy
ventromedial
v. frontal leukotomy
v. hypothalamic hamartoma
v. hypothalamic nucleus
v. nucleus
v. nucleus of hypothalamus
v. prefrontal cortex
v. prefrontal cortex of the brain
ventromedialis
nucleus hypothalamicus v.
ventroposterior medial pallidotomy
ventroposterolateral (VPL)
v. pallidotomy
venturesome
venular obstruction
VEP
visual evoked potential
VER
visual evoked response
vera
neuralgia facialis v.
polycythemia v.
Verageuth
Veraguth
fold of V.
verapamil
Veratran
Verax
verbal
v. ability
v. agraphia
v. amnesia
v. analog pain scale
v. apraxia
v. auditory agnosia
v. cue
v. deficit
v. episodic memory
v. ifiasochism
v. information
v. intellectual functioning
v. intervention
v. material
v. memory exercise
v. memory impairment
v. recall score
v. weighted sum score
Verbal-Auditory
verbalize
verbalizing
inappropriate v.
verbicide
verbigerate
verbigeration
verbomania
verborum
delirium v.
verbous
verdict
Verdun
vergae
cavum v.
Verga ventricle
verge
anal v.
vergence
v. movement
v. system
veridical memory
vermal nodulus
vermes
vermian
v. artery
v. atrophy
v. medulloblastoma
v. split
vermicular sulcus
vermilion border

NOTES

vermis
anterior v.
v. cerebelli
folium of v.
folium v.
inferior vein of v.
medullary body of v.
nodule of v.
nodulus v.
pyramid of v.
pyramis v.
superior vein of v.
tuber v.
tuber of v.
uvula v.
vena inferior v.
vena superior v.
Vermont
V. spinal fixator
V. spinal fixator articulation
vernal encephalitis
Vernet syndrome
Verneuil neuroma
vernoestival encephalitis
Verocay body
verocytotoxin
VersaPulse holmium laser
versatile
versatility
attachment v.
verse
versenate
calcium disodium v.
versican proteoglycan
versicolor
membrana v.
version
Hare Psychopathy Checklist: Screening V.
Neuropsychiatric Inventory/nursing home v.
versive seizure
VertAlign spinal support system
vertebra, pl. **vertebrae**
block v.
butterfly v.
cervical v.
coronal cleft v.
fish v.
inferior v.
lamina arcus vertebrae
limbus v.
lumbar v.
lumbosacral v.
v. spreader
thoracic v.
thoracolumbar v.
transitional v.
vertebral
v. angiogram
v. angiography
v. angioma
v. aplasia
v. artery (VA)
v. artery injury
v. artery occlusion
v. artery transposition
v. artery trauma
v. body anterior cortex
v. body anterior cortex penetration
v. body corpectomy
v. body decompression
v. body impactor
v. body tumor
v. cervical instability
v. collapse
v. column
v. dissection
v. end-plate enhancement
v. exposure
v. fascia
v. fracture
v. fusion
v. ganglion
v. hemangioendothelioma
v. hemangioma
v. level
v. marrow
v. nerve
v. origin angioplasty and stenting
v. osteosynthesis
v. osteosynthesis fusion rate
v. part
v. plate
v. plate application
v. plate bypass
v. plexus
v. pulp
v. resection
v. subluxation
v. vein
v. venography
vertebrale
ganglion v.
vertebralis
columna v.
pars v.
plexus v.
theca v.
vertebrectomy
Bohlman anterior cervical v.
cervical spondylotic myelopathy v.
microsurgical thoracoscopic v.

vertebrobasilar
v. aneurysm
v. artery
v. atherosclerosis
v. circulation
v. disease
v. infarction
v. insufficiency
v. ischemia
v. syndrome
v. system
v. transient ischemic attack
vertebrogenic
v. pain syndrome
v. symptom complex
vertebroplasty
vertebrovenous fistula
vertex
V. reconstruction system
v. sharp wave
vertical
v. conflict
v. eye movement
v. gaze
v. gaze palsy
v. gaze paresis
v. line bisection
v. midline incision
v. migration
v. nystagmus
v. ocular deviation
v. pedicle diameter
v. plane
v. ring curette
v. sharp wave
v. suspension test
v. vertigo
verticalis
sulcus v.
vertiginosus
status v.
vertiginous aura
vertigo
v. ab stomacho laeso
angiopathic v.
apoplectic v.
arteriosclerotic v.
aural v.
benign functional v.
benign paroxysmal positional v.
benign positional paroxysmal v.
benign postural v.
central v.
cerebral v.
cervical v.
Charcot v.
chronic v.
disabling positional v. (DPV)
encephalic v.
endemic paralytic v.
epidemic v.
episodic v.
galvanic v.
gastric v.
height v.
horizontal v.
labyrinthine v.
laryngeal v.
lateral v.
mechanical v.
nocturnal v.
objective v.
ocular v.
organic v.
paralyzing v.
paroxysmal v.
peripheral v.
positional v.
posttraumatic v.
postural v.
primary v.
proprioceptive v.
psychogenic v.
residual v.
rotary v.
sham-movement v.
stomachal v.
subjective v.
systematic v.
tenebric v.
toxic v.
vertical v.
vestibular v.
visual v.
voltaic v.
Vertigraft allograft product
verum
septum v.
very
v. high dose phenobarbital
v. low amplitude
v. low-density lipoprotein receptor

NOTES

very *(continued)*
v. low density syndrome
v. short Minnesota Differential Aphasia test
Vesalius
canal of V.
foramen of V.
vesania
vesanique
delire v.
vesical
v. center
v. plexus
v. reflex
vesicale
plexus v.
vesicalis
plexus v.
vesicle
cerebral v.
encephalic v.
forebrain v.
hindbrain v.
lipid-containing v.
midbrain v.
ocular v.
ophthalmic v.
optic v.
pinocytotic v.
primary brain v.
synaptic v.
telencephalic v.
vesico-sphincter dyssynergia
vesicospinal center
vesicoureteral reflux
vesicula ophthalmica
vesicular
v. eruption
v. stomatitis virus
vesiculation of the Golgi
vessel
blood v.
cerebral blood v.
collateral v.
crack-like v.
v. hyperplasia
nutrient v.
pain-sensitive v.
pial cortical v.
resistance v.
telangiectatic discectomy v.
vest
Bremer AirFlo halo v.
halo v.
Minerva v.
vestibule aqueduct of v.
vestibuli aqueductus v.
vestibular
v. apparatus
v. aqueduct
v. area
v. crest
v. deficit
v. disorder
v. end-organ nystagmus
v. fissure of cochlea
v. function
v. ganglion
v. hair cell
v. labyrinth
v. membrane
v. migraine
v. migraine headache
v. nerve examination
v. nerve section
v. neurectomy
v. neuritis
v. neuronitis
v. nucleus
v. organ
v. part of vestibulocochlear nerve
v. reflex
v. root
v. root of vestibulocochlear nerve
v. schwannoma
v. sense
v. suppressant
v. system
v. vertigo
vestibulare
ganglion v.
vestibulares
nuclei v.
vestibularis
area v.
pars caudalis nervi v.
pars inferior nervi v.
pars rostralis nervi v.
pars superior nervi v.
radix v.
ramus communicans cochlearis nervi v.
vestibule
v. aqueduct of vest
crest of v.
olfactory v.
vestibuli
aqueductus v.
v. aqueductus vest
crista v.
scala v.
vestibulocerebellar
v. ataxia
v. tract

vestibulocerebellum
vestibulocochlear
v. nerve [CN VIII]
v. neuropathy
v. nucleus
v. organ
vestibulocochleare
organum v.
vestibulocochlearis
nervus v. [CN VIII]
nuclei nervi v.
pars cochlearis nervi v.
pars vestibularis nervi v.
radix cochlearis nervi v.
radix inferior nervi v.
radix superior nervi v.
radix vestibularis nervi v.
vestibuloequilibratory control
vestibulogenic
v. epilepsy
v. seizure
vestibuloocular
v. reflex (VOR)
v. reflex suppression
vestibulopathy
idiopathic bilateral v.
vestibulospinal
v. drive
v. influence
v. input
v. reflex
v. signal
v. tract
vestibulospinalis
tractus v.
vestibulothalamic
vestibulotoxicity
Vestra
veteran
Vietnam-era v.
Vevesca
VGB
vigabatrin
VGCC
voltage-gated calcium channel
VGPT
visually guided pointing task
V-groove hollow-ground connection design
VH
variable heavy chain
VHL
von Hippel-Lindau
VHL syndrome
VI
lamina VI
viability
neuronal v.
viable
v. synapse
vibration
v. sense
v. syndrome
vibratory
v. sensibility
Vibrio parahaemolyticus
vibrometer
vibrotactile
vibrotome
vibs, VIBS, pl. **vocabulary, information, block (design), and similarities, vocabulary, information, block (design), and similarities**
vicarious violence
vice allemande
vicinity
Vicoprofen
Vicq
V. d'Azyr band
V. d'Azyr bundle
V. d'Azyr centrum semiovale
V. d'Azyr fasciculus
V. d'Azyr foramen
V. d'Azyr foramen caecum
V. d'Azyr stripe
V. d'Azyr tract
Vicryl Rapide suture
victim
v. of criminal violence
v. of domestic violence
potential suicide v.
primary v.
suicide v.
victimization
multiple v.
victimize
vidarabine
video
v. electroencephalographic monitoring
v. game epilepsy
v. game violence

V

NOTES

video *(continued)*
v. monitoring of seizure
v. therapy
video-assisted endoscopic sympathectomy
videocassette recording
videoconference
videoconferencing
video-EEG
v.-E. monitoring
videonystagmography
video-oculography (VOG)
video-polysomnographic
Videx
vidian
v. artery
v. canal
v. nerve
v. neuralgia
v. plexus
vie
Vienna encephalitis
Vietnam-era veteran
Vieussens
annulus of V.
V. ansa
V. centrum
V. ganglion
V. loop
V. valve
V. ventricle
view
field of v.
swimmer's v.
Waters v.
viewing
tachistoscopy v.
V. Wand
V. Wand image guided system
viewless
viewpoint
economic v.
genetic v.
vigabatrin (VGB)
vigil
coma v.
vigilambulism
vigilance reaction time
Vigor
Profile of Mood States, V.
vigor
Vigotsky
VIII
factor VIII
Viking II nerve monitoring device
villager
Villaret-Mackenzie syndrome
Villaret syndrome
villi, pl. **villus**
arachnoid v.
arachnoid granulation v.
choroid plexus v.
villus, pl. **villi**
viloxazine
VIM
ventral intermediate nucleus
Vim
ventrointermediate
V. thalamotomy
V. thalamus
vimentin tumor marker
vinblastine sulfate
vinca alkaloid
vincristine
v. peripheral neuropathy
procarbazine, lomustine (CCNU), v. (PCV)
v. sulfate
vincula
v. lingula
v. lingulae cerebelli
vinculum
Vineland percentile scale
Viñuela cocktail
violation
violator
norm v.
violence
graphic v.
juvenile v.
manifestation of v.
media v.
motion picture v.
origin of v.
pathogen of v.
perpetrator of v.
predatory v.
repetitive v.
risk factors for v.
vicarious v.
victim of criminal v.
victim of domestic v.
video game v.
witness to v.
witness to repetitive v.
youth v.
violent
v. conduct disorder
v. media
v. onset headache
violinist's cramp
Vioxx
VIP
vasoactive intestinal polypeptide

Viracept
viral
v. delivery
v. DNA
v. encephalitis
v. encephalomyelitis
v. infection
v. intracerebral arteritis
v. leukoencephalitis
v. meningitis
v. myelitis
v. particle
v. receptor
v. rhinitis
v. vector-mediated therapy
v. vector system
viral-mediated illness
Viramune
Virchow
V. disease
V. granulation
V. psammoma
Virchow-Robin
V.-R. space
V.-R. space of the brain
Virgoan
viridans
v. streptococci
Streptococcus v.
virile
molimen climactericum v.
v. reflex
virilescence
virilia
virilization
virtual
v. endoscopy
v. probe
v. reality therapy
V. Vision heads-up display
virtuality
virtuous
virus
Central European tick-borne encephalitis v.
cytomegalic inclusion v.
dengue v.
DNA v.
double-stranded DNA v.
ECHO v.
v. encephalomyelitis
enteric cytopathic human orphan v.
Epstein-Barr v. (EBV)
hepatropic v.
herpes simplex v. (HSV)
herpes simplex v. type 1 (HSV-1)
herpes simplex v. type 2 (HSV-2)
human immunodeficiency v. (HIV)
human T-cell leukemia v. (HTLV)
human T-cell lymphoma v.
human T-cell lymphotropic v.
inhibitory v.
Jamestown Canyon v. (JCV)
Japanese encephalitis v.
JC v.
Junin v.
Lassa fever v.
lymphocytic choriomeningitis v. (LCMV)
Machupo v.
neurotropic v.
Newcastle disease v.
Oklahoma tick fever v.
oncolytic v.
ONYX-015 v.
Powassan v.
rabies v.
Rio Bravo v.
RNA v.
rubella v.
Saint Louis encephalitis v.
Seoul v.
snowshoe hare v.
St. Louis encephalitis v. (SLEV)
Trivittatus v.
varicella zoster v.
varicella-zoster v. (VZV)
vesicular stomatitis v.
WEE v.
virus-mediated gene transfer
visceral
v. afferent fiber
v. anesthesia
v. aura
v. brain
v. crisis
v. disorder
v. efferent fiber
v. emotional state
v. epilepsy
v. larva migrans
v. lobe

NOTES

visceral *(continued)*
v. motor component
v. motor neuron
v. nerve fiber
v. nervous system
v. neurofiber
v. nuclei of oculomotor nerve
v. pain
v. plexus
v. plexuses ganglion
v. reflex
v. sense
v. sensory component
v. sympathectomy
viscerale
ganglion v.
viscerales
neurofibrae v.
visceralis
nervus v.
plexus v.
ramus v.
visceralium
ganglia plexuum v.
viscerogenic
v. referred pain
v. reflex
visceromotor
v. pathway
v. reflex
viscerosensory
v. process
v. reflex
viscerosomatic tone
viscerotome
viscoelastic action
viscosity
blood v.
social v.
visile
vision
abrupt loss of v.
v. assessment
color v.
double v.
facial v.
foveal v.
funnel v.
impaired v.
organ of v.
recovery of v.
subjective v.
tunnel v.
visionism
visionless
visit
baseline v.
clinical v.
followup v.
post baseline v.
trial v.
visitation
conjugal v.
Vista American Health 0.5 Tesla MRI scanner
Vistaril
visual
v. acuity loss
v. agnosia
v. alexia
v. allesthesia
v. amnesia
v. analog scale (VAS)
v. aphasia
v. association area
v. association cortex
v. axis
v. blurring
v. change
v. claudication
v. constructional praxis
v. cortical area
v. disturbance
v. episodic memory
v. evoked cortical potential
v. evoked potential (VEP)
v. evoked response (VER)
v. field cut
v. field defect
v. field deficit
v. field depression
v. field disorder
v. field testing
v. fixation
v. hallucination
v. image movement disorder
v. inattention
v. memory impairment
v. mismatch negativity (VMMN)
v. motor processing
v. orbicularis reflex
v. organ
v. paraneoplastic syndrome
v. pathway
v. phenomenon
v. receiving area
v. receptor cell
v. reflex epilepsy
v. region
v. representation strategy
v. shimmering with aura
v. shining with aura
v. sparkling with aura
v. spatial constructional apraxia

v. subsystem
v. symptom
v. system
v. system tumor
v. vertigo
visual-function monitoring
visualization
endoscopic v.
visualize
visual-kinetic dissociation
visually guided pointing task (VGPT)
visually-guided saccade
visual-spatial
v.-s. acalculia
v.-s. agnosia
visual-vestibular conflict
visuoauditory
visuoconstructional ability
visuoconstruction skill
visuoconstructive
visuognosis
visuomotor
Beery Developmental Test of V.
v. behavior
v. problem-solving skill
v. status
visuoperception
visuoperceptual
visuopsychic area
visuosensory area
visuospatial
v. construction
v. constructive cognition
v. disorientation
v. function
v. functioning
v. hemineglect
v. memory
v. neglect
v. skill
visuotopic
vitae arbor v.
visus
organum v.
vita
arbor v.'s
v.'s arbor visuotopic
dolce v.
VitaCarn Oral
vital
v. capacity
v. center
elan v.
v. node
noeud v.
Vitallium
V. equipment
V. plate
vitamin
v. B_6
v. B_{12}
v. B_1
v. B1 deficiency
v. B6 deficiency
v. B12 deficiency
v. B12 deficiency dementia
v. B, D, E, K
v. B12 level
v. B_{12} neuropathy
v. D deficiency
v. D malabsorption
v. E deficiency
v. K-dependent clotting factor II
v. K-dependent clotting factor IX
v. K-dependent clotting factor VII
vitrea
lamina v.
vitrectomy
vitreous
v. hemorrhage
hyperplastic primary v.
v. lamella
v. membrane
primary v.
vitritis
Vitrogen 100 collagen
vitro matrigel model
vitronectin
vituperate
vituperative
vivacious
Vivactil
vivid
vividness
vivify
viviparity
viviparous
vivipation
vivo
ex v.
vixen
vizard

NOTES

V

VJ shunt
VLA-4 adhesion
VL thalamotomy
VMETH
volumetric multiple exposure transmission holography
VMMN
visual mismatch negativity
VNS
vagal nerve stimulation
vagus nerve stimulation
VNS therapy
VNTR
variable number tandem repeat
Voa
ventralis oralis anterior
vocabulary
auditory v.
v., information, block (design), and similarities (*pl. of* vibs)
v. skill
vocal
v. cord
v. cord paralysis
v. fold approximation
v. fold paralysis
v. motor amusia
v. tic disorder
v. trill
vocalization
nocturnal v.
vocation
vocational performance
vociferate
vociferous
VOG
video-oculography
Vogt
V. disease
V. point
V. syndrome
V. triad of seizures, mental retardation, and facial angiofibroma
Vogt-Hueter point
Vogt-Koyanagi-Harada syndrome
Vogt-Spielmeyer disease
voguish
VOI
voxel of interest
voice
discordance of v.
hallucinated v.
hysterical v.'s
v. intonation
quavering v.
voiced
voice-verbal
eyes, motor, v.-v.
void
signal v.
Voigt line
voilá
Voit nucleus
VOL
volume of interest
vol
monomanie du v.
volar tip
volatile hydrocarbon
VOL-based hypothesis-driven
volitional
v. capacity
v. deficit
v. impairment
v. sleep deprivation
v. tremor
Volkmann contracture
volley
antidromic v.
Volpe criteria
voltage
transient v.
voltage-activated conductance
voltage-dependent neurotransmitter release
voltage-gated
v.-g. calcium channel (VGCC)
v.-g. potassium channel
v.-g. sodium channel
v.-g. sodium channel blocker
voltage-regulated calcium channel
voltage-sensitive
v.-s. block
v.-s. protein
voltaic vertigo
volte-face
voluble
volume
amygdala v.
blood flow v.
brain v.
caudate v.
cerebellar v.
cerebral blood v. (CBV)
cerebrospinal fluid v.
cortical v.
v. expansion
frontal lobe v.
hippocampal raw v.
infarction v.
v. of interest (VOL)
intracranial brain v.
intracranial raw v.

ischemic lesion v.
mamillary body v.
mean corpuscular v.
mean intracranial raw v.
mean normalized whole brain v.
normalized whole brain v.
prefrontal cortical v.
raw v.
regional brain parenchymal v.
v. regulation
relative cerebral blood v. (rCBV)
v. segmentation
sensitive v.
tidal v. (VT)
total fractional regional brain v.
v. transmission
tumor v.
whole-brain v.
whole brain v.
whole brain raw v.

volume-averaging error

volumetric
v. analysis
v. computed tomography
v. infusion pump
v. interstitial brachytherapy
v. loss
v. multiple exposure transmission holography (VMETH)
v. resection
v. solution (VS)
v. stereotaxy

volumetry
hippocampal v.
MRI v.

voluntary
v. mutism
v. nystagmus
v. time-out

volunteer work

voluptuous

volupty

vomer
posterior v.

vomeronasal
v. organ
v. sensory neuron (VSN)
v. zone

vomit

vomiting
anticipatory v. (AV)
v. center
cerebral v.
cyclic v.
ictal v.
v. reflex

vomitory

von
v. Ebner gland
v. Economo disease
v. Economo encephalitis
v. Eulenberg disease
v. Frey hair
v. Frey monofilament
v. Frey test
v. Gierke disease
v. Graefe sign
v. Graefe strabismus hook
v. Hippel disease
v. Hippel-Lindau (VHL)
v. Hippel-Lindau disease
v. Hippel-Lindau syndrome
v. Monakow diaschisis concept
v. Monakow fiber
v. Recklinghausen disease
v. Recklinghausen neurofibromatosis
v. Willebrand disease
v. Willebrand factor (vWF)
v. Zerssen circumplex model of premorbid personality

VONEX

voodoo

VOP, pl. **venous occlusion plethysmography, venous occlusion plethysmography**

VOR
vestibuloocular reflex

vorbeireden

votary

votive

voulu
déjà v.

vowel

voxel
contiguous v.
v. of interest (VOI)
spectroscopy v.

voxel-based morphometry

voxel-by-voxel analysis

voxel-wise analysis

voyager
brain v. 4.0

NOTES

V

voyeurism
voyeuristic
VP
vasopressin
VP shunt
VPC
vector-producing cell
VPI
velopharyngeal incompetence
ventral posteroinferior
VPL
ventral posterolateral
ventroposterolateral
VPL pallidotomy
VPM
ventral posterior medial
VR1
vanilloid VR1 receptor
VS
volumetric solution
Profile VS
VSG
variant surface glycoprotein
V-shaped incision
VSN
vomeronasal sensory neuron
VSP plate instrumentation
VT
tidal volume
VTA
ventral tegmental area
VTED
venous thromboembolic disease
V-tunnel drill system
vu
déjà vu
vulgar
vulgarism
vulgarity
vulgarize
vulnerability
danger-laden schema v.
hippocampal v.
pretraumatic v.
segmental v.
suicide v.
vulnerable
Vulpian
V. atrophy
V. effect
Vulpian-Bernhardt spinal muscular atrophy
vulpine
vulturous
vulvae
pruritus v.
vWF
von Willebrand factor
VZV
varicella-zoster virus
VZV reactivation
VZV-specific T cell

Wackenheim clivus canal line
wacky, wobbly and wet
Wada
W. language lateralization testing
W. language and memory testing
W. memory asymmetry
W. memory score
W. memory test
W. procedure
W. protocol
Waddell
W. sign
W. test
waddle
waddling gait
wafer
BCNU-impregnated polymer w.
Gliadel w.
polyanhydride biodegradable polymer w.
w. technology
waif
WAIS
Wechsler Adult Intelligence Scale
WAIS-III
WAIS-R
waiter's cramp
wake after sleep onset (WASO)
wakeful
wakefulness
w. disorder
waking
w. background EEG
w. numbness
w. paralysis
waking-NREM
Wakoz
Waldenstrom
macroglobulinemia of W.
W. macroglobulinemia
Waldeyer
W. tract
W. zonal layer
walk
scissoring w.
Walker
W. lissencephaly
W. tractotomy
Walker-Warburg syndrome
walking
w. aid
bipedal w.
chromosome w.
heel w.
w. stance
w. swing phase
wall
w. fistula
parapharyngeal w.
pharyngeal w.
ventricular w.
Wallenberg syndrome
wallerian
w. degeneration
w. law
Wallgraft endoprosthesis
wallow
Wallstent
Magic W.
W. stent
Walther ganglion
wan
wand
3-dimensional reconstruction w.
Elekta viewing w.
ISG viewing w.
NCP programming w.
Programming W.
stylus-type sensor w.
TriggerWheel W.
Viewing W.
wandering
w. cell
episodic nocturnal w.
nocturnal w.
wane
Wangensteen needle holder
waning
w. discharge
waxing and w.
wanting
wanton
war
drug w.
injury of w.
Warburg syndrome
ward
long-stay w.
wardrobe
Wardrop method
warehousing
Ware instrument
warfare
ABC w.
warfarin
w. syndrome
Waring blender syndrome
warlike

warm
w. effector
W. 'n Form lumbosacral corset
w. sensitivity
w. spot
warmhearted
warm-sensitive neuron
warmth receptor
warmup phenomenon
warm-wire anemometer
warning
black box w.
warp
Warrington Recognition Memory Test
warrior
warship
wart
brain w.
Wartenberg
W. disease
W. sign
W. symptom
wartime
wary
washboard effect
washed up
washer
plate-spacer w.
washout
drug w.
WASO
wake after sleep onset
waspish
wasted
wasting
cerebral salt w.
muscle w.
nitrogen w.
w. palsy
w. paralysis
salt w.
w. syndrome
watchful
watching
repetitive w.
watchmaker's cramp
watchword
Waterhouse-Friderichsen syndrome
water intoxication
waterjet dissection
Waters
W. view
W. view radiograph
watershed
w. area
w. area paresis
w. infarction
w. region
w. zone
water-soluble
w.-s. contrast myelography
w.-s. contrast ventriculography
watertight closure
Watson
W. angular rate sensor
W. syndrome
Watson-Schwartz test
Watson-Williams intervertebral disk rongeur
wave
A w.
alpha w.
w. analyzer
aperiodic w.
arciform w.
axon w.
beta w.
brain w.
centrotemporal sharp w.
continuous w. (CW)
delta w.
E w.
EEG alpha w.
electroencephalographic w.
expectancy w.
F w.
flat top w.
w. form
gamma w.
generalized periodic sharp w.
H w.
Hering-Traube w.
interictal sharp w.
Jewett w.
kappa w.
lambda w.
M w.
monophasic w.
mu w.
w. number
positive sharp w.
R_1 w.
R_2 w.
random w.
rho w.
sawtooth w.
sharp w.
slow frequency w.
square w.
theta w.
Traube-Hering-Mayer w.
triphasic w.
ultrasonic w.

vertex sharp w.
vertical sharp w.
waveform
abnormal w.
w. amplitude
apiculate w.
dampened w.
monophasic w.
nondampened w.
out-of-phase w.
signal voltage w.
wavelength
wavelet entropy
wavenumber
wavering light with aura
waveshape
wax
bone w.
Horsley bone w.
waxing and waning
Wayne laminectomy seat
wayward
WBC
white blood cell
WBI
whole brain irradiation
WBRT
whole-brain radiation therapy
weak-hearted
weakling
weak-minded
weakness
abduction w.
adduction w.
arm w.
bulbar muscle w.
diaphragmatic w.
eye muscle w.
facial w.
hemifacial w.
infranuclear w.
intercostal muscle w.
limb w.
neck w.
pharyngeal w.
psychological w.
sternocleidomastoid muscle w.
weaknesses
weak-willed
wealth
wealthy
wean
weaning
ventilator w.
weapon
weaponry
weapons
weariless
wearing-off phenomenon
wearisome
Weary
W. brain spatula
W. cordotomy knife
W. nerve hook
W. nerve root retractor
weary
weasling
weathered
weatherworn
web
subsynaptic w.
Weber
W. esthesiometer
W. sign
W. syndrome
W. test
Weber-Christian disease
Weber-Fergusson incision
Weber-Leyden syndrome
webspace incision
Webster needle holder
Wechsler
W. Adult Intelligence Scale (WAIS)
W. Individual Achievement Test (WIAT)
W. Intelligence Scale for Children-Revised (WISC-R)
W. Intelligence Scale for Children-Revised, Version III (WISC-III)
W. Memory Scale for Children, Russell version (WMS-R)
Wechsler-Bellevue
Weck clip
Wedensky
W. effect
W. facilitation
W. inhibition
W. phenomenon
wedge
Duo-Cline bed w.
wedge-compression fracture

NOTES

wedge-shaped
w.-s. astrocyte
w.-s. fasciculus
w.-s. tubercle
WEE
western equine encephalomyelitis
W. virus
weed
loco w.
weekend headache
Weekly
Prozac W.
weeping
overt w.
Wegener
W. granulomatosis (WG)
W. granulomatosis-associated neuropathy
Weibel-Palade body
Weigert staining
weight
w. gain potential
w. loss
w. regulation
w. sense
target w.
weighted
w. sum score
weighting
proton density w.
T1 w.
T2 w.
weight-neutral psychotic medication
Weil-Blakesley intervertebral disk rongeur
Weinberg rib spreader
Weingrow reflex
Weinstein Enhanced Sensory Test
Weiss sign
Weitbrecht cord
Weitlaner-Beckman retractor
Weitlaner retractor
Welander
W. disease
W. distal muscular atrophy
W. distal myopathy
W. muscular dystrophy
W. syndrome
welcome
welding
tissue w.
welfare
social w.
w. system
welfarism
well-advised
well-being
global w.-b.
subjective w.-b.
Wellbutrin
well-conditioned
Wellcovorin
well-defined focal brain lesion
well-formed
w.-f. electroencephalogram rhythm
well-groomed
well-motivated
wellness
w. principle
sense of w.
well-off
well-oriented
well-read
well-rounded
well-spoken
Wells stereotactic apparatus
well-timed
well-to-do
welsh
weltmerism
weltschmerz
wench
Wenzel ventricle
wept
Werdnig-Hoffmann
W.-H. disease
W.-H. spinal muscular atrophy
Wermer syndrome
Wernekinck
W. commissure
W. decussation
Wernicke
W. aphasia
W. center
W. dementia
W. disease
W. dysphasia
W. encephalopathy
W. field
W. hemianopic pupillary phenomenon
mirror of W.
W. radiation
W. reaction
W. region
W. second motor speech area
W. sign
W. syndrome
W. triangle
W. zone
Wernicke-Korsakoff
W.-K. encephalopathy
W.-K. syndrome

Wernicke-Mann spastic hemiplegia
West
W. African sleeping sickness
W. African trypanosomiasis
W. hand and foot nerve tester
W. Nile encephalitis
W. Nile fever
W. syndrome (WS)
Westco Neurostat-Mark II
Westergren method
westermani
Pargonimus w.
western
W. blot analysis
W. equine encephalitis
w. equine encephalomyelitis (WEE)
W. medicine
Weston Hurst disease
Westphal
W. disease
W. nucleus
W. phenomenon
W. pseudosclerosis
W. pupillary reflex
W. sign
W. variant
W. zone
Westphal-Erb sign
Westphal-Piltz phenomenon
Westphal-Strümpell pseudosclerosis
wet
w. beriberi
w. bipolar system
w. brain
wacky, wobbly and w.
Wever-Bray phenomenon
WFNS
World Federation of Neurosurgical Societies
WFNS scale
WG
Wegener granulomatosis
wheeze
whereabouts
whiff
whinge
whininess
whiplash
acute w.
w. injury
w. shaken infant syndrome
whipping
Whipple
W. disease
W. disease peripheral neuropathy
whispering dystonia
Whitacre spinal needle
white
w. atrophy
w. blood cell (WBC)
w. blood cell count
w. column of spinal cord
w. commissure
w. commissure of spinal cord
w. iritis
w. laminae of cerebellum
w. layer of cerebellum
w. matter
w. matter of the centrum ovale
w. matter change
w. matter degeneration
w. matter degenerative disease
w. matter hyperintensity
w. matter hypodensity
w. matter infarction
w. matter ischemia
w. matter lactate
w. matter lactate level
w. matter lesion (WML)
w. matter pathology
w. matter region
w. matter signal abnormality
w. matter structure
w. matter tissue
w. noise masking
W. and Panjabi criteria
w. rami communicantes
w. ramus
w. softening
w. substance
w. substance of cerebellum
w. substance of spinal cord
white-collar worker
white-headed
white-out syndrome
Whitesides-Kell cervical technique
whitewash
WHO
World Health Organization
WHO astrocytoma classification
WHO instrument
Who Are You

NOTES

whole
w. brain atrophy
w. brain blood flow
w. brain boundary
w. brain irradiation (WBI)
w. brain raw volume
w. brain volume
w. cranial headache
w. focus orientation
w. head
whole-body cooling
whole-brain
w.-b. mapping database
w.-b. radiation therapy (WBRT)
w.-b. volume
whole-cell
w.-c. patch-clamp
w.-c. patch clamp technique
w.-c. recording
whole-cortex MEG/EEG system
whole-head neuromagnetometer
wholeness
sense of w.
whole-spine MRI
whorl
storiform w.
whorling pattern
Whytt disease
WIAT
Wechsler Individual Achievement Test
wick
Silastic w.
wicket
w. rhythm
w. spike
wide
w. area network
w. bipole
Wide Range Achievement Test, Revised (*pl. of* WRAT-R)
wide-necked aneurysm
widespread
w. beta activity
w. distribution of activity
widowed status
widowhood
width
line w.
pulse w.
Wiener
tract of Münzer and W.
Wigraine
Wilbrand
W. knee
W. knee injury
Wilcoxon rank sum test
Wilde cord
Wildervanck syndrome
wild-type (WT)
w.-t. allele
w.-t. Parkin
will
concept of w.
willfulness
Williams
W. sequestrectomy
W. syndrome
williamsii
Lophophora w.
willingness
Willis
arterial circle of W.
W. centrum nervosum
circle of W.
W. circle aneurysm
W. circle developmental anomaly
W. cord
W. headache
W. nerve
posterior circle of W.
spontaneous occlusion of the circle of W.
W. valve
willisii
accessorius w.
chordae w.
Wilms tumor
Wilson
W. agnesis
W. disease
W. frame
W. hepatolenticular degeneration
W. rib spreader
W. syndrome
Wiltberger
W. anterior cervical approach
W. fusion
W. spinous process spreader
Wiltse
W. paraspinal approach
W. system
W. system aluminum master rod
W. system cross-bracing
W. system double-rod construct
W. system H construct
W. system single-rod construct
W. system spinal rod
Wiltse-Gelpi retractor
windage
wind contusion
window
acoustic bone w.
CT bone w.

wind-up
spinal w.-u.
wine
electric w.
wing
ashen w.
w. of central lobule
central lobule w.
w. of crista galli
gray w.
w. plate
sphenoid w.
wing-beating tremor
wingless gene
wink
anal w.
w. reflex
Winkelman disease
winking
jaw w.
w. spasm
Winquest tibial/femoral extraction system
Winquist tibial/femoral extraction system
Winslow concept
Winston-Lutz method
Wintrobe method
wire
Amplatz exchange length w.
Bentson exchange-length w.
Choice PT exchange w.
w. contour preparation
Drummond w.
w. extrusion
Fast Dasher 14 w.
guide w.
Kirschner w.
Luque w.
Mach 16 Select w.
Mullan w.
w. osteosynthesis
w. passage
w. penetration depth
w. removal technique
spinous process w.
w. stabilization
sublaminar w.
w. thrombosis
titanium w.
Transcend 14 w.
Wisconsin interspinous w.
Wisconsin spinous process w.
wiring
facet fracture stabilization w.
facet subluxation stabilization w.
posterior interspinous w.
spinous process w.
sublaminar w.
WISC-III
Wechsler Intelligence Scale for Children-Revised, Version III
Wisconsin
W. interspinous wire
W. Sleep Cohort Study
W. spinous process wire
WISC-R
Wechsler Intelligence Scale for Children-Revised
Wisniewski syndrome
withdrawal
caffeine w.
w. effect
w. emergent syndrome
emotional w.
estrogen w.
ethanol w.
neonatal opiate w.
newborn drug w.
perimenstrual progesterone w.
physical w.
w. process
w. reflex
substance w.
withdrawal-emergent dyskinesia
withdrawn
witness
w. to repetitive violence
w. to violence
Wittenborn
witzelsucht
WML
white matter lesion
WMS-R
Wechsler Memory Scale for Children, Russell version
***wnt* gene**
Wohlfart-Kugelberg-Welander
W.-K.-W. disease
W.-K.-W. syndrome
Wolf endoscope

NOTES

Wolff
W. headache
W. vasogenic theory
Wolf-Hirschhorn syndrome
Wolf-Orton body
Wolfram
W. needle electrode
W. syndrome
Wollaston theory
Wolman disease
womb
women
parkinsonian postmenopausal w.
physiology of w.
woodcutter's encephalitis
Woodson
W. dural separator
W. dural separator-spatula
W. dura packer
modification or W.
word
w. blindness
w. deafness
portmanteau w.
w. processing
w. production
w. retrieval
stimulus w.
word-finding
word-selection anomia
work
disaster w.
w. evaluation systems technology
gratifying w.
w. performance
w. schedule
volunteer w.
workaholic
worker
disaster w.
pink collar w.
white-collar w.
working
w. memory
w. memory function
workload
mental w.
workplace
work-related task
workstation
MKM w.
SUN w.
world
W. Federation of Neurological Surgeons scale (WFNS scale)
W. Federation of Neurosurgical Societies (WFNS)
W. Health Organization (WHO)
inner w.
intrapsychic w.
Worlpass Ninja balloon
wormian bone
worms
worry
severity of w.
worrying symptom
worsening
symptom w.
Wort
St. John's W.
worthlessness
wound
psychic w.
wounded
Wound-Evac drain
W-P
wrist-palm
WPPSI
wrap
cotton w.
Dura-Kold ice w.
wrapping of aneurysm
WRAT-R, pl. **Wide Range Achievement Test, Revised, Wide Range Achievement Test, Revised**
wrench
Texas Scottish Rite Hospital w.
T-handled nut w.
T-handled screw w.
T-handle nut w.
T-handle screw w.
Wright
W. Care TENS unit
W. syndrome
Wrisberg
W. ganglion
nerve of W.
W. nerve
wrist
w. clonus
w. clonus reflex
w. drop
wrist-drop
wristed
limp w.
wrist-palm (W-P)
wrist-to-abductor pollicis brevis (APB)
writer's cramp
writing
w. hand
wrongdoing
wrong-way deviation
wryneck
wry neck

WS
West syndrome
WT
wild-type
Würzburg
W. implant system
W. titanium plating system
Wyatt screening
Wyburn-Mason
W.-M. arteriovenous malformation
W.-M. syndrome
Wyler cylindrical subdural electrode

NOTES

X
X chromosome
X Knife
5.X]
X25 PCR
Xanax
xanchromatic
xanthine
x. oxidase
x. oxidase inhibitor
xanthoastrocytoma
pleomorphic x. (PXA)
xanthochromatic
xanthochromia of cerebrospinal fluid
xanthochromic
xanthocyanopsia
xanthogranuloma
xanthogranulomatous cyst
xanthoma
choroidal x.
xanthomatosis
cerebrotendinous x.
xanthomatous Rathke cleft cyst
xanthosarcoma
X-chromosome
phosphate-regulating gene with homologies to endopeptidases on the X.-c.
Xe
xenon
Xe clearance method
^{133}Xe
xenon-133
^{133}Xe intravenous injection technique
XeCT
xenon-enhanced computed tomography
X. CBF study
X. scanning
XenoDerm
xenogeneic
x. chromaffin cell
x. graft
xenograft
glioblastoma x.
xenomania
xenon (Xe)
x. computed tomography
x. CT
x. CT cerebral blood flow
x. CT measurement
x. CT scanning
x. inhalation
x. method
xenon-133 (^{133}Xe)
xenon-CT
xenon-enhanced
x.-e. computed tomography (XeCT)
x.-e. CT
x.-e. CT scanning
xeroderma pigmentosum
xerodermic idiocy
XeScan
Linde X.
^{133}XeSPECT contrast medium
***x* gradient**
Xia
X. hook system
X. spinal system
xiphodynia
xiphoidalgia
XK-95
Komet XK-95
XKnife
XL illuminator
X-linked
X-l. abnormality
X-l. anophthalmia
X-l. Charcot-Marie-Tooth disease
X-l. cortical migration disorder
X-l. hydrocephalus
X-l. lissencephaly
X-l. lymphoproliferative syndrome
X-l. recessive bulbospinal neuronopathy
X-l. recessive muscular dystrophy
X-l. recessive spinobulbar muscular atrophy
X-l. spastic paraparesis
Xomed nerve integrity monitor-2
Xomed-Treace nerve integrity monitor-2
X-O test
Xp21 myopathy
Xphoria
Xpress 100 disposable perforator burr hole drill
XR
Adderall XR
x-ray
artifact on x-r.
x-r. exposure
intraoperative x-r.
isocentric linear accelerator x-r.
x-r. localization
orthogonal x-r.

x-ray *(continued)*
plain x-r.
x-r. therapy (XRT)

XRT
x-ray therapy

X-Trel spinal cord stimulation system

X-Trozine

XXX syndrome

xyrospasm

^{90}Y
radioactive yttrium
Yale
Y. brace
Y. Global Tic Severity Scale (YGTSS)
Y. Tic Severity Scale
Yale-Brown
Yankauer suction tube
Yasargil
Y. arachnoid knife
Y. artery forceps
Y. bayonet forceps
Y. bayonet scissors
Y. carotid clamp
Y. clip-applying forceps
Y. craniotomy
Y. cross-legged clip
Y. elevator
Y. flat serrated ring forceps
Y. hypophysial forceps
Y. instrument
Y. knotting forceps
Y. Leyla retractor arm
Y. ligature carrier
Y. ligature guide
Y. microclip
Y. micro curette
Y. microcurette
Y. micro dissector
Y. microdissector
Y. micro forceps
Y. microforceps
Y. microrasp
Y. microscissors
Y. microvascular knife
Y. needle holder
Y. OptiMat floor stand
Y. pituitary rongeur
Y. rasp
Y. retractor
Y. scoop
Y. spring hook
Y. suction tube
Y. tissue lifter
Y. titanium aneurysm clip
Y. tumor forceps
Y. vessel clip
Yasargil-Aesculap
Y.-A. instrument
Y.-A. spring clip
Yasargil-Leyla
Y.-L. brain retractor
Y.-L. brain retractor z-gradient coil
Years
Disability Adjusted Life Y.
Functional Fitness Assessment for Adults over 60 Y.
yeh
yellow
y. fever
y. fever encephalitis
y. ligament
y. softening
y. spot
Yersinia enterocolitica
***y* gradient**
YGTSS
Yale Global Tic Severity Scale
Y incision
YMRS
Young Mania Rating Scale
yoga
Kundalini y.
Yohimbe
yohimbe
Pausinystalia y.
yoke
double y.
You
Who Are Y.
Young-Helmholtz trichromacy theory
Young Mania Rating Scale (YMRS)
young-old
youngster
youth
y. self support
y. violence
youthquake
yo-yo syndrome
Y-shaped reference arc
yttrium
radioactive y. (^{90}Y)
yttrium-90

Y

Z
Z coordinate
Z disk
Z score map
Z score transformation
zalcitabine
Zaleplon
zaleplon
Zanaflex
Zanarini concept
zaniness
Zantac
Zantryl
Zaraflex
Zarit burden interview
Zarontin
Zaroxolyn
Zaxopam
zazen
Z-band in nemaline myopathy
ZD
ZD frame
ZD stereotactic system
ZD-Neurosurgical localizing unit
zealousness
zebra body
Zeigarnik
Zeiss
Z. Axiovert microscope
Z. IIIRS photomicroscope
Z. Image Guided System
Z. MKM microscope
Z. operating microscope
Z. OpMi CS-NC2 surgical microscope
Z. OpMi CS-NC2 surgical microscope system
Z. OPMI Neuro/NC4 surgical microscope
Z. stereotactic tool navigator system
Z. STN surgical tool navigator
Z. Super Lux 40 light source
Zeiss-Contraves operating microscope
Zeitgeber
Zeitgebers
social Z.
Zeldox
Zellballen
Zellweger syndrome
Zen
Zenker
Z. paralysis
Z. solution
ZEPHIR system
Zephyr anterior cervical plate system
Zeppelin micro-motor system
zero
z. cerebral pseudotumor cerebri
z. drift of the sensor
z. ICP ventricle shunt
physiologic z.
protein z.
zero-order elimination kinetics
zest
Zestoretic
zeta/beta
receptor protein tyrosine phosphatase z. (RPTP zeta/beta)
RPTP z.
receptor protein tyrosine phosphatase zeta/beta
zeta-glucosaminide
zeta method
Zetran
zeugmatography
Fourier transformation z.
z-gradient
z.-g. coil
z.-g. field
***zic* gene**
zidovudine
z. and lamivudine
Ziehen-Oppenheim disease
Zielke
Z. bifid hook
Z. instrument
Z. instrumentation
Z. VDS implant
Ziemssen motor point
zifrosilone
Zika fever
Zimmer
Z. caudal hook
Z. clip
Z. microsaw
Zimmerlin atrophy
zinc
z. acetate
z. protoporphyrin level
zinc-finger
z.-f. family
z.-f. gene
Zinn
annulus of Z.
Z. corona
Z. vascular circle
Zinsser-Cole-Engman syndrome

ziprasidone
z. HCl
z. hydrochloride
z. mesylate
Zocor
zodiac
zol
zolazepam
Zollinger-Ellison syndrome
zolmitriptan
Zoloft
zolpidem tartrate
Zomaril
Zomax
zombie-like
zometapine
Zomig
Zomig-ZMT
ZON
zonisamide
zona, pl. **zonae**
z. dermatica
z. epithelioserosa
z. hypothalamicae
z. incerta
z. lateralis
z. medialis
z. medullovasculosa
z. ophthalmica
z. periventricularis
z. rolandica
zonal
z. layer of cerebral cortex
z. layer of superior colliculus
z. layer of thalamus
zonale
stratum z.
zone
active z.
analectrotonic z.
arterial border z.
chemosensitive z.
cornuradicular z.
dolorogenic z.
dorsal root entry z. (DREZ)
entry z.
ependymal z.
epileptogenic z.
Flechsig primordial z.
H z.
Head z.
hyperalgesic z.
z. of hypothalamus
ictal onset z.
intermediate z.
irritative z.
language z.
latent z.
lateral z.
Lissauer marginal z.
Marchant z.
marginal z.
medial z.
medullary inhibitory z.
motor z.
Obersteiner-Redlich z.
z. of partial preservation
periventricular z.
reflexogenic z.
root entry z.
spike-initiation z.
Spitzka marginal z.
subventricular z.
tender z.
trigger z.
vomeronasal z.
watershed z.
Wernicke z.
Westphal z.
Zonegran capsule
zonesthesia
zonifugal
zonipetal
zonisamide (ZON)
z. capsule
zonular layer
zoogonous
zoogony
zoom microscope
zoophile
zoophilic
zopiclone
ZORprin
zoster
z. encephalomyelitis
herpes z.
z. immune globulin
measles, rubella and z. (MRZ)
ophthalmic z.
z. ophthalmic
z. paresis
z. sine herpete
z. virus infection
Zostrix
zotepine
Z-plate
Z.-p. anterior thoracolumbar instrumentation
Z.-p. fixation system
z-touch laser device
Zuckerkandl
Z. convolution
organ of Z.
zuclopenthixol

Zülch
giant cell monstrocellular sarcoma of Z.
Zung Anxiety Scale
Zyban
Zydis
Z. drug delivery technology
Zyprexa Z.
zygal fissure
zygapophyseal joint
zygoma
zygomatic
z. fracture
z. nerve
z. reflex
z. resection approach
zygomatici
ramus zygomaticofacialis nervi z.
ramus zygomaticotemporalis nervi z.
zygomatico
ramus communicans nervi lacrimalis cum nervo z.
zygomaticofacial branch of zygomatic nerve
zygomaticoorbital artery
zygomaticotemporal branch of zygomatic nerve
zygomaticus
nervus z.
zygomycosis
rhinocerebral z.
zygon
zygosis
zygosity
zygote
Zyprexa Zydis

NOTES

Z

Appendix 1
Anatomical Illustrations

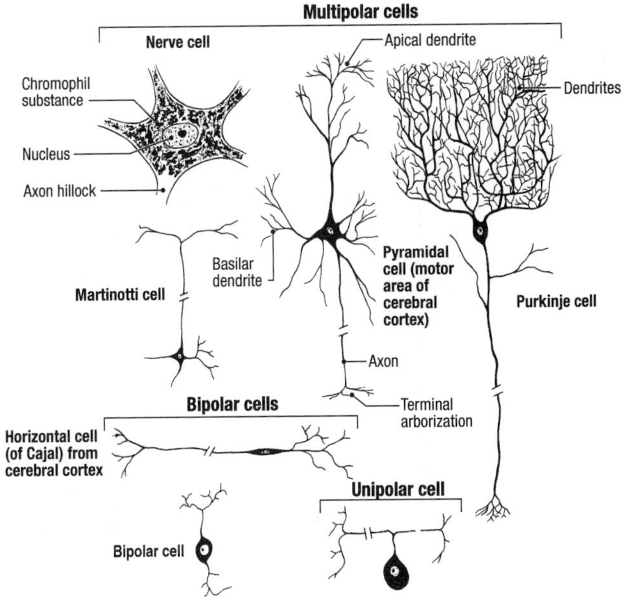

Figure 1. Types of neurons.

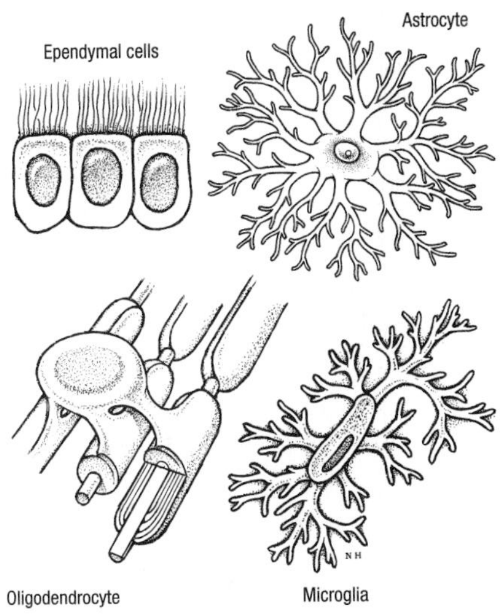

Figure 2. Neuroglia. Supporting structures of the nervous system.

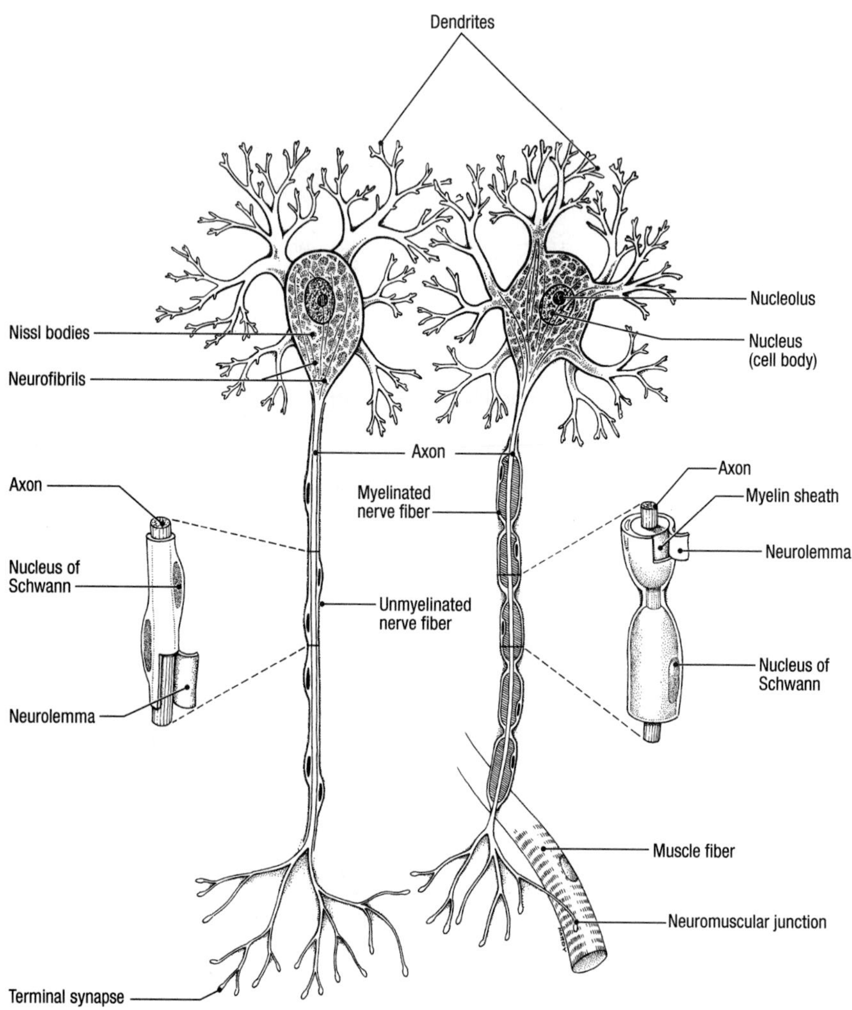

Figure 3. Myelinated and unmyelinated neurons.

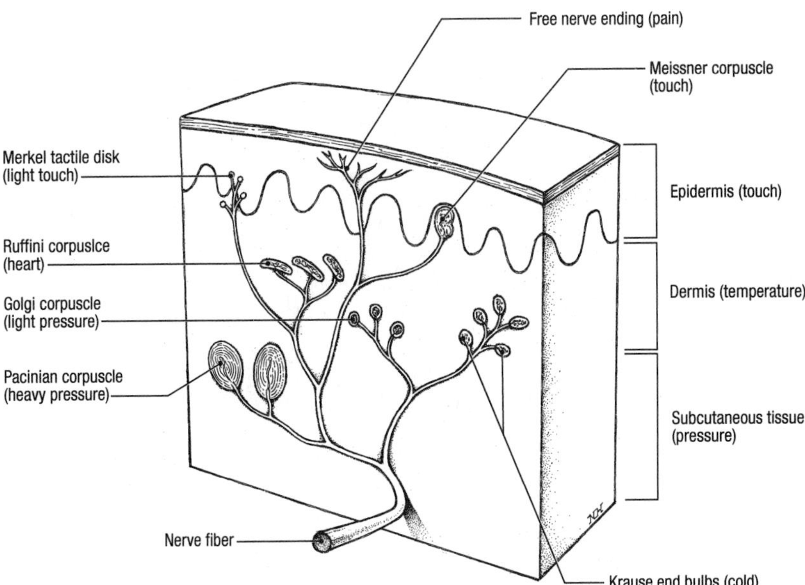

Figure 4. Sensory nerves and bodies.

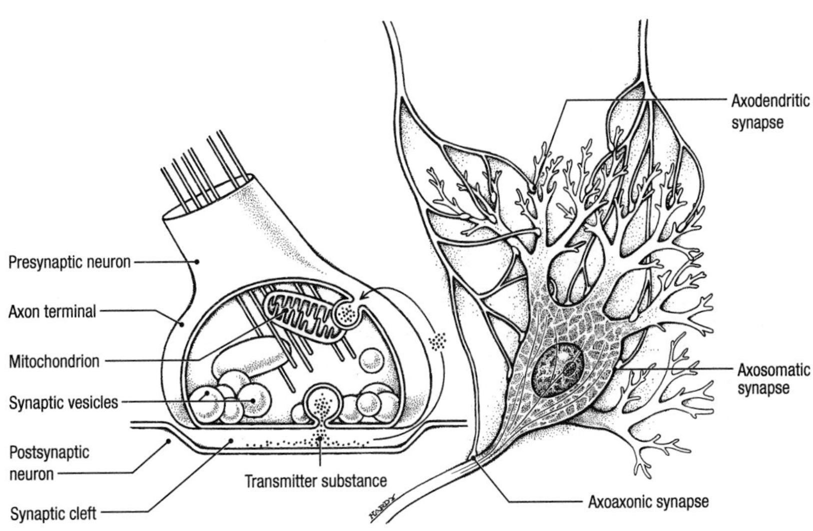

Figure 5. Nerve synapse.

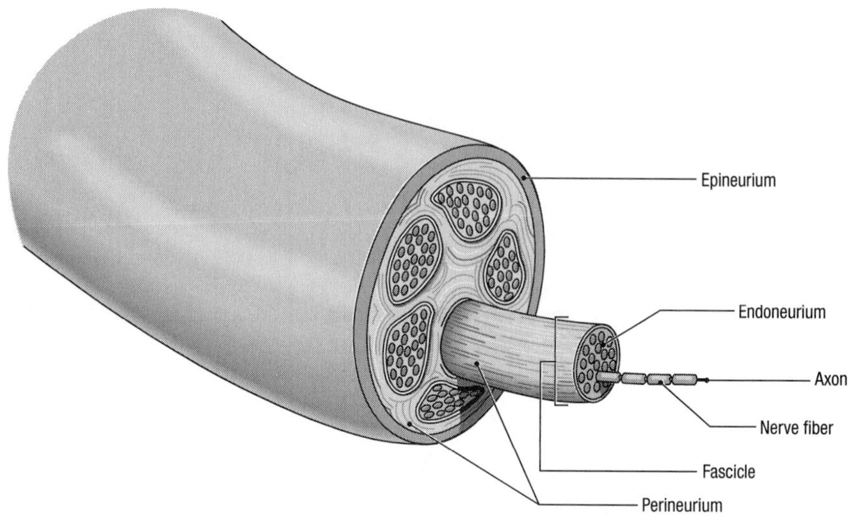

Figure 6. Peripheral nerve; outside surface or surrounding area of an organ or structure.

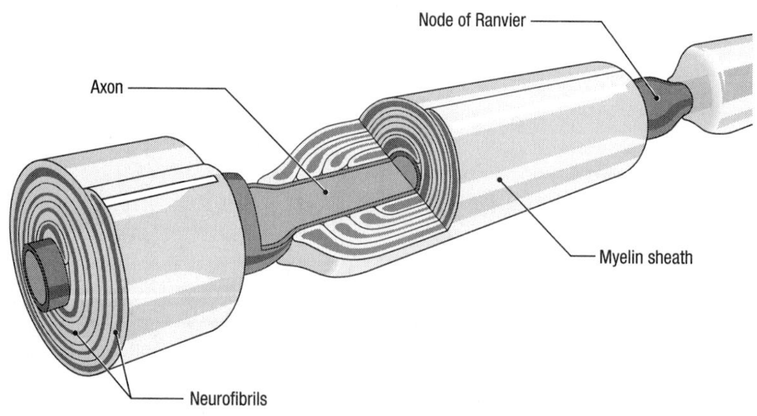

Figure 7. Axon, myelin sheath and node of Ranvier.

Diameter of fiber thickness	Histology	Fiber groups		Conduction speed	Function
1–22 μm			α	80–120 m/sec	Motor impulses, afferent impulses from muscle spindles and tendon organs.
			β	60 m/sec	Tactile impulses of the skin.
3–20 μm	Thick fibers with relatively. Thick myelin sheaths.	A	γ	40 m/sec	Efferent impulses to the contractile portions of intrafusal muscle fibers.
			δ	20 m/sec	Mechanoreceptor impulses; cold, warm, and painful sensations of the skin (fast).
1–3 μm	Thin fibers or thin myelin sheaths.	B		10 m/sec	Preganglionic vegetative fibers
1 μm	Fibers without sheaths.	C		1 m/sec	Postganglionic vegetative fibers and afferent fibers of the sympathetic trunk, impulses of mechanoreceptors, cold and warm receptors (slow).

Figure 8. Nerve fiber groups.

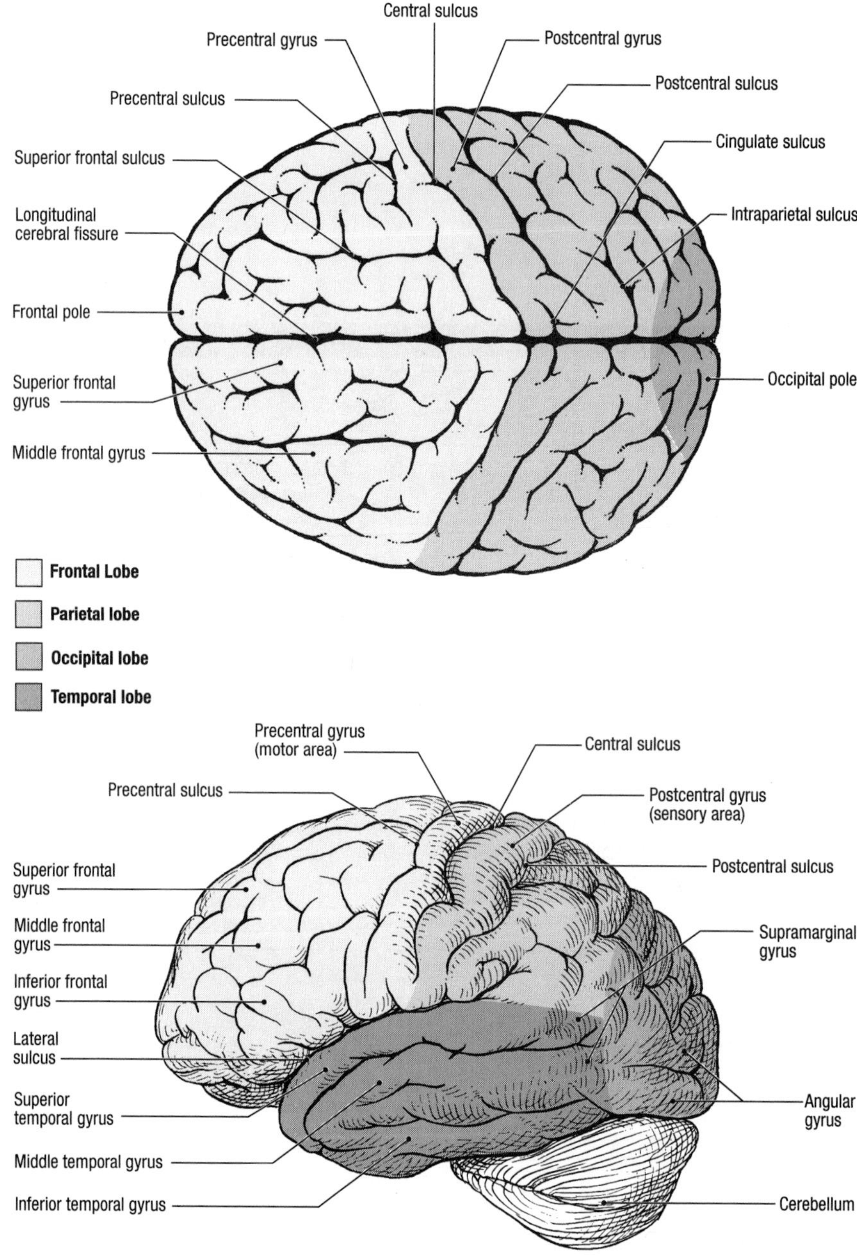

Figure 9. Brain, superior view (top) and lateral view (bottom).

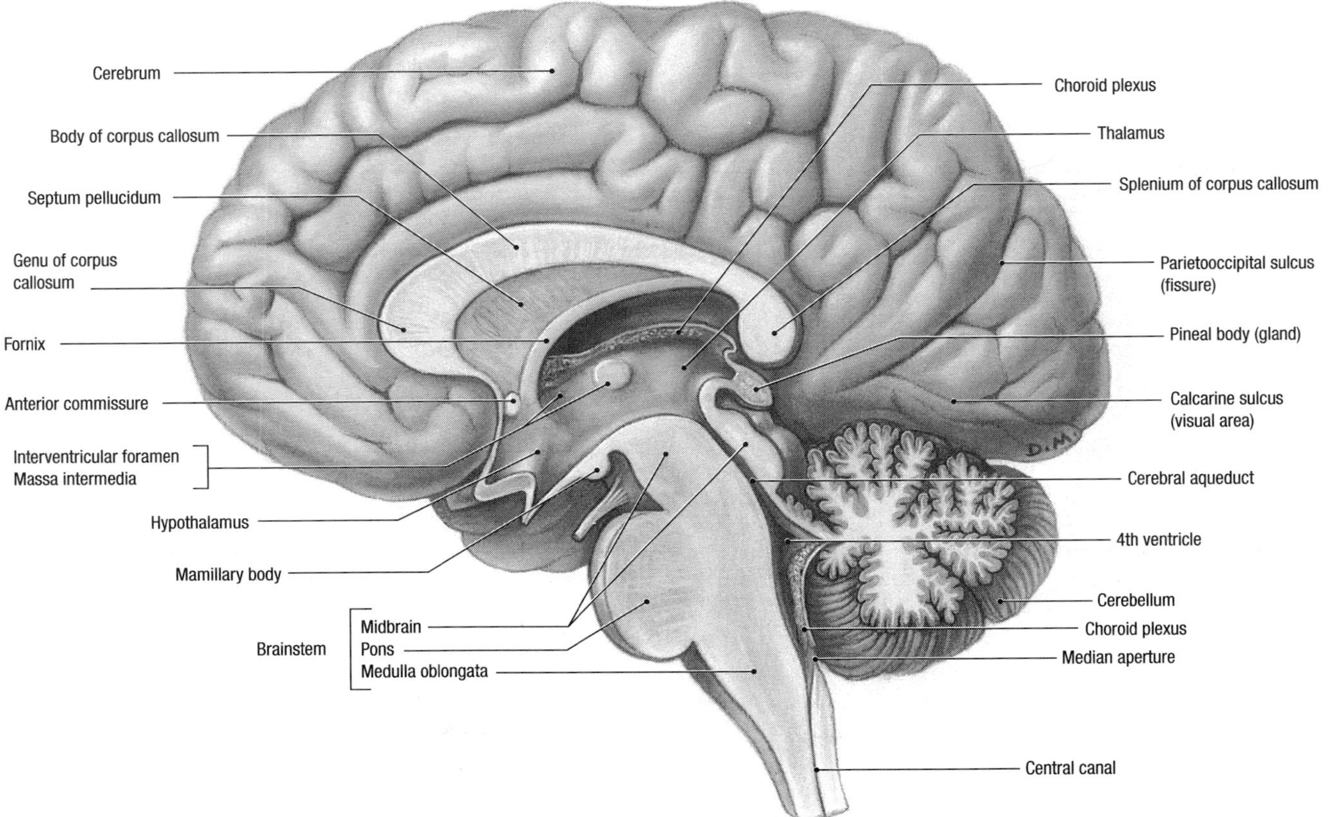

Cerebrum
Body of corpus callosum
Septum pellucidum
Genu of corpus callosum
Fornix
Anterior commissure
Interventricular foramen
Massa intermedia
Hypothalamus
Mamillary body
Brainstem
Midbrain
Pons
Medulla oblongata
Choroid plexus
Thalamus
Splenium of corpus callosum
Parietooccipital sulcus (fissure)
Pineal body (gland)
Calcarine sulcus (visual area)
Cerebral aqueduct
4th ventricle
Cerebellum
Choroid plexus
Median aperture
Central canal

Figure 10. Brain, median section.

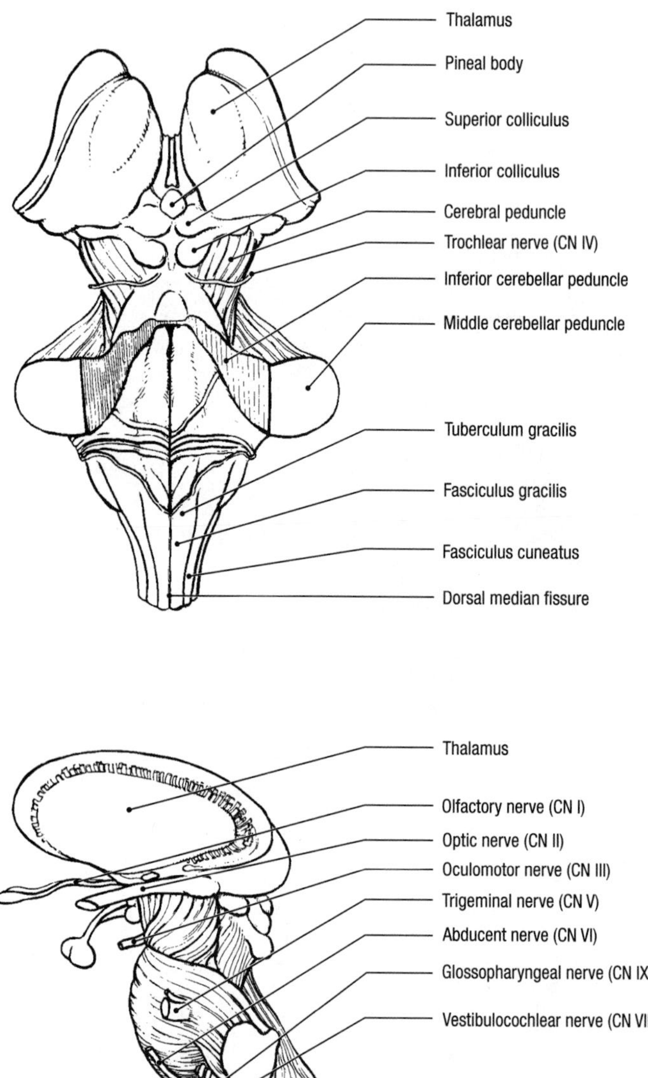

Figure 11. Brainstem, dorsal view (top) and lateral view (bottom).

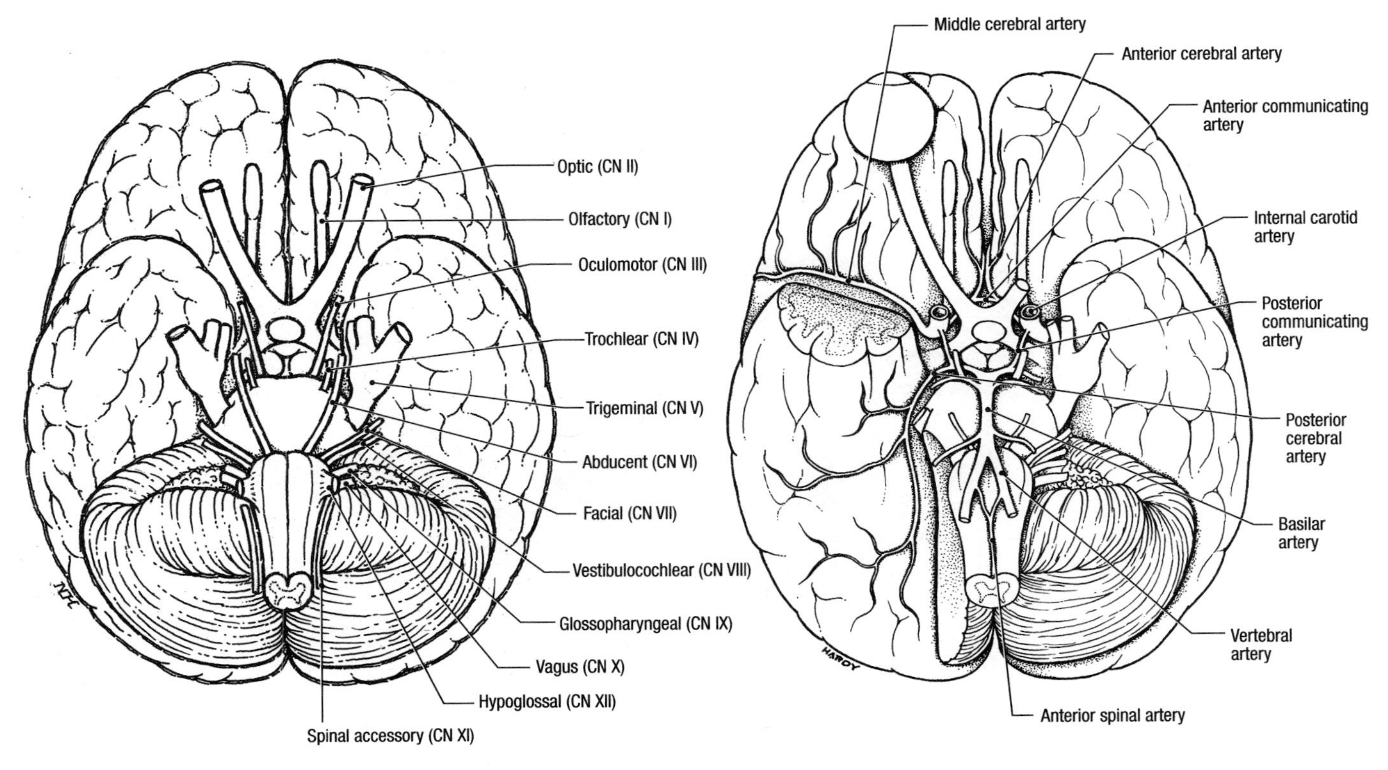

Figure 12. Cranial nerves.

Figure 13. Vascular network at the base of the brain.

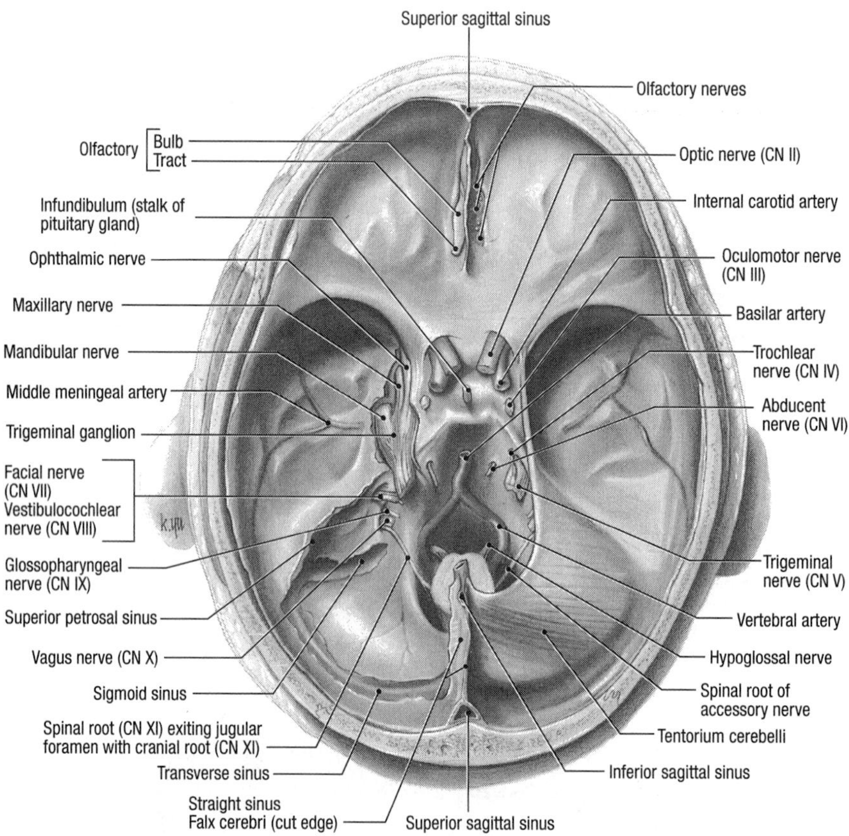

Figure 14. Nerves and vessels of the interior of base of skull, superior view.

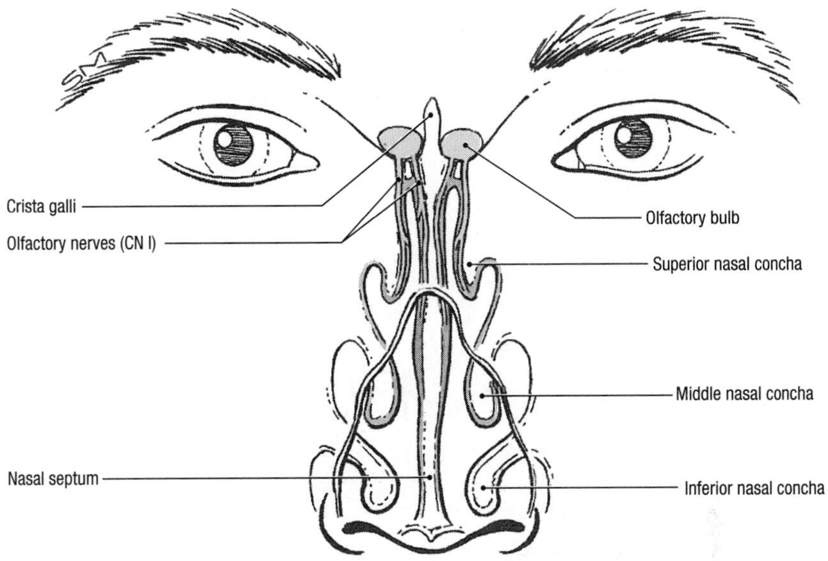

Figure 15. Olfactory nerves (CN I), anterior view.

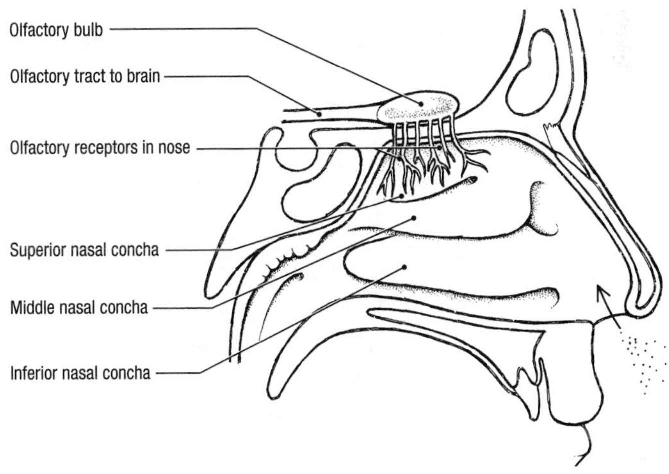

Figure 16. Olfaction.

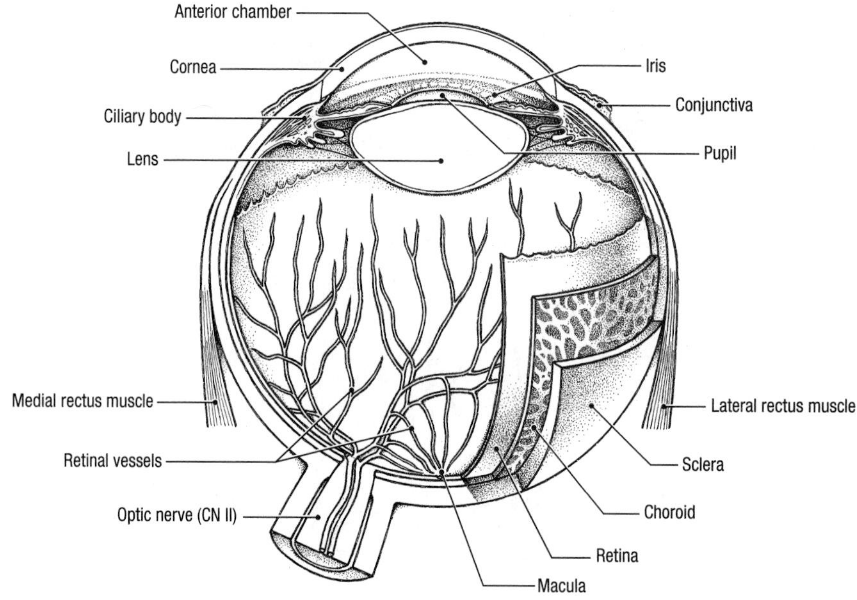

Figure 17. Optic nerve (CN II) and structures of the eye.

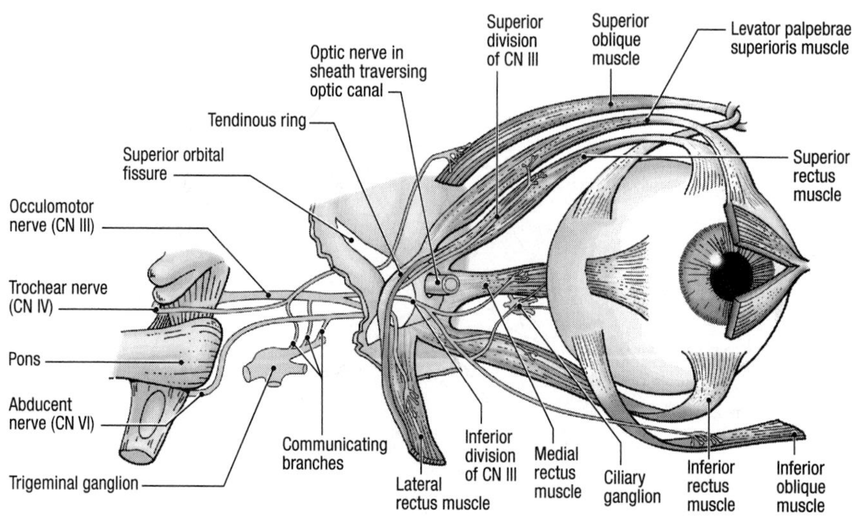

Figure 18. Oculomotor nerve (CN III), trochlear nerve (CN IV), and abducent nerve CN VI).

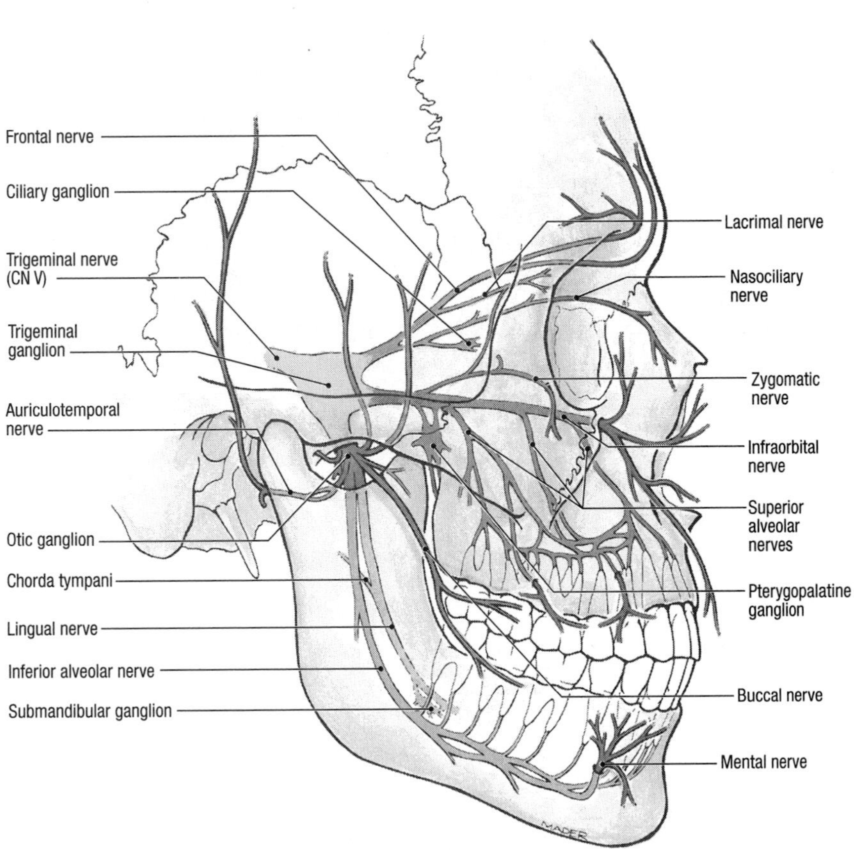

Figure 19. Distribution of the trigeminal nerve (CN V).

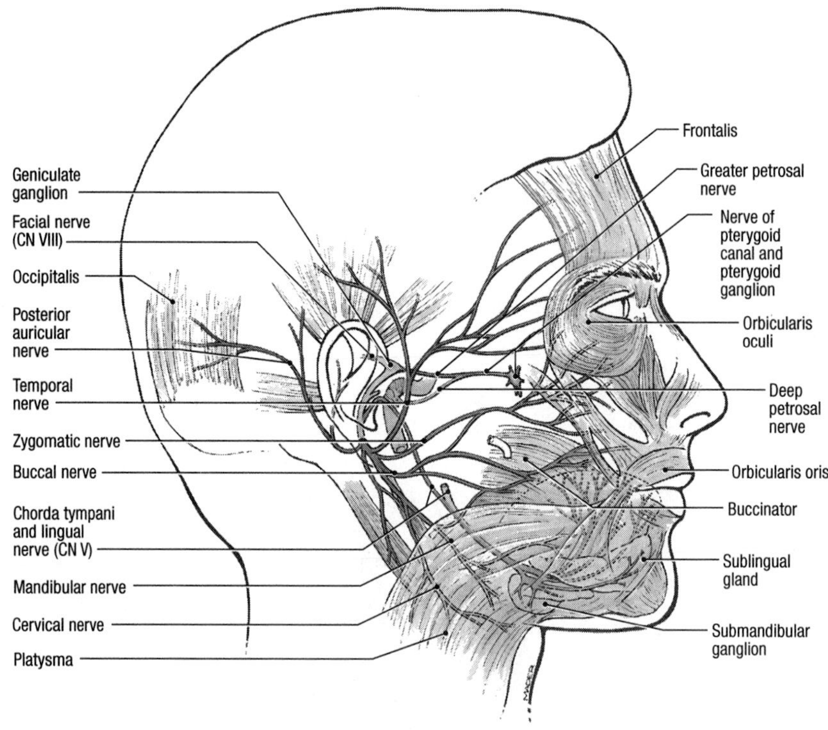

Figure 20. Facial nerve (CN VII).

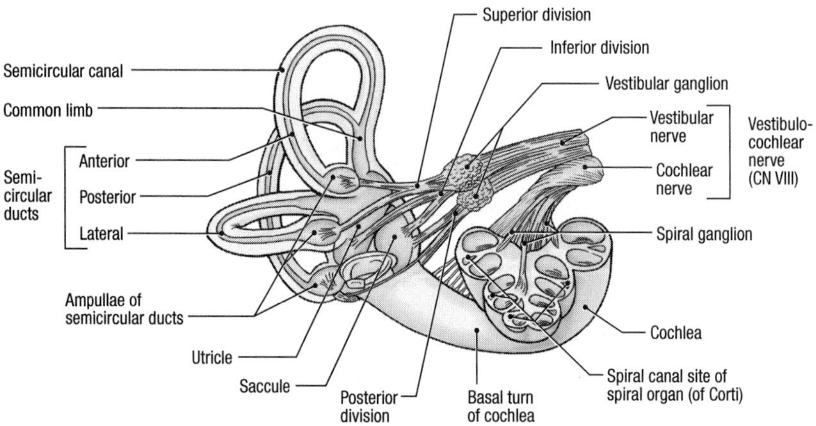

Figure 21. Vestibulocochlear nerve (CN VIII).

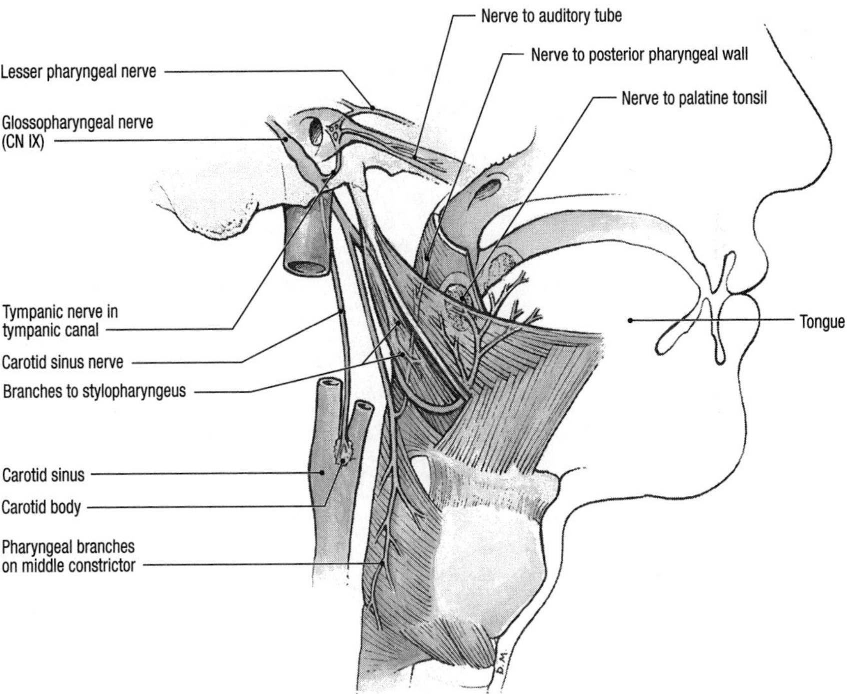

Figure 22. Glossopharyngeal nerve (CN IX).

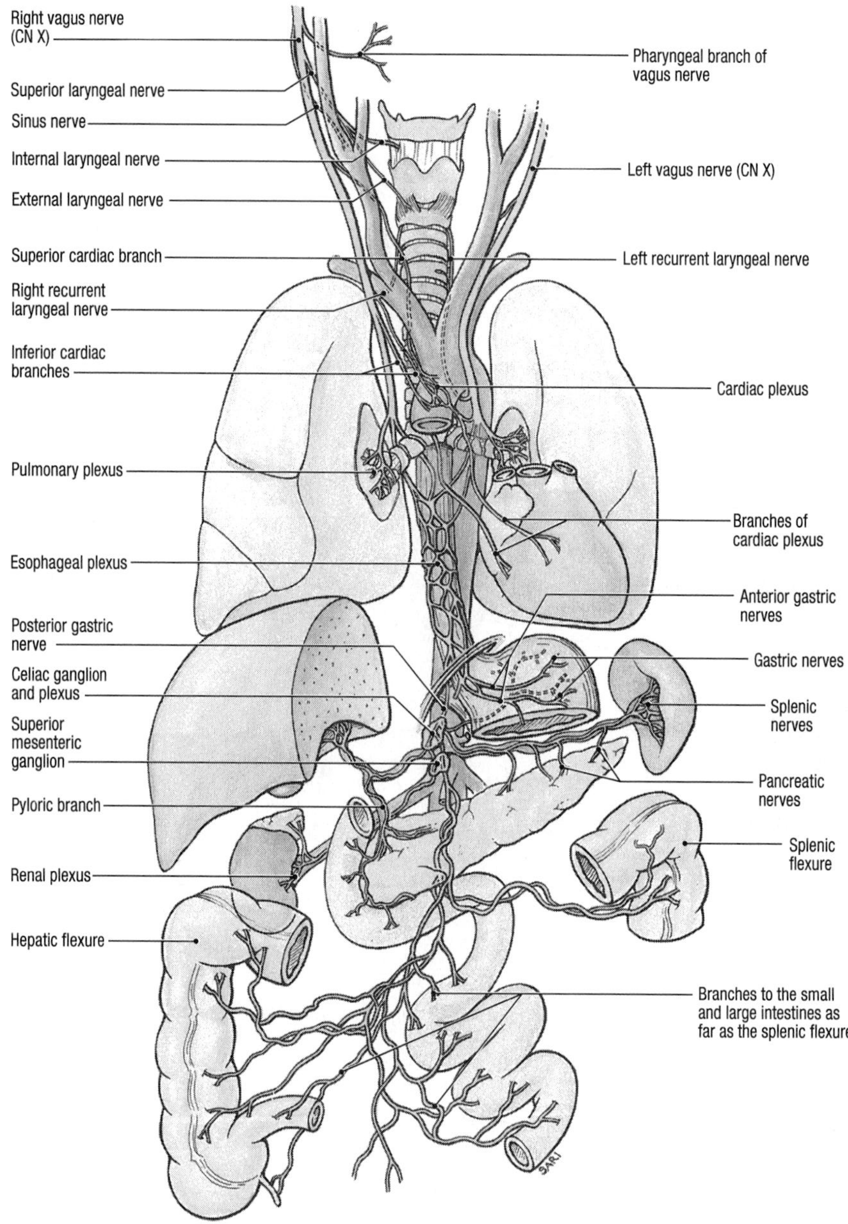

Figure 23. Distribution of the vagus nerve (CN X).

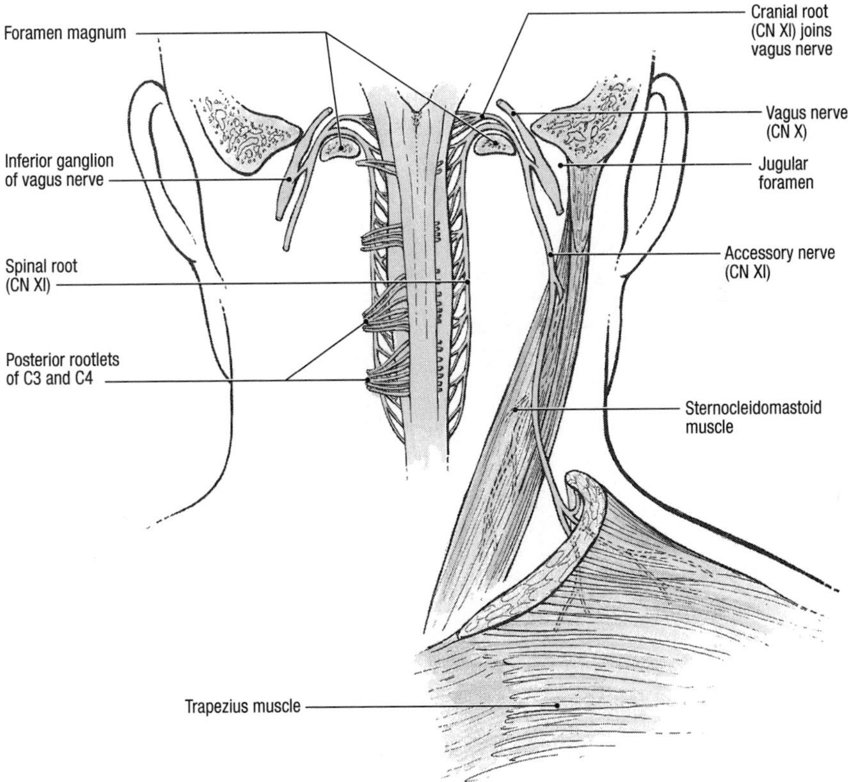

Figure 24. Distribution of the accessory nerve (CN XI).

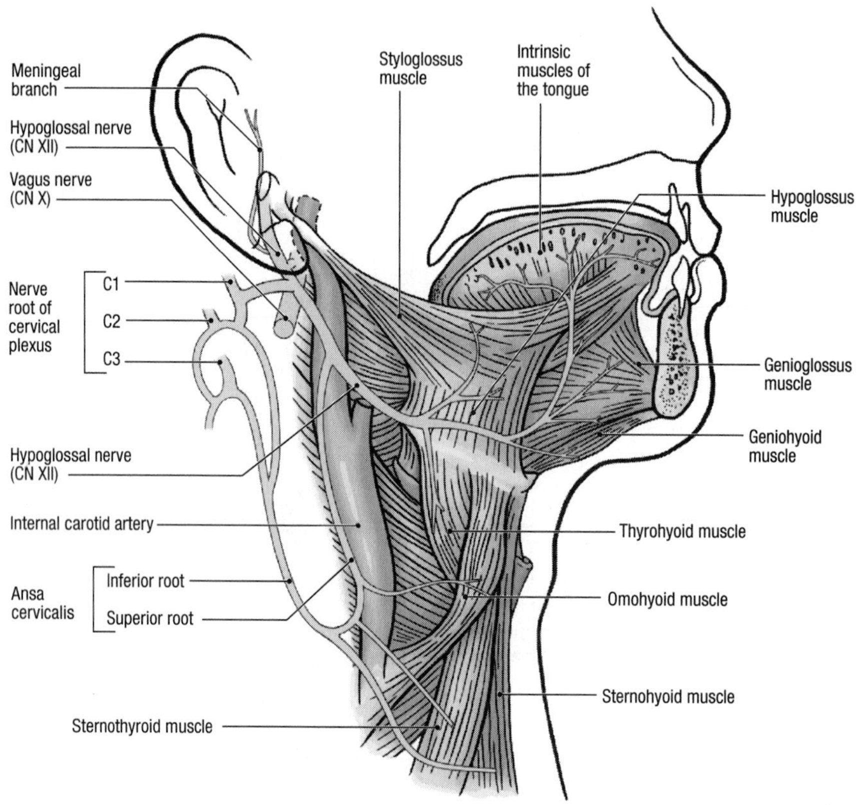

Figure 25. Distribution of the hypoglossal nerve (CN XII).

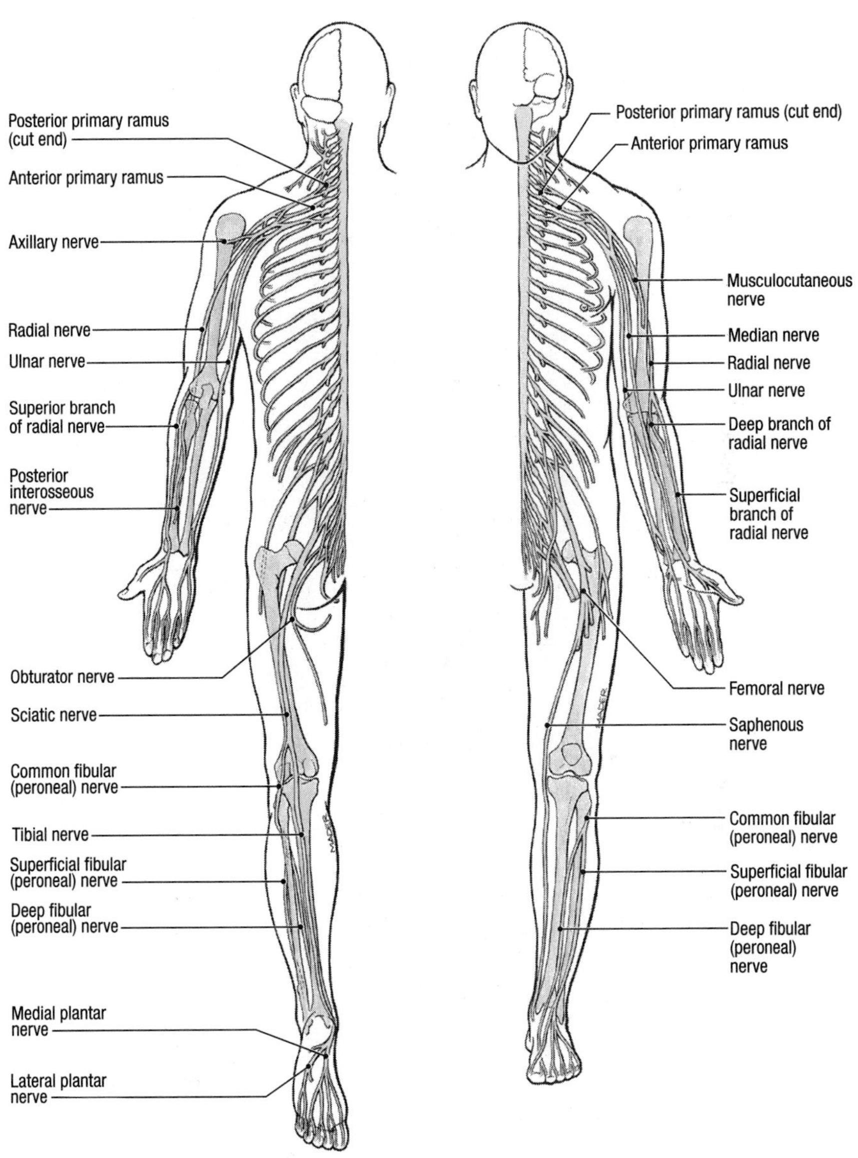

Figue 26. Overview of the nervous system, posterior view (left) and anterior view (right).

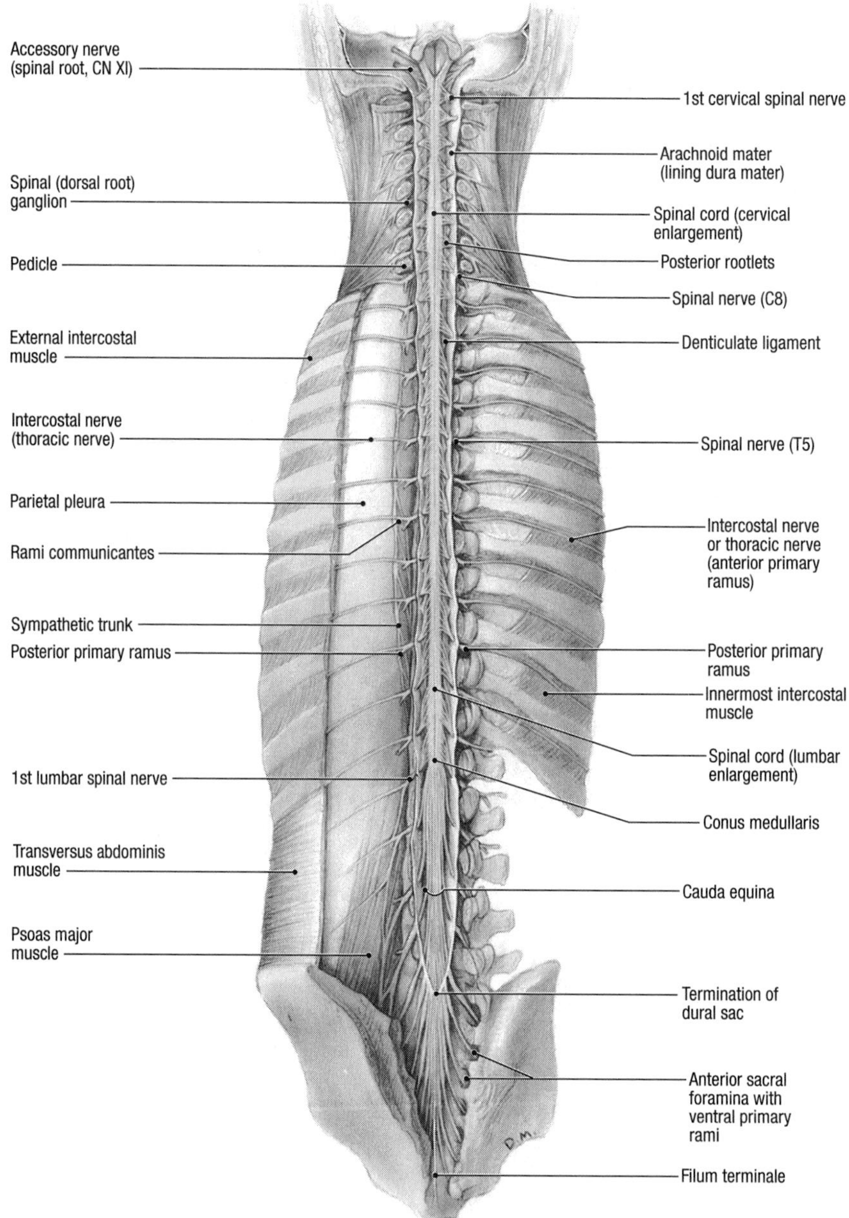
Accessory nerve
(spinal root, CN XI)
1st cervical spinal nerve
Arachnoid mater
(lining dura mater)
Spinal (dorsal root)
ganglion
Spinal cord (cervical
enlargement)
Pedicle
Posterior rootlets
Spinal nerve (C8)
External intercostal
muscle
Denticulate ligament
Intercostal nerve
(thoracic nerve)
Spinal nerve (T5)
Parietal pleura
Intercostal nerve
or thoracic nerve
(anterior primary
ramus)
Rami communicantes
Sympathetic trunk
Posterior primary ramus
Posterior primary
ramus
Innermost intercostal
muscle
Spinal cord (lumbar
enlargement)
1st lumbar spinal nerve
Conus medullaris
Transversus abdominis
muscle
Cauda equina
Psoas major
muscle
Termination of
dural sac
Anterior sacral
foramina with
ventral primary
rami
Filum terminale

Figure 27. Spinal cord and surrounding structures, posterior view

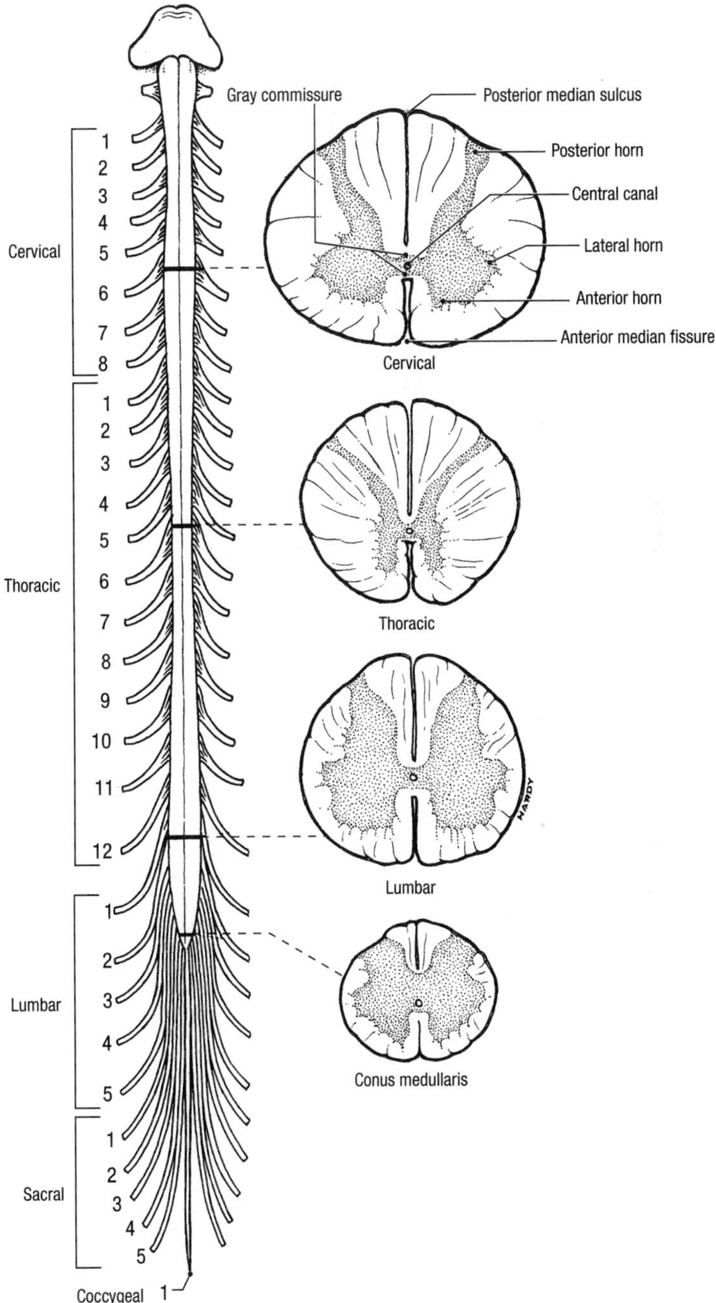

Figure 28. Spinal cord showing cross-sections at various levels.

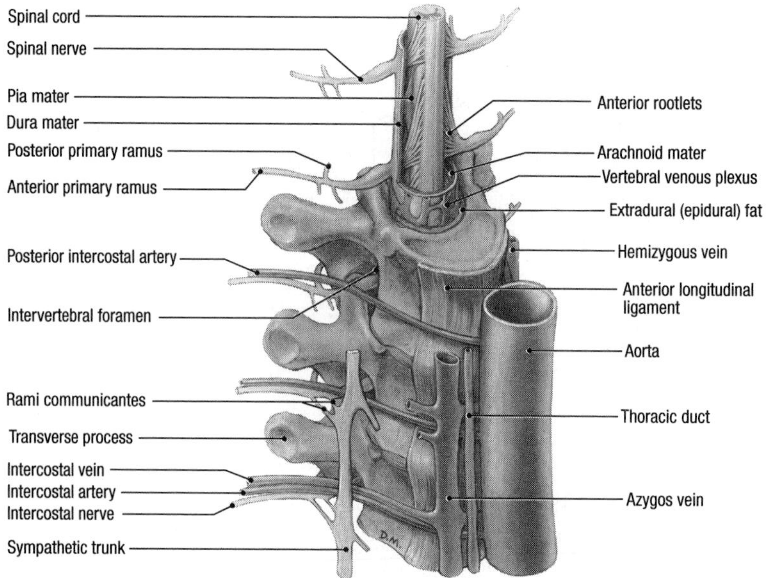

Figure 29. Spinal cord and prevertebral structures.

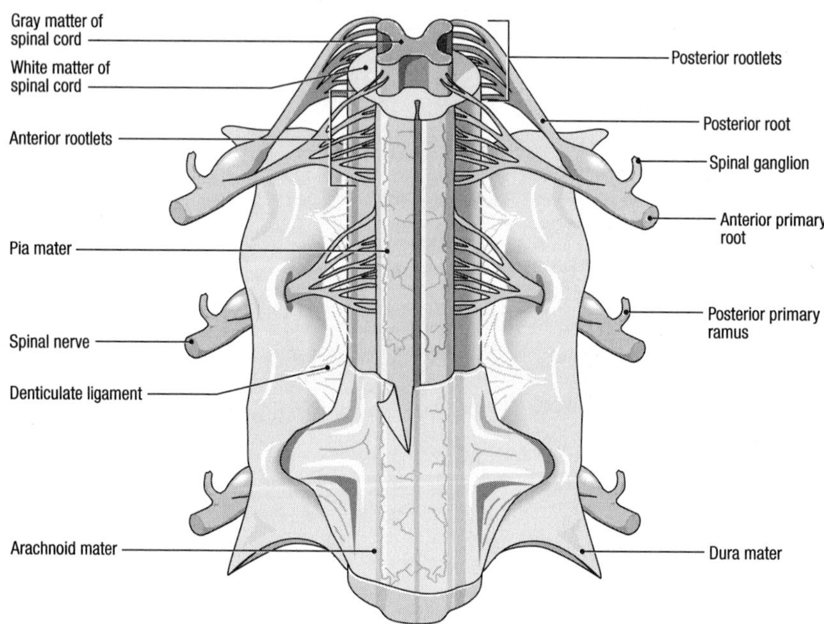

Figure 30. Open view of the compartments of the spinal cord showing the various meninges and the spinal nerves.

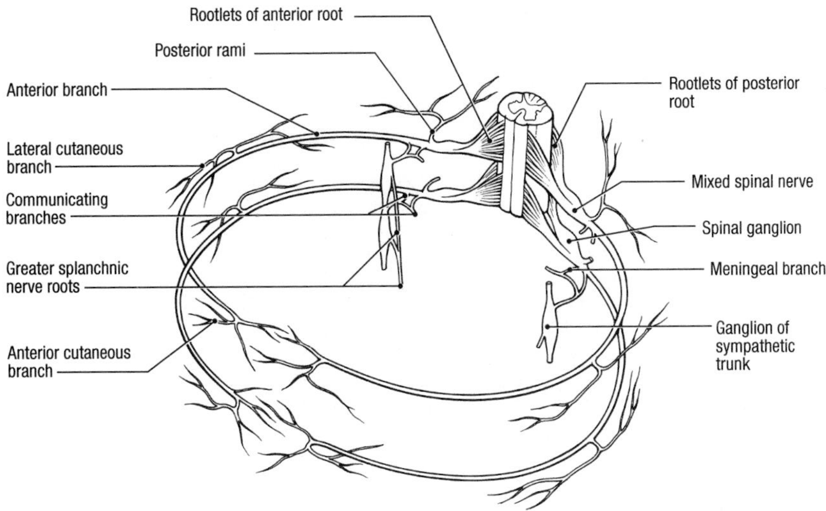

Figure 31. Spinal nerves, with roots and branches.

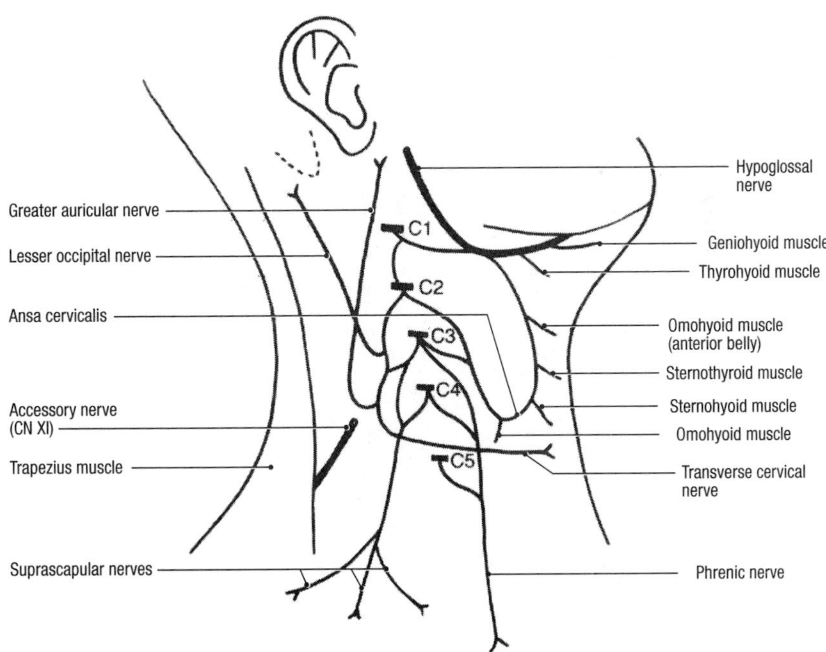

Figure 32. Cervical plexus.

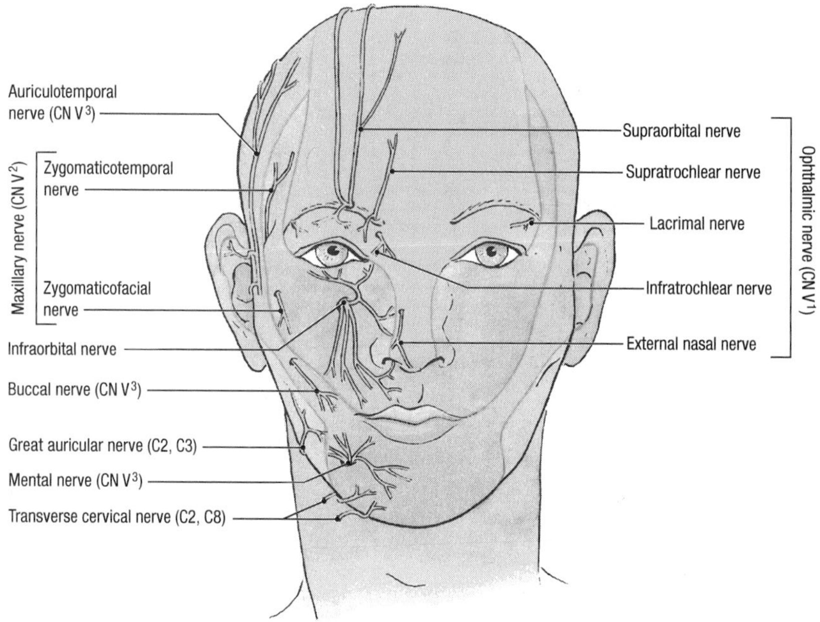

Figure 33. Sensory nerves of the face and scalp, anterior view.

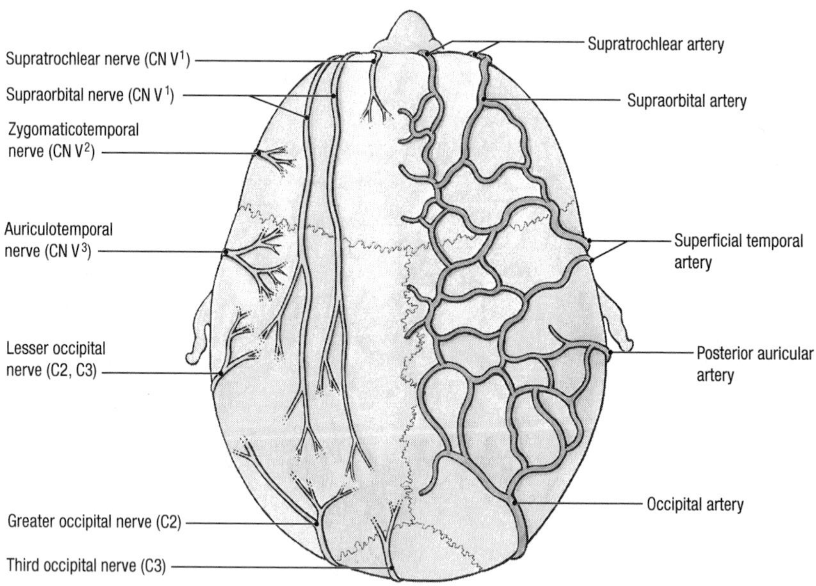

Figure 34. Sensory nerves and arteries of the face and scalp, superior view.

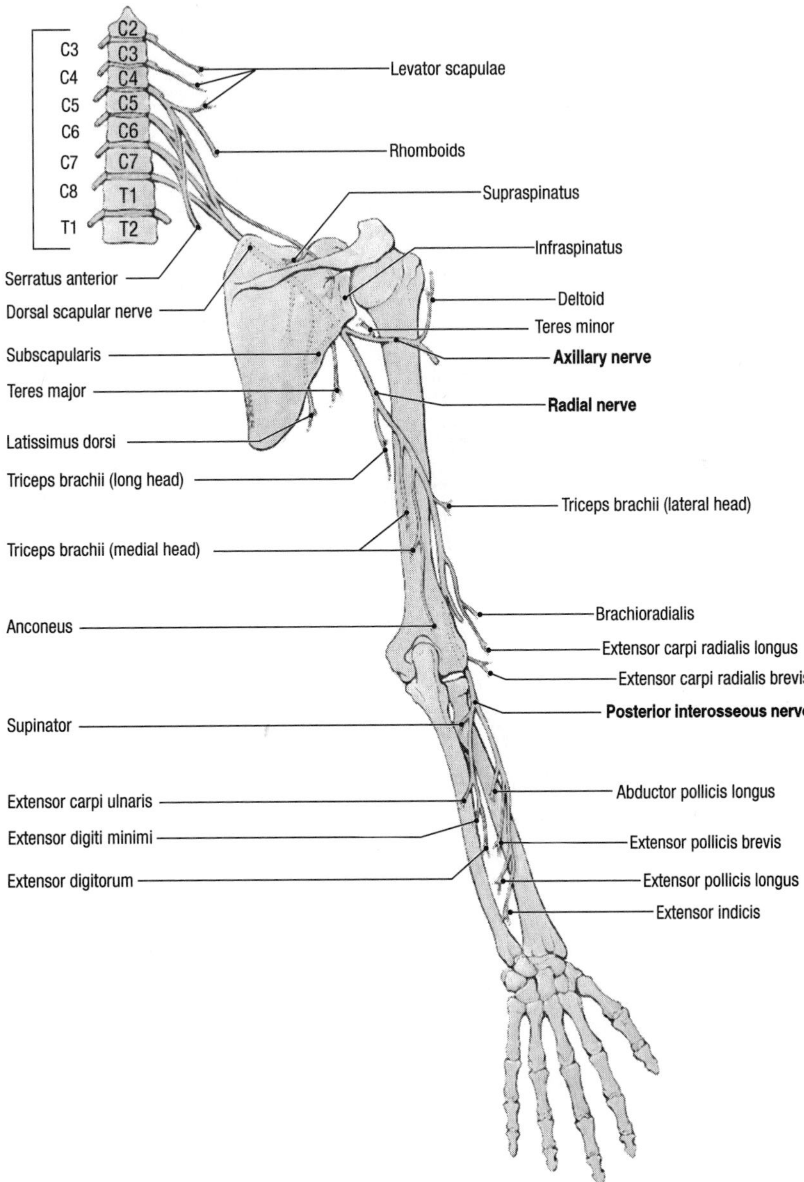

Figure 35. Innervation of the upper limb muscles, radial nerve.

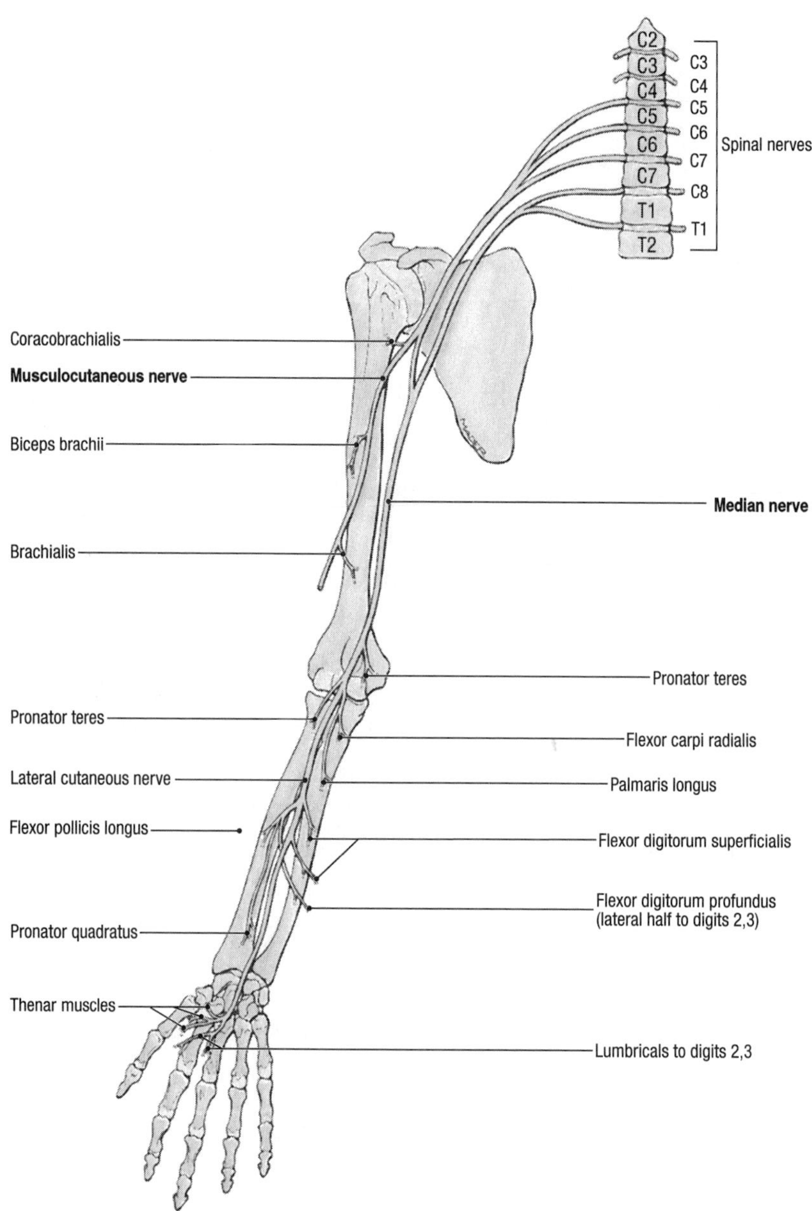

Figure 36. Innervation of the upper limb muscles, median and musculocutaneous nerves.

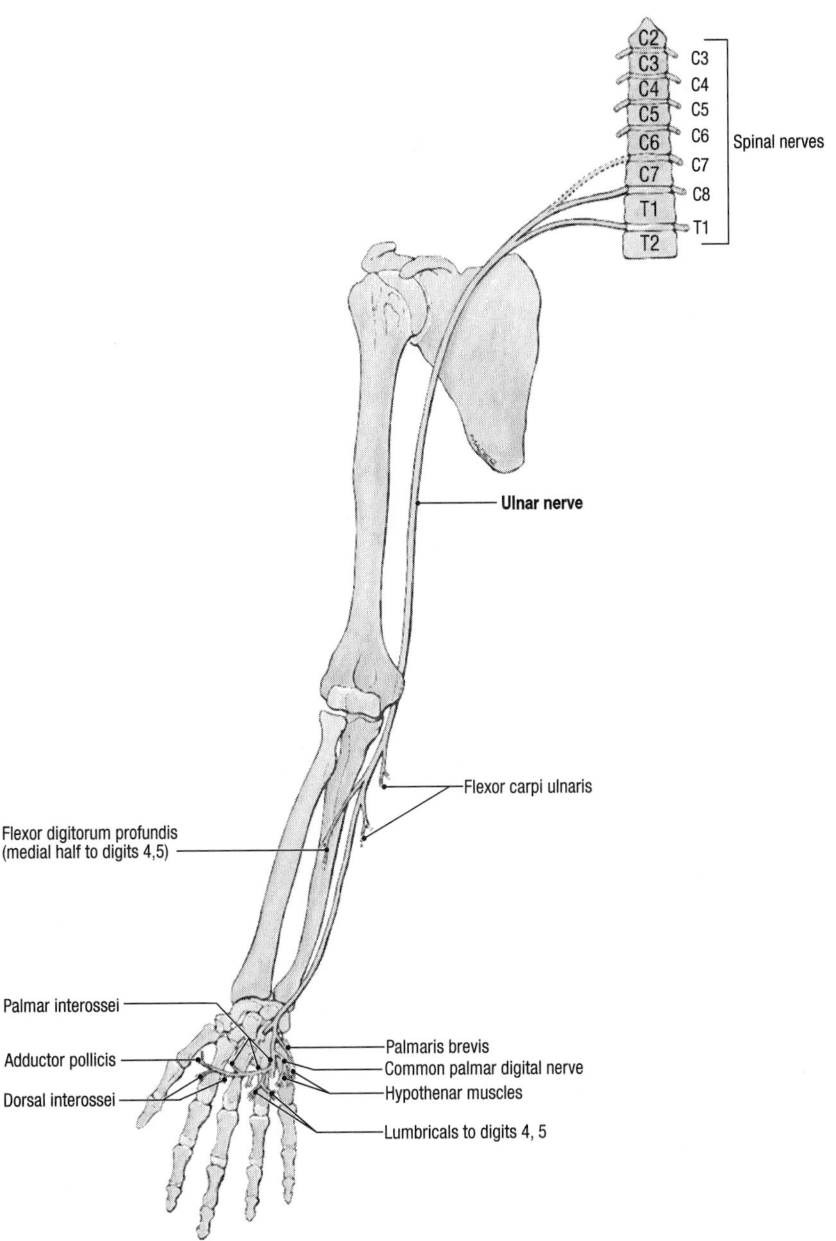

Figure 37. Innervation of the upper limb muscles, ulnar nerve.

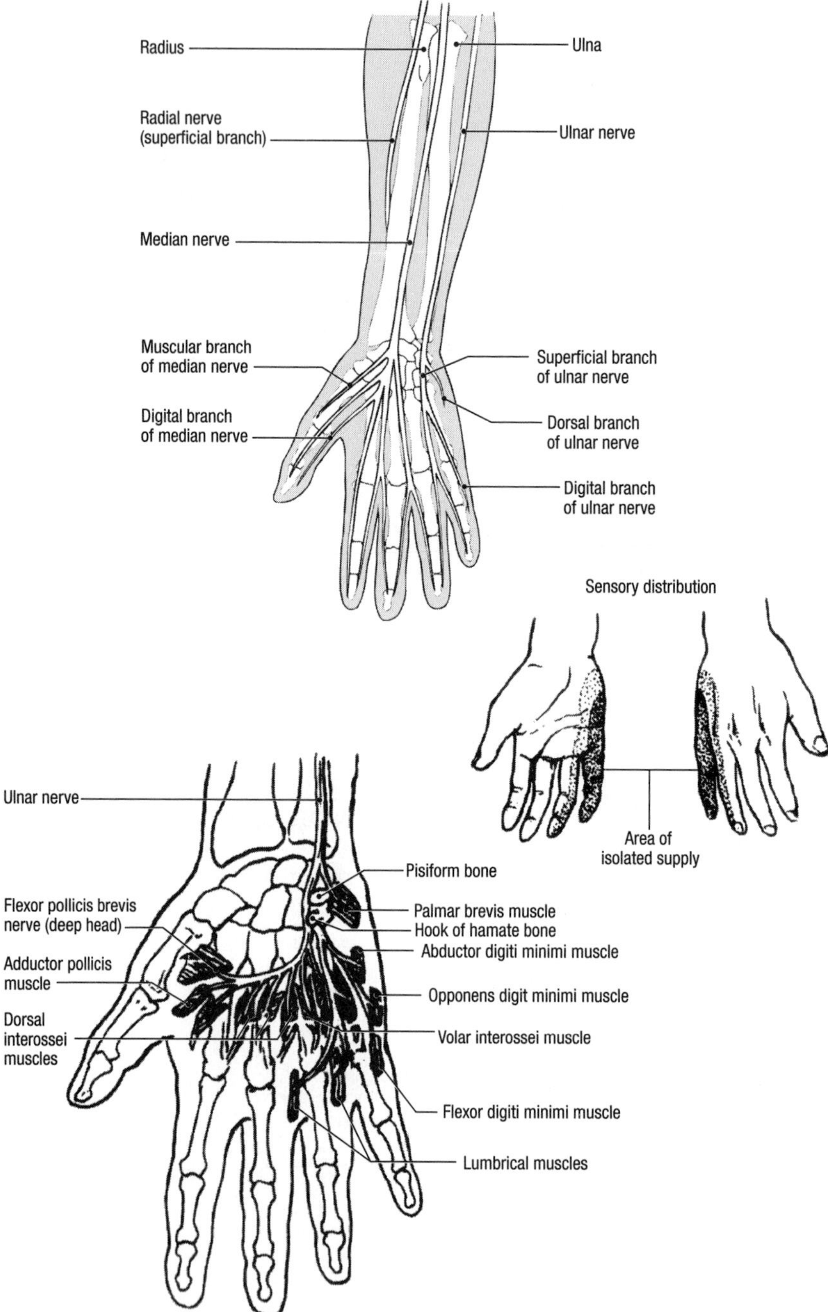

Figure 38. Nerves of the hand and sensory distribution.

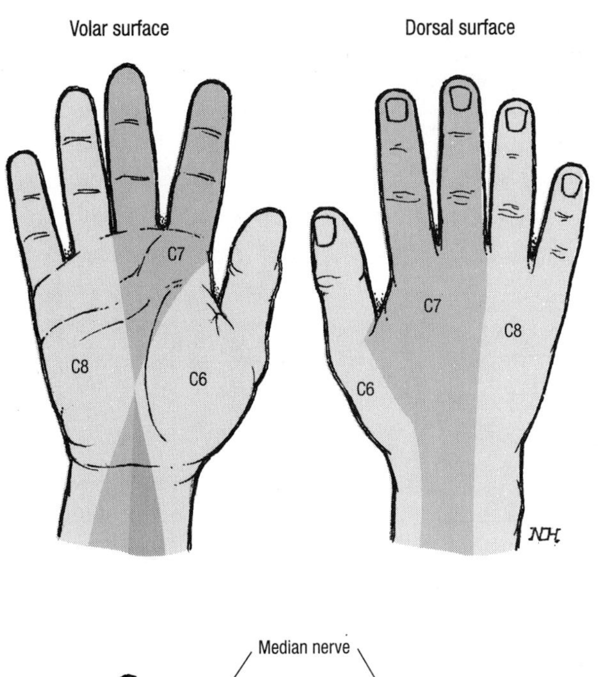

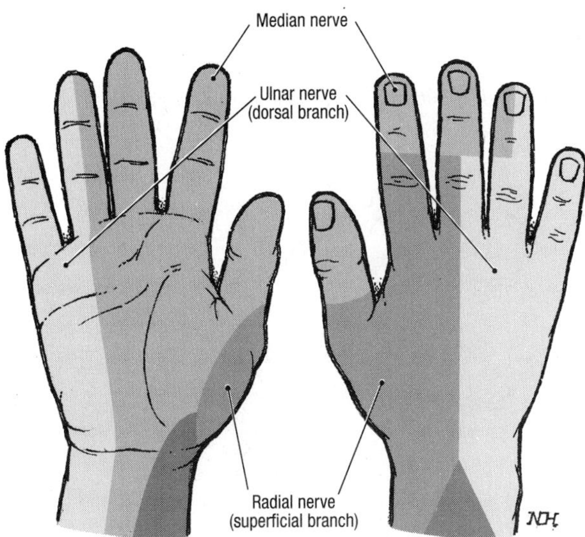

Figure 39. Innervation of hand.

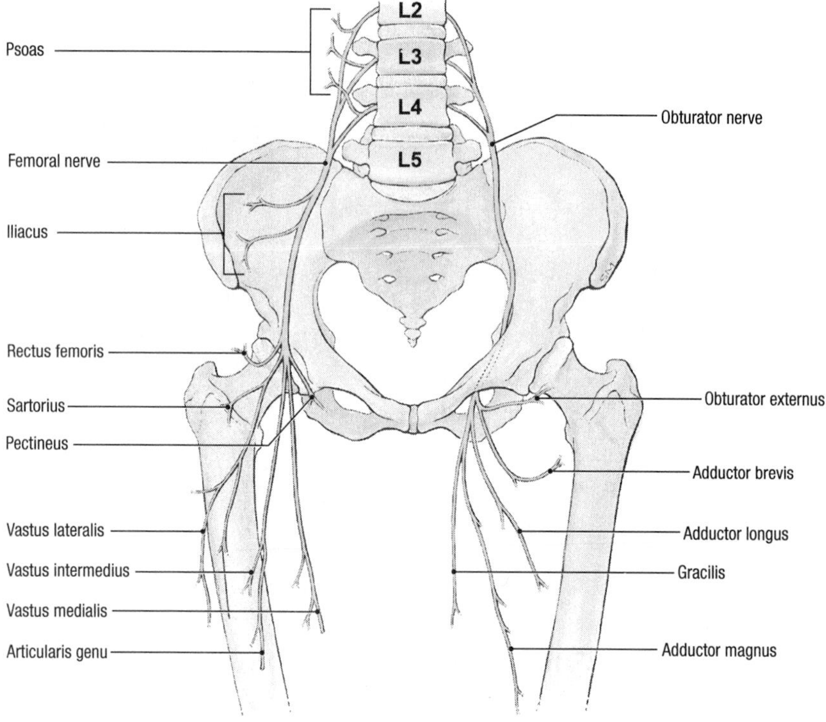

Figure 40. Motor distribution of lower limb nerves, femoral and obturator nerves.

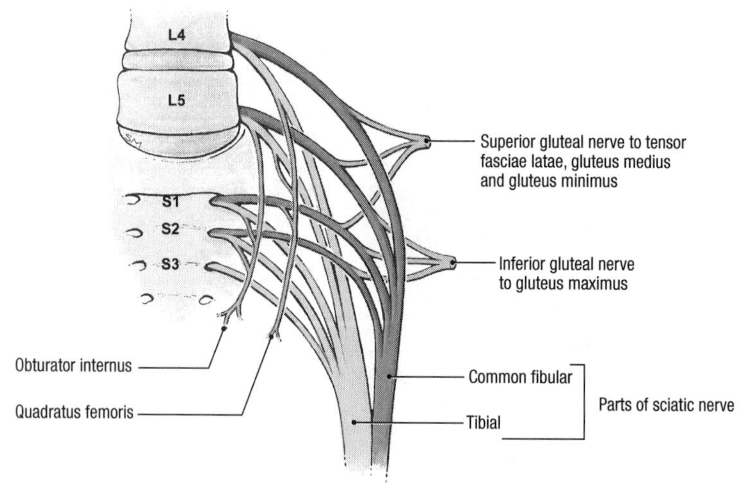

Figure 41. Motor distribution of lower limb nerves, sciatic nerve.

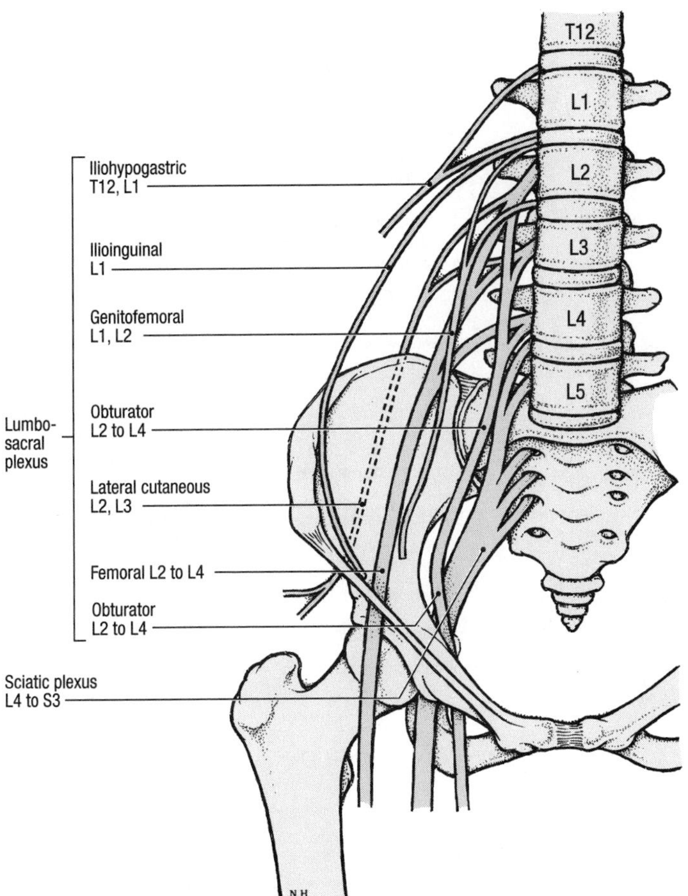

Figure 42. Lumbosacral plexus and sciatic plexus.

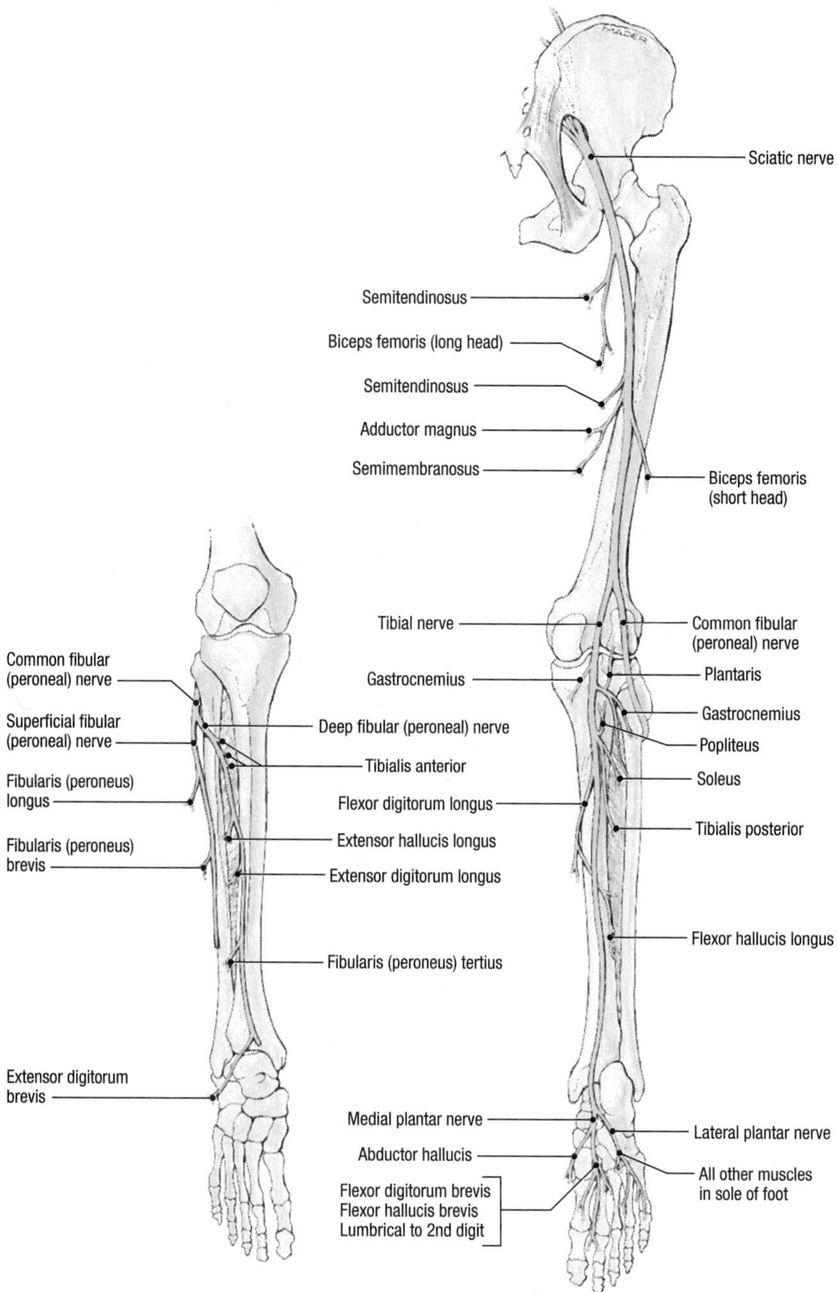

Figure 43. Motor distribution of lower limb nerves. Common fibular (peroneal) nerve (left) and sciatic nerve (right).

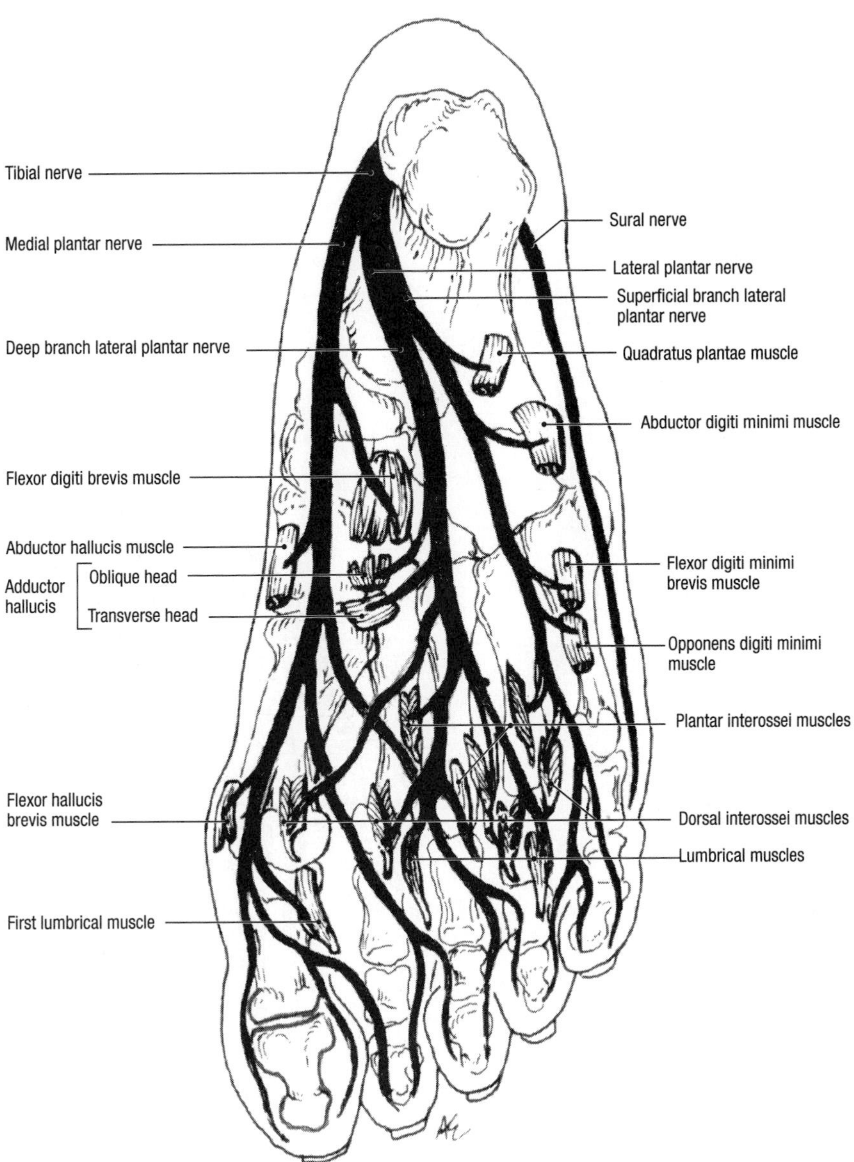

Figure 44. Nerves of the foot.

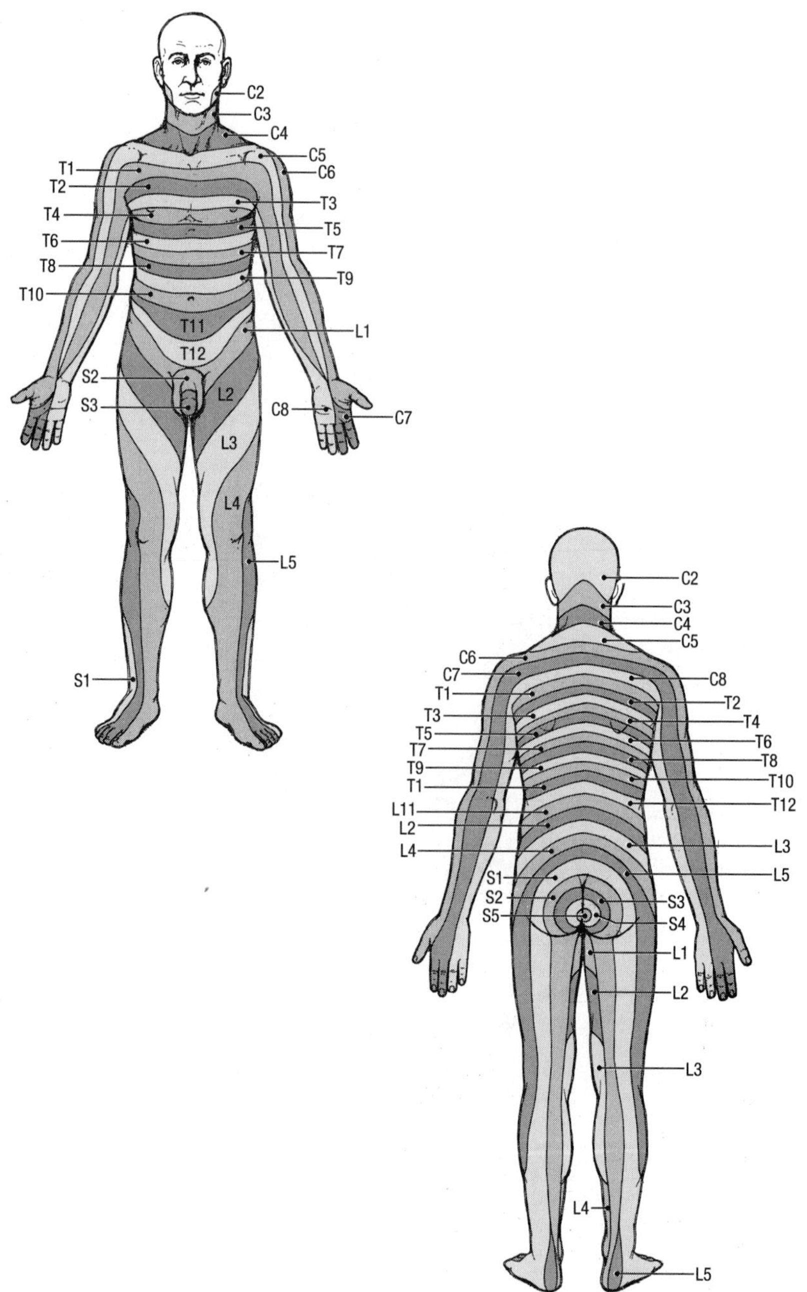

Figure 45. Dermatomes, anterior view (left) and posterior view (right). C1 nerve lacks a significant afferent component and does not supply the skin.

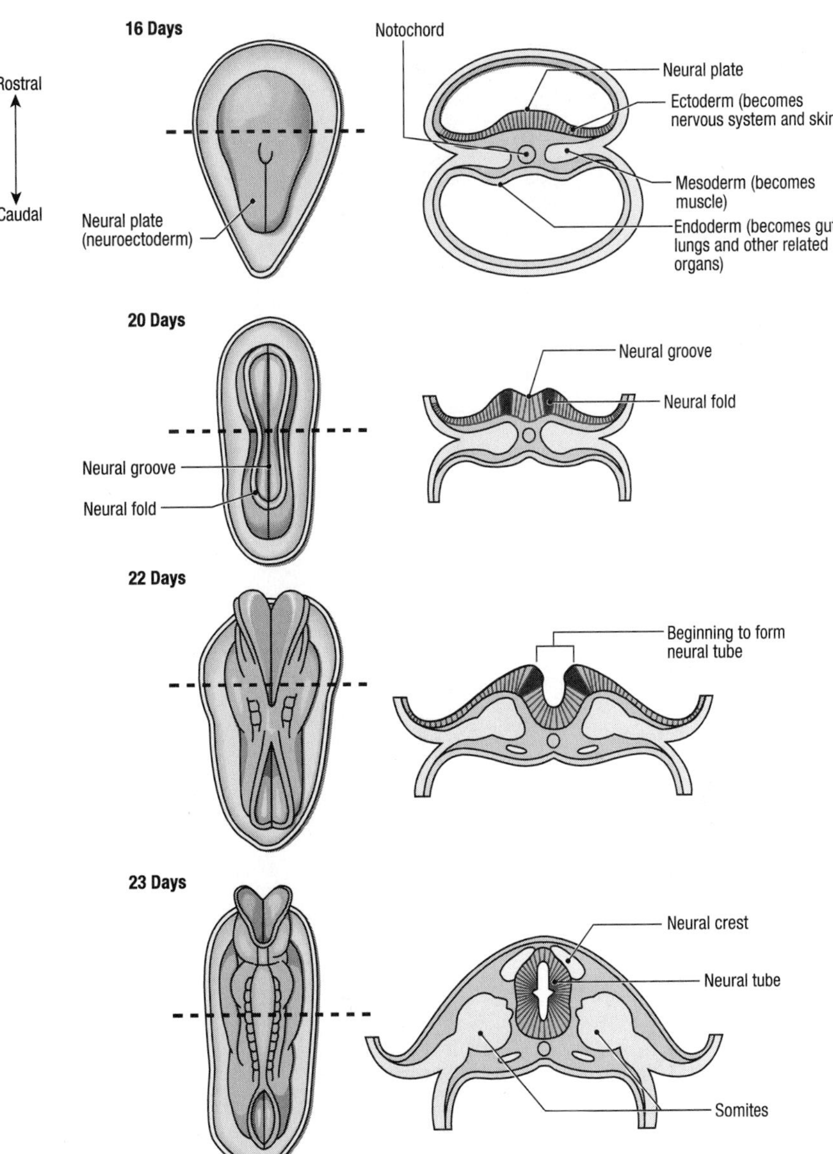

Figure 46. Progressive formation of the neural tube.

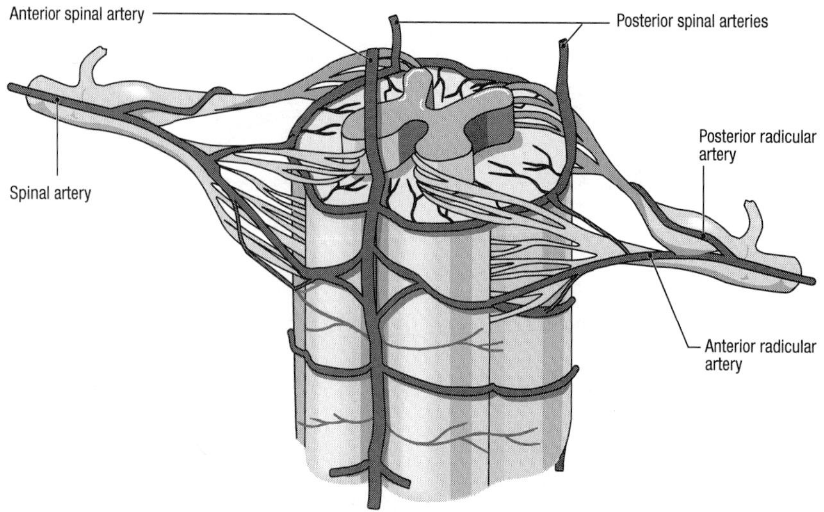

Figure 47. Arteries of the spinal cord.

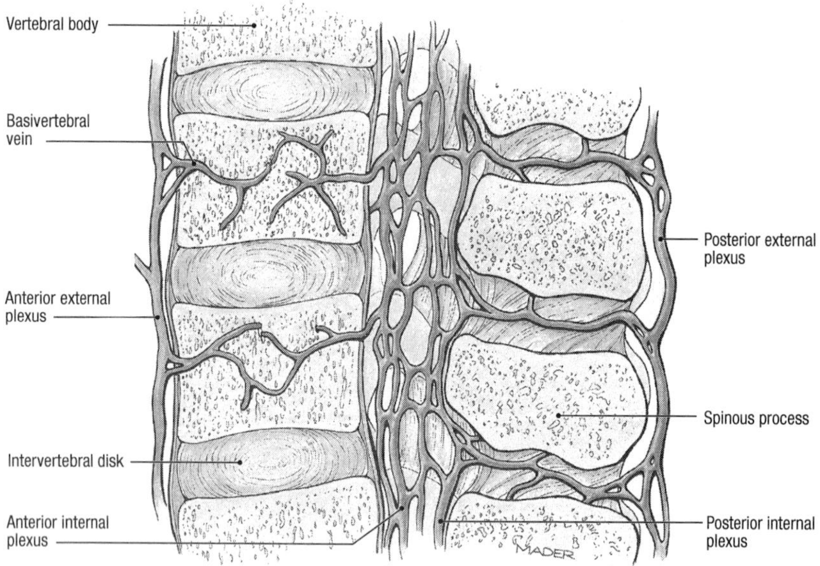

Figure 48. Vetebral venous plexus.

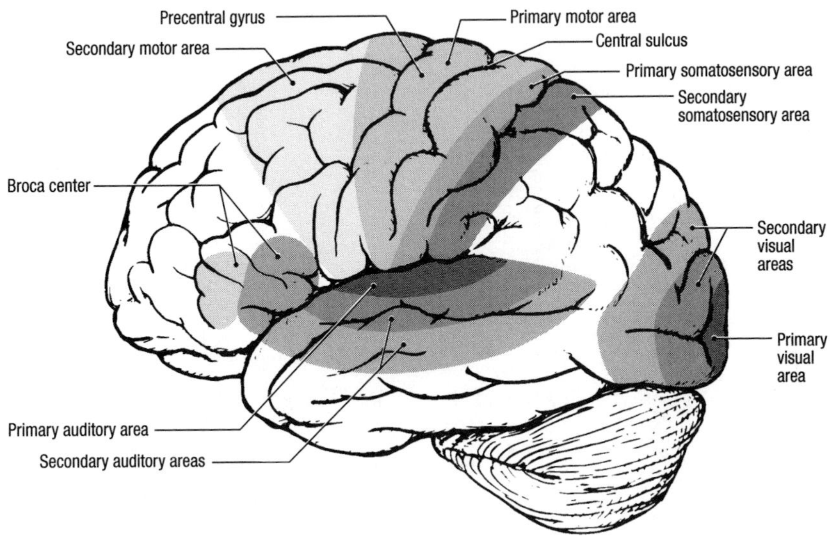

Figure 49. Cerebral cortex and its major functional areas.

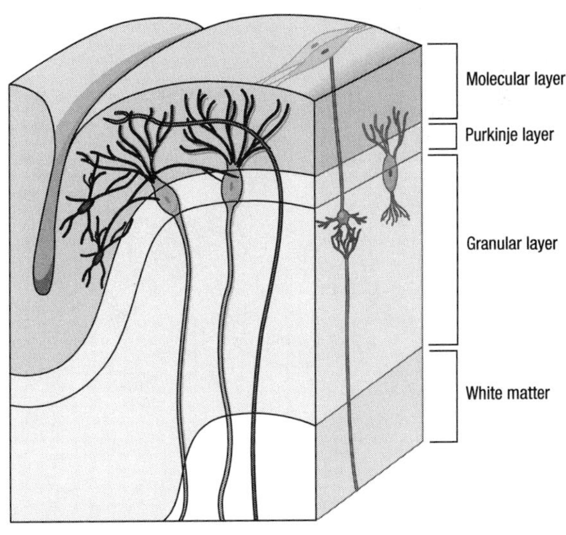

Figure 50. Cross-section of cerebellar cortex.

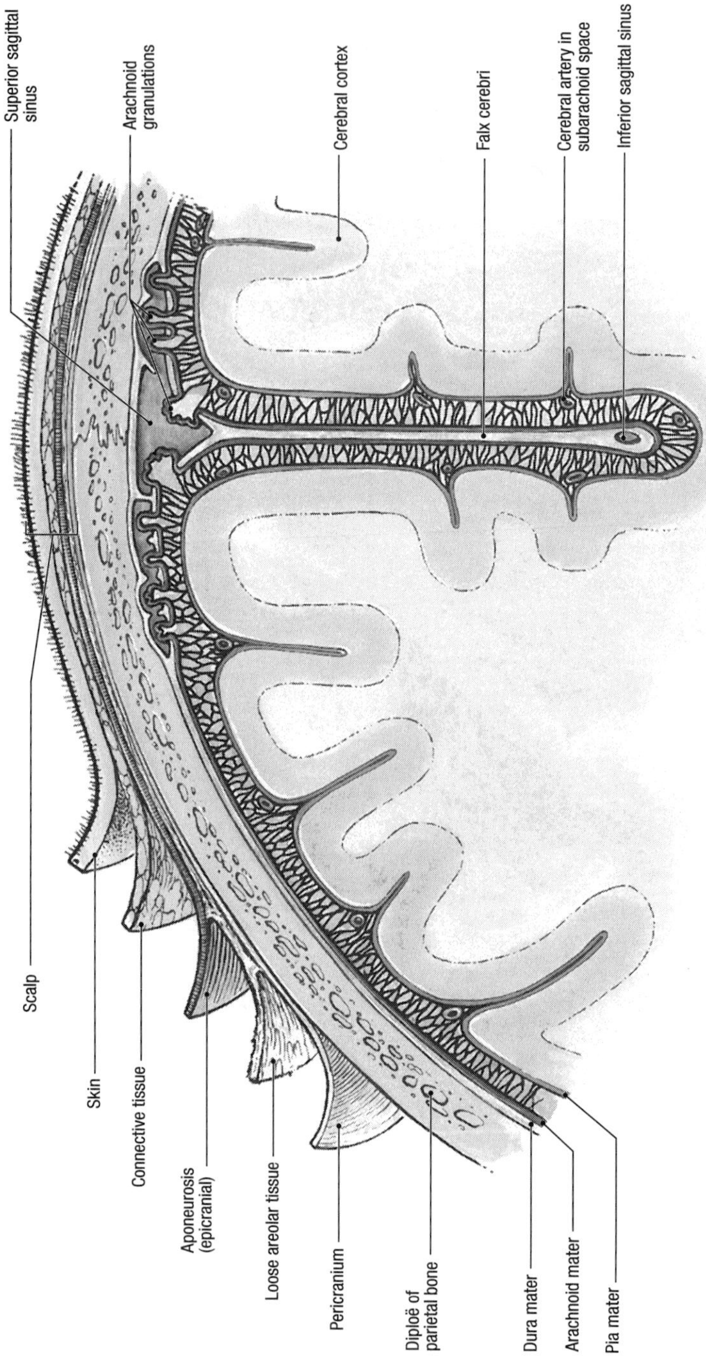

Figure 51. Scalp, skull and meninges.

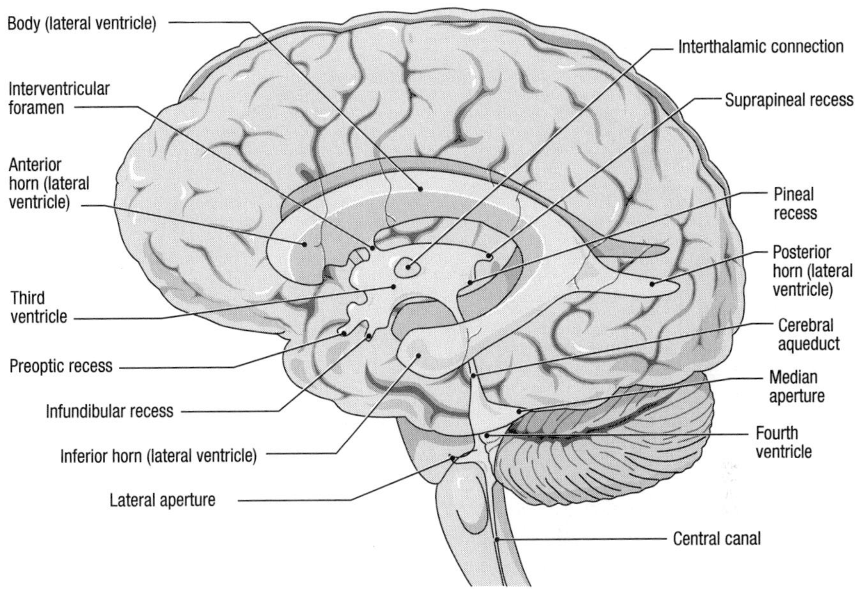

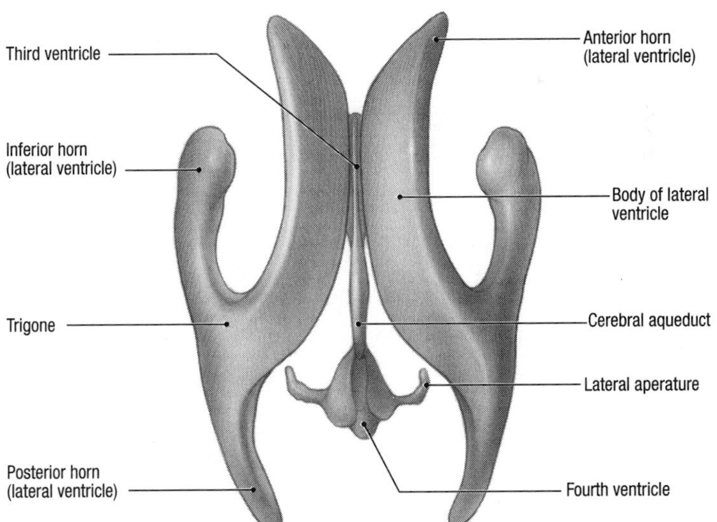

Figure 52. Ventricles of the brain, lateral view (top) and superior view (bottom).

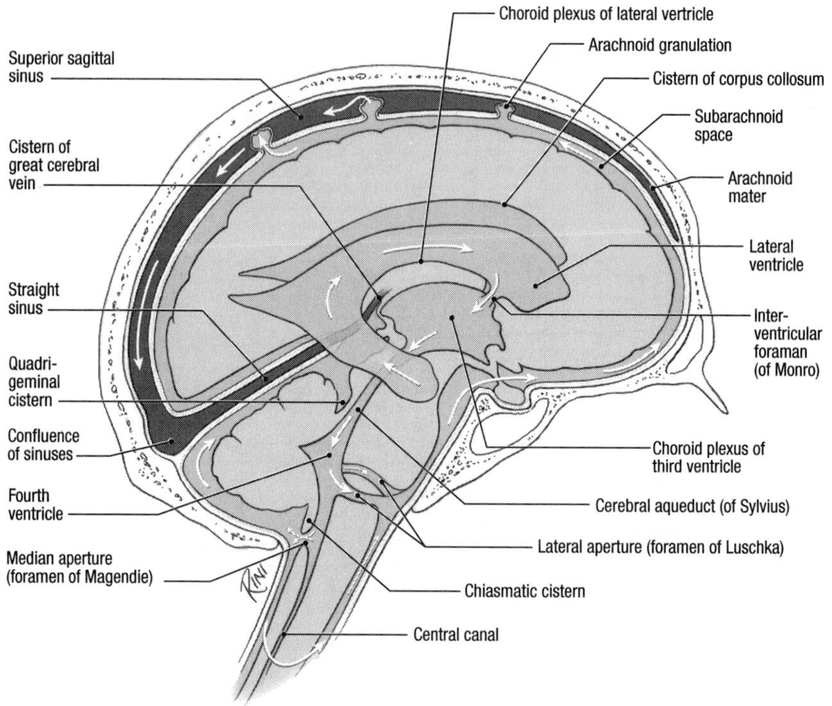

Figure 53. Circulation of cerebrospinal fluid.

Human cerebrospinal fluid (CSF)	
(Average measurements, mg/dL)	
Volume	120 – 200 ml
Specific gravity	1.006 – 1.008
Reaction	pH ca. 7.5
Freezing point depression	0.55° (0.52° – 0.58°)
Pressure (lumbar, subject reclining)	60 – 150 mm H_20
Protein	15 – 25
Glucose	50 – 75 mg/100mL
Phosphatidic acid	ca. 1.0
Cholesterol	0.3 – 0.6
Chloride	100 – 130 mEq/liter
Phosphate	3 – 5
Blood	meg/pst
Cell count	0 – 5 mononuclear cells
Protein	
Lumbar	15 – 456
Total	15 – 45
Cisternal	15 – 25 mg/100 mL
Ventricular	5 – 15 mg/100 mL

Figure 54. Human cerebrospinal fluid.

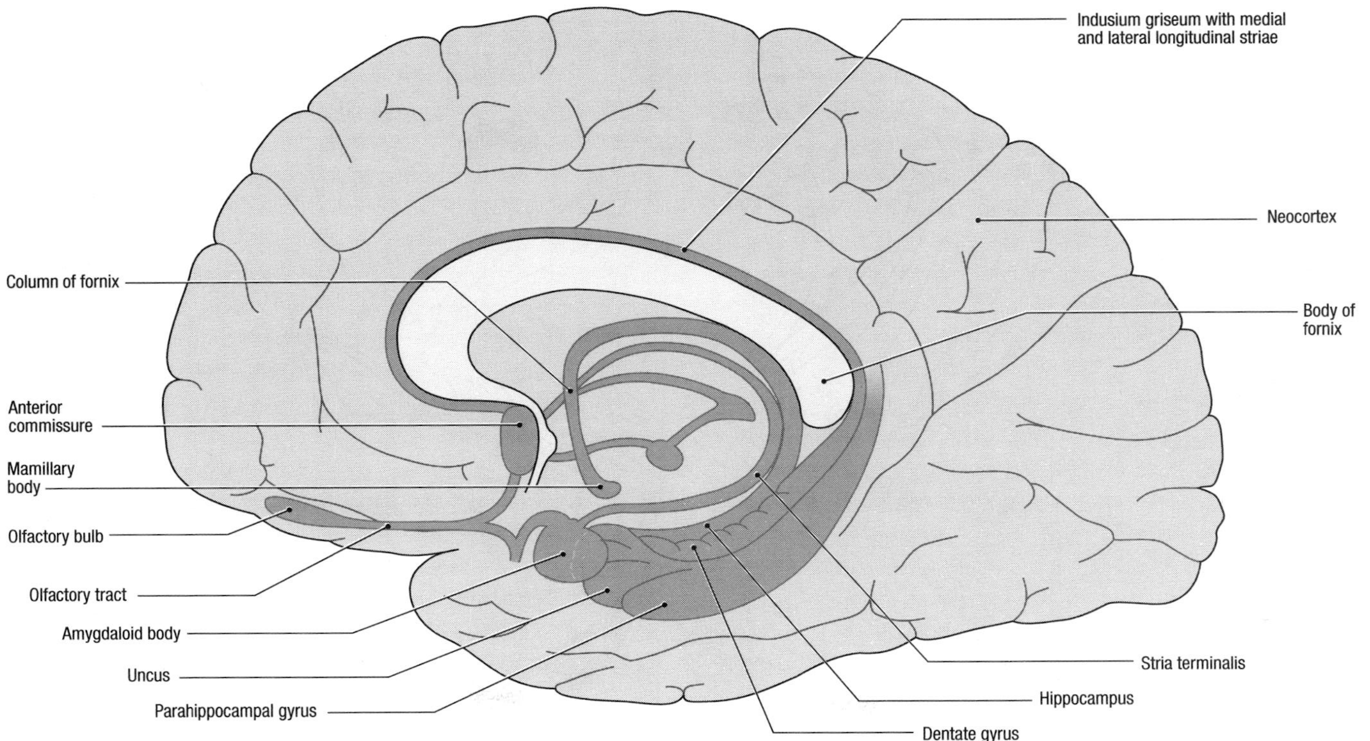

Figure 55. Limbic system (the center of emotions).

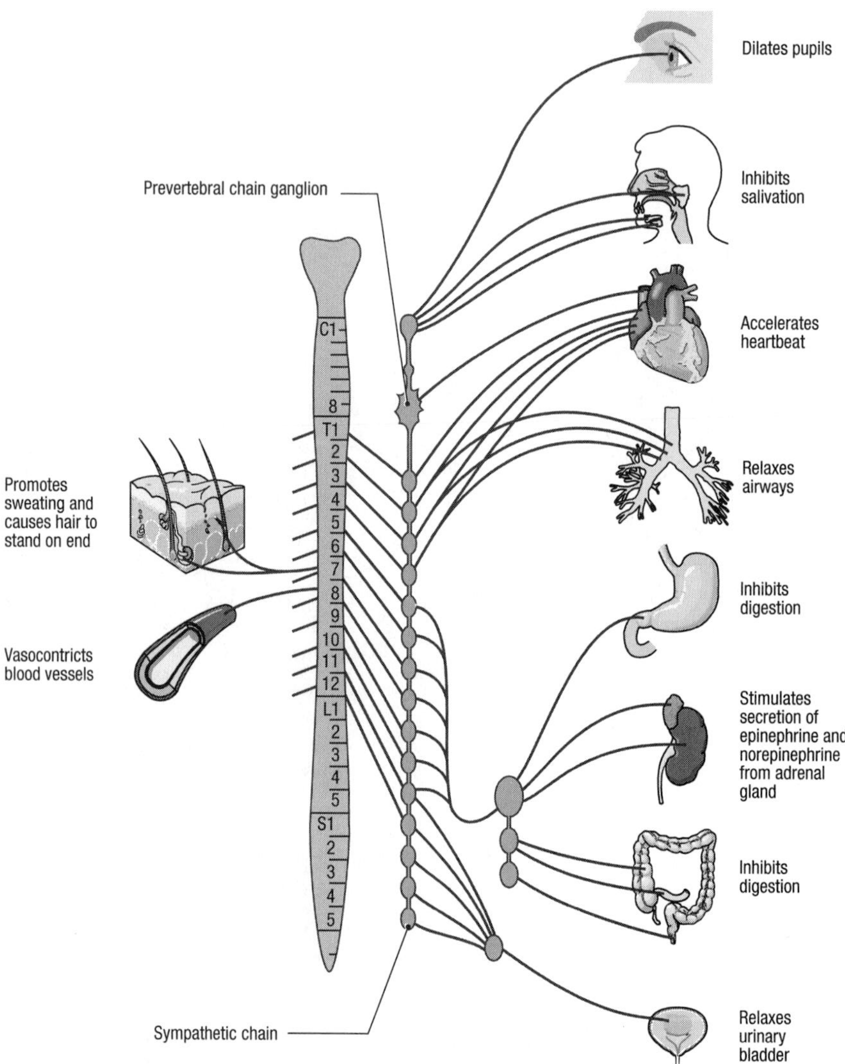

Figure 56. Components of the sympathetic nervous system. The spinal nerves and the organs they innervate. The preganglionic fibers of the sympathetic division of the autonomic nervous system arise from the thoracic and lumbar regions of the spinal cord.

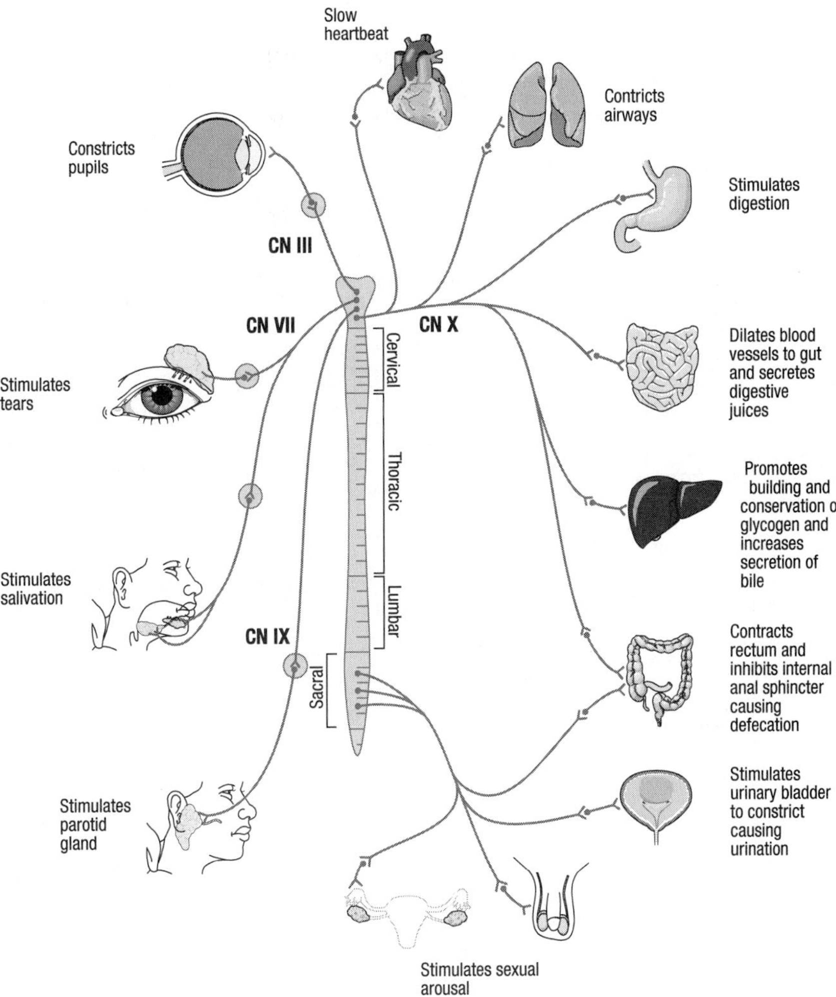

Figure 57. The parasympathetic nervous systems and the organs that are innervated by each nerve. The preganglionic fibers of the parasympathetic division of the autonomic nervous system arise from the brain and sacral region of the spinal cord.

Autonomic nervous system				
Organ	**Function of sympathetic nervous system**	**Sympathetic nerve(s)**	**Function of parasympathetic nervous system**	**Parasympathetic nerve(s)**
Eye	Pupil dilation, contraction of ciliary muscle for accommodation	Postganglionic fibers from superior cervical ganglion (internal carotid nr.)	Constriction of pupil	Postganglionic fibers from ciliary ganglion via short ciliary nerves
Lacrimal gland	Slight or no effect	Postganglionic fibers from superior cervical ganglion (external carotid nr.)	Secretion	Postganglionic fibers from pterygopalatine ganglion via zygomatico-temporal nerve
Salivary glands	Thick, viscous secretion	External carotid nerve	Abundant, watery secretion	Postganglionic fibers from submandibular ganglion and from otic ganglion
Heart	Increase of rate and strength of heartbeats, dilation of coronary vessels (indirectly), reduction of conduction time	Cervical cardiac and thoracic cardiac nerves	Contraction of coronary vessels (indirectly), increase of conduction time	Postganglionic fibers from terminal/intramural ganglia via vagus nerve
Lungs	Bronchodilation, inhibition of secretion	Pulmonary nerves	Bronchial constriction, stimulation of secretion	Postganglionic fibers from terminal/intramural ganglia via vagus nerve
Digestive tract	Peristaltic inhibition, vasoconstriction	Greater, lesser, least splanchnic nerves and branches from celiac, superior mesenteric, and inferior mesenteric ganglia	Stimulation of peristalsis and secretion	Postganglionic fibers from terminal/intramural ganglia via vagus and pelvic nerves
Liver and gallbladder	Release of glucose	Branches from celiac ganglion	Excretion of bile	Postganglionic fibers from terminal/intramural ganglia via vagus nerve
Adrenal medulla	Secretion of epinephrine	Lesser splanchnic nerve	No connection	No nerves
Kidney	Vasoconstriction, inhibition of urine formation	Branches from cortico-renal ganglion	No effect	No nerves
Bladder	Retention of urine	Branches from inferior mesenteric ganglion (via hypogastric plexus)	Release of urine	Postganglionic fibers from terminal/intramural ganglia via pelvic nerves
Genitalia	Ejaculation	Branches from inferior mesenteric ganglion (via hypogastric plexus)	Penile and clitoral erections	Postganglionic fibers from terminal/intramural ganglia via pelvic nerves
Sweat glands	Secretion	Postganglionic fibers from sympathetic chain ganglia	No connection	No nerves
Peripheral blood vessels	Constriction of smooth muscle	Postganglionic fibers from sympathetic chain ganglia	No connection, apart from dilation in the genital area	No nerves
Skeletal muscle	Constriction of smooth muscles in blood vessels	Postganglionic fibers from sympathetic chain ganglia	Dilation	No nerves

Figure 58. The autonomic nervous system.

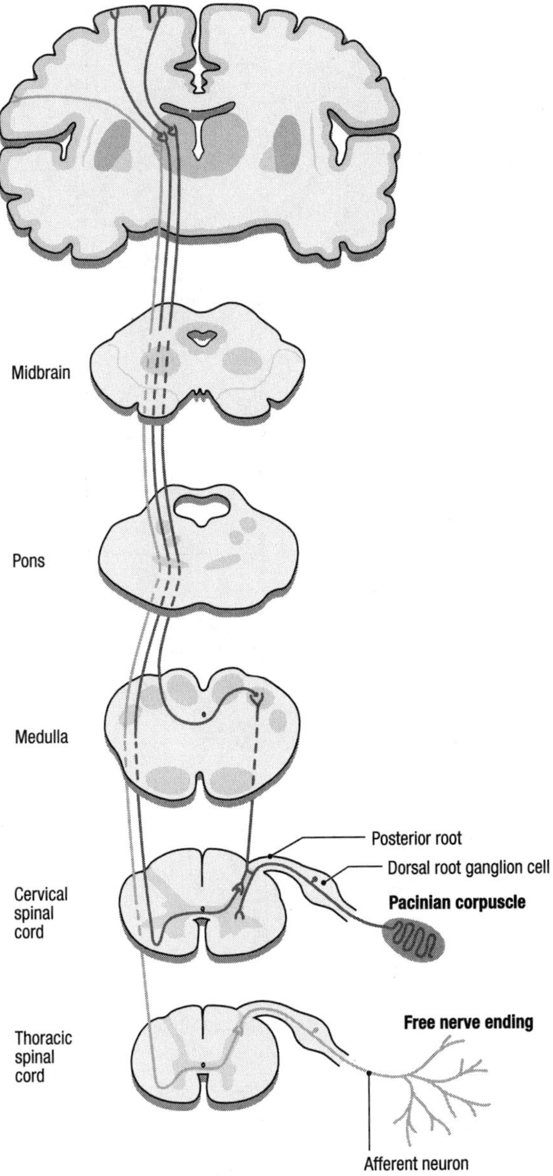

Figure 59. Afferent sensory tracts.

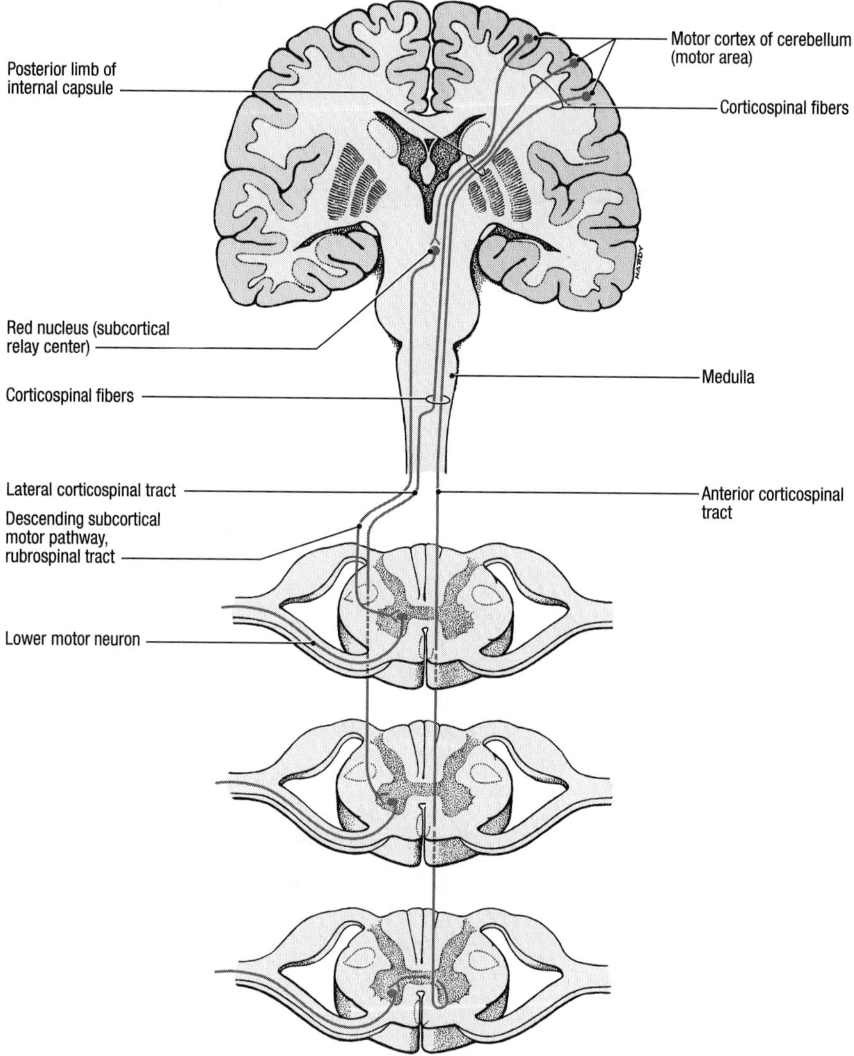
Posterior limb of
internal capsule
Motor cortex of cerebellum
(motor area)
Corticospinal fibers
HARDY
Red nucleus (subcortical
relay center)
Medulla
Corticospinal fibers
Lateral corticospinal tract
Anterior corticospinal
tract
Descending subcortical
motor pathway,
rubrospinal tract
Lower motor neuron

Figure 60. Corticospinal tract.

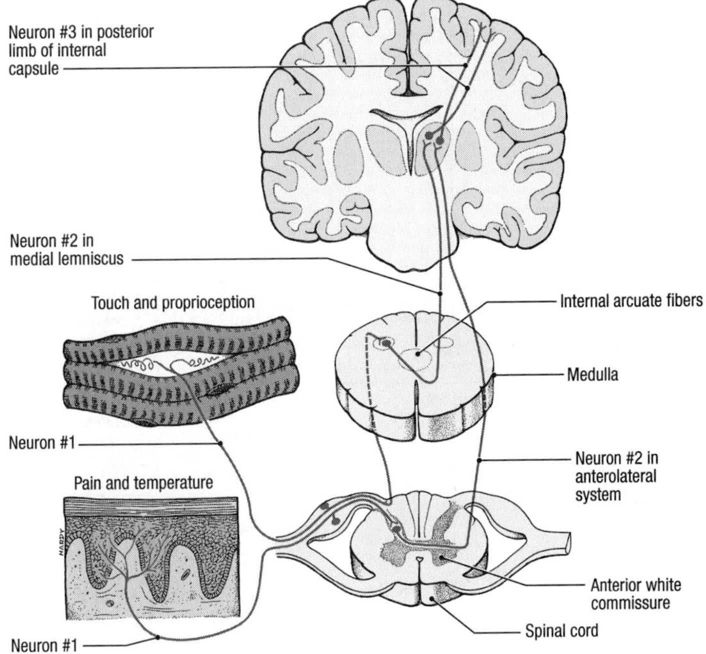

Figure 61. Decussation of nerve fibers.

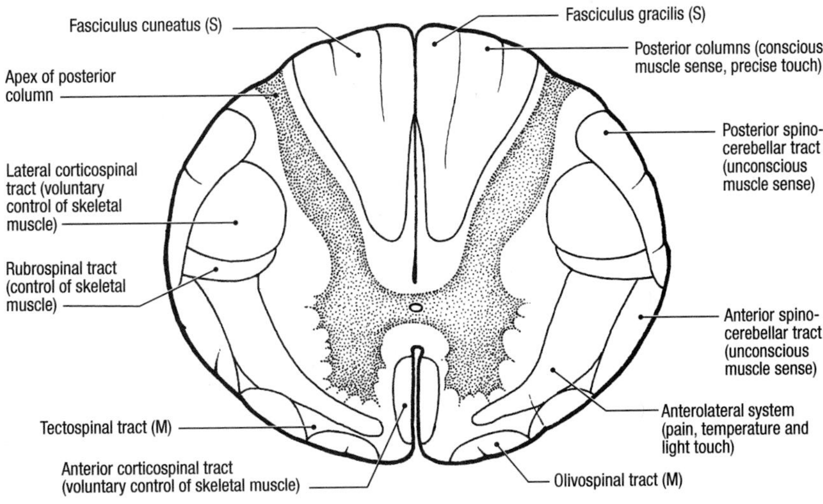

Figure 62. Principal fiber tracts of the spinal cord. Sensor (S), motor (M).

Sensation

Modality of sensation	Object of perception	Nature of stimuli	Receptor type
Sense of sight	Brightness, darkness, colors	Electromagnetic radiation 4000–7000 Å	Photo-receptors
Sense of temperature	Cold, heat	Electromagnetic radiation 7000–9000 Å, convective heat transport	Thermo-receptors
Tactile sense of skin	Pressure, touch		
Sense of hearing	Sound frequencies		
Statokinetic sense	Absolute body position, speed of body, relative body position and movement of body parts and joints, sense of strength	Modification of mechano-receptors by solid objects or transmission of air-pressure changes	Mechano-receptors
Sense of smell	Odors	Chemical substances	
Sense of taste	Sour, salty, sweet, bitter	Ions	Chemo-receptors
Sense of pain	Pain	Mechanical tissue injury	Nociceptors

Figure 63. Sensation.

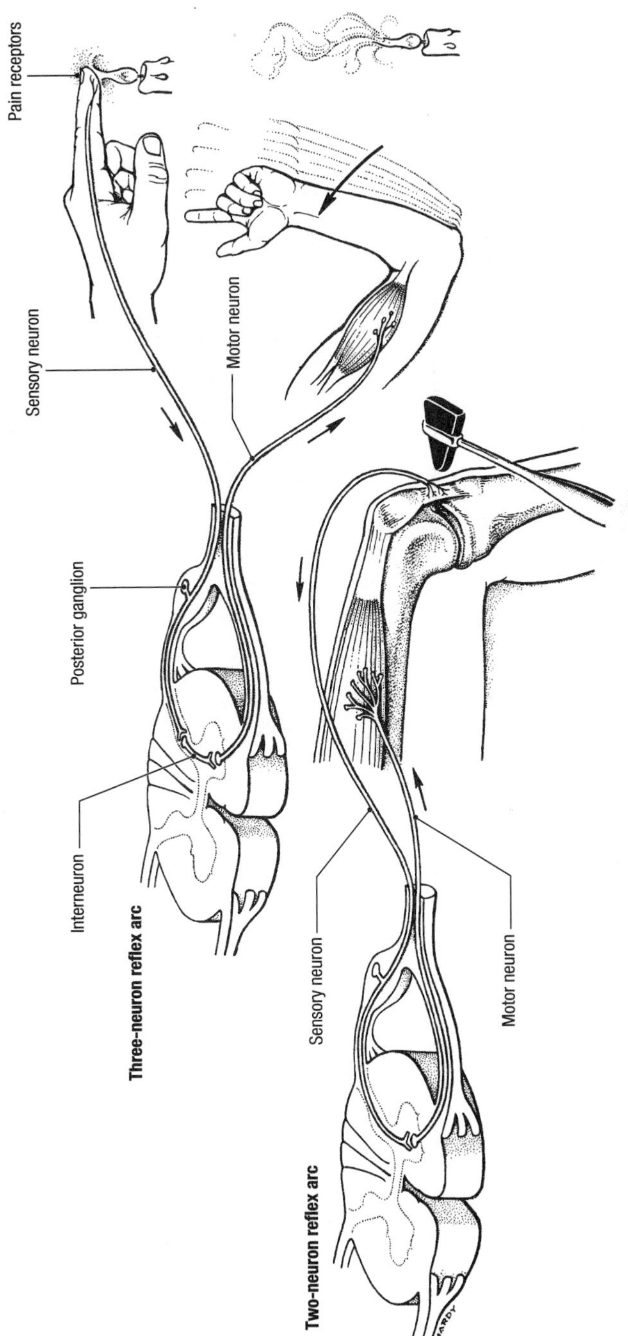

Figure 64. Reflex arcs. Flexor reflex (top) and stretch reflex (bottom).

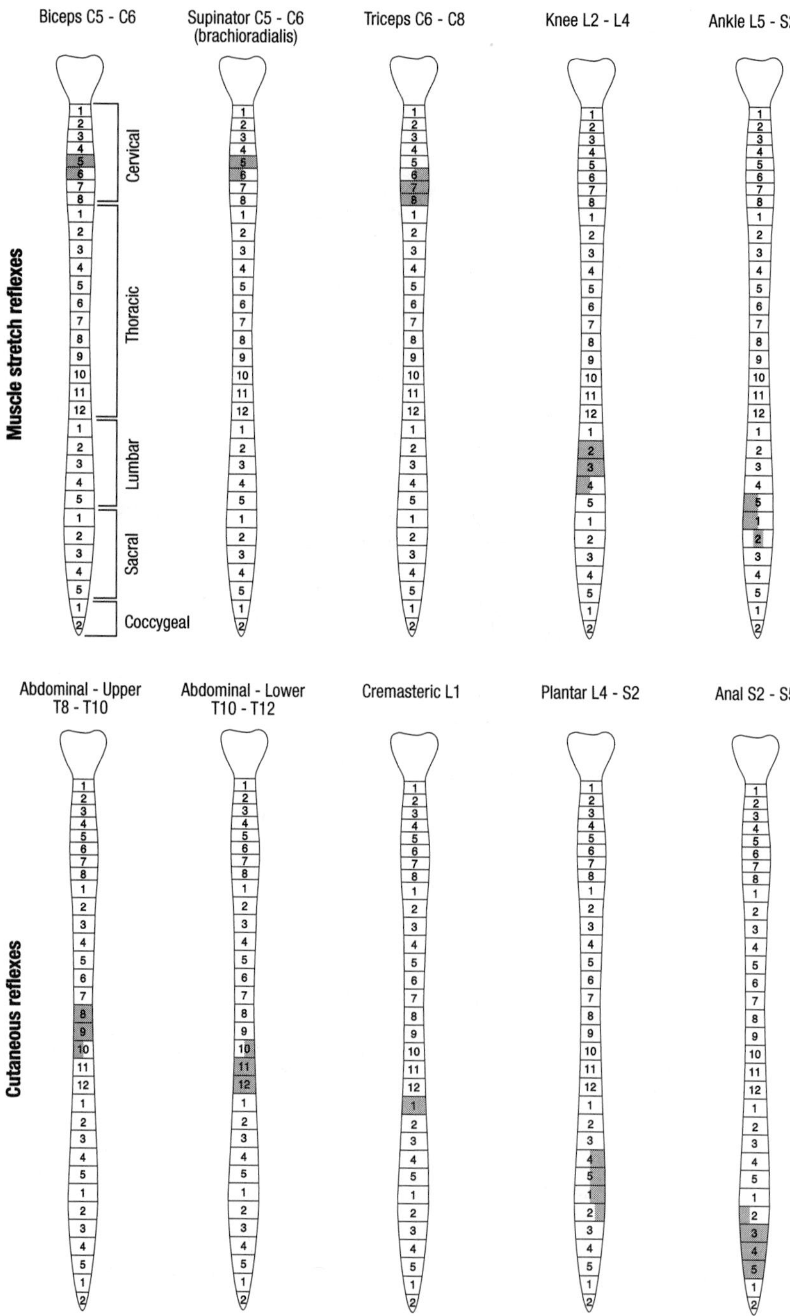

Figure 65. Spinal nerves responsible for muscle stretch reflexes and cutaneous reflexes.

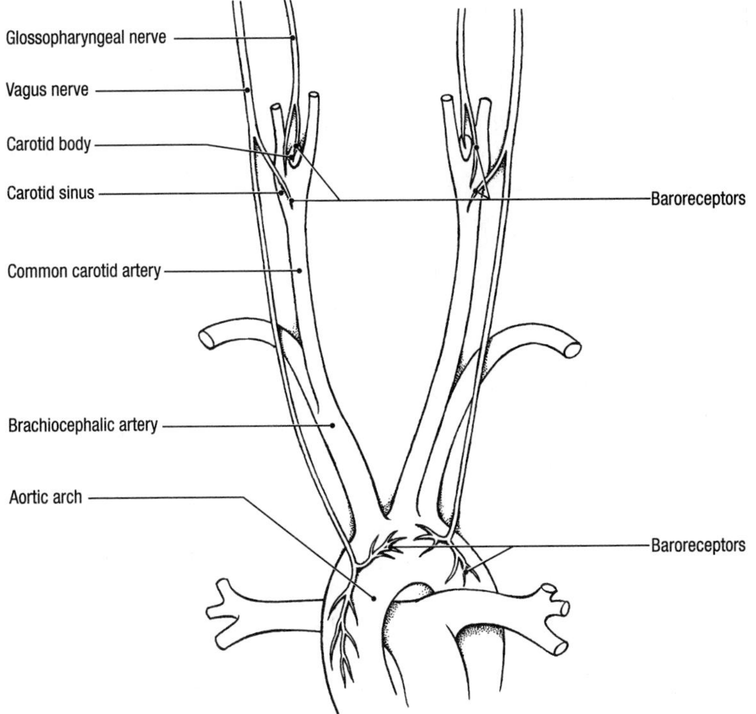

Figure 66. Baroreceptors.

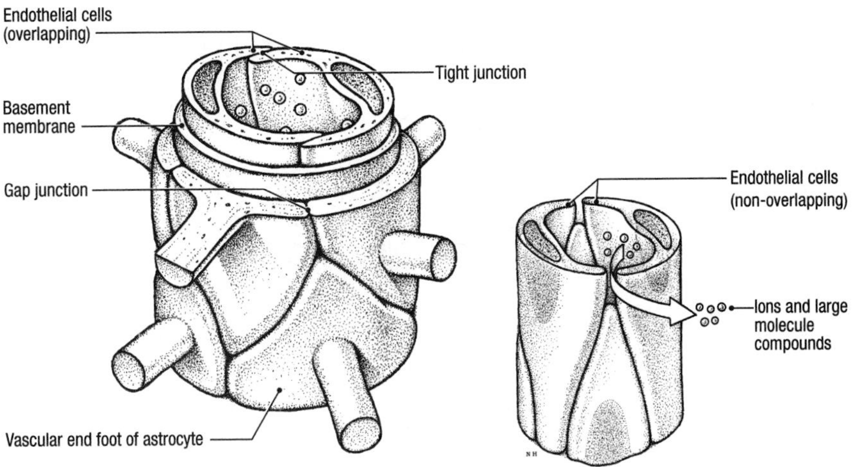

Figure 67. Blood-brain barrier.

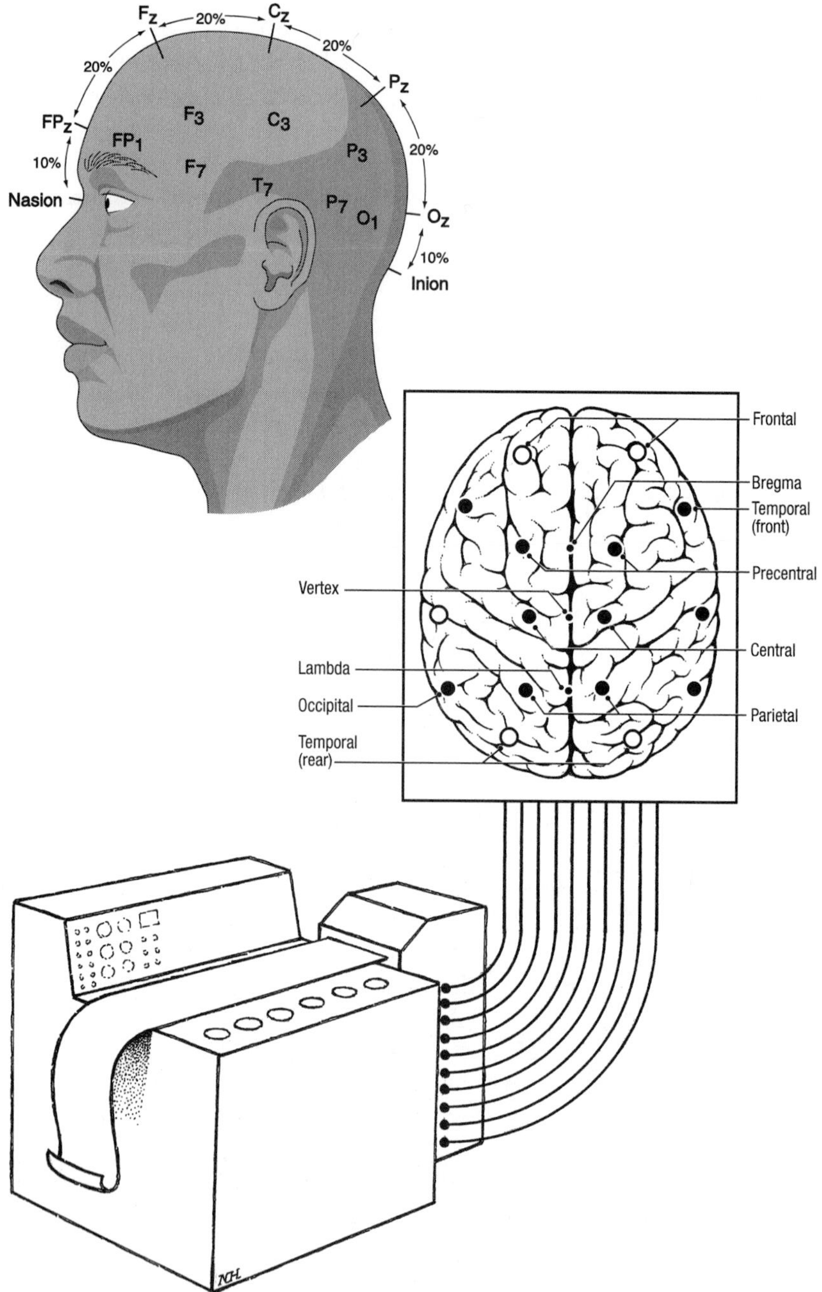

Figure 68. Electroencephalogram (EEG) and lateral view of the head showing proper EEG electrode placement.

Electroencephalogram						
				Physiologic variations of potential		
Type of wave	Shape	Frequency per sec.	Amplitude in μV	In waking EEG		In sleeping EEG
				Adult	Child	All ages
Beta		14 – 30	5 – 50	Frontal and precentral prominent, in clusters	Seldom prominent	Beta-activity ("spindles") sign of light sleep
Alpha		8 – 13	20 – 120	Predominant activity	Predominant activity, age 5 and above	Not a sign of sleep
Theta		4 – 7	20 – 100	Constant, not prominent	Predominant activity, from 18 mos. to 5 yrs.	Normal sign of sleep
Delta		0.5 – 3	5 – 250	Not prominent	Predominant activity until 18 mos.	Concomitant sign of deep sleep
Gamma	—	31 – 60	– 10	Laws governing predominance and localization not fully known		

Figure 69. Electroencephalogram.

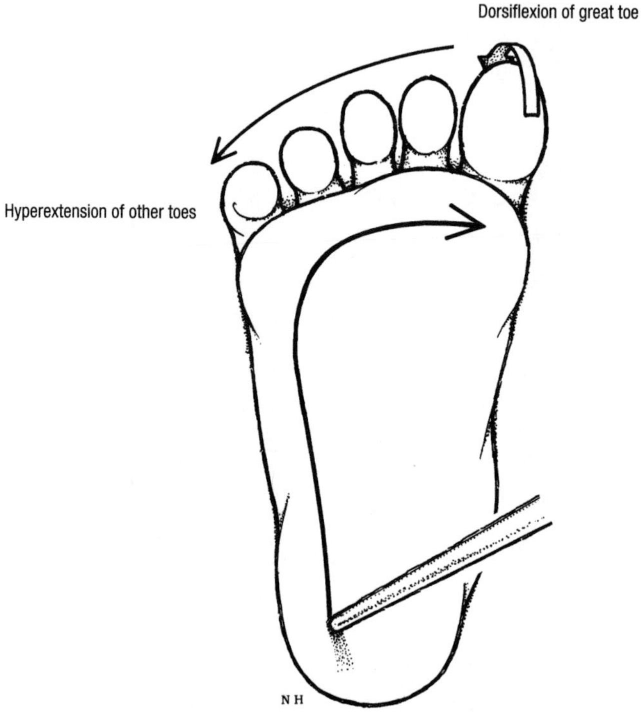

Figure 70. Babinski sign.

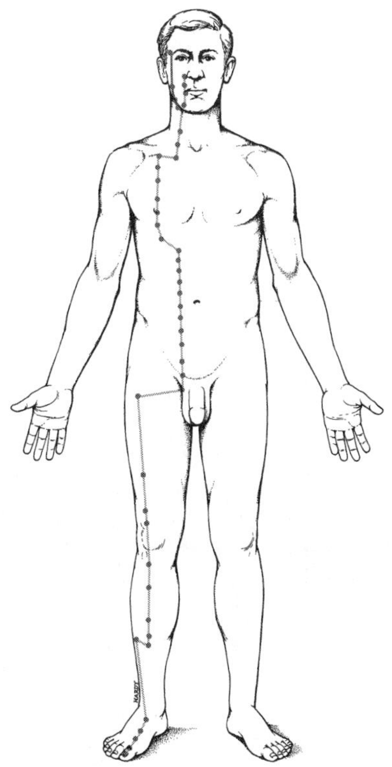

Figure 71. Acupuncture meridians.

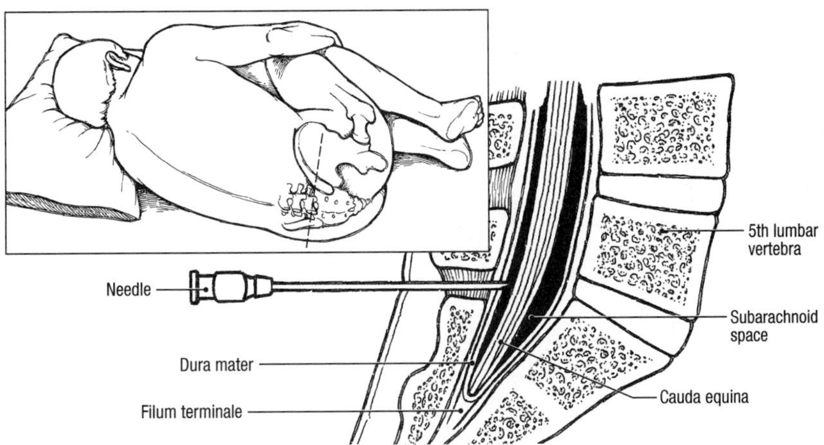

Figure 72. Lumbar puncture.

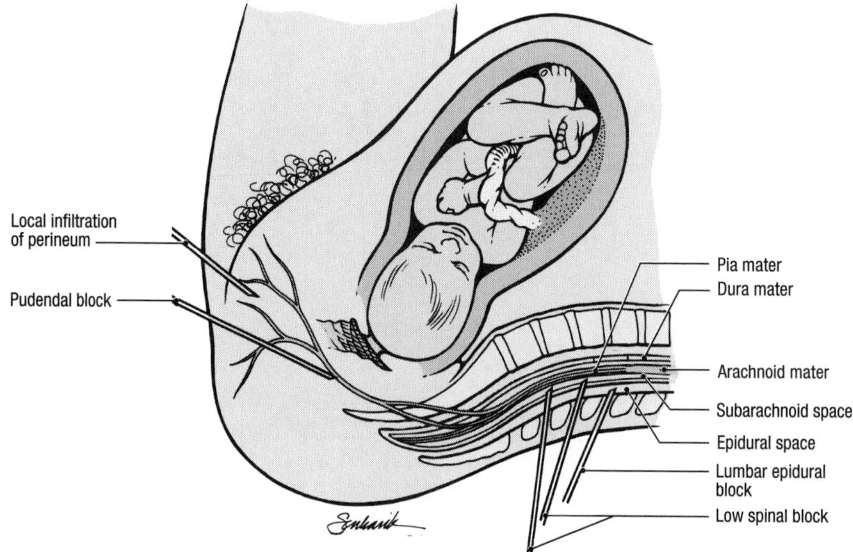

Figure 73. Regional anesthesia for childbirth (sites of injection).

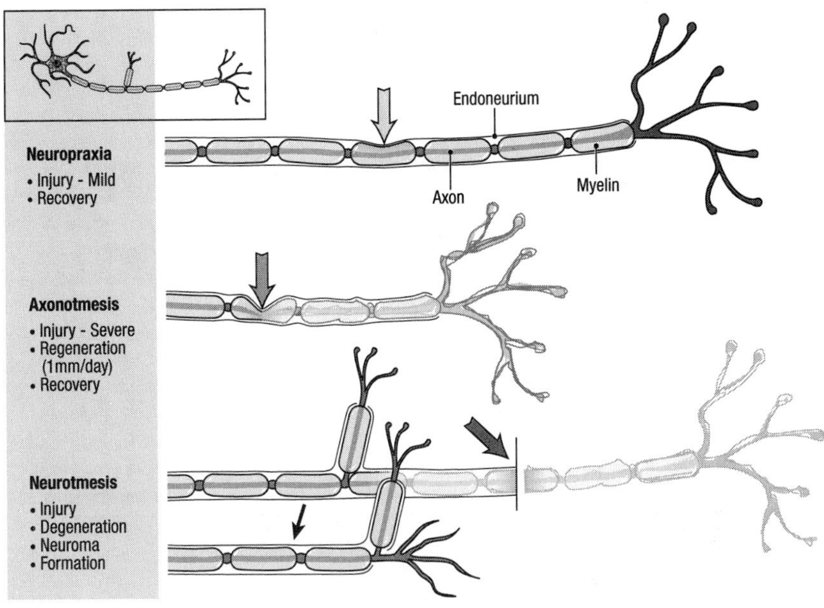

Figure 74. Nerve injuries.

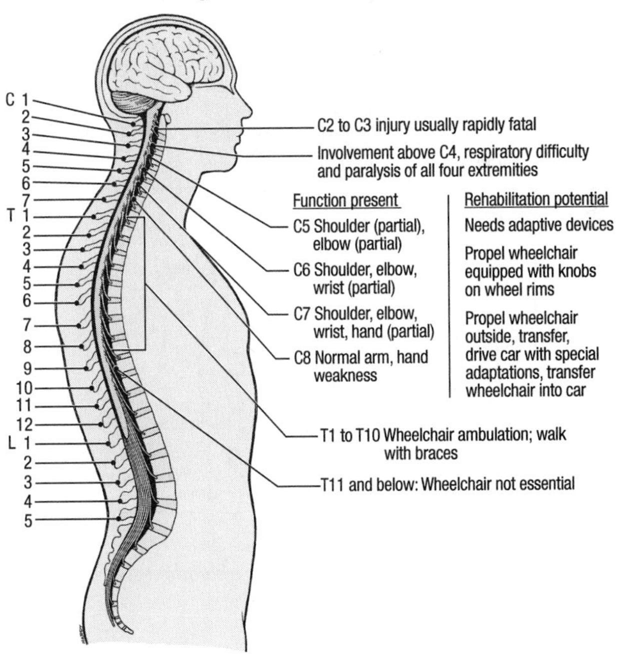

Figure 75. Spinal cord injuries.

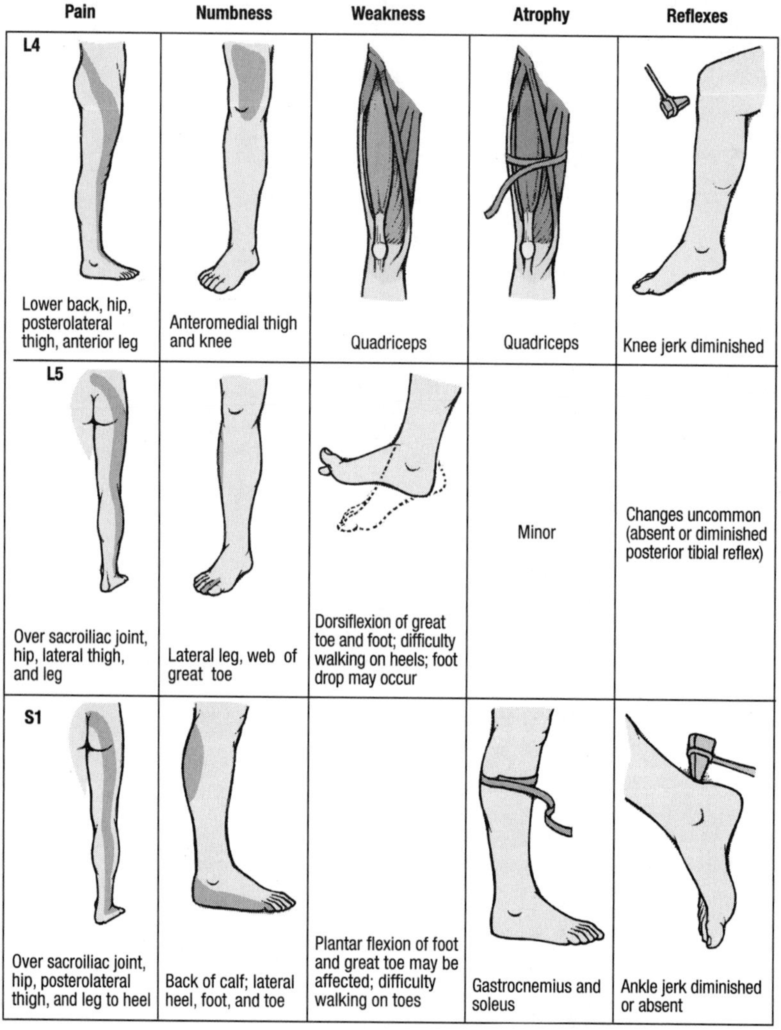

	Pain	Numbness	Weakness	Atrophy	Reflexes
L4	Lower back, hip, posterolateral thigh, anterior leg	Anteromedial thigh and knee	Quadriceps	Quadriceps	Knee jerk diminished
L5	Over sacroiliac joint, hip, lateral thigh, and leg	Lateral leg, web of great toe	Dorsiflexion of great toe and foot; difficulty walking on heels; foot drop may occur	Minor	Changes uncommon (absent or diminished posterior tibial reflex)
S1	Over sacroiliac joint, hip, posterolateral thigh, and leg to heel	Back of calf; lateral heel, foot, and toe	Plantar flexion of foot and great toe may be affected; difficulty walking on toes	Gastrocnemius and soleus	Ankle jerk diminished or absent

Figure 76. Intervertebral disk herniation (nerves compressed: L4, L5, and S1).

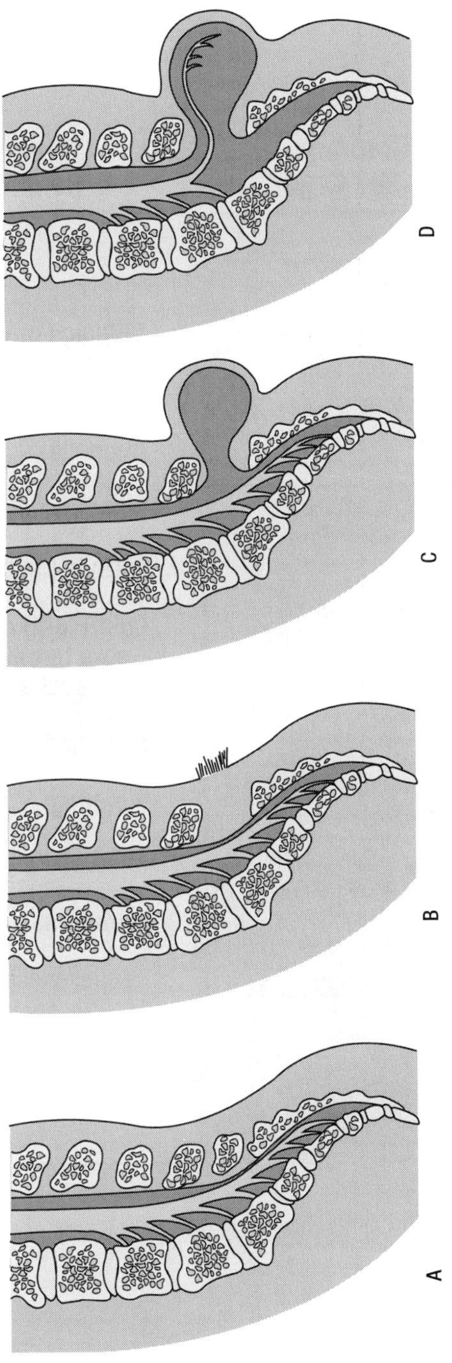

Figure 77. Four degrees of spinal cord anomalies. (A) Normal spinal cord, (B) spina bifida occulta, (C) meningocele, (D) myelomeningocele.

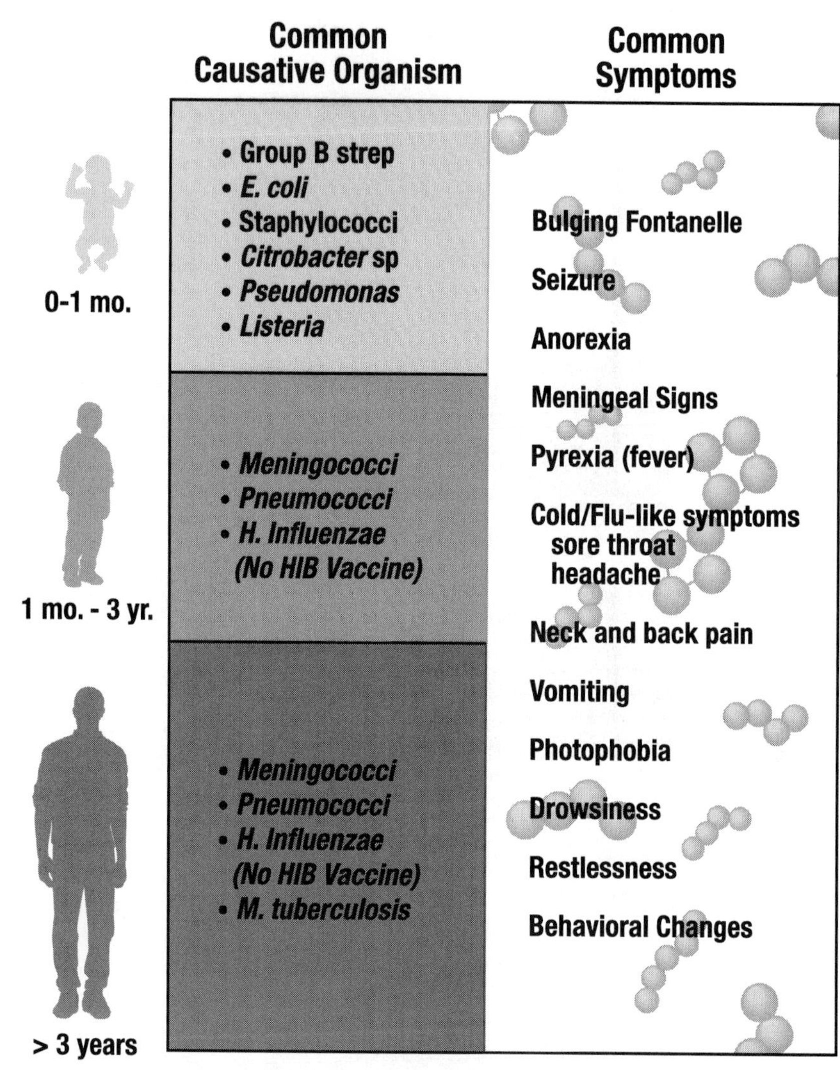

Figure 78. Causative organisms and symptoms of bacterial meningitis, arranged according to patient's age.

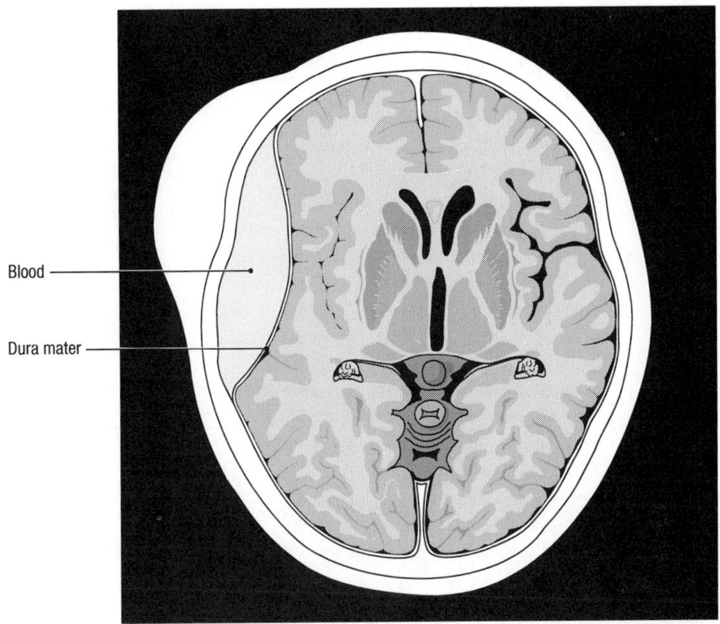

Figure 79. Epidural hematoma.

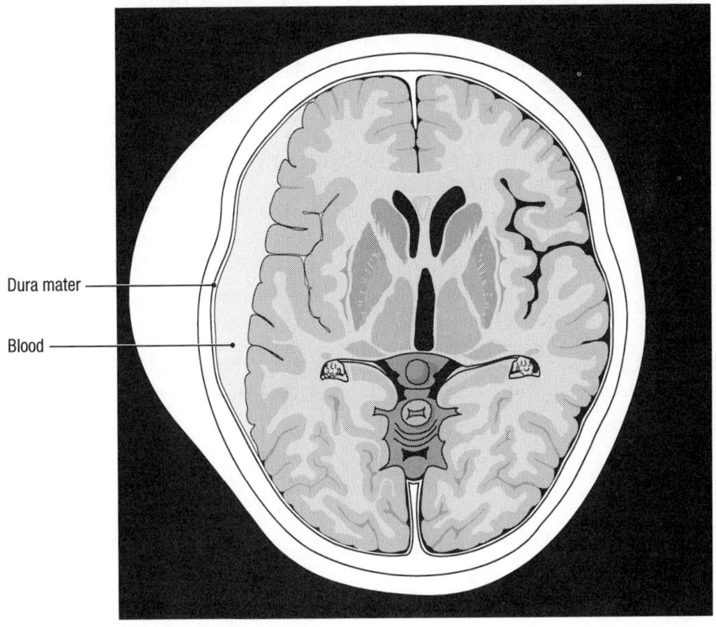

Figure 80. Subdural hematoma.

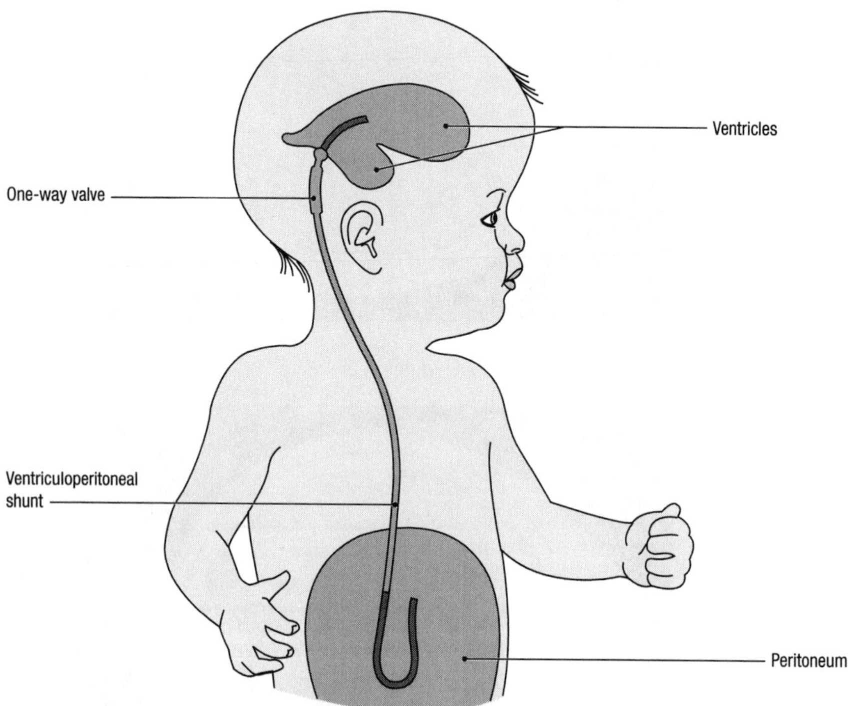

Figure 81. Infant with ventriculoperitoneal shunt. Excess cerebrospinal fluid is drained from the ventricles to the peritoneum with a one-way valve, located behind the ear, to prevent backflow.

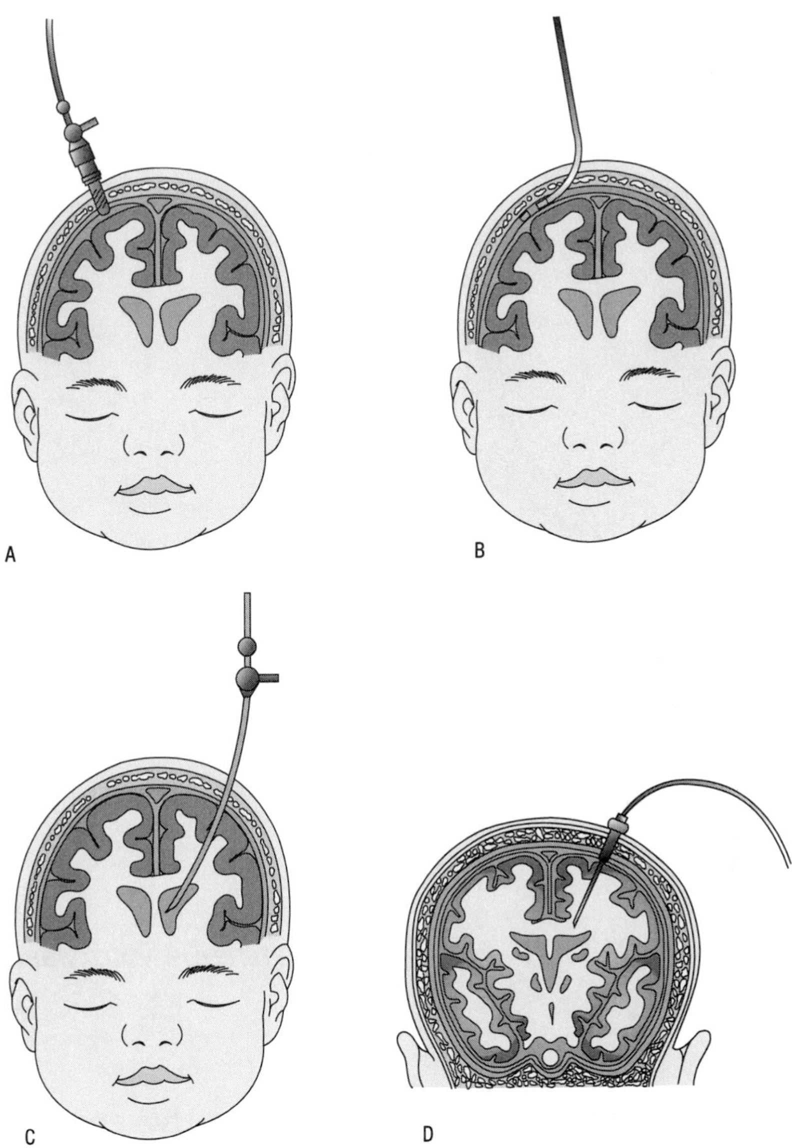

Figure 82. Placement of intracranial pressure monitor. (A) A subarachnoid screw passes through a bur hole in the skull ending in the epidural space. (B) A fiberoptic sensor is implanted into the epidural space. (C) An intraventricular catheter is inserted through the anterior fontanelle and threaded into the lateral ventricle. (D) A fiberoptic transducer-tipped catheter is inserted through a subarachnoid bolt into the white matter of the brain.

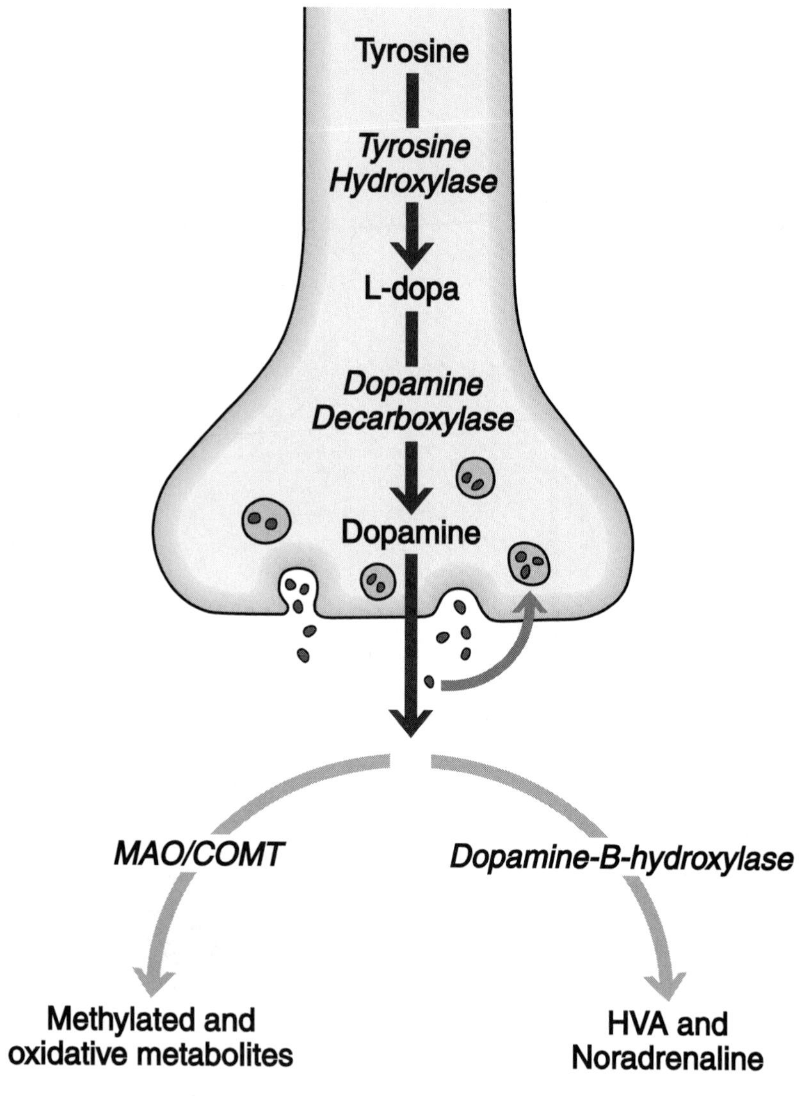

Figure 83. Process of dopamine metabolism at terminal end of axon.

Appendix 2

Table of Nerves

1. Nerves of the Head and Neck Region

Nerve	Origin	Course	Innervation
Abducent	Pons	Intradural on clivus; traverses cavernous sinus and superior orbital fissure to enter orbit	Lateral rectus
Ansa cervicalis	Hypoglossal and cervical plexus	Descends on external surface of carotid sheath	Omohyoid, sternohyoid, and sternothyroid
Deep petrosal	Internal carotid plexus	Traverses cartilage of foramen lacerum, joins greater petrosal nerve at entrance of pterygoid canal	Lacrimal gland, mucosa of nasal cavity, palate, and upper pharynx
Glossopharyngeal	Rostral end of medulla	Exits cranium via jugular foramen, passes between superior and middle constrictors of pharynx to tonsillar fossa, enters posterior third of tongue	Somatic to stylopharyngeus; visceral to parotid gland; posterior 2/3 tongue, pharynx, tympanic cavity, auditory tube, carotid body, and sinus
Great auricular	Cervical plexus	Ascends over sternocleidomastoid; anterior and parallel to external jugular	Skin of auricle, adjacent scalp over angle of jaw; parotid sheath
Greater petrosal	Genu of facial nerve	Exits facial canal via hiatus for greater petrosal nerve	Pterygoid ganglion for innervation of lacrimal, nasal, palatine, and upper pharyngeal mucous glands
Hypoglossal	Between pyramid and olive of myelencephalon	Hypoglossal canal, medial to angle of mandible, between mylohyoid and hypoglossus to muscles of tongue	Intrinsic and extrinsic muscles of tongue

(continued)

Nerve	Origin	Course	Innervation
Intermediate	Facial nerve	Internal acoustic meatus, merging with larger facial nerve	Pterygopalatine and submandibular ganglia via greater petrosal nerve, chorda tympani; tongue and palate
Lesser occipital	Cervical plexus	Parallel to anterosuperior border of sternocleidomastoid	Skin of posterior surface of auricle and adjacent scalp
Lesser petrosal	Tympanic plexus	Tympanic cavity into middle cranial fossa; descends through sphenopetrosal fissure or foramen ovale	Otic ganglion for secretomotor innervation of parotid gland
Long thoracic	Anterior rami	Distally on external surface of serratus anterior	Serratus anterior
Nerve to mylohyoid	Inferior alveolar nerve	Inferior alveolar nerve outside mandibular foramen to groove on medial aspect of ramus of mandible	Mylohyoid and anterior belly of digastric muscle
Nerve to tensor tympani	Otic ganglion	Cartilaginous portion of pharyngotympanic tube to hemicranial of tensor tympani	Tensor tympani
Nerve to tensor veli palatini	Anterior trunk mandibular nerve	Branch of nerve to medial pterygoid	Tensor veli palatini
Olfactory	Olfactory cells in olfactory epithelium of roof of nasal cavity	Foramen of cribriform plate of ethmoid to olfactory bulbs	Olfactory mucosa

(*continued*)

Nerve	Origin	Course	Innervation
Phrenic	Cervical plexus	Superior thoracic aperture between mediastinal pleura and pericardium	Diaphragm; pericardial sac, mediastinal and diaphragmatic pleura, diaphragmatic peritoneum
Posterior inferior nasal	Greater palatine	Greater palatine canal through plate of palatine bone	Mucosa of inferior concha and walls of inferior and middle meatuses
Subclavian	Brachial plexus	Posterior to clavicle, anterior to brachial plexus and subclavian artery	Subclavius; sternoclavicular joint
Supraclavicular	Cervical plexus	Center or posterior border of sternocleidomastoid; fan out as they descend onto lower neck, upper thorax, and shoulder	Skin of lower anterolateral neck, uppermost thorax, and shoulder
Supraorbital	Frontal nerve	Supraorbital foramen, breaks up into small branches	Mucous membrane of frontal sinus, conjunctivae, and skin of forehead
Suprascapular	Brachial plexus	Posterior triangle of neck; under superior transverse scapular ligament	Supraspinatus, infraspinatus muscles; superior and posterior glenohumeral joint
Supratrochlear	Frontal nerve	Supraorbital nerve, divides into two or more branches	Skin in middle of forehead to hairline
Transverse cervical	Cervical plexus	Posterior border of sternocleidomastoid muscle; runs anteriorly across muscle	Skin overlying anterior triangle of neck

(*continued*)

Nerve	Origin	Course	Innervation
Trochlear	Dorsolateral aspect of mesocephalon below inferior colliculus	Passes around brainstem to enter dura in edge of tentorium close to posterior clinoid process; runs in lateral wall of cavernous sinus, entering orbit via superior orbital fissures	Superior oblique muscle
Upper subscapular	Brachial plexus	Posteriorly enters subscapularis	Superior portion of subscapularis

2. Nerves of the Facial Region

Nerve	Origin	Course	Innervation
Auriculotemporal	Mandibular nerve	Passes between neck of mandible and external acoustic meatus to accompany superficial temporal artery	Skin anterior to auricle, posterior temporal region, tragus, helix of auricle, exterior acoustic meatus, upper tympanic membrane
Buccal	Mandibular nerve	Infratemporal fossa, passes anteriorly to reach cheek	Skin and mucosa of cheek, buccal gingiva
Chorda tympani	Facial nerve	Traverses tympanic cavity, passes between incus and malleus; exits temporal bone via petrotympanic fissure; enters infratemporal fossa, merges with lingual nerve	Submandibular and sublingual glands; taste sensation from anterior 2/3 tongue
Deep temporal	Mandibular nerve	Temporal fossa deep to temporalis muscle	Temporalis; periosteum of temporal fossa

(*continued*)

Nerve	Origin	Course	Innervation
External nasal	Anterior ethmoidal nerve	Runs in nasal cavity and emerges on face between nasal bone and lateral nasal cartilage	Skin on dorsum of nose, including tip of nose
Facial	Posterior border of pons	Runs through internal acoustic meatus and facial canal of petrous part of temporal bone, exiting via stylomastoid foramen; forms intraparotid plexus	Stapedius, posterior belly of digastric, stylohyoid, facial and scalp muscles; skin of external acoustic meatus
Greater palatine	Branch of pterygopalatine ganglion (maxillary nerve)	Passes inferiorly through greater palatine canal and foramen	Palatine glands; mucosa of hard palate
Inferior alveolar	Terminal branch of posterior mandibular nerve	Lateral and medial pterygoid muscles of infratemporal fossa to enter mandibular canal of mandible	Lower teeth, periodontium, periosteum, and gingiva of lower jaw
Infraorbital	Terminal branch of maxillary nerve	Runs in floor of orbit and emerges at infraorbital foramen	Skin of cheek, lower lid, lateral side of nose and inferior septum and upper lip, upper premolar incisors and canine teeth; mucosa of maxillary sinus and upper lip
Lesser palatine	Pterygopalatine ganglion	Passes inferiorly through palatine canal and lesser palatine foramen	Glands of soft palate; mucosa of soft palate
Lingual	Terminal branch of posterior mandibular nerve	Joins chorda tympani, passes anteroinferiorly between lateral and medial pterygoid muscles, enters oral cavity	Submandibular ganglion for submandibular and sublingual salivary glands; anterior 2/3 tongue, floor of mouth, lingual mandibular gingiva

(continued)

Nerve	Origin	Course	Innervation
Mandibular	Trigeminal ganglion	Foramen ovale into infratemporal fossa, divides into anterior and posterior trunks, ramifying into smaller branches, bifurcating into lingual and inferior alveolar nerve	Muscles of mastication, mylohyoid, anterior belly of digastric, tensor tympani, tensor veli palatini; skin overlying mandible, lower half of mouth, and temporomandibular joint
Masseteric	Mandibular nerve	Passes laterally through mandibular notch	Masseter; temporomandibular joint
Maxillary	Trigeminal nerve	Anteriorly through foramen rotundum, into pterygopalatine fossa, sensory roots to pterygopalatine ganglion; continues anteriorly through infraorbital fissures as infraorbital nerve	Pterygopalatine ganglion, lacrimal gland, mucosal glands of nasal cavity, palate and upper pharynx; skin overlying maxilla, mucosa of posteroinferior nasal cavity and maxillary sinus; upper half of mouth
Mental	Terminal branch of inferior alveolar nerve	Mandibular canal at mental foramen	Skin of chin; skin and mucosa of lower lip
Nasopalatine	Pterygopalatine ganglion	Exits pterygopalatine fossa via sphenopalatine foramen; runs anteroinferiorly across nasal septum, through incisive foramen to palate	Mucosal glands of nasal septum; mucosa of nasal septum, anterior-most hard palate
Nerve to lateral/ medial pterygoid	Anterior mandibular nerve	Arises in infratemporal fossa, inferior to foramen ovale	Lateral and medial pterygoid muscles

(*continued*)

Nerve	Origin	Course	Innervation
Nerve to pterygoid canal	Formed by merger of greater and deep petrosal nerves	Traverses pterygoid canal, to pterygopalatine ganglion in pterygopalatine fossa	Pterygopalatine ganglion
Nerve to stapedius	Facial nerve	Arises as facial nerve descends posterior to muscle in facial canal	Stapedius
Pharyngeal	Pterygopalatine ganglion	Passes posteriorly through palatovaginal canal	Supplies mucosa of nasopharynx posterior to the pharyngotympanic tubes
Superior alveolar	Maxillary nerve	Emerges from pterygomaxillary fissure into infratemporal fossa to posterior aspect of maxilla; arises from infraorbital nerve of maxillary sinus, descends walls of sinus	Mucosa of maxillary sinus, maxillary teeth and gingiva
Trigeminal	Lateral surface of pons by two roots; motor and sensory	Crosses medial part of crest of petrous part of temporal bone, trigeminal cave of dura mater lateral to body of sphenoid and cavernous sinus; motor root passes ganglion to become part of mandibular nerve	Muscles of mastication, mylohyoid, anterior belly of digastric, tensor tympani, tensor veli palatini; dura of anterior and middle cranial fossa, skin of face, teeth, gingiva, mucosa of nasal cavity, paranasal sinuses and mouth

(*continued*)

Nerve	Origin	Course	Innervation
Zygomatic	Maxillary nerve	Arises in floor of orbit, divides into zygomaticofacial and zygomaticotemporal nerves, traverses foramina of same; communicating b ranch joins lacrimal nerve	Skin over zygomatic arch, anterior temporal region; conveys secretory postsynaptic parasympathetic fibers from pterygopalatine ganglion to lacrimal gland

3. Nerves of the Eye Region

Nerve	Origin	Course	Innervation
Anterior ethmoidal	Nasociliary nerve	Arises in orbit, passes via anterior ethmoidal foramen to cranial cavity then cribriform plate of ethmoid to nasal cavity	Dura of anterior cranial fossa; mucous membranes of sphenoidal sinus, ethmoid cells and upper nasal cavity
Ciliary	Nasociliary nerve; ciliary ganglion	Passes to posterior aspect of eyeball	Cornea, conjunctiva; ciliary body and iris
Frontal	Ophthalmic nerve	Crosses orbit on superior aspect of levator palpebrae superioris; divides into supraorbital and supratrochlear branches	Skin of forehead, scalp, upper eyelid, and nose; conjunctiva of upper lid and mucosa of frontal sinus
Infratrochlear	Nasociliary nerve	Follows medial wall of orbit to upper eyelid	Skin, conjunctiva of upper eyelid
Lacrimal	Ophthalmic nerve	Palpebral fascia of upper eyelid near lateral angle of eye	Small area of skin and conjunctiva of lateral part of upper eyelid

(*continued*)

Nerve	Origin	Course	Innervation
Nasociliary	Ophthalmic nerve	Arises in superior orbital fissure, anteromedially across retrobulbar orbit, providing sensory root to ciliary ganglion, terminates as infratrochlear nerve and nasal branches	Branches of ciliary ganglion convey postsynaptic sympathetic and parasympathetic to ciliary body and iris; tactile sensation from eyeball; mucous membrane of ethmoid cells, anterosuperior nasal cavity; skin of root dorsum and apex of nose
Oculomotor	Interpeduncular fossa of mesencephalon	Dura lateral to posterior clinoid process, lateral wall of cavernous sinus, enters orbit through superior orbital fissure and divides into superior and inferior branches	All extraocular muscles except superior oblique and lateral rectus; presynaptic parasympathetic fibers to ciliary ganglion for ciliary body and sphincter pupillae
Ophthalmic	Trigeminal ganglion	Anteriorly in lateral wall of cavernous sinus to enter orbit through superior orbital fissure, branching into frontal, nasociliary, and lacrimal nerve	General sensation from eyeball; mucous membrane of ethmoid cells, frontal sinus, dura of anterior cranial fossa, falx cerebri, and tentorium cerebelli, anterosuperior nasal cavity; skin of l forehead, upper lid root, dorsum and apex of nose

(continued)

Nerve	Origin	Course	Innervation
Optic	Ganglion cells of retina	Exits orbit via optic canals; fibers from nasal half of retina, crosses to contralateral side at chiasm; passes via optic tracts to geniculate bodies, superior colliculus, and pretectum	Vision from retina
Posterior ethmoidal	Nasociliary	Leaves orbit via posterior ethmoidal foramen	Supplies ethmoidal and sphenoidal paranasal sinuses

4. Nerves of the Ear Region

Nerve	Origin	Course	Innervation
Cochlear	Division of vestibulocochlear nerve	Traverses internal acoustic meatus, enters modiolus with spiral ganglia and peripheral processes in spiral lamina	Spiral organ
Posterior auricular	As first extracranial branch of facial nerve	Passes posterior to ear, sending branch to occipital region	Posterior auricular muscle and intrinsic auricular muscles, occipital belly of occipitofrontalis
Tympanic	As first extracranial branch of glossopharyngeal nerve, from inferior glossopharyngeal ganglion	Passes into tympanic canaliculus, enters tympanic cavity, ramifies on promontory of labyrinthine wall as tympanic plexus	Otic ganglion for secretomotor innervation of parotid gland; mucosa of tympanic cavity, mastoid cells, and pharyngotympanic tube
Vestibular	As a division of the vestibulocochlear nerve	Traverses internal acoustic meatus to vestibular ganglion at fundus; branches pass to vestibule of bony labyrinth	Cristae of ampullae of semicircular ducts, maculae of saccule and utricle

(*continued*)

Nerve	Origin	Course	Innervation
Vestibulocochlear	Groove between pons and myelencephalon	Traverses internal acoustic meatus, dividing into cochlear and vestibular nerve	Spiral organ and cristae of ampullae of semicircular ducts, maculae of saccule and utricle

5. Nerves of the Thoracic Region

Nerve	Origin	Course	Innervation
Abdominopelvic splanchnic	Lower thoracic and lumbar segments of sympathetic trunk	Passes medially and inferiorly to prevertebral ganglion of paraaortic plexus	Abdominopelvic blood vessels and viscera
Cardiac plexus	Cervical and cardiac branches of vagus nerve and cardiopulmonary splanchnic nerve from sympathetic trunk	From arch of aorta, posterior surface of heart, extends along coronary arteries and to SA node	SA nodal tissue, coronary arteries; parasympathetic fibers slow rate, reduce force of heartbeat, constrict arteries; sympathetic fibers have opposite effect
Cardiopulmonary splanchnic	Cervical and upper thoracic ganglia of sympathetic trunk	Descends anteromedially to cardiac, pulmonary and esophageal plexuses	Conveys postsynaptic sympathetic fibers to nerve plexuses of thoracic viscera
Cervical splanchnic	Cervical ganglia of sympathetic trunk	Pass medially and inferiorly to cardiac and pulmonary plexuses	Conducting tissue and coronary arteries
Esophageal plexus	Vagus nerve; sympathetic ganglia, greater splanchnic nerve	Tracheal bifurcation, Vagus, and sympathetic nerve form plexus around esophagus	Vagal and sympathetic fibers to smooth muscles and glands of inferior 2/3 of esophagus
Greater splanchnic	Thoracic sympathetic ganglia	Highest abdominopelvic splanchnic nerve; anteromedially passes on bodies of thoracic vertebrae, through diaphragm to celiac trunk	Celiac ganglia, innervation of celiac arteries

(*continued*)

Nerve	Origin	Course	Innervation
Intercostal	Anterior rami of T1-T11 nerves	Intercostal spaces between internal and innermost layers of intercostal muscles	Intercostal muscles; muscles of anterolateral abdominal wall; skin overlying pleura/peritoneum deep to muscles
Lateral pectoral	Brachial plexus	Clavipectoral fascia to deep surface of pectoral muscles	Pectoralis major, medial pectoral nerve that innervates pectoralis minor
Least splanchnic	12th thoracic ganglion of sympathetic trunk	Diaphragm with sympathetic trunk, ends in renal plexus	Renal arteries and derivatives
Lesser splanchnic	10th and 11th thoracic ganglia of sympathetic trunk	Descends anteromedially to perforate diaphragm to reach aorticorenal ganglion	Prevertebral ganglia; visceral afferents from upper GI tract
Lumbar splanchnic	Lumbar ganglia of sympathetic trunk	Passes anteromedially on bodies of lumbar vertebrae to prevertebral ganglia of paraaortic plexus	Lower abdominal wall and pelvic viscera; visceral afferents from same
Medial pectoral	Medial cord of brachial plexus	Passes between axillary artery and vein, enters deep surface of pectoralis minor	Pectoralis minor and part of pectoralis major
Pulmonary plexus	Vagus nerve, cardiopulmonary splanchnic nerve from sympathetic trunk	Forms on primary bronchi, extends along root of lung and bronchial subdivisions	Parasympathetic fibers constrict bronchioles; sympathetic fibers dilate them
Recurrent laryngeal	Vagus nerve	Subclavian on right; left runs around aortic arch, ascends in tracheoesophageal groove	Intrinsic muscles of larynx (except cricothyroid); inferior to level of vocal cords

(*continued*)

Nerve	Origin	Course	Innervation
Subcostal	Anterior ramus of T12 spinal nerve	Inferior border of 12th rib in same manner as intercostal nerves	Muscles of anterolateral abdominal wall; lateral cutaneous branch supplies skin inferior to anterior iliac crest
Superior laryngeal	Vagus nerve	Descends in parapharyngeal space; lateral to thyroid cartilage divides into internal and external laryngeal nerves; inferior pierces thyrohyoid membrane; runs inferomedially to gap between cricoid and thyroid cartilages	Cricothyroid muscle; supraglottic
Thoracic splanchnic	Thoracic ganglia of sympathetic trunk	Anteromedially on thoracic vertebrae as lower cardiopulmonary splanchnic nerve to thoracic plexus; upper abdominopelvic splanchnic nerves to prevertebral ganglia of paraaortic plexuses	1st–5th splanchnic nerves; 6th–12th splanchnic nerves; thoracic ganglia; presynaptic sympathetic fibers to prevertebral ganglia
Thoracoabdominal	Lower intercostal nerve	Costal margin between 2nd and 3rd layers of abdominal muscles	Anterolateral abdominal muscles; overlying skin, underlying peritoneum, periphery of diaphragm
Thoracodorsal	Posterior cord of brachial plexus	Between upper and lower subscapular nerves, runs inferolaterally along posterior axillary wall to latissimus dorsi	Latissimus dorsi

(continued)

Nerve	Origin	Course	Innervation
Vagus	Via 8–10 rootlets from medulla of brainstem	Superior mediastinum posterior to sternoclavicular joint and brachiocephalic vein; gives rise to recurrent laryngeal nerve; continues into abdomen	Voluntary muscle of larynx and upper esophagus; involuntary muscle/glands of tracheobronchial tree, gut, and heart via pulmonary, esophageal, and cardiac plexuses; pharynx, larynx, reflex afferents from same areas as above

6. Nerves of the Back and Spinal Region

Nerve	Origin	Course	Innervation
Accessory	Medulla and cervical spinal cord	Spinal root ascends into cranial cavity via foramen magnum; exits via jugular foramen; traverses posterior triangle of neck	Sternocleidomastoid and trapezius
Dorsal scapular	Anterior ramus of C5 with contribution from C4	Scalenus medius, descends deep to levator scapulae, enters deep surface of rhomboids	Rhomboids and occasionally supplies levator scapulae
Greater occipital	Medial branch of posterior ramus of spinal nerve C2	Deep muscles of neck and trapezius to ascend posterior scalp to vertex	Multifidus cervicis, semispinalis capitis; posterior scalp
Suboccipital	Posterior ramus of C1 spinal nerve	Between occipital bone and atlas, inferior to transverse part of vertebral artery, into suboccipital triangle; communicates with occipital nerve	Suboccipital muscles

(continued)

7. Nerves of the Shoulder and Arm Region

Nerve	Origin	Course	Innervation
Anterior interosseous	Median nerve in distal cubital fossa	Inferiorly on interosseous membrane	Flexor digitorum profundus, flexor pollicis longus, pronator quadrates
Axillary	Terminal branch of posterior cord of brachial plexus	Posterior aspect of arm with posterior circumflex humeral artery; winds around surgical neck of humerus; gives rise to brachial cutaneous nerve	Teres minor and deltoid; shoulder joint and skin over inferior part of deltoid
Deep branch of radial nerve	Radial nerve distal to elbow	Neck of radius in supinator; posterior compartment of forearm, becomes posterior interosseous nerve	Extensor carpi radialis brevis and supinator
Deep branch of ulnar nerve	Ulnar nerve at wrist, passes between pisiform and hamate	Deep between muscles of hypothenar eminence, across palm with deep palmar arch	Hypothenar muscles, lumbricals of digits 4 and 5, all interossei, adductor pollicis and deep head of flexor pollicis brevis
Lateral cutaneous nerve of forearm	Musculocutaneous nerve	Descends along lateral border of forearm to wrist	Skin of lateral aspect of forearm
Lower subscapular	Posterior cord of brachial plexus	Passes inferolaterally to subscapular artery and vein, to subscapularis and teres major	Inferior portion of subscapularis and teres major
Medial cutaneous nerve of arm	Medial cord of brachial plexus	Runs along medial side of axillary vein; communicates with intercostobrachial nerve	Skin on medial side of arm
Medial cutaneous nerve of forearm	Medial cord of brachial plexus	Runs between axillary artery and vein	Skin over medial side of forearm

(continued)

Nerve	Origin	Course	Innervation
Musculocutaneous	Lateral cord of brachial plexus	Deep surface of coracobrachialis, descends between biceps brachii and brachialis	Flexor muscles of arm; lateral antebrachial cutaneous nerve
Palmar cutaneous branch of ulnar nerve	Arises from ulnar nerve near middle of forearm	Ulnar artery, perforates deep fascia in the distal third of forearm	Skin at base of medial palm, overlying medial carpals
Posterior cutaneous nerve of forearm	Arises in arm from radial nerve	Perforates lateral head of triceps, descends along lateral side of arm and posterior aspect of forearm to wrist	Skin of distal posterior arm, posterior aspect of forearm
Posterior interosseous	Terminal branch of deep branch of radial nerve	Between superficial and deep layers of posterior forearm; between extensor pollicis longus and interosseous membrane	Extensor carpi ulnaris, extensors of digits, abductor pollicis longus
Radial	Terminal branch of posterior cord of brachial plexus	Descends posterior to axillary artery; radial groove with deep brachial artery; passes between long and medial head of triceps; bifurcates in cubital fossa into superficial and deep radial nerve	Triceps brachii, anconeus, brachioradialis, extensor carpi radialis longus muscles; skin on posterior aspect of arm and forearm via posterior cutaneous nerve of arm and forearm
Superficial branch of ulnar nerve	Arises from ulnar nerve at wrist, passes between pisiform and hamate bones	Palmaris brevis, divides into two common palmar digital nerve	Palmaris brevis; skin of the palmar and distal dorsal aspects of digit 5 and medial side of digit 4, proximal portion of palm

(*continued*)

Nerve	Origin	Course	Innervation
Ulnar	Terminal branch of medial cord of brachial plexus	Runs down medial aspect of arm; does not branch in the brachium	Majority of intrinsic muscles of hand; deep head of flexor pollicis brevis; medial lumbricales for digits 4 and 5; skin of palmar and distal dorsal aspects of medial 1–1/2 digits and adjacent palm

8. Nerves of the Hand

Nerve	Origin	Course	Innervation
Common palmar digital	Median and superficial branch of ulnar nerve	Runs distally between long flexor tendons of palm, bifurcating in distal palm	Proper palmar digital nerve; skin and joints of palmar and dorsal aspect of fingers
Dorsal branch of ulnar nerve	Ulnar nerve about 5 cm proximal to flexor retinaculum	Passes distally deep to flexor carpi ulnaris, dorsally to perforate deep fascia, medial side of dorsum of hand, dividing into 2 or 3 dorsal digital nerve	Skin of medial aspect of dorsum of hand, proximal portions of little and medial half of ring finger; adjacent sides of proximal portion of ring and middle fingers
Lateral branch of median nerve	Median nerve as it enters palm of hand	Runs laterally to palmar thumb and radial side of index finger	First lumbrical; skin of palmar and distal dorsal aspects of thumb, radial half of index finger
Medial branch of median nerve	Median nerve as it enters palm	Runs medially to adjacent sides of index, middle and ring fingers	Second lumbrical; skin of palmar and distal dorsal aspects of adjacent sides of index, middle and ring fingers

(*continued*)

Nerve	Origin	Course	Innervation
Median	Arises by two roots; one from lateral cord of brachial plexus, one from medial cord; root joins lateral to axillary artery	Medial side of brachial artery; cubital fossa, between heads of pronator teres, intermediate and deep layers of anterior forearm; becomes superficial proximal to wrist; passes deep to flexor retinaculum	Flexor muscles in forearm; thenar muscles, lateral lumbricals; skin of palmar and distal dorsal aspects of lateral 3–1/2 digits and palm
Palmar cutaneous branch of ulnar nerve	Arises from ulnar nerve, near middle of forearm	Ulnar artery and deep fascia in distal third of forearm	Skin at base of medial palm overlying medial carpals
Recurrent branch of median nerve	Median nerve distal to flexor retinaculum	Distal border of flexor retinaculum, enters thenar muscles	Abductor pollicis brevis, opponens pollicis, superficial head of flexor pollicis brevis
Superficial branch of radial nerve	Radial nerve	Anterior to pronator teres, to brachioradialis; deep fascia at wrist, passes onto dorsum of hand	Skin of lateral half of dorsum of hand and thumb, proximal portions of digits 2, 3, and lateral half of 4

9. Nerves of the Abdomen and Pelvic Regions

Nerve	Origin	Course	Innervation
Cavernous nerve	Parasympathetic fibers of prostatic nerve plexus	Perforates perineal membrane to reach erectile bodies of penis	Helicine arteries of cavernous bodies; stimulation produces engorgement at arterial pressure

(continued)

Nerve	Origin	Course	Innervation
Clunial	Posterior rami of L1, L2, and L3; posterior rami of S1, S2, and S3; posterior cutaneous nerve of thigh	Superior nerves cross iliac crest: middle nerves exit through posterior sacral foramina, entering gluteal region; inferior nerves curve around inferior border of gluteus maximus	Skin of buttock or gluteal region as far as greater trochanter
Coccygeal	Conus medullaris of spinal cord	Anterior and posterior rami join adjacent rami of S4 and S5; anterior rami form coccygeal plexus, gives rise to anococcygeal nerve	Skin over coccyx
Genitofemoral	Lumbar plexus	Descends on anterior surface of psoas major, divides into genital and femoral branches	Femoral branch supplies skin over femoral triangle; genital branch supplies scrotum or labia majora; genital branch to cremaster muscle
Hypogastric	Superior hypogastric plexus into pelvis	Sacrum within hypogastric sheath, merges with pelvic splanchnic nerve in inferior hypogastric plexus	Pelvic viscera; intraperitoneal pelvic viscera
Iliohypogastric	Lumbar plexus	Traverses abdominal muscle; external oblique aponeurosis to reach inguinal and pubic regions	Internal oblique and transverse abdominal muscles; superolateral quadrant of buttock; skin over iliac crest and hypogastric region

(*continued*)

Nerve	Origin	Course	Innervation
Ilioinguinal	Lumbar plexus	Passes between 2nd and 3rd layers of abdominal muscles; inguinal canal, divides into femoral and scrotal or labial branches	Lower part of internal oblique, transverse abdominal muscles; skin over femoral triangle; mons pubis, adjacent skin of labia majora or scrotum
Inferior anal	Pudendal nerve	Pudendal canal, medially through ischioanal fat pad to anal canal	External anal sphincter; perianal skin
Inferior gluteal	Sacral plexus	Pelvis through greater sciatic foramen inferior to piriformis, divides into several branches	Gluteus maximus
Lateral cutaneous nerve of thigh	Lumbar plexus	Deep to inguinal ligament, medial to anterior superior iliac spine	Skin on anterior and lateral aspects of thigh
Nerve to obturator internus	Sacral plexus	Gluteal region, greater sciatic foramen, inferior to piriformis; descends posterior to ischial spine; lesser sciatic foramen, to obturator internus	Superior gemellus and obturator internus
Quadratus femoris	Sacral plexus	Leaves pelvis through greater sciatic foramen deep to sciatic nerve	Inferior gemellus and quadratus femoris; hip joint
Obturator	Lumbar plexus	Enters thigh through obturator foramen, divides into anterior and posterior branches	Adductor longus, adductor brevis, gracilis, and pectineus; obturator externus, adductor magnus; skin of medial thigh above knee

(*continued*)

Nerve	Origin	Course	Innervation
Pelvic splanchnic	Sacral plexus	Runs anteriorly and inferiorly to merge with inferior hypogastric plexus	Parasympathetic fibers for pelvic viscera, descending and sigmoid colon; subperitoneal pelvic viscera
Perineal	Terminal branch of pudendal nerve	Pudendal nerve from pudendal canal to superficial perineum dividing into superficial cutaneous and deep motor branch	Urogenital triangle; skin of posterior urogenital triangle
Posterior cutaneous nerve of thigh	Sacral plexus	Leaves pelvis through greater sciatic foramen inferior to piriformis, deep to gluteus maximus	Skin of buttock; skin over posterior aspect of thigh and calf; lateral perineum, upper medial thigh
Posterior labial	Perineal nerve	Pudendal canal and ramifies in subcutaneous tissue	Skin of posterior portion of labium majus
Pudendal	Sacral plexus	Enters gluteal region through greater sciatic foramen inferior to piriformis; descends to sacrospinous ligament; perineum through lesser sciatic foramen	Most motor and sensory innervation to perineum
Sciatic	Sacral plexus	Enters gluteal region through greater sciatic foramen inferior to piriformis; descends along posterior aspect of thigh, divides proximal to knee into tibial and common fibular peroneal nerves	Hamstrings; provides articular branches to hip and knee joints

(continued)

Nerve	Origin	Course	Innervation
Superior gluteal	Sacral plexus	Leaves pelvis through greater sciatic foramen, superior to piriformis, runs between gluteus medius and minimus	Gluteus medius, gluteus minimus, tensor fasciae latae

10. Nerves of the Legs and Feet

Nerve	Origin	Course	Innervation
Anterior femoral cutaneous	Femoral nerve	Arises in femoral triangle, fasciae latae of thigh along path of sartorius muscle	Skin on medial and anterior aspects of thigh
Calcaneal branches	Tibial and sacral nerves	Passes from distal part of posterior aspect of leg to skin on heel	Skin of heel
Common fibular	Terminal branch of sciatic nerve	Begins at apex of popliteal fossa; follows medial border of biceps femoris muscle to posterior aspect of head of fibula; bifurcates into superficial and deep fibular nerves	Skin on lateral part of posterior aspect of leg; knee joint via articular branch; short head of biceps femoris
Common plantar digital	Medial and lateral plantar nerves	Runs anteriorly in sole of foot between flexor tendons; bifurcates in distal sole	Proper plantar digital nerves; skin and joints of plantar and distal dorsal aspect of toes
Deep fibular	Common fibular nerve	Arises between fibularis longus and neck of fibula; extensor digitorum longus; extensor retinaculum; distal end of tibia, enters dorsum of foot	Muscles of anterior compartment of leg, dorsum of foot; skin of first interdigital cleft; sends articular branches to the joints it crosses

(*continued*)

Nerve	Origin	Course	Innervation
Femoral	Lumbar plexus	Passes deep to midpoint of inguinal ligament; lateral to femoral vessels, divides into muscular and cutaneous branches	Anterior thigh muscles; hip and knee joints; skin on anteromedial side of thigh and leg
Lateral plantar	Smaller terminal branch of tibial nerve	Passes laterally in foot between quadratus plantae, flexor digitorum brevis muscles, divides into superficial and deep branches	Quadratus plantae, abductor digiti minimi, flexor digiti minimi brevis; plantar and dorsal interossei, lateral three lumbricals, adductor hallucis; skin on sole lateral to a line splitting 4th digit
Medial cutaneous nerve of leg	Saphenous nerve	Descends medial side of leg with greater saphenous vein	Skin of antero-medial side of leg and medial side of foot
Medial dorsal cutaneous nerve	Superficial fibular nerve	Descends across ankle anteriorly running onto medial aspect of dorsum of foot	Most of skin of dorsum of foot, proximal portion of toes, except for web between great and 2nd toes
Medial plantar	Terminal branch of the tibial nerve	Passes distally in foot between abductor hallucis and flexor digitorum brevis; divides into muscular and cutaneous branches	Abductor hallucis, flexor digitorum brevis, flexor hallucis brevis and first lumbrical; skin of medial side of sole of foot and sides of first three digits
Saphenous	Femoral nerve	Descends with femoral vessels through femoral triangle and adductor canal, descends with great saphenous vein	Skin on medial side of leg and foot

(continued)

Nerve	Origin	Course	Innervation
Superficial fibular	Common fibular nerve	Arises between fibularis longus and neck of fibula, descends in lateral compartment of leg; deep fascia at distal third of leg, becomes cutaneous and sends branches to foot and digits	Fibularis longus and brevis; skin on distal third of anterior surface of leg, dorsum of foot and all digits except lateral side of 5th and adjoining sides of 1st and 2nd digits
Sural	Arises from medial and lateral sural cutaneous nerves	Descends between heads of gastrocnemius, becomes superficial at middle of leg; descends with small saphenous vein, passes posterior to lateral malleolus to lateral side of foot	Skin on posterior and lateral aspects of leg and lateral side of foot
Tibial	Sciatic nerve	Forms as sciatic, bifurcates at apex of popliteal fossa; descends through same, lies on popliteus; runs inferiorly on tibialis posterior with posterior tibial vessels; terminates beneath flexor retinaculum, dividing into medial and lateral plantar nerves	Muscles of posterior compartment of thigh; popliteal fossa, posterior compartment of leg, sole of foot; knee joint, skin of leg, sole of foot

Appendix 3

Types of Brain and Spinal Cord Tumors

Type	Location
Astrocytoma	A glioma that arises most frequently in the cerebrum of adults. Arises in the brain stem, cerebrum, and cerebellum of children. Astrocytomas can be classified as low-grade well-differentiated, anaplastic, pilocytic, and glioblastoma multiforme.
Brainstem glioma	Occurs in the lowest portion of brain.
Chordoma	Spinal cord tumor that develops from remnants of early fetal spine-like structure, which is later replaced by the spinal cord.
Craniopharyngioma	Occurs near hypothalamus, in the pituitary gland region. Usually benign, but can be considered malignant because of potential damage to the hypothalamus from pressure, affecting vital functions.
Ependymoma	Commonly develops in the lining of the ventricles; can also develop in spinal cord.
Ganglioneuroma	Occurs in the brain or spinal cord.
Germ cell tumor	Arises from developing sex cells.
Glioblastoma multiforme	Also called grade 4 astrocytoma; originates in glial cells.
Hemangioblastoma	Arises from blood vessels of the brain and spinal cord.
Medulloblastoma	Usually develops in the cerebellum, but may occur in other areas as well.
Meningioma	Develops in the medulla and can spread to the spine or to other parts of the body.
Mixed oligoastrocytoma	Comprised of oligodendrocytes and astrocytes; originates in glial cells.

Oligodendroglioma	Usually arises in the cerebrum; fewer than 10% are malignant.
Optic nerve glioma	Occurs on or near the nerves that travel between the eye and brain vision centers.
Pineal region tumor	Occurs in the pineal gland region.
Pituitary adenoma	Occurs in the pituitary gland, generally arising in adenohypophysis.
Schwannoma	May originate from a peripheral or sympathetic nerve, or from various cranial nerves, particularly the eighth nerve.

Appendix 4
Sleep Medicine Terminology

acoustic signature event (ASI)
adjustment sleep disorder
advanced sleep-phase syndrome
alcohol-dependent sleep disorder
altitude insomnia
anxiety disorder
apnea
apnea-hypopnea index (AHI)
apnea index (AI)
auto-PAP (APAP)
behavior disorder
benign neonatal sleep myoclonus
bilevel PAP (BiPAP)
body mass index (BMI)
cataplexy
central alveolar hypoventilation syndrome
central sleep apnea (CSA)
chronic obstructive pulmonary disease (COPD)
chronic insomnia
circadian rhythm
confusional arousal
congenital central hypoventilation syndrome
continuous positive airway pressure (CPAP)
cycle of sleep
delayed sleep-phase syndrome
desaturation index (DI)
disorders of excessive sleepiness
disorders of initiation and maintenance of sleep
dyssomnia
electrical status epilepticus of sleep
electrocardiogram (EKG)
electroencephalogram (EEG)
electrooculography (EOG)
environmental sleep disorder
Epworth Sleepiness Scale (ESS)
excessive daytime sleepiness
extraocular movements (EOM)
fatal familial insomnia
food allergy insomnia
full-night polysomnography
function of sleep
genioglossus advancement
hyoid advancement
hypnagogic hallucination
hypnotic-dependent sleep disorder
hypopnea
idiopathic hypersomnia
infant sleep apnea
insufficient sleep syndrome
insomnia
irregular sleep-wake pattern
laser-assisted uvulopalatoplasty (LAUP)
laser uvulopalatoplasty (LUPP)
limit-setting sleep disorder
long sleeper
lowest saturation of oxygen
maintenance of wakefulness test (MWT)
mixed sleep apnea
mood disorder
movement disorder
multiple sleep latency test (MSLT)
narcolepsy
nasal continuous positive airway pressure (NCPAP, nCPAP)
neck circumference
nightmare
nocturnal cardiac ischemia
nocturnal dyspnea
nocturnal eating syndrome
nocturnal leg cramp
nocturnal pain
nocturnal paroxysmal dystonia
nocturnal polysomnography

nonrapid eye movement sleep
obesity hypoventilation syndrome (OHS)
obstructive apnea (OA)
obstructive sleep apnea (OSA)
obstructive sleep apnea-hypopnea (OSAH)
obstructive sleep apnea-hypopnea syndrome (OSAHS)
obstructive sleep apnea syndrome (OSAS)
oral appliance therapy
oximetry
oxygen desaturation index (ODI)
panic disorder
parasomnia
periodic limb movement (PLM)
periodic limb movement disorder (PLMD)
periodic limb movements of sleep
polysomnography (PSG)
positive airway pressure (PAP)
posttraumatic insomnia
primary insomnia
primary snoring disorder (PSD)
psychophysiologic insomnia
quality of life (QOL)
rapid eye movement (REM)
recurrent insomnia
respiratory arousal index (RAI)
respiratory disturbance index (RDI)
respiratory effort-related arousal
respiratory event arousal (REA)
restless leg syndrome (RLS)
rhythmic movement disorder
saturation of oxygen (SaO_2)
short sleeper
sleep apnea (SA)
sleep apnea syndrome (SAS)
sleep architecture
sleep bruxism
sleep choking syndrome
sleep deprivation
sleep drunkenness
sleep hallucination
sleep hyperhidrosis
sleep hygiene
sleep hypopnea syndrome (SHS)
sleep inertia
sleeping sickness
sleep-onset association disorder
sleep onset period (SOP)
sleep onset of rapid eye movement
sleep paralysis
sleep-related asthma
sleep-related breathing disorder (SRBD)
sleep-related epilepsy
sleep-related headache
sleep start
sleep talking
sleep terror
sleepwalking
slow-wave sleep (SWS)
snoring
somnolence
stimulant-dependent sleep disorder
subwakefulness syndrome
sudden infant death syndrome (SIDS)
terrifying hypnagogic hallucination
toxin-induced sleep disorder
upper airway
upper airway resistance syndrome (UARS)
uvulopalatopharyngoplasty (UPPP)
uvulopalatoplasty (UPP)
velopharyngeal incompetence (VPI)
volitional sleep deprivation
wakefulness

Appendix 5
Sample Reports and Dictation

CEREBROSPINAL FLUID LEAK REPAIR

PREOPERATIVE DIAGNOSIS: Cerebrospinal fluid leak with headache secondary to dural tears.

POSTOPERATIVE DIAGNOSIS: Cerebrospinal fluid leak with headache secondary to dural tears.

PROCEDURE PERFORMED: Left L4–5 laminotomy and primary repair of tiny dural tears times two with 7–0 Prolene suture and fibrin glue.

ANESTHESIA: General endotracheal.

OPERATIVE INDICATIONS AND CONSENT: The patient is a 35-year-old female who is status post left L4–5 and right L5-S1 percutaneous microdiscectomy. She went home and was doing well, but then after being home she developed a headache, nausea, and vomiting. She was returned to the hospital with an intractable headache. She was put on bedrest with intravenous hydration and intravenous narcotics plus antiemetics. She started feeling better and I got her back up the following day and the headaches returned immediately.

At the time of the surgery, there was some CSF leakage. It was repaired with a fat graft and fibrin glue at the time. I discussed this problem with the patient and her daughter. I told her that we would have to go back and do a primary repair with suture since it is obvious clinically that the fat graft did not work. Understanding the above and the risks involved, the patient and her daughter requested the following procedure be performed.

DETAILS OF PROCEDURE: The patient was taken to the operating room after induction of general endotracheal anesthesia. The patient was placed in the prone position on the Wilson frame. The back was prepped and draped in the usual aseptic fashion and the upper portion of the old incision was reopened sharply and taken down.

The investing fascia was opened with Bovie electrocautery and a finger dissection was carried out to expose the lamina of L4 and L5, and the Aesculap retractor system was placed in the usual fashion. The microscopes were brought into place.

At this point in time, I removed the fat graft and then took down more of the ligamentum flavum dorsally and did a laminotomy of L4 and L5 with a Black Max drill using a blue 8 tip and also a 3-mm punch, being careful to keep the dura down with a Woodson. CSF was coming out through two small holes measuring a couple of millimeters each; they were adjacent to one another. These were closed with two individual interrupted 7–0 Prolene sutures. Once the second one was in place, there was no longer any CSF, and a Valsalva maneuver confirmed the same. I then placed fibrin glue over this and activated it. I then also inspected the disk space again. I found a little bit more disk material medially that I took down with a downbiting Scoville curette and then removed with pituitary rongeurs. The dura was again free, soft, and supple.

The wound was irrigated with antibiotic solution and closed in multiple layers using interrupted 0 Vicryl in the investing fascia, the second layer in the deep layer of superficial fascia, and then interrupted subcuticular closure was accomplished with 3–0 Vicryl. Benzoin and Steri-Strips were applied to the skin edges and a sterile dressing was placed over the same. Needle and sponge counts were correct. Estimated blood loss was approximately 25–50 cc. Replacement was that of crystalloid only. There were no complications. The patient was extubated and taken to the recovery room in stable condition.

Craniotomy and Hematoma Evacuation

Preoperative Diagnosis: Epidural hematoma with right temporal fracture, coma.

Postoperative Diagnosis: Epidural hematoma with right temporal fracture, coma.

Procedure Performed: Right temporal parietal craniotomy, evacuation of epidural hematoma, coagulation of middle meningeal bleeders, and right frontal bur holes through separate incision and placement of parenchymal Camino intracranial pressure monitor using Ventrix system and closure of dural laceration.

Anesthesia: General endotracheal.

Indications: The patient is a 13-year-old who had a bicycle accident where he flipped over his handlebars, hitting his head and causing a scalp laceration, hematoma. He was taken to the ER where a CAT scan was done, which showed a small epidural hematoma in the right temporal region and a small fracture. The patient was transferred to the hospital by ambulance and deteriorated en route. He was intubated en route and when he arrived he was decerebrate on the left, decorticate on the right, with dilated nonreactive pupils, right greater than left. The patient was hypertensive. He was taken immediately to the CAT scanner where the CT showed tremendous enlargement of the same epidural hematoma on the right side. He was taken immediately to the OR. I discussed the case very briefly with his mother, who accompanied us to the operating area, and discussed with her the emergent need to take care of her son.

DETAILS OF PROCEDURE: With the patient in the OR, the hair on the right side of the head was shaved. The scalp was prepared in the usual septic fashion. A hockey-stick incision was made from about the zygoma just anterior to the right ear, and this was taken a little bit posteriorly and then in a coronal fashion toward the top of the head, then brought forward. Raney clips were applied, the temporalis muscle was incised with Bovie electrocautery, and cerebellar retractors were placed. A fracture down the temporal region was noticed. A bur hole was placed in the parietal region, and an oval bone flap was obtained. This was done immediately and a very large clot was evacuated. There was a small bleeder inferiorly in the temporal region and then there was more bleeding posterior. Two more loops of bone were taken with the craniotome, and the microscope was brought into place to enable me to see back. There was a small inferior bleeder that was over the posterior aspect of the petrous bone that was coagulated and at this point in time bleeding had stopped. The wound was irrigated copiously with antibiotic solution.

The dura was tented up all the way around through multiple holes in a very snug fashion. The bone flap was reconstructed using Synthes 1.5 system titanium plates and 4-mm screws; 5-hole and 2-hole plates were used and then this was replaced using same. This was nice and solid all the way around. It should be noted that three sets of tack-up sutures were placed in the bone flap and 4–0 Prolene was used to tack the dura up. A 7 flat Jackson-Pratt drain was placed and brought through a separate stab incision superiorly, temporalis muscle closed with running 3–0 Vicryl, as was the fascia. The scalp was closed in two layers with interrupted 3–0 Vicryl on the galea and staples on the skin.

Drape was taped down, the head was again prepped in the right frontal region, skin was infiltrated with 0.5% lidocaine with epinephrine, and a parasagittal incision was made in the mid pupillary line, centered approximately 10 cm back from the glabella, 3 cm to the right of midline, and small retractor was placed. A bur hole was placed; dura was incised with a #11 blade. With the Ventrix catheter, I made two passes at the ventricle and then left it in situ at about 5-cm depth and then had it tunneled out through a separate stab incision. The pressure in the OR was running about 11 mmHg.

The wound was irrigated with antibiotic solution and closed in two layers using interrupted 3–0 Vicryl on the galea and running 3–0 Prolene to close the skin. The ICP monitor was sutured at the exit site with 3–0 Prolene. The scalp laceration on the back was irrigated with antibiotic solution and closed with running 3–0 Prolene. Sterile dressing was applied, instrument and sponge counts correct. Estimated blood loss was 200 cc. Replacement was with that of crystalloid only. No complications.

The patient was taken intubated to the ICU. It should be noted that postop the dura was nice and pulsatile, brain was pulsatile, and the pupils were now both small and equal.

Craniotomy for Clip Ligation of Posterior Communicating Artery Aneurysm

Preoperative Diagnosis: Left posterior communicating artery aneurysm.

Postoperative Diagnosis: Left posterior communicating artery aneurysm.

Procedure Performed: Left pterional craniotomy for clip ligation, posterior communicating artery aneurysm.

Anesthesia: General endotracheal.

Estimated Blood Loss: Minimal.

Complications: None.

Details of Procedure: After informed consent was obtained, the patient was brought to the operating room. General anesthesia was induced, and the patient was smoothly intubated. His head was placed in Mayfield headholder. His head was turned to the right side 20 degrees, extended in the vertex position. The left side of his head was prepped and draped sterilely.

A curvilinear incision was made from 1 cm anterior to the tragus, through the zygoma, extending superiorly and then curving anteriorly to the point of mid pupillary line on his forehead. The subgaleal space was encountered and Raney clips were placed. The skin flap was reflected inferiorly and anteriorly. A fascial splitting dissection was performed at the deep portions of the temporalis muscle. The temporalis muscle was incised just inferior to the temporal line and the muscle was cauterized. The temporalis muscle was reflected inferiorly and anteriorly using periosteal elevator, and was held in place with hooks.

Pterional craniotomy was performed and bone flap was elevated without difficulty. The dura was intact after removal of the bone. The greater wing of the sphenoid was drilled until the superior lateral orbital walls were well skeletonized. The dura was opened in a curvilinear fashion based over the coronoid process and reflected inferiorly and held in place with tack-up sutures. The sylvian fissure was opened slightly to release spinal fluid. The frontal lobe was retracted superiorly until the carotid and optic nerve cisterns were encountered. These were opened sharply to release more CSF. The medial margin of the carotid artery was carefully dissected until proximal control of the carotid artery was achieved. A large, narrow-necked aneurysm was noted along the posterior lateral wall of the carotid artery.

A straight Yasargil clip was placed after dissection of the neck of the aneurysm, deflating the aneurysm completely. Dissection after the aneurysm was clipped revealed an intact anterior carotid artery and posterior communicating artery. The third nerve was identified and noted to be free of compression. The entire subdural space was irrigated.

The dura was closed primarily and tack-up sutures were placed. The bone was replaced with three 2-hole microplates. The temporalis muscle was reattached to the fascial border and subdural space was irrigated. A 10-French round J-P drain was placed. The galea was closed with interrupted 2–0 Vicryl stitches. The skin was closed with staples. A sterile dressing was applied. The Mayfield headholder was released. The head was wrapped.

The patient was awakened from anesthesia, extubated, and transported to the recovery room in excellent condition, after tolerating the procedure well. There were no complications.

ELECTROENCEPHALOGRAM

CLINICAL HISTORY: The patient is a 76-year-old female who presents with spells consisting of tingling sensation and taste dysfunction. She also had a previous stroke. She is on Synthroid, Coumadin, Zoloft, and Cardizem.

TECHNICAL DESCRIPTION: This is a 21-channel recording with the patient in the awake and drowsy states. Eighteen channels were used for EEG, together with two channels of EOG and one channel of EKG. Referential and bipolar montages were used with the Standard 10–20 Electrode System. In addition, T1 and T2 electrodes were utilized. The patient was not sedated further.

REPORT: During wakefulness, the background activity consisted of a posteriorly dominant, relatively irregular 9 hertz alpha activity with amplitudes of up to 30 microvolts. This was reactive to eye opening and was intermixed with moderate amounts of anteriorly dominant, lower amplitude, faster frequencies in the beta band. Hyperventilation was not performed due to the patient's medical condition. Photic stimulation elicited some mild driving response symmetrically. The sleep study only showed some drowsy periods with alpha dropout. No definite spindle activity was seen. There was some fluctuating asymmetry and frequency, but no definitive focal slowing.

IMPRESSION: This electroencephalogram is within normal limits. No definite epileptiform or lateralizing activity was seen. Clinical correlation is suggested.

EVOKED POTENTIAL STUDY

CLINICAL HISTORY: The patient is a 45-year-old male who presents with back pain and sensory disturbance, particularly involving the left side of the body. Apparently, he has tingling sensation in the hands and feet. No medications are listed.

DETAILS OF PROCEDURE: Visual Evoked Potential Study: Independent stimulation of the left and right eyes with pattern reversal stimuli and other stimulating recording parameters standardized for this laboratory showed definite reproducible waveforms. There was occasionally fair signal-to-noise ratio, but attempts at different trials and check sizes were performed. On left-sided stimulation, the smaller check sizes gave a P-100 potential of 119.6 msec. Higher check sizes of the same side produced a P-100 latency of 116 msec. On right-sided stimulation, there was fair signal-to-noise ratio, and even at repeated attempts, this was difficult to determine. However, the most reliable P-100 potential was measured at 144 msec. The patient has attempted to try his best, but looked tired.

Brainstem Auditory Evoked Potential Study: Independent stimulation of the left and right ears with rarefaction clicks and other stimulating and recording parameters standardized for this laboratory showed definite reproducible waveforms. On left-sided stimulation, at 100 dB interpeak latencies were as follows: I-III 2.2 msec, III-V 2.04 msec, I-V 4.24 msec. There was minimal variability in using lower intensities at 90 dB. On right-sided stimulation, this was measured as follows: I-III 2.2 msec, III-V 2.06 msec, I-V 4.26 msec. These are within normal limits.

Median Nerve Somatosensory Evoked Potential Study: Independent stimulation of the left and right median nerves with square-wave clicks and other stimulation and recording parameters standardized for this laboratory showed reproducible obligate waveforms. There was lower amplitude fair signal-to-noise ratio cervical potential, but they were still recognizable. On left-sided stimulation, interpeak latencies were as follows: Erb point to N-13 was 3.4 msec, N-13 to N-20 was 5.3 msec, Erb point to N-20 was 8.7 msec. On right-sided stimulation, the N-13 or cervical potential was still of low amplitude for definite identification. However, the most probable waveform showed the following interpeak latencies: Erb point to N-13 of 3.5 msec, N-13 to N-20 of 5.2 msec, Erb point to N-20 of 8.7 msec. These are within normal limits.

Posterior Tibial Nerve Somatosensory Evoked Potential Study: Independent stimulation of the left and right posterior tibial nerves with square-wave clicks and other stimulating and recording parameters showed definite reproducible waveforms. There was, however, fair signal-to-noise ratio on the limbal potential for definite identification. On left-sided stimulation, the amplitude of P-37 potential was measured at 42 msec. The popliteal fossa to P-37 interpeak latency was 30.6 msec. There was poor signal-to-noise ratio for definite identification of the limbal potential. On right-sided stimulation, while there was fair to signal-to-noise ratio, there was perhaps more definite reproducible limbal potential. The popliteal fossa to limbal potential interpeak latency was 11.6 msec, while the limbal potential to P-37 interpeak latency was 19 msec. The popliteal fossa to P-37 interpeak latency was 30.6 msec. The absolute P-37 latency was 41.4 msec. These are within normal limits.

IMPRESSION: Abnormal visual evoked potential study with prolongation of the P-100 potential, worse on the right than the left. Interpretation should be made with caution, since the patient was described as being tired. Nevertheless, at least for the left side, both small and large check sizes were used, and these still showed prolongation of the P-100 potential. On right-sided stimulation, almost a sinusoidal waveform was seen for definite interpretation of the lower amplitude potential. This did not identify the exact localization in the visual axis.

Normal brainstem auditory evoked potential study.

Normal median nerve somatosensory evoked potential study.

Normal posterior tibial nerve somatosensory evoked potential study.

Clinical correlation is suggested.

HERNIATED DISK REPAIR

PREOPERATIVE DIAGNOSIS: Herniated disk with left sciatica.

POSTOPERATIVE DIAGNOSIS: Herniated disk with left sciatica.

PROCEDURE PERFORMED: Left L4–5 laminotomy, medial facetectomy, and diskectomy with microscope.

ANESTHESIA: General endotracheal anesthesia.

INDICATION AND CONSENT: The patient is a 46-year-old gentleman with severe left hip pain and left sciatica. He cannot walk very far and has to crawl. MRI shows a large disk herniation of the L4–5 level. We discussed surgical intervention, the risks involved, the pre- and postoperative course. I have answered all his questions, and in accordance with his wishes, the following has been performed.

DETAILS OF PROCEDURE: The patient was taken to the operating room. After induction of general endotracheal anesthesia, the patient was placed in the prone position on the Wilson frame. The back was shaved, prepped and draped in the usual aseptic fashion. A midline incision was made over the spinous process of L4 and L5. Subperiosteal dissection of the lamina of L4 and L5 was carried out with a Cobb periosteal dissector, and the Aesculap retractor system was placed in the usual fashion. The microscope was brought into place and Black Max drill with a blue #24 tip, which was used to perform laminotomies at L4 and L5, very small on L5, while pressure of the medial facetectomy was also carried out. The 3- and 5-mm punches were used to deepen this and also to take out the ligamentum flavum.

The nerve root was identified and teased from the disk with a #4 Penfield dissector and gently retracted medially with the Love nerve root retractor. Epineural veins were cauterized with bipolar electrocautery and the anus was cut with a #1 blade, and the disk was removed with pituitary rongeurs, straight up and downbiting. A small-diameter curette and Woodson instrument were all used to tease out a significant amount of disk from the disk space. This freed up the nerve root and dura nicely and cleaned out the disk space very nicely as well.

Wounds were irrigated with antibiotic solution. Hemostasis was achieved with bipolar electrocautery and bone wax as necessary. The wound was then closed in multiple layers using interrupted 0 Vicryl in the investing fascia, the second layer on the deep layer of superficial fascia and then an interrupted subcuticular closure was accomplished with 3–0 Vicryl. Benzoin and Steri-Strips were applied to the skin edges, and a sterile dressing was placed over the same. Needle and sponge counts were correct. Estimated blood loss was approximately 50 cc. Replacement was that of crystalloid only. There were no complications.

LAMINECTOMY WITH RESECTION OF TUMOR

PREOPERATIVE DIAGNOSIS: Likely metastatic tumor to spine, epidural T2–3 with spinal cord compression.

POSTOPERATIVE DIAGNOSIS: Metastatic epidural intraspinal tumor consistent with the lung mass, sarcomatoid carcinoma.

PROCEDURE PERFORMED: T12-L3 laminectomy and resection of epidural intraspinal metastatic tumor with microscope.

ANESTHESIA: General endotracheal.

INDICATIONS AND CONSENT: The patient is a 63-year-old gentleman with recently diagnosed sarcomatoid cancer. He underwent needle biopsy of his lung mass. This is a left pericardial mass done with a blood patch. Because of low back pain and some weakness, he had MRI of the lumbar spine which showed some abnormal signal in the L1 virtual body, but bone scan showed no evidence of uptake. This was not consistent with any tumor. He has a lot of degenerative arthritis of the lumbar spine, and he has had two previous operations in the low back many years ago. There is no cord compression at this level. Unfortunately, as he has been here he has had some neurological deterioration in terms of his ability to walk, but not in terms of being able to move his legs. They have been weak and not able to support him this past week.

MRI spinal cord evaluation was then performed with repeat of the lumbar spine, and the lesion at L2–3 was identified as an epidural mass posterior dorsal to the cord, causing cord compression. His exam does not show myelopathy, but he is unable to bear weight. I discussed the surgical approach with the patient, and he requested the following be performed.

DETAILS OF PROCEDURE: The patient was taken to the operating room. After induction of general endotracheal anesthesia, the patient was placed in the prone position on chest rolls. Head was placed in the Mayfield-Kees 3-point headholder. The upper thoracic area was prepped and draped in the usual aseptic fashion. A midline incision was made from about L1 to L3–4 and carried down through the investing fascia with Bovie electrocautery. The laminae of L1–3 were exposed with Bovie electrocautery and Cobb periosteal dissector. Cerebellar retractors were placed. Hemostasis was achieved with bipolar electrocautery and Bovie electrocautery. Spinous processes of L1, L2, and L3 were taken off, as was the base, with the Leksell rongeur. Then, using Black Max drill with a blue #24 tip under loupe magnification, the laminotomy was increased and then using microscope with 2- and 3-mm punches, the laminectomy was completed, more to the patient's left side than to the right. The tumor came into view. This was tougher and discolored tissue that was certainly different from the epidural fat. The tissue was sent off for frozen section and came back consistent with the same tissue that was obtained on the prior biopsy from his lung, specifically sarcomatoid carcinoma.

I resected all the tissue that was causing pressure on the spinal cord and chased off to the foramen on the left side, but certainly did not remove all of it. When I was done, the cord was completely decompressed and pulsating nicely. The edges of the tumor were cauterized with bipolar electrocautery. Wounds were irrigated with antibiotic solution. Hemostasis was also achieved with bone wax, as necessary.

A deep #15 round Jackson-Pratt drain was placed through a separate stab incision on the patient's right side of the wound, and then the wound was closed in multiple layers using interrupted 0 Vicryl in the muscular layer, second layer on the investing fascia, a third layer on the deep layer of superficial fascia, and then an interrupted subcuticular closure was accomplished with 3–0 Vicryl. Staples were placed to close the skin edge. A sterile dressing was applied. Needle and sponge counts were correct. Estimated blood loss was approximately 300 cc. Replacement was that of crystalloid only. There were no complications. Patient was extubated and taken to the recovery room in stable condition.

POLYSOMNOGRAPHY STUDY

CLINICAL HISTORY: The patient is a 50-year-old female who presents with a chief complaint of, "I have trouble falling asleep and staying asleep. Once I wake up at night, I have trouble going back to sleep. I often wake up with a headache." She measures 5 feet 8 inches tall, weighs 191 pounds, and has a neck circumference of 13–1/2 inches. The Epworth sleepiness scale score is 6.

REVIEW OF SLEEP QUESTIONNAIRE: Review shows that she goes to bed around 10 to 10:30 p.m., varying about 1 to 2 times a week. It takes her about an hour to go to sleep. Often, at the onset of sleep, she feels muscular tension, has an uncontrollable urge to move the legs, has some form of discomfort, has vivid dream-like scenes, and feels anxious. She sleeps for about 5 to 6 hours, awakening 2 to 3 times with some difficulty going back to sleep. At times, she may be awake 2 to 3 hours, usually in the second half of the night. Often during sleep, she feels afraid of not returning to sleep if she awakens, has a bed partner, is restless, gets up for one reason or another, and has dreams. Her sleep is often disrupted by the need to urinate and feeling like she has to move the legs. She wakes up at 6 a.m., getting out of bed at 6:05 a.m. Often she depends on the alarm clock. She often has a hard time waking up, wakes up with a headache, wakes up with a dry mouth, or within 1 to 2 hours of appointed time of awakening. She takes 5 naps a week, lasting for 1 hour, which she finds refreshing. She often is sleepy during the day, but rarely falls asleep unintentionally. She often feels muscular tension. She never feels weak when suddenly excited.

The family history is significant for a nephew who has trouble sleeping and staying asleep, and a son who has trouble falling asleep. Behaviorally, she does not drink alcoholic beverages, smoke cigarettes, or use recreational drugs. She drinks decaffeinated coffee, 1 or 2 caffeinated tea preparations a week, and 20 ounces of soda in a typical day. She has a history of headaches, depression, low blood pressure, back trouble, and allergies. She has not had any oronasal surgeries, but has had a thyroid surgery.

REVIEW OF BED PARTNER QUESTIONNAIRE: Suggests that the patient is observed every night to have loud snoring and twitching and jerking of the legs and arms. The patient is not described as being sleepy during the day.

MEDICATIONS: Synthroid, Paxil, ginkgo biloba, magnesium, Surfak, and vitamin complex preparations.

REPORT: The study was requested as a split protocol, but the patient did not satisfy criteria and only a diagnostic study is available. The patient slept for 5–1/2 hours with a sleep efficiency of 73.4%. There were increased arousals of 17 events per hour and awakenings of 1 event per hour. The sleep architecture was disrupted with reduced slow-wave sleep of 2.4% and relatively stable REM stage of 20%. There was no reduction in sleep latencies. The apnea/hypopnea index was 5.6, which in the supine position was 16.9 and during REM stage was 14.6. The patient had 6 apneic episodes and 25 hypopneic episodes. The former were mainly obstructive. The patient had soft to loud and occasionally disruptive snoring. The mean oxygenation was 93.5% SaO2 with 36 desaturations, the lowest of which was 88% SaO2. The patient spent 0.1% of the study in oxygenation of less than 89% SaO2. The mean heart rate was 63.1 beats per minute, with a minimum of 47 and maximum of 94. The periodic leg movement index was 0. No dramatic EEG changes were seen.

IMPRESSION: Sleep apnea syndrome, mainly obstructive, mild overall, with desaturation as low as SaO2 of 88%. This was exaggerated during the supine position and during rapid eye movement sleep stage. No increased periodic leg movements of sleep, with the possible historical suggestion of restless leg syndrome based on the patient's sleep questionnaire.

RECOMMENDATIONS: In general, for mild sleep apnea, conservative measures such as weight loss, appropriate sleep hygiene, avoidance of the supine position, avoidance of sedative hypnotics including alcoholic beverages at night and smoking, if applicable, are recommended. In addition, alternative approaches may also include oronasal appliances and surgical procedures. There may be a basis for using nasal CPAP in this patient's case, but a stepwise approach is suggested.

The patient has no increased periodic leg movements of sleep but may have a strong suggestion of restless leg syndrome based on the sleep questionnaire. Before treatment is to be given, however, this should be further explored in the patient's subsequent visits to determine if it is a true sleep disrupter. Restless leg syndrome may occur independently or may be associated with other comorbid states, including iron-deficiency anemia, peripheral neuropathy, uremia, vitamin deficiencies, and the like.

As mentioned previously, the study was requested as a split protocol, but the patient did not meet criteria and only a diagnostic study is available.

It is not clear whether this study alone explains the patient's chief complaint of sleep initiation and maintenance insomnia. She alludes occasionally to psychological symptoms and, as such, psychophysiologic mechanisms and psychological etiologies may need to be explored. Systemic conditions may also need to be explored.

The patient should be advised regarding safety in driving while in a somnolent condition. Clinical correlation is suggested.

STEREOTACTIC BIOPSY OF BRAIN TUMOR

PREOPERATIVE DIAGNOSIS: Malignant primary versus metastatic left parietal brain tumor.

POSTOPERATIVE DIAGNOSIS: Malignant primary versus metastatic left parietal brain tumor.

PROCEDURE PERFORMED: Left parietal bur hole and CT-guided biopsy of same with glioblastoma multiforme favored by the pathologist postoperatively on frozen section.

ANESTHESIA: General endotracheal.

INDICATION/CONSENT: The patient is a 90-year-old gentleman with a change in speech and balance problems that have been improved with Decadron. MRI was obtained and it showed an approximately 4- to 5-cm left parietal tumor that comes to the surface with a significant amount of cerebral edema. I discussed the problem with the patient and family and discussed the consideration of trying a gross total resection. The patient did not want to accept any significant risks and, therefore, requested a biopsy be performed instead. In accordance with his wishes, the following was performed.

DETAILS OF PROCEDURE: The patient was taken to the operating room, and after induction of general endotracheal anesthesia, the patient was on the CT scanner table. The stereotactic frame ring was put into place. The patient was turned left side up, right side down. He was placed into the ring and his head was supported in the usual fashion. Pillows and normal bracing were placed around his body to keep him in a somewhat lateral position and was just ever so slightly turned to the right so the left side of the head was facing upward. The hair was shaved. Markers were placed on the scalp, and the CT scan gave me the localization. I made a small needle cut in the skin at the site for the biopsy (the patient had been given contrast material). The markers were removed, and the skin scalp was further shaved, prepped and draped in the usual septic fashion.

The skin was infiltrated with 0.5% lidocaine with epinephrine, and a vertical incision was made behind the ear, centered about the point marked by CT, and small Weitlaner retractors were placed. The temporalis muscle was cauterized and opened sharply and then the bur hole was placed with a Black Max drill using an M1 tip. This was opened a little bit further with a 2-mm punch. The bone was not bleeding. The dura was cut using bipolar electrocautery and opened with an 11 blade and then the stereotatic apparatus was further placed and the biopsy probe was evaluated; it was right at the surface, as was the tumor.

Using the biopsy probe, I went below the surface and took the first biopsy, which was sent to be frozen. This came back consistent with high-grade primary tumor being favored versus metastatic. I took another freehand sample, more anterior, since this was immediately below the surface. There was a lot of good tissue that was also sent for permanent section. There was minimal bleeding. The wound was irrigated with antibiotic, and the postbiopsy CT scan showed no evidence of any blood in the tumor, but there was some air in the tumor itself, as expected.

The wound was again irrigated with antibiotic solution. A thrombin gel was placed in the bur hole site, and the scalp flap was closed in two layers using interrupted 3–0 Vicryl on the galea; running 3–0 Prolene was used to close the skin. A sterile dressing was applied. Needle and sponge counts were correct. Estimated blood loss was approximately 10 cc. Replacement was that of crystalloid only. There were no complications. The patient was extubated and taken to the recovery room in stable condition.

SUBOCCIPITAL CRANIOTOMY

PREOPERATIVE DIAGNOSIS: Left suboccipital depressed skull fracture.

POSTOPERATIVE DIAGNOSIS: Left suboccipital depressed skull fracture.

PROCEDURE PERFORMED: Left suboccipital craniotomy for elevation of depressed skull fracture.

ANESTHESIA: General endotracheal.

ESTIMATED BLOOD LOSS: Minimal.

COMPLICATIONS: None.

DETAILS OF PROCEDURE: After informed consent was obtained, the patient was brought to the operating room. General anesthesia was induced, and the patient was smoothly intubated. The Mayfield headholder was placed. He was turned in the prone position and all pressure points were carefully padded. The left suboccipital area was prepped and draped sterilely.

A linear incision was made and dissection was carried down to the bone using monopolar cautery. A depressed skull fracture was encountered. The edges of the skull fracture were carefully drilled. A small fragment of bone was removed and through that defect the dura was inspected and found to be intact. Curettes were used to elevate the remainder of the fracture into an upright position. The epidural space and the pericranial space were copiously irrigated with bacteriostatic solution. The dura was again reinspected. There was no apparent leakage of spinal fluid.

The muscle was reapproximated. The fascia was closed with Vicryl. The subcutaneous tissues were closed with Vicryl. The skin was closed with a running 4–0 chromic suture. A sterile dressing was applied. The patient was turned to the supine position, awakened from anesthesia, extubated and transported to the recovery room in excellent condition after tolerating the procedure well.

TRIGEMINAL NERVE DECOMPRESSION

PREOPERATIVE DIAGNOSIS: Left trigeminal neuralgia.

POSTOPERATIVE DIAGNOSIS: Left trigeminal neuralgia.

PROCEDURE PERFORMED: Left retrosigmoid craniotomy, microvascular decompression of left trigeminal nerve and drilling of petrous bone with microscope.

ANESTHESIA: General endotracheal.

INDICATIONS/CONSENT: The patient is a 48-year-old female with left tic douloureux, most severe in the V1 and V2 distributions, and going on for at least three years. It has gotten to the point where she is not able to get this under control with Tegretol. The pain is severely limiting all of her activities. I discussed with her the many different approaches toward treatment of this, specifically the microvascular decompression, the radiofrequency rhizotomy, the balloon rhizotomy, as well as simple avulsion procedures. We discussed the risks of each of these, the potential recurrence rate of each of these being similar, at about 17%, the risks of stroke, coma, and death as well as cranial nerve abnormalities. This was discussed with the patient in detail and all of her questions were answered. After careful consideration, the patient has requested the following be performed.

DETAILS OF PROCEDURE: The patient was taken to the operating room. After induction of general endotracheal anesthesia, a lumbar drain was placed. The patient was given mannitol. She was placed in the lateral decubitus position left side up and right side down. She is an obese woman. All pressure points were padded. An axillary roll was placed and her left shoulder was gently taped down to the side. The hair behind the left ear was shaved and the scalp was shaved and then prepped and draped in the usual septic fashion, and the skin was infiltrated with 1% lidocaine with epinephrine.

A linear, somewhat curved incision was made just posterior to the mastoid process itself, following a posterior groove, and this was opened further with Bovie electrocautery and a cerebellar retractor was placed. A bur hole was placed in the region of the asterion and this appeared to be bordering the transverse sinus. The craniotome was used to make a small bone flap and this required enlarging a little bit anterior to reach the sigmoid sinus. Once exposed, the dura was opened in a cruciate fashion.

The lumbar drain, unfortunately, was not draining adequately; therefore, the cisterna magna was opened using a #1 Penfield dissector and then a small hook and this drained CSF very nicely, which allowed excellent relaxation of the cerebellar hemisphere. It was of interest that at the superiormost portion of the cerebellar hemisphere at the junction with the tentorium there was a tremendous amount of adhesion and this required careful dissection with bipolar electrocautery to finally free this up and free up the number of small veins that drain directly in this region. Once this was accomplished, the retractor was placed.

The cerebellum was gently retracted from a more medial position, enabling us to go down directly to the region of the fifth nerve. The first thing that became apparent was that there was a very large bony protuberance from the petrous bone in the region of the trigeminal nerve. There were also very large veins. These were the superior petrosal veins. Two of these were taken, which enabled better exploration of the trigeminal nerve. There was also a vein underneath the nerve that was not taken.

The superior cerebellar artery was identified along with the bifurcation in the cranial and caudal branches, but these did not pass in the immediate vicinity of the trigeminal nerve. The nerve was explored at the exit point from the pons, and there was no evidence of any pontine artery or any aberrant vessels coming up against the nerve itself.

The drill with a diamond bur was then used to drill down the bony protuberance facing just anterior to the nerve itself. Once this was taken down, the bone eminence was waxed with bone wax. The nerve root was further explored on both sides and no more veins were taken. The retractor was removed. The cerebellar surface appeared to be intact. The wound was irrigated. The surface of the cerebellar hemisphere of the posterior fossa was irrigated copiously and carefully with sterile irrigation solution. There was no evidence of any bleeding.

The dura was closed with interrupted and running 4–0 Prolene. Two dural allografts were sutured into the dura and then with a Valsalva maneuver; there was no leakage of CSF at all. At this time fibrin glue was used over this area and another piece of AlloDerm was cut and placed over the entire exposed dural opening that had been coated with the fibrin glue. More fibrin glue was put over the outer surface and then the bone flap was replaced with three 5-hole Synthes plates. These were the 1.5 system using 4-mm screws. These held the bone graft in excellent position in the center of the opening and it held the AlloDerm graft in place. There was virtually no bleeding. No drain was placed.

The wound was closed in multiple layers using interrupted 0 Vicryl in the deep layers and also superficial layers and then staples were used to close the skin. Sterile dressing was applied. Needle and sponge counts were correct. Estimated blood loss approximately 75 to 100 cc. Replacement was that of crystalloid only. There were no complications. The patient was extubated, was moving all four extremities with no obvious cranial nerve abnormalities, and was taken to the recovery room in stable condition.

Ventricular Catheter Placement

Preoperative Diagnosis: Cerebral edema, status post evacuation of epidural hematoma.

Postoperative Diagnosis: Cerebral edema, status post evacuation of epidural hematoma.

Procedure Performed: Placement of left frontal ventricular catheter, ventriculostomy through twister.

Anesthesia: Phenobarbital coma, plus local 1% lidocaine with epinephrine.

Indications: The patient is a 13-year-old who, following a bicycling accident, was found to have skull fracture and right epidural hematoma. He was en route to the hospital when the epidural hematoma blossomed. He went into a coma, was intubated, was taken directly from the ambulance to CAT scan, where it was confirmed there was a huge clot. He was taken down to the operating room immediately, which was prepared for him. The hematoma was evacuated promptly. He had a problem with increased pressure and coagulopathy. He had a hematoma along the catheter track on the right side parenchymal catheter. Once the coagulopathy was controlled, the catheter was removed. The patient was taken off phenobarbital to see how he was generally doing, in hope that his white count and CAT scan were looking good. Once phenobarbital was sufficiently weaned, he developed cerebral edema. He was being followed with CT scans twice daily. The CT scans showed increased edema. I discussed the problem with the family, the concerns about placing another catheter, of infection, bleeding, paralysis, and seizures. The family understood and requested the following be performed.

Details of Procedure: The patient was in the pediatric intensive care unit. Hair was shaved and now, on the left side, skin was shaved and prepped with alcohol and then Betadine, and the paint was allowed to dry. After careful draping, the parasagittal incision was made approximately 3 cm left of center, about 9 to 10 cm back from the mid pupillary line from the glabella, and this was taken down to the bone. Heiss retractor was placed, and the twister was used to make the twist hole.

The dura was incised and bone was removed with forceps. Then the 35-cm ventricular catheter was advanced into the lateral ventricle without difficulty. CSF came out under what appeared to be elevated pressure; it was clear. This was then tunneled laterally and then the slack was taken out of the system. The hub was then placed and secured with 3–0 Prolene and connected to a Becker drainage system, which was primed, and the intracranial pressures were running 39 to 43.

The wound was closed with running 3–0 Prolene in a single layer and then the ventricular cavity was secured at the exit point with 3–0 Prolene. Sterile dressing was applied. We were able to drain CSF from the cavity, but after a few drops came out, it would slow down. As a result, we went back to the monitor and plan to continue this pattern to keep the catheter open. There were no complications.

VENTRICULOPERITONEAL SHUNT REVISION

PREOPERATIVE DIAGNOSIS: Ventriculoperitoneal shunt failure.

POSTOPERATIVE DIAGNOSIS: Ventriculoperitoneal shunt failure.

PROCEDURE PERFORMED: Ventriculoperitoneal shunt revision and cranioplasty.

ANESTHESIA: General endotracheal.

ESTIMATED BLOOD LOSS: Minimal.

COMPLICATIONS: None.

DETAILS OF PROCEDURE: After informed consent was obtained from the family, the patient was brought to the operating room. General anesthesia was induced. The patient was smoothly intubated. Her head was turned to the left side and her posterior scalp was prepped and draped sterilely, including her right neck, right anterior chest, and right anterior abdomen. Previous sutures were removed.

A new bur hole site was identified superior and lateral to the previous entry site to approach the lateral ventricle. Monopolar cautery dissection was used to establish the subgaleal plane. A subgaleal pocket was made.

The previous incision was opened and the shunt valve was encountered. The shunt was dismantled. There was sluggish flow through the valve into the distal system. On inspection of the valve, the valve appeared to contain some debris. Attempts were made to connect a new valve system from the new pocket to the old pocket. Because of a kink in this configuration, the entire shunt system was removed.

The abdominal incision was again explored prior to removal of the shunt. A new valve with a new distal catheter was tunneled from the new pocket. Using a ventriculoscope, the catheter was guided into the frontal horn without difficulty and connected to the distal system. Once again, a Delta performance level I valve was used. The distal catheter was cut short and then placed into the abdominal cavity without difficulty.

All wounds were copiously irrigated. The skull defect at the previous site was filled with cranioplasty material. All wounds were sutured closed. Sterile dressings were applied. The patient was awakened from anesthesia, extubated, and taken to the recovery room in excellent condition after tolerating the procedure well.

Appendix 6

Common Terms by Procedure

Cerebral Spinal Fluid Leak Repair

Aesculap retractor system
aseptic fashion
benzoin
Black Max drill
cerebrospinal fluid (CSF)
CSF leak
dural tear
fat graft
fibrin glue
finger dissection
intractable headache
investing fascia
laminotomy
ligamentum flavum
microdiscectomy
pituitary rongeur
primary repair
Scoville curette
usual aseptic fashion
Valsalva maneuver
Wilson frame
Woodson elevator

Craniotomy and Hematoma Evacuation

Bovie electrocautery
bur hole
Camino intracranial pressure monitor
epidural hematoma
galea
glabella
hockey-stick incision
ICP monitor
intracranial pressure (ICP)
Jackson-Pratt drain
parasagittal incision
stab incision
Synthes 1.5 system titanium plate
tack-up suture
temporal parietal craniotomy
titanium plate
Ventrix system
zygoma

Craniotomy for Clip Ligation of Posterior Communicating Artery Aneurysm

communicating artery aneurysm
coronoid process
curvilinear incision
frontal lobe
Mayfield headholder
microplate
narrow-necked aneurysm
optic nerve cistern
orbital wall
periosteal elevator
pterional craniotomy
Raney clip
splitting dissection
subdural space
subgaleal space
sylvian fissure
tack-up suture
temporalis muscle
Yasargil clip

Electroencephalogram

alpha activity
alpha dropout
background activity
beta band
bipolar montage
21-channel recording
driving response
electrocardiogram (EKG)
electroencephalogram (EEG)
electrooculogram (EOG)

epileptiform activity
focal slowing
lateralizing activity
microvolt
photic stimulation
rarefaction click
sleep study
spindle activity

Evoked Potential Study

amplitude potential
brainstem auditory evoked potential study
Erb point
interpeak latency
limbal potential
median nerve somatosensory evoked potential study
obligate
pattern reversal stimulus
posterior tibial nerve somatosensory evoked potential study
reproducible obligate waveform
signal-to-noise ratio
sinusoidal waveform
somatosensory evoked potential study
spindle activity
square-wave click
visual axis
visual evoked potential study
waveform

Herniated Disk Repair

Aesculap retractor system
benzoin
bipolar electrocautery
Black Max drill
Cobb periosteal dissector
crystalloid
diskectomy
disk herniation
disk space
downbiting
epineural
herniated disk
laminotomy
ligamentum flavum
Love nerve root retractor
magnetic resonance imaging (MRI)
medial facetectomy
midline incision
Penfield dissector
pituitary rongeur
sciatica
spinous process
Steri-Strips
subperiosteal dissection
superficial fascia
usual aseptic fashion
Wilson frame
Woodson instrument

Laminectomy with Resection of Tumor

abnormal signal
bipolar electrocautery
Black Max drill
bone scan
bone wax
Bovie electrocautery
cerebellar retractor
Cobb periosteal dissector
crystalloid
epidural fat
frozen section
hemostasis
intraspinal tumor
investing fascia
Jackson-Pratt drain
laminectomy
loupe magnification
lumbar spine
Mayfield-Kees 3-point headholder
metastatic tumor
3-mm punch
muscular layer
needle biopsy

neurological deterioration
pericardial mass
sarcomatoid carcinoma
spinal cord compression
subcuticular closure
superficial fascia
uptake
virtual body

Polysomnography Study

apneic episode
awakenings
continuous positive airway pressure (CPAP)
desaturation
disruptive snoring
hypopneic episode
increased arousal
maintenance insomnia
mean oxygenation
nasal CPAP
oronasal appliance
oxygen saturation (SaO_2)
periodic leg movement index
peripheral neuropathy
psychological etiology
psychophysiologic mechanism
rapid eye movement (REM)
REM stage
restless leg syndrome
SaO2
sleep apnea syndrome
sleep disrupter
sleep efficiency
sleep initiation
sleep latency
sleep stage
slow-wave sleep
uremia

Stereotactic Biopsy of Brain Tumor

biopsy probe
bipolar electrocautery
Black Max drill
bur hole
cerebral edema
computed tomography (CT)
contrast material
CT-guided biopsy
CT scanner table
dura
freehand sample
frozen section
galea
general endotracheal anesthesia
glioblastoma multiforme
gross total resection
high-grade primary tumor
lidocaine with epinephrine
magnetic resonance imaging (MRI)
malignant brain tumor
metastatic parietal brain tumor
M1 tip
parietal bur hole
parietal tumor
permanent section
scalp flap
stereotatic apparatus
stereotactic frame ring
temporalis muscle
usual aseptic fashion
Weitlaner retractor

Suboccipital Craniotomy

bacteriostatic solution
curette
depressed skull fracture
dura
epidural space
leakage of spinal fluid
linear incision
Mayfield headholder
pericranial space
pressure point
running 4–0 chromic suture
suboccipital area

suboccipital craniotomy
supine position
upright position

Trigeminal Nerve Decompression

aberrant vessel
AlloDerm graft
asterion
avulsion procedure
axillary roll
balloon rhizotomy
bifurcation
bone eminence
bone flap
bone graft
bone wax
bony protuberance
Bovie electrocautery
bur hole
caudal branch
cerebellar hemisphere
cerebellar retractor
cerebellum
cisterna magna
cranial branch
cranial nerve abnormality
craniotome
cruciate fashion
crystalloid
diamond bur
dura
dural opening
fibrin glue
lidocaine with epinephrine
mastoid process
microvascular decompression
Penfield dissector
petrosal vein
petrous bone
pontine artery
posterior fossa
posterior groove
potential recurrence
radiofrequency rhizotomy
retrosigmoid craniotomy
sigmoid sinus
superior cerebellar artery
Synthes plate
tentorium
tic douloureux
transverse sinus
trigeminal nerve
trigeminal neuralgia
Valsalva maneuver

Ventricular Catheter Placement

Becker drainage system
Betadine
CAT scan
cerebral edema
coagulopathy
computerized axial tomography (CAT)
computerized tomography (CT)
CT scan
dura
epidural hematoma
glabella
Heiss retractor
hematoma
lidocaine with epinephrine
parasagittal incision
phenobarbital
twister
twist hole
ventricular catheter
ventriculostomy

Ventriculoperitoneal Shunt Revision

bur hole site
cranioplasty
Delta performance level I valve
frontal horn
lateral ventricle

monopolar cautery
prepped and draped sterilely
shunt valve
subgaleal plane
subgaleal pocket
ventriculoperitoneal shunt failure
ventriculoperitoneal shunt revision
ventriculoscope

Appendix 7

Drugs by Indication

ALZHEIMER DISEASE

Acetylcholinesterase Inhibitor
- Aricept® [US/Can]
- Cognex® [US]
- donepezil
- Exelon® [US/Can]
- rivastigmine
- tacrine

Acetylcholinesterase Inhibitor (Central)
- galantamine
- Reminyl® [US]

Cholinergic Agent
- Exelon® [US/Can]
- rivastigmine

Ergot Alkaloid and Derivative
- ergoloid mesylates
- Germinal® [US]
- Hydergine® LC [US]
- Hydergine® [US/Can]

AMYOTROPHIC LATERAL SCLEROSIS (ALS)

Anticholinergic Agent
- atropine
- Atropine-Care® [US]
- Atropisol® [US/Can]
- Isopto® Atropine [US/Can]
- Sal-Tropine™ [US]

Cholinergic Agent
- Mestinon®-SR [Can]
- Mestinon® Timespan® [US]
- Mestinon® [US/Can]
- pyridostigmine
- Regonol® [US]

Dopaminergic Agent (Anti-Parkinson)
- levodopa

Miscellaneous Product
- Rilutek® [US]
- riluzole

Skeletal Muscle Relaxant
- Apo®-Baclofen [Can]
- baclofen
- Gen-Baclofen [Can]
- Lioresal® [US/Can]
- Liotec [Can]
- Nu-Baclo [Can]
- PMS-Baclofen [Can]

BEHÇET SYNDROME

Immunosuppressant Agent
- Alti-Azathioprine [Can]
- azathioprine
- cyclosporine
- Gen-Azathioprine [Can]
- Gengraf™ [US]
- Imuran® [US/Can]
- Neoral® [US/Can]
- Sandimmune® [US/Can]

CEREBRAL PALSY

Skeletal Muscle Relaxant
- Dantrium® [US/Can]
- dantrolene

CLAUDICATION

Blood Viscosity Reducer Agent
- Albert® Pentoxifylline [Can]
- Apo®-Pentoxifylline SR [Can]
- Nu-Pentoxifylline SR [Can]
- pentoxifylline
- Trental® [US/Can]

CUSHING SYNDROME

Antineoplastic Agent
- aminoglutethimide
- Cytadren® [US]

CUSHING SYNDROME (DIAGNOSTIC)

Diagnostic Agent
- Metopirone® [US]
- metyrapone

DEEP VEIN THROMBOSIS (DVT)

Anticoagulant (Other)
- Coumadin® [US/Can]
- dalteparin
- danaparoid
- enoxaparin
- Fragmin® [US/Can]
- Hepalean® [Can]
- Hepalean® Leo [Can]
- Hepalean®-LOK [Can]
- heparin
- Hep-Lock® [US]
- Innohep® [US/Can]
- Lovenox® [US/Can]
- Orgaran® [US/Can]
- Taro-Warfarin [Can]
- tinzaparin
- warfarin

Factor Xa Inhibitor
- Arixtra® [US]
- fondaparinux

Low Molecular Weight Heparin
- Fraxiparine™ [Can]
- nadroparin [Canada only]

DYSTONIA

Neuromuscular Blocker Agent, Toxin
- botulinum toxin type B
- Myobloc® [US]

EPICONDYLITIS

Nonsteroidal Antiinflammatory Drug (NSAID)
- Advil® Children's [US-OTC]
- Advil® Infants' Concentrated Drops [US-OTC]
- Advil® Junior [US-OTC]
- Advil® [US/Can]
- Aleve® [US-OTC]
- Anaprox® DS [US/Can]
- Anaprox® [US/Can]
- Apo®-Ibuprofen [Can]
- Apo®-Indomethacin [Can]
- Apo®-Napro-Na [Can]
- Apo®-Napro-Na DS [Can]
- Apo®-Naproxen [Can]
- Apo®-Naproxen SR [Can]
- EC-Naprosyn® [US]
- Gen-Naproxen EC [Can]
- Genpril® [US-OTC]
- Haltran® [US-OTC]
- ibuprofen
- Ibu-Tab® [US]
- Indocid® [Can]
- Indocid® P.D.A. [Can]
- Indocin® SR [US]
- Indocin® [US]
- Indo-Lemmon [Can]
- indomethacin
- Indotec [Can]
- I-Prin [US-OTC]
- Menadol® [US-OTC]
- Motrin® Children's [US/Can]
- Motrin® IB [US/Can]
- Motrin® Infants' [US-OTC]
- Motrin® Junior Strength [US-OTC]
- Motrin® [US/Can]
- Naprelan® [US]
- Naprosyn® [US/Can]
- naproxen
- Naxen® [Can]
- Novo-Methacin [Can]
- Novo-Naprox [Can]
- Novo-Naprox Sodium [Can]
- Novo-Naprox Sodium DS [Can]
- Novo-Naprox SR [Can]
- Novo-Profen® [Can]
- Nu-Ibuprofen [Can]
- Nu-Indo [Can]
- Nu-Naprox [Can]
- Rhodacine® [Can]
- Riva-Naproxen [Can]
- Synflex® [Can]
- Synflex® DS [Can]

EPILEPSY

Anticonvulsant
- acetazolamide
- Alti-Clobazam [Can]
- Alti-Divalproex [Can]
- Apo®-Acetazolamide [Can]
- Apo®-Carbamazepine [Can]
- Apo®-Divalproex [Can]
- carbamazepine
- Carbatrol® [US]
- Celontin® [US/Can]
- clobazam [Canada only]
- Depacon® [US]
- Depakene® [US/Can]
- Depakote® Delayed Release [US]
- Depakote® ER [US]
- Depakote® Sprinkle® [US]
- Diamox Sequels® [US]
- Diamox® [US/Can]
- Epitol® [US]
- Epival® I.V. [Can]
- ethosuximide
- felbamate
- Felbatol® [US]
- Frisium® [Can]
- gabapentin
- Gabitril® [US/Can]
- Gen-Carbamazepine CR [Can]
- Gen-Divalproex [Can]
- Lamictal® [US/Can]
- lamotrigine
- magnesium sulfate
- methsuximide
- Neurontin® [US/Can]
- Novo-Carbamaz [Can]
- Novo-Clobazam [Can]
- Novo-Divalproex [Can]
- Nu-Carbamazepine® [Can]
- Nu-Divalproex [Can]
- PMS-Carbamazepine [Can]
- PMS-Valproic Acid [Can]
- PMS-Valproic Acid E.C. [Can]
- Rhoxal-valproic [Can]
- Sabril® [US/Can]
- Taro-Carbamazepin [Can]
- Tegretol® [US/Can]
- Tegretol®-XR [US]
- tiagabine
- Topamax® [US/Can]
- topiramate
- valproic acid and derivatives
- vigabatrin [Canada only]
- Zarontin® [US/Can]

Anticonvulsant, Miscellaneous
- Keppra® [US/Can]
- levetiracetam
- oxcarbazepine
- Trileptal® [US/Can]

Anticonvulsant, Sulfonamide
- Zonegran™ [US/Can]
- zonisamide

Antidepressant
- Alti-Clobazam [Can]
- clobazam [Canada only]
- Frisium® [Can]
- Novo-Clobazam [Can]

Barbiturate
- amobarbital
- Amytal® [US/Can]
- Apo®-Primidone [Can]
- Luminal® Sodium [US]
- Mebaral® [US/Can]
- mephobarbital
- Mysoline® [US/Can]
- phenobarbital
- primidone

Benzodiazepine
- Alti-Clonazepam [Can]
- Apo®-Clonazepam [Can]
- Apo®-Clorazepate [Can]
- Apo®-Oxazepam [Can]
- Clonapam [Can]
- clonazepam
- clorazepate
- Gen-Clonazepam [Can]
- Klonopin™ [US/Can]

Novo-Clonazepam [Can]
Novo-Clopate [Can]
Nu-Clonazepam [Can]
oxazepam
PMS-Clonazepam [Can]
Rho-Clonazepam [Can]
Rivotril® [Can]
Serax® [US]
Tranxene® [US/Can]

Hydantoin
Cerebyx® [US/Can]
Dilantin® [US/Can]
ethotoin
fosphenytoin
Peganone® [US/Can]
Phenytek™ [US]
phenytoin

EXTRAPYRAMIDAL SYMPTOMS

Anticholinergic Agent
Akineton® [US/Can]
Apo®-Benztropine [Can]
Apo®-Trihex [Can]
Artane® [US]
benztropine
biperiden
Cogentin® [US/Can]
Kemadrin® [US/Can]
Procyclid™ [Can]
procyclidine
trihexyphenidyl

GAUCHER DISEASE

Enzyme
alglucerase
Ceredase® [US]
Cerezyme® [US]
imiglucerase

GLIOMA

Antineoplastic Agent
CeeNU® [US/Can]
lomustine

Antiviral Agent
interferon alfa-2b and ribavirin combination pack
Rebetron™ [US/Can]

Biological Response Modulator
interferon alfa-2b
interferon alfa-2b and ribavirin combination pack
Intron® A [US/Can]
Rebetron™ [US/Can]

GUILLAIN-BARRÉ SYNDROME

Immune Globulin
Carimune™ [US]
Gamimune® N [US/Can]
Gammagard® S/D [US/Can]
Gammar®-P I.V. [US]
immune globulin (intravenous)
Iveegam EN [US]
Iveegam Immuno® [Can]
Panglobulin® [US]
Polygam® S/D [US]
Venoglobulin®-S [US]

HARTNUP DISEASE

Vitamin, Water Soluble
niacinamide

HEAVY METAL POISONING

Antidote
deferoxamine
Desferal® [US/Can]

HUNTINGTON CHOREA

Monoamine Depleting Agent
Nitoman® [Can]
tetrabenazine [Canada only]

INTERMITTENT CLAUDICATION

Platelet Aggregation Inhibitor
cilostazol
Pletal® [US/Can]

INTRACRANIAL PRESSURE
Barbiturate
- Pentothal® Sodium [US/Can]
- thiopental

Diuretic, Osmotic
- mannitol
- Osmitrol® [US/Can]

JAPANESE ENCEPHALITIS
Vaccine, Inactivated Virus
- Japanese encephalitis virus vaccine (inactivated)
- JE-VAX® [US/Can]

LEAD POISONING
Chelating Agent
- BAL in Oil® [US]
- Calcium Disodium Versenate® [US]
- Chemet® [US/Can]
- Cuprimine® [US/Can]
- Depen® [US/Can]
- dimercaprol
- edetate calcium disodium
- penicillamine
- succimer

MARFAN SYNDROME
Rauwolfia Alkaloid
- reserpine

MÉNIERE DISEASE
Antihistamine
- Antivert® [US/Can]
- betahistine [Canada only]
- Bonamine™ [Can]
- Bonine® [US/Can]
- Dramamine® II [US-OTC]
- meclizine
- Meni-D® [US]
- Serc® [Can]

MERCURY POISONING
Chelating Agent
- BAL in Oil® [US]
- dimercaprol

METABOLIC BONE DISEASE
Vitamin D Analog
- calcifediol
- Calderol® [US/Can]

MULTIPLE SCLEROSIS
Antigout Agent
- colchicine

Biological, Miscellaneous
- Copaxone® [US/Can]
- glatiramer acetate

Biological Response Modulator
- Avonex® [US/Can]
- Betaseron® [US/Can]
- interferon beta-1a
- interferon beta-1b
- Rebif® [US/Can]

Skeletal Muscle Relaxant
- Apo®-Baclofen [Can]
- baclofen
- Dantrium® [US/Can]
- dantrolene
- Gen-Baclofen [Can]
- Lioresal® [US/Can]
- Liotec [Can]
- Nu-Baclo [Can]
- PMS-Baclofen [Can]

MUSCARINE POISONING
Anticholinergic Agent
- atropine

MYASTHENIA GRAVIS
Cholinergic Agent
- ambenonium
- edrophonium
- Enlon® [US/Can]
- Mestinon®-SR [Can]
- Mestinon® Timespan® [US]
- Mestinon® [US/Can]
- Mytelase® [US/Can]
- neostigmine

Prostigmin® [US/Can]
pyridostigmine
Regonol® [US]
Reversol® [US]
Tensilon® [US]
Skeletal Muscle Relaxant
tubocurarine

NARCOLEPSY

Adrenergic Agonist Agent
ephedrine
Amphetamine
Adderall® [US]
Adderall XR™ [US]
Desoxyn® Gradumet® [US]
Desoxyn® [US/Can]
Dexedrine® Spansule® [US/Can]
Dexedrine® Tablet [US/Can]
dextroamphetamine
dextroamphetamine and amphetamine
Dextrostat® [US]
methamphetamine
Central Nervous System Stimulant, Nonamphetamine
Alertec® [Can]
Concerta™ [US]
Cylert® [US]
Metadate® CD [US]
Metadate™ ER [US]
Methylin™ ER [US]
Methylin™ [US]
methylphenidate
modafinil
PemADD CT® [US]
PemADD® [US]
pemoline
PMS-Methylphenidate [Can]
Provigil® [US/Can]
Riphenidate [Can]
Ritalin® LA [US]
Ritalin-SR® [US/Can]
Ritalin® [US/Can]

NERVE BLOCK

Local Anesthetic
Ametop™ [Can]
Anestacon® [US]
bupivacaine
Carbocaine® [US/Can]
chloroprocaine
Citanest® Forte [Can]
Citanest® Plain [US/Can]
Dermaflex® Gel [US]
Duranest® [US/Can]
ELA-Max® [US-OTC]
etidocaine
Isocaine® HCl [US]
lidocaine
lidocaine and epinephrine
Lidodan™ [Can]
Lidoderm® [US/Can]
LidoPen® Auto-Injector [US]
Marcaine® Spinal [US]
Marcaine® [US/Can]
mepivacaine
Nesacaine®-CE [Can]
Nesacaine®-MPF [US]
Nesacaine® [US]
Novocain® [US/Can]
Polocaine® [US/Can]
Pontocaine® [US/Can]
Pontocaine® With Dextrose [US]
prilocaine
procaine
Sensorcaine®-MPF [US]
Sensorcaine® [US/Can]
Solarcaine® Aloe Extra Burn Relief [US-OTC]
tetracaine
tetracaine and dextrose
Xylocaine® [US/Can]
Xylocaine® With Epinephrine [US/Can]
Xylocard® [Can]
Zilactin® [Can]
Zilactin-L® [US-OTC]

NEURALGIA

Analgesic, Non-narcotic
- Arthropan® [US-OTC]
- choline salicylate
- Teejel® [Can]

Analgesic, Topical
- Antiphlogistine Rub A-535 No Odour [Can]
- Antiphlogistine Rub A-535 Capsaicin [Can]
- Arth Dr® [US]
- Arthricare Hand & Body® [US]
- Born Again Super Pain Relieving® [US]
- Caprex Plus® [US]
- Caprex® [US]
- Capsagel Extra Strength® [US]
- Capsagel Maximum Strength® [US]
- Capsagel® [US]
- Capsagesic-HP Arthritis Relief® [US]
- capsaicin
- Capsin® [US-OTC]
- D-Care Circulation Stimulator® [US]
- Double Cap® [US]
- Icy Hot Arthritis Therapy® [US]
- Myoflex® [US/Can]
- Pain Enz® [US]
- Pharmacist's Capsaicin® [US]
- Rid-A-Pain-HP® [US]
- Rid-A-Pain® [US]
- Sloan's Liniment® [US]
- Sportscreme® [US-OTC]
- Sportsmed® [US]
- Theragen HP® [US]
- Theragen® [US]
- TheraPatch Warm® [US]
- triethanolamine salicylate
- Trixaicin HP® [US]
- Trixaicin® [US]
- Zostrix High Potency® [US]
- Zostrix®-HP [US/Can]
- Zostrix Sports® [US]
- Zostrix® [US/Can]

Nonsteroidal Antiinflammatory Drug (NSAID)
- Apo®-ASA [Can]
- Asaphen [Can]
- Asaphen E.C. [Can]
- Ascriptin® Arthritis Pain [US-OTC]
- Ascriptin® Enteric [US-OTC]
- Ascriptin® Extra Strength [US-OTC]
- Ascriptin® [US-OTC]
- Aspercin Extra [US-OTC]
- Aspercin [US-OTC]
- Aspergum® [US-OTC]
- aspirin
- Bayer® Aspirin Extra Strength [US-OTC]
- Bayer® Aspirin Regimen Regular Strength [US-OTC]
- Bayer® Aspirin [US-OTC]
- Bayer® Plus Extra Strength [US-OTC]
- Bufferin® Arthritis Strength [US-OTC]
- Bufferin® Extra Strength [US-OTC]
- Bufferin® [US-OTC]
- Easprin® [US]
- Ecotrin® Maximum Strength [US-OTC]
- Ecotrin® [US-OTC]
- Entrophen® [Can]
- Novasen [Can]
- St. Joseph® Pain Reliever [US-OTC]
- ZORprin® [US]

NEURITIS (OPTIC)

Adrenal Corticosteroid
- A-HydroCort® [US/Can]
- Alti-Dexamethasone [Can]
- A-methaPred® [US]
- Apo®-Prednisone [Can]
- Aristocort® Forte Injection [US]
- Aristocort® Intralesional Injection [US]
- Aristocort® Tablet [US/Can]

Aristospan® Intra-articular Injection [US/Can]
Aristospan® Intralesional Injection [US/Can]
Betaject™ [Can]
betamethasone (systemic)
Betnesol® [Can]
Celestone® Phosphate [US]
Celestone® Soluspan® [US/Can]
Celestone® [US]
Cel-U-Jec® [US]
Cortef® [US/Can]
cortisone acetate
Cortone® [Can]
Decadron®-LA [US]
Decadron® [US/Can]
Decaject-LA® [US]
Decaject® [US]
Delta-Cortef® [US]
Deltasone® [US]
Depo-Medrol® [US/Can]
Depopred® [US]
dexamethasone (systemic)
Dexasone® L.A. [US]
Dexasone® [US/Can]
Dexone® LA [US]
Dexone® [US]
Hexadrol® [US/Can]
hydrocortisone (systemic)
Hydrocortone® Acetate [US]
Kenalog® Injection [US/Can]
Key-Pred-SP® [US]
Key-Pred® [US]
Medrol® Tablet [US/Can]
methylprednisolone
Meticorten® [US]
Orapred™ [US]
Pediapred® [US/Can]
PMS-Dexamethasone [Can]
Prednicot® [US]
prednisolone (systemic)
Prednisol® TBA [US]
prednisone
Prelone® [US]
Solu-Cortef® [US/Can]
Solu-Medrol® [US/Can]
Solurex L.A.® [US]
Sterapred® DS [US]
Sterapred® [US]
Tac™-3 Injection [US]
Triam-A® Injection [US]
triamcinolone (systemic)
Triam Forte® Injection [US]
Winpred™ [Can]

NEUROLOGIC DISEASE

Adrenal Corticosteroid

Acthar® [US]
A-HydroCort® [US/Can]
Alti-Dexamethasone [Can]
A-methaPred® [US]
Apo®-Prednisone [Can]
Aristocort® Forte Injection [US]
Aristocort® Intralesional Injection [US]
Aristocort® Tablet [US/Can]
Aristospan® Intra-articular Injection [US/Can]
Aristospan® Intralesional Injection [US/Can]
Betaject™ [Can]
betamethasone (systemic)
Betnesol® [Can]
Celestone® Phosphate [US]
Celestone® Soluspan® [US/Can]
Celestone® [US]
Cel-U-Jec® [US]
Cortef® [US/Can]
corticotropin
cortisone acetate
Cortone® [Can]
Decadron®-LA [US]
Decadron® [US/Can]
Decaject-LA® [US]
Decaject® [US]
Delta-Cortef® [US]

Deltasone® [US]
Depo-Medrol® [US/Can]
Depopred® [US]
dexamethasone (systemic)
Dexasone® L.A. [US]
Dexasone® [US/Can]
Dexone® LA [US]
Dexone® [US]
Hexadrol® [US/Can]
H.P. Acthar® Gel [US]
hydrocortisone (systemic)
Hydrocortone® Acetate [US]
Kenalog® Injection [US/Can]
Key-Pred-SP® [US]
Key-Pred® [US]
Medrol® Tablet [US/Can]
methylprednisolone
Meticorten® [US]
Orapred™ [US]
Pediapred® [US/Can]
PMS-Dexamethasone [Can]
Prednicot® [US]
prednisolone (systemic)
Prednisol® TBA [US]
prednisone
Prelone® [US]
Solu-Cortef® [US/Can]
Solu-Medrol® [US/Can]
Solurex L.A.® [US]
Sterapred® DS [US]
Sterapred® [US]
Tac™-3 Injection [US]
Triam-A® Injection [US]
triamcinolone (systemic)
Triam Forte® Injection [US]
Winpred™ [Can]

OSTEODYSTROPHY

Vitamin D Analog
calcifediol
Calciferol™ [US]
Calcijex™ [US]
calcitriol
Calderol® [US/Can]
DHT™ [US]
dihydrotachysterol
Drisdol® [US/Can]
ergocalciferol
Hytakerol® [US/Can]
Ostoforte® [Can]
Rocaltrol® [US/Can]

OSTEOMALACIA

Vitamin D Analog
Calciferol™ [US]
Drisdol® [US/Can]
ergocalciferol
Ostoforte® [Can]

OSTEOMYELITIS

Antibiotic, Miscellaneous
Alti-Clindamycin [Can]
Cleocin HCl® [US]
Cleocin Pediatric® [US]
Cleocin Phosphate® [US]
Cleocin® [US]
clindamycin
Dalacin® C [Can]
Vancocin® [US/Can]
Vancoled® [US]
vancomycin
Antifungal Agent, Systemic
Fucidin® [Can]
fusidic acid [Canada only]
Carbapenem (Antibiotic)
imipenem and cilastatin
meropenem
Merrem® I.V. [US/Can]
Primaxin® [US/Can]
Cephalosporin (First Generation)
Ancef® [US/Can]
Cefadyl® [US/Can]
cefazolin
cephalothin
cephapirin
Ceporacin® [Can]
Kefzol® [US/Can]

Cephalosporin (Second Generation)
- Cefotan® [US/Can]
- cefotetan
- cefoxitin
- Ceftin® [US/Can]
- cefuroxime
- Kefurox® [US/Can]
- Mefoxin® [US/Can]
- Zinacef® [US/Can]

Cephalosporin (Third Generation)
- Cefizox® [US/Can]
- Cefobid® [US/Can]
- cefoperazone
- cefotaxime
- ceftazidime
- ceftizoxime
- ceftriaxone
- Ceptaz® [US/Can]
- Claforan® [US/Can]
- Fortaz® [US/Can]
- Rocephin® [US/Can]
- Tazicef® [US]
- Tazidime® [US/Can]

Penicillin
- ampicillin and sulbactam
- dicloxacillin
- Dynapen® [US]
- nafcillin
- oxacillin
- ticarcillin and clavulanate potassium
- Timentin® [US/Can]
- Unasyn® [US/Can]

Quinolone
- ciprofloxacin
- Cipro® [US/Can]

OSTEOPOROSIS

Bisphosphonate Derivative
- alendronate
- Aredia® [US/Can]
- Didronel® [US/Can]
- etidronate disodium
- Fosamax® [US/Can]
- pamidronate

Electrolyte Supplement, Oral
- Calbon® [US]
- Calcionate® [US-OTC]
- Calciquid® [US-OTC]
- calcium glubionate
- calcium lactate
- calcium phosphate (dibasic)
- Cal-Lac® [US]
- Posture® [US-OTC]
- Ridactate® [US]

Estrogen and Progestin Combination
- estrogens and medroxyprogesterone
- Premphase® [US/Can]
- Prempro™ [US/Can]

Estrogen Derivative
- Alora® [US]
- Cenestin™ [US/Can]
- Climara® [US/Can]
- Congest [Can]
- Delestrogen® [US/Can]
- Depo®-Estradiol [US/Can]
- diethylstilbestrol
- Esclim® [US]
- Estinyl® [US]
- Estrace® [US/Can]
- Estraderm® [US/Can]
- estradiol
- Estratab® [US]
- Estring® [US/Can]
- Estrogel® [Can]
- estrogens (conjugated A/synthetic)
- estrogens (conjugated/equine)
- estrogens (esterified)
- ethinyl estradiol
- Gynodiol™ [US]
- Honvol® [Can]
- Menest® [US]
- Oesclim® [Can]
- PMS-Conjugated Estrogens [Can]
- Premarin® [US/Can]
- Stilphostrol® [US]

Vagifem® [US/Can]
Vivelle-Dot® [US]
Vivelle® [US/Can]
Mineral, Oral
fluoride
Polypeptide Hormone
Calcimar® [Can]
calcitonin
Caltine® [Can]
Miacalcin® [US/Can]
Selective Estrogen Receptor Modulator (SERM)
Evista® [US/Can]
raloxifene

OSTEOSARCOMA

Antineoplastic Agent
Adriamycin® [Can]
Adriamycin PFS® [US]
Adriamycin RDF® [US]
Caelyx® [Can]
cisplatin
doxorubicin
methotrexate
Platinol®-AQ [US]
Platinol® [US]
Rheumatrex® [US]
Rubex® [US]
Trexall™ [US]

PAGET DISEASE OF BONE

Antidote
Mithracin® [US/Can]
plicamycin
Bisphosphonate Derivative
alendronate
Aredia® [US/Can]
Didronel® [US/Can]
etidronate disodium
Fosamax® [US/Can]
pamidronate
Skelid® [US]
tiludronate
Polypeptide Hormone
Calcimar® [Can]
calcitonin
Caltine® [Can]
Miacalcin® [US/Can]

PARKINSONISM

Anti-Parkinson Agent
Akineton® [US/Can]
amantadine
Apo®-Benztropine [Can]
Apo® Bromocriptine [Can]
Apo®-Trihex [Can]
Artane® [US]
benserazide and levodopa [Canada only]
benztropine
biperiden
bromocriptine
Cogentin® [US/Can]
Comtan® [US/Can]
Endantadine® [Can]
entacapone
Kemadrin® [US/Can]
Parlodel® [US/Can]
PMS-Amantadine [Can]
PMS-Bromocriptine [Can]
Procyclid™ [Can]
procyclidine
Prolapa® [Can]
Requip® [US/Can]
ropinirole
Symmetrel® [US/Can]
Tasmar® [US]
tolcapone
trihexyphenidyl
Dopaminergic Agent (Anti-Parkinson)
Apo®-Levocarb [Can]
Apo®-Selegiline [Can]
Atapryl® [US]
carbidopa
Eldepryl® [US/Can]
Endo®-Levodopa/Carbidopa [Can]

Gen-Selegiline [Can]
levodopa
levodopa and carbidopa
Lodosyn® [US]
Mirapex® [US/Can]
Novo-Selegiline [Can]
Nu-Levocarb [Can]
Nu-Selegiline [Can]
pergolide
Permax® [US/Can]
pramipexole
selegiline
Selpak® [US]
Sinemet® CR [US/Can]
Sinemet® [US/Can]

Reverse COMT Inhibitor
Comtan® [US/Can]
entacapone

PARKINSON DISEASE

Anti-Parkinson Agent
ethopropazine [Canada only]
Parsitan® [Can]

POLIOMYELITIS

Vaccine, Live Virus
Orimune® [US]
poliovirus vaccine, live, trivalent, oral

Vaccine, Live Virus and Inactivated Virus
IPOL™ [US/Can]
poliovirus vaccine (inactivated)

POLYCYTHEMIA VERA

Antineoplastic Agent
busulfan
Busulfex® [US/Can]
mechlorethamine
Mustargen® [US/Can]
Myleran® [US/Can]

POLYMYOSITIS

Antineoplastic Agent
chlorambucil
cyclophosphamide
Cytoxan® [US/Can]
Leukeran® [US/Can]
methotrexate
Neosar® [US]
Procytox® [Can]
Rheumatrex® [US]
Trexall™ [US]

Immunosuppressant Agent
Alti-Azathioprine [Can]
azathioprine
Gen-Azathioprine [Can]
Imuran® [US/Can]

REYE SYNDROME

Diuretic, Osmotic
mannitol
Osmitrol® [US/Can]

Ophthalmic Agent, Miscellaneous
glycerin
Osmoglyn® [US]

Vitamin, Fat Soluble
AquaMEPHYTON® [US/Can]
Mephyton® [US/Can]
phytonadione

RHEUMATIC DISORDERS

Adrenal Corticosteroid
Acthar® [US]
A-HydroCort® [US/Can]
Alti-Dexamethasone [Can]
A-methaPred® [US]
Apo®-Prednisone [Can]
Aristocort® Forte Injection [US]
Aristocort® Intralesional Injection [US]
Aristocort® Tablet [US/Can]
Aristospan® Intra-articular Injection [US/Can]
Aristospan® Intralesional Injection [US/Can]
Betaject™ [Can]
betamethasone (systemic)
Betnesol® [Can]

Celestone® Phosphate [US]
Celestone® Soluspan® [US/Can]
Celestone® [US]
Cel-U-Jec® [US]
Cortef® [US/Can]
corticotropin
cortisone acetate
Cortone® [Can]
Decadron®-LA [US]
Decadron® [US/Can]
Decaject-LA® [US]
Decaject® [US]
Delta-Cortef® [US]
Deltasone® [US]
Depo-Medrol® [US/Can]
Depopred® [US]
dexamethasone (systemic)
Dexasone® L.A. [US]
Dexasone® [US/Can]
Dexone® LA [US]
Dexone® [US]
Hexadrol® [US/Can]
H.P. Acthar® Gel [US]
hydrocortisone (systemic)
Hydrocortone® Acetate [US]
Kenalog® Injection [US/Can]
Key-Pred-SP® [US]
Key-Pred® [US]
Medrol® Tablet [US/Can]
methylprednisolone
Meticorten® [US]
Orapred™ [US]
Pediapred® [US/Can]
PMS-Dexamethasone [Can]
Prednicot® [US]
prednisolone (systemic)
Prednisol® TBA [US]
prednisone
Prelone® [US]
Solu-Cortef® [US/Can]
Solu-Medrol® [US/Can]
Solurex L.A.® [US]
Sterapred® DS [US]
Sterapred® [US]
Tac™-3 Injection [US]
Triam-A® Injection [US]
triamcinolone (systemic)
Triam Forte® Injection [US]
Winpred™ [Can]

RHEUMATOID ARTHRITIS

Analgesic, Non-narcotic
Arthrotec® [US/Can]
diclofenac and misoprostol
Nonsteroidal Antiinflammatory Drug (NSAID), COX-2 Selective
Bextra™ [US]
valdecoxib
Prostaglandin
Arthrotec® [US/Can]
diclofenac and misoprostol

RICKETS

Vitamin D Analog
Calciferol™ [US]
Drisdol® [US/Can]
ergocalciferol
Ostoforte® [Can]

SPASTICITY

Alpha2-Adrenergic Agonist Agent
tizanidine
Zanaflex® [US/Can]
Benzodiazepine
Apo®-Diazepam [Can]
Diastat® [US/Can]
Diazemuls® [Can]
diazepam
Diazepam Intensol® [US]
Valium® [US/Can]
Skeletal Muscle Relaxant
Apo®-Baclofen [Can]
baclofen
Dantrium® [US/Can]
dantrolene
Gen-Baclofen [Can]
Lioresal® [US/Can]

Liotec [Can]
Nu-Baclo [Can]
PMS-Baclofen [Can]

SPINAL CORD INJURY

Skeletal Muscle Relaxant
Dantrium® [US/Can]
dantrolene

SPONDYLITIS (ANKYLOSING)

Nonsteroidal Antiinflammatory Drug (NSAID)
Alti-Piroxicam [Can]
Apo®-Diclo [Can]
Apo®-Diclo SR [Can]
Apo®-Piroxicam [Can]
Cataflam® [US/Can]
diclofenac
Diclotec [Can]
Feldene® [US/Can]
Gen-Piroxicam [Can]
Novo-Difenac® [Can]
Novo-Difenac-K [Can]
Novo-Difenac® SR [Can]
Novo-Pirocam® [Can]
Nu-Diclo [Can]
Nu-Diclo-SR [Can]
Nu-Pirox [Can]
Pexicam® [Can]
piroxicam
PMS-Diclofenac [Can]
PMS-Diclofenac SR [Can]
Riva-Diclofenac [Can]
Riva-Diclofenac-K [Can]
Solaraze™ [US]
Voltaren Rapide® [Can]
Voltaren® [US/Can]
Voltaren®-XR [US]
Voltaren Ophtha® [Can]

STATUS EPILEPTICUS

Anticonvulsant
paraldehyde
Paral® [US]
Barbiturate
amobarbital
Amytal® [US/Can]
Luminal® Sodium [US]
Nembutal® [US/Can]
pentobarbital
phenobarbital
Benzodiazepine
Apo®-Diazepam [Can]
Apo®-Lorazepam [Can]
Ativan® [US/Can]
Diastat® [US/Can]
Diazemuls® [Can]
diazepam
Diazepam Intensol® [US]
lorazepam
Novo-Lorazem® [Can]
Nu-Loraz [Can]
Riva-Lorazepam [Can]
Valium® [US/Can]
Hydantoin
Dilantin® [US/Can]
Phenytek™ [US]
phenytoin

STROKE

Antiplatelet Agent
Alti-Ticlopidine [Can]
Apo®-ASA [Can]
Apo®-Ticlopidine [Can]
Asaphen [Can]
Asaphen E.C. [Can]
aspirin
Bayer® Aspirin Regimen Adult Low Strength [US-OTC]
Bayer® Aspirin Regimen Adult Low Strength with Calcium [US-OTC]
Ecotrin® Low Adult Strength [US-OTC]
Halfprin® [US-OTC]
Nu-Ticlopidine [Can]
Sureprin 81™ [US-OTC]

Ticlid® [US/Can]
ticlopidine
Fibrinolytic Agent
Activase® rt-PA [Can]
Activase® [US]
alteplase
Skeletal Muscle Relaxant
Dantrium® [US/Can]
dantrolene

SUDECK ATROPHY

Calcium Channel Blocker
Adalat® CC [US]
Adalat® XL® [Can]
Apo®-Nifed [Can]
Apo®-Nifed PA [Can]
Nifedical™ XL [US]
nifedipine
Novo-Nifedin [Can]
Nu-Nifed [Can]
Procardia® [US/Can]
Procardia XL® [US]

SYPHILIS

Antibiotic, Miscellaneous
chloramphenicol
Chloromycetin® Parenteral [US/Can]
Penicillin
Bicillin® L-A [US]
penicillin G benzathine
penicillin G (parenteral/aqueous)
penicillin G procaine
Permapen® [US]
Pfizerpen® [US/Can]
Wycillin® [US/Can]
Tetracycline Derivative
Adoxa™ [US]
Apo®-Doxy [Can]
Apo®-Doxy Tabs [Can]
Apo®-Tetra [Can]
Brodspec® [US]
Doryx® [US]
Doxy-100™ [US]
Doxycin [Can]
doxycycline
Doxytec [Can]
EmTet® [US]
Monodox® [US]
Novo-Doxylin [Can]
Novo-Tetra [Can]
Nu-Doxycycline [Can]
Nu-Tetra [Can]
Periostat® [US]
Sumycin® [US]
tetracycline
Vibramycin® [US]
Vibra-Tabs® [US/Can]
Wesmycin® [US]

TOURETTE DISEASE

Antipsychotic Agent, Butyrophenone
Apo®-Haloperidol [Can]
Haldol® Decanoate [US]
Haldol® [US/Can]
haloperidol
Novo-Peridol [Can]
Peridol [Can]
PMS-Haloperidol LA [Can]
Rho®-Haloperidol Decanoate [Can]
Neuroleptic Agent
Orap™ [US/Can]
pimozide
Phenothiazine Derivative
Chlorpromanyl® [Can]
chlorpromazine
Largactil® [Can]
Thorazine® [US]

VERTIGO

Antihistamine
Antivert® [US/Can]
Apo®-Dimenhydrinate [Can]
Bonamine™ [Can]
Bonine® [US/Can]
Calm-X® Oral [US-OTC]
Compoz® Nighttime Sleep Aid [US-OTC]
dimenhydrinate

diphenhydramine
Dramamine® II [US-OTC]
Dramamine® Oral [US-OTC]
meclizine
TripTone® Caplets® [US-OTC]

WILSON DISEASE

Chelating Agent
- Syprine® [US/Can]
- trientine